P$ 50

Psychiatric Nursing

Third Edition

Psychiatric Nursing

Third Edition

Holly Skodol Wilson
RN, PhD, FAAN

Carol Ren Kneisl
RN, MS

Addison-Wesley Publishing Company
Health Sciences Division, Menlo Park, California

Reading, Massachusetts ■ Menlo Park, California ■ New York
Don Mills, Ontario ■ Wokingham, England ■ Amsterdam ■ Bonn
Sydney ■ Singapore ■ Tokyo ■ Madrid ■ San Juan

Sponsoring editor: *Debra Hunter*
Production supervisor: *Judith Johnstone*
Outside production supervisor: *Deborah Gale*
Book designer: *Detta Penna*
Cover designer: *Rudy Zehntner*
Photographers: *Holly S. Wilson, Carol R. Kneisl, Lance Brunner, Larry Lee, L. A. Takats, Sally Hutchinson, Paul Fusco, José Pruitt-Diez*
Illustrators: *AYXA, Linda Harris-Sweezy*
Copyeditors: *Antonio Padial, Loralee Windsor*
Proofreader: *Steven Sorensen*
Indexer: *Steven Sorensen*

Copyright © 1988 by Addison-Wesley Publishing Company, Inc. All rights reserved. No part of this publication may be reproduced, stored in a retrieval system, or transmitted, in any form or by any means, electronic, mechanical, photocopying, recording, or otherwise, without the prior permission of the publisher. Printed in the United States of America. Published simultaneously in Canada.

Photographs appearing on chapter opening pages in this text were taken by the authors and their friends as they traveled about the world. The photographs appear here to emphasize the universality of the human condition and human experience. In no way are the people pictured connected to the topics of the chapters in which they appear. It is assumed that all are mentally healthy and no other implication is to be drawn.

ABCDEFGHIJ—RN—891098

The authors and publishers have exerted every effort to ensure that drug selections and dosages set forth in this text are in accord with current recommendations and practice at the time of publication. However, in view of ongoing research, changes in government regulations, and the constant flow of information relating to drug therapy and drug reactions, the reader is urged to check the package insert for each drug for any change in indications of dosage and for added warnings and precautions. This is particularly important where the recommended agent is a new and/or infrequently employed drug.

Library of Congress Cataloging-in-Publication Data

Wilson, Holly Skodol.
  Psychiatric nursing.

  Includes bibliographies and index.
  1. Psychiatric nursing.   I. Kneisl, Carol Ren.
II. Title.   [DNLM: 1. Psychiatric Nursing.   WY 160 W748p]
RC440.W5   1988   610.73′68   87-37412
ISBN 0-201-11892-0

Addison-Wesley Publishing Company
Health Sciences Division
2725 Sand Hill Road
Menlo Park, California 94025

ISBN 0-201-11892-0

To Global Health and World Peace

As nurses, we are devoted to broad human values universally respected and deeply held—values of health, life, and the relief of suffering. We advocate the rights of human beings and all living creatures, unique and irreplaceable in our world, to live in peace and dignity. We are challenged with the responsibility of protecting and preserving health for our own and future generations. We believe that we must join with others in the search for ways to create a world beyond war.

We are linked by a shared vision of peace and global health. Defined most broadly, peace activism ranges from changing nations and international relations to changing people and interpersonal relationships. People at peace offer a means to a peaceful world. We dedicate this text to the ending of violence, to the wise and equitable distribution of resources, to advances in human rights and social justice, and to protection of our natural environment. We dedicate this text to a vision of global health and world peace.

About the Authors

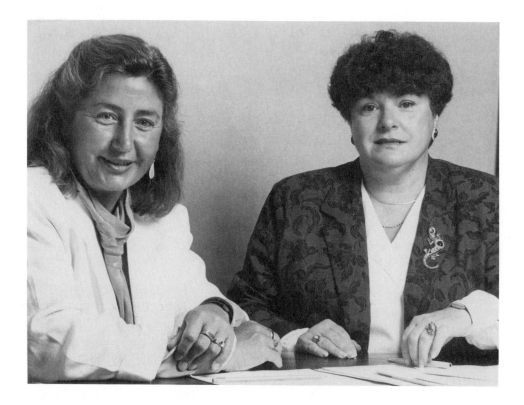

Holly Skodol Wilson, RN, PhD, FAAN, is a Professor in the Department of Mental Health, Community and Administrative Nursing, School of Nursing, University of California at San Francisco. She is also an appointed affiliated faculty member to the Women's Health and Healing Program in the Department of Social and Behavior Sciences and to the Aging Health Policy Research Unit. Her clinical and research interests are in the fields of psychogerontology, particularly community care for the demented elderly, and psychiatric nursing diagnostic practice. She has authored and coauthored nine books, has contributed chapters to three others, and has published over 50 scientific articles in professional journals. Her Addison-Wesley text *Research in Nursing* (1985) won both the *American Journal of Nursing* and *Nursing '86* Book of the Year awards. She is active as a national and international lecturer on topics ranging from research in nursing to the future of psychiatric nursing practice, education, and science.

Carol Ren Kneisl, RN, MS, a nationally and internationally known nursing author, lecturer, and consultant, is President and Educational Director of Nursing Transitions, Inc., a nursing continuing education company in Williamsville, New York. During her twenty years as a nurse educator, she taught psychiatric nursing students at the diploma and baccalaureate levels and clinical specialists in psychiatric nursing at the master's level. Actively involved in clinical practice issues, she encourages psychiatric nurses through her writing, speaking, and consultation activities to provide expert, humanistic care in psychiatric-mental health nursing and to take active leadership roles in the AIDS era. Other areas of clinical interest are group dynamics, group therapy, liaison psychiatric nursing, and stress management. She has authored and coauthored a total of nine books in nursing, six of them in psychiatric nursing.

Contributors

Lou Ellen A. Barnes, RN, MS
Doctoral Candidate
University of California at San Francisco
San Francisco, California

Carol Bradley, RN, CS, MSN
Psychiatric Clinical Nurse Specialist
Yale–New Haven Hospital
New Haven, Connecticut

Judy Banks Campbell, RN, EdD, ARNP
Professor
Palm Beach Junior College
Lake Worth, Florida

Linda Chafetz, RN, DNSc
Associate Professor
University of California at San Francisco
San Francisco, California

Catherine A. Chesla, RN, MN
Doctoral Candidate
University of California at San Francisco
San Francisco, California

Hannah Dean, RN-C, PhD
Associate Dean for Administration
UCLA School of Nursing
Los Angeles, California

Gail DeBoer, RN, MS
Samuel Merritt College
Oakland, California
Doctoral Candidate
University of California at San Francisco
San Francisco, California

Anastasia Fisher, RN, MN
Associate Director for Clinical Practice and Research
San Francisco General Hospital
San Francisco, California

Deborah I. Frank, RN, PhD
Associate Professor
Florida State University
Tallahassee, Florida

Karen Lee Fontaine, RN, MSN
Associate Professor
Purdue University, Calumet Campus
Hammond, Indiana

Susan Hunn Garritson, RN, DSN
Assistant Director, Patient Care Services
Langley Porter Psychiatric Hospital and Clinics
San Francisco, California

Janet A. Grossman, RN, CS, MSN
Research Nurse Coordinator
Center for Suicide Research and Prevention
Rush-Presbyterian–St. Lukes Medical Center
Chicago, Illinois

June Andrews Horowitz, RN, PhD
Associate Professor
Boston College
Chestnut Hill, Massachusetts

Sally Hutchinson, RN, PhD
Associate Professor
University of Florida
Jacksonville, Florida

Susan L. Jones, RN, PhD
Professor
Kent State University
Kent, Ohio

Joanne Keglovits, RN, MSN
Clinical Specialist
Pleasant Valley School District
Brodheadsville, Pennsylvania

Maxine Loomis, RN, CS, PhD, FAAN
Professor and Director
PhD Program in Nursing Science
University of South Carolina
Columbia, South Carolina

Colleen Carney Love, RN, MA
Clinical Nurse Specialist
French Hospital Medical Center
San Luis Obispo, California

Kate Mayton, RN, CS, MS
Nursing Clinical Coordinator in Child Psychiatry
Rush-Presbyterian–St. Lukes Medical Center
Chicago, Illinois

Geoffry McEnany, RN, MS
Associate Director of Nursing
Psychiatric Nursing Division
San Francisco General Hospital Medical Center
Assistant Clinical Professor
Department of Community Mental Health and Administrative Nursing
University of California at San Francisco
San Francisco, California

Beth Moscato, RN, MS
Doctoral Candidate
State University of New York at Buffalo
Buffalo, New York

Jane S. Norbeck, RN, DNSc, FAAN
Professor and Chair
Department of Mental Health
Community and Administrative Nursing
University of California at San Francisco
San Francisco, California

Anita Werner O'Toole, RN, PhD
Professor and Director
Graduate Program in Psychiatric Nursing
Kent State University
Kent, Ohio

Marilynn Petit, RN, MS
Consultant
Brockton Psychiatric Institute
Brockton, Massachusetts

Noreen King Poole, RN, CS, EdD, ARNP
Professor
Palm Beach Junior College
Lake Worth, Florida

Mary-Eve Zangari, RN, MS
Consultant
Employee Assistance of Central Virginia
Roanoke, Virginia

Reviewers

Sharon Anderson, MN, PhD
Long Island College Hospital
Brooklyn, New York

Alberta J. Boyle, BSN, MS
Oklahoma City University
Oklahoma City, Oklahoma

Katherine Buckwalter, MA, PhD
University of Iowa
Iowa City, Iowa

Merri Bunge, RN, BSN
Medical College of Ohio
Toledo, Ohio

Marilyn Bunt, PhD, MN
Loyola University
Chicago, Illinois

Lida Chase
University of Hawaii
Honolulu, Hawaii

Janet Chorpenning
Indiana University
Indianapolis, Indiana

Barbara Coldwell
Villanova University
Villanova, Pennsylvania

Phyllis Connolly, RN, MSN
San Jose State University
San Jose, California

Mary Correa, ABD, MSN
University of Cincinnati
Cincinnati, Ohio

Joann R. Cross, BSN, MSN
Wright State University
Dayton, Ohio

Kathy Dwyer, BSN, MSN
University of Akron
Akron, Ohio

Jeanne Gelman, BSN, MSN
Widener University
Chester, Pennsylvania

Sue Gottschalx, RN, PhD
Salt Lake County Mental Health
Murray, Utah

Cindy Hughes, MSN, PhD
Kent State University
Kent, Ohio

Gloria Jacobson, BSN, MS
Northern Illinois University
DeKalb, Illinois

Carolyn Kaiser
Lake Michigan College
Benton Harbor, Michigan

Patricia Lane, BSN
Rockingham Memorial Hospital
Harrisonburg, Virginia

Colleen Love, RNC, MA
French Hospital Medical Center
San Luis Obispo, California

Eileen Massura, BSN, MSN
Governor's State University
University Park, Illinois

Sheridan McCabe, MSN, PhD
University of Virginia
Charlottesville, Virginia

Rebecca McClanahan, MN
Northeast Missouri State
Kirksville, Missouri

Peggy McComb, BSN, MA
Veterans Administration Medical Center
Portland, Oregon

Nancy Opie, MSN, DNS
University of Cincinnati
Cincinnati, Ohio

Suzanne Perkins
Grand Valley State College
Allendale, Michigan

Karen Reed, BSN, MN
University of North Carolina
Greensboro, North Carolina

Suzanne Resner, MSN, DNS
American University
Washington, DC

Judith Robinson, BSN, MSN
Baptist Memorial Hospital
San Antonio, Texas

Mary Rode, PNP, MSN
University of Evansville
Evansville, Indiana

Susan Schnuerer, MN, PhD
Kent State University
Kent, Ohio

Lee Schwecke, BSN, MSN
Indiana University
Indianapolis, Indiana

Joanne Sherman
Seton Hall University
South Orange, New Jersey

Marlene K. Stroder
Southern Illinois University
Edwardsville, Illinois

Kathleen Talbot, BSN
Calgary General Hospital
Calgary, Alberta, Canada

Jackie Taylor, PhD, MS
Arizona State University
Tempe, Arizona

Marshelle Thobaben, PHN, MS
Humboldt State University
Arcata, California

Sharon Valente, RN, MN, FAAN
Wright Institute
Los Angeles, California

Patricia Ryan Wahl
University of Cincinnati
Cincinnati, Ohio

Helen Waterhouse, BSN, MeD
State University of New York
Plattsburgh, New York

Susan Yoder, BSN, MSN
University of Evansville
Evansville, Indiana

Preface

A decade ago the First Edition of *Psychiatric Nursing* changed the face of textbooks in our field. It earned professional recognition when it won the *American Journal of Nursing* Book of the Year award and was cited as a major landmark in the advancement of psychiatric nursing's unique perspective. The Second Edition, published in 1983, updated this trend-setting text by adding the American Nurses' Association Standards, the nursing process, and developments in psychiatric nursing research. By this time, *Psychiatric Nursing* had been translated into other languages and was in use throughout the world.

The same inventive energy and cutting-edge knowledge have shaped *Psychiatric Nursing's* Third Edition. Each of the following changes in the context, knowledge base, and practice of psychiatric nursing has been thoroughly integrated in this revision:

- Target populations for psychiatric care include dramatically increased numbers of elderly, chronically disabled, and physically as well as psychiatrically disordered clients.

- The diagnostic nomenclature of mental disorders in the interdisciplinary field of psychiatry has undergone a major revision with the May 1987 publication of DSM-IIIR (revised) by the American Psychiatric Association.

- The nomenclature for psychiatric nursing diagnoses has advanced significantly as a consequence of the American Nurses' Association's Phenomena Project, resulting in what we term in this text PND-I (Psychiatric Nursing Diagnosis, first edition). These are being refined for eventual inclusion in the growing NANDA taxonomy.

- Advances in neurobiology have revolutionized psychiatric nursing's body of knowledge in psychobiology, psychoendocrinology, psychoimmunology, and chronobiology, to the point where one of the nation's lead-ers challenged that psychiatric-mental health nurses must "retool or die" with respect to updating knowledge about neurotransmitters and the brain's influence on the development and treatment of many psychiatric disorders.

- Research findings are becoming the basis of nursing knowledge.

- Psychiatric nurses are carving out an important role in addressing the AIDS epidemic facing our society today.

- Consumers are rallying on an unprecedented scale around the issue of care for psychiatric clients; the National Alliance for the Mentally Ill has given consumers of psychiatric care a resounding voice.

- There are unprecedented pressures for cost containment and innovation. Prospective payment is becoming the predominant method of economic reimbursement for psychiatric care, yet the current DRGs rarely predict resource use in any meaningful way when it comes to labor-intensive interventions like therapy, counseling, and psychoeducation.

- Social support and client disability have become increasingly important areas of concern for psychiatric-mental health nurses who want to make a difference.

- Just as psychiatry is re-medicalizing, psychiatric nursing is undergoing a process of mainstreaming into the general field of nursing, where a holistic philosophy of clients as biopsychosocial entities is more reasonable to implement. Nurses have assumed leadership roles in programs designed to teach clients, families, and caregivers about the array of psychotropic medications that are now widely used.

- Psychobiologic nursing treatment plans, no longer experimental, are becoming the norm in our nation's leading centers.

- Psychiatric nurses are assuming key roles as case managers in the care of the chronically mentally ill who are homeless.

- The nursing process has become an established modus operandi for the practice of psychiatric nursing.

- Psychiatric nurses are defining political activities on behalf of meaningful causes as a necessary part of their professional role.

The Newly Revised Psychiatric Nursing, Third Edition

Psychiatric Nursing, Third Edition, has been fully revised to accommodate the sweeping changes affecting our field in the past decade. To the useful pedagogic features present in prior editions, we have added the following:

- A complete and thorough updating of *psychiatric terminology* and diagnostic criteria in all chapters to match the 1987 DSM-III Revised (DSM-IIIR) published by APA.

- Use of two psychiatric nursing diagnostic systems— *NANDA* and the new American Nurses' Association's classification of phenomena of concern to psychiatric-mental health nurses, herein called *Psychiatric Nursing Diagnoses (PND-I).*

- Tables in most chapters that show the *correspondence between the three sets of terminology* that nurses need to know: DSM-IIIR, NANDA, and PND-I diagnoses. Examples of these tables are found on pages 332, 478, and 520.

- The five steps of the *nursing process* (assessment, diagnosis, planning, implementation, and evaluation) are used to organize discussions of nursing care.

- *Nursing care plans,* presented throughout the book, are organized according to the nursing process. Examples are on pages 334 and 552.

- *Case studies* with lively clinical material. Examples are found on pages 386, 484, and 798.

- *Eleven new chapters,* including:
  Human Growth and Development Across the Life Span
  Stress, Anxiety, and Coping
  Social Support
  Psychobiology
  Research in Psychiatric Nursing
  The Chronically Mentally Ill
  Violence and Victimatology (Part I: Violence and Victimatology in the Psychiatric Setting; Part II: Rape and Intrafamily Abuse)

  The Role of Psychiatric Nursing in the AIDS Epidemic
  Stress Management
  Milieu Therapy
  Applying the Nursing Process with Dying Clients and Their Families

- *Seven psychiatric disorders chapters* (Part Three) have been expanded to be more comprehensive and up-to-date, and to fit more closely into the DSM-IIIR diagnostic system.

- A fully *biopsychosocial approach* that does not neglect cutting-edge developments in psychobiology.

- *New research notes* in every chapter cite studies in current literature, giving a brief description of the study and discussing the implications of the research for practice. Some examples are on pages 135, 309, and 821.

- *Up-to-date annotated resources* in Appendix C give specific references for hot lines, support groups, and agencies.

- *Cross references* at the beginning of each chapter refer students to other chapters for related information.

- All five axes of the DSM-IIIR, the NANDA diagnoses from the seventh national conference, the most recent rendition of the ANA classification system (PND-I), and the 1982 Standards are included in full.

- Our chapter opening captions urge psychiatric nurses and students to take courageous, informed, and articulate stances on contemporary social issues such as human rights, environmental protection, and world peace.

Supplements to Accompany Psychiatric Nursing, Third Edition

Psychosocial Nursing Concepts; An Activity Book (11895) by Holly Skodol Wilson and Carol Ren Kneisl is comprised of independent action-oriented learning activities. These activities will be useful in a number of nursing courses because they allow students to practice the various subprocesses that are key to clinical practice: communication, decision-making, teaching-learning, group dynamics, and leadership.

Available to faculty only, the *Test Bank* (11894) by Irene Russo contains over 400 questions in NCLEX format and 500 True-False and Matching Questions. Each question in the NCLEX format is presented as part of a clinical scenario, and each question is also coded by level of difficulty. Also included in the *Test Bank* is an annotated audiovisual resources list for each chapter of this text. The test items are also available from your Addison-Wesley sales representative in computer form for the IBM-PC and Apple.

Acknowledgments

There are many people we wish to thank for helping to make this Third Edition of *Psychiatric Nursing* a comprehensive, authoritative, and contemporary psychiatric nursing text.

First and foremost are our professional colleagues and friends, the contributors to this Third Edition. Their names and affiliations are listed on a separate page and we extend a hearty *thank you* to each one.

Special thanks are due to Pam Burton, Priscilla Ebersole, Joan Sayre, Andy Skodol, and Pat Underwood. Their contributions to the Second Edition continue to influence this one.

Irene Russo developed the *Test Bank* and compiled the audiovisual resources. She has been a dependable and supportive friend and a part-time saint since nursing school.

Lance Brunner and Larry Lee, Kellogg National Leadership Fellows, generously contributed some of their sensitive and very human photographs taken during their work in South America, our own country, and the Soviet Union.

Dave Rich was invaluable in compiling the Resources appendix. We were pleased to be able to work with him once again.

The thoughtful comments of nursing faculty, nursing students, and psychiatric nurses continue to be most welcome. We have tried to make this book a reflection of what they want in a psychiatric nursing text.

The talented professionals at Addison-Wesley are friends of nursing. They are responsible for pulling together what we have to say and presenting it in an appealing package. Nick Keefe, Vice President and General Manager of the Health Sciences Division, continues to support us and our work. Debra Hunter, Executive Editor and our sponsoring editor, is gracious and encouraging. Judy Johnstone, our in-house Production Supervisor, has facilitated the book-making process and provided reassuring calm.

We are especially grateful for the opportunity, once again, to work with Deborah Gale of Partners in Publishing. Deborah was our sponsoring editor for the Second Edition. This time she was responsible for shepherding our book through the complexities of the production process. She nurtured this book, and its authors, with skill, sensitivity, humor, and a warm heart.

Detta Penna created the unique and inviting design for this book. Her arresting ribbon slashes and her fine eye in arranging the photo collages on the first page of each chapter add to the book's appeal.

A book of this scope is possible only because of the dedication, openness, and support of these persons and all the others who helped to make this book a success.

Finally, we say thank you to our families—Hillary, Emily, and Molly Wilson, and Ed, Kyle, and Heidi Kneisl. They have abdicated their positions on the dedication page for this Third Edition to enable us to dedicate this book to personal and interpersonal peace as a bridge to a peaceful world.

Holly Wilson
Carol Kneisl

Contents in Brief

Part Seven
Social, Political, Cultural, and Economic Environment for Care
1049

Contents in Detail

Part Two
Processes for Psychiatric Nursing Clinical Practice
195

Part Three

Human Responses to Distress and Disorder
313

Part Four

Contemporary Clinical Concerns
581

Special Features

Boxes

PART ONE

The Theoretical Basis
for Psychiatric Nursing

ONE

Philosophical Perspectives

Holly Skodol Wilson

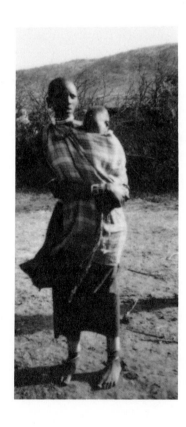

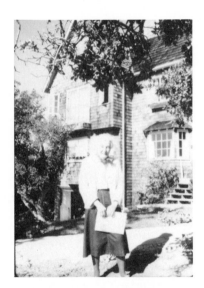

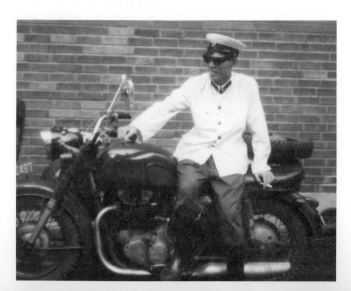

Learning Objectives

After reading this chapter, students should be able to

- Identify the major ideas of interactionism
- Identify the major principles of humanism
- Relate the premises of humanistic interactionism to the psychiatric nursing process
- Specify three characteristics of excellence exemplars in psychiatric nursing practice
- Explain six qualities associated with power and excellence under real-world conditions
- Develop a personal philosophic framework for psychiatric nursing practice

Cross References

Other topics relevant to this content are: Cultural considerations in mental health care, Chapter 38; Ethics, Chapter 10; Legal issues, Chapter 39.

This book is dedicated to the idea that a peaceful world is possible and worth working for.

Key Terms

dualism
holism
humanism

monism
symbolic interactionism

PHILOSOPHICAL PERSPECTIVES

There are many approaches to understanding people. Each is like a searchlight that illuminates some of the facts while leaving others in shadow. The practice of psychiatric nursing is grounded in certain philosophical assumptions about human nature, society, and values. Most textbook authors present a wide variety of philosophical approaches to practice. They reason that psychiatric nursing is still being defined as a specialty, and it would be inappropriate at this stage to choose only one approach; with many possible choices, the psychiatric nurse can select one that is best suited to the situation or setting. There is much to be said for this position. However, it can result in a tendency to hold on to contradictory points of view. For example, both teachers and students of psychiatric nursing tend to think of people *holistically*—as complex organisms having physical, mental, emotional, social, and cultural dimensions that are inseparable. Yet the medical model of psychiatry is *disease oriented,* and that narrower focus continues to dominate both psychiatric nursing concepts and philosophies of practice. Teachers may give mixed messages to students. On the one hand, they emphasize the well-being of the whole person and focus on individuality and freedom of choice. On the other, they continue to teach nursing interventions reflecting conformity of behavior, perception, and life-style.

A psychiatric nurse's philosophical perspective influences every aspect of practice. This chapter introduces the perspective of *humanistic interactionism.* We believe this perspective encompasses most of the variables that challenge today's psychiatric nurse, including the biologic explanations of feelings and behavior. We hope that readers will be moved to examine some basic philosophical questions and to formulate a philosophy of psychiatric nursing for their own personal and professional lives.

INTRODUCTION TO HUMANISTIC INTERACTIONISM

Scope of Practice

All nurses are concerned with the quality of human life and its relationship to health. The psychiatric nurse is especially concerned with the relationship between the individual's optimal health and feelings of self-worth, personal integrity, self-fulfillment, and creative expression. Just as important are the satisfaction of basic living needs, comfortable relations with others, and the recognition of human rights. The psychiatric nurse's scope of practice is broad enough to include issues such as alienation, identity crisis, sudden life changes, and troubled family interactions. It can encompass individual protests or mass confrontations. It deals with poverty and affluence, the experiences of birth and death, the loss of significant others, or the loss of body parts. It is concerned with sustaining and enhancing the individual and the group. This broad-ranging, humanistic, and interactional view of the scope of psychiatric nursing is dramatically different from the exclusively medical or behavioral science orientation of the last thirty years. The classic psychiatric and psychologic approaches have described and classified signs and symptoms of *illness,* then accounted for it by individual psychologic dysfunctions such as character disorder, weak ego, or failed defense mechanisms.

Concepts of "Mental Illness" and "Mental Health"

The perspective in this text differs substantially from more traditional modes of psychiatric nursing thought. In these modes, a client's "mental illness" or "mental health" is seen as arising exclusively from within the individual. We believe these concepts are interactional and derive their meaning from the definitions given to certain acts by certain audiences. We advocate looking at the social conditions under which someone is labeled "mentally ill," by whom, and with what consequences. Thus, our *interactionist approach* is inclined to view "mental illness" and "mental health" as outgrowths of interpersonal processes. Examined from this perspective, "mental illness" is not exclusively defined by particular character traits. Nor is it established purely by the nature of certain acts (*symptomatology*). Rather, it includes the individual's view of those acts, the reactions of others to them, and the overall cultural context in which they occur. In short, "mental illness" is often a matter of judgment. The appropriateness of behavior depends on whether it is judged plausible or not, based on a set of social, ethical, and legal rules that define the limits of appropriate behavior and reality. For example, if a man on a street corner says he is Napoleon, people will not believe him and will consider his statement symptomatic or disturbed. If a man at a masquerade party says he is Napoleon, people reach a different conclusion.

Mental Disorder and Psychiatric Nursing's Phenomena of Concern

With the publication of the third edition of the American Psychiatric Association's *Diagnostic and Statistical Manual of Mental Disorders* (DSM-III), psychiatric professionals accepted this definition of *mental disorder:* "A clinically significant behavioral or psychological syndrome or pattern that occurs in an individual that is typically associated with either a painful symptom (distress) or impairment in one or more important areas of functioning (disability)" (1980, p. 6). Disturbances between an individual and society are acknowledged as conditions that may require therapy or treatment but are not themselves "mental disorders." Nor are mental disorders discrete, clearly delineated entities. Psychiatric nurses are indeed concerned with care of clients with identified mental disorders. According to DSM-III and the 1987 revision of the third edition (DSM-IIIR), however, our phenomena of concern extend to the wide-ranging human responses to mental distress, disability, and disorder (ANA 1980, Loomis et al 1987).

For example, an addicted parent may suffer not only from shame, unemployment, abusive outbursts of anger, sexual impotence, tremors, family violence, hyperactivity, vomiting, diarrhea, anorexia, malnutrition, sleep disturbances, panic attacks, blackouts, and judgment impairment. He or she may also lose a sense of interconnectedness with life, lose a sense of purpose and meaning, and experience disturbed self-concept, confusion, despair, and deteriorated relationships. These responses have detrimental effects for the health of children, partners, and other significant people.

Individual, family, and community responses vary with individuality, interpretations of meaning, and culture. Faced with such a diverse array of human problems, the psychiatric nurse is challenged to synthesize a philosophy for practice that can be the basis for care.

Basic Premises of Interactionism

The approach we advocate above has come to be known as **symbolic interactionism,** a term introduced by Herbert Blumer (1969) to describe a relatively distinctive approach to the study of human conduct. It is based on three simple philosophic premises:

1. Human beings act toward things on the basis of the meaning that the things have for them. Life experiences may have different meanings to different people.

2. The meaning of things in a person's life is derived from the social interactions that person has with others. We learn meanings during our experiences with others.

3. People handle and modify the meanings of the things they encounter through an interpretive process. They come to their own conclusions.

Implications of Premises for Psychiatric Nursing

The First Premise

The notion that people's actions in a situation are based on the unique meaning that situation has for them is all but ignored in many approaches to psychiatric nursing. Instead, human conduct is treated as the product of various factors that act on passive human beings—factors such as stimuli, unconscious motives, and character traits. This emphasis on factors alleged to produce "symptoms" neglects the role of individual meaning in the formation of human behavior. We believe that all behavior has meaning. The psychiatric nurse must be wary of interventions that invalidate the meaning an experience has for the client in favor of the nurse's own definition of the situation. Thus, nurses need to develop skill in observing, interpreting, and responding to the client's experiences in the hope of arriving at a common ground of negotiated meanings and authentic communication.

The Second Premise

In many conventional approaches to psychiatric nursing, meanings—such as the meaning of "normal," "mentally healthy," and "mentally ill"—are regarded as intrinsic to the nature of the behavior, the personality, or the disease. We believe meanings arise in the *process* of interaction with others. Meanings are social products formed in and through interpersonal communication and learning. It is essential, therefore, that psychiatric nurses take into account the social and cultural environment of each client. A holistic assessment of a client accounts for the interaction patterns in that person's social world. A Mohawk haircut dyed orange, tight black leather clothing, and face paint and tattoos may appear bizarre in a milieu of upper-middle-class bankers and businesspeople, yet they represent rather strict adherence to dress and demeanor codes of the punk rock subculture. Individuals labeled "paranoid" or "neurotic" or "using alcohol or drugs as emotional crutches" cannot be understood outside their unique social context. (In Chapter 35, we are reminded that adolescents direct insults and hostile remarks at nurses for many reasons. Most of these reasons have little to do with the nurse as a person but a lot to do with the nurse as an adult or authority figure. The social context of an adolescent peer group plays a critical part in determining the meaning of such behavior.) Similarly, it is within interpersonal interaction that clients can learn new definitions for life situations and new repertoires for action. This is the heart of the psychiatric nurse's therapeutic and healing role. The sensitive, intelligent, and humanistic use of self within interpersonal relationships is a key part of the psychiatric nurse's skill. Nurses have a particular potential for helping clients rede-

fine their experiences in more satisfying ways, learn new patterns of coping with stress, and generally enhance the quality of their lives and social worlds.

The Third Premise

We believe that people handle situations in terms of what they consider vitally important about the situation. They fit their own actions to the actions of others. To understand the actions of people, the psychiatric nurse must learn to identify the meanings those actions have for them. Nurses need to keep this premise in mind when responding to an expression of human distress. A nurse may say, "I wouldn't worry about it," or "don't feel that way," "you are reacting inappropriately," or "it's not so bad." Such clichés are not usually helpful, not because they are "untherapeutic" but because in voicing them the nurse neglects the basic premise that people interpret the world in their own way in order to act in a specific situation. They deal with what they perceive. This gives their experience some meaning, which in turn becomes a basis for their behavior.

Interactionism offers psychiatric nursing a perspective of human beings as having purpose and control over their own lives. Interactionism as interpreted here provides the premises for a philosophy of healing with a strong humanistic cast and a politics of reality. It is clearly different from the position of those who interpret certain actions as purely medical problems resulting from unconscious drives and repressed conflicts. Interactionism acknowledges the interaction of psychology, biology, and sociocultural context.

Basic Premises of Humanism

The purpose of this chapter is to specify a set of premises as a basis for subsequent chapters. The three postulates of interactionism provide us with a partial orientation. A theory of life centered on human beings, termed **humanism**, rounds out the perspective.

The central proposition of humanism is that the chief end of human life is to work for well-being within the confines of life on this earth. Humanism is a philosophy of service for humanity using reason, science, and democracy.

Psychiatric nurses and students might reasonably ask why issues of philosophy should even be considered. We believe that the guiding pattern in the lives of all psychiatric nurses is their philosophy, even though that philosophy may be demonstrated primarily in actions rather than systematically thought out. Philosophy teaches people to say what they mean and to mean what they say. It is an attempt to think through the fundamental issues of life and reach reasoned conclusions about society, human nature, action, and values.

Humanism as a philosophic perspective can be clarified in eight central propositions:

1. The human being's mind is indivisibly connected with the body.
2. Human beings have the power or potential to solve their own problems.
3. All theories of universal determinism, fatalism, or predestination are false. Human beings, while influenced by the past, possess freedom of creative choice and action and are, within certain limits, masters of their own destinies.
4. Human values are grounded in life experiences and relationships, and our highest goal must be the happiness, freedom, and growth of all people.
5. Individuals attain well-being and a high quality of life by harmoniously combining personal satisfactions with activities that contribute to the welfare of the community.
6. We should develop art and awareness of beauty so that the aesthetic experience becomes a pervasive reality in people's lives.
7. We should apply reason, science, and democratic procedures in all areas of life.
8. We must continually examine our basic convictions—including those of humanism.

See Lamont (1967) for elaboration of these propositions.

The Meaning of Humanism for Psychiatric Nursing

Humanism as a philosophy of psychiatric nursing practice means devotion to the interests of human beings wherever they live and whatever their status. It reaffirms the spirit of compassion and caring toward others. It is a constructive philosophy that wholeheartedly affirms the joys, beauties, and values of human living. The subsequent chapters in this text attempt to operationalize (give specific workable meanings of) these basic premises for psychiatric nursing practice. Among such operationalizations are some fundamental concepts described briefly below.

Holistic View of Mind-Body Relations

There are two basic schools of thought about the relationship of the mind and the body. These two philosophic positions are called **monism** and **dualism**. The monistic view asserts that mind and body are one. The dualistic view asserts that mind and body are separate phenomena and may be (a) causally interrelated, (b) parallel but independent, or (c) unrelated. Our humanistic interactionist view is neither monistic nor dualistic. We maintain that physical and mental factors are interrelated and that a change in one may result in a change in another. For example, anger may result in increased blood pressure. An invading organism or toxin or structural change in the body can alter thought processes. Low self-esteem can result in hunched shoulders and severe skeletal muscle contractures. The implications for psychiatric nursing are clear. Healing and caring must be approached **holistically**. The psychiatric nurse deals with the somatic aspects of a primarily psychologic or emotional pattern and the psychologic or emotional aspects of physiologic experiences. Psychiatric nursing care transcends the bounds of "mental hospitals" to include general health care settings and may be directed toward clients whose immediate problems are primarily physical.

Expanded Role for Nurses

The humanistic interactionist perspective on "mental illness," in contrast to the medical model, implies an expanded role for psychiatric nurse practitioners. This perspective enlarges the boundaries of intervention to include political and social dimensions as well as individual client-centered work. When a person's behavior is viewed exclusively in terms of psychiatric symptoms, the emphasis is on intrapersonal variables, but we view behavior within an interpersonal field. In our opinion, no one can "have" schizophrenia all alone. We believe that psychiatric nurses should be prepared to work for change within social and political systems. Psychiatric nursing can no longer be limited to client-oriented activities designed exclusively to reduce discomfort and increase the capability of individuals to adjust satisfactorily to the existing social condition. Instead, psychiatric nursing must be involved in social goals that advance health holistically. Because psychiatric nursing has political consequences, it is essential that nurses begin to develop a philosophic and ethical framework to guide and evaluate the political outcome of therapeutic intervention. Our critical feedback on certain controversial diagnoses proposed for the revised third edition of the *Diagnostic and Statistical Manual of Mental Disorders* (DSM-IIIR) is a contemporary example. The photo essays on global health and world peace at the beginning of every chapter in this text are an even more direct example.

RESEARCH NOTE

Citation

Benner P: From Novice to Expert: Excellence and Power in Clinical Nursing Practice. *Addison-Wesley, 1984.*

Study Problem/Purpose

Nursing practice has been studied primarily from a sociologic perspective. In this qualitative study, Benner sought to portray knowledge embedded in the practice of nursing by examining the differences between practical and theoretical knowledge, providing examples of competencies in nursing practice, and outlining strategies for preserving and extending knowledge in nursing toward the goal of excellence.

Methods

To ascertain and understand the differences in clinical performance and situation appraisal of beginning and expert nurses, Benner conducted twenty-one paired interviews with each. The twenty-one pairs of nurses were selected from three hospitals. In addition to the interviews, participant observation and further interviews were conducted with fifty-one other experienced nurses, eleven newly graduated nurses, and five senior nursing students in six hospitals: two private community, two community teaching, one university medical center, and one inner-city general hospital. Textual analysis of observation and interview transcripts were accomplished according to the interpretive strategy originally based on Heideggerian phenomenology. The intent was not to come up with theoretical terms or systems but rather to identify meanings and content.

Findings

Benner identified seven "domains of nursing practice" and offered exemplars of each. The seven domains are:

1. The helping role
2. The teaching-coaching function
3. The diagnostic and patient-monitoring function
4. The effective management of rapidly changing situations
5. The administration and monitoring of therapeutic interventions and regimens
6. Monitoring to ensure the quality of health care practices
7. Organizational and work-role competencies

Implications

If we are to humanize care in the highly technical medical environment, we must master technology. We must also critique the technology and not view it as the ultimate resource in recovery, dignity, and health. As an antidote to a purely technical view of health and power, we must understand and unleash the power of caring and the power of excellence.

Decision Making

A humanistic interactionist perspective suggests a different decision-making format from that of the traditional medical model. The medical model implies that the physician is the chief decision maker. In contrast, we do not propose that any particular discipline should provide leadership in psychiatric decision making. We prefer practical collaboration among interdisciplinary team participants to generate effective strategies.

Negotiation and Advocacy

In the humanistic interactionist perspective, the model for intervention and change is one of negotiation and advocacy. The responsibility for change remains with the person who seeks psychiatric help or consultation. Clients are held accountable for their own behavior. They are not passively treated by psychiatric professionals. Instead, they are supported in the process of developing new perspectives and encouraged to weigh alternatives and make self-directed choices. Psychiatric services in this view are more consultative and advocative than directive. Implied here is a fundamental switch from the approach that upholds the values and life-style of the nurse-therapist as the image of health to an approach that helps clients find a life-style that fits in with their own cultures. When translated into practice, this approach is not entirely without conflicts and difficulties. Critics are quick to point out that Charles Manson, convicted of multiple murders, was acting in a manner consistent with his culture.

EXCELLENCE AND POWER IN PRACTICE

According to Benner (1984), the *competencies* of a psychiatric nurse can be differentiated from his or her *goals* (the way the nurse generally uses psychosocial knowledge to achieve a particular aim or realize an intention in a therapeutic relationship) and from his or her practice *strategies* (the ways in which the nurse interacts to help clients move in the direction of growth). Both goals and practice strategies are clearly influenced by the psychiatric nurse's personal and professional philosophies. Benner's exemplars of excellence revealed that psychiatric nurses:

1. Acted as psychologic and cultural mediators to help confused people "carve a path into a more shared, less idiosyncratic world" (p 67)

2. Used goals therapeutically in that goals set were realistic, workable, and aimed toward improved social and psychologic functioning

3. Worked to build and maintain a therapeutic community that can serve as an arena for working out issues of trust, conflict, and cooperation

Exemplars of excellence in practice challenge nurses to implement their caring power and professional philosophy even under conditions that act as barriers and constraints in the everyday world.

Barriers and Constraints to Excellence

It is probably naive to believe that nurses base their practice on abstract philosophies. As early as 1964, Strauss and associates found that nurses and doctors in mental hospitals negotiated their philosophies and ideologies in the context of the everyday realities of their work situations. Aspiring toward therapeutic client relationships that are caring, sensitive, holistic, meaningful, and nonjudgmental can be stressful. The nurse must work under conditions that are strongly influenced by economics, legislation, multiple levels of bureaucracy and paperwork, competition among members of the interdisciplinary mental health team, increased reliance on psychotropic medication, hasty discharges, limited follow-up care, a revolving-door pattern of hospital use, and short hospital stays (Wilson 1982). In 1983, Bunch studied how psychiatric nurses balance their professional philosophic mandate with the institutional requirements of everyday business. She found that the nurses she observed and interviewed had great difficulty, validating Kramer's finding in a 1972 study of nurses' "reality shock" upon entering the world of work.

Toward a New Entitlement

As Benner (1984) concludes, excellence under the strains of conditions described above requires philosophies of commitment and involvement, but it also requires power. She advocates six qualities of power associated with caring excellence as strategies for balancing professional/philosophic mandates with the barriers and constraints of the context in which we practice. These are:

1. *Transformative power,* in which the nurse helps a client transform his or her view of self or others

2. *Integrative caring,* in which the nurse is instrumental in helping clients continue with meaningful life activities despite disability and disorders

3. *Advocacy power* to remove obstacles or stand alongside and enable

4. *Healing power* to create a climate that mobilizes hope, to find interpretations of situations that are acceptable and clarifying to clients and families, and to help clients use sources of social, emotional, and spiritual support

5. *Participative/affirmative power,* in which engagement and involvement are sources of energy

6. *Problem-solving expertise* to grasp the problem rapidly, seeing it in relation to the past and similar as well as dissimilar situations yet not overlooking creative search and cue sensitivity (Benner 1984, pp 210–215). The chapters that follow in this text offer sources of excellence and power in the practice of humanistic interactionist psychiatric nursing.

Chapter Highlights

- The humanistic interactionist ideology is one response to a need for a framework of values and concepts in psychiatric nursing that views human beings as having purpose and control over their own lives.

- The key premises of interactionism are that people act toward things on the basis of the meanings those things have for them—that the meanings arise out of social interaction with others and are modified through the process of encountering things.

- Implications of interactionism and humanism for the practice of psychiatric nursing include the importance of finding a common ground of negotiated meaning when dealing with clients, of viewing behavior within its social context, of discovering and respecting each client's individual experience and the meaning attached to it, and of viewing physical and mental factors as interrelated.

- The key premises of humanism give rise to a holistic view of mind-body relations, an expanded role for nurses, a collaborative decision-making model, and a general posture of negotiation and advocacy in relation to clients in social, political, and individual arenas.

- Despite barriers and constraints to implementing a professional philosophy in real-world practice, psychiatric nurses can and do find sources of power.

References

American Nurses' Association: *Nursing: A Social Policy Statement.* ANA, 1980.

American Psychiatric Association: *Diagnostic and Statistical Manual of Mental Disorders,* ed 3. APA, 1980.

American Psychiatric Association: *Diagnostic and Statistical Manual,* ed 3, revised. APA, 1987.

Benner P: *From Novice to Expert: Excellence and Power in Clinical Nursing Practice.* Addison-Wesley, 1984.

Blumer H: *Symbolic Interaction: Perspective and Method.* Prentice-Hall, 1969.

Bunch EH: *Everyday Reality of the Psychiatric Nurse.* Gyldendal Norsk Forlag, 1983.

Kramer M: *Reality Shock: Why Nurses Leave Nursing.* Mosby, 1974.

Loomis M, et al: PND-I: A classification of phenomena of concern for psychiatric-mental health nursing. *Arch Psych Nursing* 1987; 1(1):16–24.

Lamont C: *The Philosophy of Humanism.* New York: Frederick Ungar Publishing, 1967.

Strauss A, et al: *Psychiatric Ideologies and Institutions.* The Free Press of Glencoe, 1964.

Wilson HS: *Deinstitutionalized Residential Care for the Mentally Disordered: The Soteria House Approach.* Grune and Stratton, 1982.

TWO

Historical Perspectives

Carol Ren Kneisl
Holly Skodol Wilson

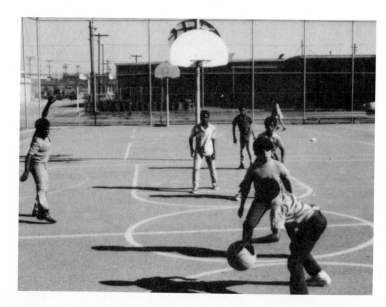

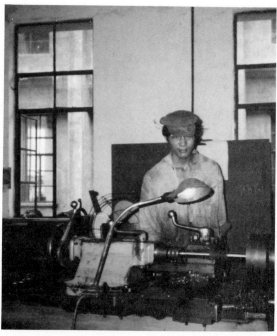

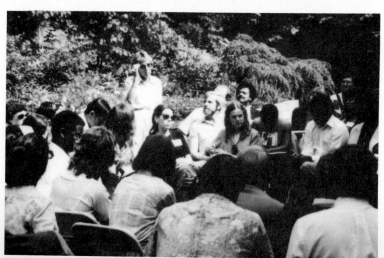

After reading this chapter, students should be able to

- Describe the history of ideas about madness
- Correlate the history of psychiatric treatment with ideas about madness
- Describe the emergence of the discipline of psychiatric nursing
- Project directions for psychiatric nursing in the 1990s.

Cross References

Other topics relevant to this content are: Community mental health movement, Chapter 40; Conceptual frameworks for psychiatric treatment, Chapter 5; Contemporary roles of psychiatric nurses, Chapter 3; Legal aspects of confinement, Chapter 39; Modern biologic treatments, Chapter 32.

This book views personal and interpersonal peace as a bridge to a peaceful world.

Key Terms

dumping	moral treatment
Malleus Maleficarum	Ship of Fools
mental hygiene movement	

Madness has been recognized by many different faces throughout history. Clearly, the meaning assigned to madness has determined whether such persons are perceived as deranged and tragic heroes, to be valued and liberated, or as criminals, to be confined and modified. Through a comparative social history, we hope to offer perspectives on the odd courses human beings have run in the past. To understand the changing faces and future directions of psychiatric nursing, we must be able to understand how it evolved as a specialty by tracing its historical development.

THE HISTORY OF IDEAS IN PSYCHIATRY

People who have been called "mentally ill" have been with us throughout history—to be feared, marveled at, ignored, banished, sheltered, laughed at, pitied, or tortured. A historical perspective on the place of the "mentally ill," however they have been defined in societies during different periods, brings up several central points:

- Dominant social attitudes and philosophic viewpoints have influenced the understanding and approach to "madness" throughout recorded history and probably before.
- Ideas that may be considered contemporary at one time often have roots centuries earlier.
- The modern medical concept of "madness" as an illness is open to the same scrutiny as other interpretations of the past, such as beliefs about witchcraft, mysticism, or the causality of substances.

Preliterate Times—Era of Magico-Religious Explanations

In preliterate cultures, mental and physical suffering were not differentiated. Both were attributed to forces acting outside the body. Consequently, medicine, magic, and religion were not distinct disciplines. All were variously directed against some mortal or superhuman force that had cruelly inflicted suffering on another. Primitive healers quite logically dealt with the spirits of torment by appeal, reverence, prayer, bribery, intimidation, appeasement, confession, and punishment. These were expressed through exorcism, magical ritual, and incantation. It is possible to perceive some of the rudiments of current psychotherapy in these practices.

Most preliterate cultures believed in:

- The liberation of immaterial (spiritual) forces by divine power or magical arts

- The principle of solidarity or contagion, which implies that human beings are continuous with, not separate from, their surroundings

- Sympathetic, imitative forms of magic occurring by telepathy and other interactions between similar elements

- The symbolism of certain elements, such as the purifying role of water

These beliefs about the nature of suffering gave rise to procedures based on the idea of *mimetic,* or imitative, magic. A medicine man would enact a person's illness and then slowly recover. This was believed to prompt the person's own recovery. The principle of continuity was the belief in continued relationship between things that were once close but now are separated. Thus, fingernail parings and afterbirths were seen as objects that could influence the lives of people from whom these things had been removed. Some approaches were based on substitution methods—i.e., transferring suffering to a scapegoat. Behavior considered to be "mental illness" by modern Western cultures was attributed in preliterate cultures to the violation of taboos, the neglect of ritual obligations, the loss of a vital substance from the body (such as the soul), the introduction of a foreign and harmful substance into the body (such as evil spirits), or witchcraft. Some of these beliefs remain part of contemporary psychiatry's definition of "mental illness."

Early Civilization— Era of Organic Explanations

There are essentially three sources of the concept of madness in Greek and Roman cultures:

1. Popular opinion continued earlier beliefs in the supernatural causation of mental suffering. This had no prescribed treatment.

2. A medical concept arose, centered on the interaction of four body "humors." It was elaborated in the writings of Hippocrates (fourth century B.C.).

3. The notion developed that violation of moral principles and subsequent punishment by the gods was part of man's destiny. This is evident in the literary and philosophic works of the period.

What might be called the professional opinion on madness was summarized by Hippocrates, who lived from about 460 to 370 B.C. He rejected demonology and proposed that psychiatric illnesses were caused mainly by disturbances of body humors—blood, black bile, yellow bile, and phlegm. These four humors were believed to influence emotional orientation. An imbalance in humors was believed to cause madness. Thus, for example, an excess of black bile caused melancholy and could be removed by purging or bloodletting. One important consequence of these beliefs was to put psychiatric suffering within the realm of the physician's medical practice.

Four ancient methods of psychotherapeutic intervention stand out because of their widespread use for many centuries in the cultures of the Near East and Mediterranean areas: the interpretation of dreams, ritual purifications, therapeutic use of the milieu, and catharsis. Both words and medicines were used in these methods. However, the need for supernatural explanations was so great that when cures were achieved, they were attributed to the interventions of the gods.

The Medieval Period—Era of Alienation

At the height of their civilization, the citizens of ancient Greece found their inner security in knowledge and reason. The Romans adopted the intellectual heritage of Greece but for their peace of mind relied more on their social institutions and the rational organization of society supported by law and military might. When these institutions disintegrated and the empire declined, fear tore apart the fabric of society. The collapse of the Roman security produced a general return to the magic, mysticism, and demonology from which people had retreated during Greek rationality. During the Middle Ages, the period between approximately 400 A.D. and the Renaissance (1300–1600), madness was seen as a dramatic encounter with secret powers. Troubled minds were thought to be influenced by the moon (*lunacy* literally means a disorder caused by the lunar body).

In the Arab world, the insane were believed to be divinely inspired and not victims of demons. An asylum for the mentally ill was built in Fez, Morocco, early in the eighth century. Other asylums in Baghdad, Cairo, and Damascus soon followed. Hospital care in these asylums was usually benevolent and kindly.

Mad people, left wandering on their own, were evidence of the greatness of God and the frailty of humans— a necessary, although sometimes annoying, part of the community. Many participated in religious wars, crusades, and long pilgrimages. Others embraced emotionally charged heretic movements, such as the dance epidemics of the fourteenth century.

By and large, through the thirteenth and fourteenth centuries, the human body and its organic afflictions were dealt with by lay physicians. During this period, the first European hospital devoted entirely to mental patients was built in 1409 in Valencia, Spain. The problems of the mind, however, remained in the domain of clerical scholars. Two Dominican monks, Johann Sprenger and Heinrich Kraemer, codified the dominant ideology of the times in their book **Malleus Maleficarum** (*The Witches' Hammer,* 1487), a textbook of both pornography and supposed psychopathology. Witch-hunts became accepted as a system to maintain the status quo. The *Malleus* details the destruction of dissenters, heretics, and the "mentally ill," most of whom were women and all of whom were labeled *witches.* The favorite way to destroy the devil was to burn his host, the witch. Any unknown disease or illness was thought to be caused by witchcraft. "All witchcraft comes from carnal lust, which is in women insatiable," warned these clerics. Theologic rationalizations and magical explanations then served as foundations for burning at the stake thousands of unfortunates.

End of the Middle Ages— Era of Ritualized Social Exclusion

A new device appeared in the imaginary landscape at the end of the Middle Ages and the beginning of the Renaissance. It was a "strange drunken boat whose crew of imaginary heroes, ethical models or social types had embarked on a symbolic voyage" (Foucault 1973). The **Ships of Fools** of the early Renaissance were boatloads of mad people sent out to sea symbolically searching for their reason. In this phase of ritualized social exclusion, social abandonment was viewed as spiritual reintegration. In the image of the Ship of Fools, madness was seen to proceed from a point within reason to a point beyond. The violent insane were shackled in prisons.

The Renaissance—Era of Confinement

The Middle Ages are generally credited with driving out or excluding the insane from community life, while the Renaissance is noted for its methods of exclusion by confinement. In the era of confinement, the Ship of Fools symbolized docks. In the Renaissance, it was no longer a ship but a hospital. Tamed, retained (on land), and maintained, madness was reduced to silence through a system of mutual obligation between the afflicted and society. Mad persons had the right to be fed but were morally constrained and physically confined.

Seventeenth-century society created enormous houses of confinement. In these asylums were gathered the mad,

the poor, and various deviants. A landmark date is 1656, when by decree the Hôpital Générale in Paris was founded. It was not a medical establishment, but rather a strange implement of power, complete with stakes, irons, prisons, and dungeons that the king established to enforce the law. The "insane" belonged to a world of almost absolute sovereignty and jurisdiction without appeal. The Hôpital Générale and others like it had little to do with any medical concept. They were institutions for the maintenance of social order. Michel Foucault (1973, p 71) describes the conditions in these terms:

> The unfortunate whose entire furniture consisted of a straw pallet, lying with his head, feet and body pressed against the wall, could not enjoy sleep without being soaked by the water that trickled from that mass of stone. . . . In winter the waters of the Seine rose . . . and cells became a refuge for a swarm of huge rats. Madwomen have been found with feet, hands, and faces torn by bites.

In London, the hospital of Saint Mary of Bethlehem became famous as *Bedlam,* where, for the entertainment of visitors on Sunday excursions, mad persons were publicly beaten and tortured.

Madness thus was given the mask of the beast. Those chained to cell walls were no longer considered people who had lost their reason, but rather beasts seized by a natural frenzy. The animality in madness was seen as evidence that the mad person was not a sick person. Madness was less than ever linked to medicine in this period. It could be mastered only by discipline and brutality.

During the 1500s, 1600s, and 1700s, some physicians again began to consider psychiatric bases for mental disorders. Johann Weyer (1515–1588), a German physician, believed that "those illnesses whose origins are attributed to witches come from natural causes." He explained a variety of so-called supernatural signs on the basis of natural factors. Weyer was a carefully observant clinician. He described a wide range of diagnostic categories with associated symptoms, including hysteria, paranoid reactions, toxic organic brain syndrome, epilepsy, folie à deux, depression, and delusions. His position on psychotherapy, however, is considered his most outstanding contribution. He insisted that the needs of individuals rather than the rules of social institutions must be given primary consideration. He recognized the importance of the therapeutic relationship and stressed not only kindness but also a benevolent attitude based on careful observation and scientific principles. His approach was radical and completely alien to the thinking of his time. As a result, his work was met with hostility at first and then was simply ignored. In retrospect, his contributions are of such importance that he is called "the first psychiatrist."

Late Eighteenth and Early Nineteenth Centuries—Era of Moral Treatment

The continuous development of scientific ideas cannot be neatly divided into centuries. It has simply become a matter of convenience to label the eighteenth century the *epoch of enlightenment.* Enlightenment there was, but the era was full of internal contradictions. Although the insane were unchained, the medical treatment they received consisted of tortures provided by special paraphernalia. In attempting to understand the incredible inhumanity with which the mentally disordered were treated in this era of enlightenment, consider the following:

- The nature of mental disorders could not be explained by any of the concepts—black humors could not be seen, demons or animal spirits could not be observed, and knowledge of anatomy could not be applied to the workings of the mind.

- Because mental disorders could not be satisfactorily explained, the deeply felt dread of the insane could not be removed.

- Mental disorders were believed to be incurable and mad persons were thought to be dangerous.

Eventually, belief in reason replaced beliefs in faith and tradition. New medical and scientific data had become so overwhelming that synthesis and systematization became necessary. The epoch of enlightenment encompassed a movement from classifying to unchaining the insane.

Eighteenth-century psychiatry typically emphasized the classification of symptoms of mental disorders. Even the most sensitive physicians failed to try to understand the sources of mental suffering. Methods of psychiatric treatment were scarcely affected by these classifiers. Because they had no way to explain or understand these disorders, classification became overextended. There was a tendency to dismiss factual data that did not fit, and the system abounded with errors. Among the classifiers was Hermann Boerhaave (1668–1738), a Dutch physician, for whom the practice of psychotherapy consisted of bloodletting, purgatives, dousing people in ice-cold water, or using other methods to put them in near shock. Boerhaave gave the medical profession one of its first shock instruments, a spinning chair that rendered its occupant unconscious. Another was William Cullen (1710–1790), who lectured at Edinburgh and was the first to use the term *neurosis* to denote diseases that are not accompanied by fever or localized pathology. Cullen believed that neurosis was due to decay, either of the intellect or of the involuntary nervous system. By his time psychiatry had discarded the concept that a demon originating outside the person caused internal disharmony. Physicians now insisted that the evil was disordered physiology.

At the same time, doctors began subscribing to another movement characteristic of the Enlightenment—a zeal for social reform and moral uplift. Rationalism, observation through experimentation, and classification were joined by a fourth approach—reform. In 1793, Philippe Pinel (1745–1826) became superintendent of the French institution Bicêtre for men and later of the Salpêtrière for women, where criminals, mentally retarded people, and the insane were housed. One of his first accomplishments was to release the inmates from their chains, abolish systematized brutality with chains and whips, open their windows, feed them nourishing food, and treat them with kindness. For this act, he himself was considered mad by his contemporaries. History reports that many of the inmates improved dramatically.

Meanwhile in England, William Tuke (1732–1822), a Quaker tea merchant unhappy about the institutions available to treat mentally disordered Quakers, founded the York Retreat in England. The goal was to reconstruct around madness a milieu resembling the community of Quakers. Tuke's work focused on liberation of the insane, suppression of constraint, and establishment of a humane milieu. With the emergence of **moral treatment**, the asylum no longer punished the mad person's guilt. It did more, it organized that guilt. By becoming aware of their guilt the mad became aware of themselves as responsible subjects and, consequently, were able to return to reason. At the York Retreat the suppression of physical constraint fostered "self-restraint" by inmates engaged in work and under the observation of others.

The insane were among the clients of the first general hospital in the United States. Pennsylvania Hospital was opened through the efforts of the Quakers, Benjamin Franklin, and others in 1756. Treatment, rather than mere confinement of the mentally ill, was the stated goal for these people, though the state of medical knowledge was such that treatment consisted of bleeding, blistering, and purging in the damp restraining cells of the hospital's cellar.

The early treatment of psychiatric clients at the Pennsylvania Hospital in the United States is closely connected with the work of Benjamin Rush (1746–1813), called "the father of American psychiatry," whose picture is reproduced on the seal of the American Psychiatric Association. Despite his association with humanitarianism and moral treatment, Rush was a major follower of Cullen's ideas in advocating bloodletting, the gyrating chair, and other inhumane devices.

The first American hospital devoted exclusively to the care and treatment of psychiatric clients opened in Williamsburg, Virginia, in 1773. The only other colony to establish a hospital that accepted mentally disordered people in the eighteenth century was New York, which began building its first general hospital in 1774. The intention was to allot the cellar of the north wing to psychiatric clients. The Revolutionary War and a fire delayed the opening until 1792. As promised, the cellar of New York Hospital received these clients.

Moral treatment, by providing an alternative to mere confinement, played a major role in the development of institutional care and treatment of the mentally disordered in the United States. The growth of the mental hospital in the early nineteenth century was not a chance occurrence but the result of numerous social factors. It arose from the general spirit of reform and humanitarianism sweeping western Europe and the United States. Scientific and technologic advances, coupled with the successful struggle for political democracy in the United States and France, were proof to many people that humanity could tackle and conquer any problem.

Private philanthropy was largely responsible for the hospital movement in the early nineteenth century. In response to the needs brought on by increases in the population, hospitals were established in urban areas. These early corporate hospitals, such as McLean Asylum in Massachusetts (opened in 1818), Friend's Asylum in Frankfort, Pennsylvania (1817), Hartford Retreat in Connecticut (1824), and Bloomingdale Asylum in New York City (1818), were small and used "moral treatment" on a homogeneous population with an astounding degree of success.

It became clear in the mid-1820s that the corporate mental hospitals would be unable to meet the needs of all those requiring services. Responsibility for psychiatric clients, then, began gradually to shift away from the corporate hospitals (just as it had, to a certain extent, shifted away from the family and to the corporate hospital). It now moved to the new institution on the horizon—the public mental hospital.

Late Nineteenth and Early Twentieth Centuries

Era of Public Mental Hospitals

Strongly influenced by optimistic and humanitarian beliefs about human nature, some community leaders took the initiative in establishing a few mental hospitals early in the nineteenth century. The most distinguished leader in generating public interest in building state mental hospitals in the United States was Dorothea L. Dix (1802–1887). Although she was not formally educated as a nurse, she devoted her life to public education concerning the needs of the mentally disordered and administered volunteer women nurses during the Civil War.

For three decades, Dix reported to state legislatures the often abominable conditions in the almshouses, jails, and mental hospitals in their states. After making her exposés, she insisted to legislators that the state had moral, humanitarian, and legal obligations toward the mentally disordered. Dix's determination about this single issue gained

her a broad base of support, and she was eventually responsible for founding or enlarging over thirty mental hospitals. J. Sanborn Bockoven (1956, p 187), an authority on moral treatment, suggests that Dix's reform movement, with its emphasis on bringing people into asylums without any planning for effective treatment, was responsible at least in part for the downfall of moral treatment in the United States.

From 1825 to 1865, the number of mental hospitals grew from nine to sixty-two. The first state institution that relied on moral treatment was Worcester State Hospital in Massachusetts, opened in 1833. It gained a national reputation for recovery of 80 to 91 percent of its acute patients. *Acute patient* usually meant a person who had been mentally ill for less than six months. The example set by the citizens of Massachusetts became a model for other states. Eventually, institutionalization had become an end in itself. As a carryover from the high rate of "cures" effected by moral treatment, people believed that once insane persons were within the walls of an asylum, they were well on their way to recovery. Moral treatment was being replaced by custodial care.

Toward the end of the nineteenth century, approaches to the "mentally ill" began to change again. Insanity was linked to faulty life habits, and separate hospital facilities were advocated for acute patients. New forms of physical therapy—diet, massage, hydrotherapy, and electroshock therapy—were introduced. Family care and the cottage system were initiated, as were training courses for psychiatric nurses and attendants.

As the twentieth century began, a few psychiatrists became interested in research, which led to the founding of the Pathological Institute of New York Hospital in 1895. Adolf Meyer (1866–1950), a Swiss psychiatrist, served on the staff of the institute from 1902 until 1913, when he became director of the newly built psychiatric clinic at Johns Hopkins Hospital. Meyer dedicated himself to improving the situation for psychiatric clients through any approach that seemed sensible and practical. He was opposed to the dualist philosophy of the separation of mind and body. He regarded each person as a biologic unit who experiences unique reactions to social and biologic influences. As his realistic, *commonsense approach* evolved, he became increasingly unwilling to believe that mental disorders were the result solely of brain dysfunction or solely of an overwhelming environment. Both had to be taken into account. He introduced the term *ergasia*, meaning integrated mental activity, and even suggested that psychiatry be called *ergasiatry*.

In 1908 another key event occurred in the development of psychiatry. Clifford Beers (1876–1943), a distinguished businessman, published *A Mind That Found Itself,* a book in which he described his intense suffering and mental anguish while receiving custodial care. This book profoundly affected the social consciousness of the nation and led to the organization of spirited groups that Meyer named the **mental hygiene movement**. Public awareness of the needs of the mentally disordered was responsible for the development of preventive psychiatry and the formation of child guidance clinics.

Era of Psychoanalysis

The eighteenth-century emphasis on clinical classification peaked in the work of Emil Kraepelin (1856–1926). This physician, like many of his time, was inclined toward an organic, neurophysiologic explanation of mental disorders. He is best known for bringing the chaotic accumulation of clinical observations into a system of distinct disease entities. He differentiated *bipolar disorder* (which he called *manic-depressive psychosis*) from *schizophrenia* (which he called *dementia praecox*) and theorized that the latter was incurable. Since then, schizophrenia and its treatment have had a fatalistic connotation, although schizophrenia can be—and has been—"cured." A Swiss psychiatrist, Eugene Bleuler (1857–1939), renamed dementia praecox *schizophrenia* and differentiated the disorder into *hebephrenic, catatonic,* and *paranoid* types. Bleuler also expressed a far more optimistic view of the treatment outcome than Kraepelin did.

The psychiatric developments of the late nineteenth century formed the background for the work of one of the most influential figures in the history of psychiatry, Sigmund Freud (1856–1939). He succeeded in explaining human behavior in psychologic terms and demonstrated that behavior can be changed under carefully constructed circumstances. Freud's contributions to psychiatry included his views on the value of catharsis (also recognized in ancient Greek culture), his notion that symptoms represented a compromise between opposing forces (life and death), his interpretations of dreams (also part of ancient traditions), his dynamic explanations of hysteria, and his studies in hypnotism and the character of psychoanalytic technique. For more than thirty years, Freud refrained from constructing a comprehensive theory of personality and instead made detailed observations. Finally, in 1929, he published the first in a series of writings compiled in his *New Introductory Lectures on Psychoanalysis.* In these he explained the logic of psychologic cause and effect. The specific premises of Freudian psychoanalytic theory are discussed in detail in Chapter 5.

The psychoanalytic concepts of personality and behavior strongly influenced treatment approaches. The aim of therapy became to extend the client's consciousness to formerly unconscious parts of the personality.

Freud's ideas also profoundly changed people's concepts of themselves. Initially, his concepts were met with a violent and almost universal rejection. But gradually Freud attracted a handful of followers, from Vienna and later from Switzerland, Hungary, and England. This group organized a small professional community devoted to the development of a new discipline, *psychoanalysis.*

- Alfred Adler (1870–1937) is known for his pioneering efforts in psychosomatic medicine, based on a concept of organ inferiority. He held to the notion that the aggressive drive is the strongest influence on personality.

- Carl Jung (1875–1961) developed various original concepts, including the notion of a collective unconscious from which universal archetypes emerge regardless of culture and historical periods. He saw the structure of the human psyche as a composite of persona (social mask), shadow (hidden personal characteristics), anima (feminine identification in man), animus (masculine identification in women), and self (the innermost center of the personality).

- Otto Rank (1884–1939) believed that creativity was a constructive outlet for neurotic conflicts. He was interested in the application of psychoanalysis to literature and art. He later separated from the psychoanalytic movement and minimized the importance of the Oedipus conflict, theorizing instead that the separation anxiety connected with birth is the most important influence on development and the source of neurosis.

- Ernest Jones (1879–1958) is considered the most faithful pupil of Freud and is best remembered for his biography of Freud (Jones 1953–1957).

- Sandor Ferenczi (1873–1933) was among the first to link homosexuality to paranoia. He also anticipated a later emphasis on *ego psychology* by advocating active therapy in which clients were encouraged to unearth unconscious material.

- Helene Deutsch, born in 1884, is mainly associated with her two-volume *Psychology of Women,* in which she described women as essentially passive and masochistic, as making a transition at puberty from a clitoral to a vaginal orientation, and as possessing an inborn maternal role.

- Karen Horney (1885–1952) believed that cultural factors play a greater part in the development of neurosis than earlier theorists believed. She also anticipated current notions of alienation.

- Anna Freud, the daughter of Sigmund Freud, was born in 1895. She devoted herself to the psychoanalytic study of children and is best known for her refinement of ideas about *ego defense mechanisms.*

Dealing with contemporary patterns is difficult, since we do not yet have the historian's hindsight to guide our judgments. Today's ideas, practices, and contributions will be subject to reappraisal in the future.

From the mid-1940s to mid-1950s, psychiatric thought in this country was characterized by a strong rift between *biologic orientation* and *dynamic orientation*. The great number of psychiatric casualties during World War II directed attention toward the problems of mental and emotional disorders in general. In 1946 the National Institute of Mental Health was opened in Bethesda, Maryland, for the purposes of research, training, and assistance to the states in providing preventive, therapeutic, and rehabilitative psychiatric services.

Dissatisfaction with the theories and methods of psychoanalysis and psychoanalytic ideology has persisted. Psychotherapy has become progressively influenced by trends toward both ego psychology and social psychology. Harry Stack Sullivan (1892–1949), the only American-born psychiatrist to found an independent school during this period, was strongly influenced by social scientists such as Ruth Benedict and Margaret Mead. Central to his thinking is an interpersonal theory of psychiatry that is at variance with the strictly individual emphasis of psychoanalysis. His pioneering psychotherapy was aimed at understanding and correcting the client's disturbed communication process in the context of a client-therapist relationship based on mutual learning.

The American trend emphasizing the social dimension of psychiatry is also seen in the emergence of both group and family psychotherapy. John Bell and Nathan Ackerman were leading proponents of treating a whole family in one place at the same time. Don Jackson, Gregory Bateson, and their colleagues extended this approach to schizophrenic people and their families. Family therapy by 1960 had become both a diagnostic tool and a mode of treatment. During this period Erik Erikson formulated his psychosocial theory of development, based on the interplay of biologic and social factors and a progressive unfolding of developmental tasks in an entire life span.

During this period of ideologic expansion, the issue of mental illness received national attention. With the strong support of the National Institute of Mental Health and many private and professional associations, the Mental Health Study Act was passed in 1955. It established the Joint Commission on Mental Illness and Health to set priorities and define adequate services for psychiatric clients throughout the country. After five years of investigation, the commission concluded that psychiatric resources and the network of mental hospitals in this country were totally inadequate. The final report of this commission, *Action for Mental Health* (1961), was essentially a proposal for a concerted attack on mental illness through a better distribution and commu-

nity orientation of psychiatric services. The commission proposed a massive program of preventive services, a shift of emphasis from institutional to community-based care, and plans for shared federal, state, and local funding of community mental health centers. (See Chapter 40.)

Between 1955 and 1975 the number of resident clients in state mental hospitals decreased from 559,000 to 193,000–almost 66 percent. Proponents of the community mental health and deinstitutionalization movements refer to "a bold new approach," while critics use less enthusiastic terms, such as **dumping**, to characterize modern trends in mental health services. In the latter view, the site of care for the chronically mentally disordered has merely been moved from a single lousy institution to multiple wretched ones.

Some experts conclude that deinstitutionalization and the principles of community psychiatry are a national disgrace and advocate the return of the old state hospital warehouse system. Others, however, prefer to rethink this approach, pointing out that criticism of the deinstitutionalization movement has merely highlighted community psychiatry's lack of true innovation. This group argues not for the desirability of the old state hospital system, but for the development of alternatives to it that emphasize self-care and self-determination for clients, rather than institutionalization (Wilson 1982).

One of our needs as we move into the 1990s is for sustained life-support systems for certain chronic client groups, not merely transitional ones. Such approaches, however, require sufficient legislation, funding continuity, and coordination to replace the current nonsystem of aftercare left in the wake of closing state mental hospitals.

EMERGENCE OF THE DISCIPLINE OF PSYCHIATRIC NURSING

Although nursing functions have existed since ancient times, the profession of nursing, particularly psychiatric nursing, is a product of the late nineteenth and twentieth centuries. Theodor and Friedericke Fliedner founded the first systematic school of nursing in Germany in 1836. It was this school at Kaiserwerth that Florence Nightingale visited in 1851 before organizing a school to educate nurses in England after the Crimean War. Her school, Saint Thomas Hospital in London, stressed the importance of providing an optimum environment for clients. Although it is true that in the context of her time she emphasized the physical environment, Nightingale's contribution to psychiatric nursing was in being among the first to note that the influence of nurses on their clients goes beyond physical care and has psychologic and social components.

Development of Early Psychiatric Nursing Education

In the early 1870s the first three American nursing schools, organized in the pattern of Saint Thomas Hospital, were opened in New York, Boston, and New Haven. Linda Richards, a graduate of the New England Hospital for Women in Boston, spent a significant part of her career developing better nursing care in psychiatric hospitals and is sometimes called "the first American psychiatric nurse." She echoed Nightingale's earlier observation about the nurse's impact.

Although the first mental hospital in the United States was established in 1773 in colonial Williamsburg, Virginia, it was more than a century before the first training program for psychiatric nurses was opened. The first American school for psychiatric nurses was opened under the direction of Linda Richards at the McLean Psychiatric Asylum in Waverly, Massachusetts in 1880. Ninety nurses graduated from its two-year course in 1882. By 1890, there were thirty-five such schools in asylums. Unlike graduates of general hospital schools of nursing, these nurses could find employment only in asylums.

By the end of the nineteenth century, trained nurses staffed some mental hospitals in the United States, but they attended mainly to the physical needs of clients and did not pursue systematic interpersonal work with them. Psychiatric theory in this period emphasized providing a physically sound environment that would promote recovery. Thus, nurses administered medications such as chloral hydrate and paraldehyde, supervised the use of hydrotherapy, and oversaw the nutritional and physical care of clients. Much of psychiatric nursing practice was custodial, mechanistic, and directed by psychiatrists. A ratio of 1 trained nurse to 140 clients was not unusual, and some large mental hospitals hired no registered nurses at all.

The trend toward preparing nurses in a general hospital to care for clients with physical disorders or in a psychiatric hospital to care for clients with mental disorders dominated nursing education for over half a century. In 1913, the school of nursing at Johns Hopkins Hospital included a psychiatric nursing component in its curriculum, heralding the beginning of a slowly developing but important change in the structure of nursing programs.

The first psychiatric nursing text, *Nursing Mental Diseases,* was written in 1920 by Harriet Bailey, the Assistant Superintendent of Nurses at the psychiatric clinic at Johns Hopkins Hospital. It was, for twenty years, the standard textbook in psychiatric nursing. Most textbooks were written by psychiatrists who devoted only a few pages to instructing psychiatric nurses in such procedures as tube and rectal feeding and preparing treatment trays.

In the years between the two world wars, mental hospitals were seriously understaffed. In an effort to cope with understaffing, mental hospitals opened schools of nursing at an incredible rate—sixty-seven in 1936 alone.

Movement of Psychiatric Nursing into the Mainstream of Nursing

It was 1937 before the National League for Nursing Education (now the National League for Nursing) recommended, but did not require, that psychiatric nursing content and clinical experience be a part of the curriculum in all basic nursing programs. The league also took over from psychiatrists the tasks of standardizing and accrediting psychiatric nursing education in single-focus schools for psychiatric nurses. The American Psychiatric Association, rather than a nursing organization, had been involved since 1906 in policing this aspect of nursing.

Psychiatric nursing moved into the mainstream of nursing in the 1940s, and nurses began to assume increasing responsibility for educating their own and taking over the teaching from physicians. However, the focus of psychiatric nursing activities continued to be the provision of kind, but custodial, nursing care. Nurses supervised or were responsible for providing housekeeping tasks such as scrubbing floors and counting mops and sheets; feeding, clothing, and bathing clients; assisting the physician with treatments; and keeping the keys to locked wards, locked cabinets, even locked toilet tissue containers.

The specialty grew slowly during the 1940s. In one West Coast state seven state hospitals housed 37,000 psychiatric clients but employed only eighteen graduate nurses: one nurse for approximately 2000 clients. In 1944, there were still fourteen states in which no psychiatric nursing course had ever been given (Kalisch and Kalisch 1987).

In the meantime, psychiatric theory expanded to encompass the interpersonal and emotional dimensions of "mental illness." During these years, Sigmund Freud published his works on *psychoanalysis,* Adolf Meyer had major impact in America and Britain through his *commonsense psychiatry,* and Harry Stack Sullivan, often called "the founder of interpersonal psychiatry," introduced the concept of *milieu therapy* as a new approach to treating hospitalized psychiatric clients. These ideologic changes in psychiatry did not have a discernible impact on psychiatric nursing care until the early 1950s.

Instead, new modes of physical treatment laid the groundwork for change. To the custodial tasks of psychiatric nurses were added specific medical-surgical procedures as psychiatry developed somatic therapies for the treatment of specific disorders. These included deep sleep therapy in 1930, insulin shock therapy in 1935, psychosurgery in 1935–1936, and electroshock therapy in 1937. Thus, it was through the use of medical-surgical skills that psychiatric nurses gained recognition as significant participants in psychiatric treatment.

Although these somatic treatments controlled dramatically bizarre client behavior and made clients more available for interpersonal interactions, it was not until 1946, with passage of the National Mental Health Act, that any systematic development of psychotherapeutic roles for nurses began. Most psychiatric clients were being cared for in large state mental hospitals where small numbers of staff were expected to manage large numbers of clients living in crowded conditions. Somatic treatments, rather than psychotherapy, were more practical in these settings. Psychotherapy was often reserved for the private clients of psychiatrists in private psychiatric hospitals or in private practice settings.

Confirmation of Psychiatric Nursing as a Specialty

Enactment of the National Mental Health Act was the government's response to growing recognition of mental illness as a national health problem. During World War II, 43 percent of all army discharges were classified as psychiatric disabilities. This created a sharp increase in the demand for psychiatric services. The National Mental Health Act provided for:

1. Establishment of the National Institute of Mental Health (NIMH)
2. Development of programs to train professional psychiatric personnel, including psychiatric nurses
3. Support for psychiatric research
4. Aid in developing mental health programs

With the establishment of the NIMH in 1946, psychiatric nursing was added to psychiatry, psychology, and social work as a field in which the highest priority became the preparation of clinically capable persons for positions of leadership. Funds administered by NIMH facilitated advanced education in psychiatric nursing. Before the 1946 act, fewer than a dozen psychiatric nurses held master's degrees in the United States and fewer than 5 percent of basic nursing education programs were at the baccalaureate level. The psychiatric nursing education given most students consisted of a few weeks of observation on a psychiatric ward. As a result of NIMH funds, nine universities received grants to expand and improve graduate programs in 1948. The number increased gradually and steadily. These programs prepared many of the nursing leaders who later developed theoretical frameworks for one-to-one relationship work.

Because of its wide-ranging effects, the National Mental Health Act of 1946 is probably the most significant piece of legislation affecting the development of psychiatric nursing.

Nursing leaders began to question the wisdom of single-focus schools of psychiatric nursing. In 1948, a report entitled *Nursing for the Future* (Brown 1948) recommended their elimination. The needs of nursing could best be served, the report indicated, if the psychiatric hospitals conducting schools of nursing made their facilities widely available instead to students in basic schools of nursing. Shortly thereafter, in 1955, the National League for Nursing made the provision of a clinical experience in psychiatric nursing a requirement for the accreditation of nursing schools. Requiring both coursework and hands-on clinical experience further cemented the mainstreaming of psychiatric nursing.

Until the early 1950s, psychiatric nurses formulated only vague concepts about how nurses might participate in one-to-one relationships with clients. Some pressed for trained postgraduate nurses to provide psychotherapy and become functioning members of an interdisciplinary treatment team that would include psychologists and social workers. Ambiguity about professional psychiatric nursing roles characterized this period.

Role Clarification in Psychiatric Nursing

The 1950s and early 1960s were a period of role clarification. Three important milestones in psychiatric nursing occurred in 1952:

- Hildegard Peplau published *Interpersonal Relations in Nursing,* the first systematic theoretical framework in psychiatric nursing. Her framework, grounded in the interpersonal psychiatry of Harry Stack Sullivan and learning theory, represents a cornerstone in the development of psychiatric nursing theory and practice. She delineated several skills, activities, and roles for psychiatric nurses. Peplau emphasized the interpersonal nature of nursing and the need for nurses to understand and use psychodynamic concepts and counseling techniques in their practice. Peplau has had greater impact on psychiatric nursing than any other nursing theoretician to date.
- Gwen Tudor Will published an article in the journal *Psychiatry* demonstrating that nurses can promote emotional growth in clients. She developed a specific nursing intervention with a sociopsychiatric base—a

unique contribution, at that time, to psychiatric nursing and to understanding the importance of milieu factors. (Will's classic sociopsychiatric nursing approach is discussed in the Research Note in this chapter.)

- Frances Sleeper, in an address to the American Psychiatric Association, advocated the use of psychiatric nurses as psychotherapists. Her advocacy ushered in a heated, ten-year controversy over caretaker versus psychotherapist roles for psychiatric nurses.

Over these next ten years, a number of developments further clarified the role of the psychiatric nurse while lending legitimacy to the counselor role. A milestone report published in 1956 (National League for Nursing 1956) introduced the concept of the psychiatric clinical nurse specialist and differentiated functions based on master's level preparation of psychiatric nurses. In this same year, the first grants were made available by NIMH to integrate mental health concepts into the basic nursing curriculum, and traineeships for graduate students in psychiatric nursing were increased.

In 1957, June Mellow introduced a system of nursing therapy based on her work with schizophrenic clients at Boston State Hospital. Her approach, designed to provide corrective emotional experiences, drew strongly from psychoanalytic theory and provided the theoretical framework for the first doctoral program in nursing in 1960 at Boston University (Mellow 1968). Unlike psychoanalysis, Mellow's nursing therapy did not investigate psychopathologic or interpersonal developmental processes. Peplau, Will, and Mellow demonstrated the effectiveness of psychiatric nurses in the counseling role.

In 1958, the American Nurses' Association (ANA) established the Conference Group on Psychiatric Nursing, now the Council on Psychiatric and Mental Health Nursing Practice, acknowledging the specialty. Ida Jean Orlando's *The Dynamic Nurse-Patient Relationship,* published in 1961, emphasized the importance of the interpersonal relationship in all aspects of nursing care, not only psychiatric nursing. Orlando advocated the involvement of nurses in prevention and in mental health. In that same year, *Action for Mental Health,* the report of the Joint Commission on Mental Illness and Mental Health, encouraged nurses to assume the counselor role. The report recommended that psychiatric nurses become skilled in group and family therapy in addition to individual therapy, nursing's primary counseling mode to this point in time.

But, perhaps the culmination of this ten-year period of role clarification was the publication in 1962 of Peplau's "Interpersonal Techniques: The Crux of Psychiatric Nursing." In this article, Peplau added to and prioritized the

psychiatric nursing roles she had identified in her 1952 book. According to Peplau, the counselor role was the primary role of the psychiatric nurse, and the others were subroles. She also predicted private practice as a legitimate role for the psychiatric nurse before the decade was over.

Confirmation of the Clinical Specialist Role

Enactment of the Community Mental Health Centers Act in 1963 further motivated a shift in psychiatric nursing to include the clinical competence required for the community care of clients and for preventive mental health programs. Psychiatric nurses broadened their practice to include schools, jails, senior citizen centers, outreach clinics, transitional services and alternative treatment settings, and private practice as well as the traditional mental hospital.

The launching in 1963 of *Perspectives in Psychiatric Care,* the journal for psychiatric nurses, was a significant event in psychiatric nursing history. Edited and published by Alice Clarke, a psychiatric nurse, this first psychiatric nursing journal provided a forum for airing issues and sharing psychiatric nursing knowledge. A second journal, the *Journal of Psychiatric Nursing and Mental Health Services* began later that same year and changed its name in 1981 to the *Journal of Psychosocial Nursing and Mental Health Services.* Clinical and research papers by psychiatric nursing leaders in these journals and in the *American Journal of Nursing* further established the counseling role as the basis of psychiatric nursing, whether it was defined as psychotherapy or not.

Shortly thereafter, the first textbook to address group therapy techniques in nursing practice was written by Shirley Armstrong and Sheila Rouslin (1963), and Shirley Burd and Margaret Marshall (1963) authored and edited what was seen as the first compilation of psychiatric nursing papers suitable for graduate students in psychiatric nursing.

The clinical specialist received the endorsement of the nursing profession to assume the role of therapist in individual, group, family, and milieu work in a 1967 ANA position paper on psychiatric nursing. By 1969, a psychiatric nurse had, as Peplau predicted a few years before, moved into private practice.

The first certification program for excellence in advanced psychiatric nursing practice was developed by the New Jersey Nurses' Association in 1971, followed in two years by the New York State Nurses Association. The psychiatric nurses who developed and implemented these early certification programs—Sheila Rouslin Welt, Carol Ren Kneisl, Marian Pettingill, Marian Krizinofski, and others—recognized the need to acknowledge expertise, distinguish generalist from specialist roles, and safeguard the public. By the mid-1970s, certification in psychiatric nursing became the responsibility of the ANA.

The first standards of psychiatric and mental health nursing practice, statements to serve as guidelines for providing the desired quality of care, were published by the ANA in 1973. These standards of practice, revised in 1982, delineate psychiatric nursing roles and functions (see Chapter 3).

The clinical specialist role was further legitimized in 1973 when the ANA formed a specialty subgroup, the Council of Specialists in Psychiatric and Mental Health Nursing. The functions of the council include the following:

- Working with and through the ANA Division of Psychiatric and Mental Health Nursing Practice to serve the need of nationwide communication among specialists in psychiatric and mental health nursing on pertinent issues confronting their field
- Promoting knowledge of its members through sharing of information about research, education, and clinical work in forums and through encouraging publications
- Formulating and aiding in the discussion of position statements
- Providing the opportunity for national discussion of controversial issues that concern any segment of council membership, formulating strategies for action, and making appropriate recommendations

Membership is limited (see Appendix C, "Resources" for membership criteria).

Psychiatric Nursing in the 1980s and 1990s

According to Osborne (1984), a significant change in psychiatric nursing textbooks and psychiatric nursing thinking was typified by the publication in 1979 of the first edition of *Psychiatric Nursing* by Holly Skodol Wilson and Carol Ren Kneisl. This was the first in a new era of comprehensive psychiatric nursing textbooks to provide and consistently use a major conceptual theme based on humanistic interactionism advocating negotiated goals between nurse and client, client advocacy, and political sensitivity, as well as caring and compassion. Since that time, other psychiatric nursing textbooks have followed in the tradition of Wilson and Kneisl. Another psychiatric nursing journal, *Issues in Mental Health Nursing,* also began in 1979.

After decades of apparently unlimited support from the NIMH in the form of money for educational programs and traineeships for psychiatric nurses at the graduate level, funding for psychiatric nursing graduate programs was cut. Programs that educated nurses to meet the needs of unserved and underserved populations (identified by an NIMH task force in 1975 as children and adolescents, the elderly, the chronically mentally ill, women, and minorities) were the only programs that were funded. The passage in 1981 of the federal Omnibus Budget Reconciliation Act further decreased the amount of funding available for even these

RESEARCH NOTE

Citation

Tudor G: A sociopsychiatric nursing approach to intervention in a problem of mutual withdrawal on a mental hospital ward. Psychiatry *1952;15:174+.*

Study Problem/Purpose

The purpose of this study was to demonstrate the effect of nursing intervention on a chronically mentally ill client. Tudor's goal was to document that nurses could not only help clients improve but could also, with less effort, make clients worse.

Methods

Tudor observed the interactional patterns among clients and staff on a busy ward of a private psychiatric hospital. She used sociopsychiatric theory to explain a mutual pattern of avoidance that emerged among the nursing staff, physicians, and one particular female client. Once the pattern had been determined to exist, Tudor determined a nursing intervention designed to disrupt the pattern of avoidance by closing the gap between herself and the client and then engaging her in activities.

To test the reliability of her intervention, Tudor taught her nursing intervention to a nursing student and supervised her in reversing a pattern of mutual withdrawal with another client.

Findings

Tudor demonstrated that:

- Psychiatric nurses can have a profoundly positive or a profoundly negative effect on the client.
- The social milieu of the psychiatric ward can maintain deviant patterns of behavior.
- The psychotherapeutic nursing role can be taught to others.
- Nurses can carry out scholarly research.

Implications

This is the classic scholarly psychiatric nursing research study. This study is significant for its dramatic impact on nursing and its contribution to an understanding of the effects of the milieu. The theoretical principles of Tudor's intervention were adapted by other nurses in other nurse-client interactions. Tudor's work was first published in the medical journal *Psychiatry* because no psychiatric nursing journals existed at the time.

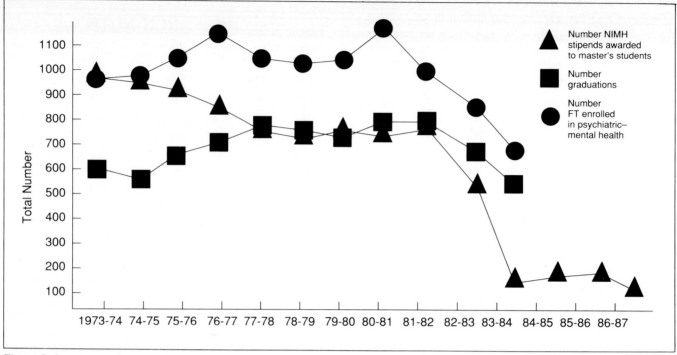

Figure 2–1

Number of full-time enrollments and graduations in master's degree programs in psychiatric-mental health nursing and number of NIMH stipends awarded to master's students between 1973–74 and 1986–87.

Source: Chamberlain JG: Update on psychiatric-mental health nursing at the federal level. Arch Psychiatr Nurs 1987;1(2):136.

training programs (see Chapter 40). Psychiatric nursing found itself on the verge of a period of retrenchment that remains in evidence today. Figure 2–1 illustrates what seems to be a causal relationship between declining enrollments in graduate programs in psychiatric-mental health nursing and the decline of federal funds supporting these programs.

Recognizing the need for a set of psychiatric nursing diagnoses to supplement those diagnoses identified by the North American Nursing Diagnoses Association (NANDA), the ANA Council of Specialists in Psychiatric and Mental Health Nursing appointed a panel of six nursing leaders (Maxine Loomis, Holly Skodol Wilson, Patricia Pothier, Anita Werner O'Toole, Marie Scott Brown, and Patricia West) to develop a classification system for the phenomena of concern for psychiatric-mental health nurses. This task force began to work on Psychiatric Nursing Diagnosis-I in 1984 and introduced the preliminary taxonomy in 1986 at the biennial ANA convention. In 1987, the task force began to synthesize its findings with those of NANDA and continues to work on the identification of relevant and useful categories for psychiatric nursing diagnosis.

The newest psychiatric nursing journal, *Archives of Psychiatric Nursing,* made its debut in early 1987. The purpose of this journal is to provide a medium in which psychiatric nurse clinician-scholars can suggest theoretical linkages between diverse areas of practice and shape public policy for the delivery of psychiatric and mental health nursing services.

According to researchers involved in an NIMH study of prevalence of mental disorders in the United States, a mental health crisis is brewing (Kramer 1983). In his keynote address at the National Forum of Graduate Program Directors in Psychiatric-Mental Health Education and Administrators of Psychiatric Nursing Services in 1984, Kramer called this crisis a pandemic of mental disorders and associated chronic and disabling conditions resulting from two phenomena: medical advances that have prolonged the lives of those who have mental disorders, and a relative increase in the numbers of young persons at high risk for developing mental disorders (U.S. Department of Health and Human Services 1986). Nationwide, the prevalence of mental disorders in those over 18 is almost 20 percent. According to Kramer, projections into the year 2005 indicate that if only 10 percent of the United States population needs mental health services, 20,000 more psychiatric nurses than were available in 1980 will be needed.

Of major concern to psychiatric nurses is the decrease in the number of nurses selecting psychiatric nursing as a specialty and a shortage of clinical training funds. Ways to encourage recruitment into the specialty are to identify psychiatric-mental health nursing content clearly, to make it highly visible in the curriculum design, and to provide role models in the persons of teaching faculty who are psychiatric nurse experts. It is basically up to psychiatric nurses to articulate who they are and what they are about to ensure the survival of psychiatric nursing in the year 2000.

Chapter Highlights

- People with mental disorders have been viewed differently at different times in history; at times such persons were perceived as tragic figures to be liberated and at times as dangerous persons to be confined.

- Some contemporary ideas about mental disorders have their origins in earlier centuries.

- Conflicts about the nature of mental dysfunction have always existed; two age-old issues are biologic versus nonbiologic causes and the individual's responsibility or lack of responsibility for actions.

- To understand the present and future directions of psychiatric nursing, one needs to understand its historical development as a specialty.

- The profession of psychiatric nursing is a product of the late nineteenth and twentieth centuries and was brought about by ideologic changes, interest in reform, attention to the importance of milieu, and the introduction of physical modes of treatment.

- Nightingale was among the first to note that nursing care has a psychosocial as well as biologic component.

- The focus of psychiatric nursing activities continued to be the provision of kind but custodial nursing care until the early 1950s, when Peplau published the first systematic theoretical framework in psychiatric nursing and emphasized psychotherapeutic roles for nurses.

- In the 1960s and 1970s, psychiatric nurses broadened their roles and functions to include individual, group, family, and milieu work as well as community mental health nursing.

- In the 1980s, psychiatric nursing found itself on the verge of a period of retrenchment that remains in evidence today; fewer funds are available for clinical training programs in the specialty.

- Although there has been a decrease in the number of nurses selecting psychiatric nursing as a specialty, research indicates that 20,000 more psychiatric nurses will be needed in the United States in the year 2005 than were needed in 1980.

References

Alexander FG, Selesnick ST: *The History of Psychiatry: An Evaluation of Psychiatric Thought and Practice from Prehistoric Times to the Present.* Harper & Row, 1966.

American Nurses' Association: *Statement on Psychiatric Nursing Practice.* ANA, 1967.

Armstrong SW, Rouslin S: *Group Psychotherapy in Nursing Practice.* Macmillan, 1963.

Beers CW: *A Mind That Found Itself,* rev ed. Doubleday, 1948.

Blain D, Barton D: *The History of American Psychiatry: A Teaching and Research Guide.* American Psychiatric Association, 1979.

Bockoven JS: Moral treatment in American psychiatry. *J Nerv Ment Dis* 1956;125:167–194, 292–321.

Brown EL: *Nursing for the Future.* Russell Sage Foundation, 1948.

Burd S, Marshall M (eds): *Some Clinical Approaches to Psychiatric Nursing.* Macmillan, 1963.

Chamberlain JG: The role of the federal government in development of psychiatric nursing. *J Psychosoc Nurs Ment Health Serv* 1983;21(4):11–17.

Chamberlain JG: Update on psychiatric-mental health nursing education at the federal level. *Arch Psychiatr Nurs* 1987;1(2):132–138.

Church O: From custody to community in psychiatric nursing. *Nurs Res* 1987;36(1):48–55.

Deutsch A: *The Mentally Ill in America,* ed 2. Columbia University Press, 1948.

Doona ME: At least as well cared for . . . Linda Richards and the mentally ill. *Image* 1984;16(2):51–56.

Fagin CM: Psychiatric nursing at the crossroads: Quo vadis. *Perspect Psychiatr Care* 1981;14:99–104.

Fagin CM: Concepts for the future: Competition and substitution. *J Psychosoc Nurs* 1983;21(3):36–41.

Foucault M: *Madness and Civilization.* Vintage Books, 1973.

Greenblatt M, York RH, Brown EL: *From Custodial to Therapeutic Care in the Mental Hospital.* Russell Sage Foundation, 1955.

Howells JG: *World History of Psychiatry.* Brunner/Mazel, 1975.

Joint Commission on Mental Illness and Health: *Action for Mental Health.* Basic Books, 1961.

Jones E: *The Life and Work of Sigmund Freud.* 3 volumes. Basic Books, 1953–1957.

Kalisch PA, Kalisch BJ: *The Changing Image of the Nurse.* Addison-Wesley, 1987.

Kramer M: The continuing challenge: The rising prevalence of mental disorders, associated chronic diseases and disabling conditions. *Am J Soc Psychiatry* 1983;3(4):13–23.

Mark B: From "lunatic" to "client": 300 years of psychiatric patienthood. *J Psychiatr Nurs Ment Health Serv* 1980;18(3):32–36.

Martin EJ: A specialty in decline? Psychiatric-mental health nursing, past, present and future. *J Prof Nurs* (January–February) 1985;48–53.

Mellow J: Nursing therapy. *Am J Nurs* 1968;68:2365–2369.

Mitsunaga BI: Designing psychiatric/mental health nursing for the future: Problems and prospects. *J Psychosoc Nurs* 1982;20(12):15–18.

Mora G: History of psychiatry, in Kaplan HI, Sadock BJ (eds): *Comprehensive Textbook of Psychiatry,* ed 4. Williams & Wilkins, 1985, pp 2034–2054.

National League for Nursing: *The Education of the Clinical Specialist in Psychiatric Nursing: Report of a National Working Conference.* Williamsburg, Virginia, November 26–30, 1956.

Neaman JS: *Suggestion of the Devil: The Origins of Madness.* Anchor Press/Doubleday, 1975.

Orlando IJ: *The Dynamic Nurse-Patient Relationship.* Putnam, 1961.

Osborne OH: Intellectual traditions in psychiatric mental health nursing: A review of selected textbooks. *J Psychosoc Nurs* 1984;22(11):27–32.

Peplau HE: *Interpersonal Relations in Nursing.* Putnam, 1952.

Peplau HE: Interpersonal techniques: The crux of psychiatric nursing. *Am J Nurs* 1962;62:50–54.

Peplau HE: Historical development of psychiatric nursing: A preliminary statement of some facts and trends, in Smoyak S, Rouslin S (eds): *Collection of Classics in Psychiatric Nursing Literature.* Charles B. Slack, 1982, pp 10–46.

Rosen G: *Madness in Society.* Harper & Row, 1968.

Slavinsky A: Psychiatric nursing to the year 2000: From a nonsystem of caring to a caring system. *Image* 1984;16(1):17–20.

Slavinsky A, Krauss J: Mutual withdrawal or Gwen Tudor revisited. *Perspect Psychiatr Care* 1980;18(5):194–203.

United States Department of Health and Human Services, Public Health Service, Alcohol, Drug Abuse, and Mental Health Administration: *Psychiatric-Mental Health Nursing: Proceedings of Two Conferences on Future Directions.* DHHS Publication no. (ADM) 86-1449, 1986, pp 4–6.

Wilson HS: *Deinstitutionalized Residential Care for the Severely Mentally Disordered.* Grune & Stratton, 1982.

THREE

The Psychiatric Nurse and the Interdisciplinary Mental Health Team: Personal Integration and Professional Role

Carol Ren Kneisl
Holly Skodol Wilson

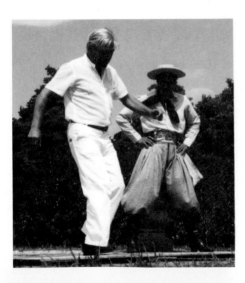

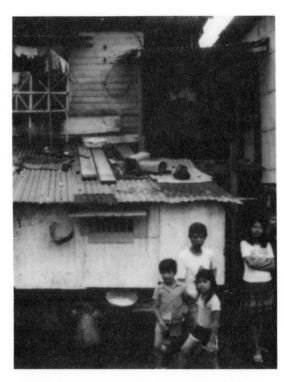

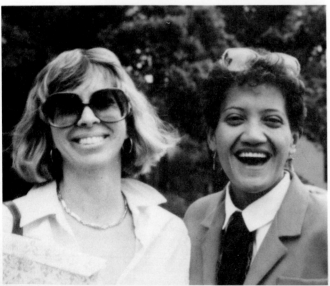

After reading this chapter, students should be able to

- Explore the concept of personal integration as it relates to the self and to psychiatric nursing practice

- Identify problems that influence personal integration

- Relate these problems to some strategies for coping

- Discuss the qualities that enable psychiatric nurses to practice the use of self artfully in therapeutic relationships

- Discuss the use of empathy in psychiatric nursing practice

- Describe the roles of the psychiatric nurse and other members of the mental health team

- Identify the means by which collaboration on the mental health team is achieved

Cross References

Other topics relevant to this content are: Ethics, Chapter 10; Liaison role of the nurse, Chapter 24; Nurses' role with the chronically mentally ill, Chapter 22; Nurses' role in family therapy, Chapter 33; Nurses' role in groups, Chapter 30; Nurses' role in milieu therapy, Chapter 31; Nurses' role in one-to-one relationships, Chapter 27; Relaxation and stress management techniques, Chapter 28; Therapeutic use of self, Chapter 27.

This book considers personal, interpersonal, and world peace as part of the nurse's commitment to global health.

Key Terms

advocacy
aggressive behavior
assertive behavior
assertiveness training
burnout
certification
clinical specialist in psychiatric nursing

empathy
negotiated reality
nonassertive behavior
psychiatric nurse
psychiatric nursing
role taking
self-awareness
values clarification

The value of self-knowledge is a recurring theme in both the popular and the professional literature. Libraries are stocked with volumes dealing with the undiscovered self, expanding human awareness, values clarification, strategies for self-realization, and the like. Common to all these references is the idea that the quality and nature of a person's relationships with others are strongly influenced by the ways in which those interactions fit with the person's self-view. Consider the following comments made by students in their psychiatric nursing clinical experience.

I just can't take it. . . . I feel myself getting confused about who is the crazy one. There's such a fine line. Sometimes I think I'll be a patient here.

I hated psych—it just didn't seem like nursing to me. I really like to keep busy. When you change someone's dressing, you really feel like you've helped them. Here it's all so uncertain.

All I kept thinking about was that a lot of the patients had done really weird things. This one guy had lived in an apartment with his dead mother's body for three months before they brought him in. Another had tried to shoot the governor. I never felt safe even turning my back on them.

This chapter helps nursing students and practitioners explore some dimensions of self-knowledge through an examination of the concepts of personal integration and professional role. Specifically, we will examine recurring problems that intersect with the nurse's identity and some strategies for coping with them. Our goal is to enhance the nurse's interactions with persons who may be labeled psychiatric clients.

THE NURSE'S PERSONAL INTEGRATION

Many students and practitioners faced with relating to people whose behavior they view as offensive, frightening, curious, or socially inappropriate find that their personal attitudes, expectations, myths, and values make it difficult for them to fulfill their professional roles. This was the case in the following example.

Penny, a baccalaureate nursing student, had selected a clinical placement at a methadone clinic in the community. Despite her initial interest, she developed a pattern of absences from the clinic. When her faculty adviser discussed this observation with her, she blurted out that, much to her surprise, she was unable to assist with the group meetings for pregnant heroin addicts. The thought of addicting babies before their births— babies who would ultimately suffer because of their mothers' self-indulgence—was horrifying to Penny. She found herself judging their choices constantly and avoiding interaction with them. "I feel like they should be shot instead of given all this free support and sympathy."

For many nurses, confrontation with deviance reinforces a personal sense of stability. Others are threatened by such confrontation.

One psychiatric nurse, in recalling her childhood experiences with community deviants, commented on the intense and sometimes morbid excitement that she and her friends found in taunting "Crazy Helen" to run out on her porch and shout incoherently at the neighborhood children or in telling bizarre stories about a grotesque old man called "Charlie-No-Face," who walked along a road late at night chain smoking from the gaping hole that had once been a mouth.

The interest these characters held for the children, along with "Vince-the-Window-Peeper," "Red-the-Bum," and the other small-town deviants, was reawakened in her as she approached her first psychiatric nursing experience. It was all very frightening, yet seductive and stimulating at the same time. The nursing students gossiped about the bizarre histories of their assigned clients as if to reaffirm their separateness from them—their sense of being normal and OK.

Dealing with people whose personal integration is fragmented, dissolving, divided, or alienated puts the nurse's own identity on the line as well. To respond with both compassion and the critical distance necessary to be effective, psychiatric professionals must confront their own identity; separate it from another's identity, which may indeed be dissolving; and finally integrate different values and behaviors comfortably in the therapeutic relationships they develop with clients.

This personal quality has been called *detached concern*—the ability to distance oneself in order to help others. It is an essential quality not only in avoiding *burnout*, a problem discussed later in this chapter, but also in **values clarification**, in ethical dilemmas, in using appropriate *assertiveness* when collaborating with colleagues, and in maintaining *empathic abilities* in highly stressful situations.

In the conventional focus on the client, the nurse is regarded as the caregiver, the provider of services, the therapist. Little attention is paid to the stresses psychiatric nurses experience attempting to relate fully to clients while maintaining their own personal integration. This chapter is an attempt to explore that aspect of psychiatric nursing.

Negotiated Reality

Nurses often find that encounters with psychiatric clients are distancing experiences. The nurses become acutely aware of their difference and separateness from clients. They reaffirm their own subjective view of reality and rationalize their actions to keep these actions consistent with their sense of self as healthy, normal people.

Since people are all constantly building and protecting their own self-images, they try to get others to see their image of themselves. However, it is impossible to see another's self-image or world view exactly as that person experiences it. Despite this fact, psychiatry has traditionally attempted to get certain people, labeled *crazy*, to assume the perspective of certain other people, called *therapists*.

A more acceptable alternative seems to lie in the creation of some common ground, a mutually understood, **negotiated reality**. Even to this common ground the nurse and the client bring their own conceptions, feelings, and attitudes toward and images of each other and themselves. In many instances the nurse's image of the client—how the nurse expects the client to act or feel—is not the same as the client's self-image. This causes a lot of confusion and hinders the establishment of therapeutic relationships and effective communication.

Feelings: The Affective Self

The ultimate effectiveness of efforts to relate to and communicate with others depends on how well people know themselves and develop the capacity for empathy. Self-awareness and empathic caring seem to go hand in hand. The fact that human beings are capable of empathizing with each other and trying to understand each other's attitudes and feelings makes social life possible. The fact that each human being is unique makes empathizing a difficult and challenging task. One way to develop this ability is to practice it. Learning to be aware of one's responses to expression of feelings from another person is a starting point.

Josh is a middle-aged man who sought out nursing as a career. Although he is highly proficient in technical skills and charming and engaging in relationships with most clients, he discovers a surprising intolerance for some of the tears, complaints, and self-preoccupation of depressed clients. He finds himself responding with admonitions to stop it, to bite the bullet, to grow up. He personally has seldom allowed himself to experience his own sadnesses but jokingly characterizes himself as a firm believer in repression and denial. The need to empathize with people unable to control their feelings evoked such discomfort that he found himself unable to work with such clients.

Self-Awareness of Feelings

Feelings seem like icebergs—only the tips stick up into consciousness, while the deeper parts are submerged. One such feeling is fear (see Figure 3–1). The conscious part may be experienced as dislike, avoidance, or reluctance. At a deeper level, the feeling is reported as anxiety. Even deeper, the person may acknowledge, "I feel scared." Deeper yet, the person may experience genuine panic. Such an iceberg may well explain Josh's attitude toward tearful, depressed clients. His annoyance, irritation, sarcasm, and disdain may represent the tip of the iceberg of Josh's fear of depression.

Other feelings, such as love, hurt, and guilt, also occur in iceberg depths. A person feeling love may be aware only of a liking or attraction for another. Beneath the tip of that iceberg are feelings of warmth and affection. Deeper are feelings of love, and at the deepest level may be feelings of fusion or ecstasy.

Problems with Submerged Feelings

One characteristic of icebergs of feeling is that at the tip the feelings lose their experiential quality and become translated into impulses to act. For example, a person with a lot of submerged guilt may express it by doing a lot of worrying and explaining and may be completely unaware of the underlying feelings. The behavior is the only outward manifestation. Being out of touch with their feelings lessens people's control over some of their behavior.

People lose touch with their feelings over time as they shape their sense of self. They hear messages saying "boys don't cry" or "girls are too sensitive," and they incorporate these injunctions into their emerging self-system—espe-

---

RESEARCH NOTE

Citation

Bunch EH: *Everyday Reality of the Psychiatric Nurse.* Gyldendal Norsk Forlag, 1983.

Study Problem/Purpose

The everyday reality of a psychiatric hospital ward may mean inadequate staffing, an overload of clients who can be belligerent and difficult to understand, and demanding doctors. To complete the everyday institutional business, the nurse must learn to balance many demands. The purpose of this study was to explore and describe how psychiatric nurses are affected by the communication used by schizophrenic clients in the everyday work world of a hospital ward.

Methods

Data were collected from approximately 150 hours of observations on a locked psychiatric ward in a county hospital in the western United States and from four in-depth interviews with nurses from that unit. Qualitative comparative analysis was used for both data collection and analysis. This analysis yielded a theory or explanatory scheme grounded in the empirical reality of the participants in the field.

Findings

Nurses engaged more in talking business, administering medication, and implementing control measures such as secluding clients rather than in therapeutic interventions that would derive from their professional philosophies and mandate. In the everyday work world, institutional requirements seem to take precedence over professional philosophic commitments.

Implications

Given that nurses in this study had great difficulty operationalizing their professional philosophies and mandates in the face of institutional demands, nurses must learn where controls lie and how to deal with them. If nurses are to avoid burnout and reality shock, educational programs and materials must prepare them to manage the task of balancing professional and bureaucratic mandates, particularly in this era of short hospital stays and increased regulatory requirements.

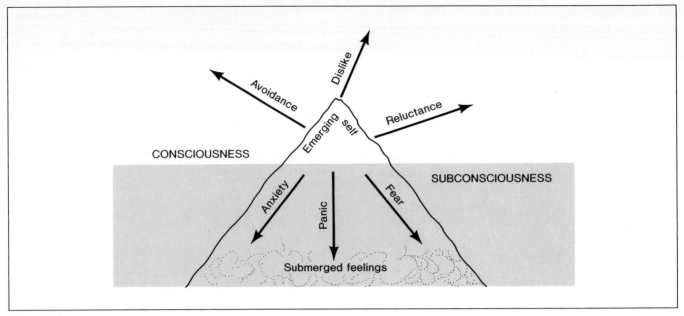

Figure 3–1
Self-awareness of feelings.

cially into the "me" or "self for others." Not being sufficiently aware of one's feelings has several disadvantages:

- What people don't know *can* hurt them. Repressed feelings may reappear in behaviors that are difficult to alter. For example, hidden anger may emerge in migraine headaches or a tendency to use sarcasm that alienates other people.

- When people are not aware of their feelings, it is more difficult for them to make decisions. It is hard to tell a "should" from a "wish." Without some awareness of their real wants, they may have trouble saying "no" or requesting something they need. They are more likely to rely on others—experts, authorities, rules and regulations, and so forth—for guidance.

- When people are "out of touch with" or unaware of their feelings, they, like Josh, the nurse in the example, may find it difficult to be really close and empathic toward others. Intimacy and empathy demand the expression of here-and-now feelings, whether positive or negative.

Most people realize the value of thinking clearly. They understand that it is a learned ability and takes practice. Feeling clearly (authentically) can also be practiced and learned. Most writers acknowledge that feelings are as important as facts, because they shape people's versions of reality as much as facts do. Becoming more aware of feel-

ings begins with the search for one's dominant emotional themes.

Dominant Emotional Themes

Nurses need to ask themselves what are the dominant emotional themes in their personalities. If they find that they respond to many situations with the same feelings, they are probably narrowing their range of potential feelings.

Whatever the occasion, Marge used it to be tired or bored. Fatigue and chronically depressed states were routine for her. Holidays, vacations, dinner engagements all evoked the same predictable response.

Joan was afraid of everything. When she met her brother at the plane, her first question was, "Aren't you afraid of flying?" She was afraid driving home from the airport. The prospect of starting back to school scared her. She was fearful about wearing a bikini to the swimming club.

When people feel the same way in a variety of situations, they may be missing a lot of what is happening in those situations. They look for and perceive only what will fit a narrowed range of feelings. Becoming aware of limited emotional themes is a way to begin to widen the range of feelings.

Acceptance of Disapproved Feelings

Most people have been taught to block off their awareness and expression of certain feelings. Children are taught that being rude or ungrateful or cranky is rarely acceptable to significant others. To retain love and approval, they usually comply, not by stopping the feelings but by acting as if they didn't have them. Nursing students often get similar messages from teachers. It is not acceptable to find a client repulsive, to dislike someone who is sick and dependent, to express anger at or criticism of the teacher. Positive feelings of attraction and love may also seem unacceptable. Failure to recognize these feelings can interfere with interactions.

Recognizing and accepting their own feelings makes nurses less vulnerable to other people's ideas about how they should feel. Instead of feeling guilty when they don't feel what others imply they should feel, nurses come to realize that others merely disapprove of the way they do feel. When nurses can allow themselves the right to their own feelings more fully, they can allow clients the right to have and express their own feelings as well.

Beliefs and Values

Beliefs and values take three major forms:

1. Rational beliefs are beliefs supported by available evidence.
2. Blind belief is belief in the absence of evidence.
3. Irrational belief is belief held despite available evidence to the contrary.

Dogmatism includes both blind and irrational belief. Dogmatically held beliefs are not based on personal experience. Operating on the basis of dogmatically held beliefs often causes nurses to distort their personal experiences of the world to fit their preconceptions. The following are examples of strongly held beliefs about behaviors that are labeled "mental illness" and about the people who do and don't engage in those behaviors:

- Most clients in mental hospitals are dangerous.
- People who are mentally disordered let their emotions control them.
- Normal people think things out.
- If parents loved their children more, there would be fewer mental disorders.
- When a person has a worry, it is best not to think about it.

- Many people become mentally disordered just to avoid the problems of life.
- Most psychiatric clients are lazy.
- People would not become mentally disordered if they avoided bad thoughts.
- A woman would be foolish to marry a man who has had a mental disorder.
- Anyone who is in a hospital for a mental disorder should not be allowed to vote.
- To become a psychiatric client is to become a failure in life.
- If a man in a mental hospital attacks someone, he should be punished so that he doesn't do it again.
- Most clients in mental hospitals don't care how they look.
- One of the main causes of mental disorders is a lack of moral strength.

Most research on strongly held beliefs indicates that people usually know more about the statements they believe than about those they don't believe. The process works like this: If people let themselves find out about those things they don't believe, they might find some validity in the statements. Then they would have to question the beliefs and disbeliefs they already hold. By staying ignorant about anything they don't already agree with, they can avoid changing. This posture cuts off personal growth and learning that could be derived from the unknown.

Attitudes and Opinions

A feeling is a transitory experience. A feeling held over a period of time is called an attitude. An attitude linked to an idea or belief becomes an opinion. An opinion, then, involves both thinking and feeling. Research in this area has shown that people are more comfortable when their beliefs and attitudes are consistent with each other. People do several things to keep their attitudes and beliefs consistent:

- They repress the belief or attitude that seems inconsistent.
- They distract their awareness from conflict either physically (e.g., by leaving the room) or psychologically (e.g., by daydreaming).
- They distort their perceptions to fit an existing attitude or belief.

Similar maneuvers take place to keep actions consistent

Table 3–1 Subprocesses of Valuing	
Subprocess	**Indicator**
Choosing beliefs and behaviors	Choosing from alternatives
	Choosing after considering consequences
	Choosing freely
Prizing beliefs and behaviors	Cherishing
	Publicly affirming
Acting on beliefs	Taking action
	Demonstrating a pattern of action that is consistent and repetitive

Source: Adapted from Raths L, Harmin M, Simon S: Values and Teaching, *ed 2. Charles E. Merrill, 1978. Copyright © 1978. Reprinted by permission of Merrill Harmin.*

with attitudes or beliefs. Nurses often justify treating psychiatric clients inhumanely or unkindly by arguing that the clients deserved it or were asking for it.

Nurses need to be careful that their self-image—as people who act intelligently—does not keep them from seeing the world clearly. Some attitudes are inconsistent with beliefs or actions. It is probably preferable to acknowledge this point than to engage in the elaborate self-deceptions necessary to avoid it.

Arriving at Values

Every day, each person meets life situations that call for thought, opinion forming, decision making, and action. At every turn in their personal and professional lives, nurses are faced with choices. Their choices are based on the values they hold, but often those values are not really clear. People actively value something to the degree that they are willing to put energy into doing something about it. Their values are shown in their interests, preferences, decisions, and actions.

In talking with colleagues, Susan, a psychiatric nurse, claims to value interacting with clients more than doing paperwork. Yet a quick assessment of how she spends her time—all excuses taken into account—reveals that she acts on other values.

Mel, a nurse working in a state hospital ward for pro-

foundly retarded children, claims that he believes these clients are human beings, despite their uncommunicative, immobile forms. He demonstrates this value in the hours he spends trying to communicate his presence and concern for them, using acupressure and touch performed slowly and with genuine feeling.

The distinction in the above examples is between *cognitive* and *active values.* Susan verbally subscribed to values but failed to act on them. These were cognitive values. Mel's actions demonstrated more than lip service for his respect for the dignity of all living beings. He was following active values.

Valuing, according to most authorities, is composed of several hierarchically ordered subprocesses. These are presented, along with their behavioral indicators, in Table 3–1. The behavioral indicators in the phases move from those reflecting moderately held values to those that represent internalized philosophic commitments.

People may learn values in a number of ways:

- Moralizing is a direct, although sometimes subtle, method of inculcating desired values in someone else.

- The laissez-faire approach leaves people alone to forge their own set of values. This may create unnecessary frustration, conflict, and confusion, especially in young people or people being socialized into a profession such as nursing.

- Modeling, in which actions follow professed values, transmits values by setting a living example for a learner to follow.

- Values clarification is a systematic, widely applicable method of teaching the process of valuing rather than the content of any specific values. It uses strategies and exercises (see Wilson and Kneisl, 1988) to engage learners in becoming aware of their beliefs and values, choosing among alternatives, and matching stated beliefs with actions.

The small amount of research comparing these four methods of learning values highlights the advantages of the fourth method. People who engage in values clarification are more zestful and energetic, more critical in their thinking, and more likely to follow through on their decisions than those who learn values in other ways. However, values clarification must be undertaken in circumstances that allow for sufficient follow-up with students who may uncover uncomfortable or disturbing values.

TAKING CARE OF THE SELF

Knowing who they are is just a beginning for nurses. Taking care of others requires that nurses respect and care for themselves. Assertiveness, the need for solitude, maintaining physical health, and attending to cues of personal stress are actions crucial to preserving the nurse's personal integration.

Assertiveness

Have you ever had difficulty expressing yourself in a staff meeting? Did you find yourself feeling hopeless, resentful, angry? Were you wishing you had the courage to speak up? Hoping someone else would?

Are you intimidated by the high-pressure tactics of supervisors, physicians, teachers? Do you have trouble standing up to these sacred cows? Do you remain silent but seething? Do you speak up but sound defensive? Do you say yes when you mean no?

Have you ever needed to give someone counseling? Did you avoid the problem, hoping things would change? Did you find yourself beating around the bush? Or did you find yourself being overly harsh when you finally gave the correction?

These questions are from a manual written specifically to help nurses cope with on-the-job stressors (Muff 1984, pp 239–240) by using assertiveness techniques to express themselves more effectively. Often people are either so timid that they do not get what they want or so aggressive and belligerent that they offend and alienate others. Assertiveness is asking for what one wants or acting to get it in a way that respects other people. It is the middle way between timid holding back and inconsiderate, offensive aggression.

Assertiveness training exercises are designed to teach people to ask for what they want and also to refuse someone without feeling guilty.

Compare the nonassertive, aggressive, and assertive behaviors listed in Table 3–2 to see which descriptions best characterize your behavior with others. Fortunately, old behaviors can be unlearned, and new behaviors can be learned.

Recognizing one's rights as a nurse is necessary before one is able to assume responsibility for asserting them. The list below (Chenevert 1983) was originally designed to help women health professionals recognize their rights. They are, however, applicable to any health professional regardless of sex.

- You have the right to be treated with respect.
- You have the right to a reasonable workload.
- You have the right to an equitable wage.
- You have the right to determine your own priorities.
- You have the right to ask for what you want.
- You have the right to refuse without making excuses or feeling guilty.
- You have the right to make mistakes and be responsible for them.
- You have the right to give and receive information as a professional.
- You have the right to act in the best interest of the client.
- You have the right to be human.

Table 3–2
Comparison of Nonassertive, Aggressive, and Assertive Behaviors

Nonassertive	Aggressive	Assertive
Denies anger/experiences fear	Denies fear/experiences anger	Recognizes both fear and anger
Does not respect self	Does not respect others	Respects both self and others
Destroys relationships as avoidance and resentment build	Destroys relationships through angry outbursts, self-aggrandizement, and need to control	Builds relationships
Wastes energy by repeating situations that were not adequately resolved	Wastes energy in bluster and argument	Uses energy constructively
Fails to achieve goals	Occasionally achieves goals through intimidation	Achieves goals
Is stressful (low self-esteem, helplessness, hopelessness, depression)	Is stressful (power struggles, painful arguments, need to be ever vigilant)	Is stressful (defying traditional stereotypes; pain of being conscious)

Source: Muff J: Balancing communication: Assertive skills, in Smythe EEM: Surviving Nursing. Addison Wesley, 1984, p 248.

Remembering that you have rights is not enough; you must assert them.

Solitude

Most people need time to be alone to assimilate what has happened in time spent with other people. They also need it for relief from responding to the demands of others. Aloneness need not mean physical distance. People can be alone in a crowded library. What is crucial is that they are making no demands on others and no one is making demands on them. Most people return to their relationships, work, and usual circumstances refreshed from a sanctioned time-out. Planning for time alone is highly preferable to reaching a breaking point and then aggressively and irresponsibly running away from others.

Personal Physical Health

An important way in which nurses take care of themselves is by providing for the physical health of their bodies. A proper diet, adequate rest, and exercise rejuvenate and restore the body. All these activities potentially make nurses more alive and better able to share this quality of aliveness with their clients.

Attending to Internal Stress Signals

Nursing students encountering emotionally disturbed clients commonly begin seeing in themselves all the "symptoms" about which they are learning. This is probably due more to heightened awareness of and attention to emotional aspects of their lives than to anything else. However, it is important for nurses to learn to recognize and respond to their own genuine stress signals. All people have times in their lives when they feel a little crazy. They may become very upset at small disturbances or see things out of proportion to their ultimate importance. These feelings are significant warning signals that the person is not coping adequately with stress.

"Crazy" times can be important turning points in people's lives. They are strong messages that change is needed. It is foolish to ignore these messages. British psychiatrist R. D. Laing has found that if people who have "gone crazy" are given supportive and nurturing conditions, they can often work through important matters while they are in this altered state of consciousness. According to Laing,

these individuals emerge "saner than sane" and resume functioning at a higher level than people who are given heavy doses of suppressive drugs.

In their daily lives, nurses are often tempted to handle their own symptoms of stress by suppressing them with tranquilizers or other drugs. They could serve themselves better by really experiencing their feelings and attending to what the signals are saying.

Pain and suffering are sources of some of the most intensely experienced stresses in life. Events such as death of loved ones, divorce, illness, separation from loved ones, and failure are all part of the cycle of life's experience. Being told that they deserve it, or that they really don't have it so bad and therefore have no right to feel the way they feel does not help people cope with pain and suffering. They need to find ways of handling their suffering without being destroyed by it.

There is an old Buddhist teaching that a third of people's suffering is inevitable but they themselves create the rest of it. Realizing that pain and hardship are part of what it is to be a human being makes the pain a bit gentler. Frequently pain centers around losing or being afraid of losing something or someone valued—a job, mate, money, self-respect. People want to continue what was instead of living with what is. It is important to attend to genuine feelings about the loss or prospective loss. These feelings give messages about what the sufferer needs to do. Some people need to replace what they have lost with something similar. Others need to explore a new dimension in their lives.

The alternative to experiencing pain is to live on the surface, out of touch with the real peak experiences in life as well as the painful ones. A more life-enhancing approach is to experience all of life.

QUALITIES OF EFFECTIVE PSYCHIATRIC NURSING

Psychiatric nursing, according to the American Nurses' Association (ANA) Congress for Nursing Practice, is "a specialized area of nursing emphasizing theories of human behavior as its scientific aspect and purposeful use of self as its art." Self-awareness, empathy, and moral integrity all enable psychiatric nurses to practice the use of self artfully in therapeutic relationships. Some characteristics of artful therapeutic practice are respect for the client, availability, spontaneity, hope, acceptance, sensitivity, vision, and accountability.

Respect for the Client

Many psychiatric clients behave in ways that indicate their loss of self-respect. Some may appear dirty and disheveled. Others may plead, beg, or cry. Still others may try to do themselves physical harm. A relationship in which they experience a sense of dignity and receive messages that they are respected by the nurse is of inestimable value. The nurse can convey respect in relationships with clients by:

- Taking the time and energy to listen
- Avoiding invalidating their experience of their world with comments such as, "It's not so bad," "Don't be that way," "Time heals all wounds," or "Keep a stiff upper lip"
- Giving clients as much privacy as possible during examinations or treatments or when they are upset
- Minimizing experiences that humiliate clients and strip them of identity—allowing them to make as many of their own choices and be in control of as much of their own lives as possible
- Being honest with clients about medicines, privileges, length of stay, etc., even when the truth may be difficult to handle

Availability

Of all the members of the psychiatric team, the nurse has the richest opportunity to be available to clients when needed, at any time of day or night. Being with clients on a relatively constant basis places responsibility in the nurse's hands for:

- Creating a nurturing, healing milieu in the unit
- Assisting suffering clients to meet their basic human needs
- Collecting and conveying crucial data about clients that will influence decisions about them

Spontaneity

Many nurses have come to believe that therapeutic relationships with psychiatric clients require them to be stiff, stilted robots uttering clichés from a list of unnatural-sounding communication "techniques." Nurses who are comfortable with themselves, aware of therapeutic goals, and flexible about using a repertoire of possible interventions for any particular clinical problem find that being natural and spontaneous is their most effective "technique." Clients experience such nurses as authentic. Each nurse is unique and necessarily brings a different personal style to practice. We have different ways of putting the words together to convey to clients that we accept and care about them. Sometimes we say it with nonverbal behavior: keeping promises, coming on time, touching, and staying with a client who needs someone. We need to trust our own natural styles in working toward therapeutic goals.

Hope

Effective psychiatric nursing practice is characterized by hope and optimism that all clients, no matter how debilitated, have the capacity for growth and change. Even clients whose most marked attributes are chronicity and deterioration can be helped to some optimal level of well-being by a nurse who believes in their possibilities and is willing to search for some strengths to build on. In one locked ward of a huge government psychiatric hospital, a chronic client joined in a partnership with a creative nurse to assist less able clients toward self-care. It is not unusual in such a situation for the healing to become a source of help to the healer-client.

Acceptance

There is a distinction between acceptance and approval. Acceptance means refraining from judging and rejecting a client who may behave in a way the nurse dislikes. Therapeutic work requires that clients be able to examine, explore, and understand their coping mechanisms without feeling the need to cover up or disguise them to avoid negative judgments or punishments. Nurses who tell clients what they should say or do or feel deny these clients the acceptance they need to explore their problems.

Sensitivity

Genuine interest and concern provide the basis for a therapeutic alliance. Clients recognize the falseness of memorized phrases and assumed postures considered indicative of sensitive behavior. The nurse conveys general interest and concern by trying to understand the client's perspective, working with the client on mutually formulated goals, and persisting even when breakthroughs and improvements are subtle and slow instead of dramatic and quick.

Vision

Because psychiatric nurses focus their work on enhancing the quality of life for all human beings, they must come to terms with a personal and professional vision of what quality means. Conditions of life associated with high quality by some writers are: influence or power, freedom, accountability, self-determinism, openness to gratifying experience, action, mastery, a sense of purpose or meaning, privacy, hope, stability, nonviolence, and intimacy.

Accountability

According to Peplau (1980), the need for personal account-ability—professional integrity—is greater in psychiatric practice than in any other type of health care. Clients in mental health settings are usually more vulnerable and defenseless than clients in other health care settings, particularly since their psychopathologies hinder their thinking processes and their relationships with others. Psychiatric nurses are accountable for the nature of the effort they make on behalf of clients and answerable to clients for the quality of their efforts. As Peplau puts it, "Personal accountability is an attitude—a quality of the heart and mind of those professionals who are competent and determined that every psychiatric patient will have the best problem-resolving assistance possible" (Peplau 1980, p 133).

Psychiatric nurses are also accountable to themselves, their peers, their profession, and the public. Accountability to self involves bringing personal behavior under conscious control so that the nurse becomes the person-as-nurse she or he wants to be. Accountability to peers involves engaging in peer review with nurse colleagues to give and receive feedback intended to improve the quality of care. Accountability to the profession involves participating in the work of the profession by continuing to clarify the role of the psychiatric nurse and encouraging self-regulation within the profession to protect the public and enhance the quality of care. Accountability to the public requires keeping abreast of the knowledge in the field, becoming credentialed according to level of competence, applying the ANA Standards of Psychiatric-Mental Health Nursing Practice, and protecting the rights of clients and their families.

EMPATHY

The Value of Empathy in Nursing

Psychiatric nurses are instructed to engage in "therapeutic use of self." They are told that their "relationship" with a client is the primary therapeutic tool, that they should demonstrate qualities of sensitivity and caring. For many beginning students, these instructions are mysterious jargon quite unlike the clear-cut step-by-step procedures they learn for some physical treatments.

I found myself watching the nurses on the unit and my instructors closely when they talked with the clients. Somehow I thought maybe by imitating things that they did or said I'd figure out what "being therapeutic" was supposed to mean. I knew it had something to do with things the nurse said or didn't say when she talked with the clients. But it all got very fuzzy to me beyond that very elementary grasp of it. I used to latch onto ideas like "Agreeing is untherapeutic. So is giving advice or opinions." The only entries I felt safe in putting down in my process-recording were stiff-sounding reflections, like "You sound angry."

Comprehension of and ability to use the process of empathy give the nurse one strategy for responding to the feelings of aloneness often experienced by persons labeled psychiatric clients. Nurses are taught skills of active listening. But listening is not enough without empathy. Empathic understanding not only increases the nurse's grasp of the client's difficulties but also provides a basis for offering feedback on how the client affects others. Perhaps its most important function is to enable the nurse to give the client the very precious feeling of being understood and cared about.

Definition of Empathy

Empathy is a pervasive phenomenon in the life experience of all people. It allows people to feel the feelings of another and respond to and understand that person's experience on his or her terms. A nurse who empathizes with a client momentarily abandons the personal self and relives the emotions and responses of someone else. People in everyday life tend to empathize most with those to whom they feel closest. In psychiatric practice, nurses often seek to empathize with persons from whom they feel most separate or whose closeness threatens their own sense of integration.

Empathy has been defined as a subtle imitation through which people assume an alien personality. They become aware of how it feels to behave in a certain way and then feed back into the other person's consciousness this awareness and sensitivity to what the behavior feels like. Empathy characteristically develops early in an infant's pattern of relating to its parents. Tension or anxiety in the parent, for example, induces anxiety in the baby.

Psychiatric Concepts of Empathy

Intimacy is closely related to empathy. Psychoanalytic theory postulates the development of empathy as a process of "mutual incorporation." The mother compensates for her loss of biologic oneness with the infant at birth by establishing a primitive unity with the child during the first weeks and months of life—an emotional bonding. The child likewise views the mothering parent as incorporated into its sense of self. Once the child begins to see the mothering parent as a being separate from itself, identification replaces incorporation, and the child experiences the mother as one to imitate in order to secure love and comfort. From identification comes the capacity for empathy. Identification enables human beings to achieve a clearer sense of self, to gain another person's point of view, and to establish an intimate association with others.

People have the capacity to identify not only with contemporaries but also with those who have been significant in the past. Adults can empathize through past, present, and future identifications. Psychiatric nurses must be able to shift from one identity to another without losing their own sense of integration.

Social interactionists discuss empathy as **role taking**, a process through which people feel with one another. They are able to sense the feelings of another because they have aroused in themselves the attitude of the person to whom they are relating. Role taking among children is a necessary part of social life. It is a means for developing the sense of self and of learning methods for adjusting to society. Role taking can be likened to learning to play games, in which children not only learn to enact their own roles but also become fully aware of the roles of others.

People form an image of themselves because they have learned to assume the roles of others and have developed the ability to see themselves as others see them. The other, then, is like a mirror in which they see themselves, and that mirror becomes the source of their own image of themselves as persons. Faulty ability to take roles is the result of limited opportunity for role experimentation. Individuals who have not experimented enough fail to develop a clear sense of their own integration and thus cannot shift from the role of participant to that of observer.

The capacity for empathy relies on personal integration. Whether problems with empathy are seen as the loss of primitive instincts for imitation in the psychoanalytic framework or as the result of inadequate opportunities for role experimentation in the social psychologist's view, the conclusion is the same. A firm sense of self is necessary for a person to be a good empathizer. As people continue to interact with others, they learn to be sensitive to others without losing their own integration.

Therapeutic Use of Empathy

From time to time, we hear accounts of dramatic and surprising breakthroughs with psychiatric clients. There are instances in which the usual tools of systematic, logical problem solving and the application of theory seem to be getting nowhere. Instead therapists fall back for a moment on their empathic sensitivity and get an inside comprehension of some complex emotion. This empathic understanding may be a key to establishing trust with a sullen, withdrawn, suspicious adolescent, or beginning verbal interaction with a chronically mute institutionalized person, or controlling the violent flailing rage of an emotion-

ally disturbed child. In all these instances, empathy is used as a therapeutic tool.

The term *empathy* is often mistakenly used synonymously with *sympathy,* and this confusion is misleading. Empathy contains no elements of condolence, agreement, or pity. When nurses sympathize, they assume that there is a parallel between their feelings and those of the client. The analogy between them makes good judgment and objectivity difficult. Empathy also should be differentiated from *identification.* Identification is generally thought to be an unconscious process and only the initial phase of the empathizing process.

Steps in Therapeutic Empathizing

The process of empathic understanding has four phases:

1. *Identification:* Through relaxation of conscious controls, we allow ourselves to become absorbed in contemplating the client and the client's experiences.

2. *Incorporation:* We take in the experiences of the client rather than attribute our own experiences and feelings to the client.

3. *Reverberation:* We interplay the internalized feelings of the client and our own experiences or fantasies. While fully absorbed in the identity of the client, we still experience ourselves as separate personalities.

4. *Detachment:* We withdraw from subjective involvement and totally resume our own identity. We use the insight gained from the reverberation phase as well as reason and objectivity to offer responses that are useful to the client.

Burnout as a Consequence of Empathy

After hours, days, and months of listening to other people's problems, something inside you can go dead and you don't care anymore. That's when you'd rather sit at the desk and do the paperwork than be out talking to clients on the floor.

This nurse verbalizes one of the possible consequences of using empathy when working intensely with troubled people. **Burnout** is the name given this phenomenon, and it happens to poverty lawyers, social workers, clinical psychologists, child-care workers, prison personnel, and others who struggle to retain both their objectivity and their empathic concern for the people with whom they work.

Burnout is a condition in which health professionals lose their concern and feelings for their clients and come to treat them in detached or even dehumanized ways. It is an attempt to cope with the stresses of intense interpersonal work by a form of distancing. It hurts not only clients but also psychiatric professionals, in that they become ineffective and dissatisfied.

One nurse noted that her emotions shifted dramatically, first toward cynical feelings, then negative ones about her clients. "I began to despise every one of them and couldn't conceal my contempt for them." Another reported, "I found myself caring less and less and feeling really negative about the clients here." In many cases, burning out involves not only thinking in derogatory terms about the clients but also believing that somehow they deserve any problem they have.

There is little doubt that burnout plays a major role in the poor delivery of psychiatric care. It is also a key factor in low staff morale, absenteeism, and high job turnover.

Cues to Burnout

Cues to burnout can be found in the language used to depict clients. Burnout victims may refer to their clients as "crocks," "vegetables," "wackos," "brown baggers," and so forth, or they may become highly analytic and abstract: "That's just a manifestation of his primary process thinking."

Another cue is lack of involvement with clients. Some nurses "hide" in the nurses' station or staff conference room to avoid interacting. Some openly reject bids for human contact.

A newly admitted client tearfully pleads at the nurses' desk. "Will you listen to me! Can't you come down to my room to sit with me? I want to lie down. I need somebody." The nurse replies, "No, I'm not going to send somebody to babysit you and hold your hand. Are you an infant?" The client replies, "No, I'm just scared." The nurse retorts, "Then stay out of your room. Doesn't that make sense?"

Another withdrawal technique involves "going by the book" rather than considering the unique factors in a situation. It is a way of minimizing personal involvement with the client. By rigidly applying the rules, the nurse can avoid having to think about the client's specific problems. Burnout can transform an original and creative nurse into a mechanical bureaucrat.

Another cue to burnout is joking put-downs among staff members, which makes their work less frightening and overwhelming.

When the nurse is asked where Mr. G is, she laughingly reports that he's taking a shower in preparation for his MMPI test. Everyone in the nurses' station breaks up in gales of laughter.

Staff members on one psychiatric ward referred to their morning meeting as the "laugh-in" show and their discussions of the clients as their sociopathy.

In a discharge conference, the psychiatrist says he'd like to discharge E, a young male client with a history of violent outbursts. The nurse replies, "With or without baseball bat?" and everyone chuckles.

Reducing Burnout

Most research indicates that the causes of professional burnout are rooted not in the permanent psychologic characteristics of individuals but rather in the social context of their work. Most nurses usually expect the presence of negative conditions—large client loads, time pressures, and daily confrontation with suffering, pain, and death. It is the absence of positive factors—a sense of significance, rewarding interpersonal relationships, being appreciated, challenge, and variety—that is most distressing (Pines and Kanner 1982). The disequilibrium created in the health care system by burnout is illustrated in Figure 3–2. The strategies listed below can be used to reduce and modify the occurrence of burnout:

- Keep staff-client ratios low. Staff members can then give more attention to each client and have time to focus on the positive, nonproblem aspects of the client's life.

- Provide for sanctioned breaks rather than guilt-arousing escapes from the work situation for staff members.

- Provide some relief from prolonged direct client contact, through shorter work shifts or rotating work responsibilities, so that certain staff members are not always working directly with clients.

- Set up formal or informal programs in which staff members can talk over their problems to get advice and support when they need it.

- Encourage staff members to express, analyze, and share their feelings about burning out. This lets them get things off their chests and gives them the chance to get constructive feedback from others and perhaps a new perspective as well.

- Encourage staff members to understand their own motivations in pursuing a psychiatric career and to recognize their expectations for work with clients. Nurses can be on a variety of "ego trips," in which their primary purpose is to deal with their own personal problems, not those of the clients.

Empathic involvement with troubled clients can have a number of stressful consequences for the nurse in addition to burnout. Problems can arise at any phase in the empathy process. The nurse may overidentify and lapse into sympathy for the client. The nurse may fail to incorporate the client's feelings and instead project personal ones. The nurse may bypass the reverberation phase and substitute gut-level intuitions for rational problem solving. At the detachment phase, the nurse may experience overdistancing or burnout. Each of the common obstacles to achieving an empathic concern for clients can be understood as a failure to cope with one of the four phases of achieving empathy. Burning out has been given particular attention here because it is common and is less psychologic than circumstantial. It therefore is not inevitable and can be prevented with thoughtful planning.

THE NURSE'S PROFESSIONAL ROLE

As society and society's needs change, so too do the roles and functions of the psychiatric nurse. The role of **psychiatric nurses** has changed over the years from that of custodian to a multifaceted role that includes the following:

- Providing direct client and family care
- Using the environment constructively

- Teaching self-care
- Coordinating the diverse aspects of care
- Providing continuity of care
- Advocating on the behalf of clients and their families
- Engaging in primary prevention activities
- Rehumanizing psychiatric care

Providing direct client and family care involves using the nursing process in many settings: the community, the in-patient psychiatric setting, walk-in clinics or health maintenance organizations, private practice, schools, industry, general hospital settings, and others. Because nurses are often considered the experts on the environment, helping clients and their families to use the environment constructively is a natural function for the nurse. Psychiatric nurses teach not only the traditional aspects of self-care—e.g., medications and health care—but also those emphasized in psychiatric settings. Among the latter are how to relate to others, how to solve problems, how to communicate clearly, and how to try out new ways of being. Two crucial roles for the psychiatric nurse are coordinating the diverse aspects of client care and evaluating how the components are functioning. The nurse is often the only professional with a complete appreciation of the client's round-the-clock activities. For this reason, the psychiatric nurse often provides the glue that cements continuity. Psychiatric nurses help to make sure that clients do not fall through the cracks in the health care system and that clients progress toward less restrictive living situations and less restrictive environments for care.

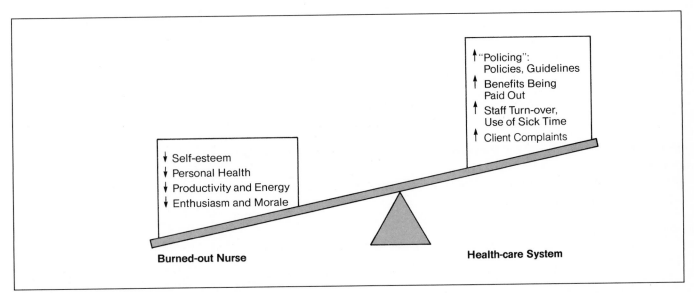

Figure 3–2
Burnout toll: disequilibrium in the health care system.
Source: Smythe EEM: Surviving Nursing. Addison-Wesley, 1984, p 54.

Being an advocate for clients and their families involves more than educating them about their rights and their responsibilities. Nurses must also work to influence local, state, national, and international policy in their dual roles as citizen and mental health professionals. It is important to negotiate for the mental health services that individuals and the community need. Teaching primary prevention is yet another psychiatric nursing role. Psychiatric nurses can inform the public about available mental health facilities, the nature of psychiatric illness, treatment approaches, and the prevention or reduction of stress. Finally, rehumanizing psychiatric care involves providing humane care in an increasingly technologic society. It requires a judicious blending of "high touch" with "high tech," a person-to-person human experience.

Guidelines for psychiatric nursing and mental health nursing practice were revised by the ANA in 1982. These professional practice and performance standards are given in Box 3–1.

THE MEMBERS OF THE MENTAL HEALTH TEAM

Role definitions have become increasingly blurred among mental health workers as various members of the mental health team have taken on tasks traditionally assigned to other disciplines. Traditionally assigned tasks are illustrated in Figure 3–3. This role blurring is perceived as

having positive consequences at times and negative ones at others. It has increased the quantity and raised the quality of one-to-one care in mental health settings. Some of the role changes have created anxiety among nurses who have become more interpersonally involved, more autonomous, and more responsible for the quality of mental health services delivered to the consumer. Psychiatrists, the traditional heads of mental health teams, have suffered some anxiety as other mental health workers and clients have sought to share in decision making and as other capable professionals have assumed administrative functions. In many settings, clinical nurse specialists, social workers, and psychologists, among others, have more direct influence than ever before. Roles are less specifically defined, and in many settings, mental health professionals take on whichever functions they do best.

The descriptions below of the education and tasks of mental health team members reflect more traditional lines. Students should keep in mind that many of the functions are now shared across disciplines when the team member has been educated for the task and when laws permit the sharing of functions.

The Psychiatric Nursing Generalist

The *psychiatric nursing generalist* may have received basic nursing preparation in a diploma, associate degree, or baccalaureate program. Basically a generalist who works in a specialized setting, this nurse provides the bulk of the nursing care to clients in in-patient settings. Registered nurses offer direct and indirect care through the nurse-client relationship, although they are not prepared at the psychotherapy level. They have major responsibility for the

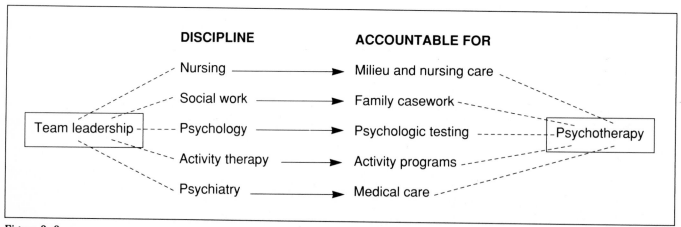

Figure 3–3
Traditionally assigned tasks for mental health team members.
Source: Benfer BA: Defining the role and function of the psychiatric nurse as a member of the team. Perspect Psychiatr Care *1980;18(4):167.*

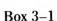
Box 3–1

1982 ANA STANDARDS OF PSYCHIATRIC AND MENTAL HEALTH NURSING PRACTICE

Professional Practice Standards

Standard 1   Theory

The nurse applies appropriate theory that is scientifically sound as a basis for decisions regarding nursing practice.

Standard 2   Data Collection

The nurse continuously collects data that are comprehensive, accurate, and systematic.

Standard 3   Diagnosis

The nurse utilizes nursing diagnoses and/or standard classification of mental disorders to express conclusions supported by recorded assessment data and current scientific premises.

Standard 4   Planning

The nurse develops a nursing care plan with specific goals and interventions delineating nursing actions unique to each client's needs.

Standard 5   Intervention

The nurse intervenes as guided by the nursing care plan to implement nursing actions that promote, maintain, or restore physical and mental health, prevent illness, and effect rehabilitation.

Standard 5A   Psychotherapeutic Interventions

The nurse uses psychotherapeutic interventions to assist clients in regaining or improving their previous coping abilities and to prevent further disability.

Standard 5B   Health Teaching

The nurse assists clients, families, and groups to achieve satisfying and productive patterns of living through health teaching.

Standard 5C   Activities of Daily Living

The nurse uses the activities of daily living in a goal-directed way to foster adequate self-care and physical and mental well-being of clients.

Standard 5D   Somatic Therapies

The nurse uses knowledge of somatic therapies and applies related clinical skills in working with clients.

Standard 5E   Therapeutic Environment

The nurse provides, structures, and maintains a therapeutic environment in collaboration with the client and other health care providers.

Standard 5F   Psychotherapy*

The nurse utilizes advanced clinical expertise in individual, group, and family psychotherapy, child psychotherapy, and other treatment modalities to function as a psychotherapist, and recognizes professional accountability for nursing practice.

Standard 6   Evaluation

The nurse evaluates client responses to nursing action in order to revise the data base, nursing diagnoses, and nursing care plan.

Professional Performance Standards

Standard 7   Peer Review

The nurse participates in peer review and other means of evaluation to assure quality of nursing care provided for clients.

Standard 8   Continuing Education

The nurse assumes responsibility for continuing education and professional development and contributes to the professional growth of others.

Standard 9   Interdisciplinary Collaboration

The nurse collaborates with other health care providers in assessing, planning, implementing, and evaluating programs and other mental health activities.

Standard 10   Utilization of Community Health Systems*

The nurse participates with other members of the community in assessing, planning, implementing, and evaluating mental health services and community systems that include the promotion of the broad continuum of primary, secondary, and tertiary prevention of mental illness.

Standard 11   Research

The nurse contributes to nursing and the mental health field through innovations in theory and practice and participation in research.

Standards 5F and 10 are specific to clinical specialists with a master's degree in the specialty of psychiatric/mental health nursing.

Source: ANA Standards of Psychiatric and Mental Health Nursing Practice. *Published by the American Nurses' Association and reprinted by permission.*

milieu and have contact with clients at all stages of daily life. Nurses at this level may be certified as generalists through the ANA.

Colleagues who are clinical nursing specialists may provide supervision of and consultation in the registered nurse's therapeutic work.

The Psychiatric Nursing Clinical Specialist

The clinical specialist in psychiatric nursing is a graduate of a master's program providing specialization in the clinical area. A number of colleges and universities provide graduate study in adult, child, adolescent, and family psychiatric nursing and in community mental health as well. Nurses may also pursue the doctoral degree in two to four more years of study. The National Institute of Mental Health funds some programs, providing stipends and tuition-free study for qualified full-time students.

Clinical specialists may also seek certification by a professional nursing body. Such certification attests to advanced level competence and is a means of protecting consumers. Certification at the advanced level exists nationally through the ANA. Although other mental health professions, such as psychiatry, psychology, and social work have well-established certification programs, certification for psychiatric nurses is relatively recent.

Clinical specialists in psychiatric settings provide individual, family, and group psychotherapy in in-patient, out-patient, community mental health, and private practice milieus. They also provide indirect services, teach, consult, administer, and do research. The liaison psychiatric nurse provides these services in general hospital settings.

The Psychiatrist

The psychiatrist is a physician whose specialty area is mental disorders or mental diseases. Certification in psychiatry by the American Board of Psychiatry and Neurology requires that the physician serve a three-year approved psychiatric residency, engage in two years of clinical psychiatric practice, and successfully complete an examination. Certification in neurology requires further preparation through a two-year neurology residency and an additional examination.

Psychiatrists are responsible for diagnosis and treatment. Some are oriented primarily toward biologic therapies, others are psychotherapeutically oriented, and a few are chiefly interested in community psychiatry. In traditional medical model settings and in many in-patient settings, the psychiatrist is usually the team leader or administrator. This is not so in milieus where role distinctions are less clearly defined.

The Psychoanalyst

In the United States, a person must be a physician in order to become a psychoanalyst. Analysts are trained at psychoanalytic institutes that provide training programs in psychoanalysis only. The majority of psychoanalysts are in private practice in large urban settings. They may also be certified in the practice of psychiatry, neurology, and/or psychoanalysis. There are nonphysician analysts, called lay analysts, who are also trained at psychoanalytic institutes. Some nurses have become lay analysts.

The Clinical Psychologist

The clinical psychologist is a psychologist specially educated and trained in the area of mental health. To be certified, the clinical psychologist must hold a doctoral degree from a program approved by the American Psychological Association and must have completed a one-year psychology internship at an approved clinical facility.

Clinical psychologists perform psychotherapy; plan and implement programs of behavior modification; select, administer, and interpret psychologic tests; and carry out research.

The Psychiatric Social Worker

The psychiatric social worker is a graduate of a two-year master's program in social work with an emphasis in the field of psychiatry. Social workers deal with the full range of social problems that confront clients and their families. Their goal is to help clients and their families cope more effectively. The social worker may also help identify appropriate community resources for clients.

Traditionally, the social worker has helped the hospitalized person maintain relationships with family, friends, and the community and has facilitated the client's return to the community. With the blurring of traditional mental health roles, social workers have undertaken counseling and psychotherapeutic roles in various settings, including private practice.

The Mental Health/Human Service Worker

The newest addition to the roster of persons on the psychiatric team is the mental health/human service worker. These "indigenous nonprofessionals" were initially recruited into the mental health delivery system to bridge the gap between middle-class-oriented professionals and clients from lower socioeconomic or otherwise disadvantaged populations (drug addicts, alcoholics, the aged, the chronically mentally ill) and rural communities.

The growing need for mental health services, the manpower crisis, the widespread popularity and economy of community college programs, and the documented effectiveness of these workers are responsible for the emergence of more than 400 mental health/human service training programs at the certificate, associate, and baccalaureate levels.

The Psychiatric Aide or Attendant

Paraprofessionals provide much of the direct service to hospitalized persons, particularly in large public facilities. These nonprofessional workers are known by a variety of titles, including *psychiatric aide, psychiatric technician,* and *psychiatric attendant*. Most agencies that employ psychiatric aides provide in-service training programs to help them use their interpersonal potential. Because a large number of the personnel who work in in-patient settings are psychiatric aides, it is extremely important that they maintain a therapeutic milieu under the supervision of professional nurses.

The Occupational Therapist

Occupational therapists in mental health settings use manual and creative techniques to elicit desired interpersonal and intrapsychic responses. They focus on the psychologic aspects of rehabilitation through arts and crafts. In some settings they may participate in preparing clients for return to community living by teaching self-help activities or, in sheltered workshop settings, help clients prepare to seek employment. Occupational therapists prepare for their careers in college and university programs. The Occupational Therapist, Registered (OTR) has completed a baccalaureate degree in occupational therapy or a master's degree in occupational therapy after receiving a baccalaureate in another field. The OTR may also participate in research and administration and supervises Certified Occupational Therapy Assistants (COTA). A COTA is a graduate of an associate degree program and helps clients follow treatment plans.

The Recreational Therapist

The *recreational therapist* plans and guides recreational activities to provide not only socialization and healthful recreation but also desirable interpersonal and intrapsychic experiences. Recreational activities are based on the therapeutic needs of clients. With increasing fre-

quency, recreational therapists are being prepared in university physical education and health education programs.

The Creative Arts Therapist

Creative arts therapists use art, music, dance, and poetry to facilitate personal experiences and increase social responses and self-esteem. Although creative arts therapists are not found in all settings, they are becoming valued and recognized members of the mental health team. Programs of study are available in universities to prepare art, music, dance, or poetry therapists. Creative arts therapists have their own professional organizations, such as the Americana Art Therapy Association, the American Dance Therapy Association, and the National Association for Music Therapy. Chapter 30 discusses art, music, dance, and poetry therapy groups.

COLLABORATING ON THE MENTAL HEALTH TEAM

Mental health personnel should seldom function totally autonomously. Psychiatric nursing practice, whether in institutions or in private practice settings, requires planning and sharing with others to deliver maximum mental health services to clients. The purpose of collaboration is to use the different abilities of mental health team members to give the client the most effective service available. Relationship problems among mental health team members must be worked through to avoid distorting the team's efforts in behalf of the client.

Cooperation versus Competition

Working together on a common problem for a common purpose is best facilitated by cooperation rather than competition. Cooperation ensures movement toward the common goal, while inappropriate competition hinders goal achievement and may be destructive to the competing individuals.

Most of the present understanding of cooperative and competitive behavior has come from the efforts of game theorists, who have researched player behavior. Players have been categorized as:

- Maximizers—those interested only in their own gain
- Rivalists—those interested only in defeating their partners

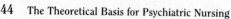

- Cooperators—those interested in helping both themselves and their partners.

Maximizers and rivalists jeopardize the client's welfare because they put themselves first and the client last. Rivalists direct their energies toward being "one up" through put-downs of others. They are concerned not with the client but with the process of winning. Cooperators are interested in helping both themselves and their colleagues to aid the client. Participants who actively recognize the importance of each individual member of the mental health team can influence maximizers and rivalists to become cooperators.

Respect for the Positions of Others

Most nursing textbooks and nursing instructors emphasize the need to respect and accept the client and to act in ways that demonstrate personal trustworthiness. They less often consider the need to respect, accept, and demonstrate trust in one's colleagues. Yet effective collaboration is based on respect for the position from which another participant acts. Our values and our culture direct our beliefs and the climate in which we operate. Knowing this, we can become aware of the values and culture of others and, in turn, respect them.

Unfortunately, the process of socialization into a profession may make it difficult for a person to respect, accept, and trust the position of another. As students become committed to a profession through the process of socialization they tend to view members of other disciplines with suspicion. Nursing is particularly susceptible in this regard because nurses have had to struggle to become colleagues with other health professionals. They may not yet have gained the degree of comfort and professional self-esteem that permits nonthreatened respect, acceptance, and trust of others. Of course, the same holds true for other members of the mental health team. As lines become blurred and once-sacred tasks and functions are shared, other colleagues may experience anxiety about respecting, accepting, and trusting the psychiatric nurse.

Supervision, support, and self-exploration are recommended for the expansion of nursing roles within and beyond traditional relationships. Clinical supervision of nurses by nurses can help pinpoint times when traditional caretaking roles are appropriate and when they inhibit growth. Administrative and peer support creates an atmosphere in which nurses are free to share their knowledge, skills, and evolving ideas. Such support increases creativity, depth, and perspective in nursing. Self-exploration and self-assessment, through reading and dialogue with other

nurses, can help nurses to consider alternatives to traditional stereotypic roles.

Engaging the Client in Collaboration

It is best to include clients in the collaboration of the mental health team whenever possible. This allows clients to participate in their health care and assures nurses that their clients are informed consumers of mental health services.

Clients can also be invited to participate in case conferences. These conferences often have an important place in the functioning of mental health agencies and may have a number of purposes. The client should be invited to participate in case conferences that involve collaboration among a number of agencies or a number of mental health workers moving toward similar goals with the client.

The client should be consulted about the information the nurse shares with other members of the mental health team. Exactly how much should be shared and with whom are not always clear. When the question of confidentiality is not clear, the nurse should also confer with the supervisor or a colleague to determine what should be shared. Decisions should take into consideration what agreement exists between nurse and client about sharing information and how the person or agency receiving information will use that information in the client's best interests.

Chapter Highlights

- The psychiatric nurse's capacity for empathy and ability to collaborate on the mental health team are related to his or her consciousness of meaning, use of language, willingness to negotiate, definitions of reality, awareness of feelings, ability to take care of self, and own self-view.

- Psychiatric nurses experience significant stresses in attempting to relate fully to clients and still maintain their own personal integration.

- Burning out is an attempt to cope with the stresses of intense interpersonal work by a form of distancing.

- The causes of professional burnout are most likely rooted in the social context of the individual's work situation, not in his or her permanent psychologic characteristics.

- Methods the nurse may use to preserve personal integration include development of assertiveness, recognizing and planning for some time alone, maintaining personal physical health, and attending to cues of personal stress.

- Characteristics of artful therapeutic practice include respect for the client, availability, spontaneity, hope, acceptance, sensitivity, vision, accountability, and empathy.

- Phases in the development of empathic understanding are identification, incorporation, reverberation, and detachment.

- The psychiatric nurse's professional role includes providing direct client and family care, using the environment constructively, teaching self-care, coordinating the diverse aspects of care, providing continuity of care, advocating on behalf of clients and their families, engaging in primary prevention activities, and rehumanizing psychiatric care.

- Members of the mental health team frequently practicing in contemporary United States settings include the psychiatric nursing generalist, the psychiatric nursing clinical specialist, the psychiatrist, the psychoanalyst, the clinical psychologist, the psychiatric social worker, the mental health/human service worker, the psychiatric aide or attendant, the occupational therapist, and the creative arts therapist.

- Quality of mental health services depends on cooperation among health team members and across disciplines, knowledge about each member's contribution, inclusion of the client in decision making, and respect for the position of others.

References

American Nurses' Association. *Standards of Psychiatric and Mental Health Nursing Practice.* ANA, 1982.

Benfer B: Defining the role and function of the psychiatric nurse as a member of the team. *Perspect Psychiatr Care* 1980;18:166–177.

Benner P: *From Novice to Expert: Excellence and Power in Clinical Nursing Practice.* Addison-Wesley, 1984.

Bunch EH: *Everyday Reality of the Psychiatric Nurse.* Gyldendal Norsk Forlag, 1983.

Chenevert M: *STAT: Special Techniques in Assertiveness Training for Women in the Health Professions,* ed 2. Mosby, 1983.

Cohen, H: *The Nurse's Quest for a Professional Identity.* Addison-Wesley, 1981.

Cohen S, McQuade K: Developing empathy with co-workers. *Am J Nurs* 1983;83:1573–1588.

Cronin-Stubbs D, Brophy EB: Burnout: Can social support save the psychiatric nurse? *J Psychosoc Nurs* 1985;23(7):8–13.

Edelwich J, Brodsky A: *Burn-out: Stages of Disillusionment in the Helping Professions.* Human Sciences Press, 1980.

Henderson FC, McGettigan BO: *Managing Your Career in Nursing.* Addison-Wesley, 1986.

Kalisch P, Kalisch BJ: *The Changing Image of the Nurse.* Addison-Wesley, 1987.

Mason DJ, Talbott SW: *Political Action Handbook for Nurses.* Addison-Wesley, 1985.

Mericle BP: The male as psychiatric nurse. *J Psychosoc Nurs* 1983;21(11):28–34.

McConnell EA: *Burnout in the Nursing Profession.* Mosby, 1982.

Muff J: Handmaiden, battle axe, whore: An exploration into the fantasies, myths, and stereotypes about nursing, in Muff J (ed): *Socialization, Sexism and Stereotyping.* Mosby, 1982.

Muff J: Balancing communication, in Smythe EEM: *Surviving Nursing.* Addison-Wesley, 1984.

Peplau HE: The psychiatric nurse—accountable? To whom? For what? *Perspect Psychiatr Care* 1980;18(3):128–134.

Pines AM, Kanner AD: Burnout: Lack of positive conditions and presence of negative conditions as two independent sources of stress. *J Psychiatr Nurs Ment Health Serv* 1982;20(8):30.

Raths L, Harmin M, Simon S: *Values and Teaching.* Merrill Publishing, 1966.

Smythe EEM: *Surviving Nursing.* Addison-Wesley, 1984.

Thomas S, Witt D: Mental health nursing clinical specialization: Extinction or adaptation? *Issues Mental Health Nurs* 1986;8(1):1–13.

Wilson HS, Kneisl CR: *Learning Activities in Psychiatric Nursing,* ed 3. Addison-Wesley, 1988.

FOUR

Applying the Nursing Process and Nursing Theory

Holly Skodol Wilson

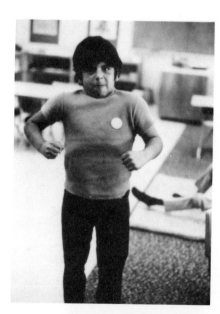

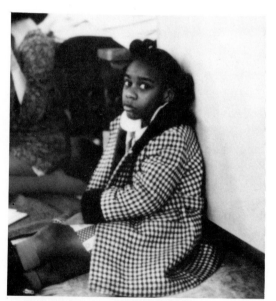

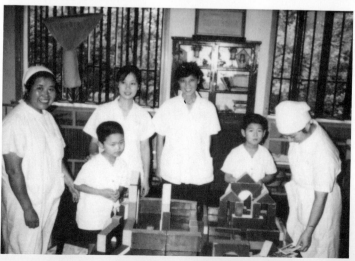

Learning Objectives

After reading this chapter, students should be able to

- Discuss the steps of the nursing process in relation to the 1982 Standards of Psychiatric Mental Health Nursing Practice
- Apply the nursing process to situations involving clients with psychiatric/mental health diagnoses
- Comprehend key concepts in selected contemporary nursing theories
- Evaluate the usefulness of selected contemporary nursing theories for organizing data and guiding the practice of psychiatric nursing

Key Terms

Diagnostic and Statistical Manual of Mental Disorders, third edition revised (DSM-IIIR)
metatheory
North American Nursing Diagnosis Association (NANDA)
nursing diagnosis
nursing process
objective data
primary data source

professional standards review organization (PSRO)
Psychiatric Nursing Diagnoses, first edition (PND-I)
secondary data source
subjective data
theory
theory for practice
theory of nursing

Cross References

Other topics relevant to this content are: Assessment, Chapter 12 and Research, Chapter 14.

Diane S, a 23-year-old woman, is admitted to a medical unit with severe anorexia nervosa and thoughts of suicide. She is agitated and tearful and says life looks so bad that she just wants to get out of it.

B.J. is a 27-year-old man who walked into the hospital emergency room because he sees the walls sparkling and weaving around, he feels like people are laughing at him, and he tastes petroleum in his mouth, which he describes as the "taste of afterbirth." He was on his way to jump off the George Washington Bridge when he saw the hospital and decided to come in for help.

The client is a 52-year-old, disheveled woman dressed in ragged street clothes and wearing a turban on her head. She believes that there are radio waves in her teeth reporting of a plot to have her committed to mental hospitals. She has lived on the streets of Berkeley for the past two years with all her possessions and clothing in four large brown paper bags. She speaks in an uninterrupted monotone and is hostile toward the nurse.

How does a nurse approach the clinical problems above? Obviously no quick and easy cookbook formulas are adequate for responding to such genuine human complexities. The 1982 ANA Standards of Psychiatric and Mental Health Nursing Practice reflect the current state of knowledge in the field and offer some guidance in providing nursing care to clients like those described above.

The six standards of psychiatric and mental health nursing presented in Box 4–1 are the focus of this chapter. Together they guide the nurse in the use of the nursing process and nursing theory in the practice of psychiatric-

This book is dedicated to the restoration and preservation of the human rights of oppressed people because without social justice, a world without war is not possible.

mental health nursing. The nursing process steps are as follows:

- Assessment
- Diagnosis
- Planning
- Intervention
- Evaluation

Each of these steps and the six standards are discussed in detail in the sections that follow.

Box 4–1

1982 ANA STANDARDS OF PSYCHIATRIC AND MENTAL HEALTH NURSING

Professional Practice Standards

Standard 1   Theory

The nurse applies appropriate theory that is scientifically sound as a basis for decisions regarding nursing practice.

Standard 2   Data Collection

The nurse continuously collects data that is comprehensive, accurate, and systematic.

Standard 3   Diagnosis

The nurse utilizes nursing diagnoses and standard classification of mental disorders to express conclusions supported by recorded assessment data and current scientific premises.

Standard 4   Planning

The nurse develops a nursing care plan with specific goals and interventions delineating nursing actions unique to each client's needs.

Standard 5   Intervention

The nurse intervenes as guided by the nursing care plan to implement nursing actions that promote, maintain, or restore physical and mental health, prevent illness, and effect rehabilitation.

Standard 6   Evaluation

The nurse evaluates client responses to nursing actions in order to revise the data base, nursing diagnoses, and nursing care plan.

Source: ANA Standards of Psychiatric and Mental Health Nursing Practice. *Published by the American Nurses' Association and reprinted by permission.*

APPLYING THE NURSING PROCESS

Process suggests movement toward a goal in phases or stages. The **nursing process** is the conscious, systematic set of cognitive and behavioral steps that comprise the clinical act of nursing practice. The steps include:

1. Assessment of the client's health status based on objective and subjective data
2. Formulation of a psychiatric nursing diagnosis
3. Development of a plan for nursing intervention
4. Implementation of the planned interventions
5. Evaluation of the nursing care

This chapter describes the ways in which the nursing process approach is applied to psychiatric nursing practice. We urge that the nursing process become the way in which nurses think about clients with the human responses discussed in other chapters of this text. The nursing process is flexible and adaptable. It can be applied in a variety of settings with individual clients, families, groups, and aggregates. It requires that the nurse use judgment and creativity in caring for clients in an organized and systematic way.

Assessment

Standard 2 of the 1982 Standards of Psychiatric and Mental Health Nursing Practice states that

> The nurse continuously collects data that are comprehensive, accurate, and systematic.

Rationale

The rationale for including assessment among the standards of quality in nursing derives from a belief that effective nursing depends on comprehensive, accurate, systematic, and continuous data collection that enables the nurse to reach sound conclusions about the client's human responses to actual and potential mental health problems. From these data, the nurse plans fitting interventions.

Process Criteria

1. The nurse informs the clients that data collection is their mutual responsibility.
2. The nurse seeks data in at least the following categories:

    - Biophysical, developmental, emotional, and mental status
    - Spiritual resources and beliefs
    - Family, social, cultural, and community systems

- Daily activities, interactions with others, and coping patterns
- Economic, environmental, and political factors affecting the client's health
- Personally significant support systems including those that are available in the community but not yet used
- Knowledge, satisfaction, and motivation for change of health practice and status
- Strengths that can be used in reaching health goals
- Knowledge pertinent to legal rights
- Contribution from the family, significant others, and members of the mental health care team

Outcome Criteria

1. Clients and their significant others participate in and affirm that the data-gathering process was beneficial to them.
2. Data are recorded in a standard format.

Data collection requires astute observation, purposeful listening, broad knowledge of human behavior, and understanding of what needs to be known and where to obtain the information. The tools used in psychiatric assessment of individual clients include:

- Psychiatric history
- Mental status examination
- Psychosocial assessment
- Neurologic assessment
- Psychologic testing

Subjective Data

Subjective data are reported by the client and significant others in their own words. An example is the chief complaint expressed by clients in the course of an intake interview or psychiatric history. Here are some examples of chief complaints:

I was in "warp 5" and pretending to be an undercover cop.

My brother doesn't think I take good enough care of myself.

My husband has been beating me and I think I am losing my mind.

Objective Data

Objective data are collected and verified by people other than the client and family. Examples include:

- Physical examination findings, e.g., hearing loss
- Neurologic examination findings, e.g., those observed when testing for reflexes or observing for tremors
- Results of psychometric tests, e.g., the Temporal and Personal Orientation Test or the Global Cognitive Function and Language Comprehension Tests used to assess functional status among the elderly
- Scores on rating scales developed to quantify the severity of disabilities among the chronically mentally ill
- Laboratory test results including complete blood count, sedimentation rate, blood chemistry, thyroid function studies, serum vitamin B_{12}, folate levels, computed tomography, brain scan, chest x-ray films, and electrocardiograms

The Nursing History

The nursing history is the foremost method of collecting data from the primary source (the client). Nursing histories summarize holistic information about clients that can be used by the nurse to individualize care. They differ from medical or psychiatric histories, which are records of previous illness and hospitalizations, in that they focus on the *clients' perceptions and expectations* related to their illness, hospitalization, and care. See Figure 4–1 for a sample guide for a holistic nursing history.

The **primary** subjective and objective **data source** is the client. Secondary data sources include laboratory and psychologic test results, family members, and other members of the mental health team. Together, these data sources provide a rationale for determining the client's nursing diagnosis and a basis for planning, implementing, and evaluating nursing care. The assessment phase of the nursing process culminates in the formulation of a nursing diagnosis.

Nursing Diagnosis

Standard 3 of the 1982 Standards of Psychiatric and Mental Health Nursing Practice states that

The nurse utilizes nursing diagnoses and standard classification of mental disorders to express conclusions supported by recorded assessment data and current scientific premises.

A. General Information

Client's name, age, medical diagnosis, occupation (client's and spouse), religion, educational level, residence, marital status

B. Guide Questions

1. Family situation
   a. With whom do you live?
   b. How many children do you have, if any?
   c. Who is caring for them while you are here?
   d. How many brothers and sisters do you have?
   e. Do your parents live nearby?
   f. Was there anything that happened to you or your family in the past year other than this illness that was upsetting to you?

2. Work situation (including financial aspect)
   a. What type of work do you do?
   b. How long have you done this type of work?
   c. Are you on sick leave from work?
   d. Do you think your illness will interfere with your work?
   e. Do you have health insurance?

3. Client's activities
   a. What kind of environment and pace are you used to?
   b. What are your feelings concerning your activity schedule in the hospital?
   c. Do you have any special interests or hobbies that you would like to pursue, if feasible, while you are here?
   d. What habits have you had to change here?

4. Eating habits
   a. Are you on a restricted diet?
   b. Are you allergic to any foods?
   c. Are there any particular foods you like or dislike?
   d. Do you eat breakfast?
   e. Do you need an early morning cup of coffee or the like?
   f. How many times do you eat each day?
   g. When do you usually eat your meals?
   h. Has being sick affected your eating habits? How?
   i. Do you foresee any difficulty with hospital food?
   j. Do you prefer plain or ice water?
   k. Are you accustomed to eating snacks? At regular times?

5. Sleeping habits
   a. How long do you usually sleep? Between what hours?
   b. Do you sleep well at home?
   c. Do you nap? Occasionally? Regularly? Rarely?
   d. Are you an early riser?
   e. Do you need medication to sleep?
   f. Do you get up at intervals?
   g. Does light or noise disturb you?
   h. If you are awakened at night, can you go back to sleep?
   i. Do you sleep with a night light on?
   j. Do you like an extra blanket at night?
   k. Do you usually sleep with a window closed or open?
   l. Have you found that strange surroundings decrease your ability to sleep soundly?
   m. How many pillows do you use?

6. Elimination habits
   a. What are your elimination habits at home?
   b. Do you have any difficulty with elimination?
   c. Do you take laxatives? If so, how often?
   d. Do you take any special foods to aid in elimination?

7. Allergies
   a. Do you have any allergies to drugs, food, adhesive tape, etc.?

8. Drugs or special diets
   a. Were you on any medications before you came to the hospital?
   b. Do you routinely take any nonprescription medicines?
   c. Did you bring any of these medications with you?

9. Previous illnesses or hospitalizations
   a. Have you had other experiences when you or members of your family were ill?
      1) What kind of experience was it—good, bad, indifferent?
      2) What problems, if any, did you or they encounter?
   b. Have you ever been sick before?
      1) What was wrong?
      2) Were you in the hospital?
      3) How long were you sick?
      4) What do you remember most about being hospitalized?
      5) What did you like most about the hospital care, routines, etc.?
   c. Do you have any disability, other than your present illness, that may restrict your normal activity?
   d. Who cares for you when you are sick at home?

Figure 4–1

Sample psychiatric nursing history guide.

Source: Lamonica EL: *The Nursing Process: A Humanistic Approach:* Addison-Wesley, 1979. Jones & Bartlett Publishers, Inc., Boston.

e. What can you do when you are sick at home that makes you feel better.

10. Current illness
   a. Why are you in the hospital?
   b. What do you think made you will?
   c. How long have you been ill?
   d. Can you tell me what you feel about your illness?
   e. What kinds of things usually make you feel better when you are sick?
   f. Were there other things that happened when you first became ill?
   g. What do you feel about the outcome of your illness?
   h. What is causing you the most discomfort at this time?

11. Current hospitalization
   a. What do you think you need done for you while you are here?
   b. What do you feel about being here in the hospital?
   c. What do you miss most by being in this hospital?
   d. Are there things at home that you would like to have here with you? If so, what?
   e. Are there things at home that might bother or worry you while you are here?

12. Personal preferences regarding visitors— family and friends
   a. If feasible, would you prefer to be alone or with other clients during the day?
   b. Would you like to have visitors?
      1) Just family?
      2) Just friends?
      3) Both family and friends?
      4) Just certain individuals? Who?
   c. How many visitors would you like at one time and how frequently?
   d. Is it possible for your family or friends to visit you if you so desire?
   e. Has anyone visited you yet, or did anyone come with you when you were admitted?
   f. (For persons with serious illness, or as hospital policy allows) Would you feel better if it was possible for some of your family to stay here with you overnight?

13. Expectations of hospital personnel and physician by client
   a. Would you like your doctor and nurses to explain everything that is going on with you?
   b. Would you be comfortable enough to ask them questions if they do not explain?

c. Would you like someone to come in frequently during the day just to talk or be with you?
d. Is there anything special you expect or would like me to do for you or see that it gets done, if feasible, while you are here?
e. What do you expect from nurses?
g. What has your doctor told you about your illness and what to expect while you are in the hospital?
h. What do you expect from your doctor?
i. What do you expect from the hospital?
j. What do you expect from hospital policy or routine?
k. Would you like a minister to visit with you, if possible?
l. How best can we help you while you are in the hospital?

C. Visual Observation on General Appearance
1. Immediate general impression of appearance:
2. Overall physical appearance:
3. Motor activity/posture:
4. Build and weight:
5. Prosthesis/limitations/debilitations:
6. Complexion and appearance of skin:
   a. Color
   b. Lesions
   c. Abrasions
   d. Rash
7. Subjective symptoms:
   a. Watery eyes
   b. Running nose
   c. Cough
8. Mouth:
   a. Oral hygiene
   b. Dentures
9. Eyes:
   a. Eye glasses
   b. Contact lenses
10. Age group:
11. Clothing:
12. Belongings and objects in environment:
13. Speech:
14. Apparent cultural, educational, and intellectual levels:
15. Other pertinent factors:

D. Nonverbal Behavior Observations
1. Emotional tone, facial expression, attitude:
2. Gestures, movements, or activities during interview:
3. Main theme of client's conversation and behavior:
4. Topics the client seemed to avoid:
5. Client's response to interviewer:
6. Interviewer's response to client:
7. Other pertinent factors:

E. Summary

Rationale

The rationale for inclusion of Standard 3 is that nurses' logical basis for providing care rests on recognition and identification of actual or potential health problems within the scope of nursing practice. In other words, formulation of nursing diagnoses makes it possible to identify the specific contribution of nurses to the health team. A diagnostic classification system for psychiatric nursing practice that applies diagnoses specific to nursing interventions enhances our ability to define the scope of nursing and answer the question, "What do psychiatric nurses do that is different from what social workers, psychologists, and psychiatrists do?"

Process Criteria

- Peer validation of nursing diagnoses
- Peer exchange, education, and research regarding the scientific and humanistic premises underlying nursing diagnoses
- Nursing diagnoses for psychiatric clients that identify actual or potential health problems in respect to the categories outlined in Box 4–2

Box 4–2
CATEGORIES OF NURSING DIAGNOSES FOR PSYCHIATRIC CLIENTS ACCORDING TO ANA STANDARDS

- Self-care limitations or impaired functioning with general etiologies, such as mental and emotional distress, deficits in the ways significant systems are functioning, and internal psychic or developmental issues relevant to health
- Emotional stress or crisis components of illness, pain, self-concept changes, and life process changes
- Emotional problems related to daily experiences such as anxiety, aggression, loss, loneliness, and grief
- Physical symptoms, such as altered intestinal functioning or anorexia, which occur simultaneously with altered psychic functioning
- Alterations in thinking, perceiving, symbolizing, communication, and decision-making abilities
- Behaviors and mental states that indicate that the client is a danger to self or others or is gravely disabled

---

Outcome Criteria

The outcome criteria for meeting this standard are that nursing diagnoses are validated by the client or the client's significant others and recorded to facilitate nursing research.

Guidelines recommended by members of the First National Conference on the Classification of Nursing Diagnoses (Gebbie and Lavin 1975) further guide the nurse in this process. They include the following:

- People should be viewed as whole, worthwhile, dignified beings regardless of their degree of dysfunction or level of competence.
- Nursing diagnoses should involve the client and should be validated with the client.
- Nursing diagnoses should be stated in terms of concerns and levels of competence or dysfunction.
- Nursing diagnoses should always be referred to as "nursing" diagnoses to avoid confusion with medical diagnoses.

Nursing Diagnosis Defined

Several definitions of **nursing diagnosis** exist in the nursing literature, including the following:

- "Nursing diagnosis made by professional nurses describes actual or potential health problems that nurses, by virtue of their education and experience, are capable and licensed to treat" (Gordon 1976, p 1299).
- "A nursing diagnosis is a concise phrase or term summarizing a cluster or set of empirical indicators, representing normal variations and altered patterns (actual or potential) of human functioning which nurses by virtue of education and experience are capable and licensed to treat" (McLane 1979, p 33).
- "A nursing diagnosis is the statement of a patient's response which is actually or potentially unhealthful and which nursing intervention can help to change in the direction of health" (Mundinger and Jauron 1975, p 97).

The Two-Component Statement of Nursing Diagnosis

Most authorities, including the above, propose that the nursing diagnosis statement have two components:

1. The client's potential or actual unhealthful response
2. The reasons for or etiology of the client's unhealthful response

These authorities believe that incorporating both components gives clearer direction to the planning, implementation, and evaluation steps of the nursing process. Others maintain that cause-and-effect relationships are premature given the current state of nursing research and that the etiology component of the diagnosis statement is therefore purely speculative. This text acknowledges the lack of consensus on the issue of etiology and presents nursing diagnosis as a name for a perceived difficulty (ANA 1980, p 11) organized by a classification system.

Toward a Classification System for Psychiatric Nursing Diagnoses

NANDA

The North American Nursing Diagnosis Association (NANDA) solicits proposed new nursing diagnoses for review by the association. Such proposed diagnoses undergo a systematic review that concludes with a mail vote by the entire membership. If the proposed diagnosis is accepted, it is included in NANDA's official list of diagnoses. Such acceptance indicates NANDA's view that the diagnosis is ready for use and continuing development.

To assist interested parties in submitting proposed diagnoses, the NANDA Diagnoses Review Committee has prepared a set of guidelines for submission. These guidelines ensure consistency, clarity, and completeness of submissions. Submitted diagnoses that do not meet the guidelines are returned to the person submitting them for revision so that the review process can begin. Proposed diagnoses are reviewed by the Diagnoses Review Committee, the Clinical Technical Review Task Forces, and the NANDA board prior to review and comment by the General Assembly and membership vote. An example of a proposed nursing diagnosis in the required NANDA format appears in Box 4–3.

The alphabetical list of NANDA nursing diagnoses (see Box 4–4) is organized into nine "human response patterns." These are:

1. Exchanging—mutual giving and receiving
2. Communicating—sending messages
3. Relating—establishing bonds
4. Valuing—assigning relative worth
5. Choosing—selecting alternatives
6. Moving—activity
7. Perceiving—receiving information
8. Knowing—meaning associated with information
9. Feeling—subjective awareness of information

NANDA nursing diagnoses have the following components:

● Definition
● Etiology
● Defining characteristics

Box 4–3
NANDA NURSING DIAGNOSIS: HOPELESSNESS*

Definition

A subjective state in which an individual sees no alternatives or personal choices available and cannot mobilize energy on own behalf.

Defining Characteristics

Major: Passivity, decreased verbalization
Minor: Lack of initiative; decreased response to stimuli; decreased affect; verbal cues (hopeless content, "I can't," sighing); turning away from speaker; closing eyes; shrugging in response to speaker; decreased appetite, increased sleep; lack of involvement in care/passively allowing care

Substantiating/Supportive Materials

Eisman, R. (1971). Why did Joe die? *American Journal of Nursing,* March.

Farbertow, N. LO. (1981). Suicide prevention in the hospital. *Hospital and Community Psychiatry, 32*(2), 99–104.

Jolowiec, A., Powers, M.J. (1981). Stress and coping in hypertensive and ER patients. *Nursing Research,* January–February.

Jourad. (1970). Suicide, an invitation to die. *American Journal of Nursing,* February.

Kritek, P. (1981). Patient power and powerlessness. *Supervisor Nurse, 12*(6), 26–29, 32–34.

Lambert, Lambert. (1981). Role theory and the concept of powerlessness. *Journal Psychosocial Nursing,* September.

Miller, C., Denner, P., Richardson, V. (1976). Assisting the psychosocial problems of cancer patients: A review of current research. *International Journal of Nursing Studies.*

Related Factors

Prolonged activity restriction creating isolation; failing or deteriorating physiologic condition; long-term stress; abandonment; lost belief in transcendent values/God.

One of twenty-two diagnoses proposed for review and comment by the General Assembly of the Seventh Conference.

Source: NANDA Diagnosis Review Committee Correspondence, February 15, 1986.

NANDA nursing diagnoses are in the process of being organized into a provisional taxonomy structure. Numeric codes are being established for diagnostic entities and qualifying

Box 4–4
APPROVED NURSING DIAGNOSES

Activity intolerance
Activity intolerance, potential
Adjustment, impaired*
Airway clearance, ineffective
Anxiety
Body temperature, altered: potential*
Bowel elimination, altered: constipation
Bowel elimination, altered: diarrhea
Bowel elimination, altered: incontinence
Breathing pattern, ineffective
Cardiac output, altered: decreased
Comfort, altered: pain
Comfort, altered: chronic pain*
Communication, impaired: verbal
Coping, family: potential for growth
Coping, ineffective family: compromised
Coping, ineffective family: disabled
Coping, ineffective individual
Diversional activity, deficit
Family processes, altered
Fear
Fluid volume deficit: actual (1)
Fluid volume deficit: actual (2)
Fluid volume deficit: potential
Fluid volume excess
Gas exchange, impaired
Grieving, anticipatory
Grieving, dysfunctional
Growth and development, altered*
Health maintenance, altered
Home maintenance management, impaired
Hopelessness*
Hyperthermia*
Hypothermia*
Incontinence, functional*
Incontinence, reflex*
Incontinence, stress*
Incontinence, total*
Incontinence, urge*
Infection: potential for*
Injury, potential for
Injury, potential for: suffocating
Injury, potential for: poisoning
Injury, potential for: trauma
Knowledge deficit (specify)

Mobility, impaired physical
Noncompliance (specify)
Nutrition, altered: less than body requirements
Nutrition, altered: more than body requirements
Nutrition, altered: potential for more than body requirement
Parenting, altered: actual
Parenting, altered: potential
Post-trauma response*
Powerlessness
Rape-trauma syndrome: compound reaction
Rape-trauma syndrome: silent reaction
Role performance, altered
Self-care deficit: bathing/hygiene
Self-care deficit: dressing/grooming
Self-care deficit: toileting
Self-care deficit: feeding
Self-concept, disturbance in: body image
Self-concept, disturbance in: self-esteem
Self-concept, disturbance in: personal identity
Sensory/perceptual alterations: visual, auditory, kines-
    thetic, gustatory, tactile, olfactory
Sexual dysfunction
Sexuality, altered patterns*
Skin integrity, impaired: actual
Skin integrity, impaired: potential
Sleep pattern disturbance
Social interaction, impaired*
Social isolation
Spiritual distress (distress of the human spirit)
Swallowing, impaired*
Thermoregulation, ineffective*
Thought processes, altered
Tissue integrity, impaired*
Tissue integrity, impaired: oral mucous membrane
Tissue perfusion, altered: renal, cerebral, cardiopulmon-
    ary, gastrointestinal, peripheral
Unilateral neglect*
Urinary elimination, altered patterns
Urinary retention*
Violence, potential for: self-directed or directed at others

*Diagnoses accepted in 1986.

Source: North American Nursing Diagnosis Association
(NANDA), 1986.

information. Furthermore, additional diagnoses continue to be proposed for inclusion in the official NANDA classification.

PND-I

From its inception in 1973 as the National Group for the Generation and Classification of Nursing Diagnosis, NANDA has taken a strong public position on the incompleteness of its first and even seventh list. Nurses have been invited to describe, label, and contribute their phenomena of concern to the collaborative goal of increased scientific growth in the discipline. In such a proactive spirit, the former Division of Psychiatric and Mental Health Nursing Practice of ANA authorized support for a project to identify the phenomena of specific concern for psychiatric-mental health nursing. This action reflected an awareness that such identification was essential for implementing the 1980 ANA Social Policy Statement. The objective was to develop a comprehensive working list of the phenomena of concern for psychiatric-mental health nursing. The strategy was to convene a panel of specialists with expertise in specific age and diagnostic client groups. The outcome of the first stage of work was a conceptual classification system organized according to the following three generic response classes:

1. The individual response class
2. The interpersonal/family response class
3. The community/environment response class

The classification system, called the ANA Classification of Phenomena of Concern to Psychiatric and Mental Health Nursing, is also referred to as **Psychiatric Nursing Diagnoses, First Edition, or PND-I**. The individual response class has been refined to include the human response patterns presented in Box 4–5.

Toward a NANDA–PND-I Synthesis

Recognizing the need for the development of a single, comprehensive system for classification, representatives from NANDA and PND-I collaborated to produce the classification system for nursing diagnosis presented in Box 4–5, and used throughout this text. This collaborative diagnostic classification system in its first draft has been submitted to the World Health Organization for inclusion in the tenth edition of the *International Classification of Disease.* This system, and its subsequent drafts, represent the cutting edge in the nosology (classification of disorder) of nursing (Loomis et al 1987). The names of phenomena from this system may or may not be augmented with associated risk, predictive data, or etiologic data, depending on what is known when one formulates the diagnosis. If an etiologic or risk factor is included in a nursing diagnosis, that factor should be identified by the name of the diagnosis and its code number, e.g., 02.06.02 delirium, secondary to pneumonia.

DSM-IIIR and Psychiatric Nursing Diagnoses

The standard interdisciplinary psychiatric diagnosis is the mental health team's way of labeling a client's psychiatric disorder. A nursing diagnosis for a psychiatric client is the conceptualization of a client's human response from the unique nursing perspective. Such conceptualizations are abstractions or concepts either generated by the clinician or adapted from existing theory to organize, categorize, and ultimately make sense of the data collected during the assessment phase of the nursing process. The PND-I and DSM-IIIR purposely advocate an atheoretical stance, while NANDA seeks to ground nursing diagnoses in nursing theory or view the labels themselves as an early step in theory generation. Selected nursing theories are discussed later in this chapter. Psychiatric nurses must be knowledgeable about both psychiatric diagnostic nomenclature as well as the expanding efforts of nurses to develop our own diagnostic nomenclature. Both are essential for communication with colleagues and for developing an individualized nursing care plan. Table 4–1 (page 58) compares a sample DSM-IIIR diagnosis and related psychiatric nursing diagnoses according to PND-I and NANDA.

Nursing Care Planning

Standard 4 states that

> The nurse develops a nursing care plan with specific goals and interventions delineating nursing actions unique to each client's needs.

Rationale

The rationale for inclusion of this standard is that the nursing care plan is used to guide therapeutic intervention and to achieve desired goals or outcomes effectively and affirmatively.

Process Criteria

Structural criteria for this standard are:

- Tools and mechanisms for communicating nursing diagnoses and nursing care plans, progress, and evaluation to colleagues and to the client

Text continues on p. 58

Box 4–5
CLASSIFICATION OF HUMAN RESPONSES OF CONCERN FOR PSYCHIATRIC MENTAL HEALTH NURSING PRACTICE (PND-I)*

01. Human response patterns in activity processes
  01.01 Altered motor behavior
    01.01.01 Bizarre motor behavior
    01.01.02 Catatonia
    01.01.03 Impaired coordination
    01.01.04 Hyperactivity
    01.01.05 Hypoactivity
    01.01.06 Muscular rigidity
    01.01.07 Psychomotor retardation
  01.02 Altered recreation patterns
    01.02.01 Inadequate diversional activity
  01.03 Altered self-care
    01.03.01 Altered eating
    *01.03.02 Altered grooming
    01.03.03 Altered health maintenance
    *01.03.04 Altered hygiene
    01.03.05 Altered participation in health care
    *01.03.06 Altered toileting
  01.04 Altered sleep/arousal patterns
    01.04.01 Difficult transition to and from sleep
    01.04.02 Hypersomnia
    01.04.03 Insomnia
    01.04.04 Nightmares
    01.04.05 Somnolence
  01.97 Undeveloped activity processes
  01.98 Altered activity processes not otherwise specified
  01.99 Potential for altered activity/processes

02. Human response patterns in cognition processes
  02.01 Altered decision making
  02.02 Altered judgment
  *02.03 Altered knowledge processes
    02.03.01 Agnosia
    02.03.02 Altered intellectual functioning
    *02.03.03 Knowledge deficit
  02.04 Altered learning processes
  02.05 Altered memory
    02.05.01 Amnesia
    02.05.02 Distorted memory
    02.05.03 Long-term memory loss
    02.05.04 Short-term memory loss
  02.06 Altered orientation
    02.06.01 Confusion
    02.06.02 Delirium
    02.06.03 Disorientation
  02.07 Altered thought content
    02.07.01 Delusions
    02.07.02 Ideas of reference
    02.07.03 Magical thinking

    02.07.04 Obsessions
  *02.08 Altered thought processes
    02.08.01 Altered abstract thinking
    02.08.02 Altered concentration
    02.08.03 Altered problem solving
    02.08.04 Thought insertion
  02.97 Undeveloped cognition processes
  02.98 Altered cognition processes not otherwise specified
  02.99 Potential for altered cognition processes

03. Human response patterns in ecological processes
  03.01 Altered community maintenance
    03.01.01 Community safety hazards
    03.01.02 Community sanitation hazards
  03.02 Altered environmental integrity
  *03.03 Altered home maintenance
    03.03.01 Home safety hazards
    03.03.02 Home sanitation hazards

04. Human response patterns in emotional processes
  04.01 Abuse response patterns
    *04.01.01 Rape-trauma syndrome
  04.02 Altered feeling patterns
    04.02.01 Anger
    *04.02.02 Anxiety
    04.02.03 Elation
    04.02.04 Envy
    *04.02.05 Fear
    *04.02.06 Grief
    04.02.07 Guilt
    04.02.08 Sadness
    04.02.09 Shame
  04.03 Undifferentiated feeling pattern
  04.97 Undeveloped emotional responses
  04.98 Altered emotional processes not otherwise specified
  04.99 Potential for altered emotional processes

05. Human response patterns in interpersonal processes
  *05.01 Altered communication processes
    05.01.01 Altered nonverbal communication
    *05.01.02 Altered verbal communication
  05.02 Altered conduct/impulse processes
    05.02.01 Aggressive/violent behaviors
      05.02.01.01 Aggressive/violent behaviors toward environment
      05.02.01.02 Aggressive/violent behaviors toward others
      05.02.01.03 Aggressive/violent behaviors toward self

05.02.02 Dysfunctional behaviors
  05.02.02.01 Age-inappropriate behaviors
  05.02.02.02 Bizarre behaviors
  05.02.02.03 Compulsive behaviors
  05.02.02.04 Disorganized behaviors
  05.02.02.05 Unpredictable behaviors
05.03 Altered role performance
  05.03.01 Altered family role
  05.03.02 Altered leisure role
  *05.03.03 Altered parenting role
  05.03.04 Altered play role
  05.03.05 Altered student role
  05.03.06 Altered work role
05.04 Altered sexuality processes
05.05 Altered social interaction
  05.05.01 Social intrusiveness
  *05.05.02 Social isolation/withdrawal
05.97 Undeveloped interpersonal processes
05.98 Altered interpersonal processes not otherwise specified
05.99 Potential for altered interpersonal processes
  *05.99.01 Potential for violence

06. Human response patterns in perception processes
06.01 Altered attention
  06.01.01. Distractibility
  06.01.02. Hyperalertness
  06.01.03. Inattention
  06.01.04. Selective attention
*06.02 Altered comfort patterns
  06.02.01 Discomfort
  06.02.02 Distress
  06.02.03 Pain
06.03 Altered self-concept
  *06.03.01 Altered body image
  06.03.02 Altered gender identity
  *06.03.03 Altered personal identity
  *06.03.04 Altered self-esteem
  06.03.05 Altered social identity
  06.03.06 Undeveloped self-concept
06.04 Altered sensory perception
  *06.04.01 Auditory
  *06.04.02 Gustatory
  06.04.03 Hallucinations
  06.04.04 Illusions
  *06.04.05 Kinesthetic
  *06.04.06 Olfactory
  *06.04.07 Tactile
  *06.04.08 Visual
06.97 Undeveloped perception processes
06.98 Altered perception processes not otherwise specified
06.99 Potential for altered perception processes

07. Human response patterns in physiological processes
07.01 Altered circulation processes

07.01.01 Altered vascular circulation
  *07.01.01.01 Tissue perfusion
  *07.01.01.02 Altered fluid volume
07.01.02 Altered cardiac circulation
07.02 Altered elimination processes
*07.02.01 Altered bowel elimination
  *07.02.01.01 Constipation
  *07.02.01.02 Diarrhea
  *07.02.01.03 Incontinence
  07.02.01.04 Encopresis
*07.02.02 Altered urinary elimination
  *07.02.02.01 Incontinence
  *07.02.02.02 Retention
  07.02.02.03 Enuresis
07.02.03 Altered skin elimination
07.03 Altered endocrine/metabolic processes
  07.03.01 Altered growth
  07.03.02 Altered hormone regulation
    07.03.02.01 Premenstrual stress syndrome
07.04 Altered gastrointestinal processes
  07.04.01 Altered absorption
  07.04.02 Altered digestion
07.05 Altered neurosensory processes
  07.05.01 Altered levels of consciousness
  07.05.02 Altered sensory acuity
  07.05.03 Altered sensory processing
  07.05.04 Altered sensory integration
    07.05.04.01 Learning disabilities
07.06 Altered nutrition processes
  07.06.01 Altered cellular processes
  07.06.02 Altered systemic processes
    *07.06.02.01 More than body requirements
    *07.06.02.02 Less than body requirements
  07.06.03 Altered eating processes
    07.06.03.01 Anorexia
    07.06.03.02 Pica
07.07 Altered oxygenation processes
  07.07.01 Altered respiration
    07.07.01.01 Altered gas exchange
    *07.07.01.02 Ineffective airway clearance
    *07.07.01.03 Ineffective breathing pattern
07.08 Altered physical integrity processes
  *07.08.01 Altered skin integrity
  *07.08.02 Altered tissue integrity
07.09 Altered physical regulation processes
  07.09.01 Altered immune responses
    07.09.01.01 Infection
07.10 Altered body temperature
  *07.10.01 Hypothermia
  *07.10.02 Hyperthermia
  *07.10.03 Ineffective thermoregulation
07.97 Undeveloped physiological processes
07.98 Altered physiological processes not otherwise specified

continued

Box 4–5 (continued)

07.99 Potential for altered physiological processes
08. Human response patterns in valuation processes
   *08.01 Altered meaningfulness
     *08.01.01 Hopelessness
     08.01.02 Helplessness
     08.01.03 Loneliness
     *08.01.04 Powerlessness
   08.02 Altered Spirituality
     *08.02.01 Spiritual distress
     08.02.02 Spiritual despair
   08.03 Altered values
     08.03.01 Conflict with social order
     08.03.02 Inability to internalize values
     08.03.03 Unclarified values

08.97 Undeveloped valuation processes
08.98 Altered valuation processes not otherwise specified
08.99 Potential for altered valuation processes

NANDA diagnosis.

Source: ANA Classification of Individual Human Responses by M. Loomis, A. O'Toole, M. Brown, P. Pothier, P. West, H. S. Wilson. Copyright 1986. Published by the American Nurses' Association and reprinted with permission.

This classification is based on previous work of the Phenomenon Task Force and the Advisory Panel on Classifications for Nursing Practice of the American Nurses' Association. The abbreviation, PND-I, is used by this text's authors.

- Evidence of a collaborative team effort to plan care so that the client's needs are addressed in a consistent way

The well-developed nursing care plan conforms to the qualities outlined in Box 4–6.

Format of the Plan

A nursing care plan usually has at least four components:

- A diagnostic formulation that communicates the phenomena of concern according to nomenclature accepted in the discipline

---

Table 4–1
Comparison of DSM-IIIR and Psychiatric Nursing Diagnoses

DSM-IIIR Diagnosis	Psychiatric Nursing Diagnosis, First Edition (PND-I)*		North American Nursing Diagnosis Association (NANDA)
209.1x Primary degenerative dementia Alzheimer's type, presensile onset	01.03	Altered self-care[†]	Self-care deficits
	02.08.01	Altered abstract thinking	Thought processes, altered
	02.03.01	Agnosia	
	02.05	Altered memory	Coping, ineffective individual
	05.02.02.05	Unpredictable behaviors	
	05.03	Altered role performance[†]	Role performance, altered
	05.05	Altered social interaction[†]	Social interaction, impaired
	02.06.01	Confusion	

*Four-digit codes (00.00) are primarily generalist diagnoses. Six-digit (00.00.00) and eight-digit codes (00.00.00.00) are primarily specialist diagnoses.

[†]PND-1 diagnosis also in NANDA list.

- Short- and long-term client care goals stated in measurable terms and accompanied by a time deadline
- Nursing orders or interventions that specify what nurses or other mental health team members will do to address clients' diagnosed needs or problems
- Outcome criteria stated in observable terms on which to base a judgment about the effectiveness of the intervention in achieving client goals

Nursing care plans have various formats depending on the resources and constraints of a setting and the operating conceptual framework or philosophy for practice. A sample nursing care plan is presented on page 60.

Outcome Criteria

The ultimate outcome criterion for this standard is evidence that regardless what format is used for the care plan, it is revised as goals are achieved, changed, or updated. Such goals should be:

- Stated in clear, concise, measurable terms
- Accompanied by a time frame
- Not in conflict with the multidisciplinary team's goals

Planning nursing care requires that both short- and long-term goals be set for the client. Such goals, however, must reflect the client's own goals, and when the two sets of goals are not compatible, negotiation should occur.

Hints in Negotiating Goals

The first step is to determine whether to try to convince the client that the nurse's goals are the right goals or to alter the nurse's goals. One way to do so is to ask clients what their goals are and how the psychiatric professional can help them achieve their goals. Some clients respond that they just came along to appease a significant other who is the one with the real problem. Others believe they are there for a "rest" or a "checkup." Some want to be taken care of and protected, and some believe they have been tricked or betrayed and locked up against their will. Having asked, the nurse must *listen*. Sometimes the simple experience of being heard and understood without being invalidated and dismissed out of hand becomes the ground for subsequent negotiations and eventual agreement about mutually determined goals.

Once a nursing diagnosis has been identified and clear, unambiguous goals have been set and listed in order of priority, the nurse can consider possible solutions by using what are known as "predictive principles." Bower (1985) calls predictive principles "guides for developing realistic alternatives of action or action hypotheses that tell the nurse what will promote or inhibit progress toward a desired goal." The nurse selects one intervention from many choices

---

Box 4–6

PROPERTIES OF AN EFFECTIVE NURSING CARE PLAN

1. Identifies priorities of care
2. States realistic goals in measurable terms with an expected date of accomplishment
3. Is based on identifiable psychotherapeutic principles
4. Indicates which client needs are the primary responsibility of the psychiatric nurse and which will be referred to others with appropriate expertise
5. Reflects mutual goal setting and shared responsibility for goal attainment at the level of the client's abilities
6. Forms the basis for client care activities done by others under the nurse's supervision

---

based on a prediction of the likely or probable consequences of each option. The use of predictive principles cuts down on trial-and-error and the rigid use of standard operating procedures. Figure 4–2 illustrates the sequences of decision-making process for a depressed client.

Implementing Nursing Interventions

Interventions are the actions to be taken to achieve the stated goals. The actions may be independent, collaborative, or dependent and include orders from nursing, medicine, and other disciplines. The following are the major categories of nursing intervention with psychiatric clients:

- Psychotherapeutic interventions: individual, family, and group
- Health teaching
- Self-care activities of daily living
- Biologic therapies including medications
- Therapeutic environment
- Psychobiologic nursing prescriptions regarding diet, nutrition, and exercise

Each of these areas is taken up specifically in a subsequent chapter of this text.

Yura and Walsh (1978) characterize the implementation phase of the nursing process as a time when the nurse continues to collect data about the client's condition, prob-

Text continues on p. 62

Sample Nursing Care Plan

Nursing Diagnoses (PND-I/NANDA)	Client Care Goals	Nursing Planning/ Intervention	Evaluation
05.05 Altered social interaction* /Social interaction, impaired	Client will be able to tolerate limited interaction with staff (at least 5 minutes 3 times/shift).	Nurse will do the following: Introduce self each shift. Attempt to meet needs despite his inability to verbalize them. Set up 3 times/shift to be with client. Spend the time in structured ways, e.g., do grooming tasks, go for a walk. Client does not tolerate intense verbal interaction and becomes more inappropriate with direct questions. If he starts to giggle, allow him time to be alone. Help him join activities as tolerated. Verbally redirect client from situations with too many stimuli. Give encouragement and positive feedback when appropriate. Role model social interaction and use group activities to increase social skills. Use nurse-client relationship to help him learn new social skills.	On discharge, client will be able to tolerate limited interaction with others in a structured environment as evidenced by his ability to follow his schedule.
01.03 Altered self-care* /Self-care deficit 01.03.04 Altered hygiene /Self-care deficit: bathing/ hygiene 01.03.02 Altered grooming /Self-care deficit: dressing/ grooming 01.03.06 Altered toileting /Self-care deficit: toileting	Client will: Be up, dressed, and shaved by 9:00 A.M. Make bed and clean area by 9:30 A.M. Do laundry Monday and Thursday P.M. Shower Monday, Wednesday, and Friday P.M.	Nurse will: Arrange hygiene schedule with client. Review schedule early in the shift and give reminders as necessary of tasks to be done. Monitor and give further assistance if needed. Give positive feedback for all tasks accomplished. Allow him to do as much as possible for himself. Be alert for progress and allow the client as much independence as he tolerates.	At discharge, client will do self-care tasks independently.

*PND-I diagnoses also in NANDA list.

NURSING PROBLEM	PREDICTIVE PRINCIPLES (guides to action)	ALTERNATIVES	CONSEQUENCES	PROBABILITY	VALUE	RISK	NURSING DECISION
How to increase Mr. Fox's sense of self-esteem, self-respect, and self-worth	• The level of depression determines the type of nursing action. • An open and accepting attitude facilitates a development of trust.	1. Sit next to Mr. Fox and try to get him to verbalize his feelings.	He will verbalize his feelings. He will not verbalize his feelings.	0.2 0.8	+ −	Low High	...
How to get Mr. Fox to take fluids and food.	• The outward expression of aggression and hostile feelings decreases the possibility that these feelings will be turned inward and thus lower self-esteem. • Believing someone cares promotes feelings of worth.	2. Say, "You must feel very uncomfortable in those wet clothes, come with me and let's get you more comfortable." Get a *male nurse* or orderly if necessary.	He will know you care. He will feel cleaner. His dignity will have been preserved. His skin will be clean and less liable to breakdown.	0.8 0.9 0.9 0.8	+ + + +	Low Low Low Low	Alternative 2
	• Nursing interventions that encourage severely depressed persons toward acts of daily care protect that person from further deterioration. • Feelings of self-esteem, self-respect, and acceptance enhance a positive and realistic self-concept, thus lifting feelings of depression.	3. In the privacy of his room, offer Mr. Fox sips of fruit juice and selections of food.	He will take juice and food. He will not take juice and food. His dignity and self-respect will be preserved since he has privacy.	0.7 0.3 0.8	+ − +	Low Moderate Low	Alternative 3

Figure 4–2

Decision-making sequence for a depressed client.

Source: Reproduced by permission from *Bower FL:* The Process of Planning Nursing Care, *ed 4.* Mosby, 1985.

lems, reactions, and feelings. The plan is not carried out blindly as if all decision-making phases have been completed. Changes in identified goals will alter the effectiveness of intervention strategies. Therefore, the nurse must be alert, observant, attentive, thoughtful, and caring, continually using decision-making skills to evaluate and modify intervention strategies and use of available resources.

Evaluation

Standard 6 states that

> The nurse evaluates client responses to nursing actions in order to revise the data base, nursing diagnoses, and nursing care plan.

Rationale

The rationale for inclusion of this standard is that psychotherapeutic nursing care is a dynamic process with events that sometimes alter data, diagnoses, or plans previously made.

Structural Criteria

Criteria that facilitate achievement of Standard 6 include supervision or consultation with colleagues to help the nurse analyze the effectiveness of care given.

Process Criteria

- The nurse pursues validation, suggestions, and new information that is subsequently discussed with colleagues.
- The nurse documents results of the evaluation of nursing care.

Outcome Criteria

The outcome criteria for this standard are that nursing care plans are revised based on evaluations and that evaluation recordings promote refinement of psychiatric nursing theory.

Evaluation is a judgment of merit or worth. It is the natural intellectual activity to complete the phases of the nursing process, because it indicates the degree to which the nursing diagnosis and nursing actions have been correct. As in all other phases, clients and their significant others are involved in evaluation.

Since Isobel Stewart first developed guidelines in 1919 to measure the quality of nursing care, numerous others have been tested. Methods for monitoring the quality of nursing care have been developed that simultaneously consider people, activities, and environmental elements, as well as the administrative and organizational structure for delivery of care. Instruments to evaluate client care while the care is in process have been developed and tested. Periodic nursing audits are used increasingly by nurses to inspect or review records and other accounts of nursing transactions. Betts (1978) has related the psychiatric audit to a model for quality assurance in nursing.

Bower (1985) urges nurses to recognize the importance and necessity of structuring evaluation outcome criteria in client-centered behavioral terms. Nurses may have to discard the attitude that nursing care is composed of ethereal, well-meaning qualities or that certain aspects of the clinical act and its art "just can't be evaluated." The 1980s and 1990s are a time of resource retrenchment and accountability among consumers of health care, and psychiatric nurses are experiencing the challenges of the era. We are challenged to provide cost and quality accountability for our practice and to demonstrate that nursing is a profession capable of in-depth self-study sufficient to prove quality performance by its practitioners. If we do not maintain the confidence of the public, we will soon cease to be a social force.

Professional standards review organizations (PSRO), mandated by Congress in 1972, require that professionals and health care delivery systems implement quality control methods if they wish to maintain professional autonomy. This legislation was the source of evaluation by peer review. The ANA has defined peer review as evaluation against the stated norms or standards of the profession. These standards have been presented as a framework for relating the nursing process to practice with psychiatric clients. The first of these standards, however, requires that

> Nurses base practice decisions on the application of theory to clinical phenomena.

Standard 1 is the focus of the remainder of this chapter.

APPLYING NURSING THEORY

Professional nursing knowledge consists of three elements:

1. Basic natural, social, and behavioral sciences
2. The tools, skills, and attitudes that comprise the clinical act in nursing, such as communication, assessment, and ethical reflectiveness
3. The theories for and of nursing

A theory of **nursing** is a grand general theory that addresses the definition of the domain and scope of nursing. A theory **for** practice is a set of interrelated propositions that specify actions and intended consequences in a situation. In other words, a theory for practice guides the clinician in deciding what to do to achieve certain results.

Historical Antecedents of Contemporary Theory

Our first era might well be described as the *magico-religious era.* Nursing took place within the confines of huge institutions where nursing practice was shaped by values of self-sacrifice and dedication. Nursing ceremonies formalized these values and attitudes, and remnants of these ceremonies, such as capping rituals, are still familiar to us today. Educational programs for nurses were based on assumptions of passivity and sameness among nursing students.

With the publication of the Sue Barton and Cherry Ames books, nursing moved into another phase in relation to its guiding perspective, a perspective termed *romanticism* by some. The image of the nurse was idealized, open, simplistic, and glamorous, but nursing was seen as a temporary job en route to every woman's true goal: marriage and motherhood.

As a result of the two world wars, nursing moved into an era of *pragmatism.* The emphasis was on tools, tasks, and procedures; the goal was efficiency. Hospital geography dominated the organization of nursing knowledge. In our educational programs, we rotated through the emergency room, the operating room, the nursery, the clinics, central supply, and even formula lab, which was thought to be essential learning experience in every student's curriculum. Watered-down medicine, modeled after the disease and body systems paradigms used by physicians, organized both the curriculum and the practice of nursing. We learned and delivered diabetes nursing, cancer nursing, rare tropical disease nursing, and so on.

Since approximately the early 1950s, however, nursing has moved away from such dualistic approaches. Contemporary conceptual schemes are more *holistic and humanistic.* Changes in technology, other disciplines, and health care needs have all contributed to this development. Even the image of the nurse has changed.

The concept of nursing as primarily technologic (e.g., hypodermics, bedpans, and other tools of the trade) has been replaced by the idea that nursing is theory based. Still, nursing remains more divergent than convergent when it comes to identifying the theories to be applied. Most authorities concur that *theoretical pluralism*—that is the simultaneous refinement and testing of numerous contenders for nursing's dominant theory—is highly appropriate for the present early phase in nursing's scientific and intellectual history. Let's briefly examine a few of the best-known contenders and attempt to identify the concepts and principles most relevant to psychiatric nursing.

Overview of Nursing Theories

In the early 1950s, Lydia Hall, Virginia Henderson, and Hildegard Peplau had already published precursors to contemporary nursing theories, and Faye Abdellah had begun empirical observations that led to the formulation of her theory by 1955.

RESEARCH NOTE

Citation

Corcoran, SA: Task complexity and nursing expertise as factors in decision making. Nurs Res 1986; 35(2):107–112.

Study Problem/Purpose

This study described the initial and overall approaches to planning drug administration for clients in pain used by expert and novice nurses when cases varied in complexity.

Methods

Sample. Two groups of volunteer subjects were formed: six expert and five novice nurses in a hospice care situation. Sample selection for each group was based on specified criteria.

Materials. Three written cases were developed for study purposes representing three types of severe and chronic pain and three levels of complexity for decision making.

Procedure. Each subject was asked to develop and write a drug administration plan for a case and to think aloud through the planning process. The written plans and tape-recorded verbal protocols were coded and scored according to rules for deciding about type of planning approach. Coding and scoring were done by two independent judges.

Findings

Findings supported existing information-processing literature in that no relationship was found between overall approach to planning and the quality of the plan and that the task itself is the major determinant of decision-making behavior among nurses.

Implications

The finding that decision-making across tasks is not necessarily systematic among either experts or novices in nursing has implications for teaching the nursing process. More needs to be learned about how nurses make decisions when planning and implementing nursing care under practice conditions.

Hall

Lydia Hall's (1959) theory is best represented by three interlocking circles depicting what she called the "aspects of nursing." Hall's three aspects of nursing were The Person (the Core), The Disease (the Cure), and The Body (the Care). She developed her theory at the Loeb Center for Rehabilitation primarily for the adult client recuperating from a physical illness in a residential treatment center. She showed relationships among the three concepts by varying the size of the three circles to represent the amount or proportion of nursing time focused on each. See Figure 4–3. Most psychiatric nursing practice would focus on the Core component of her model.

Henderson

Virginia Henderson (1966) contributed the now famous definition of nursing:

> Nursing is primarily assisting the individual (sick or well) in the performance of those activities contributing to health or its recovery (or a peaceful death) that he would perform unaided if he had the necessary strength, will, or knowledge.

Henderson went on to identify a list of fourteen components of basic nursing care with the notion that nurses either helped the client with the activities or provided conditions under which the client would perform them unaided. The categories are:

1. Breathe normally.
2. Eat and drink adequately.
3. Eliminate body wastes.
4. Move and maintain desirable postures.
5. Sleep and rest.
6. Select suitable clothing—dress and undress.
7. Maintain body temperature within normal range by adjusting clothing and modifying the environment.
8. Keep the body clean and well-groomed and protect the integument.
9. Avoid dangers in the environment and avoid injuring others.
10. Communicate with others in expressing emotions, needs, fears, or opinions.
11. Worship according to one's faith.
12. Work in such a way that there is a sense of accomplishment.

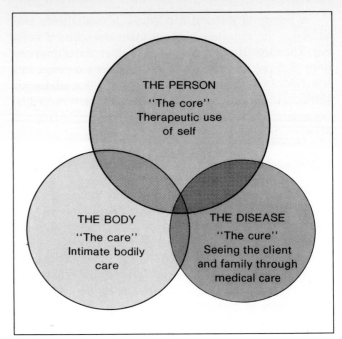

Figure 4–3
Hall's three aspects of nursing.
Source: Adapted from Hall L: Nursing—What Is It? *Publication of the Virginia State Nurses' Association, Winter 1959.*

13. Play or participate in various forms of recreation.
14. Learn, discover, or satisfy the curiosity that leads to normal development and health and use of the available health facilities.

The first nine activities encompass a version of basic physiologic human needs. The remaining five include needs for communication, spirituality, work, play, and learning—the categories that are emphasized by psychiatric nurses.

Peplau

Hildegard Peplau published her nursing theory in the classic book *Interpersonal Relations in Nursing* (1952). She defined nursing as a significant therapeutic interpersonal process, and the core concepts of her theory were the four phases of the nurse-client relationship.

1. Orientation
2. Identification
3. Exploitation (or Working)
4. Resolution

Some say that these phases are ancestors of the phases of the nursing process. Psychiatric nurses continue to use Peplau's theory to understand and guide decisions in the one-to-one relationship.

Abdellah

Faye Abdellah (1960) presented a list of twenty-one nursing problems that she developed over a five-year period in the late 1950s. The list, presented in Box 4–7, includes physiologic as well as sociopsychologic needs and resembles both Henderson's fourteen nursing care components and Maslow's hierarchy of needs.

Orem

Dorothea Orem's (1971) theory of self-care was originally introduced around 1959 and identified ten Universal Self-care Requisites, which are divided into six categories that encompass both physical and psychosocial human needs. Orem also introduced a second order of concepts originally called Health Deviation Self-care Demands to refer to care required in the event of illness, injury, or disease. Nursing, a second key component of her scheme, was divided into Wholly Compensatory, Partially Compensatory, and Supportive-Educational Systems of Care that could be matched to the client's assessed level of self-care functioning in each area (see Figure 4–4). This theory firmly established the notion of a goal of self-care as integral to the discipline of nursing's perspective on the meaning of health. Orem's theory is particularly well adapted to meeting nursing care needs of the severely and chronically mentally disordered.

Rogers

Martha Rogers (1970) drew on knowledge from anthropology, sociology, religion, philosophy, mythology, and general systems theory to define nursing as a holistic science of human nature and development. Rogers's key nursing principles are called the Principles of Homeodynamics. Subprinciples of homeodynamics are:

- The principle of complementarity, which refers to the continuous, simultaneous interaction process between human and environmental fields

- The principle of resonancy, which refers to the tendency of humans to function according to patterns that can be studied

- The principle of helicy, according to which the nature and direction of human and environmental change are continuous, innovative, probabilistic, and diverse but also evolutionary and goal directed

These three principles are ways of viewing human beings holistically. Changes in life processes are irreversible, nonrepeatable, and rhythmic and indicate patterns of increasing complexity and organization. Most of her concepts have counterparts in general systems theory, but she has added the notions of life processes, change, and human-environmental interaction to the concepts central to nursing. Rog-

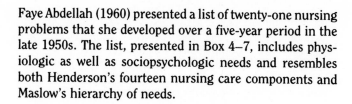

Box 4–7
THE TWENTY-ONE NURSING PROBLEMS

1. To maintain good hygiene and physical comfort
2. To promote optimal activity: exercise, rest, and sleep
3. To promote safety through the prevention of accidents, injury or other trauma, and infection
4. To maintain good body mechanics and prevent and correct deformities
5. To maintain a supply of oxygen to all body cells
6. To maintain nutrition of all body cells
7. To facilitate elimination
8. To maintain fluid and electrolyte balance
9. To recognize the pathological, physiological, and compensatory responses of the body to disease conditions
10. To maintain regulatory mechanisms and functions
11. To maintain sensory function
12. To identify and accept positive and negative expressions, feelings, and reactions
13. To identify and accept the interrelatedness of emotions and organic illness
14. To maintain effective verbal and nonverbal communication
15. To promote the development of productive interpersonal relationships
16. To facilitate progress toward achievement of personal spiritual goals
17. To create or maintain a therapeutic environment
18. To facilitate awareness of self as an individual with varying physical, emotional, and developmental needs
19. To accept the optimum possible goals in the light of physical and emotional limitations
20. To use community resources in resolving problems arising from illness
21. To understand the role of social problems as influencing factors in the cause of illness

Source: Reprinted with permission of Macmillan Publishing Co., Inc., from Patient-Centered Approaches to Nursing *by Faye G. Abdellah, Almeda Martin, Irene L. Beland, and Ruth V. Matheney. © Copyright, Macmillan Publishing Co., Inc., 1960.*

---

ers requires that psychiatric nurses use such holistic principles to guide their practice and consider physical as well as psychosocial problems and needs.

Roy

Sister Callista Roy's (1976) adaptation theory views people as constantly faced with the need to adapt to focal, contextual, and residual stimuli. She identifies four modes of human adapting: (1) *physiologic needs,* (2) *self-concept,* (3) *role function,* and (4) *interdependence.* Obviously, these adaptive modes again include physiologic, psychologic, and social aspects of people. The notion of coping or adapting to stimuli again relates nursing to people in interaction with their environment. Self-concept, role function, and interdependent areas of coping all lend themselves to the conceptualization of the practice of psychiatric nursing.

Others

The theories presented in the past few pages in no way represent the entire universe of contenders. Ida Jean Orlando (1961) stresses the interaction of meanings between nurse and client. Ernestine Wiedenbach's (1964) work presents an example of a "situation-producing" theory that conceptualizes a goal and a nursing prescription for fulfilling the goal. Myra Levine (1967) uses four conservation principles to conceptualize nursing interventions: (1) *conservation of energy,* (2) *conservation of structural integrity,* (3) *conservation of personal integrity,* and (4) *conservation of social integrity.* Imogene King (1971) discusses concepts of social systems, perceptions, interpersonal relations, and health and their impact on people.

A review of these theories indicates some clear differences in emphasis and perspective and some intriguing similarities. From these theories are emerging the parameters of our discipline. Such parameters provide the beginnings for directing practice, focusing nursing research, and providing a framework of concepts integral to the teaching of professional students.

Evaluating Nursing Theories

Although it is premature to close the question of which among the array of contending paradigms will dominate the discipline of nursing and which is best suited to psychiatric nursing, we can and should assess each according to a framework of questions derived from metatheory (Chinn 1987, Fawcett 1984, Fitzpatrick 1982, Meleis 1984). Problems of metatheory raise general issues, provide criteria of choice or standards, and should be discussed in any serious consideration of the construction of theory and its proper

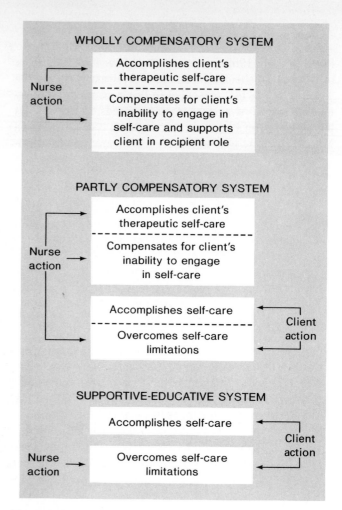

Figure 4–4
Orem's self-care deficit theory.
Source: Adapted from Orem DE: Nursing: Concepts of Practice. McGraw-Hill, 1971.

application. Three metatheoretical questions are used to assess the value of nursing theories for psychiatric nursing practice.

- Is it a theory? What definition of theory should prevail in our shared understanding?

- Is it a nursing theory? What, if any, theoretical orientations comprise and inform nursing's unique body of knowledge?

- Is it any good? What standards might we select to evaluate a theory or a fragment of a theory?

Is It a Theory?

There seem to be almost as many definitions of what a theory should be as there are contemporary theorists in nursing. However, most authorities agree that a theory should describe, explain, and predict truths about the world or that part of the world on which the theory focuses. Furthermore, most theorists accept the focal concepts for nursing as *people, nursing, health,* and *society.*

A **theory** can be defined as "a system of propositions containing interrelated concepts." A nursing theory must include the concept of nursing and explain and predict how nursing actions affect or interrelate with the person and the environment to produce a desired health-related outcome.

Components of a Theory

Practically, a theory is considered fairly complete if it contains:

- Concepts to describe and classify empirical facts
- Definitions that allow for consensual meaning and potential measurement
- Propositions that connect two or more concepts and allow for beginning explanations and predictions
- Linkages between the propositions forming a system or scheme

The ordering of these propositions into some specific inductive or deductive arrangement is an elegance achieved slowly, and it characterizes only mature sciences. A final point bearing on our definition of a theory is its distinction from a model. A *model* is a concrete rendition of the theory that can be used to help visualize and understand the abstraction that cannot be directly observed. Models may be replicas, analogies, or symbols.

Is It a Nursing Theory?

Our second metatheoretical problem concerns the debate about the existence of any unique nursing theory. In science there are often boundary disputes about the proper focus of a discipline that claims to be a science. Many humanists and philosophers of science are opposed to what they called "disciplinary territorialism." They urge scholars to acquire the skills to investigate any question that arouses their curiosity. Yet Immanual Kant (1900) suggests a contrasting point of view. He wrote:

> To yield to every whim of curiosity and to allow our passions for inquiry to be restrained by nothing but the limits of our ability shows an eagerness of mind not unbecoming to scholarship. But it is wisdom that has the merit of selecting from among the innumerable problems which present themselves, those whose solution is important to mankind.

In the view of many nurses, it is on such wisdom that the definition, refinement, and growth of nursing theory will depend.

The debate boils down to one question. Can and should we develop nursing theories? Those opposed claim that there are no phenomena unique to nursing and therefore nurses have nothing about which to develop theories. Those who believe that nurses should develop nursing theories base their argument on the need for a systematically organized body of knowledge on which to base practice. A related assertion is that nurses have a great need for knowledge that scientists in other fields may not be interested in developing, and therefore nurses must take responsibility for developing the knowledge themselves.

Is It Any Good?

Our final question is: How can we judge or evaluate a theory or theory fragment? Nine conventional standards used for this purpose are:

1. Clarity. Is the theory understandable? Are the key concepts and propositions clear in both their connotative and denotative meanings?

2. Consistency. Is the theory internally consistent in the meanings of terms, interpretations of concepts, inclusion of principles, implications for method, and basic assumptions?

3. Logical development. Do the premises logically warrant the conclusion? In other words, does the theory's development follow the rules of logic?

4. Utility. Is the theory useful in education, research, or practice? Can the concepts of the theory be operationalized in ways that allow for application and testing?

5. Significance. Does the theory address essential issues and genuinely contribute to the development of the knowledge base in the discipline?

6. Scope. How many of the basic problems in a discipline or specialty can be handled by the theory?

7. Parsimony. Does the theory explain as much as possible with the fewest possible variables?

8. Precision of prediction. Does the theory provide reasonable, precise prediction of outcomes?

9. Accurate explanation. Is the theory right or true? Obviously, this is a place where empirical verification through research plays a vital role.

Applying Nursing Theories to Practice

We have discussed the question: What is a good theory? Selma Fraiberg (1959) asks: What good is a theory? She challenges us to explain what practical use all this research and theorizing have. To do so, we must consider the application of theory to clinical practice in psychiatric nursing.

There are many ways of knowing what to do in the clinical act. Some of us rely on authority, others on past experience. Trial and error is a time-tested method, and some of us yearn for divine inspiration. Scientists, however, are governed by rules of empirical research methodology. They must deductively test a theory to confirm or refute it or inductively generate theories from data.

Most nurses acknowledge that principles govern their actions regardless of how practical the nurse's orientation. Without the concepts and propositions of nursing theory we cannot categorize data acquired through assessment, formulate nursing rather than medical diagnoses, and select from possible nursing actions those with the greatest probability of achieving the desired goal.

Some of our colleagues challenge us to demonstrate how nursing theory is more than mere restatement of well-known psychologic, physiologic, systems, or medical principles in a special jargon. If all nursing theory exists ultimately for the sake of practice, the theory developed to guide psychiatric nursing practice ought to be clearly distinguishable from mental health practice based on borrowed theories in other disciplines. Colleagues in other disciplines cannot be expected to learn and apply new terms to describe familiar phenomena just because we in nursing choose to use them. Nursing theories must have both intellectual and practical coherence if they are to achieve a foothold in the knowledge base of the mental health team.

Chapter Highlights

- The nursing process and contemporary nursing theories based on research organize knowledge and provide a scientific way of knowing what to do with psychiatric clients.

- Phases of the nursing process include assessment, nursing diagnosis, planning, intervention, and evaluation.

- The 1982 ANA Standards for Psychiatric and Mental Health Nursing Practice reflect the current state of knowledge and base practice on theory.

- The nursing process is a conscious, deliberate, yet flexible and adaptable systematic set of cognitive and behavioral steps that describe the clinical act in nursing practice with individuals, families, groups, and aggregates.

- Effective nursing depends on accurate, systematic, and continuous data collection.

- Nursing diagnoses express conclusions about clients' human responses supported by recorded assessment data, current scientific premises, and humanistic principles.

- The nursing care plan is used to guide therapeutic intervention, achieve desired goals; it should reflect agreement between client and professional on short- and long-term goals.

- The implementation phase of nursing process is characterized by continued data collection and observation as well as modification in intervention strategy and timing, if necessary.

- Evaluation completes the phases of the nursing process and occurs so that the data base, nursing diagnosis, and nursing care plan can be revised.

- Concepts serving as focus for contemporary nursing theories are people, nursing, health, and society.

- Contemporary debate in nursing theory includes questions as to what a theory of nursing should be, whether any unique nursing theory exists, and how it might be evaluated.

References

Abdellah FG, et al: *Patient-Centered Approaches to Nursing*. Macmillan, 1960.

American Nurses' Association: *Standards of Psychiatric and Mental Health Nursing Practice*. ANA, 1982.

Betts V: Using psychiatric audit as one aspect of a quality assurance program, in Kneisl CR, Wilson HS (eds): *Current Perspectives in Psychiatric Nursing*. Mosby, 1978, vol 2.

Bower F: *The Process of Planning Nursing Care*, ed 4. Mosby, 1985.

Chinn PL, Jacobs MK: *Theory and Nursing*, ed 2. Mosby, 1987.

Fawcett J: *Analysis and Evaluation of Conceptual Models of Nursing*. FA Davis, 1984.

Fitzpatrick J, Whall A, Johnston R, Floyd J: *Nursing Models and Their Psychiatric Mental Health Applications*. Prentice-Hall, 1982.

Fraiberg S: *The Magic Years*. Charles Scribners' Sons, 1959.

Gebbie KM, Lavin MA (eds): *Classification of Nursing Diagnoses*. Mosby, 1975.

Gordon M: Nursing diagnosis and the diagnostic process. *Am J Nurs* 1976;76:1298–1299.

Hall L: *Nursing—What Is It?* Publication of the Virginia State Nurses' Association, Winter 1959.

Henderson V: *The Nature of Nursing.* Macmillan, 1966.

Kant I: *Dreams of a Ghost Seer.* Macmillan, 1900.

Kim MJ, McFarland GR, McLane AM: *Classification of Nursing Diagnosis.* Mosby, 1984.

King IM: *Toward a Theory of Nursing: General Concepts of Human Behavior.* Wiley, 1971.

Levine ME: The four conservation principles of nursing. *Nurs Forum* 1967;6:45–59.

Loomis M, et al: A classification of phenomena of concern for psychiatric-mental health nursing. *Arch Psychiatr Nurs* 1987;1(1):16–24.

McLane AM: A taxonomy of nursing diagnoses: toward a science of nursing. *Milw Prof Nurse* 1979;20:33.

Meleis A: *Theoretical Nursing: Development and Progress.* Lippincott, 1984.

Mundinger M, Jauron GO: Developing a nursing diagnosis. *Nurs Outlook* 1975;23(2):94–97.

Orem DE: *Nursing: Concepts of Practice.* McGraw-Hill, 1971.

Orlando IJ: *The Dynamic Nurse-Patient Relationship: Function, Process and Principles.* Putnam, 1961.

Peplau HE: *Interpersonal Relations in Nursing.* Putnam, 1952.

Rogers ME: *The Theoretical Basis of Nursing.* FA Davis, 1970.

Roy C: *Introduction to Nursing: An Adaptation Model.* Prentice-Hall, 1976.

Stevens BJ: *Nursing Theory,* ed 2. Little, Brown, 1984.

Wiedenbach E: *Clinical Nursing, A Helping Art.* Springer, 1964.

Yura H, Walsh M: *The Nursing Process.* Appleton-Century-Crofts, 1978.

FIVE

Conceptual Frameworks for Interdisciplinary Psychiatric Care

Holly Skodol Wilson

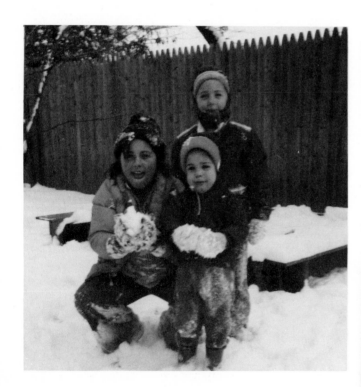

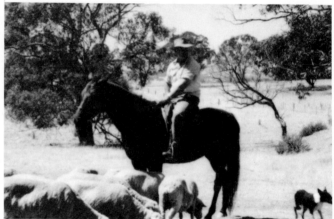

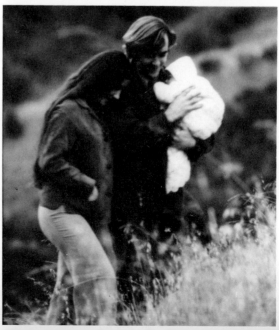

After reading this chapter, students should be able to

● Identify the assumptions and key ideas of the medical-biologic, the psychoanalytic, the behavioral, and the social-interpersonal frameworks

● Discuss the implications each framework has for psychiatric nursing practice

● Assess the strengths and weaknesses of each of the four frameworks

● Relate their framework to the four models presented

Cross References

Other topics relevant to this content are: Community mental health, Chapter 40; Cultural considerations, Chapter 38; Ethics, Chapter 10; Historical perspectives, Chapter 2; Philosophic perspectives, Chapter 1; and Psychobiology, Chapter 9.

Key Terms

behaviorist model
bioperiodicities
cathexis
chronobiology
circadian
conditioned reflex
defense mechanism
desensitization
ego
general systems theory
homeostasis
id
infradian
libido
medical-biologic model
negative reinforcement
neurosis
neurotic conflict
pleasure principle
positive reinforcement
psychic determinism
psychoanalysis
psychoanalytic model
psychosis
reality principle
reflected appraisals
reinforcement
residual deviance
response
self-system
shaping
social-interpersonal model
stimulus
superego
transference
ultradian
unconscious

This book celebrates efforts to protect the habitats of all earth's creatures.

To practice psychiatric nursing humanistically, nurses must devote themselves to understanding what makes people human, how they express their joy of living, their sadness, their desire to love, their hopes for growth. Understanding these phenomena becomes even more crucial when psychiatric nurses must explain how the joy of living suddenly turns to the desire to die, how love of self and others turns to violence and hate, and how the hope for growth turns to withdrawal and despair.

In Chapter 1 we described one philosophic framework for understanding the human responses with which psychiatric nurses work. However, what is called psychiatric-mental health nursing may undergo far-reaching changes depending on how we define it. The framework presented in Chapter 1 is by no means the only conceptual view nurses use in caring for clients. In this chapter we offer a comparative analysis of the basic assumptions and implications for practice inherent in four dominant models of interdisciplinary psychiatric care. These are the **medical-biologic model**, the **psychoanalytic model**, the **behaviorist model**, and the **social-interpersonal model**. Either explicitly or implicitly clinicians choose one or a combination of frameworks from these models in determining what information to assess about clients, what intervention goals and approaches to recommend, and what ultimate evaluation criteria to set. In this chapter, we attempt a critique of these models. By *critique* we mean an inquiry that reveals the hidden assumptions of a model, that grounds it in history, and that involves a systematic appraisal (Wilson 1985). The chapter reflects the humanistic interactionist perspective outlined in Chapter 1, since it is from that perspective that the authors view the study and practice of psychiatric nursing.

People base their actions on the meaning they attribute to the behavior and situations they confront. Suppose a 20-year-old woman hears and uses a private language and relates more to her paintings than to her peers. If nurses view this woman as having an illness called *schizophrenia* with identifiable symptoms such as hallucinations, it is likely that her treatment program will include the use of phenothiazine medications such as Prolixin, Thorazine, or Haldol. The therapeutic emphasis will be on treating and curing a person who has been identified as mentally disordered. If, however, nurses view this woman as "withdrawing into *primary process thinking* to defend against an unconscious conflict rooted in traumatic childhood experiences," the therapeutic approach may emphasize individual psychotherapy designed to bring the conflict to the surface and resolve it. If nurses view this woman's behavior as a learned pattern that has been reinforced by significant others throughout her life, intervention is more likely to follow a behaviorist approach. In this case, the therapist may engage members of the woman's family in planning and learning a new mode of interacting with her, carefully prescribed to extinguish old patterns of behavior and to reinforce new, more functional ones. Finally, nurses may not view the young woman as having an illness or an exclusively intrapsychic personal problem at all. Rather, they may view her as one participant in a network of interpersonal relationships that includes her immediate family and extends to her cultural context. In this case the "client" may include the whole constellation of social variables bearing on the young woman's human responses and the meaning assigned to them by significant others. "Therapy" then may include interventions ranging from family counseling to political action. Applying a nursing process approach may require data and ideas that integrate all four approaches.

Consider the different actions that a therapist might recommend to this client. She can:

- Take a trip to avoid what is making her anxious
- Take a rest and strengthen her inner defenses
- Yell, scream, cry, and reduce inner pressure
- Have sex if it reassures her
- Avoid having sex if it worsens her anxiety
- Learn sexual techniques that she has avoided out of anxiety, if the sex she is having is unfulfilling and tension producing
- Breathe deeply or try a massage to relieve tension
- Work harder and get a reward, if her narcissism is low
- Fail and get punished, if her guilt is high

- Join a religious cult
- Take a drink
- Calm down and try medication
- Attack the ruling class
- Join the ruling class or work for it
- Be a double agent
- Leave her family
- Make up with her family
- Commit a crime
- Enlighten herself, meditate
- Share her experience with others in a group and try to work out her problem-raising patterns in dealing with others
- Go to an analyst and try to obtain insight into mastery over her unconscious world
- Watch television
- Eat a special diet
- Enroll in an exercise class

If any of these maneuvers tips the balance so that the woman is better able to deal with destructive forces in her life, it may be called *therapeutic*. However, changes cannot be measured by any absolute standard. They can be measured only by the standards of the individual. One person's inner peace is the inertia of a zombie to another. Integrity to one may be rigidity to another.

What, then, are the predominant models of therapy? To answer this question, we must begin by noting that a particular strategy is seldom carried out in isolation. A therapeutic model fits therapeutic strategies with an ideology. Each model is based on a certain view of the human world, a theory of madness and health, a set of practices, qualifications for practitioners, and so forth. Each of the four dominant conceptual models for interdisciplinary psychiatric care is discussed in detail below. We will present the basic assumptions of each, its implications for psychiatric nursing, and a summary of our critique of it.

THE MEDICAL-BIOLOGIC MODEL

The medical-biologic model in psychiatry originated in the era of classification. The classification of mental disturbances brought the emotional and behavioral aspects of people into the domain of the medical doctor. During this period, the systematic observation, naming, and classification of symptoms were emphasized. Long-standing and somewhat barbaric treatment approaches were all but overlooked. As diagnostic designations became the rage, doctors began to search for the causes of mental illness in an organ or organ system. Emil Kraepelin's monumental descriptive diagnostic classification system is acknowledged as the first comprehensive medical model. It included the notions that the cause of mental illness was organic, that it was located in the central nervous system, that the disease followed a predictable course, and that treatment should be based on accurate diagnosis. Contemporary research findings in the field of psychobiology lend support to some of these early ideas.

Assumptions and Key Ideas

Proponents of the medical-biologic model view emotional and behavioral disturbances in the same way as they view any physical disease. Thus abnormal behavior is directly attributable to a disease process, a lesion, a neuropathologic condition, a toxin introduced from outside the human body, or most recently a biochemical abnormality of neurotransmitters and enzymes. This position might be summarized as follows:

- The individual suffering from emotional disturbances is sick and has an illness or defect.
- The illness can, at least presumably, be located in some part of the body (usually the brain's limbic system and the central nervous system's synapse receptor sites).
- The illness has characteristic structural, biochemical, and mental symptoms that can be diagnosed, classified, and labeled.
- Mental diseases run a characteristic course and have or haven't a particular prognosis for recovery.
- Mental disorders respond to physical or somatic treatments, e.g., drugs, chemicals, hormones, diet, or surgery.
- The behavioral disorders called "mental illnesses" are properly within the charge of physicians and should be treated following general medical practice. In other words, take the client's history, give a general physical exam, conduct laboratory tests, make a diagnosis, and select a treatment method in keeping with the diagnosis.

Implications for Psychiatric Nursing Practice

When nurses first became involved in the care of psychiatric clients, they were primarily responsible for the client's physical well-being. Their responsibilities included administering drugs prescribed by the physician and caring for clients undergoing treatments such as insulin shock, electroshock therapy, or hydrotherapy. Although in retrospect the medical model is associated with a comparatively limited view of people and a limited role for nurses, in the DRG era, it is still the major mode of naming phenomena of concern even among nurses in search of more appropriate alternatives.

The biologic-medical model is the conceptual basis for the continued use of biologic therapies in the care of psy-

chiatric clients, the hospital as the setting for care, research into genetic transmission of mental illness, research on biochemical and metabolic variables among diagnosed psychiatric clients, and dominance of the medical doctor in the psychiatric treatment team. Yet, as long as psychiatric clients are admitted to and reimbursed for care according to medical diagnoses, knowledge of this framework is crucial.

Understanding Medical Nomenclature

The psychiatric nurse clearly needs to be knowledgeable about current medical nomenclature and emerging research. Before the publication of the third edition of the *Diagnostic and Statistical Manual of Mental Disorders* (DSM-III) and the 1987 revision (DSM-IIIR) by the American Psychiatric Association (APA), the agreement about psychiatric diagnoses was amazingly low (five clinicians examining the same client using the medical model approach tended to reach at least three different diagnoses). Yet the APA's nomenclature predominated. It is still the most frequently used system of classifying behaviorally disturbed people, and its validity and reliability statistics have been considerably improved. Therefore, even psychiatric nurses who disagree with the mental disorder approach must be generally familiar with this system in order to communicate with peers on the psychiatric team. Knowledge of the system is also needed for identifying human responses associated with disorders so that the nurse can plan care.

It has been said that neurotics build dream houses, psychotics live in them, and psychiatrists collect the rent. This adage hints at how the diagnostic labeling of clients was done in the past. Minor distortions of reality, e.g., excessive fantasizing, inability to cope, and worrying, supposedly all lead the diagnostician to consider a broad category of disorders that were called neurotic disorders or **neuroses** before DSM-IIIR. Major alterations in perceptions of reality (such as hallucinations and delusions), massive withdrawal, and major disturbances of affect (feelings), lead to the consideration of psychotic disorders or **psychoses**. The basic difference between neuroses and psychoses presumably depended on how clients perceive the world and how they behave in light of these perceptions. The research of noted social scientists, however, has demonstrated that the distinction may be based on socioeconomic or other factors. In particular, Hollingshead and Redlich (1958) in their classic study found that neurotic diagnostic labels were applied significantly more often to clients at the higher levels of social class structure and that psychoses were attributed more often to the lower classes.

In his study on diagnostic screening associated with court orders, Thomas Scheff (1966), another sociologist, concludes that mental disorder is more a social status than a disease (and an ascribed rather than achieved social status). Problems of definition and diagnosis occur in part because behavior arises in variable social and cultural contexts, and the frames of reference of those making the judgments are not always comparable. Thus, as David Mechanic (1968) points out in his research, the behaviors defined as symptoms of illness may be as much characteristic of some particular situation or group setting as they are enduring attributes of the individual client. Consider the following historic account of a clinical examination conducted by Emil Kraepelin and described in his own words:

> Gentlemen, the cases I have to place before you today are peculiar. First of all, you see a servant-girl, aged twenty-four. In spite of her emaciation the patient is in continual movement. On attempting to stop her movement, we meet with unexpectedly strong resistance; if I place myself in front of her with my arms spread out in order to stop her, she suddenly turns and slips through under my arms so as to continue her way. If one takes firm hold of her, she distorts her face and weeps. She holds a crushed piece of bread in her left hand which she will not allow to be forced from her. If you prick her in the forehead with a needle, she scarcely winces or turns away. To questions she answers almost nothing. . . . [Quoted in Laing 1967, p 107.]

British psychiatrist R. D. Laing used this illustration to point out that practitioners tend to view such situations primarily from the psychiatrist's point of view. In this context, Kraepelin is sane, and the woman insane; he is rational, she is irrational. This conclusion entails looking at the client's behavior out of the context of the social situation as she experiences it. From the woman's point of view, the psychiatrist's actions are quite extraordinary: He tries to stop her movements by standing in front of her with arms spread out, tries to force a piece of bread out of her hand, sticks a needle in her forehead, and so on. Recent diagnostic systems have attempted to respond to these classic studies by making the psychiatric professionals' point of view explicit.

Psychiatric nurses need to interpret and appraise the contributions of biologic sciences to the understanding of human feelings and behavior. Genetics, biochemistry, and biorhythms are prominent areas of current research. Best known among the classic studies in psychiatric genetics is Kallman's (1953) work conducted in Berlin in 1938. His research supports the theory that genetic factors are always at least partially involved in the development (*pathogenesis*) of schizophrenia. Subsequent "twin" studies, which found that schizophrenia is likely to occur in both twins, especially if they were identical, have been cited by pro-

ponents of the biologic model as evidence of the role of heredity in schizophrenia. Similar family and twin studies were conducted throughout the world in relation to the occurrence of behaviors then labeled *manic-depressive reaction, involutional psychosis, neurosis, male homosexuality, criminal behavior,* and *disorders of aging.*

Biochemistry

Biochemistry is another area of active, biologically oriented psychiatric research. Certain biochemical changes are demonstrably associated with particular behavior disorders. For example, a defect in the metabolism of serotonin is currently being investigated as a possible cause of schizophrenia. Seymour Kety (1959) notes that schizophrenia may result from abnormal transmethylation of catecholamines yielding DMPEA, a compound closely related to mescaline. Wise and Stein (1973) provide evidence that 6-hydroxydopamine (6HD), an aberrant dopamine metabolite, produces schizophrenic symptoms by causing "a prolonged or permanent depletion of brain catecholamine." Evidence of a protein called taraxein in the blood of schizophrenics has also been reported. This agent blocks the action of acetylcholine in the limbic system, resulting in the client's inability to experience pleasure or pain. Carlsson and Lindqvist (1973) note that central dopaminergic receptors are blocked by all effective antipsychotic drugs, such as chlorpromazine. In sum, it is hypothesized that biochemical neurotransmission may eventually explain schizophrenia.

Medical-biologic research has also found relationships between mood disorders and biochemical changes. Some, if not all, depressions are associated with an absolute or relative deficiency of catecholamines, particularly norepinephrine, at functionally important receptor sites in the brain. Conversely, elation may be associated with an excess of such amines. However, the catecholamines have such complex relationships with enzymes and other elements of body chemistry that this hypothesis may be an oversimplification.

Chronobiology

A relatively new avenue of biologic research in psychiatry is the area called **chronobiology**. Implicit in much of this research is the hypothesis that disturbances in periodic processes (biorhythms) may contribute to psychopathology. These disturbances may not be apparent at the surface level of clinical description and observation. Measurement of such latent periodic processes may therefore be crucial in advancing the psychobiologic understanding of psychiatric illness. Rhythms underlie much of the range of homeostasis (the steady state) in people and in the world. A healthy human being's appearance of stability cloaks an inner symphony of biologic rhythms ranging from microseconds for biochemical reactions, milliseconds for nerve activity, a second for heart rhythm, the twenty-four-hour rest-activity cycle, and the twenty-seven-day menstrual cycle to the entire life span cycle.

Figure 5–1 provides a schematic spectrum of these rhythms, called **bioperiodicities**. Rhythms that are shorter than 24 hours have been designated **ultradian**, those longer than 24 hours **infradian**. In view of documented **circadian** (daily) fluctuations in human levels of consciousness and liver and kidney function, it is not unreasonable to think that the body also varies cyclically in its ability to tolerate stress or to detoxify and excrete harmful substances. Study of these cycles is the focus of psychophysiologic chronotography. If this line of research continues to yield promising findings, it could provide a new precision in preventive psychiatry—perhaps improving and complementing the traditional retrospective approach of psychoanalysis and the here-and-now emphasis of other therapeutic techniques.

Catherine Norris's (1975) studies on restlessness represent one example of how human rhythmicity can apply to a client problem. Norris noted that all human life is characterized by rhythmicity. Although some rhythms are learned and others are genetically determined, one of the first indicators of a threat to biologic rhythms may be the feeling of restlessness. Her concept of the relationship between rhythmicity and restlessness is portrayed on a continuum between "health" and "illness," as shown in Figure 5–2.

Critique

Perhaps the best known critic of the medical-biologic model is psychiatrist Thomas Szasz (1974), who argues that the concept of mental illness or mental disease, like the explanatory concepts of gods and witches, has outlived its usefulness and now functions merely as a convenient myth. Szasz and others contend that the medical model deals basically with the inner workings of the self, whereas disturbed behavior most often occurs in relationships with others. Since behaviors that are currently referred to as psychiatric symptoms are more likely to be aspects of communication with others, real or illusory, or legal problems about conformity, the medical model overlooks half the data. When vocabulary and concepts developed to describe intrapersonal processes are applied to interactional fields the result is strain, ambiguity, and obscurity.

Szasz bases his case against the medical model on several central premises:

- If mental symptoms were manifestations of disease of the central nervous system, they would correspond

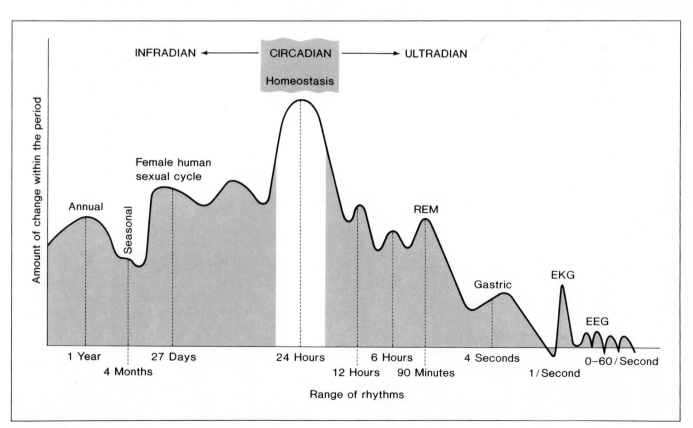

Figure 5–1
Schematic spectrum of human biologic rhythms.

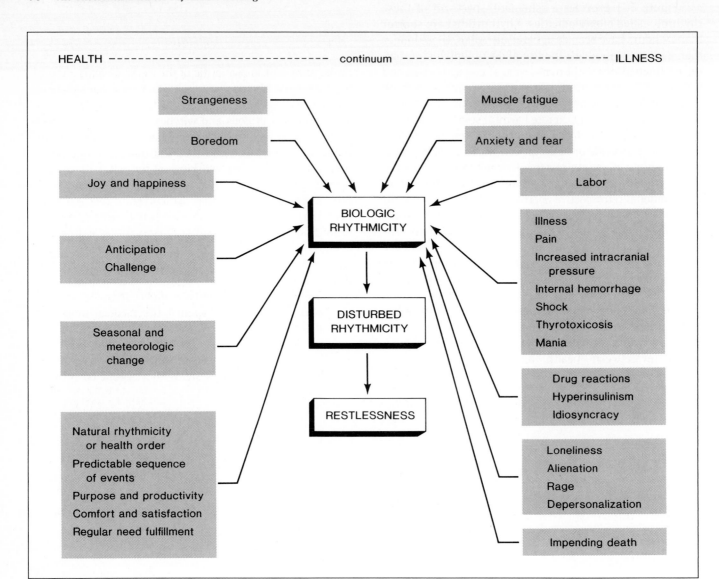

Figure 5–2
Rhythmicity and restlessness.
Source: C. Norris, "Restlessness: A nursing phenomenon in search of meaning." Copyright © 1975, American Journal of Nursing Company. Reproduced with permission from Nursing Outlook, Vol. 23, No. 2, February.

more to symptoms that result from diseases of the body, such as blindness or paralysis, rather than problems in living or relating to others.

- The medical model's view of mental and physical symptoms is not supported by observations. For example, when practitioners speak of physical symptoms, they mean either signs (such as fever) or symptoms (such as pain). When they speak of mental symptoms, they mean clients' communications about themselves, others, and the world. Practitioners have to judge whether a client's statements correspond with their

own and society's ideas, concepts, or beliefs. In short, the notion of a mental symptom is inextricably tied to the social and ethical context in which it occurs. Some studies have shown that knowledge about the orientation and education of the clinician is a better predictor of diagnostic outcome than the client's behavior.

- The medical model of mental illness concerns the role of illness in excusing conduct. The idea that serious disease is beyond the control and responsibility of the individual has long been accepted. With the emergence of self-healing practices and evidence that life-style choices, such as diet and exercise, affect physical disease, this notion is coming into question. To relieve people of ethical responsibility for their behavior because they have a disease seems even more questionable. The symptoms of "mental illness" are often behaviors that are associated with the very heart of responsibility—the mind and the character. They are, therefore, quite reasonably beyond excuses.

In his critique of the medical model, Szasz concludes that "mental illness" is a name for problems in living according to certain psychosocial, ethical, and legal norms. The idea, for example, that hostility, vengefulness, or rape is indicative of mental disorder is based on the cultural value attached to love, forgiveness, or consensual sexual relationships. The irony, then, is that a remedy is sought in terms of medical measures, and even the medical diagnostic labels currently in use provide no indication of the specific treatment that will be tried. A diagnosis of schizophrenia may be followed by any one or a combination of treatments, including drugs, electroshock therapy, psychotherapy, group therapy, milieu therapy, or family therapy. The policies of the clinical setting and the client's age, place within the family structure, socioeconomic status, and (often) sex usually are better predictors of the treatment that will be advised than the diagnosis is.

Human behavior is complex. A change in body structure or body chemistry results in a change in behavior. An organism or a toxin can initiate and ultimately alter thought processes. Similarly, a problem in feelings, such as low self-esteem, can produce structural body changes, such as hunched shoulders or muscle contractions. It is likely that there is no single "cause" of the troubled and troublesome behavior called mental illness and the human responses to it. The medical model's attempt to find one is often unnecessarily limiting. It obscures the relevance of interpersonal and cultural factors and challenges nursing to articulate and develop them.

The publication of the American Psychiatric Associations' third edition of the *Diagnostic and Statistical Manual of Mental Disorders* (DSM-III) in 1980 and its 1987 revision reflects efforts to respond to these criticisms in several important ways:

- Psychiatric diagnoses according to DSM-IIIR are based on specified, empirical criteria not linked to any particular theory of etiology.

- The diagnostic criteria have been field-tested for reliability and validity, with encouraging results.

- A DSM-IIIR diagnosis is multifaceted in that it assesses the presence or absence of an individual's biologic, psychologic, and social pathology.

- The diagnosis includes a client's strengths or level of adaptive functioning and contextual stresses.

- The "V-codes" allow the clinician to note the presence of a problem in living that does not represent a psychiatric disorder (Williams and Wilson 1982).

THE PSYCHOANALYTIC MODEL

The psychoanalytic model is usually credited to the Viennese physician Sigmund Freud (1962b). Freud's premise was that all psychologic and emotional events, however obscure, were understandable. For the meanings behind behavior he looked to childhood experiences that he believed caused adult neuroses. Therapy in this model consists of clarifying the meaning of events, feelings, and behavior and thereby gaining insight about them. Freud's work shifted the focus of psychiatry from classification to a dynamic

RESEARCH NOTE

Citation

Norris C: Restlessness: A nursing phenomenon in search of meaning. Nurs Outlook 1975;23:103–107.

Study Problem/Purpose

In this classic inductive clinical study, Norris set out to observe and describe the clinical phenomenon of human restlessness. Study questions included: What is restless? When does it occur? How does one experience restlessness?

Methods

The investigator observed migratory land and sea animals, reviewed related literature, drew on her own practice experience with clients, interviewed nurse colleagues about their experiences, and engaged in purposeful observation under diverse conditions associated with restlessness. These conditions included biologic changes (hemorrhage or toxicity), perception of changes (new or strange experiences), disruption of biologic rhythmicity, fatigue, boredom, and role deprivation. She also observed clients in pain and clients suffering anxiety.

Findings

Although her method was relatively unsystematic, Norris concluded that restlessness may be a person's first response to change, strangeness, or threat.

Implications

If additional research confirms these early findings, restlessness may belong to a group of disturbances in rhythmicity that have a warning function. Although the activity may seem random and without purpose, it may generate the energy needed to cope with a perceived threat. The author urges other clinicians to document and describe such clinical phenomena from their practice to build nursing science.

view of mental phenomena. Psychoanalytic concepts have so widely permeated the education and practice of psychiatric clinicians that they have come to be regarded as a fundamental part of understanding and approaching emotional disorders. Psychoanalysis has emerged as a method of investigation, as a therapeutic technique, and as a body of scientific concepts and propositions.

Assumptions and Key Ideas

Psychic Determinism

A fundamental concept associated with the psychoanalytic model is **psychic determinism.** The psychic determinist believes that no human behavior is accidental. Each psychic event is determined by the ones that preceded it. Events in people's mental lives that seem random or unrelated to what went before are only apparently so. Thus, psychoanalysts never dismiss any mental phenomenon as meaningless or accidental. They always search for what caused it, why it happened. For example, people commonly forget or mislay something. They usually view this as just an accident. Psychoanalysts, on the contrary, seek to demonstrate that the accident was caused by a wish or intent of the person involved. Psychoanalysts also view dreams as subject to the principle of psychic determinism, each dream and each image in each dream bearing some relationship to the rest of the dreamer's life.

Role of the Unconscious

A second fundamental concept in the psychoanalytic model is that significant unconscious mental processes occur frequently in normal as well as abnormal mental functioning. These processes are called simply the **unconscious.** The unconscious is so intimately related to the premise of psychic determinism that it is hard to discuss one without the other. According to psychoanalysts, the fact that much of what goes on in people's minds is unknown to them accounts for the apparent discontinuities in their mental lives. If the unconscious cause or causes of some behavioral symptoms are discovered, then the apparent discontinuities disappear, and the causal sequence becomes clear.

Psychoanalysis

The most powerful and reliable method for studying the unconscious is the technique that Freud evolved over several years, called **psychoanalysis.** The basic logic behind psychoanalysis is:

- The client has undergone a *traumatic experience* that stirred up intense and painful emotion.

- The traumatic experience represented to the client some ideas that were incompatible with the dominant ideas constituting his or her ego. Thus a **neurotic conflict** was experienced.

- The incompatible idea and the neurotic conflict associated with it force the ego to bring into action **defense mechanisms** that manifest themselves in the client as neurotic symptoms.

- Therapy is directed toward resolving the conflict by uncovering its roots in the unconscious. If the client is able to release the *repressed feelings* associated with the conflict, the symptoms will disappear.

Among the strategies used in psychoanalysis are: (a) hypnosis, (b) the interpretation of dreams, and (c) free association, in which the client is encouraged to express every idea that comes to mind—no matter how insignificant, irrelevant, shameful, or embarrassing—ignoring all self-censorship and suspending all judgment.

In the initial phase of psychoanalysis, the analyst's task is to facilitate establishing a *therapeutic alliance.* In the transition to the middle phase of analysis, **transference** occurs and the analyst uses techniques calculated to induce *regression* in the client. In this stage the analyst remains relatively passive to avoid giving either permissive or authoritarian expressions and to limit observations to interpretations of the client's mental dynamics as heard in the free associations. In the long-range course of analysis, the client undergoes two basic processes—remembering and reliving. *Remembering* refers to the gradual extension of consciousness back to early childhood, when the core of the neurosis was formed. *Reliving* refers to the actual reexperiencing of past events and feelings in the context of the client's relationship with the analyst. The alleviation of symptoms is not usually regarded as the most significant factor for evaluating therapeutic change. Instead the chief basis of evaluation is the client's capacity to attain reasonable happiness, to contribute to the happiness of others, and to deal adequately with the stresses of life. In short, the most important criterion for successful analysis is the extent to which it releases the client's normal potential, which had been blocked by neurotic conflicts.

Topography of the Mind

Freud classified mental operations according to regions or systems of the mind in a body of thought now referred to as *topographic theory.* Any mental event that occurred outside of conscious awareness represented the *unconscious region.* Mental events that could be brought into conscious awareness through an act of attention were said to be *preconscious.* Those that occurred in conscious awareness were regarded as the *conscious surface* of the mind. This topographic model, although still used to classify mental events in terms of the quality and degree of awareness, has been supplanted by the structural model.

Structure of the Mind

Freud abandoned the topographic model of the mind for the *structural model* with the publication of *The Ego and the Id* (1962a) in 1923. The structural model of the mind contends that there are three distinct entities—the id, the ego, and the superego. The id was seen as a completely unorganized reservoir of energy derived from drives and instincts. The **ego** controls action and perception, controls contact with reality, and, through the defense mechanisms, inhibits primary instinctual drives. One of its fundamental functions is also the capacity for developing mutually satisfying relationships with others. The **superego** is concerned with moral behavior. Frequently, the superego allies itself with the ego against the id, imposing demands in the form of conscience or guilt feelings. The id in a child operates according to what Freud called the **pleasure principle**—the tendency to seek pleasure and avoid pain. This is not always possible, so the demands of the pleasure principle have to be modified by the **reality principle**. The reality principle is largely a learned ego function by which people develop the capacity to delay the immediate release of tension or achievement of pleasure.

Drives

Freud believed that psychic energy was derived from *drives.* Instincts or drives were genetically determined psychic constituents. He used the word **cathexis** to refer to the attachment of psychic energy to a person or a thing. The greater the cathexis, the greater the psychologic importance of the person or object. Initially Freud postulated a life and death instinct, but by 1920, in *Beyond the Pleasure Principle* (1975), he had revised these ideas to accord with the theory of drives accepted by or modified by analysts today. In the later formulation, Freud accounted for the instinctual aspects of people's mental lives by assuming the existence of two drives—*the sexual drive* and *the aggressive drive.* The former gives rise to the erotic component of mental activity, and the latter gives rise to the destructive component. The two drives can be fused, for example, when an act of intentional cruelty also has some unconscious sexual meaning for the actor and provides a degree of unconscious gratification. The sexual drive has come to be known as the **libido**.

Implications for Psychiatric Nursing Practice

The psychoanalytic model has historically provided a very limited treatment role for the nurse. Psychoanalytic clients are usually seen in the analyst's office as private clients.

With the emergence of psychoanalytically oriented settings such as Chestnut Lodge in Rockville, Maryland, nurses became somewhat more involved, sharing at least in the psychoanalytic language, concepts, and speculations about client dynamics. In the United States a nurse needs a medical degree as well as psychoanalytic training in order to practice as a psychoanalyst. Some nurses have sought preparation as lay analysts at settings such as the William Alanson White Institute and the Chicago Psychoanalytic Institute. However, the nurse has served more frequently as an adjunct therapist focusing on here-and-now issues with clients undergoing psychoanalysis or in a supportive role to family members.

Acknowledging that the psychoanalytic model has provided few clear-cut therapeutic roles for nurses does not suggest that nurses have failed to do useful work with clients undergoing psychoanalytic treatment or that knowledge of psychoanalytic theory is irrelevant to psychiatric nurses. Concepts derived from the psychoanalytic model, such as the unconscious, pervade not only the field of psychiatry but also the entire culture. These concepts are understood by the educated public and are useful in comprehending fields of human endeavor ranging from public relations to art and literature. The psychoanalytic vocabulary has crept into everyday speech through college courses in psychology, personal therapy, and pervasive use in the popular culture. Ordinary people think about being conflicted. They check their ids periodically for death wishes and their egos for weaknesses. People who are rejecting are considered egocentric. Castration complexes, sibling rivalry, and phallic symbols are recognized everywhere. Marital and divorce court proceedings are conducted in "psychoanalese." Certainly if nurses are to participate as equal members of the psychiatric team, and if they are to be valued as theorists, they must learn the language of and ideas about psychodynamics that are the common heritage of many psychiatric professionals.

Critique

We criticize Freudian psychoanalysis somewhat uneasily. As one authority put it, "Who knows, they might be right. All of us hardy souls who persist in our skepticism might be 'resisting'—the very evidence of our sickness." Yet some critical analyses of the psychoanalytic movement have emerged. Several differ with small sections of Freud's work (Adler and Horney, for example, disapproved of psychic determinism, the instinct theory, and the structural approach of id, ego, and superego). Others go so far as to found a whole empirical school of behaviorism in opposition to Freudianism, attacking the "absurdities" of the whole.

Perhaps the most compelling synthesis of critical arguments launched against the psychoanalytic model can be found in the literature of feminism. Feminists have pointed out that

1. Psychoanalytic theory's emphasis on early childhood determinism underrates the effects of environmental systems on dynamic processes in people.

2. The psychoanalytic model tends to accept as unchangeable the social context in which repression and resulting neurosis must develop.

3. Freud's ideas were rooted in the social and political culture of his time (that is, early twentieth-century Viennese society).

These critics have noted further that the psychoanalytic framework is blatantly antifemale. Shulamith Firestone (1971), for instance, comments that Freud's theory about women is limited to analyzing them only as negative males (e.g., the Electra complex is an inverse Oedipus complex). His concept of two types of female orgasms, clitoral and vaginal, was refuted as myth in the research of Masters and Johnson. Widespread acceptance of Freudian theory has promoted social adjustment for women instead of feminist revolt, contends Firestone. In short, she sees psychoanalysis as patching up with Band-Aids casualties of the immense social unrest and role confusion associated with the rigid, patriarchal, nuclear family. As evidence of psychoanalytic insensitivity to the objective difference in women's and men's social situations, Firestone cites some of the work of the neo-Freudians. The attitude that almost all women are afraid that the man they love will leave them, but hardly any man is afraid that a woman will leave him, is apparent as a consistent theme. Other examples are the beliefs that girls find their own genitals ugly compared to those of boys, that women devote great effort to adorning their bodies in order to compensate for this physical deficiency, and that women are insecure and self-conscious because they lack penises. Firestone notes examples of such analysts' misinterpretations of client interactions based on these notions.

Helene Deutsch, trained in psychoanalysis by Freud and author of a monumental two-volume work on women (1944–1945), expounded the following ideas in her theories of "normal femininity":

- Preadolescent girls have masochistic longings to be raped.

- Women find enjoyment through childbirth, forced intercourse, and lost causes.

- Women with "masculinity complexes," whom Deutsch "unmasked" in therapy, were cases of thwarted femininity, since women cannot compete successfully with men.

- Motherhood is the only true fulfillment for all women.

Deutsch describes truly "feminine" women as the loveliest and most unaggressive of helpmates, women who do not insist on their own rights but are easy to handle in every way if one just loves them. Most critics view such theories of "normal femininity" as representing a traditional perspective that has limited women's choices.

Freud, Deutsch, Erikson, and Reik view the difference in genital apparatus between the sexes as the critical variable affecting personality development in men and women. These theorists posit a separate psychology of women linking all traits, interests, attitudes, emotions, and neuroses to an anatomic "defect." Erik Erikson (1968), a neo-Freudian, makes a valiant attempt to wed cultural relativity with innate biologic differences, but he still ends up with the advocates of "anatomy as destiny." Most feminists argue that, even if an anatomic theory did explain human behavior, birth and breast envy ought to be given equal time with the penis envy so dominant in Freud's essays.

Other feminists writing about psychoanalysis point out that, although adult mental health in American society is masculine centered, most psychoanalytic theory has been written about women. Phyllis Chesler (1972) criticizes Freud's vision of women as essentially "breeders and bearers," potentially warmhearted creatures, but cranky children with uteruses, forever mourning the loss of male organs and male identity. The headaches, fatigue, chronic depression, frigidity, paranoia, and overwhelming sense of inferiority that Freud noted in so many of his female clients were never viewed by him as the indirect communications characteristic of slave psychologies. Instead, such symptoms were viewed as hysterical and neurotic productions manufactured by spiteful, self-pitying, and generally unpleasant women. Their inability to be happy as women, Freud concluded, stemmed from unresolved penis envy, unresolved Electra complexes, or general mysterious female stubbornness.

Freud's views about women have been extensively reviewed, criticized, and rejected wholly or partially by such female theoreticians as Karen Horney, Clara Thompson, Margaret Mead, Eva Figes, Simone de Beauvoir, Betty Friedan, Kate Millett, and Germaine Greer. Male theoreticians such as Bronislav Malinowski, Alfred Alder, Harry Stack Sullivan, Wilhelm Reich, Ronald Laing, David Cooper, and Thomas Szasz have also refuted Freudian theory but not necessarily or primarily because of its premises about women.

Those who do emphasize Freud's psychology of women as the basis for their critique argue that biologic differences between the sexes have been overemphasized and that all mammals show a vast array of bisexual or unisex behaviors. These theorists modify Freud's libido concept to refer to forces in both sexes that lead to experimentation and growth. They conclude that curiosity, aggressiveness, dependence, expressiveness, interest in the body, self-esteem, and the need for growth, security, and creativity are all part of a common human repertoire that transcends anatomy. These givens, however, can be elaborated, drastically altered, or suppressed as each individual comes into contact with his or her immediate family environment and total culture.

THE BEHAVIORIST MODEL

The behaviorist model in psychiatry has its roots in psychology and neurophysiology. To the behaviorist, symptoms associated with neuroses and psychoses are clusters of learned behaviors that persist because they are somehow rewarding to the individual. One of the most important conceptual contributions to this framework was made by Pavlov (1849–1936), who in 1902 discovered a phenomenon he called the **conditioned reflex** in a famous experiment with a dog and a bell. The basic principle of the conditioned reflex is this:

- A **response** is a reaction to a **stimulus**.
- If a new and different stimulus is presented with or just before the original stimulating event, the same response reaction can be obtained.
- Eventually the new stimulus can replace the original one, so that the response occurs to the new stimulus alone.

The conditioned or learned response has come to be viewed as the basic unit of all learning, the unit on which more complex behavioral patterns are constructed. Such construction occurs through a process called **reinforcement**, in which behaviors are rewarded and persist. Pavlov's theories have continued into the present, valued for their simplicity, concreteness, and objectivity. Some behaviorists see them as the key to comprehension and control of the whole range of problematic human behavior.

Assumptions and Key Ideas

The fundamental premises of the behaviorist perspective can be summarized as follows:

- Human beings are merely complex animals. The difference between human and animal is one of degree and not kind. Human powers of conceptual thought, propositional language, and abstraction are fully attributable to physiologic complexity rather than some nonmaterial source. Thus the use of animal experience as an analogue to human experience is clearly justifiable.
- The self in humans is the sum or repository of past conditionings or simply the behavioral repertoire. Therapists can know clients only by the clients' behav-

ior. The concepts of consciousness and self and the belief in subjective reality are products of human pride rather than scientific discovery. If they are real, they can be inferred only from observable behavior.

- Behavior is what the organism does. It can be observed, described, and recorded.
- There is, properly speaking, no autonomous person. People are what they do and what they are reinforced for doing by conditions in their environment.
- The self is a structure of stimulus-response chains or hierarchies of habit. It is possible to know and predict conditions under which behavior will occur.
- The symptoms of a person's disorders are, in fact, the substance of that person's troubles. There is no hidden motive, no underlying cause, no internal pathogenic process. There is only the symptom or the behavior, and the aim of behaviorist therapy is to change the behavior.
- The classification of mental diseases is meaningful only to provide legal labels. It provides little or no assistance in prescribing a treatment program.
- People can control others whether others want to be controlled or not. Control is neither good nor bad in and of itself.
- The therapist determines what behavior should be changed and what plan should be followed. Change is effected by identifying events in the client's life that have been critical stimuli for the behavior and then arranging interventions for *extinguishing* those behaviors. A changed way of acting precedes a changed way of thinking, according to behaviorist theory.

Both Joseph Wolpe (1956) and B. F. Skinner (1953, 1971) are associated with psychiatric treatment approaches that represent one form of *conditioning* and reflect the above assumptions. Wolpe defined *neurotic behavior* as unadaptive learned behavior acquired in anxiety-generating situations. He based his therapeutics on the introduction of a response that inhibits anxiety when situations occur that ordinarily evoke anxiety. Relaxation, for example, was considered incompatible with anxiety and, therefore, effective in inhibiting it. Thus, Wolpe would direct his intervention to a counter-conditioning technique, usually putting the client under hypnosis and using various techniques for gradual **desensitization**. For example, a man with a fear of dying might gradually attempt to overcome his anxiety at the sight of a coffin, the attendance of a funeral, and so on, by trying to relax in the face of these situations.

Skinner's approach, called *operant conditioning*, emphasizes discovering why the behavioral response was elicited in the first place and what current variables actively reinforce it. The key concept in operant conditioning is reinforcement. Skinner originally used the term **positive reinforcement** to describe an event that increases the probability that the response will recur—a reward for behavior. A **negative reinforcement** was defined as an event likely to decrease the probability of recurrence because it penalizes the behavior.

Other contemporary behaviorists have redefined Skinner's original terms and introduced some new ones. Positive reinforcement is still an environmental event that rewards and thus increases the probability of a behavioral response. Negative reinforcement can mean removal of an adverse stimulus (e.g., an electric shock to animals or the restriction of people's privileges) to increase the likelihood of a behavior's recurrence. *Positive punishment,* in contrast, is the introduction of aversive stimuli to decrease the likelihood of recurrence of a behavior. *Negative punishment* removes something that has been a prior reinforcer, thus again decreasing the likelihood of such behaviors as smoking, drug abuse, truancy, temper outbursts, and abuse. Table 5–1 contains examples of each of these neobehaviorist concepts.

The frequency with which a response is given is a clear, observable measure of behavior. Most people exhibit aggressive behavior at some time. To say that a client is hostile suggests that this class of response occurs more frequently than usual. The term given to an intervention designed to change a client's behavior is **shaping.** It is a procedure of manipulating reinforcement to bring the person closer to the chosen behavior. There are, according to Skinner, times in a client's life when responses are accidentally reinforced by a coincidental pairing of response and reinforcement. This accidental pairing may play a role in the development of phobias (irrational fears) and other distressing and/or dysfunctional behaviors.

Most psychiatric nurses acknowledge that the application of principles of behavior modification to clients is quite complex, since such interventions are powerful tools with a heavy philosophic overlay. The use of this approach raises issues of control, responsibility for behavior, and the morality of using negative or punitive stimuli in a therapeutic context, to name only a few. Consider the notion of the nurse as "behavioral engineer." Therapists who successfully resolve such basic philosophic issues have designed and implemented successful behavior modification plans with disturbed, overtly aggressive children, developmentally disabled clients, and violently self-destructive people.

In many institutional environments, clients follow prescribed schedules for daily living that include a token economy. Clients are rewarded for desired behavior by token reinforcers, such as food, candy, and verbal approval. The movement toward community-based psychiatric treatment has made plain some of the shortcomings and economic realities of therapies aimed toward resolving everyone's intrapsychic conflicts. The movement has instead attempted to replace maladaptive behavior with behavior that will enable people to function effectively within their natural environment. When parents or others in the client's environment are taught to implement the behavior change procedures, therapy moves away from the partial and artificial situation of the therapist's office into the client's total environment. It no longer requires the presence of highly trained, often expensive experts and thus makes treatment more affordable.

Some behaviorists envision a future in which behavior therapy based on learning theory will become the dominant mode of psychiatric intervention. This would move psychiatry out of the hospitals and into adaptive function learning centers.

Psychiatric nurses have had a special role in teaching behaviorist principles to people with little training so that they can act as change agents. Nonprofessional staff on psychiatric wards can be taught effective use of behaviorist principles to eliminate chronic, maladaptive behavior by

Table 5–1
Examples of Behaviorist Concepts

Concept	Purpose	Example
Positive reinforcer	Increase recurrence of the behavior through reward	Leave of absence from hospital as per contract with client
Negative reinforcer	Increase recurrence of the behavior by removing aversive consequences	Removal of restrictions on phone calls or visitors as per contract with client
Positive punishment	Decrease behavior by adding aversive consequences	Quiet time
Negative punishment	Decrease behavior by withdrawing a reinforcer or reward	Withdrawal of privileges, such as recreational outings in a residential milieu

long-term psychiatric clients. Hyperactive children or children with borderline intelligence can be treated in the home by their parents when nurses teach the parents to use approaches such as frequency counts on specific behaviors to be modified, time-outs (short periods of isolation) for undesired behavior, and the bestowal of attention, praise, and affectionate physical contact as rewards.

In general, behavior modification offers a rapid, efficient, and effective system of intervention congruent both with psychiatric nurses' conventional roles as planners and teachers and with trends in community psychiatry. However, it may not always be in accord with a nurse's personal philosophy.

Critique

Intervention based on the behaviorist model has proved effective in the treatment of persons so alienated from society, functionally incapacitated, or destructive that they are unable to interact with or respond to others. Nonetheless, criticism has been leveled against this model. The criticism fundamentally rests on ethical concerns about people's rights, dignity, and freedom. The model has been criticized for its simplistic explanation of human feelings and behavior and for its authoritarian therapist-client relationship.

Advocates of behaviorism contend that without a strict, logical, reductionist methodology, psychiatric practice will be plagued with all sorts of methodologic and logical improprieties. Without a strict reduction to empirical or observable content, they believe, therapists are left with a discipline based on emotions, introspection, and subjective feelings.

Humanistic social scientists, in contrast, contend that ignoring emotions, introspection, and subjective feelings distorts the creative role of people in shaping their environments instead of merely adapting to them. Humanists further argue that these qualities differentiate humans from animals. People are self-aware. They can step outside themselves and reflect on their subjective inner lives. Their ability to think about themselves enables them to talk about themselves and to contemplate their future possibilities. Such self-consciousness is the genius of human individuality. No other animal is burdened with this gift. Crucial to this quality, of course, are the abilities to comprehend meaning and to use language.

If Freud's theories challenged the rationality of human beings, many critics find that behaviorist learning theories reduce humans to little more than cogs in a machine that can be conditioned to do almost anything. Such a conception of human beings ignores uniquely human abilities—the ability to be self-conscious, to act intentionally, to experience reality differently from each other, and to create images, dreams, fantasies, and a private inner life. Many clinicians value certain interventions generated according to principles of stimulus-response learning, but the behaviorists' most basic assumptions about people and their

environments contrast harshly with the image of humans and society offered by other theoretical schools. Yet problems such as an abusive parent or spouse, a self-mutilating adolescent, or a fire-setting child urge that we keep an open but ethical mind on this approach.

THE SOCIAL-INTERPERSONAL MODEL

The social-interpersonal model of psychiatry grew out of a general dissatisfaction with approaches that account for "mental illness" in terms of either intrapersonal mechanisms (e.g., the symptoms of a disease) or individual personality dynamics such as anxiety, ego strength, and libido. Advocates of this model assert that other models neglect the crucial social processes and cultural variation involved in the development, identification, and resolution of disturbed human responses. The social-interpersonal perspective is advanced as more logical, more appropriate, more encompassing of the issues involved, and more readily substantiated by research. It focuses on the larger and more general context of deviance and on the processes by which an individual comes to be labeled as deviant. The humanistic interactionist philosophic base for this text represents an extension and refinement of the social-interpersonal model. It is a synthesis particularly of the sociologic and social interpersonal models for explaining human responses to mental distress and dysfunction.

Assumptions and Key Ideas

Three somewhat separate schools of thought that are philosophically congruent make up the social-interpersonal model. These are the sociocultural, the interpersonal-psychiatric, and the general systems approaches. The assumptions and key ideas of each are discussed below.

The Sociocultural School

The sociocultural approach is summarized partially by sociologist Kai Erikson (1962): "Deviance is not a property inherent in certain forms of behavior; it is a property conferred upon these forms by audiences which directly or indirectly witness them." A similar view is proposed by Howard Becker (1963, p 9): "Deviance is not a quality of the act a person commits, but a consequence of the application by others of rules and sanctions to an 'offender.'"

Thus, mental illness is a *label* earned by certain behaviors that violate the rules of conduct imposed by various significant others. The focus for psychiatry is on the interplay between the deviant and the audience—the person and the social context. Sociologically, the critical variable in the study of the forms of deviance labeled *mental illness* is the social audience rather than the individual person, since it is the audience that eventually decides whether any given action will be labeled deviant. Included in the study of "mental illness," then, are various aspects of audience reactions to behavior, the labeling process, the criteria used in labeling, the extent of consensus on such criteria, the consequences for an individual so labeled, etc. The criteria of DSM-IIIR represent a move in this direction.

A well-known example of this approach is the research of Thomas Scheff (1966), who concludes that "mental illness" is a label given to diverse forms of deviance that do not fit under any other explicit label, such as delinquency. In this regard, he views mental disorders as a form of **residual deviance**—a label given to nonconforming behavior. The label reinforces and stabilizes that behavior and enters the labeled client into a deviant role of "mental patient." Once a person has been labeled deviant and societal reactions have become organized, Scheff argues, the deviant may incorporate the definitions of others into his or her own self-concept.

Scheff's research confirms many of the early ideas of sociologist Edwin Lemert (1951), who proposes that mental illness bears a greater similarity to other forms of social deviance than it does to medical disease. Lemert introduced the ideas of primary and secondary deviation to differentiate between occasional or situational lapses from normal behavior and deviation that becomes a life-style or established social role. Lemert argues that, when society becomes the active labeler, occasionally nonconforming primary deviants are cut off from their nondeviant status and begin life as full-time secondary deviants. Hospitalization, commitment, and psychiatric diagnostic classifications are all ways of forbidding the temporarily lapsed person (such as the daydreamer or the person who goes on a bender but is not yet an alcoholic) from reentering the community with "normal" status intact. When the individual begins to develop behavior that fits the new status and finds the new role gratifying, he or she adopts a deviant life-style.

In the view of the sociologic school, then, behaviors that are often called symptoms acquire meaning only when considered within their social context. This view emphasized the social system consisting of the client, others reacting to the client, and the official agencies of psychiatric control and treatment. It de-emphasizes individual personal dynamics.

The Interpersonal Psychiatric School

Significant contributions were made to the social-interpersonal model by psychiatrists Adolf Meyer (1948–1952) and Harry Stack Sullivan (1953) in the first half of the twentieth century. Sullivan trained with William Alanson White and Adolf Meyer rather than Freud. He is viewed as the least reductionist of psychiatric theorists and emphasizes modes of interaction as the real focus of psychiatric inquiry. Sullivan argues that psychiatry should renounce the futile attempt to define isolated individuals and instead define the significant interpersonal aspects of situations. His main theoretical concern is with the integration of organism and milieu. Sullivan became the theoretical and ideologic leader of the interpersonal school of psychiatry often associated with the William Alanson White Foundation, which sponsors the well-known journal *Psychiatry*. The sociologic theorists differ on some points from those adhering to the interpersonal school of psychiatry (for example, on the relative importance of the self and individual psychology). They are bound together, however, by a number of fundamentally compatible ideas.

One concept that plays a crucial role in the organization of behavior, according to Sullivan, is the **self-system** or *self-dynamism*. The self is a construct built from the child's experience. It is made up of **reflected appraisals** the person learns in contacts with other significant people. The self develops in the process of seeking physical satisfaction of bodily needs and security. To feel secure, the self essentially requires feelings of approval and prestige as protection against anxiety. In summary, Sullivan emphasizes the pervasive interaction between organism and personal environment. He objects in principle to the concept that organized psychologic impulses, drives, and goals belong to the person as an individual. He feels instead that the person cannot be distinguished from the person-in-the-interpersonal-situation.

Despite the environmentalist phrasing of many of his key concepts and a certain emphasis on the effects of cultural configurations on the development and functioning of the personality, Sullivan has comparatively little to say about the impact on behavior of specific variations in the social or cultural scene. Like Sullivan, other advocates of the interpersonal school of psychiatry, such as Karen Horney (1950) and Erich Fromm (1941), stress the general climate in the immediate family. Alfred Adler (1971), however, attempts to understand more of the social and cultural conditions influencing behavior. The interpersonal school of psychiatry in general focuses less on social context than the sociologic perspective and takes basically a developmental-interpersonal view of the self.

The General Systems Theory School

General systems theory, when applied to living systems (people), provides a conceptual framework within which the content of the biologic and social sciences can be logically integrated with that of the physical sciences. In psychiatry it offers a new resolution of the mind-matter dichotomy, a new integration of biologic and social approaches to the nature of human beings, and a new approach to psychopathology, diagnosis, and therapy.

The personality theory proposed by Karl Menninger (1963) presents normal personality functioning and psychopathology in general systems theory terms. His theory deals with four major issues:

1. Adjustment or individual-environment interaction
2. The organization of living systems
3. Psychologic regulation and control, known as *ego theory* in psychoanalysis
4. Motivation, which is often called *instinct* or *drive* in the psychoanalytic framework

A salient point of Menninger's theory is the idea of homeostasis (human balance). He asserts further that the greater the threat or stress on a system, the greater the number of system components involved in coping with or adapting to it. Therefore pathology can exist at various levels, from the cell and organ level to the group and community level. An example of the former might be the behavioral changes that follow cellular alterations due to addictive drugs, to a blood clot, or to a tumor. Examples of pathology at the group level include family conflicts. At the community level, overpopulation, pollution, homelessness, and poverty are instances of pathology. In systems theory, all represent abnormalities or stresses on matter-energy processes and would be included within the domain of psychiatric professionals.

In Menninger's view, then, a system's well-being depends on the amount of stress on it and the effectiveness of its coping mechanisms. He asserts that "mental illness" is an impairment of self-regulation in which comfort, growth, and production are surrendered for the sake of survival at the best level possible but at the sacrifice of emergency coping devices (1963, pp 526–527). Psychiatric clients are described as "obliged to make awkward and expensive maneuvers to maintain themselves, somewhat isolated from their fellows, harassed by faulty techniques of living, uncomfortable themselves and often to others" (Menninger 1963, p 5). Emphasis in therapy according to the general systems approach is on current conflicts, restoration of impaired systems of functioning, and subsequent reintegration of the restored function into future coping strategies.

Implications for Psychiatric Nursing Practice

The social-interpersonal framework gives independent and collaborative psychiatric nursing clear theoretical direction and support. Nursing roles are associated with shifts

in the delivery of psychiatric services variously termed *social psychiatry, community psychiatry, psychoeducation,* and *milieu therapy.* All are associated with efforts to provide psychiatric services more efficiently to large groups of people, particularly those previously neglected, and attempts to counteract the debilitating effects of long-term institutionalization. All are also associated with a political and ideologic movement to address the client's social context in providing psychiatric care. According to these orientations, all social, psychologic, and biologic activity affecting the mental health of the population is of interest to professionals in community psychiatry. Therapeutic interventions may include programs for social change, political involvement, community organization, social planning, family support groups, and education. The implications for practice derived from this theoretical model are many:

- Clients are approached in a holistic way, reflecting the interrelation and interaction of the biophysical, psychologic, and socioeconomic-cultural dimensions of human life. This increases the number of factors that must be assessed when caring for a client.

- Because of the increased number and diversity of variables to be considered, graduate and undergraduate content in psychiatric nursing education must be revised. Curricula must include concepts, theories, and research findings to support extended and new thinking about mental health, culture, social systems, ethnicity, deviant behavior, social support, psychobiology, and the human condition. These new content areas drawn from the social and natural sciences must then be integrated with conventional psychiatric nursing content to form an internal coherent knowledge base.

- Definitions of the client expand to include the concept of client system. A family, a couple, an aggregate, or even a community may be the client.

- Intervention strategies include primary prevention roles of psychoeducation, social change agent, and researcher. The goals are to help individuals cope with stresses in their environment, alter environments that contribute to pathology, and conduct research to establish the logical basis for preventive and adaptive measures.

- The yardsticks for measuring "normality" are revised to reflect several notions. First, some deviant behaviors resemble physical illness and others do not. Second, applying psychiatric labels on the basis of selective and flimsy evidence often has destructive consequences. Third, goals for therapy or treatment should not be set without first investigating the client's interpersonal and sociocultural situations.

- Therapy focuses on helping troubled persons to gain a useful perspective on their life-styles and social environments, rather than on exclusively repressing and controlling symptoms. Psychiatric nurses need to acknowledge the political and moral implications of involuntary drug therapy and behavior modification therapy.

- The psychiatric nurse must be prepared to function as an autonomous member of the psychiatric team and to assume more responsibilities. There is a shift away from the dominance of the physician in decision making and toward diffusion of roles. Practitioners' roles are based less on background discipline than on availability and interest in helping the client. For example, a cadre of mental health professionals who could become chronic care experts is direly needed.

In short, once clients are viewed as becoming disturbed and/or dysfunctional in the context of unhealthy or problem-filled interpersonal relationships, establishing healthy, constructive interpersonal relationships becomes important in their care. Psychiatric nurses can work milieu therapy, primary prevention, social psychiatry, and community psychiatry to implement this fundamental idea. The following case example illustrates this idea:

Mrs. S is a 67-year-old, upper-middle-class woman in good physical health. She has become increasingly untidy, forgetful, seclusive, sad, and suspicious since the death of her aggressive, bank president husband from a heart attack six months ago. She recently sold the large Tudor house where she had lived for the past 45 years, and she moved into a two-bedroom apartment in a nearby town. Because of apartment rules, she was unable to take her 12-year-old cat. She sold the house because her husband had told his lawyers that she should do so. (He had made all the family decisions while he lived.) Mrs. S has taken to skipping meals except for candy bars, since she must rely on a friend to drive her to the grocery store. (Her husband never felt she needed to learn to drive.) Her younger sister (age 59), seeking advice about Mrs. S's behavior, phoned the community mental health center on the suggestion of the family physician.

The social-interpersonal psychiatric nurse assessing Mrs. S's situation would tend not to focus on her symptoms as psychologic conflicts due to ambivalence toward her dead husband or as manifestations of a psychiatric disease such

as major, single-episode depression. Such a nurse would instead focus on the way Mrs. S is functioning in her current interpersonal situation and her human responses to it. In this analysis Mrs. S is not seen as diseased and therefore in exclusive need of a somatic treatment such as medication. Instead treatment consists of helping Mrs. S to develop strategies for coping with her new situation and satisfying her needs. The nurse will want to see the younger sister and other family members in an attempt to enhance Mrs. S's social support network. Efforts may be directed toward mobilizing other environmental forces (including the nurse) to provide company, stimulation, and proper nutrition for Mrs. S, since the absence of all three contributes to her symptoms and discomfort. Such a clinical situation will undoubtedly reinforce the psychiatric nurse's political efforts to point out the potential consequences of lifelong passive dependence of some adult women. The nurse may also become involved in community organizations working for better services for the elderly.

Critique

The social-interpersonal model has been criticized on three major fronts: conceptual, philosophic, and practical. Conceptual criticisms are brought most squarely to bear on Sullivan's interpersonal psychiatric theory. Writers such as Ruth Munroe (1955) view interpersonal psychiatric formulations as *word-building*—thinking up new names for old psychoanalytic concepts. Sullivan's theory is perceived as "losing a lot" when contrasted with the richness of Freudian analysis. Sullivan and the other interpersonal theorists, such as Adler, Horney, and Fromm, underplay the role of the biologic demands of the organism and tend to limit social psychiatry to the immediate family of significant others, neglecting the impact of culture and social structure. Furthermore, according to the critics, if the Freudians have neglected the dynamic importance of the self-system, the self-theories have given the concept too global a role. In sum, the concept does not usually add much to the clinical understanding of any living client. Finally, Munroe proposes that Sullivan's neglect and repudiation of the sexual systems are more a reflection of his era, a reaction against narrow Freudianism, than an intrinsic part of the interpersonal theoretical approach.

Thomas Szasz (1971) emerges as both a proponent and a critic of the social-interpersonal model, at least on a philosophic level. He argues that this model in community psychiatry looks to public health and preventive medicine for both its theoretical model and its moral justification for using the control power of the state. This is an error, says Szasz. If preventive psychiatry is a logical extension of traditional medical practice, psychiatric professionals can justify promoting their own business. Community psychiatry extends the control and power of mental health workers by asserting that psychiatric professionals have responsibility not only for persons who come for help but also for those who do not. Szasz points out the political implications of looking to public health medicine as the model for community psychiatry. Hypothetically, laws could be passed enacting compulsory mental health measures supposedly designed to protect the community "from psychologic contamination." Like public health laws concerning control of communicable disease, these mental health laws would be presented as value free and nonpolitical. Szasz concludes that once community psychiatric practice is commissioned and paid for by the state, the crusading psychiatric professional will owe the same unswerving loyalty to the government that the priest owed to the medieval church during the witch-hunts. Through crisis intervention and other methods of environmental manipulation, community mental health programs aim to eliminate known producers of stress. These include urban slums, rural depressed areas, and all other potential breeding grounds for mental disturbance. According to Szasz, preoccupation with "mental health" has the potential of victimizing individuals or groups who may be identified as "producers of stress" for the majority culture. In summary, Szasz attacks the model for its inclusiveness, its posture of condescending benevolence and righteous paternalism, and its covert potential for political repression.

Finally, criticism is brought to bear on the social-interpersonal model from real-world mental health workers who must cope with the stressful clinical realities, e.g., the window smashing, verbal abuse, and self-destructiveness of a young man brought to the psychiatric ward for threatening to assassinate the governor; the incoherent bizarre ravings of a vagrant, drunk on cheap wine, brought to the psychiatric emergency room of a New York City hospital from the snowy doorways of Broadway; or the mute, motionless living death of a catatonic woman found hidden away in an attic. To complicate matters further, sociocultural diagnoses are not currently among the categories being considered for psychiatric diagnostic reimbursement groups (DRGs). In our economic reality, they would not qualify a client for financial reimbursement. For these critics, the social-interpersonal model is impractical, idealistic, economically naive, and ill-suited to the realities of psychiatric care—where time is limited, money and supplies are even more so, and immediate problems of symptom control must be solved.

THE CHOICE OF A
CONCEPTUAL FRAMEWORK

Psychiatric nurses use one or a combination of theoretical frameworks, either implicitly or explicitly, to guide the application of the nursing process to their practice. In this text, we use the humanistic interactionist philosophic approach elaborated in Chapter 1 as the primary basis for subsequent ideas about human responses. As acknowledged earlier, it represents a synthesis of strengths derived primarily from the social-interpersonal conceptual model

and allows for the evolution of nursing theories as our body of knowledge grows. In clinical work, however, the selection of a conceptual framework may be influenced by various factors. Among them are the practitioner's education, the philosophy of the setting in which clients are treated, the nature of the client's present problem, the available treatment, the need to be efficient and practical, and even client attributes such as social class and gender. For example, in most cases physicians are inclined to view clients according to the medical model, the approach stressed in their education. This is particularly likely when the client's problem is identified as one of the syndromes for which somatic treatment is readily available and effective in symptom control, such as major depression or bipolar affective disorder, manic type. The former syndrome has been shown to respond to antidepressant medication and electroshock therapy, and the latter to lithium carbonate. The choice of a biologic-medical model is even more likely when the client is from a lower or lower-middle-class background, or elderly, or not highly intelligent or verbal. These characteristics are often used to rule out candidacy for psychotherapy. If the setting must respond to large numbers of clients on a short-term basis, the decision to label, sort, patch up with medicines, and dispatch back into the community often seems the only realistic alternative.

The social-interpersonal framework is more likely to be chosen as a basis for assessment and planning of client care under the following conditions: The clinician is a psychiatric nurse or social worker; the client's problem is one of relating to others or adjusting to a situation in life; the client is relatively verbal, intelligent, young, motivated, and from an upper-middle-class background; and the setting one in which long-term residential milieu therapy or group or individual psychotherapy is possible.

The failure of any model to "cure" a client may induce clinicians to recast the problem in a different framework with different treatment options. For example, a psychotic client who does not respond to medication may respond to a well-planned behavior modification program. Approaches associated with two or more different models are often used in combination. For example, bizarre, self-destructive behavior may be controlled with medications so that the client is more available for group or individual therapy. Such a combined or eclectic approach demands that a clinician be capable of functioning within any and all models of care, depending on which is best for the client and fits the resources and limitations of the situation. Yet conceptual models often remain implicit and unacknowledged, rather than being knowledgeably, explicitly, and systematically employed. If nurses give adequate consideration to the conceptual framework of their psychiatric nursing, they will foster practice-oriented research and clinical judgments that can be articulated and taught to others. Table

Table 5–2
A Comparative Analysis of Major Features of Four Conceptual Frameworks

Conceptual Framework	Assessment Base	Problem Statement	Goal	Dominant Intervention
Medical-biologic	Individual client symptoms	Disease	Symptom control Cure	Somatotherapies
Psychoanalytic	Intrapsychic Unconscious	Conflict	Insight	Psychoanalysis
Behavioristic	Behavior	Learning deficit	Behavior change	Behavior modification or conditioning
Social-interpersonal	Interactions of individual and social context	Dysfunction	Enhanced awareness and quality of interactions	Group and milieu therapies

5–2 summarizes the major features of each of the conceptual frameworks discussed in this chapter. Research is a tool for developing psychiatric nursing theory that synthesizes the most useful elements of these frameworks.

Chapter Highlights

- The choice of a conceptual framework for psychiatric nursing treatment determines information assessed, goals and interventions recommended, and evaluation criteria set.

- Therapeutic models for interdisciplinary mental health practice traditionally include the medical-biologic model, the psychoanalytic model, the behaviorist model, and the social-interpersonal model.

- In the medical-biologic model, emotional and behavioral disturbances are viewed as diseases. This view tends to limit the nurse's role to administration of somatic treatments and observation.

- Critics of the medical model of mental illness suggest that (a) social, ethical, interpersonal, and cultural factors are overlooked or obscured; (b) labeling behavior or "illness" relieves people of responsibility for their behavior; (c) mental symptoms correspond more to problems in living and relating to others than to diseases of the body.

- Psychoanalytic theory developed by Freud purports that all psychologic events have meaning and are understandable.

- Psychoanalytic theory states that much of what goes on in people's minds is unknown to them, or unconscious, and accounts for apparent discontinuities in their lives that are due to unresolved conflicts in stages of psychosexual development.

- In the psychoanalytic model, the nurse usually functions in a supportive therapeutic role.

- Criticism of Freudian psychoanalytic theory has come from feminists, behaviorists, and ego psychologists.

- In the behaviorist model, the self and mental symptoms are viewed as learned behaviors that persist because they are rewarding to the individual.

- In the behaviorist model, the nurse's role is expanded to planner, counselor, and educator, but therapeutic goals are limited to symptom control through behavior modification techniques that raise ethical issues.

- The behaviorist model has been criticized for its ethics, its reductionist explanation of human feelings and behavior, and its controlling, authoritarian therapist-client relationship.

- In the social-interpersonal model, (a) treatment occurs within an interpersonal context; (b) social processes (e.g., labeling by those involved in disturbed behavior) are assessed; (c) the focus is on the broader context of deviant behavior and integrates biologic and sociocultural sciences through a general systems perspective.

- In the social-interpersonal framework treatment is likely to include helping clients develop strategies for coping, mobilizing social support networks, and therapist involvement in community organization and planning.

- The psychiatric nurse's role in the social-interpersonal framework is expanded to include social and political action and community intervention as well as direct intervention with individuals, families, and groups.

- Research that develops nursing theory can synthesize the most useful ideas from all the dominant theoretical frameworks for psychiatric care.

References

Adler A: *The Practice and Theory of Individual Psychology.* Translated by P. Radin. 1929; reprint edition, Humanities Press, 1971.

Becker HS: *Outsiders: Studies in the Sociology of Deviance.* Free Press, 1963.

Carlsson A, Lindqvist M: Effects of chlorpromazine or haloperidol on formation of 3-methoxytyramine and normetanephrine in mouse brain. *Acta Pharmacolog Toxicol* 1973;20:140.

Chesler P: *Women and Madness.* Doubleday, 1972.

Deutsch H: *Psychology of Women.* Grune and Stratton, 1944–1945, 2 vols.

Erikson EN: *Identity, Youth and Crisis.* W. W. Norton, 1968.

Erikson K: Notes on the sociology of deviance. *Soc Prob* 1962;9:308.

Firestone S: *The Dialectic of Sex.* William Morrow, 1971.

Freud S: *The Ego and the Id.* W. W. Norton, 1962 (a).

Freud S: *The Standard Edition of the Complete Psychological Works of Sigmund Freud.* Hogarth Press, 1962 (b), 24 vols.

Freud S: *Beyond the Pleasure Principle.* W. W. Norton, 1975.

Fromm E: *Escape from Freedom.* Irvington Publishers, 1941.

Hollingshead AB, Redlich FC: *Social Class and Mental Illness.* John Wiley, 1958.

Horney K: *Neurosis and Human Growth.* W. W. Norton, 1950.

Kallman FG: *Heredity in Health and Mental Disorder.* W. W. Norton, 1953.

Kety SS: Biochemical theories of schizophrenia. *Science* 1959;129:1528,1590.

Laing RD: *The Politics of Experience.* Ballantine Books, 1967.

Lemert E: *Social Pathology.* McGraw-Hill, 1951.

Mechanic D: Some factors in identifying and defining mental illness, in Spitzer S, Denzin NK (eds): *The Mental Patient: Studies in the Sociology of Deviance.* McGraw-Hill, 1968.

Menninger K: *The Vital Balance.* Viking Press, 1963.

Meyer A: *Collected Papers of Adolf Meyer.* Johns Hopkins University Press, 1948–1952, 4 vols.

Munroe RL: *Schools of Psychoanalytic Thought.* Holt, Rinehart and Winston, 1955.

Norris C: Restlessness: A nursing phenomenon in search of meaning. *Nurs Outlook* 1975;23:103–107.

Scheff T: *Being Mentally Ill: A Sociological Theory.* Aldine, 1966.

Skinner BF: *Science and Human Behavior.* Macmillan, 1953.

Skinner BF: *Beyond Freedom and Dignity.* Knopf, 1971.

Sullivan HS: *The Interpersonal Theory of Psychiatry,* Perry HS, Gawel ML (eds). W. W. Norton, 1953.

Szasz TS: *The Myth of Mental Illness: Foundations of a Theory of Personal Conduct.* Harper and Row, 1974.

Szasz TS (ed): *The Manufacture of Madness.* Dell Publishing, 1971.

Williams JBW, Wilson HS: A psychiatric nursing perspective on DSM-III. *J Psychosoc Nurs* 1982;20:14–20.

Wilson HS: *Research in Nursing.* Addison-Wesley, 1985.

Wise CD, Stein L: L dopamine beta-hydroxylase deficits in the brains of schizophrenic patients. *Science* 1973;181:384.

Wolpe J: Learning versus lesions as the basis of neurotic behavior. *Am J Psychiatry* 1956;112:923–931.

SIX

Human Growth and Development Across the Life Span

June Andrews Horowitz

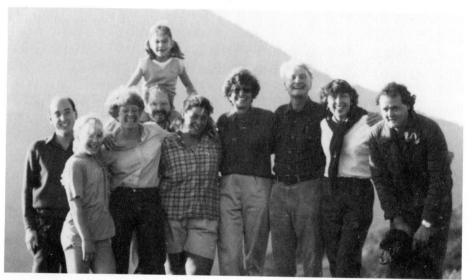

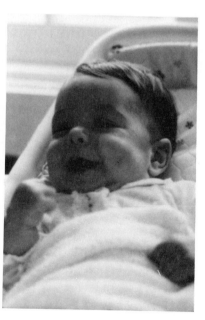

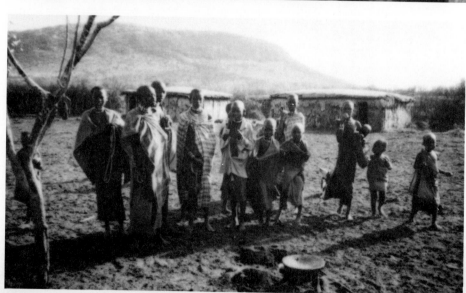

Learning Objectives

After reading this chapter, students should be able to

- Recognize that knowledge of growth and development is an integral component of nursing assessment and nursing diagnosis

- Examine historical changes in ideas about growth and development

- Compare major developmental theories

- Differentiate between developmental stages along the entire life cycle

- Discuss physical, cognitive, and psychosocial development in each life stage

- Describe developmental tasks for each stage

- Incorporate knowledge of growth and development in the nursing process

Cross References

Other topics relevant to this content are: Adolescents, Chapter 35; Children, Chapter 34; Developmental crises and crisis management, Chapter 29; Elderly, Chapter 36; Families, Chapter 33; Medical-biologic, psychoanalytic, behavioral, and social-interpersonal frameworks for understanding growth and development, Chapter 5.

Key Terms

accommodation	epigenetic principle
adaptation	mid-life crisis
animism	Oedipus complex
assimilation	parataxic mode
cephalocaudal principle	prototaxic mode
developmental/maturational crisis	proximal-distal principle
	schema
developmental phases/stages	self-actualizing people
developmental task	self-system
egocentric thought	symbiosis
Electra complex	syntaxic mode

The fabric of human life is woven in patterns of growth and development. Individuals are shaped by a continuous developmental process that progresses in the direction of increasing complexity and diversity. This process involves continuous interaction with the environment. Concepts of human growth and development have evolved over time in concert with changes in social structure and historical events. Many thinkers have made major contributions to our understanding of how people move through the phases of life and what developmental tasks characterize each stage. Because patterns of growth and development are central factors in people's mental health, nurses must recognize milestones, anticipate tasks and maturational crises, and understand the importance of helping clients negotiate the many challenges of the life cycle.

HISTORICAL FOUNDATIONS

An appreciation of history enriches our perspective of the present and future. Current thinking about growth and development has evolved from social and cultural changes.

Thirteenth Through Seventeenth Centuries

The idea that childhood is a distinct developmental stage is now basic to Western scientific thought; however, it is a relatively new concept in human history. In medieval society, the idea of childhood did not exist. As soon as the infant could live without the constant attention of the mother figure, the child belonged to adult society (Aries 1962).

This book supports those organizations and individuals working to end the torture of political prisoners.

Portions of the material in this chapter were contributed to the second edition of this text by Joan Sayre and Carol Bradley.

From this medieval view, conceptions of childhood emerged as schools were created outside the home to teach the skills needed in the marketplace of early industrial society. Childhood became, in part, a time for preparation for the adult world of work. The roots for seeing childhood as a separate life phase were established.

This embryonic view of childhood as a stage was shaped by the various environmental pressures on families to prepare children for changing adult roles and by beliefs concerning the basic nature of the child. These beliefs were influenced by thinkers of the day. John Locke (1632–1704) believed that children were incomplete adults. He rejected the concept of the genetic determination of development. Locke compared the mind of an infant to a *tabula rasa,* or "blank slate." According to this view, the child's mind is empty at birth and is gradually filled by knowledge gained by experience. Simple ideas are formed from direct sensory experience, and more complex ideas develop from associations between these simple ideas. Personality is formed through an accumulation of knowledge. Locke considered the early experiences of childhood crucial to the formation of personality. He believed that infants were significantly influenced by even very small impressions, which might completely alter the direction of their lives. This idea that children are extremely easy to influence and open to experience is still significant in developmental psychology.

Eighteenth and Nineteenth Centuries

The belief that children needed to be properly molded was evident in the colonial American family. The family had the responsibility to teach children religious values and to promote work skills through family chores or apprenticeships as preparation for later adult roles. In this environment, life was likened to a highway over which people traveled. Childhood was the beginning of the journey, but its course did not necessarily determine later development. Horowitz, Hughes, and Perdue (1982, pp. 21–22) summarize these views of growth and development:

> The historical record and subsequent analyses of seventeenth- and eighteenth-century notions of childhood and life stages indicate that children were not really considered miniature adults. Rather, children were seen as persons with fewer capacities than adults who required guidance, education, and strict disciplinary measures in order to grow into competent adults. Ideas of childhood were less deterministic than they are today—that is, problems during the early years were not considered automatic determinants of later difficulties. Children were expected to contribute to work of the household and to learn skills important in the adult world. Respect for parental author-

ity and God was a primary parenting concern, yet parents cared for their children.

Thinkers like Rousseau (1712–1778) suggested that children were qualitatively different from adults. Rousseau rejected the ideas that the infant was a formless being created through the accidents of experience, that the child was an incomplete adult, and that the child's reasoning processes were an imitation of adult thinking. Rousseau thought that from the moment of birth the infant was actively engaged in exploring and constructing a personal knowledge of the world. If left to nature, development would occur in an orderly progression, and at each stage the individual would be complete. The implication of this view for child rearing was that the adult should not interfere too much with the spontaneous process of development. The child is a "noble savage," endowed by nature with moral values. Adults who try to alter a child's behavior to conform to their own values distort the child's development. Rousseau's ideas remain influential today. They account for the emphasis placed on discovery, rather than on didactic education, in the teaching methods of Dewey and Montessori.

Much of the early speculation on the nature of childhood was purely philosophic. It was not based on actual observations of children. The emergence of psychology as a scientific discipline in the nineteenth century focused attention on direct observations of behavior. G. Stanley Hall (1844–1924), influenced by Darwin's evolutionary thesis, adopted a recapitulation theory of growth. He postulated that each individual's development reflected the growth of the species through its various evolutionary stages. Although this theory was later abandoned by developmental psychologists, Hall's systematic method of observing development established him as the founder of developmental psychology in the United States.

Several other psychologists did influential work in this field during the nineteenth century. Gesell described in detail the development of children at different ages. Watson attempted to explain the development of behavior through the principles of classical conditioning. Freud theorized that the experiences of infancy and childhood largely determined the adult personality.

Twentieth Century

Twentieth-century thinkers clearly differentiated childhood as a distinct stage with special developmental needs and tasks. Theorists and researchers began to study childhood and adult stages in great detail. The increasing knowledge of growth and development that has emerged is critical to the nurse's understanding of mental health.

The potential impact of ideas is illustrated when applied to a hypothetical nursing situation. Consider the nurse's assessment of a preschool child who is having behavioral problems at home and at nursery school following the birth of a sibling. A nurse who has adopted previously accepted notions about the nature of childhood might see the behavior as pathologic because the child is not acting as a little adult should, i.e., being thrilled by the awaited addition to the family and responsibly handling the infant. Or, the nurse might assess the problem to be one of needing to mold this blank slate of a child into the proper type of sibling. In contrast, by thoughtfully selecting and applying current research and theory, the nurse can understand the developmental needs of the child and help the parents and others such as the teacher provide the needed support and guidance during this difficult transition.

THEORETICAL FOUNDATIONS

Theoretical perspectives provide a foundation for examining the stages and developmental tasks of life. Theory is the lens through which the nurse can focus attention on various facets of a client's behavior and history. Theory also provides probable explanations and predictions of developmental phenomena that serve as guides for research. It is important to note, however, that theory is not fact. No one theory is sufficient to explain the complexities of human growth and development.

Freud's Psychosexual Developmental Theory

Sigmund Freud (1856–1939), the founder of psychoanalytic theory and one of the earliest developmental theorists, revolutionized modern thinking about developmental processes. Working in detective-like fashion, Freud sought to discover the hidden causes of various symptoms of his clients. His explorations led to a complex theory with many offshoots in psychoanalytic treatment today. Portions of his theory of development have been challenged, particularly as it relates to females. However, several of his fundamental concepts are important because they continue to influence thinking about developmental processes and stages.

Id, Ego, and Superego

Freud theorized that mental life was the function of several parts: the id, ego, and superego (Freud 1949). All inherited psychic properties, most notably the instincts, were seen as the id. Thus people are born with the id already present. The id finds expression in forms not known to the person. The newborn infant whose world revolves around instinctual gratification of such physical needs as eating, sleeping, and comforting provides a good example of the operation of the id.

The ego was thought to have developed from the id to receive and screen stimuli from the external world. As such, it functions as a shield and intermediary between the id

and the outside world. Its primary task is self-preservation of the person. The ego has become a central concept in psychoanalytic and developmental theory because it is seen as the seat of human functioning.

Emergence of the ego marks a major developmental task of infancy and childhood. It is first marked by the baby's recognizing separateness from others and learning to tolerate small delays in gratification of needs, e.g., being able to wait without crying while food is being prepared. The ego then evolves into the special intermediary between the child's wishes and impulses and the limits and demands of the external world. Identification of these ego functions is an important aspect of any nursing assessment.

During the long period of childhood, a special agency in the ego, the superego, results from parental influence and the contributions of later parental figures, such as teachers. The superego embodies the rules and values concerning what should not be done (the conscience) and what should be done (the ego ideal). The disciplinary function of the superego is experienced through feelings of pride for correct action and guilt for wrongdoing. The nurse who identifies an absent or excessively vigilant conscience during a nursing assessment is likely to find that the client also experiences difficulties in relating to others and functioning in a society based on rules and behavioral norms.

Stages of Psychosexual Development

Freud's developmental stages are outlined in Table 6–1. The first phase of development is the oral stage from birth to about 18 months. The infant derives satisfaction from and copes with discomfort or anxiety through oral activity, such as sucking.

The anal stage follows from approximately 18 months to 3 years. In Freud's view, this stage represents a major developmental challenge. The young child needs to learn to delay gratification and to exert the muscle control required in toilet training. Parents can attest to the importance of control during this period. This control is exerted not only in toileting but also in many aspects of daily life with a toddler, who is struggling to gain some mastery and separateness. The parental expectations and limits that are internalized at this time are the foundations of the superego.

The phallic stage follows from approximately 3 to 6 years. Although the genitals are thought to be emphasized during this phase, the processes of note involve identification with the same-sex parent, incestuous feelings toward the parent of the opposite sex, growing awareness of the genital area, and gender identification. The hallmark of this period is the Oedipus conflict (based on the ancient Greek myth) in which boys are thought to have incestuous feelings toward their mothers and hostile feelings toward

Table 6-1
Freud's Psychosexual Stages

Stage	Age Span	Task	Key Concept
Oral	0–18 months	Satisfaction and anxiety management from oral activity	Oral activity gives pleasure and is source for learning
Anal	18 months–3 years	Learning muscle control for toilet training	Delayed gratification and rule internalization
Phallic	3–6 years	Gender identification and genital awareness	Repression of attraction to opposite-sex parent leading to proper same-sex identification
Latency	6–12 years	Repression of sexuality	Oedipal conflict resolved with shift to other interests and friends
Genital	12–young adult years	Channeling sexuality into relationships with opposite sex	Reemerging sexuality to motivate behavior

their fathers as they vie for their mother's affection. Freud hypothesized that fear of castration motivates boys to repress sexual feelings toward their mothers and to shift identification appropriately to their fathers. The **Electra complex** is thought to be a parallel phenomenon in girls, who during this time have incestuous feelings for the father. Although the formulations concerning girls' development during this period are not clearly delineated, both boys and girls are thought to have sexual feelings that they need to learn to channel appropriately. Identification with the parent of the same sex is the desired outcome. Examples of this process are the 5-year-old boy who tells his mother that he will take care of her if Daddy fails to return from a business trip and the 3-year-old girl who wants to sleep on Mommy's side of the bed while she is away for a conference. These children show their identification with the same-sex parent when the boy enthusiastically mimics his father's lawn mowing and the girl pretends to play office and go to work as her mother does. Parents with children at this stage often hear their own words and see their actions played back with perfect accuracy in their children's play.

During the latency stage, from roughly 6 to 12 years, sexual energy is repressed or latent. According to Freud, the major developmental goal is to sublimate sexual energy by achieving skill mastery. The enthusiasm of school-age children for competitive sports, games, and learning in the classroom or playground illustrates this process.

The next period, the genital stage, is for Freud the period of complete personality organization. A reemergence of sexual urges motivates masturbation and heterosexual attraction. The adolescent seeks relationships with the opposite sex to satisfy these sexual feelings. According to Freud (1949), homosexual attraction is a perversion resulting from an object-tie fixation, a failure to resolve an

earlier identification appropriately. Although many aspects of Freud's view of the genital period have been challenged, particularly his ideas concerning homosexuality, his notion of sexuality as a motivating force remains an important contribution.

Freud's theory fails to map out any phases of adult development. In his theory, retrospective reviews of clients' lives were the basis for correcting present problems, not investigation of the unique challenges of adulthood. However, his theory has enhanced understanding of human development through concepts such as the unconscious, ego formation, and psychosexual stages.

Erikson's Developmental Phases

Erik Erikson's (1963) most significant contribution is his conception of the life cycle as a series of developmental phases, each with a major developmental task. A **developmental task** is a challenge that arises during predictable life periods calling for the individual to use available skills, resources, and supports to achieve the goal inherent in the task. Successful resolution promotes movement to later developmental stages by providing a foundation for accomplishing upcoming tasks. For example, the infant who learns to trust that a parenting figure will meet her needs consistently is ready to tackle the challenge of autonomy versus shame and doubt through such tasks as toileting during the toddler period. An infant who has not learned to trust will not feel safe enough to develop independent skills.

Developmental phases or **stages** are a universally experienced sequence of biologic, social, and psychologic events.

The individual's personality is constantly redeveloping in response to changing inner and outer requirements. This developmental process is governed by the **epigenetic principle**, a concept Erikson adapted from embryology. According to this principle, physical and psychosocial growth are regulated by a plan that is innate in the capacities of the individual on the one hand and arises in relation to others through social expectations on the other. The innate capacity for development of intellectual skills arises most dramatically during school age. It is also encouraged by parents' and teachers' expectations that children will apply themselves to learning at this age.

Within each developmental phase are a series of normative conflicts or specific psychosocial tasks with which every person must deal. During each developmental period, two opposing energies—a positive and a negative force—occur together and must be synthesized. For instance, in the first stage of development in infancy, the potential for trust and the potential for mistrust exist side by side. Infants who experience a feeling of physical comfort and minimal fear will jeopardize some of their feeling of safety to gain new experience. Each experience of having this sense of trust validated tends to produce positive expectations for new experience.

However, in infancy, as in all phases of life, there are physical and psychologic hazards. The rapid physical changes in infancy can in themselves foster mistrust as the infant experiences continual change. The infant learns to sit up, crawl, kneel, and walk within a period of months. If he or she has many unsatisfactory physical and psychologic experiences, the feeling of mistrust will predominate, leading the infant to fear the future. Such infants also find it hard to trust others. If the synthesis between trust and mistrust is basically positive because the parent nurtures the infant, a sense of trust will pervade the individual's life.

However, the potential for mistrust will still exist to some degree and must continue to be worked out in future developmental phases. For example, in early childhood the individual must maintain a sense of trust while dealing with the frustrations of toilet training and parental discipline.

The subjective feeling of having accomplished or having failed to accomplish the tasks appropriate to a specific phase influences the progress of development to the next phase. Achievement of a sense of trust must take place during infancy. At the age of 1 to 1½, childhood begins, bringing with it the new task of resolving a sense of autonomy and a sense of shame and doubt. Children who have not already accomplished the earlier task of achieving trust will be handicapped in dealing with the next developmental phase. This principle is obvious in the growth of the fetus. Each organ system must develop during its own crucial time, or defects will result. The same principle applies after birth in the achievement of psychosocial tasks. Thus, developmental phases are a kind of timetable for personality development.

Significant others help to resolve **developmental crises** (turning points during which usual coping patterns are ineffective and the opportunity for finding new adaptive

patterns exists) by satisfying the person's interpersonal needs and by conveying their interpretations of the meaning of the crisis. People who have enough opportunities to realize their developmental potential during the crucial period grow out of the crisis with important new abilities. If the crisis is not resolved in a constructive way, the person develops attitudes that are not helpful in future developmental tasks.

Thus, Erikson conceived of the life cycle as a series of building blocks, one influencing the next as the individual grows progressively more or less capable of dealing with life. This progression is depicted in Table 6–2.

Developmental tasks also reflect the structure of the society, since the culture dictates the desirable rate of development and favors certain aspects of development at the expense of others. American culture, for instance, stresses competition and achievement. These are appropriate concerns for young adults. However, American culture devalues the tasks of later years. These include the wisdom and contemplation that characterize the successful resolution of the last phase of life. Therefore, people in American culture may not experience a sense of achievement in fulfilling their potential in this phase. Although all the people in a given culture face similar developmental tasks, Erikson recognizes that each person resolves these tasks in an individual way. For example, some people may resolve the task of generativity, the task of adulthood, by nurturing children. Others may do so by producing artistic or scientific works.

A special contribution is Erikson's demonstration that development does not end in adulthood but continues until death. He also demonstrates reciprocity of development. For instance, to meet the infant's need to develop trust, a parent must successfully resolve the dichotomy of adulthood—that of generativity versus stagnation. Parents who cannot focus on their children's development will not be able to provide experiences that allow them to trust the world. Erikson's concepts of development remain very important in explaining personality.

Piaget's Cognitive Developmental Theory

As the concept of developmental phases became an integral part of psychologic theory, attention was given to examination of specific developmental phenomena, such as perception, abstract thinking, and memory. Jean Piaget (1896–1980) was a pioneer in cognitive theory formulation. Piaget (1952, 1958) viewed development as a constant process of interaction between environmental influences and the innate, genetically determined attributes of the individual.

Table 6–2
Erikson's Eight Stages

Age	Stage of Development	Task/Area of Resolution	Concepts/Basic Attitudes
Birth–18 months	Infancy	Trust versus mistrust	Ability to trust others and a sense of one's own trustworthiness; a sense of hope Withdrawal and estrangement
18 months–3 years	Early childhood	Autonomy versus shame and doubt	Self-control without loss of self-esteem; ability to cooperate and to express oneself Compulsive self-restraint or compliance; defiance, willfulness
3–5 years	Late childhood	Initiative versus guilt	Realistic sense of purpose; some ability to evaluate one's own behavior Self-denial and self-restriction
6–12 years	School age	Industry versus inferiority	Realization of competence, perseverance Feeling that one will never be "any good," withdrawal from school and peers
12–20 years	Adolescence	Identity versus role diffusion	Coherent sense of self; plans to actualize one's abilities Feelings of confusion, indecisiveness, possibly antisocial behavior
18–25 years	Young adulthood	Intimacy versus isolation	Capacity for love as mutual devotion; commitment to work and relationships Impersonal relationships, prejudice
25–65 years	Adulthood	Generativity versus stagnation	Creativity, productivity, concern for others Self-indulgence, impoverishment of self
65 years to death	Old age	Integrity versus despair	Acceptance of the worth and uniqueness of one's life Sense of loss, contempt for others

Source: From Childhood and Society, *2nd ed. by Erik H. Erikson, by W. W. Norton & Company, Inc. Copyright © 1950, 1963. Renewed 1978 by Erik H. Erikson.*

His basic theory is that the development of knowledge involves not only learning new things but also gaining the ability to reason abstractly and think logically. Children inherit a mode of intellectual functioning that remains essentially the same throughout life. However, cognitive structures are not inherited; they are formed through intellectual development. According to Piaget, in order to grow, individuals must adapt their cognitive structures to the demands of the environment. Intelligent behavior facilitates this adaptive process.

The structure of the intellect consists of schemata and operations. A **schema** is the internal representation of some specific action. The infant has a number of innate schemata for sucking, grasping, crying, seeing, and so on. During the course of development, these schemata become integrated and further elaborated. They are the fundamental structure of knowing. Operational schemata are mental structures of a higher order. They are not usually acquired until adolescence, when abstract thinking becomes possible.

Another key concept in Piagetian theory is adaptation. **Adaptation** occurs whenever an interchange between the organism and the environment results in a change in the organism that enhances its capacity for further interchange. Adaptation involves two interlocking components—assimilation and accommodation. **Assimilation** means the adjustment of an object to the structure of the organism. **Accommodation** means the adjustment of the organism to an object in the environment. Assimilation and accommodation operate simultaneously in the mutual adaptation between the individual and the environment.

The process of ingesting food offers a prototype of adaptation. Adaptation of the food to the needs of the individual occurs through a mutual transformation. The food is chewed and digested (assimilation). The body makes the necessary adjustments to facilitate the process, such as opening the mouth, secreting gastric juices, and so on (accommodation).

If one applies the concept of adaptation to cognitive

development, one begins to understand that every cognitive encounter involves a structuring process. This process meshes the individual's particular intellectual organization with the special characteristics of the object that is perceived. For instance, a child playing with a ball will first make a series of exploratory accommodations, such as looking and touching or rolling the ball back and forth. These accommodations are directed by concepts of touching and rolling, which are already part of the child's cognitive organization. These actions with respect to the ball are both accommodations to the roundness and size of the ball and assimilations of the ball to the child's cognitive organization.

Piaget's work in the definition of the fundamental characteristics of intelligence is still being developed. His key concepts are summarized below:

- Developmental processes occur in absolute continuity.

- This continuity proceeds by a continuous unfolding of capacities.

- The development of each new capacity has its origins in a previous phase and continues into the next phase.

- Each developmental phase entails a repetition of the processes of the previous level of development in a different form of organization or schema.

- The continuous development of more highly differentiated schemata creates a hierarchy of experience and action. Previous behavioral patterns are seen as inferior to present levels of behavior.

- Assimilation is the adaptation of the environment to oneself, the taking in of as much experience as the individual can integrate.

- Accommodation is the incorporation of an experience as it actually is—the taking in of the actual impact of the environment.

The cognitive stages and central developmental tasks according to Piaget's theory are outlined in Table 6–3.

Maslow's Hierarchy of Needs as Developmental Stages

Abraham Maslow's theory of self-actualization follows the premise of other theorists. Maslow believes that growth and development proceed in an orderly fashion through a set sequence of stages. His view of these stages differs, however, because the stages are need driven and not tied to age periods. Maslow's hierarchy of needs appears in Table 6–4.

Maslow's theory makes another significant contribution to our understanding of human development through its focus on mental *health.* Maslow was one of the first writers to criticize the emphasis on the study of disordered emotional functioning (Maslow 1962). He believed that mental illness cannot be understood without a prior knowledge of mental health. Maslow focused his attention on the positive aspects of human behavior, such as happiness, contentment, and elation. His studies of self-actualizing people—those he considered to be exceptionally healthy and mature—resulted in a more comprehensive, multidisciplinary approach to human problems. He saw mental health as involving every aspect of the individual's functioning.

Maslow defined **self-actualizing people** as those who make full use of their talents and potentialities, those who are doing the best they can do. Self-actualizing people are characterized by the ability to see life as it is rather than as they wish it were. Self-actualizing people are less emotional and more objective than those who have not achieved this level of development. They see people clearly, for they do not allow their own hopes and wishes to distort their judgment. Self-actualizing people understand themselves better than other people do. This enables them to consider

Table 6–3 Piaget's Cognitive Developmental Stages		
Age	**Stage**	**Task/Key Concept**
Birth–24 months	Sensorimotor	Learns about self as separate from world and about environment through manipulation and exploration; object permanence develops
2–4 years	Preoperational/preconceptual	Expressive language develops; symbolic play, thinking in mental images and egocentric thought emerge
4–7 years	Preoperational/intuitive	Learns to make rudimentary classifications; language expands; egocentric thought decreases slightly
From 6 or 8–12 years	Concrete operations	Systematic reasoning, application of rules, abstract thought, and reversible operations develop
12 years–adulthood	Formal operations	Learns to think using abstract, logical, conceptual operations; sees multiple relationships among things, properties, and classes

Table 6–4
Maslow's Hierarchy of Needs

Need	Definition
Physiologic	Biologic needs for food, shelter, water, sleep, oxygen, sexual expression
Safety	Avoiding harm; attaining security, order, and physical safety
Love and belonging	Giving and receiving affection; companionship; and identification with a group
Esteem and recognition	Self-esteem and the respect of others; success in work; prestige
Self-actualization	Fulfillment of unique potential
Aesthetic	Search for beauty and spiritual goals

the opinions of others and to admit their own lack of knowledge. Self-actualizing people are dedicated to some duty or vocation. They are creative, which allows them to be spontaneous, open, and experimental in their work and relationships. They are not in conflict with themselves, for their personalities are integrated around important values and life goals. Though they enjoy relationships with others, they may give the impression of remoteness, since they rely fully on their own capacities and do not need other people to complete their personalities. They are governed far more by their own nature and goals than by the opinions of others.

The basic difference Maslow saw between these people and the average person is that people who are not self-actualizing are motivated by deficiencies. Much of their energy is focused on fulfilling basic needs for safety, belonging, love, respect, and self-esteem. Self-actualizing people have met these security needs.

Sullivan's Interpersonal Theory

An important shift in analytic theory occurred with the work of Harry Stack Sullivan (1892–1949). As a neo-Freudian, Sullivan saw the reduction of anxiety as a prime motivator of behavior and shaper of personality. However, rather than emphasize the major concepts postulated by Freud, such as id, ego, and superego, Sullivan (1953) focused on the role of the environment and interpersonal relations as

the most significant influences on an individual's development.

Although essential, the interpersonal environment is also the source of anxiety, the nonspecific, unpleasant feeling of apprehension and discomfort. From a developmental perspective, anxiety is aroused by emotional disturbance in the significant person with whom the infant is interacting, such as the parent. Sullivan suggests that the significant other's inability to fulfill a need of the infant, such as feeding, or the significant other's own experience of anxiety makes the infant feel anxious. Inherent here is the concept that anxiety is communicated interpersonally.

Sullivan described three modes through which the environment is perceived: the prototaxic, parataxic, and syntaxic. The prototaxic mode refers to the earliest experiences of the infant in which all the baby knows consists of momentary experiences, undifferentiated feeling states in which no connections or sequences exist and there is no sense of self as a separate being. The parataxic mode appears as the infant matures so that parts of experience are recognized; however, there is still no ability to see connections or logical relationships. When the child learns to use language in a consensually validated way, i.e., with reference to meaning accepted by the listener, the child has acquired the ability to use the syntaxic mode of experience. These modes are important influences on the person's development and integration of experience.

The interpersonal experience of anxiety and its relief and the modes of perception shape the child's development through what Sullivan called the self-system, the constellation of tools or behaviors designed to avoid anxiety and establish security. The self-system operates interpersonally, leading to beginning personifications of the self or me. Sullivan describes three aspects of the self: the good-me that results from pleasant, rewarding experiences with the mothering one; the bad-me that results from increasing degrees of anxiety associated with interaction with the mothering one; and the not-me that occurs in the parataxic mode of experience, such as in dreams for all of us and in everyday existence for severely disturbed individuals. The not-me is made up of dreadful, poorly grasped aspects of living that are later differentiated into experiences associated with feelings of awe, horror, loathing, and dread (Sullivan 1953). These aspects of the self evolve from early parental influences but can be altered through interactions with others, i.e., via reflected appraisals, as new experience is incorporated.

Sullivan maps out these interpersonal processes in age-related stages. His emphasis on the interpersonal, rather than intrapersonal or intrapsychic, nature of development is a hallmark of his contribution to developmental theory. His stages of interpersonal development are outlined in Table 6–5. The importance of Sullivan's theory for nurses is increased by his influence on Hildegarde Peplau's (1951) explication of the interpersonal relationship as the central feature of nursing. Peplau's stamp on psychiatric nursing

Table 6–5
Sullivan's Stages of Interpersonal Development

Age	Stage	Task/Key Concept
Birth–18 months (to appearance of speech)	Infancy	Experiences anxiety in interaction with mothering one; learns to use maternal tenderness to gain security and avoid anxiety
18 months–6 years (from first speech to need for playmates)	Childhood	Learns to delay gratification in response to interpersonal demands; uses language and action to avoid anxiety
6–9 years	Juvenile	Develops peer relationships and uses environment outside the family to shape self
9–12 years	Preadolescence	Develops caring relationship with same-sex peer, chum relationship
12–14 years	Early adolescence	Develops interest in opposite-sex relationships
14–21 years	Late adolescence	Has satisfying relationships; directs sexual impulses
21 years +	Adulthood	Establishes love relationship

practice is demonstrated throughout this text in such principles as:

- Thought and language are intimately linked.
- Clarification of the client's meaning via verbal communication with the nurse leads to greater clarity in thought processes.
- Consistency is demonstrated by all the nurse's behavior and is the basis for trust.
- The nurse-client relationship offers some opportunity to relive and alter difficult aspects of the client's past relationships with significant others.
- This corrective experience can help the client master developmental tasks from earlier stages of life.

Themes from Developmental Theories

The theorists discussed in this chapter differ in their focus and their explanations of developmental processes. For example, Freud emphasizes internal psychosexual processes, whereas Sullivan stresses interpersonal forces that shape individual patterns. Most theorists do see development as age-related and sequential. However, Maslow views human development in terms of a needs hierarchy not related to specific ages. The predominant theme shared by all the theorists is that human development is directional and understandable.

People who examine and apply any developmental theory need to remember that theories are human creations—efforts to make complex phenomena meaningful and predictable. The risk in using theories is that they become so accepted that they gain a reality of their own; it becomes assumed that theories represent truth about our world. Rather, the nurse needs to use theories as road maps for organizing observations, perceptions, and other data in ways that increase understanding of people.

The nurse needs to recognize that people interact within and among themselves and with the environment. This recognition allows the nurse to examine multiple factors that contribute to anyone's development. Rigid norms thought to be orchestrated by fixed factors, such as age and heredity, give way to principles of human development that are shaped by many aspects of living, including the intrapsychic, interpersonal, and situational contexts. From this perspective, the nurse is better equipped to see the uniqueness of the person and to adapt the nursing process.

Assessment is done with milestones in mind; however, individuality is valued rather than labeled as deviant when it is not dysfunctional. Developmental theory guides the nurse's analysis and diagnosis in a manner that reflects an appreciation for the person's innate values, relationships, and context such as cultural heritage. Planning in relation to developmental goals includes the person and significant others, as appropriate; the nurse does not select goals in isolation. The individual and frequently the family are active players in the intervention process; the nurse does not do something to clients to promote their development but works with them. Evaluation of care outcomes includes clients' views in addition to objective measures of how developmental tasks have been achieved. Applying a humanistic interactionist model calls for nurses to use their analytic and interpersonal skills and to appreciate and nurture their own development as professionals and people.

THE HUMAN LIFE CYCLE

Developmental theories provide the foundation for identifying the significant processes and tasks in each major period of the life cycle.

The Prenatal Period

In the prenatal period, both the mother and embryo-fetus undergo development. Although there is no agreement about when the embryo-fetus truly becomes a person (opinion ranges from conception to viability or birth), embryonic-fetal development is always an important nursing concern. At the same time, mothers experience many emotional and physical changes and fathers also undergo psychosocial change. Looking at pregnancy as a developmental crisis can be helpful in understanding its tremendous impact on people's lives. Moore (1983) identifies four factors that affect the developmental processes of pregnancy:

- The meaning of the pregnancy for the individual
- The individual's stage of development, i.e., readiness for pregnancy
- Acceptance or denial of the pregnancy
- Resources that the individual has to deal with the pregnancy (Moore 1983, p 219)

These factors influence the expectant parents' successful accomplishment of the developmental tasks of pregnancy. The process of meeting these developmental tasks is illustrated in comments shared by expectant parents.

One pregnant woman described her awe at realizing that a developing separate person lived inside her—

she felt connected yet recognized the fetus as a separate being.

Another woman who became pregnant after previous problems with infertility reported that in her dreams she grappled with her fears that she would not be able to produce a normal baby. In one such dream, she gave birth to a hydatidiform mole.

An expectant father found he was spending much more time worrying about financial responsibilities and reflecting on his relationship with his own father as the birth of his first child approached.

The expectant parents are not alone in experiencing change. Throughout the pregnancy, the embryo-fetus undergoes tremendous developmental changes. The transformation from fertilized ovum to a living infant at birth is miraculous.

Infancy

Infancy extends from birth to 18 months. It is a time of rapid change in all areas of the baby's functioning. Major tasks of infancy are learning to trust, to use comforting from parenting figures to manage anxiety, and to begin to differentiate the self from the outside world.

Physical Development

Physical development during infancy is greater than at any other time in the life cycle and proceeds in predictable patterns. The **cephalocaudal principle** guides physical development. That is, development progresses first from the head and proceeds to lower body parts. For example, newborns quickly master sucking skills but do not gain motor control of the hands for many months; it is still later that sphincter control and coordination of leg muscles required for tasks like crawling and walking are achieved. The **proximal-distal principle** also governs the infant's physical progress; mastery proceeds in an inward to outward direction. To illustrate, the infant can move an entire arm in a desired direction before he or she is able to grasp with the hand (Mott, Fazekas, and James 1985).

A significant physical development during infancy is the gradual regulation of bodily patterns. Neuromuscular development proceeds to help the infant integrate processes such as sleeping, eating, eliminating, moving, and perceiving. Critical to this process is the interplay of the infant's own subsystems, and interaction of the infant with the human and physical environments. For the newborn, physiologic needs (e.g., hunger) create tension. When the parenting figure meets these needs consistently, satisfaction results, and the infant gradually learns to predict comfort in response to need tension. Rhythmic patterns are then established and the foundation for security established, as emphasized in Sullivan's theory.

Motor development is dramatic during this stage. The newborn steadily refines seemingly uncoordinated, gross motor efforts as he or she masters a series of skills, culminating in the toddler's ability to walk by the end of this stage. Physical progress coordinates with cognitive and psychosocial development; as babies gain some ability to control bodily processes and direct their own movement, interaction with the world grows to promote overall development.

Cognitive Development

Cognitive development during infancy has been the subject of extensive research. Piaget's (1952, 1958) work presents the infant's cognition primarily as rudimentary reflexive activity. Gradually, the infant creates a repertoire of behaviors to accommodate present schemata to novel situations. The sensorimotor stage, from birth to about 24 months, includes substages that further delineate the infant's cognitive development.

In the first month, the infant uses reflexive behaviors (schemata), like sucking, for survival. While beginning bodily control is evident, the infant has no concept of cause and effect at this point. From 1 to 4 months, the infant's behaviors continue to be random, but the infant learns to associate pleasure with certain actions, e.g., thumb sucking, and repeats them. This period is called the *primary circular reaction stage.* In the *secondary circular reaction stage,* from 4 to 8 months, the infant's interests shift from exclusive focus on the body to a focus on the environment. A major cognitive accomplishment at this time is the infant's realization that behavior can create an outcome in the world. Babies at this stage may be able to connect such events as an accidental kicking of a hanging toy and the resultant movement or noise.

In the next stage, *purposeful coordination of means and ends,* from 8 to 12 months, the infant uses multiple schemata to reach a goal. The infant sees and moves toward a desired toy and then reaches to pick it up. Objects are purposefully manipulated. Babies at this stage love to throw things from highchairs and playpens, delighting at the game of having someone else pick up the objects and repeating the process. Piaget observed that children do not search for hidden objects at this stage; from this he concluded that object permanence was absent. However, there is variation in this cognitive ability. For example, one 10-month-old girl was observed finding a little human figure toy after it had been hidden under a cup. Also, babies typically experience stranger anxiety during this stage, e.g., crying when new people appear. This behavior indicates the infant's ability to differentiate familiar parenting figures from others.

The *tertiary circular reaction stage,* from 12 to 18 months, marks the baby's ability to accommodate. Behav-

ior repetition now includes modification to produce a new outcome. For example, the infant may use a hammer to hit different objects to hear novel sounds.

The role of reinforcement in learning has also been emphasized by behaviorists and social learning theorists. Pleasant reinforcers become associated with specific actions far earlier than Piaget's stages would allow. Mothers frequently report that very young infants, those only a few weeks old, give them real social smiles and become quiet in response to their voices, indicating the infant's ability to associate pleasure with mother's presence.

Language also emerges during this period. First the infant communicates through nonverbal communication. Parents and siblings become adept at translating the infant's unique messages in which a groan, sound, motion, or laugh has distinct meaning. From around 10 to 12 months, the infant typically begins to use words to communicate. A few months later, infants usually begin to use very basic phrases, e.g., "All gone" to signal the end of a meal. Although there is great variation in the timing of infants' use of verbal communication, a steady increase in understanding and effort to use language should be seen between 12 and 18 months.

Psychosocial Development

Theorists emphasize different aspects of psychosocial development during infancy; however, the goal of gaining a sense of self clearly emerges as the key developmental task (Figure 6–1). Establishing trust, as Erikson stresses, is the basis of distinguishing the self from the environment.

Mahler (1975) identifies two stages in the separation-individuation process: the symbiotic stage and the separation-individuation stage. The symbiotic stage, from birth to 4 or 5 months, involves a normal undifferentiated state in which the infant does not see the self as separate from the world and the mothering figure. Toward the end of this period, **symbiosis** occurs, in which the mother and infant are psychologically fused. One mother described this process as "falling in love with my baby"; symbiosis is a reciprocal venture.

The separation-individuation phase extends from 4 or 5 months to 3 years; however, two important subphases occur during infancy. The differentiation subphase, from 4 or 5 months to 7 to 10 months, involves continuation of the mother-infant symbiotic bond, but movement into the environment also occurs as the infant begins to sit and crawl. The infant also begins to discriminate between mother and other objects and people.

The practicing subphase, from 7 to 10 months to 16 to 18 months, involves increasing awareness of the self as

Physical Development

Physical growth slows after infancy but continues at a steady rate. In early childhood, the chubby, bowlegged toddler changes into the taller, slimmer preschooler. Awkward locomotion with frequent falls is replaced by greater agility in walking, running, and climbing. Neuromuscular coordination increases and is demonstrated in gains in gross and fine motor skills.

Cognitive Development

Major strides in cognition are evident during early childhood. The period of mental representation from about 18 to 24 months is the final phase of Piaget's sensorimotor stage. Young children no longer need to rely on trial and error to see the outcome of their actions. They can internalize representations of events to anticipate what will happen in a sequence of events. In the preoperational preconceptual phase that follows from 2 to 4 years, the child learns to think in mental images and develops symbolic play and language. Children at this age may begin to act out the characters in a favorite story.

Language development is one of the most important abilities to emerge during early childhood. By the end of the second year, the child typically has an active vocabulary of 50 words. Nouns and verbs are the usual speech components, but adjectives are used occasionally. Such speech has been called telegraphic and is illustrated by messages such as "where Mommy," "take dolly," and "juice all gone." By 3 years, the child's vocabulary has expanded to about 1000 words, with 80 percent of verbal communication being understandable to others. Grammatical construction becomes more complex, although errors are common as the child mimics adults and tries to learn the rules. Often errors actually reflect the child's application of a rule at the wrong time, for example, the word *mine's* to indicate possessive case. Language is well established by the end of the early childhood period.

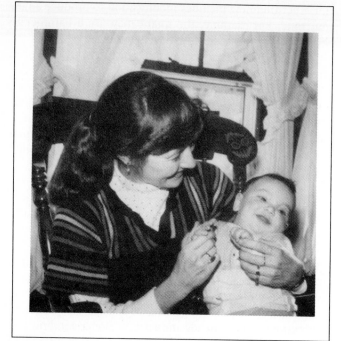

Figure 6–1
Interaction of mother and infant promotes accomplishment of the developmental tasks of trust for the baby and generativity for the mother.

distinct from others. The ability to move away from mother and explore the world is a major factor in this development. Infants in this stage typically toddle away from the mothering person in order to explore and then return for physical contact that provides emotional support through a renewed sense of connectedness. The links between physical, cognitive, and psychosocial growth in this process are readily apparent. In addition, the parents' ability to balance feelings of caring and concern with sound judgment concerning the infant's growing skills and need for realistic limits, and to suppress their own needs in favor of the infant's are critical factors in successful completion of the tasks of infancy (Horowitz, Hughes, and Perdue 1982). Table 6–6 highlights developmental challenges and infant and parental stressors of this stage.

Early Childhood

The transition from infancy to childhood occurs during the early childhood phase from 18 months to 5 years. During this stage, the child struggles to achieve a sense of autonomy, self-reliance, and self as clearly separate from others.

Psychosocial Development

In early childhood, issues of autonomy and learning to relate to others are developmental milestones (Figure 6–2). The final substages of Mahler's (1975) model outline the completion of the separation-individuation process.

In the rapprochement phase from between 16 to 18 months to 25 months, the young child is keenly aware of being separate from the mothering figure. This awareness leads to a renewed desire for closeness with mother, and fears related to separation and helplessness are common. The feeling is intense, as illustrated by the 20-month-old boy who screamed the instant his mother picked up his infant cousin. The boy had never seen his mother pick up another child and registered his upset at the threat of sep-

Table 6–6
Developmental Stressors in Parenting During Infancy and Early Childhood

Area of Concern	Stage in Growth		
	Up to 1 year	Up to 2 years	Up to 5 years
Eating	Establishing nursing routine. Establishing optimum pattern of weight gain. Dealing with "gassy" or colicky baby. Introducing solids. Dealing with food allergies. Weaning.	Establishing optimum pattern of weight gain. Weaning. Dealing with food fads, pickiness, refusal to eat certain foods, appetite lapses. Trying not to establish poor food habits such as using food as bribe or way to control child.	Maintaining well-balanced diet. Curtailing sweets. (Plus the stressors listed at left.)
Sleeping	Dealing with wakefulness during night. Dealing with a diminished need for sleep. Learning to enforce parent/child separation at night.	Dealing with wakefulness during night. Dealing with unwillingness to go to bed. Dealing with rocking, head banging, nightmares. Enforcing parent/child separation at night.	Dealing with wakefulness during night. Enforcing parent/child separation at night. Dealing with nightmares/night terrors, night wandering. Dealing with bedwetting if it disrupts sleep.
Security/Autonomy	Dealing with difficulty in establishing attachment bonds with baby because of fatigue, illness, not having wanted the baby, having to care for other children, temperamental misfit between parent and child, and so on. Managing temperamental responses of infant, such as high activity level, withdrawal from new situations, intense reaction to situations, lack of adaptability to new situations, irregular habits. Trying to provide child with multiple security outlets— feeding, sucking, holding, playing.	Dealing with temper tantrums and other negative reactions to separation from parent. Dealing with child who clings excessively. Trying to replace infantile security outlets such as the bottle with more mature ones. Encouraging self-esteem.	Promoting independence in play, self-care. Dealing with separation anxiety from parent. Dealing with habits such as thumbsucking, attachment to security objects, fear of animals. Dealing with child who seeks much parental attention.
Health/Sickness	Learning to recognize minor illness from that requiring medical attention. Treating illness in the infant. Dealing with the disruption to family and work caused by illness. Dealing with the child who has unusual number of illnesses.	Preventing accidents. Learning to maintain balance between underconcern and overconcern regarding normal illness. Developing health-promoting habits and environment that minimizes the risk of illness. Dealing with child's fears regarding going to doctor or nurse practitioner. (Plus the stressors listed at left.)	Helping child deal with threats to body integrity. Dealing with child's fears regarding going to dentist. (Plus the stressors listed at left.)

Continued

Table 6–6 *(Continued)*
Developmental Stressors in Parenting During Infancy and Early Childhood

Area of Concern	Stage in Growth		
	Up to 1 year	Up to 2 years	Up to 5 years
Discipline	Understanding the limits of an infant's ability to control behavior. Approaching infant control and safety with flexibility and range of techniques	Using a variety of techniques to control behavior rather than relying on one method such as physical punishment. Understanding when to ignore behavior and when to intervene actively. Deciding beforehand how certain situations (for example, temper tantrums) will be handled. Avoiding excessive negative interactions with child. Maintaining limits with consistency, firmness, and assertiveness. Dealing with sibling fighting.	Understanding that certain behaviors (such as boasting, "lying," use of "bad" words, exuberant and aggressive play, and tattling) are part of a child's development and should not be harshly punished. (Plus the stressors listed at left.)
Sexuality	Dealing with and understanding infant's touching of genitalia.	Dealing with child's curiosity regarding anatomic parts. Dealing with and understanding child's interest in touching genitalia.	Dealing with curiosity regarding anatomy and function of genitalia and breasts. Dealing with child-child exploration and play involving genitalia. Providing child with sexual information appropriate to interest and capabilities. Dealing with tensions and relationships within family that result from sexuality and gender, such as father-daughter attraction. (Plus the stressors listed at left.)
Play/Socialization	Providing adequate parent-infant play time.	Resolving sibling hostility and competition with active, intrusive toddler. Dealing with aggressiveness (biting, hitting), shyness, sharing problems, excessive crying with peers or siblings. Providing opportunities for peer play. Providing appropriate play environment.	Dealing with name calling, being left out, excluding others, tattling, shyness, bullying others. Dealing with child who shows lack of interest in peer play. Allowing child independence in working out peer problems, yet understanding when to intervene.

Source: From Parenting Reassessed: A Nursing Perspective, *pp 116–117 by JA Horowitz, CB Hughes, BJ Perdue. Copyright © 1982 by permission of Appleton & Lange Publishing Co.*

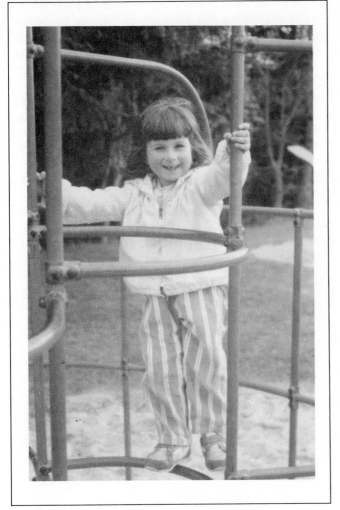

Figure 6–2
Enjoyment of activity and exploration assist the young child to develop autonomy.

aration. In addition, mental representations of "good-mother" and "bad-mother" develop now without the child's being able to integrate the dual images into a cohesive whole.

In the object constancy period from 25 to 36 months, the child's trust and confidence are stronger, allowing the child to develop a firm sense of self with established boundaries. Object images, such as good-mother and bad-mother, are integrated to form a stable mental image. The successful negotiation of the separation-individuation process is influenced by the parent's ability to be nurturing, consistent, responsive, and emotionally available.

The young child's sense of self and autonomy are evident through many activities, most particularly toilet training. Once sphincter control is present, toileting becomes dependent on the child's ability to feel and predict sensations and to master this new complex skill without a struggle of wills between parent and child. Most parenting experts recommend that parents first observe for signs of physical readiness and then encourage readiness by modeling and

providing opportunity to practice toileting behaviors. However, many parents can attest to how easy it was to become frustrated when their child never seemed to be ready to learn. The young child is struggling to master a new independent skill and give up a part of babyhood. This struggle provides a ripe opportunity for the child to exert control by not doing what anxious parents would like. Although it is difficult to do so, it is usually best for parents to encourage but wait until the child takes the initiative in using the toilet.

During this period, the child also learns basic interactive skills. The child's world expands from home and parent and siblings to include peers. Struggles over toys with other children are common as the child begins to learn to share and participate with others in activities. Interaction with other children helps the child learn basic rules for socializing and tools for self-control. These skills assist the child to establish a clear sense of autonomy without shame and doubt and provide the basis for achieving later developmental tasks. Developmental stressors for child and parent in the early childhood stage are discussed in Table 6–6.

Middle Childhood

During the middle childhood period, from 5 to 8 years, children learn to consolidate their sense of self in a social world that extends beyond the family and to use their growing abilities.

Physical Development

Children's physical growth slows during middle childhood, and fine and gross motor abilities are further developed. Children become more athletic as their skill in manipulating objects and their own bodies increases steadily. They learn writing skills and draw representative figures. Team and group activities are often begun during this time and can help the child to learn new activities. The risk is that young children who are less skilled than others may feel pressured to compete.

Cognitive Development

Children make the transition to Piaget's preoperational intuitive stage of cognition during this period. They begin to group similar objects and separate different objects according to basic classification systems. Symbolic reasoning increases. At the same time, children also show **egocentric thought**, i.e., everything is considered from their point of view. Any parent who has tried to reason with a 5-year-old in order to coax the child away from a favorite activity to avoid being late for some other event can testify to the young child's inability to take the parent's perspective. Rules tend to be a more effective means of helping children at this stage to organize and regulate behavior. Egocentric thought extends to **animism**—attributing human attributes to objects, e.g., thinking that a flower hurts when its stem is cut.

Imitative behavior typifies this era. Identification with adult figures and reinforcement probably work together to promote imitation. Children model parents, older children, and other figures, such as teachers and sports figures. For example, girls typically enjoy dressing up like Mommy and playing house with dolls and friends. Boys often like to mimic a favorite athlete by practicing a particular sport. Although many of these behaviors tend to be gender-related at this time, children of both sexes enjoy modeling physical activities and feel free to imitate a wider range of behavior when such variety is encouraged. For instance, girls may imitate adult women working outside the home and boys may try nurturing behaviors with pets or in imaginative play.

The period of concrete operations, according to Piaget's model, begins between 6 and 8 years. Children now can represent mentally what has been seen and view the self, others, and actions more objectively. Reason is used systematically to apply rules to new events. The ability to classify according to more abstract and complex characteristics and relationships emerges. Conservation is an important principle that is mastered at this time. Children come to understand that the volume of a substance does not vary simply because it takes a new shape. This ability is essential to learning mathematical skills. By age 8, egocentric and animistic thought should disappear, and interest in causation increases.

Language development also progresses during this era. The 5-year-old typically has a vocabulary of 2500 words and is understandable to adults. Vocabulary continues to grow and assists children to decrease egocentric thought and to increase the ability to classify as this stage proceeds. Reading skills are learned during these years. Reading is an essential foundation for more complex learning in the school years to come and greatly enhances language development.

Psychosocial Development

Socialization and learning are hallmarks of this era. According to Erikson, initiative and industry are the devel-

opmental tasks of this stage. Sullivan stresses the importance of establishing peer relationships. Early in the period, children typically engage in parallel play: a group of children play alongside each other rather than cooperatively. It is important to note, however, that children often can mix modes of play, interspersing interactive symbolic play, like a tea party, with parallel play. Later in this stage, children are far more interactive in their play, organizing team and group activities and using rules to govern action. Through play, children learn to give and receive feedback, empathize, share, cooperate, and enjoy peer contact. Interaction with peers also helps children broaden their views of the world beyond the family boundary.

School becomes a major focus of children's lives. In the school setting, physical, cognitive, and psychosocial development all contribute to children's ability to learn. In this arena, children clearly have the opportunity to meet the developmental tasks of initiative and industry. Table 6–7 illustrates developmental stressors for children and parents during the middle childhood period.

Late Childhood

During late childhood, from 8 to 12 years, children build on the accomplishments of the previous stage with even greater emphasis on friendships and skill mastery as sources of self-esteem.

Physical Development

Individual and gender differences in growth patterns are more evident during this period. Boys tend to be somewhat taller and heavier at the start of this stage, but girls typically have a growth spurt around age 10. Boys later catch up around age 13 or 14, during their own growth spurt. Gains in gross and fine motor skills continue, but children from 8 to 12 years tend to be more controlled and purposeful in their activity. The child usually becomes more graceful and stronger, and ability to engage in sports increases. Competition typifies this era; children match and measure skills in the playground and through organized team endeavors, such as soccer and Little League, fulfilling the latency age developmental task identified by Freud. As sex-role stereotypes have decreased, girls have become more active participants in team sports.

Cognitive Development

Sometime from age 8 to 12, the child makes a transition from Piaget's period of concrete operations to the stage of formal operations. Children show interest in rules of behavior and causation. Abstract thinking and the ability to classify and to see various connections mark a major cognitive shift toward what is considered more adult styles of reasoning.

Table 6–7		
Developmental Stressors in Parenting During Middle and Late Childhood		
Area of Concern	**Stage in Growth**	
	5–8 Years	8–12 Years
Eating	Maintaining optimum pattern of weight gain. Learning to deal with normative "bad" table manners—eating with fingers, dawdling, awkwardness at table, criticism of family members. Maintaining well-balanced diet. Curtailing sweets. Adjusting to appetite extremes.	See stressors at left.
Sleeping	Allowing for individual needs of sleep/rest. Maintaining bedtime hour. Dealing with nightmares, fear of the dark, strange noises. Learning to help child who is still bedwetting.	See stressors at left.
Security/Autonomy	Working with child to promote tolerance for longer, more continuous separations such as those that occur in school day, sleep-overs. Dealing with child's separation anxiety as manifested in somatizations, school phobia. Promoting child's interest in "work." Dealing with threats to child's self-esteem and methods for releasing tension, such as thumbsucking, temper tantrums, stuttering, biting nails, blinking. Dealing with the numerous normal fears of this age—fear of loud noises, the supernatural, being lost or hurt.	Tolerating comparisons with outsiders. Encouraging and allowing child to "succeed" at individual endeavors at school, home, and play. Dealing with child who has poor self-image and feels inadequate and inferior. Dealing with numerous fears associated with this age. Dealing with child who has not accomplished the developmental tasks of self-care, self-protection, ability to use time, and ability to select friends and activities.
Discipline	Adjusting disciplinary methods to suit increasing age of child—for example, forfeiture of privileges, logical consequences. Maintaining fair limits with consistency and firmness. Dealing with typical behaviors of this age including stealing, lying, sibling jealousy, labile feelings toward mother.	Learning to deal with rebelliousness and challenges to parental demands. Learning not to overreact to lability of child's emotional system. Dealing with child who has not yet learned internal controls in behavior, or feelings of guilt about behavior, or ideas of good and bad.
Sexuality	Providing age-appropriate sex education. Understanding and learning to deal with mutual investigation by both sexes, mild sex play, exhibitionism, and peeping. Providing for privacy of child as desired. Understanding role of masturbation in child's sexual development.	Understanding sex swearing, sex poems, and smutty jokes as developmentally normative. Understanding and dealing with same-sex relationships as foundation of later heterosexual ones. Making available to child further information regarding sexuality. Dealing with feelings of shame, fear, and guilt with regard to pubertal changes. Avoiding creating a climate where sex is viewed as dirty or taboo.
Play/Socialization	Providing active, rigorous play. Acknowledging importance of peer play and acceptance by peers to normal growth and development.	Avoiding the formation of excessively high expectations for child regarding athletics, school work, and so on.

Continued

Table 6–7 *(Continued)*
Developmental Stressors in Parenting During Middle and Late Childhood

Area of Concern	Stage in Growth	
	5–8 Years	8–12 Years
Play/Socialization	Providing active, rigorous play. Acknowledging importance of peer play and acceptance by peers to normal growth and development. Avoiding defining play to child as primarily competitive. Dealing with child who has not learned to compete, compromise, cooperate, and collaborate with peers. Encouraging age-appropriate play. Providing appropriate amount of supervision.	Avoiding the formation of excessively high expectations for child regarding athletics, school work, and so on. Dealing with child who has not gained peer success, acceptance, or friendship. (Plus the stressors listed at left.)
Health/Sickness	Learning to deal with child's increased susceptibility to infection. Learning to differentiate somatic complaint from real illness. Promoting safety and preventing accidents, particularly fractures, drowning, automobile-related accidents, and injuries to eyes. Promoting personal hygiene. Enforcing good dental hygiene and supervision.	Promoting and enforcing personal hygiene standards. Helping child deal with physical changes associated with puberty. Promoting balance of activity and rest.

Source: From Parenting Reassessed: A Nursing Perspective, *pp 116–117 by JA Horowitz, CB Hughes, BJ Perdue. Copyright © 1982 by permission of Appleton & Lange Publishing Co.*

Many children demonstrate this cognitive gain by a keen interest in school, particularly in subjects that require application of logic, such as arithmetic, and application of principles and discussion of differences, such as social studies.

Moral judgment is another area of major change. Children begin to question parental guidelines for behavior, no longer content to follow automatically the moral or religious rules given to them earlier. Children can now discriminate between societal norms for right and wrong behavior but cannot be expected to have complete control over their own behavior. They are likely to make moral judgments according to categories, such as "good-boy" or "nice-girl" concepts, or later according to rules that enforce law and order (Kohlberg 1969). Opportunities to question and to make choices in a supportive environment help children to progress to higher levels of moral reasoning.

Psychosocial Development

Industry is the key developmental task of this era, according to Erikson. Sullivan stresses the importance of establishing a chum relationship. Thus, the abilities to perform and relate become the primary basis for self-concept. Positive feedback in school, at home, and from friends reinforces a strong self-image. When these opportunities for positive appraisal are missing, children are prone to low self-esteem.

Social relationships during this phase are marked by competition, compromise, and cooperation (Sullivan 1953). The goal is for children to learn a balance in these elements to feel competent in relating and achieving. Establishing and using rules help children in this process. Peer relationships provide opportunity for children to extend their views of the world beyond their family boundaries. They use friendships as safe arenas for comparison and exploration. Children can use friendships to obtain satisfactions and to learn to see the other's point of view. Trust in a peer reinforces a positive self-image and provides a feeling of acceptance. Such chum relationships provide a basis for later intimate relationships during adolescence and adulthood.

Kimberly, age 9, had little self-confidence in social situations. Her parents stressed scholastic performance but thought that sports and play were unimportant. Thus, as an only child with no close friends, she felt left out and inadequate. When a new girl, Katherine, moved into her neighborhood, Kimberly had a chance to make a friend. Katherine liked the way Kimberly used her imagination to make up stories. Kimberly began to feel safe enough to share confidences and try new activities, increasing her confidence among school peers. The acceptance shown by Katherine helped Kimberly to see herself in a new light, to broaden her scope beyond her nuclear family, and to develop a trusting chum relationship.

Sexuality was thought to lie dormant or latent, according to psychoanalytic theorists such as Freud, who called this period latency. However, more recent work with children indicates that they are interested in their developing bodies and in sexuality, particularly in relation to procreation and sexual activity. Bodily changes typically happen for girls first; many begin menses sometime between the middle to end of this stage, and secondary sex characteristics often develop. Thus, girls need specific information concerning their developing sexuality, and children of both sexes need support as they struggle with changing emotions, changing bodies, and beginning levels of knowledge concerning sexuality and appropriate limits. Table 6–7 illustrates developmental stressors and child and parental goals for the late childhood period.

Adolescence

Adolescence begins with puberty around 12 or 13 and extends to around age 20. Adolescence is not just a time of physical and sexual growth. It is a stormy period in life, an interruption between the docility of the latency years and the acclimation of adulthood. Adolescence is a time when the individual is confronted with conflicting ideas and feelings, when inconsistency and disharmony are the norm. In comparison to adult behavior, the adolescent's incongruous activity does seem to warrant professional attention. In fact, a steady state during this period of reawakening and redefining could be considered deviant.

With the onset of puberty, spectacular physical and sexual changes occur. A boy may grow 4 or 5 inches in a single year. Over the course of a summer vacation, a girl may reach menarche and begin to develop breasts. Although the pubertal changes have actually been going on for some time, they seem sudden to the adolescent. The timing and the extent of these changes are unpredictable. The degree to which the adolescent can adapt to them and to the upsurge in sexual capacity is equally unpredictable. Table 6–8 summarizes the many physical changes that occur during this time.

As adolescents attempt to adjust to physical changes,

their behavior and attitudes change. Up to now the child has been preoccupied with developing a congenial role. Often these preoccupations assume an unconventional nature. Nurses who can recollect their own experiences and reactions during this tumultuous time will better appreciate the adolescent's dilemma.

Cognitive Development

People make great strides on all intellectual fronts during the adolescent years. They gain in intellectual capacity and power. They exhibit increasing progress in forming concepts, understanding time, generalizing, and abstracting. Like a child, the adolescent lives in the present, but unlike the child, also lives in the future in the realm of the hypothetical. Piaget notes that the adolescent's conceptual world is full of informal theories about self and about life. These theories include idealistic plans for the individual's and society's future. This egocentrism in adolescence motivates the individual toward a naïve idealism, dedicated to the reshaping and perfecting of reality. It is not unusual to hear an adolescent making grandiose plans to reorganize the structure of the federal government or to eradicate poverty.

During adolescence, the formal operations stage of cognitive development is more fully realized (Piaget 1952). This is the highest stage of intellectual development that provides the basis for adult cognition. In this stage, the adolescent learns to use propositional thinking or to hypothesize, an ability that frees the person from the restriction of experience only, as in the previous concrete operations stage. The person is now able to consider several alternative solutions to problems, multiple combinations of cause and effect, and variations of spatial position and concepts seen from others' perspectives. Thinking in this stage is more abstract and complex, reflecting a cognitive developmental level that is not reached by all adolescents or even all adults.

Psychosocial Development

This period of conflict and disharmony is an emotionally labile time, when numerous doubts, uncertainties, and fears surface. The 14-year-old who was happily listening to her favorite song on the radio five minutes ago may now be uncontrollably sobbing about a fantasized love loss because she hasn't yet received an expected telephone call. However, her feelings of loss are as real as if her boyfriend had actually rejected her.

Table 6–8
Physical Changes During Puberty

Characteristic	In Males	In Females
Maturation of genitals and accessory reproductive organs	Acceleration of growth of penis and testes Development of breasts, which is usually transitory and subsides Occurrence of seminal emissions	Development of skin and tissue surrounding vulval region Rapid increase in growth of uterus and ovaries Development of breasts Ovulation and beginning of menses
Development of the secondary sex characteristics	Development of pubic hair Appearance of axillary hair and facial hair approximately two years after development of pubic hair Rapid increase in growth of larynx, resulting in "breaking" of voice	Development of pubic hair approximately two years prior to menarche Appearance of axillary hair approximately two years after onset of pubic hair Increase in growth of larynx, less pronounced in females
	Axillary sweat glands becoming functional in both sexes Appearance of acne common, especially in males	
	Increased pigmentation of skin, particularly darkening of areola in males Loss of scalp hair toward end of puberty	Increased pigmentation of skin, particularly darkening of areola (although to lesser extent than in males, except during and after pregnancy)
Development of the skeleton	Dramatic acceleration of growth in both height and weight, beginning at approximately 12½ to 13 years; pubertal spurt greater than in females	Acceleration of growth in both height and weight, beginning approximately at 10½ to 11 years, pubertal spurt less than in males
	Generally, growth of skeleton begins with feet and hands, followed by calf and forearm, followed by hips and chest, and finally by shoulders	
	Shoulders grow more than pelvis	Pelvis becomes wider, shallower, and roomier than in male
Development of teeth	Acquisition of full dentition by the end of puberty	

The individual's relationship to others of the same age becomes increasingly important during adolescence. Becoming competent in social skills, developing bonds of mutual trust, attaining peer acceptance, and establishing a unique form of communication all become tantamount to achieving success and happiness. Attempts to do this take many forms. These include formulating esoteric words or terms understood only by companions, forming exclusive groups or cliques, sharing a multitude of secrets, and generally establishing ways to identify the adolescent's own group as unique. It is particularly important to be recognized as separate from the world of the adult. In developing this sense of belonging, adolescents ward off the fear of loneliness and rejection. They are secure in the belief that their newfound feelings and images are acceptable to the group and therefore acceptable to themselves. Establishing

close ties and identifying with the group make it easier for adolescents to cope with their physical changes, sexual urges, social adjustment, and competitive feelings (Figure 6–3).

During late adolescence, individuals usually begin to establish an intimate relationship with someone of the opposite sex in an eager attempt to fuse the facets of their own developing identity with that of another. These social attempts with the group and with another individual create alternating excitement and fear, skillfulness and awkwardness, elation and despair.

The ideas of the three masters of developmental theory offer insights into the adolescent's quest for maturity. Although Freud offers little explanation for adolescent growth other than the reemergence of the Oedipal conflict, the significance of the parental figures in this context cannot

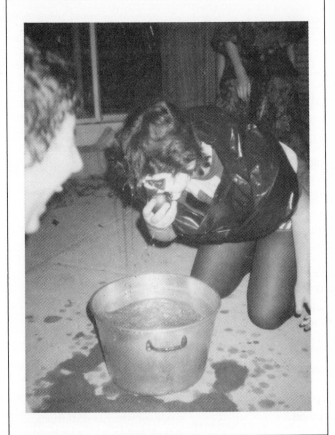

Figure 6–3
Bobbing for apples at a Halloween party provides teenagers with the opportunity to hone their group socializing skills.

ships if individuals cannot resolve the psychologic strain caused by the interplay among their conflicting feelings. Intimacy and sexual closeness are less closely related in Sullivan's theory. Sullivan even asserts that in the beginning stages of development, sexual activity is not considered. He defines intimacy as a situation that involves closeness and a validation of the other's worth. At the point when the genital drive appears, the change from a similar to a different object occurs.

As for love, Freud defines it as a sublimated sexuality. Sullivan believes that love evolves only if one feels as strongly about the love object's welfare as one does about one's own. The object of Sullivan's love is a person. The object of Freud's sexuality is the release of a physical tension. Erikson does not even seriously consider love in the adolescent years. He believes that adolescent love is merely a projection of one's diffused self-image onto another in an attempt to define one's identity.

Regardless of the theory one chooses to use in practice, the value and relatedness of the others cannot be overlooked. The similarities as well as the contrasts among them offer nurses insights into the many complex facets of adolescent psychosocial development. Table 6–9 outlines areas of development and adolescent and parental stressors.

Young Adulthood

The period following adolescence, called postadolescence or young adulthood, extends from approximately age 20 to 29 years. It is a period during which young men and women consolidate the sense of identity forged during late adolescence and face the challenge of realizing independence from parents and other guardians. The worlds of work, college, or family can present risks and opportunities. Although some are not ready to create independent lives early in this stage and need a longer period to examine their options, most begin to establish adult roles by training for and starting in an occupation, moving away from the family of origin, and developing the capacity to have an intimate relationship. For many, this last task includes marriage.

Physical and Cognitive Development

Healthy young adults have completed the major gains expected in physical and cognitive development; however, males may continue to have some physical growth early in this stage. Normally, this is the healthiest period of life, characterized by peaks in muscular strength and repro-

be ignored. Sullivan agrees with Freud that the parental figures are important but disagrees about the sexual nature of their role.

Erikson and Sullivan hold similar views concerning the stages of development. Erikson focuses on conflicts that must be resolved throughout life. Both Erikson and Sullivan view the completion of each stage as necessary to optimal development. Therefore they agree that abnormalities arise whenever a stage is not completed. For example, Sullivan believes that failure to move from a similar to a different object of intimacy may lead to overt or covert homosexual tendencies. Abnormalities also arise whenever a crisis is not resolved.

Erikson and Sullivan disagree about the ultimate goal of development. Erikson believes this goal to be the formation of identity. He is therefore primarily concerned with the origin of identity in the adolescent period. For Sullivan, the ultimate goal is satisfactory genital activity.

Intimacy also plays an important role in the developmental theories of both Erikson and Sullivan. Attempts to attain intimacy, sexual or otherwise, are significant in Erikson's identity formation. The results of these attempts can lead to isolation or superficiality in personal relation-

Table 6–9
Developmental Stressors in Parenting During Adolescence

Area of Development	Stage in Growth		
	Early Adolescence (12–14 years)	Middle Adolescence (15–16 years)	Late Adolescence (17–adulthood)
Sexuality	Facilitating formation of close friendships with members of the same sex. Dealing with differences and extremes in grooming, i.e., females may be neat dressers while males may dress sloppily.	Allowing both sexes to move toward heterosexual relationships. Dealing with sexually active child. Allowing need to engage in great deal of fantasy.	Dealing with young adult who does not seek intimate relations with significant other, or who does not perceive sexuality as part of entire body, image, and goals.
Cognitive thinking	Dealing with child's descriptive view of world and comments on current events and circumstances.	Dealing with child who has ability to maintain an argument.	Promoting synthesis of data from a variety of sources and use of both inductive and deductive reasoning.
Body image	Dealing with child who has less stability of self, lowered self-esteem, heightened self-consciousness.	Dealing with females' concern with physical attractiveness; and males' preoccupation with physical fitness.	Dealing with young adult who has not integrated adult physical maturity with self-image, or who has distortions in body image, e.g., obesity or thinness.
Personal value system	Dealing with child who adopts values from peers and is heavily influenced by current fads.	Dealing with rejection of parental value system as superficial and hypocritical.	Dealing with personal values that fluctuate, concern about finding the right mate, males' and females' concern about career.
Preparation for productive citizenship	Dealing with child who may view school as irrelevant.	Dealing with child who may fantasize about a mate, job, and material possessions. Dealing with a child who is concerned about choosing a life-style and vocation, and desires work skills and employment. Dealing with child who associates parent with all society's ills.	Encouraging young adult's natural interest in getting ahead; selecting the right job, the right mate, and the right school. Helping young adult come to terms with many of the ills blamed on society.
Achievement of independence from parents	Dealing with strong same-sex peer identification as a means to separate from parent. Dealing with child who is socially isolated from peers. Dealing with changes in family life-style resulting from increasing independence of child.	Understanding that heterosexual relationships may substitute for relationship with parents. Encouraging part-time jobs and financial responsibility associated with job.	Allowing the young adult to move away from home, to develop intimate and other relationships with the opposite sex.

Source: From Parenting Reassessed: A Nursing Perspective, pp 116–17 by JA Horowitz, CB Hughes, BJ Perdue. Copyright © 1982 by permission of Appleton & Lange Publishing Co.

ductive ability (Edelman and Mandle 1986). According to Piaget's stages, cognitive development should be completed. The young adult typically refines use of cognitive ability to meet educational and employment goals and to solve problems of living.

Psychosocial Development

This is a period in which the young adult struggles to synthesize the identity that emerged during adolescence and to choose a life-style. In his discussion of identity formation, Erikson speaks of prolonged adolescence and characterizes this stage as a second period of delay after adolescence. Many young adults see this time as an opportunity to try out different roles, jobs, or adventures before settling down to the serious business of adulthood. An ideal version of life may be shaped and colored by the illusion that anything is possible in coexistence with contrasting fears that choices made now might be irrevocable.

This period, sometimes called the *psychosocial moratorium,* is crucial for some people. Even though they may have consolidated their social roles, selected their life tasks, and disengaged from their parents during adolescence, young adults may not be completely integrated. The psychologic purpose of the moratorium is to harmonize the component parts of the personality. People must assimilate adolescence completely to achieve an adult functioning identity. Sheehy (1976) and others believe that such a process is necessary to fix the identity completely.

Not all young adults are able to use this stage to explore roles and to forge their identities. Financial pressures, responsibilities for others such as a baby, and problems in living can disrupt the process of identity consolidation. (Further discussion of parental roles is found in the section on adulthood and the case study in the final section; the content is also applicable to parenting during young adulthood.)

According to Erikson, people achieve intimacy with others only after developing the capacities associated with identity development. This intimacy involves true mutuality. In true mutuality we can merge ourselves in friendships or sexual relationships without fear of losing our sense of self. The ability to love results in a new and shared identity.

The counterpart of intimacy is isolation. Isolation manifests itself in withdrawal from relationships or in an active repudiation of people and ideas that seem foreign to the self. Isolated people may avoid close relationships or involve themselves in a series of highly stereotyped relationships that lack any sense of fusion.

Sheehy (1976) describes the "urge to merge" that occurs during the end of the psychosocial moratorium. Women have a more difficult time with identity formation than men do. There is a general cultural expectation that they will marry and share in the prestige of the identity earned by their husbands. Some women may wish to marry to be

as safe and secure as they were in their parents' home. These women may give birth to a child to prove their worth. Sheehy believes that many women are immature because early marriage has foreclosed their identities. However, the recent increased tolerance for a diversity of life-styles supports a variety of forms of commitment and intimacy. Living together, marriage without children, less stereotyped roles, and pursuit of a career all are situations in which women have a greater variety of ways to demonstrate their worth.

Gilligan (1982) raises another fascinating point concerning possible differences in developmental milestones for young women and men that challenges traditional theory. She proposes that male gender identity is tied to separation and individuation and female identity is linked to attachment. Thus, according to Gilligan, masculinity is threatened by intimacy, and femininity is threatened by separation. This hypothesized difference becomes troublesome when theorists and clinicians blindly apply the developmental tasks of adolescence and young adulthood that call for increasing levels of differentiation (as measured by independence or separateness) as indicators of health. Women who fail to achieve total separation but achieve intimacy risk being seen as failures. Although Gilligan's ideas are not universally accepted, they clearly help alert us that sexist attitudes may be distorting views of female development.

Men may also marry for reasons of conformity, or they may marry so that they will have someone to depend on emotionally. They hope their wives will help them define and carry out their career ambitions. Whether the decision is made on the basis of genuine wishes for intimacy or is simply a matter of conforming to societal expectations largely depends on the degree of identity formation. Male roles have also changed in recent years to include greater participation in parenting and more freedom to express a range of emotions and to engage in roles formerly associated with females.

Adulthood and the Mid-Life Crisis

From about age 30 to 42 years, adults typically consolidate relationships and occupational status and goals. It is a time of decision making during which individuals struggle with conflicting urges to settle down as well as to make needed changes now while still young enough. People in this period are recognized as full members of the adult community and are expected to accept the responsibility inherent in the many adult roles of a society, such as parent, spouse, worker, and community leader.

Physical and Cognitive Development

Although there is great variation in physical changes during this period, some signs of aging typically appear. Changes in muscle strength, skin, and hair are most common, although life-style, physical conditioning, diet, and genetic heritage all can slow or speed their course. Some professional athletes are able to polish skills and adapt to physical changes and thus preserve ability well into their thirties; other adults develop early signs of aging—loss of stamina, expanded waistlines, wrinkles, or hair loss or graying. Many adults find this period to be one of greater emotional maturity and stability so that they are able to take care of their bodies and enjoy good physical health and vitality.

Cognitive development during this period of adulthood is not characterized by new abilities but rather by enhanced ability to apply abstract and logical thinking to a wide range of problems. Typically, this time is a very productive one in the arenas of work and family.

Psychosocial Development

In adulthood the ideal person is a responsible independent agent who can make decisions and maintain relationships. Clearly those who have failed to complete the developmental tasks of previous stages do not attain this ideal. This time can also be marked by turmoil as people try to change patterns established during their twenties. Sheehy's investigations of adults from 29 to 32 revealed that they wanted to make major changes such as starting a new career, finding a mate, or leaving one. In the early thirties, adults typically feel more settled as many life-style decisions have been made.

Parenting as a Major Task

Parenting represents a major task of adulthood for many. The birth of a first child is often a happy event of this period but also may constitute a crisis due to the massive shifts in roles and responsibilities. Men frequently feel an added sense of responsibility. Today, large numbers of women work outside the home following the birth of children. The strains of employment and motherhood are compounded when traditional sex-role expectations dictate that the mother maintain responsibility for the bulk of household and childrearing tasks. Single parents who have no partner to help them are at even greater risk to be stressed by the competing demands of the work world and children. Until there is far greater support for quality day care, equality in wages earned by men and women, and greater flexibility in employment situations, parents will continue to feel the stress of balancing multiple roles.

The relationship of multiple roles to mental health has been the subject of a growing number of research studies in nursing and social science research. A good example is Woods's (1985) study to investigate if the complement of women's multiple roles is associated with negative effects on mental health in a particular social context. She found that the complement of employment and family roles was not associated with mental ill health, nor was there a clear The context for role performance, however, did have an influence on mental health. See the Research Note in this chapter.

Adjusting to the maternal role is a process that interests nurses whose role it is to assess, teach, and support mothers during the period following the birth of a child. Mercer's (1985) research concerning the pattern of maternal role attainment indicates that learning and coping evolve and feelings of associated competence shift as new challenges arise in concert with changes in the baby's development. This study suggests that a nursing assessment should focus on the developmental tasks, abilities, and needs of both mother and baby, and on the interaction between them. Helping mothers anticipate the developmental stages, identify potential difficulties, and plan ways to manage the problems and find support are important nursing interventions.

Although the birth of children is discussed as a frequent event in adulthood, it is important to stress that variations in this pattern are many. Parenthood can occur anytime from adolescence to mid-life for women and even later for many men. Additionally, some adults do not choose to become parents and instead devote great energy to other goals, such as career achievement. Others find they cannot become biologic parents and do not opt to become parents via adoption. Additionally, not all families with children are headed by two parents. As the rates of divorce and teenage pregnancy mount, the numbers of single parents continue to grow. Recent statistics show that increasingly women are heads of household (in 9.4 million families according to the latest census); young adult women between the ages of 25 and 34 are particularly likely to find themselves solely responsible for their families (the number of female heads of household in this age group grew 170 percent from 1970 to 1982).

A parent may be single for many reasons—among them teenage pregnancy outside of marriage, death of a spouse, and planned pregnancy by unmarried self-supporting career women—but single parent status is increasingly the result of divorce (Griffith-Kenney 1986). All these life-styles are common and viable alternatives during the adult phase of development. In their effort to understand the developmental tasks of adulthood, nurses must guard against setting expectations concerning the married parent as the sole healthy role choice for adults. Nurses should appreciate the special challenges and rewards that can come to adults choosing a variety of roles.

At the age of 40 we are impressed by the fact that we are at the midpoint of life. As we enter what may be the stage of greatest occupational and interpersonal fulfillment, we become vividly aware that death lies ahead. At 40 we are no longer promising young people with potential. The degree of affirmation we have received professionally thus far is a good indicator of the amount of success that we will achieve, and current interpersonal commitments may represent the degree of intimacy we will attain.

During the years between 39 and 42, people pass through a period of acute discomfort as they face the discrepancy between their youthful ambitions and their actual achievement. The period has been called the **mid-life crisis.** Until recently, developmental psychologists have generally ignored middle age. Now interest in this period is increasing. The mid-life crisis is important because it marks the passage between early maturity and middle age. The onset and duration of this crisis vary with the individual. Most women pass through it between 35 and 40, and most men between 40 and 45.

The mid-life crisis is characterized by feelings of boredom, dissatisfaction with the way life has developed, and ambivalence and uncertainty about the future. During this time we reevaluate what we have done to date and assess our goals. We may view with dismay the signs of aging—graying hair, wrinkled skin, and changes in eyesight. Women may anticipate the onset of menopause.

At 40 we must reconsider life in the light of the reality of aging and death. The optimism of earlier years that enabled us to shrug off disappointments gives way to depression. We recognize that our productive time is limited and fear that we cannot accomplish all we had hoped to accomplish before time runs out. Teenage children may suddenly seem intellectually and sexually mature and may challenge our sense of omnipotence. Parents—whom we looked to once for security and comfort—may now need taking care of. When a parent contracts a terminal illness or dies, we become next in line in the generational progression. Now we directly confront the threat of aging and death.

As we face early signs of physical deterioration and question social roles we used to take for granted, our personality changes.

This is a time when some make decisions to alter their lives, feeling that time is running out. For example, Elaine, the woman in the case study at the end of this chapter, had devoted her full attention to pursuing a career. She saw her late thirties as the last chance to decide whether or not to try to have a baby. For her, the biologic clock forced her to tackle the issue of whether or not she wanted to be a mother and how she could blend parenting with a demanding career. Clients facing such decisions at midlife can be helped by a nurse who guides them to list their possible choices and to consider the pros and cons of each. Planning ways to handle expected outcomes of differing

---

RESEARCH NOTE

Citation

Woods NF: Employment, family roles, and mental ill health in young married women. Nurs Res 1985;34:4–9.

Study Problem/Purpose

The purpose of this study was to determine if the complement of women's roles was associated with negative mental health effects.

Methods

A sample of 140 married women was selected randomly from registrants at a family health clinic. The subjects were interviewed about their roles and mental health. Specific measures of the independent variables (the complement of women's roles and support) were the Index of Sex Role Orientation to measure sex role norm traditionalism and two sets of questions concerning emotional support, task-oriented support, and sharing of household responsibilities. The dependent variable (mental ill health) was measured by the Cornell Medical Index.

Findings

The complement of women's roles was not associated with mental ill health, nor was there a significant relationship between parenting or employment and mental health. In this sample, the context for role performance had a stronger relationship to mental health than did the actual roles performed. The following variables had a protective effect on mental health: Confiding support (having someone to confide in) was most important for women who were both spouse and parent; task-sharing support was most important for women who were employed but not parents; and nontraditional sex role norms were the most important for women who were spouse, employee, and mother.

Implications

The results of this study suggest that nurses assess both the actual roles held and the context of those roles. Role conflict and resultant ill effects on mental health may arise from the situation in which the woman performs her roles, the particular combination of roles, or the types of support that are lacking. Interventions to improve the mental health of young married women might be fruitful if these factors are addressed in order to produce changes that mirror the findings. The limitations of this study, particularly the sampling and one-time-only measurement, suggest the need for future research featuring a longitudinal investigation of role transitions and selection of a more heterogeneous sample.

decisions helps clients to make realistic choices. Some people make changes that drastically alter their lives and the lives of significant others.

Melissa, 39, called the mental health center requesting a therapist to see her family after discovering that her husband, Jim, had quit his job and planned to move to another state with a younger woman he met at work. At the age of 40, Jim faced the mid-life crisis by abruptly changing everything about his life. Marital counseling did not alter his decision. Melissa used the nurse therapist to assist her with parenting her two adolescent children following her husband's departure. In addition, she used therapy as an arena for gaining needed support and problem solving. Two years after Jim left, she met the former therapist and told her of the many positive ways her life had improved despite the pain resulting from Jim's leaving. This woman used a personal and family crisis to improve the quality of her life.

Middle Age

Middle age is generally placed from between 40–45 to 65–70 years of age. When the mid-life crisis is negotiated successfully as a transition to middle age, the adult can focus attention on the tasks of economic productivity and planning for the future, maintenance of personal health or treatment of physical problems, and family responsibility and transition of roles as children are launched from the home toward independent living.

Physical Development

Many physical changes become evident during this life phase. Typically there is a physical slowing down and gradual decrease in the functional capacity of all organ systems. Although life expectancy has increased past age 70, physical problems during the middle years continue to be common and some, such as cardiovascular disease and cancer, remain life-threatening. However, health promotion and better detection and treatment of many illnesses have enabled millions of adults to enjoy a more robust middle age. An

important physical change for women between ages 45 and 55 is menopause with accompanying changes in secondary sex characteristics, e.g., decrease in breast size, shrinking of reproductive organs, and decrease in vaginal secretions. Libido does not typically decrease. Psychologic reactions may include feelings of loss of youth and one's ability to have children. Men at this stage usually experience a plateau of sexual responsiveness as a result of stable testosterone levels with a decrease in the later part of middle age (Edelman and Mandle 1986).

Cognitive Development

Cognitive ability may stabilize or even peak as middle-aged adults of both sexes achieve career goals or move into new arenas. Women who had not worked outside the home when their children were young may decide to return to school or the job market after children spend more time at school or leave home. For middle-aged adults who have consolidated earlier developmental tasks and reached some life goals, there can be a freedom to pursue intellectual and career challenges, to produce the best contributions to professional fields. For others who reach middle age with less personal success, it can be a time of stability without major cognitive gains and emphasis on maintaining jobs until retirement.

Psychosocial Development

The person in the mid-life crisis is very different from the person who has restabilized around middle age. People in the mid-life crisis define their situation in relation to others. They relate their career plans to competition with younger people. They maintain their physical attractiveness in the face of what they see as a struggle to keep up with younger rivals. Their marriage partner or lover is crucial to their self-definition. These people feel they are at their peak in ability. But as we reach middle age, we look back on the mid-life crisis as only a stage in the ongoing life cycle. We cease to blame our marriage partner for our problems, and we relax our sense of competitiveness. A new freedom to be independent and follow our individual interests opens up. Sheehy defines this change as a movement from "us-ness" to "me-ness." We can now enjoy the prerogatives of middle age without making invidious comparisons with others, and fears of aging and death ease a bit.

Generativity versus Stagnation

In Erikson's view, the developmental choice in middle age is between generativity and stagnation. Erikson defines generativity as a concern for establishing and guiding the next generation. We evaluate our productiveness and make inferences about what we can look forward to accomplishing. If we have been able to contribute something to society or care for dependents, we have resolved the issue of generativity in a positive way. If we refuse to assume the power and responsibility of middle age, we become stagnant. Erikson thinks that people who cannot expand their interests at this point in life suffer a pervading sense of boredom and impoverishment. If the crisis is resolved constructively, we will have a greater capacity for responsible involvement and will shift our values away from physical attractiveness and strength to intellectual abilities. A corresponding shift from sexuality to platonic relationships may widen our circle of acquaintances in the community and vocational world. Our stature as an experienced person may provide contacts with people over a wide age range, and relationships may become more varied and differentiated.

The Productivity of Middle Age

People who have done the work of self-confrontation and change in the early forties enter what may be the most productive period of their lives. Sheehy describes the period between 43 and 50 as a time of restabilization and flowering. We come to terms with the fact that our life is finite and reconcile what is with what might have been. Children previously loved as extensions of ourselves are respected as individuals, and we are able to modify early illusions about our capacities. A well-developed sense of judgment makes more efficient and well-reasoned decisions possible.

In middle age interests left dormant during early struggles to establish a family and a career can be redeveloped. Previous hobbies or secondary interests can blossom into serious work. A teacher can retire and turn her hobby of weaving into a small business. A lawyer can concentrate on his interest in photography. Development of alternative abilities releases new energies.

The cues for changes associated with middle age vary according to the predominant roles held. Sheehy found that cues varied by sex: Men took their cues from career and health changes while women took theirs from family events, such as the marriage of children and the birth of grandchildren (Figure 6–4). This model is appropriate only in traditional family structures in which roles are defined by gender; that is, father works outside the home and mother raises children and manages the home. For adults who have varied this pattern by adopting more androgynous roles, such as women who maintain active careers outside the home or who are not married, cues differ or overlap. For example, both men and women who are parents and employed are likely to react to their children's departure for jobs or college and the simultaneous loss of a promotion to a younger colleague with concern about aging. Alternatively, many middle-aged adults find this period a refreshing break from the constant responsibilities and worries of childrearing and career building that are frequently hallmarks of the young adult years. Certainly, greater life-style options lessen the stereotype of middle age as a time of decline or preoccupation with physical complaints.

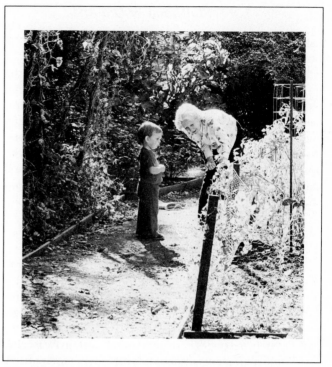

Figure 6–4
During middle and late adulthood, new roles like being a grandparent can offer fulfillment.

Emphasis on One's Own Values

Experience brings with it certain psychologic benefits. Other people's opinions become less important as the middle-aged person becomes more preoccupied with inner life and philosophic and religious concerns. We may come to approve of ourselves ethically and morally in a way that is independent of the standards of others. The early habit of trying to please everyone, a particularly difficult problem for women, may be overcome. A woman may find she can tell the truth more often, instead of hiding her thoughts to protect other people's feelings.

We may understand, finally, that even if we have not achieved what we hoped for, we are good enough or successful enough. This feeling comes with self-respect. Outward manifestations of success, such as physical strength and material possessions, become less important. We appreciate everyday human experience more as we relinquish the search for glamour and power. The awareness of death may cause some individuals to value life in a deeper way.

Late Adulthood or Old Age

Late adulthood spans from age 65 or 70 until death. In the United States older adults make up roughly 11.5 percent of the population. Estimates predict steady increases in the number of elderly, particularly in the next century when today's adult baby boomers reach old age. The large numbers of older people, coupled with their increased physical, cognitive, and psychologic vulnerability and risk factors, make it particularly important to understand the developmental challenges of this population. Understanding and gains in knowledge can assist us to strip away stereotypes and promote the quality of life for older people.

Physical Development

There is great variability in physical and cognitive functioning of the elderly. Age alone does not predict an individual's state of health. However, there is a typical pattern of degenerative changes in structural and functional capacity.

While all systems undergo change, some are particularly marked and common. Bones lose mass and density, resulting in decrease in height, risk of bone compression and breakage, and posture changes. Postmenopausal women, with less bone mass and density than men and lowered estrogen levels, are particularly at risk for osteoporosis. Cartilage changes and joint disease decrease joint mobility and can cause pain.

Perceptual changes are typified by declines in visual and hearing acuity. A diminishing sense of taste and smell contribute to appetite loss with potential risks for malnutrition when poor financial resources, decreased mobility, and isolation also limit food availability and the desire to eat well.

Changes in other body systems are also seen. Cardiovascular and respiratory function and capacity decline with aging, resulting in less efficient oxygen utilization. Gastrointestinal functioning is characterized by a decrease in secretions and motility. If there is loss of teeth, digestive difficulties may be compounded. Thus, constipation and poor nutrition are risks. Renal function also decreases, and the bladder usually loses tone and capacity. Skin wrinkles due to lost elasticity, becomes more dry and thin, and develops "age spots" from pigmentation changes. The sex drive may decrease, and reproductive function is lost for women and diminished or also lost for men. Sexual relations may remain a source of affection and pleasure, however. The many physical changes are reflected in the five leading causes of death among the elderly: heart disease, malignant neoplasms, cerebrovascular accident (CVA or stroke), influenza, and pneumonia. The five most common

chronic illnesses are arthritis, hearing and visual problems, hypertension, and heart conditions (Edelman and Mandle 1986).

Cognitive Development

Cognitive changes are normal in aging. People lose brain cells from youth to old age, but we have more cells than are truly needed and only 10 to 20 percent of the elderly experience cognitive impairment. Typical changes are:

- Diminished spatial perceptual organization
- Slower retrieval from memory
- Slower learning
- Increased caution in making decisions
- Continued creativity when demonstrated throughout previous life stages

When cognitive dysfunction does occur, the following problems are seen:

- Confusion
- Disorientation in reference to time, place, or person
- Confabulation (filling in imaginary content to cover memory gaps)
- Dementia (permanent personality disorganization and loss of cerebral function, often the result of Alzheimer's disease)
- Transient ischemic attacks (TIAs) resulting from inadequate flow of blood to the brain

Psychosocial Development

Changes in roles and relationships are hallmarks of psychosocial development in old age. Erikson sees the developmental task of this period as integrity versus despair. Positive resolution involves acceptance of one's life and accomplishments as being meaningful and worthwhile, expansion of relationships and interests compatible with one's life situation, and provision of a legacy for the following generations. Negative resolution, in contrast, involves preoccupation with fears of death, feelings of loss, and a sense of life's meaninglessness.

A major role change that typically marks the transition to late adulthood is retirement. For people who have held jobs throughout all or most of their adult lives, leaving work can create a real identity crisis as the sense of self is no longer tied to a job title. Work is central to human beings. People work not only for physical sustenance, but also for social reasons. Various writers have described the moral, economic, and social dimensions of work. Some say that work is a bond with the community; others, that it is simply the best way to fill up a lot of time. Most agree that work fulfills a basic and profound human need. Because it plays a pervasive and powerful role in the psychologic, social, and economic aspects of people's lives, work can be called a basic or central institution. The example below illustrates some of the disruptive effects of early retirement from work.

"My God, what'll Lorraine do with Howard around all day? I'd go crazy if Alan retired early," said Eleanor. The talk of this upper-middle-income suburban community was Howard's retirement at age 50 from his job as an aviation engineer. Howard, the sole heir of his two aunts, came into a large sum of money when they died. Eleanor's reaction echoed that of many of her female friends and neighbors.

As it turned out, Howard and Lorraine discovered that their interests were not shared. Whereas Howard had devoted most of his energy to success at his job, Lorraine had devoted hers to being the perfect home-maker. Their house was spotless, and Lorraine saw that it was kept that way. She baked, cooked, and grew and canned her own vegetables. With all three children away from home, the couple had little to say to each other and even less to do together.

Howard found he did not enjoy hobbies, sports, reading, or other leisure activities. As their unhappiness with each other escalated, Howard purchased a small vending machine business. He viewed this as a hobby, an interesting way to spend his time. But the business soon proved unsuccessful, and Howard and Lorraine were back where they started. This time, however, they enrolled in an adult education course on the pursuit of leisure at a local college. Through this they discovered an interest they could both enjoy. Howard's aunts had left him two old Victorian homes in a nearby small community, and both were completely furnished in antiques. It seemed natural to open a small antique store. Lorraine and Howard soon found they were able to value each other's skills and abilities in an enjoyable activity that was satisfying to both.

In our culture, a person may opt for early retirement, but most people find themselves faced with forced retirement. Some view retirement as a pleasurable experience. To others, it is a distressing, painful time of life, signaling old age and the approach of death. Most often, it is a time of stress when people feel unwanted, unvalued, and unproductive.

A person's life-style influences how that person approaches retirement. For example, hobbies and interests that are primarily pleasure-related rather than work-related help persons look forward to retirement. A specifically planned retirement project, such as travel, a course of study, or learning to play a musical instrument, provides a pos-

itive reason for retirement. Another major influencing factor is the degree of comfort or ease with which a person can retire. Retirement is less stressful when health, income, and living environment are sufficient to make the person comfortable.

Losses in physical or cognitive abilities and loss of family members and friends compound the adjustments of role transitions during this life stage. The reality of loss and appropriate feelings of sadness are communicated in one 70-year-old woman's comment, "Thirty people have died in my building since I moved in a few years ago. I've lost so many friends and loved ones. . . ." The elderly sometimes also face loss of financial resources and the ability to live independently, placing them at risk for abuse and decreased self-esteem. These stresses are associated with increased rates of depression and suicide among the elderly.

Successful completion of the developmental tasks of old age helps older persons to counteract difficulties and diminish the risk of mental health problems. In a classic work on aging, Havighurst and Albrecht (1953) outline the following challenges:

- Preparing for retirement
- Obtaining satisfaction from leisure time
- Nurturing relationships with members of younger generations, e.g., grandchildren and greatgrandchildren
- Adjusting to changes in physical health, retirement, and loss of loved ones
- Developing a connection with one's age group
- Taking on new social roles
- Creating a satisfactory and appropriate living situation

An additional task that might be added is to cope with dependence on others, particularly one's children. A role reversal often takes place during this period, and adult children may need to function as parents for their aging parents. When this occurs, it is important for the nurse to assist the older adult to maintain integrity and dignity (Griffith-Kenney 1986). Resolution of the developmental challenges of late adulthood can enable the elderly to achieve integrity, self-actualization, meaning, and happiness despite the potential difficulties of aging.

The Family Life Cycle

Understanding individual developmental phases can be enhanced when the context of the family's life cycle is considered. Although there is variation in family patterns (e.g., some couples do not have children), the bulk of nuclear families follow a predictable course. Individual develop-

Table 6–10
Stage-Sensitive Family Developmental Tasks Through the Family Life Cycle

Stage of the Family Life Cycle	Positions in the Family	Stage-Sensitive Family Developmental Tasks
Married couple	Wife Husband	Establishing a mutually satisfying marriage Adjusting to pregnancy and the promise of parenthood Fitting into the kin network
Childbearing	Wife-mother Husband-father Infant daughter or son or both	Having, adjusting to, and encouraging the development of infants Establishing a satisfying home for both parents and infant(s)
Preschool-age	Wife-mother Husband-father Daughter-sister Son-brother	Adapting to the critical needs and interests of preschool children in stimulating, growth-promoting ways Coping with energy depletion and lack of privacy as parents
School-age	Wife-mother Husband-father Daughter-sister Son-brother	Fitting into the community of school-age families in constructive ways Encouraging children's educational achievement
Teenage	Wife-mother Husband-father Daughter-sister Son-brother	Balancing freedom with responsibility as teenagers mature and emancipate themselves Establishing postparental interests and careers as growing parents
Launching center	Wife-mother-grandmother Husband-father-grandfather Daughter-sister-aunt Son-brother-uncle	Releasing young adults into work, military service, college, marriage, and so on with appropriate rituals and assistance Maintaining a supportive home base
Middle-aged parents	Wife-mother-grandmother Husband-father-grandfather	Refocusing on the marriage relationship Maintaining kin ties with older and younger generations
Aging family members	Widow or widower Wife-mother-grandmother Husband-father-grandfather	Coping with bereavement and living alone Closing the family home or adapting it to aging Adjusting to retirement

Source: From Marriage and Family Development, *by Evelyn Millis Duval and Brent C. Miller. Table 3.5, p. 62. Copyright © 1985 by Harper & Row, Publishers Inc. Reprinted by permission of Harper & Row Publishers, Inc.*

ment of the members overlaps with the family's cycle. Duvall and Miller (1985) describe eight stages in the family life cycle with corresponding tasks. Table 6–10 outlines the family life cycle stages and tasks.

These tasks serve as a helpful guide during a nursing assessment. As the example below illustrates, when individual members' developmental tasks conflict with those of the family as a whole at a given time, problems in coping and interpersonal relations may arise.

Jim entered into his second marriage at age 47. His new wife, Carla, was 32 and had never had children;

Jim had two grown children. The couple decided to have two children within the next five years. No major conflict between family and developmental tasks occurred until the "launching phase" of the family life cycle. Jim was ready to retire from his job but found the financial burden of helping two more children attend college would require that he continue to work when he felt it was time to enjoy leisure time with his wife. Jim developed hypertension, and he and Carla began to quarrel.

A nursing assessment would reveal the conflict between individual and family developmental tasks. Once the problem was diagnosed, possible solutions could be planned to ease the financial stress. For example, Jim and Carla could work part-time, investigate ways that the children could help to pay some of the tuition costs, and consider a variety of schools to weigh their costs in light of the benefits. Such plans would give the couple and the children options to ease the fit between individual and family developmental phases.

APPLYING THE NURSING PROCESS

Throughout this chapter, developmental theory has been discussed in relation to the life cycle. Brief examples have illustrated how theory is applied, and some implications for nursing have been suggested. This final section is a synopsis of the major goals for each phase of the nursing process in light of human growth and development and correlates a clinical example to each step in the nursing process.

Assessment

The primary goal for assessment of growth and development is the determination of the client's progress toward mastery of the milestones and tasks for the appropriate developmental stage. The first step in reaching this goal is to collect an essential piece of data—the age of the client (or ages of family members when the family is the focus). Age is the starting point for placing the client within a life cycle phase. To allow for individual variation, the nurse should use developmental milestones only as guides. Nonetheless, the major phases and related tasks and accomplishments are age-related. The developmental tasks identified by the major theorists discussed earlier should be reviewed and compared to the client's achievements. Physical, cognitive, and psychosocial aspects of the client's development are to be measured according to age-related norms. Observation, interview including the history, and measurement by instruments are all ways to collect assessment data.

Consider the following questions when assessing a client's growth and development:

- What is the client's age?
- Where is the client's physical, cognitive, and psychosocial development in relation to the norms for his or her age group?
- What developmental tasks have been met or remain to be completed in relation to the client's age? What progress has been made?
- What intrapersonal, interpersonal, and environmental factors influence the client's development?
- What steps need to be taken to complete the appropriate developmental tasks?

Nursing Diagnosis

Diagnosis requires an analysis of the assessment data. Patterns are detected and human responses are categorized. Once a label of an actual or potential problem is assigned, the nurse tries to understand the etiology, i.e., explain how the difficulty arose. In their research concerning the cause and evolution of behavioral problems from infancy through early adult life, Thomas and Chess (1984) found that three factors were sufficient to explain the root of problem behavior:

- Objective, overt characteristics of the child
- Patterns of parental functioning
- Specific environmental influences

Other factors, such as anxiety, were clearly secondary. In other words, these factors were a consequence rather than a cause of the problem. Once present, however, anxiety frequently has a profound effect on the subsequent course of difficulties.

When nurses develop diagnoses related to individual developmental patterns, the concept of "goodness of fit" and the related ideas of consonance and dissonance are most useful. "Goodness of fit results when the properties of the environment and its expectations and demands are in accord with the organism's own capacities, motivations, and style of behaving. When this *consonance* between individual and environment is present, optimal development is possible. Conversely, poorness of fit involves *dissonance* between individual and environment, so that distorted development and maladaptive functioning occur" (Thomas and Chess 1984).

Maladaptive development can be categorized according to DSM-IIIR, PND-1, and NANDA diagnostic systems. Table 6–11 compares diagnoses from these different systems in relation to the clinical example on pages 122–124.

Planning and Implementing Intervention

The major goal is for the client to master the unmet developmental tasks of the current and previous stages. This long-term goal is modified according to the client's abilities. Short-term goals constitute small steps in the completion of simple developmental tasks, leading to successful mastery of the major tasks. The nurse assists the client to reach this goal by enhancing the consonance between the individual and environment. Change in individual, interpersonal, or environmental factors is used to improve the "goodness of fit."

Evaluation

The nurse evaluates the outcome of the previous steps in the nursing process by measuring the progress made toward achieving the designated developmental tasks. When the client has not made satisfactory progress, a review of the earlier steps in the nursing process may lead to a reassessment, different diagnosis, or new plans and interventions.

Clinical Example

Assessment

Elaine, 37, and Rick, 35, had spent the first ten years of their marriage building their respective careers of law and dentistry. When Elaine tried to become pregnant at age 34, she discovered infertility problems. A round of tests and surgery cost three years of time on her biologic clock. At 37, she finally became pregnant.

Elaine planned the standard six-week maternity leave from her practice, and Rick took off a long weekend following the birth of their daughter, Jessica. During the leave period, Elaine felt disoriented and unable to organize the various aspects of her new role. She felt tired following nights of getting up to feed the baby. Rick spent longer hours at work in an effort to increase the size of his dental practice in case Elaine decided to take off more time from work. Elaine felt criticized by her relatives, who told her she should bottle-feed rather than breast-feed so that she would be less tired. They warned Elaine that a swift return to work would deprive Jessica of needed mothering during the important early years. As the date for her return to work approached, Elaine felt depressed, still thought she was disorganized, and had no one to care for the baby while she worked. When Rick came home late one evening, he found Elaine crying with the baby in her arms. She stated, "I'm falling apart. I never knew it would be so hard. I don't know how to be a good mother. I'm so scared." Elaine's sense of desperation signaled the need for intervention. In Elaine's call for help, Rick recognized his own mounting anxiety. The couple scheduled six counseling sessions with the psychiatric nurse clinician at their health maintenance organization.

Nursing Diagnosis

Clearly, the couple faced a major developmental crisis. Driscoll (1986) labels the period of 9 to 12 months following giving birth as probably the most difficult time in a woman's life. This transition time requires learning by both parents so that their coping mechanisms can be applied in their new roles.

Conflicting role demands coupled with inadequate support, information, and feedback led to Elaine's feelings of failure and anxiety. Rick spent more time at work to avoid Elaine's difficulties and his own anxiety about being a good father coupled with feelings of inadequacy. Table 6–11 summarizes the analysis of the case through a listing and comparison of the diagnoses for Rick and Elaine.

Planning and Implementing Interventions

The nurse helped Elaine and Rick to list the problems from small to large, to state what they expected life with a new baby to be like in comparison to the reality, and to identify their strengths and support systems. In this manner, the couple were active participants in the assessment and diagnostic processes. They were able to identify the uncomfortable feelings and to connect them to specific expectations and difficult situations. The nurse provided needed information concerning the everyday realities of child care during the first year. The nurse's description of this time as a developmental crisis in which their feelings were normal was very helpful.

More realistic goals were developed together: to share parenting responsibilities, to reduce time devoted to careers, to build a support system, and to feel successful in the new parental roles. Implicit in the last goal was the expectation that Jessica would be successful in reaching her own developmental milestones. These goals were to be met by the following interventions:

- Open discussion of feelings and problems daily to give support and feedback to each other

- Designation of family jobs to each partner and plans to obtain housecleaning and other affordable services to reduce stress and improve sharing

- Extension of Elaine's leave for two months to allow time for the family to reorganize and find needed supports, e.g., child care and meeting other parents of infants

- Limits on what advice will be tolerated from family members to reduce intrusiveness and negative feedback

- Time planned for the couple to be alone to shift the focus from an exclusive concern with parenting roles to a more balanced view of their lives

Evaluation

After three months, Elaine and Rick met with the nurse to evaluate their progress. Life still felt disorganized, especially in the morning before work, but they had ways to manage better. Child care had been set up, and both Elaine and Rick had decided to reduce their work hours after

Table 6–11
Comparison of Diagnoses for the Clinical Example

DSM-IIIR	PND-I Diagnoses	NANDA Diagnoses
For Elaine		
309.28 Adjustment disorder with mixed emotional features (Axis I)	05.03 Altered role performance 05.03.01 Altered family role	Adjustment, impaired
	04.02 Altered feeling patterns 04.02.02 Anxiety*	Anxiety
	02.02 Altered decision making	Coping, ineffective individual
V62.89[†] Phase of life problem		Growth and development, altered Home maintenance management, impaired Hopelessness
	02.03 Altered knowledge processes 02.02.03 Knowledge deficit*	Knowledge deficit (related to parenting) Parenting, alteration in: potential
	06.03 Altered self-concept* 06.03.04 Altered self-esteem 06.06.03 Altered personal identity	Self-concept, disturbance in (self-esteem, role performance, and personal identity)
For Rick		
309.24 Adjustment disorder with anxious mood (Axis I)	05.03 Altered role performance 05.03.01 Altered family role 05.03.06 Altered work role	Adjustment, impaired
	04.02 Altered feeling patterns 04.02.02 Anxiety*	Anxiety
		Coping, ineffective individual
		Home maintenance management, impaired Parenting, alteration in: potential
V62.89 Phase of life problem	06.03 Altered self-concept* 06.03.03 Altered personal identity	Self-concept, disturbance in (role performance)
For both Elaine and Rick		

Axis II: V71.09 No diagnosis
Axis III: No diagnosis
Axis IV: Severity of psychosocial
    Stressor = 5 (severe)
    Event = birth of child
    Type = predominantly acute event
Axis V: GAF = 70 for present (some difficulty or mild symptoms); GAF = 90 for recent past (good in all areas)
		Coping, family: potential for growth

*PND-I diagnosis also in NANDA list.
[†]V-codes are for conditions not attributable to a mental disorder that are a focus of treatment.

realizing that the bills could still be paid. They accepted that their careers need not always proceed at full speed; Jessica needed time with both parents, and they needed some time to nurture the marital relationship. Both felt there was a better balance in their lives and saw themselves as doing a good job together. Jessica's growth and development was normal, another important indicator that the parents were coping well. All agreed that they felt happier now and believed that the challenges of this phase of personal and family development could be mastered, even if it took time and help. Plans for follow-up were made to provide support for the couple in anticipation of the crises expected during Jessica's rapid changes in the months to come. The nurse felt satisfied that this couple had moved toward successful mastery of the individual and family tasks involved in the transition to parenthood and were now better equipped to nurture their daughter's and their own growth and development.

Chapter Highlights

- Individuals are shaped by a continuous developmental process from birth until death.

- Although the idea that people progress through developmental stages with distinct characteristics is relatively new, its origin can be traced to the Middle Ages and Renaissance.

- Most current developmental theorists identify age-related and sequential stages throughout the life cycle.

- The life cycle is a complex series of events with predictable physical, cognitive, and psychosocial changes.

- Developmental stages have specific challenges or tasks to be met.

- Successful resolution of the tasks from one stage is an important foundation for coping with the challenges of subsequent stages.

- Multiple factors contribute to a person's growth and development.

- According to a humanistic-interactionist model, the complexities of human growth and development cannot be predicted or understood according to any one theory.

- Although there are norms of physical, cognitive, and psychosocial development, there is great variation among people's healthy development.

- Knowledge of growth and development is an essential prerequisite to any thorough nursing assessment.

- Nurses can use developmental theories and stage-related norms in assessing individuals and families by identifying tasks that have been resolved successfully and identifying potential difficulties related to an expected developmental challenge.

- Application of norms for growth and development uncovers potential and existing problems, leads to nursing diagnoses, provides the basis for planning client goals and implementing interventions, and becomes the measure for evaluating the outcomes of intervention.

References

Aries P: *Centuries of Childhood: A Social History of Family Life.* Vintage Books, 1962.

Driscoll J: How to survive the first nine months and the second nine months. Presentation sponsored by the Massachusetts Nurses Association, District V, Boston, November 13, 1986.

Duvall EM, Miller BC: *Marriage and Family Development,* ed 6. Harper & Row, 1985.

Edelman C, Mandle, CL: *Health Promotion throughout the Lifespan.* Mosby, 1986.

Erikson EH: *Childhood and Society,* ed 2. W. W. Norton, 1963.

Freud S: *An Outline of Psycho-Analysis,* rev ed. W. W. Norton, 1949.

Gilligan, C: *In a Different Voice: Psychological Theory and Women's Development.* Harvard University Press, 1982.

Griffith-Kenney J: *Contemporary Women's Health: A Nursing Advocacy Approach.* Addison-Wesley, 1986.

Havighurst RJ, Albrecht R: *Older People.* Longmans, 1953.

Horowitz JA, Hughes CB, Perdue, BJ: *Parenting Reassessed: A Nursing Perspective.* Prentice-Hall, 1982.

Kohlberg L: The cognitive-developmental approach to socialization, in Goslin D (ed): *Handbook of Socialization.* Rand-McNally, 1969.

Mahler M: *The Psychological Birth of the Human Infant: Symbiosis and Individuation.* Basic Books, 1975.

Maslow A: *Toward a Psychology of Being.* D. Van Nostrand, 1962.

Mercer RT: The process of maternal role attainment over the first year. *Nurs Res* 1985;34:198–203.

Moore ML: *Realities in Childbearing,* ed 2. Saunders, 1983.

Mott SM, Fazekas NF, James SR: *Nursing Care of Children and Families: A Holistic Approach.* Addison-Wesley, 1985.

Peplau H: *Interpersonal Relations in Nursing.* Putnam, 1951.

Piaget J: *The Origins of Intelligence in Children.* International Universities Press, 1952.

Piaget J: *The Growth of Logical Thinking from Childhood to Adolescence.* Basic Books, 1958.

Sheehy G: *Passages.* Dutton, 1976.

Sullivan HS: *The Interpersonal Theory of Psychiatry.* W. W. Norton, 1953.

Thomas A, Chess S: Genesis and evolution of behavioral disorders: from infancy to early adult life. *Am J Psychiatry* 1984;141:2–9.

Woods NF: Employment, family roles, and mental ill health in young married women. *Nurs Res* 1985;34:4–9.

SEVEN

Stress, Anxiety, and Coping

Carol Ren Kneisl

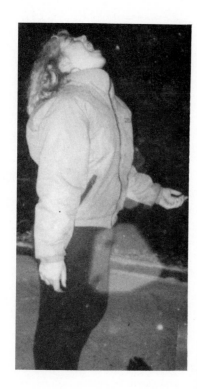

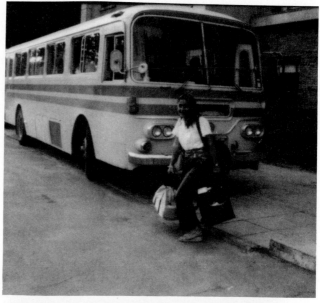

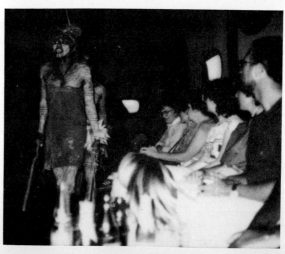

This book is committed to ending racism and sexism because without their end, global health and a peaceful world are not possible.

Learning Objectives

After reading this chapter, students should be able to

- Describe the effects of stress on an individual
- Compare three theories that purport to explain stress
- Discuss the sources of anxiety
- Describe the effects of anxiety on an individual
- Explain everyday methods for coping with stress and anxiety
- Explain the resources that help people resist stress
- Discuss constructive and destructive coping strategies
- Define common defense-oriented behaviors and give examples of them

Cross References

Other topics relevant to this content are: Applying the nursing process to the care of anxious clients, Chapter 19; Assessing the severity of stress according to Axis IV of DSM-IIIR, Chapter 12 and Appendix B; Nursing intervention for intellectualization and denial, section on intervention into detachment in Chapter 27; Posttraumatic stress disorder, Chapter 19; Psychophysiologic conditions thought to result from stress, Chapter 23; Relaxation and stress-management techniques, Chapter 28; Social support systems, Chapter 8.

Key Terms

anxiety
conflict
coping strategies
defense mechanisms
denial
displacement
dissociation
fantasy
fight-flight
frustration
general adaptation syndrome (GAS)

identification
intellectualization
introjection
panic
projection
rationalization
reaction formation
repression
selective inattention
stress
stressor
suppression

Health care professionals have long been interested in stress and anxiety and in the ways that healthy and dysfunctional persons cope or fail to cope with them. Stress and anxiety affect the person's well-being. Various behavioral and physiologic disorders have been linked to stress and anxiety. Some behavioral manifestations are discussed here and elaborated in later chapters. The cost of stress and anxiety can be quite high: They can cost a woman her job, a man the love and respect of his family. When sufficiently prolonged, stress can kill.

STRESS

Stress is a part of being alive. Standing erect stresses the muscles and bones that must work together to keep the body erect; eating stresses the digestive system, which must produce enzymes and absorb nutrients; and breathing stresses the respiratory system, which must exchange carbon dioxide and oxygen. More broadly and holistically, **stress** designates a broad class of experiences in which a demanding situation taxes a person's resources or coping capabilities, causing a negative effect. This broader definition approximates the humanistic perspective of this textbook. In this view, stress is a person-environment interaction. The source of the stress, the demanding situation, is known as a **stressor**. The internal state the stress produces is one of tension, anxiety, or strain.

There is no universally accepted definition of stress among stress theorists and researchers. An interactional view of stress, such as the one given above, is consistent

---

Portions of the material in this chapter were contributed to the second edition of this text by Joan Sayre. Other portions of this chapter appeared in Ames SW, Kneisl CR: How illness develops; and Kneisl CR: Coping with illness, in Kneisl CR, Ames SW: *Adult Health Nursing.* Addison-Wesley, 1986.

with how nurses view human experiences. The theories of stress that follow are the perspectives in common use. Although they do tell us a great deal about responses to stressful situations, it is crucial for nurses to recognize that these explanations are not necessarily consistent with nursing's orientation. Such factors as cause, the situational context in which the stressful event occurs, and the psychologic interpretation of the demanding situation must be considered in a holistic, humanistic approach to the client. Axis IV of DSM-IIIR offers some general parameters for assessing the severity of stress.

The Fight-Flight Response to Stress

Beyond the routine and essential stress of everyday life, humans risk encountering undesirable or excess stress that threatens well-being and may even be life threatening. They cope with such threats through either a **fight** (aggression) or **flight** (withdrawal) response. The fight-flight response was first discussed by Walter Cannon, a physician, in 1932 when he identified stress as an actual cause of disease. Consider the following situation of extreme stress: A woman is walking down a dark, deserted street when a man with a knife emerges from the shadows just in front of her. Does she try to defend herself? Does she run away? Whichever action she takes is a result of a variety of physiologic responses to extreme danger. According to Mason (1980), when a person faces such a situation:

- The heartbeat increases to pump blood throughout the necessary tissues with greater speed, carrying oxygen and nutrients to cells and clearing away waste products more quickly.

- As the heart rate increases, the blood pressure rises.

- Breathing becomes rapid and shallow.

- Epinephrine and other hormones are released into the blood.

- The liver releases stored sugar into the blood to meet the increased energy needs of survival.

- The pupils dilate to let in more light; all the senses are heightened.

- Muscles tense for movement, either for flight or protective actions, particularly the skeletal muscles of the thighs, hips, back, shoulders, arms, jaw, and face.

- Blood flow to the digestive organs is greatly constricted.

- Blood flow increases to the brain and major muscles.

- Blood flow to the extremities is constricted, and the hands and feet become cold. This is protection from bleeding to death quickly if the hands or feet are injured in fight or flight and allows blood to be diverted to more important areas of the body.

- The body perspires to cool itself, because increased metabolism generates more heat.

Although these physiologic responses seem appropriate for the situation described, imagine the wear and tear on the body if humans responded to all stress in these ways.

Selye's Stress-Adaptation Theory

Hans Selye, a Canadian endocrinologist and the most well known and widely recognized stress researcher, developed another framework for understanding how persons respond to stress. According to him, each person has a limited amount of energy to use in dealing with stress. How quickly it is used and, therefore, how quickly one adapts to stress depend on several factors such as heredity, mental attitude, and life-style, among others.

Selye defines stress as the rate of wear and tear on the body. He disputes the idea that only serious disease or injury causes stress. Selye thinks that any emotion or activity requires a response or change in the individual. Stressors can be physical, chemical, physiologic, developmental, or emotional. Playing a game of tennis, going out in the rain without an umbrella, having an argument, or getting a promotion are all examples of stressful events. Life itself is basically stressful, since it involves a process of adaptation to continual change. Though the experience of adaptation is stressful, it is not necessarily harmful. Indeed, it can be exciting and rewarding under certain circumstances, and although we cannot avoid the stress of living, we can learn to minimize its damaging effects.

While a medical student, Selye made an interesting and important observation that became the cornerstone of his stress-adaptation theory. He observed that, regardless of the diagnosis, most clients had certain symptoms in common—they lost their appetites, they lost weight, they felt and looked ill, they were anxious and fatigued, and they had aches and pains in their joints and muscles. He introduced his observations and the general adaptation syndrome concept in 1936 in a letter to the editor of the journal *Nature*. A long series of experiments (1956) led to more objective evidence of actual body damage—enlargement of the adrenal glands; shrinkage of the thymus, spleen, and lymph nodes; and the appearance of bleeding gastric ulcers.

Feelings of anxiety, fatigue, or illness are subjective aspects of stress. Though stress itself cannot be perceived, Selye found that it can be appraised by the objectively measurable structural and chemical changes that it produces in the body. These changes are called the **general adaptation syndrome (GAS)** because when stress affects the whole person, the whole person must adjust to the changes. The GAS occurs in three stages: alarm, resistance, and exhaustion. An example of the GAS can be found in combat

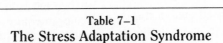

Table 7–1
The Stress Adaptation Syndrome

Stage	Physical Change	Psychosocial Changes
Stage I: Alarm reaction Mobilization of the body's defensive forces and activation of the "fight-or-flight" mechanism	Release of norepinephrine and epinephrine causing vasoconstriction, increased blood pressure, and increased rate and force of cardiac contraction Increased hormone levels Enlargement of adrenal cortex Marked loss of body weight Shrinkage of the thymus, spleen, and lymph nodes Irritation of the gastric mucosa	Increased level of alertness Increased level of anxiety Task-oriented, defense-oriented, inefficient, or maladaptive behavior may occur
Stage II: Stage of resistance Optimal adaptation to stress within the person's capabilities	Hormone levels readjust Reduction in activity and size of adrenal cortex Lymph nodes return to normal size Weight returns to normal	Increased and intensified use of coping mechanisms Tendency to rely on defense-oriented behavior
Stage III: Stage of exhaustion Loss of ability to resist stress because of depletion of body resources	Decreased immune response with suppression of T cells and atrophy of thymus Depletion of adrenal glands and hormone production Weight loss Enlargement of lymph nodes and dysfunction of lymphatic system If exposure to the stressor continues, cardiac failure, renal failure, or death may occur	Defense-oriented behaviors become exaggerated Disorganization of thinking Disorganization of personality Sensory stimuli may be misperceived with appearance of illusion Reality contact may be reduced with appearance of delusions or hallucinations If exposure to the stressor continues, stupor or violence may occur

Source: Kneisl CR, Ames SW: Adult Health Nursing: A Biopsychosocial Approach. Addison-Wesley, 1986, p 20.

soldiers. These men are exposed to ever-present threats of death and mutilation. They also experience the severe psychologic shock of witnessing the destructiveness of war. Other psychologic and interpersonal factors contribute to their overall stress load. One such factor is the reduction of personal freedom and gratification. Another is separation from loved ones. The experiences of combat soldiers can be used to illustrate the three stages of the GAS. The three stages of the GAS are summarized above in Table 7–1.

Alarm Reaction

When the soldier first encounters the stress of war, he experiences the *alarm* reaction. In alarm the body undergoes biochemical reactions as the adaptive hormones are stimulated. These adaptive hormones fall into two basic groups. The anti-inflammatory hormones include the

adrenocorticotropic hormone (ACTH), cortisone, and cortisol. The proinflammatory hormones include the somatotropic hormones, aldosterone and desoxycorticosterone. The biochemical reactions that occur during alarm result in an enlargement of the adrenal cortex and lymph nodes and increases in hormonal levels. These changes lower the subject's overall resistance. For example, soldiers may show such behavioral changes as increasing irritability, disturbances of sleep, and recurrent nightmares. Soldiers are described as being hypersensitive to minor stimuli. For instance, they will leap up in fright at the sound of a branch cracking. This behavior generally indicates failure to maintain psychologic integration.

Stage of Resistance

Many men are able to adjust to combat. As they do so, the next stage, *resistance*, occurs. In the stage of resistance the biologic changes in hormonal levels, adrenal cortex, and lymph nodes are reversed. These men can maintain their psychologic integrity. They may become used to killing and may even take pride in it. They may be able to maintain a fatalistic attitude about their own and their comrades' survival. A soldier who has made this adjustment may be able to resign himself to fate and believe that his role has an important purpose, even though he cannot fully understand it. He may take comfort in hoping that the combat will not last long, or that he will soon be rotated out of the combat area to a less stressful role. The nature of this adaptation seems to depend on many psychologic and social factors. These include the stability of the soldier's personality, the morale of the combat unit, the sense of security and control provided by the leadership, and the friendships the soldier forms with other soldiers, which provide emotional support.

Exhaustion

The third stage, *exhaustion,* occurs if stress continues over a prolonged period of time. It also occurs when multiple stressors are active simultaneously, or when the person undergoes repeated or overwhelming stress. When too many life changes occur within a short time, there is not enough time for the body to accommodate and adjust. When this situation occurs, adaptive energy is exhausted, and the body surrenders to stress. The adrenal glands again enlarge and then are depleted. The lymph nodes enlarge, producing a subsequent dysfunction of the lymph system. There is an increase and then a decrease in hormonal levels.

The longer a soldier is in combat, the more vulnerable and anxious he is likely to feel. Prolonged combat lowers stress tolerance. It may produce increased anxiety, depression, tremulousness, and impairment of judgment and self-confidence. This decompensation results in disturbances in interpersonal relationships. The soldier may lose all sense of loyalty to his comrades. In some cases, the residual effects of combat exhaustion persist for a long time. Combat experience may continue to disturb a former soldier after he has returned to civilian life. He may experience guilt about killing and have nightmares about his war experiences.

Exhaustion may be reversible if the total body is not affected and if the individual is eventually able to eliminate the source of stress. However, if stress is unrelieved, or if the body's defenses are totally involved, the individual may not regain psychologic stability.

Most people are accustomed to thinking of untoward events as stressful, but they do not realize that desirable events such as job promotions, vacations, or outstanding personal achievements may also prove stressful. Holmes and Rahe (1967) studied life changes as stressful events to learn the amount of social readjustment required to cope with them. These authors believe that the life events that require coping behavior tend to decrease a person's ability to handle illness or subsequent stress.

Their research assigned ratings to forty-three different life changes, called *life change units* (LCUs). They asked subjects to indicate what life changes had occurred in the past year and then add up the points assigned to each identified life event. According to these researchers, a low score indicated that the subject was not likely to have an adverse reaction. A "mild" score meant that there was a 30 percent chance that the impact of stress would be experienced through physical symptoms. Persons in the "moderate" category had a 50 percent chance of a change in health status, and a "high" score meant an 80 percent chance of major illness in the next two years. High LCU scores also correlated with an increased probability of accidental injury. The example given below demonstrates how this model could be applied in understanding one individual's situation.

Marcia M, a 22-year-old woman in group therapy, had recently been divorced from her husband (LCU 73) after attempting to achieve a marital reconciliation (LCU 45). Marcia's pregnancy (LCU 40) earlier in the year was uneventful, and the Ms' healthy son was born on June 2 (LCU 39). At 6 weeks of age, the child suddenly and unexpectedly died in his crib (LCU 63). The Ms began to argue frequently (LCU 35) before they made the decision to divorce. After the divorce, Marcia found herself short of funds (LCU 38) and went to work as a waitress in a pizza restaurant (LCU 36). She found it necessary to move to a smaller and less expensive apartment (LCU 20). In the short period of one year, Marcia accumulated an LCU score of 390 and was in the high-risk group.

In the early 1970s, other researchers correlated life stress events and mental health. In a study of 720 households in a metropolitan area, J. Meyers and his associates (1972) found a relationship between a high number of life changes and changes in the mental status of individuals. For example, an increase in the number of life changes preceded worsening of psychiatric symptoms, while a

Table 7–2	
Coping Methods	
Affect-Oriented Coping Methods	**Problem-Oriented Coping Methods**
Hope things will get better	Try to maintain some control over the situation
Eat, smoke, chew gum, drink alcoholic beverages, take drugs	Find out more about the situation so you can handle it better
Pray, trust in God	Think through different ways to handle the situation
Get nervous; worry	Look at the problem objectively
Seek comfort or help from family or friends	Get an objective opinion
Want to be alone	Try out different ways of solving the problem to see which works the best
Laugh it off, figure things could be worse	Draw on experience to help you handle the situation
Try to put the problem out of your mind	Try to find meaning in the situation
Daydream, fantasize	Seek advice
Prepare to expect the worst	Set specific goals to help solve the problem
Get mad, curse, swear, shout	Accept the situation as it is
Cry, get depressed	Talk the problem over with someone who has been in the same type of situation
Go to sleep, figure things will look better in the morning	Settle for the next best thing
Don't worry about it; everything will probably work out fine	Do anything just to do something
Withdraw from the situation	Let someone else solve the problem
Work off tension with physical activity	
Take out your tensions on someone or something else	
Resign yourself to the situation because things look hopeless or because it's your fate	
Deny the situation	
Do nothing in the hope that the problem will take care of itself	
Blame someone else for your problems	
Do meditation, yoga, biofeedback, self-hypnosis	

Source: Compiled from Jalowiec A, Powers MJ: Stress and coping in hypertensive and emergency room patients. Nurs Res *1981;30:13; and Ziemer MM: Coping behavior: A response to stress.* Top Clin Nurs *1982;2(4):8.*

decrease in life changes brought improvement. The more stressful the life changes, the greater the likelihood of mental ill health. Meyers and his associates also found that entrance-related life events (those involving the addition of a new person into one's social sphere, perhaps through marriage or the birth of a child) produced less symptomatology than did exit-related life events (those associated with the loss of a valued individual or status). A number of nurse researchers have been involved in studying life changes and hospitalization as stressful events. However, applying this model in nursing practice should be based on the following cautions:

This model is based on several assumptions that depict a person as a passive recipient of stress. It assumes that events affect all people in the same way, regardless of how the individuals perceive the event. It also assumes that there is a common threshold beyond which disruption occurs. In addition, it assumes that the same amount of adaptation is required for each event among all persons. Further, it equates "change" with "stress" (Lyon and Werner 1987).

Jalowiec and Powers (1980), the nurse researchers who studied affect-oriented and problem-oriented coping strategies (see Table 7–2), did not find a relationship between the number of life events experienced by hypertensive and emergency room clients and these clients' rating of the stress level.

Thoughtful nursing care requires identifying what each individual perceives as stressful in order to understand the effects of life changes on health. Once this has been done, the Holmes and Rahe model can be used to help people become aware of the stress they face in their lives. It is also useful in planning for the future. To return to the example of Marcia M:

During the course of group therapy, Marcia shared her desire to return to college and complete the junior and senior years of a medical technology program in which she had been enrolled before her marriage. To do so, she would have to make a number of changes—move to an apartment close to the college because she could not afford to own a car, change her working hours or job so that she could attend day classes, change her sleeping habits, change her recreational and social activities, and reduce her other expenses to pay school-related costs. The changes required would add almost 200 LCUs to her score.

In group, Marcia was able to consider this information and reevaluate her goals. She decided to delay her return to school until she could get on her feet financially. She chose not to make any other changes in her life for the present time.

Clients can use this information, much as Marcia did, to decide when it is advantageous or disadvantageous to engage in life change. This knowledge helps them make responsible decisions about the directions their lives will take. Nurses can assist clients by incorporating the guidelines below in their practice:

- Help clients to recognize when a life change occurs.
- Encourage clients to think about the meaning of the change and identify some of the feelings experienced.
- Discuss with clients the different ways they might best adjust to the event.
- Encourage them to take time in arriving at decisions.
- If possible, encourage clients to anticipate life changes and plan for them well in advance.
- Encourage clients to pace themselves. It can be done, even if they are in a hurry.

- Encourage clients to look at the accomplishment of a task as a part of daily living and to avoid looking at such an achievement as a stopping point or a time for letting down.

Stress as an Interaction

Richard Lazarus, a pioneering theorist and researcher in stress, coping, and health, is known for his interactional approach to understanding stress. Lazarus (1966, 1976) sees *perceived* threat as the central characteristic of stressful situations, and in particular, threat to a person's most important goals and values. His view is reflected in the definition of stress given at the beginning of this chapter. He believes that stress depends not only on external conditions but also on the constitutional vulnerability of the person and the adequacy of that person's coping styles. Attention is also given to the role of frustration and conflict in producing stress. **Frustration** is the thwarting or the delaying of some important ongoing activity or the attainment of some important goal. **Conflict** is a state in which opposing desires, feelings, or goals coexist. Conflict, of necessity, leads to frustration because activity designed to achieve one goal frustrates the attainment of the other. Satisfactory resolution of conflict is impossible as long as the person remains committed to both courses of action or both goals. This imbalance gives rise to the experience of stress.

The major points of Lazarus's theory are discussed below.

Conflict as a Stressor

The concept of conflict is useful in identifying the stresses that help cause disturbed coping patterns. Conflict often explains such observable behaviors as hesitation, vacillation, blocking, and fatigue. Conflict is frequently seen in the behavior of psychotic clients, who may have difficulty making even the simplest decisions.

The following conflicts are the most likely to cause stress:

- Conflicts that involve social relations with significant people
- Conflicts that involve ethical standards
- Conflicts that involve meeting unconscious needs
- Conflicts that involve the problems of everyday family living

A conflict proceeds according to the following four steps:

1.   The person holds two goals simultaneously.

2. The person moves in relation to both of the goals, using
   a. Approach-avoidance movements, or
   b. Avoidance-avoidance movements.
3. The person shows hesitation, vacillation, blocking, or fatigue.
4. Resolution occurs either temporarily or permanently.

Conflict with Approach-Avoidance Movements

When a person holds two incompatible goals at the same time, the goals usually constitute an either-or situation. If the person chooses one goal, the other goal is rejected or abolished automatically. This situation is called a double approach-avoidance conflict. Here is an example:

Mrs. R holds two goals. She wants to talk with the nurse about her fears of going back to work. At the same time, she wants not to be perceived as weak or "a bother." Mrs. R makes a movement in relation to her first goal—talking to the nurse—by walking up to her. When the nurse stops and turns toward her, Mrs. R asks some superficial question about her supper. In this way she avoids discussing her real concerns. When the nurse offers an opening to talk further, Mrs. R avoids the conversation she needs by saying she wants to rest. An hour later, she rings the bell with an apologetic but vague question about her medication.

Vacillation describes Mrs. R's behavior.

Principles That Explain Vacillation

To understand how vacillation comes to be the manifest behavior and what is going on during a conflict situation like the one described above, one needs to understand four key principles.

1. As you near a desirable goal, the approach tendency is strengthened.
2. As you near an undesirable goal, the avoidance tendency is strengthened.
3. The strength of the avoidance tendency always increases more rapidly with nearness to the goal than does the strength of the approach tendency.
4. The strength of both tendencies varies with the strength of the need basic to the tendencies. That is, an increased need can strengthen both tendencies and intensify the conflict, while a decreased need can weaken both tendencies and lessen the conflict.

Avoidance-Avoidance Conflict

In avoidance-avoidance conflict, a person is faced with two undesirable goals at the same time. The person attempts to avoid the nearer of these two goals, but with the retreat from the nearer goal, the tendency to avoid the second goal increases. Unless the tendency to avoid one of the goals overpowers the tendency to avoid the other, or unless there is a third way out of the conflict, the person feels trapped by the conflict.

Robert P, the 35-year-old son of well-to-do parents, was strongly attracted to "the good life." He wanted to live in a creative, esthetic environment, read good books, attend the opera, drink quality wine. Simultaneously he wanted both to avoid working to earn the money for the life-style he desired and not to depend on his parents for support. His life-style became one of waiting to find a resolution to his conflict. He neither worked nor accepted "handouts" from his family, but his preferred life-style became one that he talked about rather than lived.

ANXIETY

Anxiety is a state of uneasiness or discomfort experienced to varying degrees. It is frequently coupled with guilt, doubts, fears, and obsessions. Beyond the mild level, anxiety is often described as a feeling of terror or dread; anxiety is believed to be the most uncomfortable feeling a person can experience. In fact, anxiety is so uncomfortable that most persons try to get rid of it as soon as possible.

Anxiety is a potent force, for the energy it provides can be converted into destructive or constructive action. When it is used destructively, anxiety can immobilize a person with problems. When it is used constructively, anxiety can stimulate the action necessary to alter the stressful situation, fill a painful need, arrange a compromise, and so forth. It is easier to use anxiety constructively when a client understands its source.

Sources of Anxiety

Anxiety is an inevitable condition of human existence in the attempt to maintain equilibrium in a changing world.

People experience anxiety in many different kinds of situations and interpersonal relationships. The stimulus varies with the individual. However, the general causes of anxiety have been classified into two major kinds of threats:

1. Threats to biologic integrity: actual or impending interference with basic human needs such as the need for food, drink, or warmth
2. Threats to the security of the self:
    a. Unmet expectations important to self-integrity
    b. Unmet needs for status and prestige
    c. Anticipated disapproval by significant others
    d. Inability to gain or reinforce self-respect or to gain recognition from others
    e. Guilt, or discrepancies between self-view and actual behavior

It is crucial to understand that either actual *or* impending interference may cause anxiety (i.e., actual interference with a biologic or psychosocial need is not a necessary condition). All that is necessary for anxiety to arise is the *anticipation* of one of these major threats.

Threats to biologic integrity or to the fulfillment of such basic human needs as food, drink, warmth, and shelter are a general cause of anxiety. Threats to the security of self are not as easily categorized. In some instances, they are obvious; in others, they are more obscure because each person's sense of self is unique. To one person, power and prestige may be essential; to another, independence; to a third, being of service to others.

Consider the last category—being of service to others. Suppose that Mrs. C, a nurse, is convinced that a particular client would feel much better if he expressed his fears to her. But no matter how often she provides the opportunity, he insists, "This is not the time to talk about it," and thwarts her attempt. She is not able to help him in a way that is important to her sense of self. In addition, she believes that the unit's head nurse (whose communication skills she admires) expects her to have been successful in this endeavor. When unmet needs or expectations related to essential values (e.g., being of service to the client) are coupled with the actual or anticipated disapproval of others who are important (the head nurse), anxiety is generated.

Anxiety as a Continuum

Many theorists conceptualize anxiety as a continuum. Mild to moderate anxiety can be functionally effective in that it helps us focus our attention and generates energy and

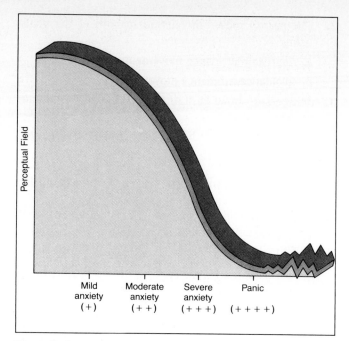

Figure 7–1
The effect of anxiety on the perceptual field.
Source: Adapted from Kneisl CR, Ames SW: Adult Health Nursing: A Biopsychosocial Approach. *Addison-Wesley, 1986, p 119.*

motivation. Thus, anxiety is an aspect of problem solving in that it alerts us to the need to concentrate our resources. However, severe anxiety and panic narrow our attention to a crippling degree. Under these conditions alertness is greatly reduced, and learning does not usually take place.

Mild Anxiety

Mild anxiety (+) helps one deal constructively with stress. A mildly anxious person has a broad perceptual field because mild anxiety heightens the ability to take in sensory stimuli. Such a person is more alert to what is going on and can make better sense of what is happening with others and the environment. The senses take in more—the person hears better, sees better, and makes logical connections between events (Figure 7–1). The person feels relatively safe and comfortable. Because learning is easier when one is mildly anxious, mild anxiety helps clients learn how best to give their own insulin. Mild anxiety can also help a nursing student review psychiatric-mental health nursing before a final examination.

Moderate Anxiety

In moderate anxiety (+ +), a person remains alert, but the perceptual field narrows (see Figure 7–1). The moderately anxious person shuts out the events on the periphery while focusing on central concerns. For example, the nursing student who is moderately anxious about the final examination may be able to focus so intently on studying that she or he is not distracted by an argument between roommates, loud music on the stereo, and a rousing chase scene on television. The student shuts out the chaos in the environment and focuses on what is of central personal importance—preparing for the exam. This process of taking in some sensory stimuli while excluding others is called selective inattention.

Selective inattention may also be used to cope with anxiety-provoking stimuli. This phenomenon may account for the anxious preoperative client who fails to remember what the nurse said about postoperative pain or the need to cough and deep breathe after surgery.

Although the perceptual field is narrowed and the person sees, hears, and grasps less, there is an element of voluntary control. The moderately anxious individual can, with direction, focus on what has previously been inattended.

Severe Anxiety

In severe anxiety ($+++$), sensory reception is greatly reduced (see Figure 7–1). Severely anxious persons focus on small or scattered details of an experience. They have

difficulty in problem solving, and their ability to organize is also reduced. They seldom have the complete picture. Selective inattention may be increased and may be less amenable to voluntary control. The person may be unable to focus on events in the environment. New stimuli may be experienced as overwhelming and may cause the anxiety level to rise even higher.

The sympathetic nervous system is activated in severe anxiety, causing an increase in pulse, blood pressure, and respiration and an increase in epinephrine secretion, vasoconstriction, and even body temperature. A multitude of physiologic changes may be observed, which are described in the section that follows.

Panic

The panic level of anxiety ($++++$) is characterized by a completely disrupted perceptual field (see Figure 7–1). Panic has been described as a disintegration of the person-

---

RESEARCH NOTE

Citation

Scott DW: Anxiety, critical thinking and information processing during and after breast biopsy. Nurs Res 1983;32:24–28.

Study Problem/Purpose

The purpose of this study was to examine how an individual's level of anxiety, critical-thinking ability, and capacity to process information (time perception) were affected during times of stress.

Methods

The subjects in the study were eighty-five women who were admitted to a large urban hospital for breast biopsy. The ranged in age from 18 to 60. No subject had a previous diagnosis of cancer. Subjects were tested after hospitalization but before test results were known. The surgical procedure was performed under general anesthesia, and only those subjects who were found to have a benign condition continued in the study. These subjects were retested in the postcrisis period, six to eight weeks after biopsy.

Anxiety was measured by the administration of a twenty-item paper-and-pencil inventory, the State-Trait Anxiety Inventory (STAI). Critical thinking ability was measured by the Watson-Glaser Critical Thinking Appraisal (CTA). Scott used judged duration to measure the estimated time it took for a subject to process information.

Findings

Anxiety levels of subjects prior to their knowledge of diagnosis was extremely high. With high levels of anxiety, subjects had increasing difficulty in reasoning and decision making.

Critical thinking or general reasoning ability was substantially reduced at the time of hospitalization when compared with six to eight weeks after discharge.

Although not statistically significant, judged duration, a measure of information processing, tended to be greater during crisis than at a time six to eight weeks later.

Implications

These subjects with high anxiety, low critical-thinking ability, and low capacity for information processing constitute a high-risk group in need of special support measures. The reasoning ability of these clients may be compromised at a time when critical decisions are required, e.g., decisions relating to surgical procedures, informed consent, and other therapeutic actions. When planning care, the nurse should consider these variables and pay particular attention to the period of early hospitalization when the client may be least able to make responsible decisions. The nurse may then provide the needed education, clarification, or consultation.

ality that is experienced as intense terror. Details may be enlarged, scattered, or distorted. Logical thinking and effective decision making may be impossible. The person in panic is unable to initiate or maintain goal-directed action. Behavior may appear purposeless, and communication may be unintelligible.

Not all those in panic behave alike. At the scene of an auto accident in which an elderly couple lost control of the travel trailer they were towing, the husband remained immobile in the driver's seat, hands firmly fixed to the steering wheel, eyes focused on some distant spot despite the threat of explosion from the smoking car. The wife ran around in circles. Having lost her shoes in the accident, she was unaware she was running through the broken glass of the windshield in her bare feet despite numerous bleeding cuts.

Recognizing Anxiety

Anxiety can be assessed in the physiologic, cognitive, and emotional/behavioral dimensions. This observation illustrates the relationship between the mind and the body. Anxiety is a multidimensional phenomenon in that the total person is involved in every aspect of it. Objective data, particularly nursing observations, may be critical because of the nature of anxiety. Selective inattention and dissociation interfere with the client's awareness of anxiety and ability to give accurate reports. Families and friends also can contribute data useful to the assessment of anxiety.

Physiologic Dimension

Observations of the client's physiologic state are likely to indicate autonomic nervous system responses, particularly sympathetic effects. Various organs may be affected, such as the adrenal medulla, heart, blood vessels, lungs, stomach, colon, rectum, salivary glands, liver, pupils of the eyes, and sweat glands (Figure 7–2). Anxious clients may have an increased heart rate, increased blood pressure, difficulty in breathing, sweaty palms, trembling, dry mouth, "butterflies in the stomach" or a "lump in the throat," as well as other symptoms.

Laboratory tests are not routinely done to evaluate anxiety because observation is faster and more accurate, but anxiety affects the results of laboratory tests. Blood studies may show increased adrenal function, elevated levels of glucose and lactic acid, and decreased parathyroid function and oxygen and calcium levels. Urinary studies

may indicate increased levels of epinephrine and norepinephrine.

Cognitive Dimension

Assessment of cognitive function may indicate difficulty in logical thinking, narrowed or distorted perceptual field, selective inattention or dissociation, lack of attention to details, difficulty in concentrating, or difficulty in focusing. The extent to which cognitive function is affected is determined by the level of anxiety. Mild, moderate, severe, or panic level of anxiety is assessed according to the descriptions earlier in this chapter.

Emotional/Behavioral Dimension

In the emotional/behavioral dimension, clients may be irritable, angry, withdrawn, and restless, or they may cry. The affective response can often be assessed through the client's subjective description. Clients may describe themselves as "on edge," "uptight," "jittery," "nervous," "worried," or "tense." They may feel dizzy or faint and may experience a feeling of impending doom as if something terrible were about to happen.

COPING WITH STRESS AND ANXIETY

Nurses can be helpful if they understand the changes the client is undergoing. Reactions to threatening situations, such as illness and hospitalization, can be divided into two general categories: task-oriented and defense-oriented responses. When we feel competent to deal with stress and the situation is not too threatening to our sense of self, our behavior tends to be task oriented. Task-oriented behavior is geared toward problem solving. A student who is majoring in mathematics fails his courses. If he is not too frightened by the possibility that he may not be suited for a career in this field, he can assess the situation and change his major. This is a task-oriented reaction. It is based on a realistic appraisal of the situation and involves a series of carefully thought-out judgments about what course of behavior would be most effective.

When we feel inadequate to cope with stress and the situation is extremely threatening to our sense of self, we tend to engage in defense-oriented reactions. The diagnosis of a terminal illness, for instance, may be so overwhelming that a person must temporarily defend against acknowledging this reality. Everyone uses defense-oriented behavior from time to time as a protective measure. Such behavior becomes harmful only when it is the predominant means of coping with stress. In such cases, problem-solving and reality-based behavior are continually avoided.

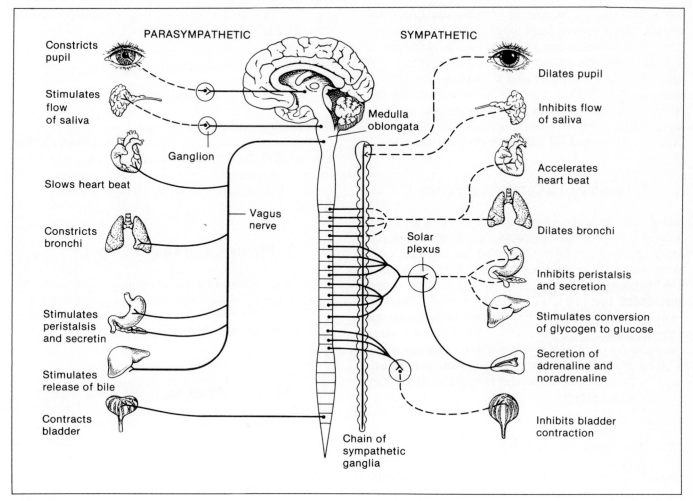

Figure 7–2
The autonomic nervous system and some of the organs it innervates. In anxiety,
sympathetic nervous system responses are most common.
Source: Ramsey JM: Basic Pathophysiology: Modern Stress and the Disease Process. *Addison-Wesley,
1982, p 46.*

Coping strategies are a set of behaviors persons under stress use in struggling to improve their situations. Coping strategies can be thought of simply as ways of getting along in the world.

Everyday Ways of Coping with Stress

Everyday coping strategies offer an immense repertoire of defenses to maintain control and balance in the face of stress. A person can cope on different levels, including the physical, social, cognitive, and emotional levels. However,

the devices people choose to cope with stress depend on many factors. Among them are the external circumstances, the suddenness and intensity of the stress, the resources available to the person, and the person's predisposition to one or another coping pattern. Certain coping patterns are established in the course of one's development. One man who is late for an appointment because he gets caught in a traffic jam may react with a furious outburst of anger. Another may begin to daydream and forget where he is going. A third may use the time to solve some problem.

Most often, individuals use behaviors that have worked well for them in the past. Sometimes they behave in a certain way because it is the only method they have of coping with stress or because other coping strategies failed to work. Some persons learn to turn to others for protection and nurturance; some learn to turn to chemicals or to food; some rely on self-discipline and keeping a stiff upper lip; others feel better after the intense expression of feelings; some withdraw physically and/or emotionally; still others work out or talk the problem out. Table 7–2 lists some of the common coping methods identified in the literature. Some general categories are discussed below.

Turning to a Comforting Person

No doubt the earliest coping strategy is the familiar method of turning to a mothering figure for soothing and protecting. To get love is to be reassured that one is lovable. Love from supportive others may take the form of physical touching, rocking, patting, or verbal reassurances of various kinds ("Don't be afraid, I'll stay with you"). This category also includes the function of eating in times of stress and for general support. Alcohol, nicotine, and other chemicals are often used to enhance well-being in the face of stress. Many theorists view these alternatives as substitutes for the dependent comfort of being a baby in the care of a mothering parent.

Relying on Self-Discipline

Whereas some people under stress tend to turn to the comfort of friendly company, food, or alcohol—all of which are reminiscent of childhood dependency—others rely on self-discipline. Self-control ranks high in the value system of many cultures and subcultures. This coping style involves pride in the ability to laugh off problems, endure frustrations, and discount anxiety. Keep a stiff upper lip, bite the bullet, and get over it are all admonitions that people address to themselves when self-discipline is their patterned response to stress. These people are unlikely to want the company of supportive others and may even push them away. They are often unresponsive when others seek comfort from them, for they see such dependency as weak.

Intense Expression of Feeling

Crying, swearing, and laughing all tend to relieve tension. Swearing loses its usefulness as an escape valve if it becomes a habit. This is less likely to be true of crying and of laughing. Crying and laughing tend to release energy and exert a soothing effect on a person who is experiencing tension.

Avoidance and Withdrawal

While some people find it hard to sleep when they are under tension, others react to worries, bad news, or an argument with somnolence. Still others respond with a form of waking sleep like apathy or emotional withdrawal, which accomplishes the same thing.

Talking It Out

Many people relieve tension by talking it out. Talking implies establishing and maintaining a contact of sorts with another human being. In addition, it enables new ideas to emerge and new perspectives to be entertained. Obviously, this device is the medium of most therapeutic intervention.

Privately Thinking It Through

Some people believe that the unexamined life is not worth living. When faced with a problem that causes them anxiety, these individuals become introspective about it. The rationalizations that emerge serve as effective tension relievers.

Working It Off

Acting to relieve tension may range from pointless activity such as finger tapping, floor pacing, and door slamming to activities purposely designed to alter the tension-producing circumstances. In addition, some tense individuals feel a lot of aggressive energy. Physical exertion in the form of demanding sports, like soccer or tennis, or manual labor, like washing walls or scrubbing the floor, is a way to use this energy constructively.

Using Symbolic Substitutes

Stress may be relieved by ascribing symbolic values to acts or objects. These acts or objects may or may not have other meanings. There are symbolic devices for the management of tensions in religious conventions like meditation, confession, prayer, or sacrifice. For some people, the automobile has a symbolic significance; others ascribe symbolic significance to their annual income or their physical appearance.

The list is almost endless, but the principle is always the same. Some people attach a meaning beyond the obvious one to objects, experiences, and people. Through their involvement with these meanings, they find a means to reduce their tensions.

Somatizing

Many organs have an expression and communication function. This is sometimes known as *somatizing* or *organ language.* Some organs communicate their messages only to their owner. For example, the heart may communicate by means of palpitation. Other demonstrations are public, e.g., blushing or stuttering. Urination and defecation, increased sweating, and altered sexual activity are other familiar examples of organ language.

Coping Resources

Early classic research on coping was concerned with how individuals respond to specific stresses in a laboratory setting. More recent studies that consider the whole being in interaction with the environment have helped in viewing coping as a dynamic process that involves the demands and restrictions on a client as well as the resources available. For example, according to Antonovsky (1980), persons stay healthy or cope adequately with stress because they possess what he calls *generalized resistance resources* (GRRs). A GRR is any factor in the person, group, or organization that helps in managing tension.

Physical and biochemical GRRs are physiologic characteristics, such as genetic features and levels of immunity. These GRRs also include interaction of the nervous and endocrine systems that help in adaptation (e.g., interactions involving adrenocorticotropic hormone or ACTH, thyroid-stimulating hormone or TSH, vasopressin, norepinephrine, and insulin and their influence on human behavior). Not only are individuals different in their genetic and biochemical makeup, but the physiologic effects of illness and stress may also alter the person's ability to use physical and biochemical GRRs positively.

Material goods and relative wealth constitute the *artifactual and material* GRRs; having these attributes makes it easier to cope with illness. Money helps to ensure the best health care available. Effective coping is often interrelated with one's socioeconomic status simply because the higher the socioeconomic status, the greater the resources to help the person cope. For example, household help not only relieves an ill person's worries but also reduces the practical burden.

Cognitive GRRs have to do with intelligence and knowledge. When persons know about stressors, they can avoid them. They can also predict when periods of stress are imminent and thus reduce their impact. Knowing what community services are available is also a cognitive GRR.

Emotional GRRs are possessed by those who are self-aware—who know their own capacities and potentials and have a well-developed sense of themselves. Emotional GRRs determine the extent of psychologic hardiness. In general, they have to do with how competent and self-assured one feels.

Valuative and attitudinal GRRs are the products of a person's culture and environment. Persons are apt to respond in learned ways. The attitudinal aspect also is related to how flexible, rational, and farsighted the person is. The more rational or accurate one's appraisal of a threatening situation and the more flexible one is in approaching the situation and envisioning the consequences, the greater one's resources for coping.

Interpersonal-relational GRRs are available social support systems. The greater a person's social contacts, the greater the social resources available to augment the ability to deal with stress. Love, affection, and nurturance are hallmarks of interpersonal-relational GRRs.

Institutional structures that facilitate coping are called *macrosociocultural* GRRs. These resources include governmental programs such as Aid to Dependent Children as well as cultural institutions such as death and funeral rites, religious rituals, and ceremonies.

According to this model, the ability to cope is determined by the extent and effectiveness of each person's generalized resistance resources. Yet the actual process of coping remains unclear. Exactly which personal resources should be mobilized and under which conditions still is not fully understood.

Little research has been performed on the preferred coping methods of "normal" subjects (those not facing a crisis). Ziemer (1982) found that over 50 percent of the study population reported that their preferred method of coping was to talk to someone. This finding has profound implications for nursing, because nurses are the health care providers who spend the most time with clients. It also has profound implications for clients whose communication is dysfunctional or whose ability to communicate freely is restricted. Psychiatric clients generally fall into these categories.

Defense-Oriented Ways of Coping

The coping strategies described above are considered normal. They are simply ways of getting along. In some people, however, what passes for a normal adjustment is actually a very tenuous one with few outlets for controlled aggression, few sublimations, few love objects, few opportunities for satisfaction and growth. These people find it more and more difficult to cope with additional stress. Ultimately the external stress that the person is trying unsuccessfully to ward off is matched by a mounting internal stress. The person suffers both from increased anxiety and from the strain on overworked stabilizers. And, what happens to the client who has no one to talk with, who can't jog 5 miles, or who can't laugh off the problem?

When a person is unable to ward off stress or reduce tension in the usual way, anxiety mounts as the client feels increasingly inadequate to cope with the situation. Under these circumstances, the person is more likely to engage in *defense-oriented behavior.* Defense-oriented behavior is not a specific attempt to solve a problem. It consists of using mental mechanisms to lessen uncomfortable feelings of anxiety and to prevent pain regardless of cost. These characteristic mental mechanisms are commonly called **defense mechanisms.** They protect the self by enabling us to deny or distort a stressful event or by restricting awareness and reducing the sense of emotional involvement. But they can also interfere with rational decision-making. People who use defense mechanisms are excluding some information about the situation they are in. They are also denying their own feelings about it.

Defense mechanisms are primarily unconscious and often inflexible coping patterns that protect a person through intrapsychic distortions that are really self-deceptions. The person usually has little awareness of what is happening or even less control over events. Although these reactions may help keep the lid on anxiety, they also limit the ability to grow from and savor the experience, they interfere with rational decision making and the ability to work productively, and they impair and erode interpersonal relationships. Even adaptive devices can go wrong.

Because human behavior is so complex and various, classification of defense mechanisms is necessarily incomplete. Often, they are classified according to whether they are simple or complex, whether they are most likely to arise in a specific phase of development, or whether they are commonly associated with a particular form of psychopathology. Definitions of various defense mechanisms overlap, and the same observed behavior may often be explained by more than one type of defense. People do not use one method of defense at a time. Usually they rely on a combination of defenses. For study purposes, the common defense mechanisms discussed here are: repression, suppression, disassociation, identification, introjection, projection, denial, fantasy, rationalization, reaction formation, displacement, and intellectualization. They are summarized in Table 7–3.

Repression

Repression, the basis of all defense mechanisms, is the dynamic behind much of "forgetting." When persons repress, they unconsciously exclude distressing emotions, thoughts, or experiences from awareness. It is initiated to bar access to consciousness of feelings and thoughts that would cause anxiety and thus disrupt the self-concept. It also affords protection from sudden, traumatic experience until the individual is able to deal with the shock. From the individual's point of view, a repressed memory is "forgotten" and cannot be deliberately brought to awareness. The repressed feelings remain out of awareness but continue to exert pressure for expression. The self must exert energy to maintain the repression and in instances of extreme stress may not be able to sustain repression. In situations of extreme anxiety and in febrile or toxic states, repression may begin to fail. Clients who are intoxicated by alcohol or drugs or who are emerging from anesthesia may verbalize feelings that they usually repress.

Susan was raped. She was brought to an outpatient clinic by her roommate. Susan said she felt very anxious and could not recall the circumstances surrounding the rape or what the rapist looked like. Her use of repression protected her from facing her fears and humiliation.

Nursing intervention in such cases should be supportive and protective of the client's defenses. After the initial shock has lessened and the client's anxiety level has been reduced, the client can be helped to examine the traumatic event.

Suppression

Suppression is an intentional act that helps to keep thoughts, feelings, wishes, or actions that cause anxiety out of conscious awareness. Suppression is the conscious analog of repression.

A middle-aged male business executive discovers bright red rectal bleeding the day before he is to leave for a visit to his company's international offices in three European countries. Worrying about the bleeding interferes with his concentration and his ability to complete a report about the division he heads. His decision to put off worrying about the bleeding until he returns in three weeks is an example of using suppression to deal with the emotional discomfort of this discovery.

A client may refuse to consider his difficulties by saying that he "doesn't want to talk about it" or that he will "think about it some other time." This, too, is suppression. Suppression can be dealt with in the same way as repression. Suppression is generally easier to deal with because the material remains conscious. We can be somewhat more directive in assessing why the client avoids talking about a situation, and we can suggest that the client try to look

Table 7–3
Defense Mechanisms

Name	Definition	Example
Repression	Unconsciously keeping unacceptable feelings out of awareness	A man is jealous of a good friend's success but is unaware of his feelings.
Suppression	Consciously keeping unacceptable feelings and thoughts out of awareness	A student taking an examination is upset about an argument with her boyfriend but puts it out of her mind so she can finish the test.
Dissociation	Handling emotional conflicts, or internal or external stressors, by a temporary alteration of consciousness or identity	A woman has amnesia for the events surrounding a fatal automobile accident in which she was the speeding driver.
Identification	Unconscious assumption of similarity between oneself and another	After hospitalization for minor surgery a girl decides to be a nurse.
Introjection	Acceptance of another's values and opinions as one's own	A woman who prefers a simple life-style assumes the materialistic, prestige-oriented values of her husband.
Projection	Attributing one's own unacceptable feelings and thoughts to others	A man who is quite critical of others thinks that people are joking about his appearance.
Denial	Blocking out painful or anxiety-inducing events or feelings	A boss tells an employee he may have to fire him. On the way home the employee shops for a new car.
Fantasy	Symbolic satisfaction of wishes through nonrational thought	A student struggling through graduate school thinks about a prestigious, high-paying job he wants.
Rationalization	Falsification of experience through the construction of logical or socially approved explanations of behavior	A man cheats on his income tax return and tells himself it's all right because everyone does it.
Reaction formation	Unacceptable feelings disguised by repression of the real feeling and by reinforcement of the opposite feeling	A woman who dislikes her mother-in-law is always very nice to her.
Displacement	Discharging of pent-up feelings on persons less dangerous than those who initially aroused the emotion	A student who has received a low grade on a term paper blows up at his girl friend when she asks about his grade.
Intellectualization	Separating an emotion from an idea or thought because the emotional reaction is too painful to be acknowledged	A man learns from his doctor that he has cancer. He studies the physiology and treatment of cancer without experiencing any emotion.

at the situation because it affects future plans. Offering him information about rectal bleeding may enable him to look at his situation objectively. As he learns more about his condition, it may become less threatening to him.

Dissociation

In **dissociation**, the individual handles emotional conflicts, or internal or external stressors, by a temporary alteration

of consciousness or identity (see Chapter 19 for specific mental dysfunctions in which dissociation is the major mental mechanism). Dissociation resembles repression, but it has a different origin. The self is formed through the process of disapproval and approval from significant other people. Therefore the self *dissociates* or refuses awareness to the expression of personal qualities and experiences that significant other people disapprove of. These feelings come to exist separately from the person's self-concept. A little girl with latent artistic abilities that are not validated by her parents will not think of herself as artistic. She may deny her abilities even when other people point them out.

People who express dissociated feelings or qualities do not "notice" what they are doing. This limitation of awareness is maintained because the person experiences anxiety whenever permissible levels for the self are trespassed.

Ms T consciously believes that sexual overtures are wrong, yet she behaves seductively toward men. She cannot understand why men see her behavior as a sexual invitation. The use of repression or dissociation complicates Ms T's problems. She needs to ignore or deny aspects of her situation in order to feel comfortable in it. Other people notice and point out Ms T's seductive behavior, but she cannot recognize it because it is not a part of her self-concept. If Ms T admitted her sexual feelings she would experience severe anxiety and personality disorganization.

Identification

Identification is the wish to be like another person and to assume the characteristics of that person's personality. It represents an estrangement from our own personality. Identification is unconscious. In this it differs from *imitation,* which is the conscious copying of another person's qualities. Identification with admired persons can serve an important function in maturation by evoking latent qualities. The little girl identifies with her mother and sisters and thus learns the behavioral characteristics of womanhood.

The most primitive type of identification is seen in the infant's relationship with the mother. Infants seem to perceive no difference between their mothers and themselves and only gradually become aware that their mothers exist apart from them. Small children deal with people in terms of how these people meet their needs. They do not see them as separate persons with needs of their own. Such identifications may persist into adult life in people who have not differentiated themselves psychologically from seemingly powerful parents.

One specific manifestation of identification is an attitude of passive receptivity rather than reciprocity in relationships. People who feel they have no resources of their own will overvalue the resources of others and expect to be taken care of. People who are most identified with their parents tend to be people who were not allowed to develop their own individuality. Part of the process of self-realization occurs in adolescence, when we discard, with much anxiety and insecurity, our identification with the parents on whom we have been so dependent. Some clients may not have achieved a degree of self-identity sufficient to enable them to do this. Continuing the process of identification can inhibit our usefulness, because it prevents us from focusing on our own capacities.

Identification can be seen in clients who rely heavily on the nurse's advice and support. They expect that all their needs will be met and that nothing will be expected of them.

Mr. L is diabetic. He is not interested in learning about the diet he must follow and the medication he must take. He expects the nurse to take the responsibility for seeing that he gets the right food and medicine. Identification prevents him from being self-reliant.

Nurses who work with clients like Mr. L should clarify what the client's expectations of the nurse are and then correct any misperceptions about the nurse's role. It is important to help the client increase his own skills and to take responsibility for his own care. Initially, the nurse can offer the client collaboration and interdependence. The long-term goal in dealing with identification is for the client to formulate a self-care plan independently of the nurse.

Introjection

Introjection is closely related to identification. It is the process of accepting another's values and opinions as one's own even if they contradict the values one had previously held. A man whose employer engages in shoddy workmanship may introject his employer's values even though they are contrary to his own moral beliefs because he is afraid of losing his job. Introjection also occurs in severe depression following the death of a loved person. The depressed person may assume many of the deceased person's characteristics and in so doing lose some self-awareness. The nurse can treat introjection like identification, remembering that introjection is more primitive and more intractable. It originates in our experience of being fed as infants. We incorporated people and objects into ourselves in the same way that we swallowed food. We felt a sense of oneness with everything in the external world and could not differentiate ourselves from others. Because thinking processes are not involved in the first experience of introjection, this defense tends to be difficult to explore on the verbal level.

Projection

Projection is an unconscious means of dealing with personal difficulties or unacceptable wishes by attributing them to others. We blame other people for our shortcomings or see them as harboring our own unacceptable feelings or thoughts. In the course of development, the child, who needs the parents' approval, will identify with them and will also deny what they seem to condemn or fail to acknowledge. For instance, if her parents do not openly express and recognize angry feelings, a little girl will tend to regard anger as dangerous. She will then deny awareness of her own anger. Anger in others will disturb her, and she will tend to condemn in others the anger she cannot accept in herself. It is common knowledge that people often tend to criticize others for their own unacknowledged inferiorities. The person who fears being taken advantage of is often an opportunist.

In adult life, projection can be destructive if it interferes with our ability to acknowledge our own feelings. The tendency to attribute our own undesired feelings to others also blurs the boundaries between ourselves and others. This, in turn, makes it difficult to understand other people's feelings. People who make excessive use of projection tend to attribute to others hostile or seductive motives that do not actually exist. This prevents them from forming trusting and reciprocal relationships. A tendency to projection may also interfere with problem solving. A young woman who believes she is failing a course because of her teacher will not focus her energies on her studies.

Clients who must deal with the stress of serious illness may shift the blame for their condition onto the nurse. They may complain of poor nursing care to a nurse who is actually very skillful. These clients may actually fear that they have caused their own problems by neglecting their health. They may believe that they are being "paid back" for wrongdoing in the past. If nurses feel that such a client is accusing them falsely, they should not show anger or retaliate but should show, through consistency and attention, that they respect these clients and are concerned about their welfare. As clients feel more secure in the nurse-client relationship, nurses can encourage these clients to explore the realistic aspects of their situation. For example, a man who blames his family for his alcoholism can be helped to explore objectively what is known about the etiology of alcoholism. This may help him come to terms with his feelings of guilt and anger. This type of intervention helps the client to separate his own feelings from the objective facts of the situation.

Denial

Denial of reality is one of the simplest of the defense mechanisms. In denial, painful or anxiety-producing aspects of awareness are blocked out of consciousness. The reality of a situation is either completely disregarded or transformed so that it is no longer threatening. Denial is one of the commonest defenses against the stress of diagnosis and illness and is typically present in the first few minutes of adjustment to the death of a loved person. It may be helpful as a temporary protection against the full impact of a traumatic event.

A father reacts with denial when he shouts, "No, it can't be true; there must be a mistake," when told his 8-year-old son has just died in the trauma unit of injuries incurred when his bicycle collided with an automobile.

A young woman admitted to a psychiatric hospital because of acute anxiety and frightening hallucinations says she just "needs a rest."

Sometimes denial is the best solution for the client. In such situations, the defense should be supported. A terminally ill client who believes she will soon recover and who cannot think about her illness should be allowed the protection of denial. Not all clients need to face up to reality. The nurse should recognize that denial may be preventing serious personality disorganization.

Sometimes, however, denial is directly harmful to the client, as when a man refuses to take medication that is crucial to his survival. In such cases, the motivation for the client's behavior should be assessed. Once the particular protective function the denial is serving has been discovered, the nurse can focus attention on helping the client meet these needs in a way that is not self-destructive. The nurse can also help by taking care not to reinforce patterns of denial but rather to focus on instances when the client seems to be dealing with reality.

Fantasy

Fantasy is a form of nonrational mental activity that enables the individual to escape temporarily the demands of the everyday world. Fantasies are not confined by the reality consideration of cause and effect and time and space. Fantasy normally characterizes the thinking of children before they are able to engage in consensually validated communication. Adults revert to fantasy during times of stress to obtain a symbolic satisfaction of wishes.

A businesswoman facing financial difficulties temporarily escapes by daydreaming that she is enjoying a luxurious vacation on a Caribbean island.

Another woman with advanced multiple sclerosis imagines herself a famous ballerina with complete control of her body.

A man whose wife has told him she wants a divorce imagines how much his wife will appreciate him now that he has been diagnosed with cancer.

Fantasy may offer temporary relief from pressures, but people who spend too much time in fantasy may be unable to meet the requirements of reality.

Clients who are very ill may fantasize that when they recover many good things will happen to them. They may imagine that they will receive special recognition in their work or that they will get along better with their families. These fantasies may help such clients deal with the deprivations caused by illness. However, they may also cause unrealistic expectations. Such clients may expect to be paid back for their suffering. They may cherish "suffering hero" fantasies. These fantasies provide some measure of compensatory gratification but interfere with problem solving.

Clients who are engaging in fantasy related to their illness need gradual help in assessing the responses others are likely to make and the achievements they themselves may realistically expect. Clients who fail to adjust to reality will be very disappointed when their grandiose expectations are not met.

A helpful approach that will not devastate clients who need to hold onto some fantasy is to ask them to discuss their specific future plans. Examining the details of work and interpersonal adjustment may help a person to relinquish unrealistic expectations and make more realistic plans. For example, the man who believes that a diagnosis of cancer will improve his marriage because his wife will appreciate him more fully must recognize that this is improbable. He needs to examine the real effects his illness will have on her. He must plan how to make specific improvements in their communication by anticipating problem areas.

Imagination does have a creative aspect, however. Fantasies have a richness and variety that is lacking in the everyday world. Certain artists, such as Dali and Picasso, enrich their works of art through fantasy. Evidence also exists that insights into scientific discovery do not come about as the result of step-by-step logical thinking. Rather, they are created through fantasy.

Rationalization

Rationalization is the substitution of "good" or plausible reasons for questionable behavior to justify it or to deal with disappointment. Rationalizing helps to avoid social disapproval and to bolster flagging self-esteem.

A nurse fails to return to the bedside of the elderly nursing home client despite a promise to do so before leaving work. She feels her behavior is justified because the client has problems with recent memory and probably wouldn't remember anyway.

Many people use rationalization because they wish to prove to themselves or others that their actions are governed by reason and common sense—even though they may not fully understand the reasons for their own behavior. Such explanations may be essential to maintain personal integrity. They are not destructive as long as they do not prevent one from solving everyday problems.

Rationalization becomes more of a hindrance when it prevents us from making necessary changes in our behavior by interfering with our ability to examine that behavior. One sign of rationalization is an active search for reasons to justify our behavior or beliefs. Another is an inability to recognize inconsistencies in our beliefs. A third is being upset when our reasons are questioned, since such questioning threatens our defenses.

Clients may use rationalization to soften the blow of losses caused by illness. Work interrupted by illness may be given up prematurely if the client rationalizes that he or she wouldn't have been successful in that field anyway. Such unnecessary restrictions deprive us of possible achievements.

Nurses must respect their clients' need to rationalize fears and insecurities they cannot face. However, nurses must hold open the possibility for change. Such clients must be helped to face the reality of their situation by being encouraged to explore ways in which they can change to deal with it more effectively. One way is to help them explore in detail past instances in which they did change to cope with a stressful situation. Believing that we have real strengths helps us to face areas of insecurity.

Reaction Formation

Reaction formation is a means of defense whereby an undesirable impulse is kept out of awareness by emphasizing its opposite. To protect ourselves from recognizing dangerous feelings, we develop conscious attitudes and behavior patterns that are just the opposite of those feelings. Hostility may be concealed behind a facade of love and kindness. The desire to be sexually promiscuous may be concealed behind a moralistic demeanor. People who use this defense are not conscious of their true feelings.

People who crusade passionately against alcohol, pornography, or cruelty to animals may be dealing with an underlying wish to enjoy these things. Of course, this is not true of everyone who is devoted to a cause. Clues that reaction formation is occurring are an inappropriate intensity of feeling and the inability to consider alternative points of view. The person who is always unnaturally sweet and loving and cannot consider the possibility of being angry is probably using this excess of feeling to counteract an unacceptable anger.

Reaction formation can be useful. It can help us maintain socially approved behavior and avoid awareness of desires that are not socially acceptable. But this defense, too, results in self-deception, because it is not under conscious control. Therefore, it may result in exaggerated or rigid behaviors that leave us ill equipped to deal with crisis. People who feel they can never express annoyance and discomfort may need to be "good" clients, who never question their care or make demands. Such clients may not be able to allow themselves to depend on others. They may not be able to acknowledge their needs and seek fulfillment. This rigid stance is a reaction formation against the unconscious wish to be completely dependent. It is destructive because it masks the individual's needs. It also prevents the person from meeting a crisis with flexibility, because many possible actions are blocked from awareness. People who use this particular defense may also be excessively harsh in dealing with other people's weaknesses. They may be unable or unwilling to help others because they think everyone should be able to solve their own problems.

Coping with reaction formation requires essentially the same approach as coping with repression. The nurse should respect and support the client's defenses while providing a secure relationship in which to explore feelings and new behavioral alternatives. Nurses must also be aware that it is easy to be annoyed at clients who cannot face their true feelings. The rigid and excessive display of what seems to be an insincere emotion can be frustrating. It is important for nurses to remember that these clients are not "lying" or pretending. They are unconsciously protecting themselves against having to recognize threatening feelings.

Displacement

Displacement is the discharging of pent-up feelings, generally hostility, on an object less dangerous than the object that aroused the feelings. This defense is used when emotions are aroused in a situation where it would be dangerous to express them.

John has just failed an important examination. He believes his failure was the instructor's fault. He cannot express the full extent of his anger, because that would get him into worse trouble with the instructor. John goes quietly back to the dormitory. But when his roommate turns the stereo on too loud, John explodes. He doesn't fear retaliation from his roommate—they are peers and friends.

In some cases, anger aroused by another person may be turned inward on the self. When this happens, the individual experiences exaggerated self-accusations and guilt.

Clients may express inappropriate anger to the nurse when they are actually angry at someone or something else. The client may feel more secure with the nurse, who offers a safe target for displaced feelings. Displacement differs from projection in that people who use displacement are not distorting their feelings and attributing them to someone else. The feelings are clear, and the person acknowledges them. They are simply being directed at the wrong person. Therefore, it may be easier to help these clients acknowledge the real situation. This may be achieved by remaining calm and accepting during an angry outburst. An example of what the nurse can say after the outburst is over, is: "You seem so angry. I wonder if you really are angry that your breakfast is cold or if there might be some other reason." Opening up the possibility for a discussion of anger may help these clients to sort out just who they are angry at and why.

Intellectualization

Intellectualization is the process of separating the emotion aroused by an event from ideas or opinions about the event because the emotion itself is too painful to acknowledge. The painful emotion is avoided by means of a rational explanation that divests the event of any personal significance. Failures are made less significant by telling oneself that the situation could have been worse. A woman may deal with her husband's death by saying objectively that sudden death is better than chronic illness. A boy who breaks his pelvis skiing seeks consolation by reminding himself that he could have broken his neck.

Clients may use intellectualization to blunt the emotional impact of their problems. This may be difficult for the nurse to perceive, because such clients often seem to know a great deal about their condition. They may be able to discuss in great detail the metabolic processes in dia-

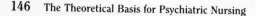

betes or the psychodynamics of anxiety. At the same time they cannot apply these concepts to their own situation in an emotional sense.

Intellectualization resembles rationalization in that it provides a verbal means of dealing with anxiety. Its use closes off the possibility of accepting and working out problems. Clients often use intellectualization at the onset of a crisis, and the need for this defense may decrease in a supportive nurse-client relationship. The nurse can help the client relate emotionally to a problem by not forcing the expression of feeling. This will only frighten the client further. Asking these clients to explain how their knowledge relates to them personally may encourage them to accept and explore their emotional reactions.

Chapter Highlights

- Stressful situations are those that tax a person's resources or coping capabilities, causing a negative effect. The source of the stress is known as a stressor.

- Selye's stress adaptation theory can be used to explain the physiologic effects of stress.

- A humanistic interactionist view of stress depends not only on external conditions but also on the constitutional vulnerability of the person and the adequacy of that person's coping styles. The humanistic interactionist view is consistent with how nurses view human experiences.

- Anxiety is an uncomfortable feeling that stems from threats to biologic integrity and the security of the self.

- Nurses can expect clients and their families to become anxious in the face of unknown or potentially painful, dangerous, or disfiguring events.

- Stress, changes, and threats to one's self-concept cause anxiety and place additional coping demands on the individual.

- The choice of coping strategy often depends on external circumstances, the suddenness and intensity of the stress, the resources available to the person, and a predisposition to a certain coping pattern.

- Persons cope with stress in a variety of ways that seem to have worked in the past. Some talk it over with others; some jog; others pray or laugh off the problem.

- When someone is unable to ward off stress or reduce anxiety in the usual way, tension mounts. Persons may have to rely on largely unconscious and inflexible coping patterns that are self-deceptive.

- Defense mechanisms may be used by anyone to cope with anxiety or stress, but a healthy person will more often use problem-solving methods.

- Defense mechanisms include repression, suppression, dissociation, identification, introjection, projection, denial, fantasy, rationalization, reaction formation, displacement, and intellectualization.

References

Antonovsky A: *Health, Stress, and Coping.* Jossey-Bass, 1980.

Cox T: *Stress.* University Park Press, 1979.

Dohrenwend BS, Dohrenwend BP (eds): *Stressful Life Events and Their Contexts.* Rutgers University Press, 1984.

Garber J, Seligman MEP: *Human Helplessness: Theory and Applications.* Academic Press, 1980.

Graydon JE: Measuring patient coping. *Nurs Papers* 1984;16:3–12.

Holmes TH, Rahe RH: The social readjustment rating scale. *J Psychosom Res* 1967;11:213–218.

Hopping B: Physiologic response to stress: A nursing concern. *Nurs Forum* 1980;19:259–269.

Jalowiec A, Powers MJ: Stress and coping in hypertensive and emergency room patients. *Nurs Res* 1980;30:13.

Kneisl CR, Ames SW: *Adult Health Nursing: A Biopsychosocial Approach.* Addison-Wesley, 1986.

Kobasa SC, Maddi SR, Kan S: Hardiness and health: A prospective study. *J Pers Soc Psychol* 1982;42:168–177.

Lazarus RS: *Patterns of Adjustment.* McGraw-Hill, 1976.

Lazarus RS: *Psychological Stress and the Coping Process.* McGraw-Hill, 1966.

Lazarus RS, Folkman S: An analysis of coping in a middle-aged community sample. *J Health Soc Behav* 1980; 21:219–239.

Lazarus RS, Folkman S: *Stress, Appraisal, and Coping.* Springer, 1984.

Lyon BL, Werner J: Stress: Ten years of practice-relevant research, in Werley H, Fitzpatrick J (eds): *Annual Review of Nursing Research.* Springer, 1987.

Mason LJ: *Guide to Stress Reduction.* Peace Press, 1980.

Meyers J, et al: Life events and mental status. *J Health Human Behav* 1972;1:398–406.

Mishel MH: Perceived uncertainty and stress in illness. *Res Nurs Health* 1984;7:163–171.

Murphy L, Moriarty A: *Vulnerability, Coping, and Growth.* Yale University Press, 1976.

Norbeck JS: Modification of life event questionnaires for use with female respondents. *Res Nurs Health* 1984;7:61–71.

Pelletier KR: *Healthy People in Unhealthy Places: Stress and Fitness at Work.* Doubleday, 1984.

Perley NZ: Problems in self-consistency: Anxiety, in Roy C: *Introduction to Nursing: An Adaptation Model.* Prentice-Hall, 1984.

Rahe RH: Life change events and mental illness: An overview. *J Human Stress* 1979;5:2–10.

Robinson KM, Bridgewater SC, Molla PM, Wathen CA: Concepts of stress for nursing. *Issues Ment Health Nurs* 1982;4:167–176.

Selye H: *The Stress of Life.* McGraw-Hill, 1956.

Selye H: *The Stress of Life.* McGraw-Hill, 1976.

Selye H: *Stress without Distress.* American Library, 1974.

Sutterley DC, Donnelley GF (eds): *Coping with Stress: A Nursing Perspective.* Aspen, 1982.

Tache J, Selye J: On stress and coping mechanisms. *Issues Ment Health Nurs* 1985:7:3–24.

Ziemer MM: Coping behavior: A response to stress. *Top Clin Nurs* 1982;2(4):8.

EIGHT

Social Support

Jane S. Norbeck
Lou Ellen A. Barnes

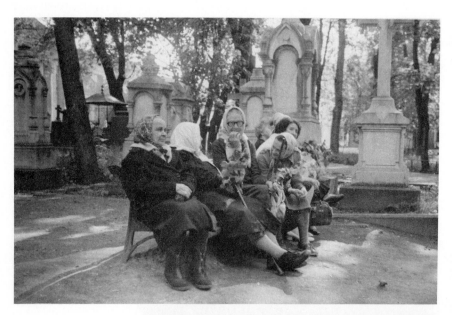

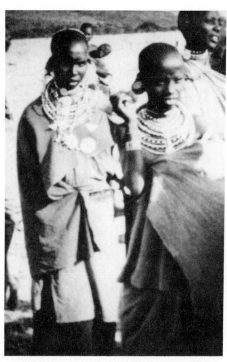

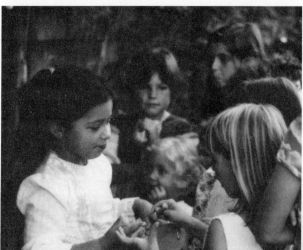

After reading this chapter, students should be able to

- Identify similarities and differences among definitions of social support

- Differentiate between the concepts of social support and social network

- Describe how social support is related to health or mental health outcomes in the simplified and more complex social support models

- Describe study findings supporting the hypothesis that social support is related to health outcomes

- Contrast the social network characteristics of the mentally ill and normal populations

- Describe how research has demonstrated the effects of family interaction on the relapse rates of schizophrenic clients

- Identify at least three properties of the person that influence the need for social support

- Differentiate between the effects of developmental versus situational crises on the availability of social support

- Discuss the relevance of Axes IV and V of the DSM-IIIR to the assessment of social support

- Name three interventions that are designed to enhance the support laypersons give to a person in crisis

- Give the rationale for situations in which a professional might provide support directly rather than attempt to increase the support from the naturally occurring network

- Name three community programs designed to provide support to the chronically mentally ill and/or their families

- Explain characteristics of persons with schizophrenic disorder that influence the unique social support needs of this population

- Appreciate the relevance of subjective and objective factors in understanding individuals' perceptions of their needs for social support

Cross References

Other topics relevant to this content are: Assessment, Chapter 12; Chronic mental illness, Chapter 23; Crisis management, Chapter 29; Family burden, Chapter 17; Nursing process and nursing theory, Chapter 4; Psychoeducation of family caregivers, Chapter 40; and Research, Chapter 14.

This book encourages psychiatric nurses to seek alternative modes of conflict resolution for individuals, groups, communities, and nations.

Key Terms

focus person	reciprocity
multiplex relationship	social network
mutual self-help groups	social support
negative expressed emotion	uniplex relationship
network density	volunteer linking

HISTORICAL FOUNDATIONS

The topic of social support has emerged recently as an interdisciplinary focus for research and clinical practice. Researchers and clinicians from the fields of anthropology, epidemiology, medicine, nursing, psychiatry, psychology, social work, and sociology have contributed to the literature in this field. Because nursing has been concerned with the social environment of the client for decades, the term *social support* might be seen as pouring old wine into new bottles. Yet the emergence of the term is important because a clearly defined concept can be studied and applied to practice with greater understanding and precision than a more vaguely stated concern. We begin our exploration of this concept with a review of how social support has been defined.

How Is Social Support Defined?

Two early writers introduced the concept of social support in the 1970s. The epidemiologist John Cassel (1974) reviewed studies of the effects of rapid social change, social and family disorganization, family competence and cohesiveness, cross-cultural migration, and psychosocial assets on health outcomes. Cassel sees a common theme in these and other studies as a deprivation of meaningful social contact. Such lack of social support was shown in the studies he reviewed as contributing to diminished health or well-being.

The community psychiatrist Gerald Caplan (1974) expands on the work by Cassel to discuss how social support facilitates dealing with a crisis. In Caplan's view, the outcome of the crisis is influenced not only by the characteristics of the stress and the ego strength of the individual but also by the quality of emotional and task-oriented support available from the person's social network. Caplan speculates that social support consists of three elements: "They [support persons] help the individual mobilize his psychological resources and master his emotional burdens; they share his tasks; and they provide him with extra supplies of money, material, tools, skills, and cognitive guidance to improve his handling of his situation" (p 6). Caplan describes two additional functions of support systems: collecting and storing information about the outside world to offer guidance and direction and acting as a refuge or sanctuary for the individual to rest and recuperate.

The work of Robert Weiss (1974) has been used as a starting point for defining social support. Weiss studied what he called the provisions of social relationships and identifies six categories that describe specific complementary functions of social relationships. Each provision is distinct from the others, and one type of provision cannot substitute for another. These are: (a) attachment or the sense of security and place; (b) social integration in which participants share concerns, information, ideas, services, and events; (c) opportunity for nurturance in which one can develop a sense of being needed; (d) reassurance of worth or confirmation of an individual's worth in a social role; (e) sense of reliable alliance in which one can expect continuing assistance even without reciprocating; and (f) guidance from a trustworthy and authoritative person in stressful situations.

Weiss's six provisions are listed on Table 8–1 along the left column as a basis for comparison with definitions from four other authors discussed in this chapter. Similar ideas are listed in parallel rows; e.g., Caplan's idea of a refuge or sanctuary for stability and comfort is similar to Weiss's concept of attachment. These similarities illustrate common features among the various definitions of social support; however, they gloss over some distinct meanings and unique ideas. The central idea underlying each author's list of support elements is shown at the top of the table (e.g., Weiss's "provisions of social relationships").

Sidney Cobb (1976) defines social support in terms of information—that one is cared for and loved, that one is esteemed and valued, and that one belongs to a network of communication and mutual obligation. In this definition, actual goods and services are not considered social

Table 8–1
Comparison of Social Support Definitions

Weiss (1974)	Caplan (1974)	Cobb (1976)	Kahn (1979)	House (1981)
Provisions of social relationships	Support from continuing relationships	Information leading people to believe:	Interpersonal transactions including:	Supportive behaviors or acts
Attachment or sense of security	A refuge or sanctuary for stability and comfort	That they are cared for and loved	Affect (feeling liked or loved)	Emotional
Social integration	Information, guidance, and feedback	That they belong to a network of communication	Affirmation of behaviors, perceptions, and views	Appraisal informational
Opportunity for nurturance	(Notion of reciprocal relationships with mutual need satisfaction)		(Notion that social support involves giving or receiving)	
Reassurance of worth	Help in mobilizing psychologic resources and mastering emotional burdens	That they are esteemed and valued	Affect (feeling respected or admired)	Appraisal
Sense of reliable alliance	Provision of material supplies and skills; help with tasks	That they belong to a network of mutual obligation (excluding tangible services or material aid)	Aid (material)	Instrumental
Obtaining of guidance	Provision of cognitive guidance		Aid (symbolic)	Informational

Source: Adapted from Lindsey AM, Norbeck JS, Carrieri VL, Perry E: Social support and health outcomes for postmastectory women: A review. Cancer Nurs 1981;4:378. Reproduced with permission.

support. As Table 8–1 shows, Cobb is the only author who excludes tangible services or material aid from the definition of social support.

Two more recent definitions of social support contain similar elements. Robert Kahn (1979) defines social support as interpersonal transactions that include one or more of three components: "the expression of positive affect of one person toward another, the affirmation or endorsement of another person's behaviors, perceptions, or expressed views, and the giving of symbolic or material aid to another" (p 85). Finally, James House (1981) proposes four components of social support: emotional support, instrumental support, informational support, and appraisal support.

These definitions of social support help us arrive at a common meaning of the concept; however, the actual number or types of components remain to be determined empirically. Although there seem to be distinct elements (e.g., emotional versus tangible support), it is unlikely that any one type of support is given or received without aspects of other types. For example, if someone offers the tangible support of giving another person a ride to the doctor, it is likely that some emotional support is embedded or perceived in the process.

Social Support and Social Networks

Social support is usually given and received by persons who know one another and who come into contact on a regular basis rather than by strangers. The term **social network** refers to all those persons known personally by the **focus person**. Some of these relationships are very close and intimate, such as a best friend, spouse or partner, and certain members of the nuclear family. Other relationships arise out of the roles a person assumes, such as friendships and acquaintances acquired at work or at school. Networks also include relatives in the extended family, neighbors, and people who participate in the same activities, such as churches, clubs, and teams. Finally, networks include people met simply through other network members.

With this large list of potential members in a person's network, it seems that everyone should have ample sources of social support. An important distinction must be made between social networks and social support. Not every person in the social network provides social support. In fact, some network members are sources of interpersonal stress rather than support. Figure 8–1 shows that the social network (circle 1) is much larger than the social support system (circle 2). The social support system is almost entirely enclosed by the larger social network, because most of our social support comes from our network members. The small section of the social support system (ellipse 3) represents potential sources of social support from persons who are not in our social networks, such as the chance conversation with the person seated next to us on the bus. Finally, the section outside these circles represents the larger society.

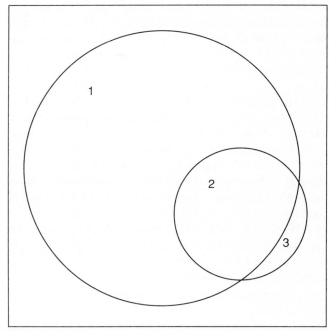

Figure 8–1
Social network and social support system. The larger circle (circle 1) represents the entire social network. Circle 2 represents the social support system within the social network. Ellipse 3 represents the small amount of social support that might be exchanged between strangers.

People can move in or out of these circles as we interact with them. We either incorporate them into our social networks or social support systems or we do not.

Characteristics of Social Networks

Many characteristics of social networks can be measured or described. Anthropologists and sociologists have defined several terms to describe and study social networks. Among these terms, those that are most important to the study of social support are (a) reciprocity, (b) size of network, (c) uniplex or multiplex relationships, and (d) network density.

Reciprocity refers to the extent to which each person gives and receives in the exchanges that occur between the two persons. Most close friendships are approximately equivalent in giving and receiving social support, although the exact form of the support might not be the same. For example, one friend might be a good listener who provides emotional support to the other, whereas the other friend might provide more in the area of initiating activities that the two enjoy. Some relationships, like the parent-child relationship, are not balanced in giving and receiving as usually defined; however, many parents describe a more abstract form of receiving that comes from parenting. Furthermore, over the course of the life span, the balance of giving might shift as the child takes care of an elderly parent.

The size of the network is an important consideration in whether or not the person has potential sources of social support. Those with very small networks might not have sufficient resources to receive the social support that they need, either on a day-to-day basis or during a crisis. In contrast, a large network may place overwhelming demands on the person to give support or simply to maintain the relationships.

Whether a relationship is uniplex or multiplex depends on how many different types of functions or activities occur in the relationship. In **uniplex relationships**, only one function or type of activity is shared; e.g., two persons have contact only at work. In **multiplex relationships**, more than one function or type of activity is shared. Most friendships are highly multiplex: The two persons enjoy talking about many shared interests; they participate in activities together; and they provide both emotional and tangible support to each other.

Finally, the concept of **network density** refers to the extent to which other members in the network know one another. In a hypothetical network with 100 percent density, every member of the network would know every other member. Most networks have a density of about 20 percent; however, this varies with the extent to which the network is comprised of relatives, with the size of the community, and with the length of time the people have lived in proximity. A network with high density may have advantages for situations in which the focus person requires help over a long time, e.g., in caring for an invalid family member. In such a situation, a dense network might function well because the members talk among themselves and are aware of what role each network member is playing. In contrast, highly dense networks are a disadvantage in situations in which the focus person wants to make a change in his or her behavior or life. First, the sources of information to help the person change are limited. Second, a dense network is likely to discourage change.

Figure 8–2 illustrates a social network of a typical size and density. There are distinct clusters within the network, representing perhaps a highly dense subset of relationships with relatives, a less dense cluster of work associates, and loose ties with persons who share common interests. When we examine the research on the network characteristics of psychiatric clients, we will discuss how the concepts of reciprocity, network size, multiplexity, and network density affect well-being or functioning.

THEORETICAL MODELS FOR RESEARCH AND PRACTICE

Simplified Social Support Model

Most of the early writings on social support emphasized the stress-buffering role of social support. In this view, lack of social support would theoretically not be a problem in the absence of stress. Conversely, social support may have a direct effect on health outcomes, regardless of stress level. In this view, everyone needs some social support to function on a day-to-day basis. These two views can be synthesized in a model that incorporates both direct and buffering effects, as illustrated in Figure 8–3. The direct effect of social support on health is shown by arrow c, and the buffering effect by the dotted arrow b. Research findings support direct, buffering, and combined effects of social support but not in a consistent pattern as yet.

The model in Figure 8–3 is greatly oversimplified because the arrows show movement in only one direction. Actually, each of the elements affects the other elements over time in a circular fashion. For example, a man who becomes depressed because of overwhelming life stress and little social support might subsequently experience even less social support because network members are discouraged from interacting with him. A depressed woman might also fail to ward off impending negative life events because of her low energy level. Thus, the depressive symptoms can affect subsequent stress and social support, thereby perpetuating the cycle of high stress, low support, and depression.

More Comprehensive Models

Other models of social support take other factors into account, particularly the personal resources of the individual (Gottlieb 1983) or other individual variables. The model depicted in Figure 8–4, developed by James House (1981), is congruent with stress and coping theory. This model has both direct and buffering or conditioning effects and incorporates coping and defenses in the stress process. Furthermore, the effects of stress and social support on health are mediated through short-term responses to stress. Thus, in childhood autism, for example, brain damage (an enduring health outcome) might occur because of short-term responses to stress such as head banging.

A Nursing Process Model

When we move from predictive research models to clinical application, a model that incorporates assessment and intervention is needed. Figure 8–5 presents a model devel-

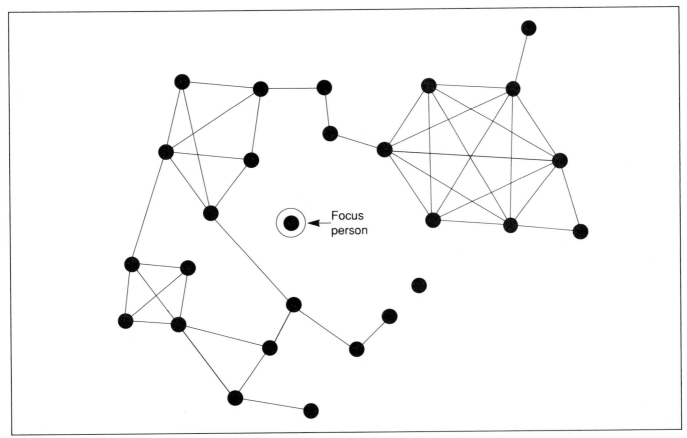

Figure 8–2
Network map with size and density illustrated. The focus person in the center knows
every person in this network (for simplicity, the lines between the focus person and the
other network members are not drawn). The lines between network members represent
those persons who know one another. This hypothetical network depicts a typical size
and density (20 percent) for an adult from the general population.

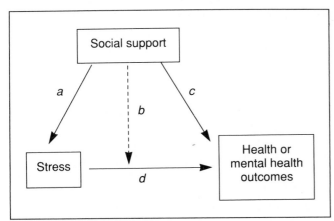

Figure 8–3
Simplified model of the main and buffering effects of social
support on health. The solid arrows depict direct or main
effects between variables, and the dotted arrow depicts a
buffering effect. That is, arrow b buffers the effect of arrow d.

oped by Norbeck (1981) in which the nursing process activities of assessment, planning, intervention, and evaluation are integrated into the stress, support, and outcome model.

In this model the quantity or quality of social support that is needed depends on both the individual and the situation, including stressors. Many health-related situations present unique demands that affect the kind and amount of social support that are needed, and this is an important area for nursing research.

The quantity or quality of support that is needed is weighed against the social support available. Again, properties of the individual (e.g., social skills) and properties of the situation (e.g., a commonly understood crisis or a unique and stigmatized event) jointly influence what social support is available. This assessment is the basis for planning strategies to augment social support or to provide surrogate support if needed. Such interventions are discussed in greater detail later in the chapter, as are personal and situational factors that affect assessment.

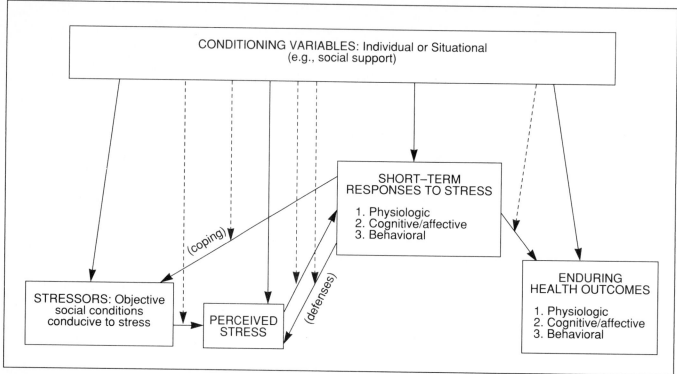

Figure 8–4

A paradigm of stress research. Solid arrows between boxes indicate presumed causal relationships among variables. Dotted arrows from the box labeled "conditioning variable" intersect solid arrows, indicating an interaction between the conditioning variables in the box at the beginning of the solid arrow in predicting variables in the box at the head of the solid arrow.

Source: House JS: Work Stress and Social Support. *Copyright © 1981 by Addison-Wesley Publishing Company, Reading, MA. p. 36.*

Evaluation is a necessary component of the model to determine (a) whether an intervention actually increased social support and (b) whether improved or augmented social support had a beneficial effect.

Just how important is social support? In the next section we outline a few of the hundreds of studies that have demonstrated beneficial effects from social support, and we examine studies with the mentally disordered.

EMPIRICAL STUDIES

Studies with General Populations

Many of the studies in the social support field are descriptive, correlational studies that demonstrate significant relationships between social support and health, mental health, or other measures of well-being. These studies make an important contribution, but they cannot prove causality. Prospective studies are needed to demonstrate causal relationships. The two research studies presented next are prospective studies that demonstrate the deleterious effects of low social support resources.

Berkman and Syme (1979) studied nearly 5000 adults and found that people who lacked social and community ties were two to three times more likely to die during the nine-year follow-up period than people with more extensive contacts. These findings held even when socioeconomic status, prior health status, and health practices were controlled. This study suggests the direct, rather than buffering, effect of social support because stress was not studied.

A second study offers support for the stress-buffering hypothesis. Norbeck and Tilden (1983) studied eighty-one medically normal pregnant women and found that the combination of high stress during pregnancy and low social support predicted complications of gestation, labor, and

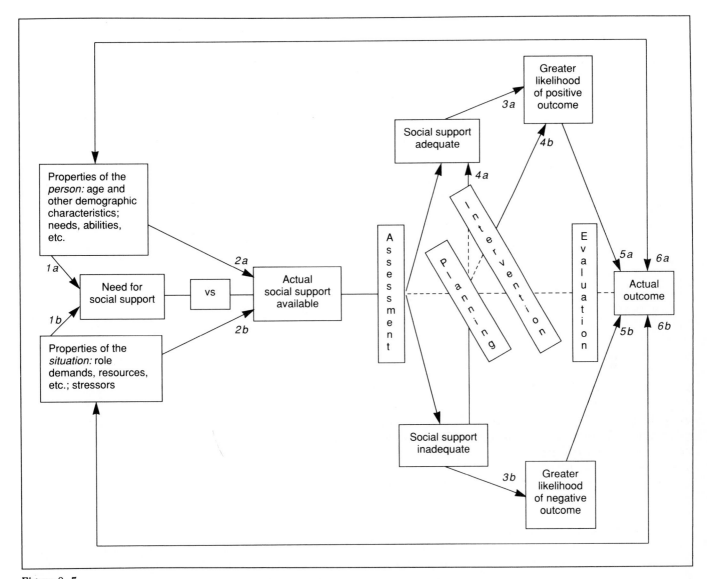

Figure 8–5
Clinical practice model of social support. This model illustrates the elements and relationships that must be considered to incorporate social support into nursing practices. Arrows *1a, 1b, 2a,* and *2b* demonstrate that properties of the person and the situation jointly determine the need for social support, as well as the actual support available. The situation can produce both resources and stressors. After assessment of the adequacy of social support, one can predict whether a positive or negative outcome will result (arrows *3a* and *3b*). The actual outcome is determined through evaluation of the social support intervention (arrows *5a* and *5b*). Additional influences from the person, situation, or other sources may affect the actual outcome (arrows *6a* and *6b*).
Source: Norbeck JS: Social support: A model for clinical research and application. Adv Nurs Sci 1981;3(4):46. Reproduced with permission of Aspen Publishers, Inc.

delivery and the condition of the infant at birth. These findings were over and above the effects of parity, age, race, social class, and marital status.

Studies with the Mentally Disordered

Networks of the Mentally Disordered

Deinstitutionalization of the mentally disordered has directed attention to the importance of the client's social network. Consequently, research studies have been conducted to examine and analyze the characteristics of psychiatric clients' social networks systematically. These features include the number of people with whom the client has contact, the composition of the group (i.e., family, friends, neighbors), interrelationships among the members, and the degree to which the social network provides support to its members.

Consideration of both the quantitative and qualitative aspects of the social network is necessary. The number of people in a person's network or the frequency of interactions does not necessarily indicate the presence of socially supportive relationships. The quality of the social interactions between network members determines whether these relationships are a source of support or distress, or both, for an individual.

Researchers have applied a variety of social network analyses to define and describe the characteristics and qualities of the social networks of psychiatric clients. In an early study, Hammer (1963–1964) explored the social networks of schizophrenic and manic-depressive clients through interviews with these clients and their families. In this preliminary work, the promptness of hospitalization was studied in terms of three network characteristics: symmetry (reciprocal relationships), interconnectedness (density), and the client's position in the network (e.g., breadwinner, homemaker). She found that clients who held critical positions in the network and had symmetrical ties to the persons with whom they had daily contact received greater assistance and were more likely to be hospitalized sooner. Also, networks with greater interconnectedness were more effective in sustaining their relationships with the client.

Pattison et al. (1975) compared interpersonal relationships in groups of neurotic and psychotic clients to those in groups of normal individuals. Table 8–2 summarizes their findings. They found that the psychotic clients not only had the smallest number of persons in their networks but also that the network rarely extended beyond family members. The relationships in the psychotic persons' networks were uniformly ambivalent and nonreciprocal. These results illustrate that both quantity and quality of social relationships differ between psychiatric clients and normal individuals.

Tolsdorf (1976) compared the social networks of a sample of ten hospitalized schizophrenic clients with ten nonpsychiatric, medical clients in terms of network characteristics, coping styles, and recent histories. He reported that psychiatric clients had fewer intimate relationships within their networks and that their networks were dominated by family members, with few nonkin members. The psychiatric clients' relationships were more frequently characterized by hostile, rejecting, domineering, or possessive mothers and belligerent, uninvolved, or alcoholic fathers.

Tolsdorf also found that the psychiatric clients had a negative orientation to their network characterized by the belief that it is "inadvisable, impossible, useless, or potentially dangerous to draw on network resources" (p 413). Holding such a belief, psychiatric clients might be reluctant to use sources of support that are potentially available to them. These negative orientations may be due, in part, to the lack of support that psychiatric clients experience, leading to dissatisfaction with their networks and reluctance to seek help from their relatives.

In a psychiatric nursing study of the functioning of persons with schizophrenia, Turner (1979) found distinctive patterns of social support for the group with troublesome behavior and poor social functioning. The poorly functioning group had lower social support scores, more lived with their parents, fewer had extrahousehold contacts or friends, fewer could name a helping person, more denied having a confidant, and fewer had helping persons or confidants outside the home than the group with better social functioning. These findings are important because the two groups were similar in age, sex, race, and psychiatric treatment history; thus, the associations between the current behavior and social functioning and the social support variables appear to be upheld.

Other research illustrates that even schizophrenics who do not live with their families are affected by the characteristics of their social networks. The structure of the personal networks of schizophrenics who resided in an urban, single-room occupancy hotel was studied by Sokolovsky et al. (1978). These investigators found that schizophrenics, as compared with nonpsychiatric residents, had fewer reciprocal relationships and more dependent interactions. Schizophrenics who did not develop a complex of relationships outside the hotel and who failed to link with a matrix of social organization within the hotel, such as a group that shared meals, were more likely to be rehospitalized.

Each of these studies has shown that the networks of schizophrenics differ in many ways from those of nonpsychiatric populations; however, they do not indicate whether these differences existed prior to the illness or resulted because of the illness. Lipton et al. (1981) studied the changes that occur in social networks of schizophrenics over the course of their disease by comparing the networks of clients who were hospitalized for their first schizophrenic break with clients who had a history of multiple hospitalizations for schizophrenia. Compared with the networks of clients experiencing their first hospitalization for schizophrenia, individuals with multiple admissions had fewer persons in their networks, had a higher percentage of relatives in their networks, and perceived their network members as less important than did the first admission group. Although Lipton and colleagues did not follow individuals across time, the findings suggest that networks change as a consequence of the chronic course of schizophrenia, resulting in a marked decrease in social ties and resources. It is interesting to note that while the multiple admission group had a higher percentage of relatives in their networks, they were more dependent on nonkin network members for instrumental aid, such as money, housing, food, and professional help.

Network characteristics also appear to affect how readily the patient receives professional help when symptoms increase. Perrucci and Targ (1982) studied the social network characteristics of psychiatric clients who were hospitalized for the first time to determine how network members respond to a client's symptom changes and the need for rehospitalization. In networks with certain characteristics, members more accurately interpreted and responded to the increases in the client's psychotic symptomatology. These network attributes include positive social-emotional bonds, extensive interaction ties among members, and identifiable decision-making and leadership roles. The investigators summarized that close, supportive networks with substantial knowledge of, and favorable attitudes toward, mental illness are more likely to assist the psychiatric network member to seek professional assistance quickly when required.

If the course of the illness results in a decrease in social ties and resources, what happens to those clients who stop living with their families and move to community settings? Parks and Pilisuk (1984) analyzed the personal support networks of formerly hospitalized psychiatric clients who resided in board-and-care homes. The psychiatric clients identified their family and board-and-care operators as their primary sources of emotional support. Although the family was most frequently named as meeting the client's material and instrumental needs, a high proportion of social companionship contacts were with fellow residents. These findings indicate that these former mental clients are socially

and psychologically removed from the mainstream community. Isolation has been identified as a risk factor contributing to physical and psychologic problems. Therefore these researchers suggest that such psychiatric clients be encouraged to establish relationships outside of the board-and-care home to reduce the possibility of their developing overly dependent relationships and becoming isolated.

Overall, these studies show that the social networks of schizophrenics and other psychiatric clients are less supportive and less functional than the networks of nonpsychiatric clients. Although studies investigated a variety of network characteristics, overall the networks of schizophrenics were smaller and had more relatives than friends, neighbors, or work associates. Also, network relationships were more dependent and less reciprocal than relationships in ordinary networks. Researchers who examined these changes over time concur that after the first hospitalization of a schizophrenic the network size tends to decrease.

What are the possible causes for the disruptions and dysfunctions in the social networks of schizophrenics? Goffman (1963) asserts that the label of mental illness is stigmatizing. This stigma causes former friends and neighbors to remove themselves from the labeled person's environment. Beels (1981) describes the labeling process as redefining the social position of the mentally ill person. The relationships that exist in the network before the illness change to include fellow psychiatric clients and only a core of relatives. As a result of this network change, the person's social confidence and competence decrease significantly.

Other factors influence social performance. For instance, schizophrenic persons who are chronically ill have marked cognitive impairment that may result in distortions of reality. This cognitive disorganization is manifested by psychotic symptoms such as delusions, hallucinations, and thought process disorders. The schizophrenic may also misperceive boundaries of self and other persons. These

---

Table 8–2

Social Support and Network Properties for Normal, Neurotic, and Psychotic Clients According to Pattison et al. (1975)

Groups	Size	Composition	Density	Quality of Interaction
Normal	20–30	kin and nonkin	60%	Rated positive or neutral symmetric relationships
Neurotic	10–12	fewer nonkin	30%	More negative ratings
Psychotic	4–5	mostly kin	90%	Ambivalent ratings Asymmetric (dependent) relationships

Source: Norbeck JS: The use of social support in clinical practice. J Psych Nurs 1982;20(12):25. Reproduced with permission. Charles B. Slack, Inc.

perceptual distortions influence the schizophrenic person's ability to communicate with others. The result is disturbed communication and poor social skills.

Perceptual disturbances influence how persons use the support that may be available and how satisfied they feel with that support. Psychotic persons may reorganize their world around delusions. As a result, satisfaction with support varies according to the reality that they create, leading to problems in communicating, giving and receiving, and perceiving support.

An additional factor is that schizophrenic persons are extremely sensitive to stimuli from their social environment. Wing (1977) describes the delicate balance that a schizophrenic person must maintain between too much and too little social stimulation. Too much social stimulation, such as the intrusiveness of others, can result in relapse of psychotic symptoms. Too little social stimulation can result in social withdrawal, slowness, and decreased motivation. Thus, the schizophrenic's equilibrium between the need for social involvement and social distance is tenuous. Therefore, networks that present too many demands may be stressful, whereas social withdrawal may prevent the person from seeking the support needed to cope with daily life and crisis situations.

The finding that social networks of schizophrenics are inadequate to support these persons has clinical implications. Gottlieb (1983) recommends that clinicians comprehensively assess the client's social network by (a) identifying the primary network members, (b) determining the degree of support or distress that exists in the network, and (c) determining the level of understanding, attitudes, and responses that the primary network members have concerning the illness and treatment. Then efforts can be directed to designing beneficial interventions.

Practitioners must be cautious when interpreting the research findings that the networks of schizophrenic clients are small. Increasing network size may not prove beneficial. Expanding the number and types of network members may create increased demands on the schizophrenic person who already has limited social skills and resources. Although social isolation in normal persons has been associated with poor mental health, social isolation, up to a point, may be protective for persons with schizophrenia.

In a similar fashion, findings about differences in the quality of relationships between schizophrenic and normal individuals should not be used to shape the relationships of schizophrenics. Unlike nonschizophrenics, who benefit from close, intimate relationships, schizophrenics appear to benefit most from supportive but casual and brief interactions.

A further caution in applying research findings to schizophrenic clients concerns the fact that schizophrenia is a spectrum disorder in which symptoms may range from mild to severe psychotic symptoms. Thus, nurses assessing and planning interventions must integrate these group characteristics with individual characteristics to understand the types and degrees of support that are most appropriate for each client.

Studies of Negative Expressed Emotion

Goldman (1982) estimates that 65 percent of all of the clients discharged from psychiatric hospitals return to their families. Not all of these clients are severely disabled or chronically mentally ill. For those who are, however, the influence of family life on the course of mental illness is an important area for study. Researchers studying the effects of family members on schizophrenics have developed the term **negative expressed emotion (EE)** to describe family members' negative responses that adversely influence the relapse rates of clients.

Negative expressed emotion refers to the extent that a key relative makes critical or hostile comments about the client or comments that indicate emotional overinvolvement with the client during the intake interview for psychiatric hospitalization. High negative expressed emotion by relatives of schizophrenics means that these relatives made more negative comments about their schizophrenic member as compared with relatives who were evaluated as being low in negative expressed emotion.

High negative expressed emotion affects the recurrence of psychotic symptoms and rehospitalization. Vaughn and Leff (1976) replicated an earlier study by Brown et al. (1972) by interviewing relatives at the time of admission and at a nine-month follow-up (see the Research Note). When compared with schizophrenics whose relatives demonstrated low negative expressed emotion, a significant percentage of the schizophrenic persons who lived with relatives with high negative expressed emotion had more florid psychotic symptoms—e.g., delusions, hallucinations, and disturbed behaviors—and were rehospitalized at a greater rate during the follow-up period. These findings were independent of other factors, such as length of psychiatric history, type of symptoms, or the severity of previous behavioral disturbance.

Figure 8–6 shows that schizophrenic relapse in clients who lived with relatives who were high in negative expressed emotion was associated with two additional factors: greater time in close proximity to their relatives and discontinuation of maintenance antipsychotic medications. However, neither time spent in close proximity to relatives nor maintenance on medications were related to schizophrenic relapse in clients whose families demonstrated low negative expressed emotion. Thus, the effect of negative expressed emotion is an independent factor in contributing to relapse. For those clients living among family with high negative expressed emotion, reducing the amount of face-to-face

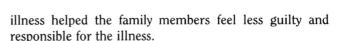

contact with their negative relative and maintaining their antipsychotic medication have a protective function.

Vaughn and Leff (1981) suggest possible explanations for why relatives with high negative expressed emotion were more intolerant, emotionally reactive, and intrusive than relatives with low negative expressed emotion. They propose that high negative expressed emotion by parents and spouses may be a reflection of the disappointment they feel with the schizophrenic family member when their social performance expectations are not met. Interviews with such relatives indicated that they did not understand the true nature of the mental illness as genuine and chronic and that they thought the client could control his or her symptoms. Thus, the relatives had unrealistic expectations of the client and tended to hold the client responsible for behaviors that are actually out of his or her control. Although relatives with high negative expressed emotion seemed disappointed in the client, relatives with low negative expressed emotion seemed to accept the social and psychologic limitations of the schizophrenic family member.

The intrusiveness of the relatives with high negative expressed emotion was attributed to an unrealistic expectation of mutual exchange of support from their schizophrenic member. The relatives with low negative expressed emotion, however, seemed more sensitive to the schizophrenic member's need for social distance: They allowed the client more personal space and autonomy.

Psychoeducation for Families of Schizophrenics

The findings of the Vaughn and Leff study indicate that inclusion of family members in the treatment of the schizophrenic member is crucial. Education about the nature and course of the illness is essential so that relatives can understand and support their schizophrenic member. Family members can learn that giving too much support can lead to dependence and regression, whereas not making enough demands can result in lack of motivation and underachievement in their relative with schizophrenia. In addition to individual sessions with family members about their relative's illness and treatment, Leff (1979) recommends a professionally led family therapy group that includes relatives with both high and low negative expressed emotion but not the client. Through professional guidance and feedback, these family therapy sessions can give the family members with high negative expressed emotion the opportunity to learn more effective coping skills from the participants with low negative expressed emotion.

McLean et al. (1982) conducted multiple family groups for families of adult chronically mentally ill individuals. The purpose of these groups was to provide the families with information, coping skills, and support. As a part of the group, a team of nurses, psychologists, and social workers presented ideas about theories and treatment of schizophrenia. Knowledge about the possible etiologies of the

illness helped the family members feel less guilty and responsible for the illness.

In addition, family members were taught the skill of setting clear but firm behavioral limits with their schizophrenic member. For example, the family members learned how to set limits on violent or acting-out behaviors through role-playing these situations within the group. The family members were taught to increase the autonomy and independence of their mentally ill member by being less intrusive and by encouraging the mentally ill person to spend more time physically away from relatives.

Through education and group support, the family members felt less socially isolated and stigmatized. Reduc-

---

RESEARCH NOTE

Citation

Vaughn CE, Leff JP: The influence of family and social factors on the course of psychiatric illness: A comparison of schizophrenic and depressed neurotic patients. Br J Psychiatry *1976;129:125–137.*

Study Problem/Purpose

To replicate and extend the work of Brown, Birley, and Wing (1972) concerning the effect of family behavior on psychotic relapse in schizophrenia.

Methods

Negative expressed emotion was rated by counting the critical, hostile, or overprotective comments made about the client during an interview with relatives at the time of psychiatric admission.

Findings

Schizophrenic persons who live with relatives who are high in negative expressed emotion, spend more than 35 hours in close contact with these relatives per week, and are not on an antipsychotic drug, have the highest relapse rate (92 percent). In families with low negative expressed emotion, how much time the client spent with relatives and whether the schizophrenic person was on drugs were unrelated to psychotic relapse (13 percent relapse rate).

Implications

Schizophrenic persons who live with relatives who are high in negative expressed emotion may be protected from psychotic symptom relapse by having less direct contact with these relatives and by taking antipsychotic medications.

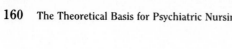
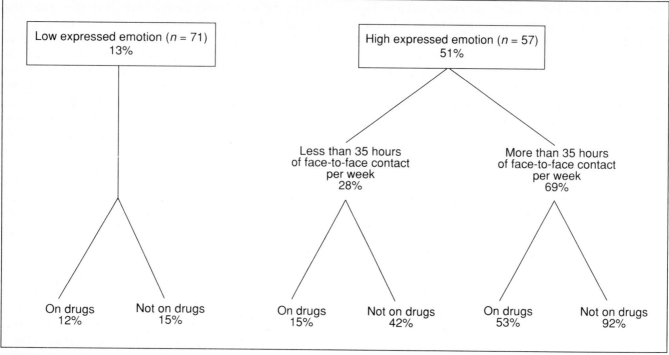

Figure 8–6
Nine-month relapse rates of schizophrenics for different levels of expressed emotion, face-to-face contact, and medication use.

Source: Vaughn CE, Leff JP: The influence of family and social factors on the course of psychiatric illness. Br J Psychiatry 1981;129:132. Reproduced with permission.

ing the family's sense of isolation and stigmatization enabled them to help the schizophrenic member.

ASSESSMENT

Writers of social support theory differ in whether they view social support as an important factor at all times in our lives or only during times of crisis. In this chapter, we take the view that there are universal needs for social support, both on a day-to-day basis and in times of crisis. There are, however, differences both in the amount and the expression of social support required by individuals and groups; thus, the assessment of social support needs for the individual is complicated by individual differences, situational differences, and cultural patterns. The left portion of the model in Figure 8–5 shows that both the need for social support and the availability of social support are determined by properties of the person and by properties of the situation.

Properties of the Person Influencing Social Support

Individual differences in the need for social support appear to vary greatly, ranging from the so-called lifelong isolates (Lowenthal and Haven 1968) to people who need large and extensive networks to feel that they are adequately integrated into a social system. The concept *need for affiliation* might help explain this difference in need for social support. This need level might be shaped both by personality traits and socialization patterns.

Age or developmental stage is another factor that the nurse must take into account when evaluating a person's need for social support. This is particularly true when the person is at either extreme of the developmental spectrum, when dependency needs are greatest. Along the developmental continuum, the most appropriate sources of support appear to change from parents in infancy and young childhood, to peers in late childhood and adolescence, to intimate partner in adulthood, and perhaps to adult children in later years.

Individual differences influence how much social support is potentially available to a person. Social skills are important in developing and maintaining a network. The abilities to maintain reciprocity in relationships and to initiate contacts with others are two examples of social skills needed in this process. Perhaps the concept of interpersonal attraction is also influential.

Gender differences also contribute to the availability of social support. Males and females seem to elicit social support in different ways. Two common examples of these differences embody the idea of role competency: Women more often receive help from passersby when their car is stalled, and men more often receive practical help from neighbors (e.g., a hot casserole) when they are taking care of their children by themselves. In general, women tend to have larger social networks than men; however, they are not more satisfied with the support that they receive. Women are thought to provide more social support for both men and women; perhaps women's somewhat larger networks are at the expense of having to provide more support to others.

Properties of the Situation Influencing Social Support

The developmental and situational crises that arise in our lives require additional coping and resources beyond that needed to cope with normal role demands. Table 8–3 outlines the duration and intensity of social support that might be required for various situations, including changes along the health-illness continuum. The assumption that every-

one needs social support even when no crisis is occurring is reflected in the lower left box, which shows that low-intensity support is required continuously to maintain individual well-being and performance in major social roles (e.g., worker role, parent role). Long-term support of greater intensity is required for persons who are coping with chronic stressors or illnesses.

At the other extreme, high-intensity support is required by people experiencing acute stressors (e.g., a fire in one's home or an illness or injury), but this high-intensity support is required for only a short period. Between these extremes is the medium-intensity support required for an intermediate period of time for other life changes or transitions (e.g., birth of a first baby). Research is needed to validate the exact intensity and duration of social support required for various situations that can occur in the life course.

Situational properties also influence the availability of social support. Certain situations, particularly developmental crises, are familiar to network members, and formalized mechanisms have been developed to assist in the provision of support. Baby showers, housewarming parties, and graduation celebrations all provide interaction that acknowledges the transition, allows people to talk about the transition, and in many cases, provides additional material resources for dealing with the transition.

Situational crises—e.g., a serious illness, a death in the family, or unemployment—are not "expected" matu-

Table 8–3
Grid for Predicting the Intensity and Duration of Support Required for Situational Demands and Stressors

Duration of Support Required	Intensity of Support Required		
	Low	Medium	High
Short-term			Support needed for acute stressors or illnesses
Intermediate		Support needed for managing life changes and transitions and for facilitating rehabilitation from major illnesses or surgery	
Long-term or continuous	Support needed for day-to-day living for individual well-being and performance in the major social roles	Support needed to cope with chronic stressors or illnesses	

Source: Norbeck JS: Social support: A model for clinical research and application. Adv Nurs Sci 1981;3(4):50. Reproduced with permission of Aspen Publishers, Inc.

rational or normative crises, but unexpected and perhaps unfamiliar events in the experience of the network members. When no one in the person's network has had prior experience with a crisis event, network members can offer only limited advice or help. In these situations, the value of a less dense network with looser ties can be evident: A "friend of a friend" might be able to provide assistance that the network members cannot.

When the network loses a member through death, divorce, or the like, other members not only require additional coping and resources but also lose one of the sources of social support that would ordinarily be called on for help at such a time. Thus, losses of key social support members could be doubly stressful. By contrast, the loss of a non-supportive or disruptive network member could be beneficial, and such a loss may be experienced with minimal stress.

The stigma attached to a crisis also influences the availability of social support. When an event, e.g., being raped, is considered too embarrassing to disclose to others, support is not provided because key network members are not aware of the event. Depending on the values of the individual and the network members, situations such as unwed pregnancy, unemployment, diagnosis of cancer, psychiatric problems, and many other events might be outside the range of what the network either can or is willing to respond to in helpful ways.

Incorporating Social Support Assessment into DSM-IIIR

The psychologic and social information considered in Axes IV and V of the DSM-IIIR provide guidelines for assessing the client's need for social support. Axis IV provides a rating scale of the severity of psychosocial stressors that may be associated with a client's disorder. This axis helps nurses to identify the properties of the situation (e.g., psychosocial stressors) that might influence the need for social support. This scale ranges from no apparent psychologic stressor to extreme, catastrophic stressors that have occurred in the year preceding the disorder. Identifying psychosocial stressors can help nurses recognize possible disruptions in the client's social relationships. For example, a minor argument with a family member might be a mild social stressor. The death of a significant relative is an extreme social stressor. Assessing severity of psychosocial stressors according to DSM-IIIR also involves specifying if the stressor(s) is predominantly acute (duration less than six months) or predominantly enduring (duration greater than six months).

Axis V of the DSM-IIIR provides a guideline for establishing the person's highest level of psychologic, social,

and occupational functioning currently and during the past year. This information provides a baseline for inferring that person's resources, e.g., social relations, occupational or school functioning, and use of leisure time. Axis V reflects a global assessment of functioning and is a revision of the Global Assessment Scale designed to measure overall severity of psychiatric disturbance.

Guidelines for Assessment

Clinical assessment instruments have not been developed to measure social support. Two research instruments are being used widely in nursing research: the Personal Resources Questionnaire (PRQ) developed by Brandt and Weinert (1981) and the Norbeck Social Support Questionnaire (NSSQ) developed by Norbeck, Lindsey, and Carrieri (1981, 1983). Findings from these instruments are contributing to our understanding of patterns of social support for different clinical populations. Research instruments are not valid for clinical assessment, however, until large-scale normative data are available and the predictive ability of the instrument is tested extensively.

Until instruments appropriate for clinical assessment are available, the psychiatric nurse must rely on questions that elicit descriptive information that can be interpreted in relation to individual and situational differences affecting the particular client. Brandt (1984), Ellison (1983), and Norbeck (1982) suggest that important considerations in this assessment include questions to determine (a) the size of the client's support network; (b) the relationship between the client and each support person, e.g., parent, friend, or coworker; (c) the potential availability of each support person based on factors such as geographic distance or frequency of contact; (d) the kinds of help that are available, e.g., emotional support, direct or tangible support, or information; (e) the client's satisfaction with the support he or she receives; and (f) whether the client reciprocates the help given by network members. Because clients' specific support needs depend in part on their life situations, questions about social support should include both general support needs and special needs related to these situations. The need to confide in another person is an example of a general support need. The need to develop shared living arrangements is a specific need of psychiatric clients who are adjusting to discharge from in-patient hospitalization. Support that the psychiatric client might need in this situation includes information regarding available apartments and potential roommates, tangible help in moving or locating personal possessions, and problem-solving help to resolve difficulties that arise in learning to live with another person. Thus, the skilled clinician anticipates areas of support that the client might need and inquires about several facets of the client's situation to obtain a complete picture of the social support that is needed and available. Areas of unmet need that are identified guide the planning of specific interventions.

INTERVENTION

Many of the considerations related to assessment are mirrored in planning interventions for people with inadequate social support. Just as assessment is based on properties of the person and properties of the situation, intervention strategies must take into account both individual and situational factors.

We begin by considering situational factors that arise from the various crises that people experience. Individual factors, e.g., inadequate social skills, are discussed in relation to interventions appropriate for psychiatric clients.

Interventions for Coping with Crises

When people who have adequate social support systems experience normal developmental crises, they usually receive the support they need because the network members have experience with the types of events that occur over the life span. Unplanned or situational crises, however, often leave people without the support they need because (a) the network members do not know what to do in this unusual situation, (b) the stigma associated with the event makes others reluctant to get involved, or (c) the crisis has involved the loss of an important support person. Of course, there can be overlap among these reasons for inadequate support, as in the case of parents surviving the death of an adolescent child because of an impulsive suicide. In this case, the parents lose a key network person and at the same time receive less support from the network because of the stigma attached to suicide.

Supporting the Supporters

In those crises that exceed the network's experience or capacity to respond, the professional can take several approaches after determining that the client has inadequate support. It is sometimes possible to work with a key network member to increase the capacity of that person to provide support. For example, key network members might be helped to support a bereaved person by teaching them the phases of the grief process. Without this knowledge, network members commonly do not allow the grieving person to continue to express feelings of loss after a few weeks because they do not understand that this phase is normally much longer.

Volunteer Linking

If a network member cannot be influenced to provide the needed support in a particular situation, another strategy is to obtain temporary support from someone who has undergone a similar crisis. This strategy is called **volunteer linking**, and it can involve either someone who is currently experiencing the same situation (a fellow traveler) or someone who has successfully experienced this situation in the past (a veteran). Helmrath and Steinitz (1978) recommended volunteer linking when they discovered that couples did not receive any support from their network members following the death of their newborn even though these couples had normal networks. Couples who had successfully weathered this experience could not only provide guidance for the grief process but also help the grieving couple to understand the isolation that they felt in this process.

Mutual Self-Help Groups

Extensions of the volunteer linking concept can be seen in **mutual self-help groups** that have formed to help people cope with situations as diverse as having a schizophrenic family member to dealing with the death by suicide of an adolescent child. Some of these groups are formed by professionals. Others, such as Alcoholics Anonymous, one of the earliest and most effective of the mutual self-help groups, are formed without any professional guidance.

Mutual self-help groups, whether initiated by lay people or by professionals, can be very effective for crises involving stigma. Young women who have experienced rape or sexual abuse frequently feel people can tell by looking at them that they have been victimized. When they see other victims in the group who look normal, they can begin the normalization process as they work through their psychologic trauma.

Supplemental Professional Support

In the situations involving the loss of a key support person, whether through death, divorce, geographic relocation, or other reasons, professionals might offer temporary support directly until the client has had the opportunity to "repeople" the network. The client might need assistance not only with expanding the network, but also while experiencing acute grief.

In other situations, it might be preferable for the professional to provide support directly rather than focusing on improving the capacity of the network to respond appropriately. Short-term crises require immediate support. After the crisis is over, the professional might explore with the client ways to improve the social support system if it is inadequate. Direct support by professionals is also appropriate if effective support cannot be made available through the client's network, volunteer linking, or mutual aid groups.

Professionals who provide support to clients in these situations constitute the formal support system, as distinguished from the informal support system. The informal support system is the naturally occurring social network. There are three reasons why professional support from the formal support system is different from social support from the informal support system. First, the helping relationship is not reciprocal—professionals do not turn to clients for help. Second, the helping functions are limited to expected role-related functions. Clients do not call on the professional for help in nonpsychiatric or medical emergencies, such as having car trouble on the freeway. Third, the relationship is likely to disappear when the service is no longer needed; there are no other functions that maintain the relationship. Although clients acknowledge how essential support from professionals was, clients do not regard professional helpers as part of their networks. Instead, they feel that giving good advice, for example, is the professional's job. Thus, regardless of satisfaction with the service, professional support is best thought of as surrogate support that extends or replaces support that is not available in the client's network.

An example of professional support for discharged clients who refused continuing treatment illustrates the effectiveness of even brief and limited contacts by professionals in sustaining suicidal clients. Motto et al. (1981) developed a suicide prevention program for persons who were admitted to the hospital because they were depressed or suicidal. At discharge, clients who refused posthospital therapy were divided into contact and no-contact groups. The contact group received a telephone call or letter from a staff member who had interviewed them in the hospital every one to three months. During a two-year period, the persons who were contacted by a staff member had lower rates of death by suicide. These results illustrate the value of ongoing professional support to clients at risk for suicide through contacts, although the professionals were not providing therapy as such.

Intervention with Chronically Mentally Ill People

How do psychiatric nurses intervene to improve the social support resources of the chronically mentally ill? Both in hospital and community settings, the nurse focuses on two major areas of social support intervention. According to Ellison (1983), these areas include: (a) strengthening and maintaining existing social network relationships and (b) improving the person's network-building skills. Nursing intervention in these two areas begins with establishing a therapeutic relationship with the client.

In the therapeutic relationship, the nurse provides a safe environment in which sensitive and nonthreatening supportive interaction between the nurse and the client can occur. The nurse's initiation of this relationship is important because the chronically mentally ill person may be socially isolated or without family, friends, or even casual acquaintances. This therapeutic relationship with the nurse can provide an opportunity for the client to gradually increase his or her social confidence and skills.

As the nurse-client relationship develops, the nurse can begin to reconnect the client with existing network members and link the client to new relationships. During hospitalization, the nurse can introduce the client to other people. As the client becomes more comfortable with the setting, the nurse may set a goal with the client that he initiate interaction with others at least once a day. The nurse also includes the client's family in the treatment plan through counseling and education.

Psychiatric nurses also provide social skills training through experiences designed to assist the chronically mentally ill person to develop more satisfying interpersonal relationships and to achieve material support, such as money, food, and lodging. Many clients have underdeveloped and ineffective social skills; therefore, their social isolation continues. They typically experience difficulty in initiating casual conversations with others, expressing ideas or feelings appropriately, maintaining social contacts, or pursuing social or vocational activities (Brady 1984).

Nurses teach social skills through the use of role-playing or role-modeling to help the client deal more effectively with difficult interpersonal situations. The client role-plays these difficult situations (e.g., interviewing for a job) in a one-to-one session or in a social skills training group. Specific instructive feedback and praise are given for appropriate responses. Guidance, practice, and goal setting should result in successful experiences that increase confidence and self-esteem.

In addition to interventions through the nurse-client relationship, there are a variety of community support treatment approaches that provide support systems for mentally ill clients and their families. Treatment programs may focus on the client alone, on the client's family, or on both client and family. Although support from the natural network is preferred, professionals may intervene to provide, augment, or supplement support as necessary.

Halfway houses ease the transition from psychiatric in-patient hospitalization to the community. These houses are staffed by nurses and other mental health professionals to provide a wide range of services. In these environments, staff provide emotional and material support, including assistance with problem-solving, reality testing, and finding a job. In addition, new social contacts can be developed with peers.

Day treatment centers for the chronically mentally ill provide opportunities for clients in the community to build a social network outside of their living situations. For clients living with high negative expressed emotion, these centers provide a means of reducing the hours of face-to-face contact with their relative. The focus of these centers is to provide a social environment that accepts the client. In these centers, mentally ill clients have the opportunity to converse informally with other clients and staff and perhaps to gain support in this way.

Respite care programs can provide a relief for the families who experience stress due to caring for a chronically ill member at home. Respite care involves routine, prescheduled short-term hospitalization of the chronically mentally ill person to ensure that the medication program is monitored. At the same time, the family gets time away from the client and the demands of caregiving. Chronic illnesses such as schizophrenia are disruptive because the family focuses mainly on the support needs of the schizophrenic member. As a result, family members spend less time in leisure or social activities outside the home and are themselves at risk for increased isolation and reduced support.

UNRESOLVED ISSUES

The social support field is an exciting area that continues to stimulate creative research in several disciplines. Nonetheless, there are critical questions that have not been answered, and we need to continue to update our evaluation of the usefulness of this concept for our practice.

First, we must remember that social support is a relatively new field, and research findings are incomplete. Most of the research has been descriptive, and only a few controlled studies demonstrate the effectiveness of support interventions. Although research has clearly demonstrated the beneficial effects of social support across many health outcomes, research has not answered important questions about how social support actually works. Beginning efforts in this direction address what types of support or sources of support were most effective in specific situations. These types and sources are likely to vary among people from different socioeconomic and cultural backgrounds.

Second, several important conceptual issues have not been resolved. For example, the term *social support* may be too broad to be useful in all contexts. This term does not reflect the complexities of helping behavior, particularly efforts to help that are not regarded by recipients as helpful at the time but that are later acknowledged as pivotal experiences.

Third, there is the possibility that there are negative consequences of help, particularly when the help offered is perceived as inappropriate by the recipient. For example, a young woman with schizophrenia who lived in a halfway house began to withdraw from other residents because she felt increasingly anxious when they urged her to join a dancing group. This suggestion was potentially helpful because she needed more social interaction; however, participating in dancing was not an appropriate suggestion for her because she had always felt extremely awkward and self-conscious in such activities. When help—even needed and appropriate help—is provided to people who have no opportunity to reciprocate, the result might be stress, lowered self-esteem, or loss of autonomy. The provision of direct support by professionals must be weighed against the possibility of increasing a person's dependency upon health care providers.

Finally, untested assumptions need to be examined. For example, the beneficial effects of the social support that occurs spontaneously in a person's naturally occurring network might not result from artificially contrived support provided through intervention programs. The assumption that all people need at least a small amount of social support to function in daily life does not appear to hold for lifelong isolates—those fiercely independent people who value self-sufficiency to the extreme.

Research in social support is moving steadily closer to answering these and other questions of vital importance to clinicians. In turn, insights from clinicians play a valuable role in shaping the research questions that need to be studied. Collaborative research by academic scientists and practicing clinicians can perhaps provide the most useful findings for guiding practice.

HUMANISTIC INTERACTIONIST IMPLICATIONS

The balance between objective and subjective reality tips toward the subjective. Supportive acts are not truly supportive if the potential recipient does not perceive them as such. Thus, there is a need for a phenomenologic approach in this field, both in research and in clinical application.

As researchers and clinicians, we need to work as partners with clients who can tell us more accurately than we can judge what their life situations are like and what is supportive to them. There are no easy prescriptions, as the absurd recommendation for stomach pain illustrates: "Make two new friends and come back for a checkup in four weeks." Instead, each individual and each situation is unique, in relation to both assessment and intervention.

Professionals can share ideas that have worked for others and information about potential resources (e.g., a mutual self-help group), but ultimately the proposed solution must be acceptable to the client. Even clients who are seriously lacking in social support have valuable ideas about what might be helpful to them. Instead of our prescriptions, they might need our help in working through a solution themselves. For many clients, insight alone often leads to corrective action when they become aware of the imbalance between the stressors they are coping with and the availability of social support.

Chapter Highlights

- Social support is a relatively new area of research that is of interest to researchers and clinicians from many disciplines.

- Definitions of social support identify both psychologically supportive behaviors, such as emotional support, informational support, and appraisal or affirmation support, and tangible forms of support, such as assistance with tasks or material resources.

- The concepts of social support and social network have related, but distinct meanings. The social support system is a smaller portion of the overall social network that actually provides social support to the person.

- Effective support relationships are usually reciprocal; each person shares approximately equally in the giving and the receiving of social support.

- Uniplex relationships—those that have only one function or shared activity—are less effective forms of social support.

- The extent to which a social network is interconnected (its density) affects the type of social support that is likely to be provided. In some situations, a highly dense network is desirable; in others, a network with lower density is more suitable.

- Social support appears to have both direct and buffering effects on health or mental health outcomes.

- Clinical application of social support concepts requires individualized assessment and planning that takes into account unique properties of the person and the situation.

- Studies with mentally ill populations have found differences in network size, network density, reciprocity, multiplexity of relationships, and quality of relationships compared with normal populations, and these differences are related to clients' well-being.

- Negative expressed emotion exhibited by relatives of hospitalized schizophrenic clients was a major factor in predicting subsequent relapse rates. The influence of high negative expressed emotion was reduced when the client had less face-to-face contact with the negative relative and when the client maintained antipsychotic medication therapy.

- Age, gender, and other individual differences influence both how much social support is needed and how much is available.

- Normative developmental crises are events that the social support system can usually respond to positively; however, situational crises that are unexpected or associated with stigma are more difficult for the social support system to understand or respond to appropriately.

- Axes IV and V of the DSM-IIIR provide information relevant to assessing clients' social support needs.

- When planning interventions for persons with little support, the nurse must consider the reason for the inadequate support. Possible interventions include assisting a key network member to provide support, volunteer linking, mutual self-help groups, and supplemental professional support.

- Interventions to increase the social support for the chronically mentally ill include halfway houses, day treatment centers, and respite care programs.

- Research is needed to move from descriptive research findings to studies that test the effectiveness of social support interventions for various client groups.

- In the area of social support, the individual's perceptions must be taken into account in interpreting his or her needs for social support and in discovering what types or sources might be most helpful.

References

Beels C: Social support and schizophrenia. *Schizophr Bull* 1981;7:58–72.

Berkman LF, Syme SL: Social networks, host resistance, and mortality: A nine year follow-up study of Alameda County residents. *Am J Epidemiol* 1979;109:186–204.

Brady JP: Social skills training for psychiatric patients, I: Concepts, methods, and clinical results. *Am J Psychiatr* 1984;141:333–339.

Brandt PA: Clinical assessment of the social support of families with handicapped children. *Issues Compr Ped Nurs* 1984;7:187–201.

Brandt PA, Weinert C: The PRQ—A social support measure. *Nurs Res* 1981;30:277–280.

Brown GW, Birley JL, Wing JK: Influence of family life on the course of schizophrenic disorders: A replication. *Br J Psychiatry* 1972;21:241–258.

Caplan G: Support systems, in Caplan, G (ed): *Support Systems and Community Mental Health.* Behavioral Publications, 1974, pp 1–40.

Cassel JC: Psychiatric epidemiology, in *American Handbook of Psychiatry. Child and Adolescent Psychiatry, Sociocultural and Community Psychiatry,* ed 2, Caplan, G (ed). Basic Books, 1974, vol 2, pp 401–410.

Cobb S: Social support as a moderator of life stress. *Psychosom Med* 1976;38:300–314.

Ellison ES: Social networks and the mental health caregiving system: Implications for psychiatric nursing practice. *J Psychosoc Nurs Mental Health Serv* 1983;21:18–24.

Goffman E: *Stigma*. Prentice-Hall, 1963.

Goldman RH: Mental illness and family burden: A public health perspective. *Hosp Community Psychiatry* 1982; 33: 557–560.

Gottlieb BH: Social support as a focus for integrative research in psychology. *Am Psychol* 1983;38:278–287.

Hammer M: Influence of small social networks as factors on mental hospital admission. *Hum Organization* 1963–1964;22:243–251.

Helmrath TA, Steinitz EM: Death of an infant: Parental grieving and the failure of social support. *J Fam Pract* 1978;6:787–790.

House JS: *Work Stress and Social Support*. Addison-Wesley, 1981.

Kahn RL: Aging and social support, in Riley MW (ed): *Aging from Birth to Death: Interdisciplinary Perspectives*. Westview Press, 1979, pp 77–99.

Leff JP: Developments in family treatment of schizophrenia. *Psychiatr Q* 1979;51:216–232.

Lipton FR et al: Schizophrenia: A network crisis. *Schizophr Bull* 1981;7:144–151.

Lowenthal MF, Haven C: Interaction and adaptation: Intimacy as a critical variable. *Am Sociol Rev* 1968;33:20–30.

McLean CS et al: Group treatment for parents of the adult mentally ill. *Hosp Community Psychiatry* 1982;33:564–568.

Motto JA et al: Communication as a suicide prevention program, in Soubrier JP, Vedrinne J (eds): *Depression and Suicide*. Pergamon Press, 1981, pp 148–154.

Mullis N, Byers P: Social Support in suicidal inpatients. *J Psychiatr Nurs* 1987;25(4):16–19.

Norbeck JS: Social support: A model for clinical research and application. *Adv Nurs Sci* 1981;3:43–59.

Norbeck JS: The use of social support in clinical practice. *J Psychosoc Nurs* 1982;20:22–29.

Norbeck JS, Lindsey AM, Carrieri VL: The development of an instrument to measure social support. *Nurs Res* 1981;30:264–269.

Norbeck JS, Lindsey AM, Carrieri VL: Further development of the Norbeck social support questionnaire: Normative data and validity testing. *Nurs Res* 1983;32:4–9.

Norbeck JS, Tilden VP: Life stress, social support, and emotional disequilibrium in complications of pregnancy: A prospective, multivariate study. *J Health Soc Behav* 1983; 24:30–46.

Parks SH, Pilisuk M: Personal support systems of former mental patients residing in board-and-care facilities. *J Community Psychol* 1984;12:230–244.

Pattison EM et al: A psychosocial kinship model for family therapy. *Am J Psychiatry* 1975;132:1246–1251.

Perrucci R, Targ DB: Network structure and reactions to primary deviance of mental patients. *J Health Soc Behav* 1982;23:2–17.

Sokolovsky J et al: Personal networks of ex-mental patients in a Manhattan SRO hotel. *Hum Organization* 1978;37:5–15.

Tolsdorf CC: Social networks, support, and coping: An exploratory study. *Fam Process* 1976;15:407–417.

Turner SL: Disability among schizophrenics in a rural community: Services and social support. *Res Nurs Health* 1979;2:151–161.

Vaughn CE, Leff JP: The influence of family and social factors on the course of psychiatric illness: A comparison of schizophrenic and depressed neurotic patients. *Br J Psychiatry* 1976;129:125–137.

Vaughn CE, Leff, JP: Patterns of emotional response in relatives of schizophrenic patients. *Schizophr Bull* 1981;7:43–44.

Weiss RS: The provisions of social relationships, in Rubin Z (ed): *Doing Unto Others*. Prentice-Hall, 1974.

Wing JK: The social context of schizophrenia. *Am J Psychiatry* 1977;135:1333–1339.

NINE

Psychobiology

Geoffry McEnany

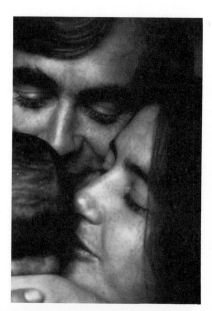

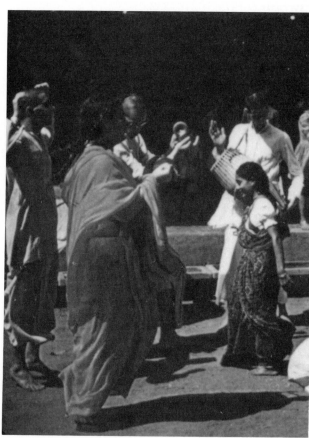

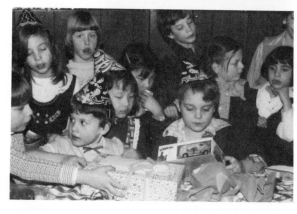

Learning Objectives

Upon completion of this chapter, the student will

- Identify the historical roots of the psychobiologic tradition

- List and describe gross neuroanatomic structures and their functions

- Discuss the role of neurotransmitters in health and disease

- Analyze the role of stress on psychobiologic functioning

- Discuss one biologic theory of schizophrenia, mood disorders, and anxiety disorders

- Enumerate two basic principles upon which clinical ecology is based

- Discuss three areas of nursing care for psychiatric clients that are amenable to psychobiologic assessment

- List and describe two psychobiologic nursing interventions

Cross References

Other topics relevant to this content are: Biologic therapies, Chapter 32; History, Chapter 2; Mood disorders, Chapter 18; Organic mental syndromes and disorders, Chapter 15; Philosophy, Chapter 1; and Schizophrenia, Chapter 16.

Key Terms

axon
cerebellum
cerebrum
circadian rhythms
clinical ecology
complex partial seizure
dendrite
diencephalon
dualism
extrapyramidal system
holism
limbic system
medulla oblongata
midbrain
neuron
neurotransmitter
pons
psychobiology
psychoendocrinology
psychoimmunology
reticular activating system
synapse
synaptic vesicles

A HISTORICAL PERSPECTIVE ON PSYCHOBIOLOGY

Psychobiology—the word brings to mind some ultramodern, high-tech future. But psychobiology is neither a new concept nor a recent discovery. It has existed since the birth of humankind and has been a subject of discussion for at least the last 2000 years. What *is* new in psychobiology is a broader understanding of the biologic basis of the mind and behavior. Contemporary knowledge of the biologic components of behavior is revolutionizing not only psychiatry but also our view of so-called mental illness and its treatment.

Defining the Concept

A comprehensive definition of psychobiology is difficult at best. Psychobiology encompasses an enormous body of information that is growing almost exponentially. For this reason, the conceptual "face" of psychobiology is changing. With these thoughts in mind, we can offer the following definition: **Psychobiology** is the study of the biochemical foundations of thought, mood, emotion, affect, and behavior. It takes into consideration both internal and external influences such as genetics, the effects of other body systems such as the endocrine and immune systems, and the external environment across the life span of an individual.

When students study the neurologic system in an anatomy and physiology class, they are likely to look at the material through the "lens" of an anatomist or physiologist. Similarly, when they study psychosis in a psychology or psychiatric nursing class, they probably explore the behavioral or psychodynamic aspects of psychosis, not really

This book views humanitarian and political action as appropriate and important aspects of nurses' professional responsibilities.

169

knowing how they will use the knowledge from an anatomy and physiology class in the psychology classroom or in clinical work. In this chapter we strive to give students an overview of psychobiology and make them aware of how psychobiology principles dovetail with those of nursing. It is impossible in one chapter to even touch upon all of the facets of psychobiology in any detail; this chapter is an attempt to motivate students to apply psychobiologic principles in professional work.

From Hippocrates to the Present

Every achievement that people perceive as great or spectacular—the seven wonders of the world, the Roman Empire, the landing of men on the moon, a Mozart concerto, test-tube babies, artificial hearts, computers, telecommunications—is due to the capacity of the human brain. Extraordinarily complex in its composition and functioning, the human brain is the source of all creativity, logic, thought, and emotion.

The brain has been regarded as a mysterious wonder throughout history. Hippocrates (460 B.C.) the "father of medicine," postulated that the brain is the central organ of intellectual functioning and that mental disorders are secondary to brain pathology:

> Men ought to know that from the brain, and from the brain only, arise pleasures, joys, laughters, jests, and our sorrows, pains, griefs or fears. . . . It is the same thing that makes us mad or delirious, inspires us with dread or fear, whether by night or by day, brings sleeplessness, inopportune mistakes, aimless anxieties, absent-mindedness, and acts that are contrary to habit.

In light of the Greek belief that mental disorders were of supernatural origin, Hippocrates' biologic model of illness must have seemed shocking. Nonetheless, it established a differentiation between mind and body in the Greek thought of Hippocrates' era.

Plato and Aristotle also influenced the concept of mental illness. Plato (ca. 400 B.C.) was more supportive of what might be termed today as a psychologic rather than biologic notion of "mental" illness. For example, in *The Republic,* Plato discussed three subdivisions of the soul, which have been compared to the id, ego, and superego. In contrast, Aristotle (ca. 350 B.C.) believed that disturbed mental functioning was secondary to an imbalance in the four body humors (blood, phlegm, black bile, and yellow bile) postulated by Hippocrates, thus associating states of the mind with body function.

Ancient Romans furthered the idea that mental illness had a biologic base and was not due to supernatural influences. Asclepiades, founder of a Roman school of medicine, described phrenitis and mania, noting physical aspects of each condition. Additionally, Asclepiades recommended coarse biologic treatments, e.g., placing clients with certain mental conditions in rooms filled with light, rather than in the dark. Today, exposure to light is known to influence the reticular activating system, a part of the brain that controls various states of wakefulness. Additionally, exposure to full spectrum light is used today to treat conditions such as seasonal affective disorder.

During the Dark Ages (400–1200) there was little support for the notion that mental illness has a biologic basis. However, some important ideas emerged about the classification of psychobiopathologic states. Several descriptions of illness, including cyclic patterns of mood, melancholia, mania, psychotic behaviors, epilepsy, and dementia were written during this period. Treatments of mental disorders were physical, e.g., bloodletting and trepanation. Others were spiritual, as evidenced by the popularity of exorcisms during that period.

The Renaissance contributed a miscellaneous collection of explanations about the cause of mental disorders and varied treatments. One school of thought held closely to the belief that mental disorders were the result of spiritual imbalance or witchcraft. Another group, led mainly by Johann Weyer, viewed psychopathology as the result of interacting physical and spiritual factors. Weyer expanded on the descriptive classifications of mental disorders and emphasized the importance of accurate assessment and close observation during treatment.

During the seventeenth and eighteenth centuries, a marked shift in thought occurred, as the mind-body explanation of illness reemerged. During this era mental disorders came under the domain of medicine, and many physicians believed that doctors should be the sole caretakers of the mentally disordered. During this period great attention was given to the physical manifestations of "hysterical" conditions, which were perhaps the beginnings of what has come to be known as psychosomatics.

Between the nineteenth century and the present, the greatest strides have been made toward understanding mental disorders from a biologic perspective. A clearly biologic model began to emerge. In the latter part of the nineteenth century, physicians began to view psychopathology as a result of changes in the nervous system. Eventually other causes were considered, e.g., genetic predisposition and the role of endocrine dysfunction in various states of mental illness.

Of course, during the late nineteenth and early twentieth centuries, Sigmund Freud developed his theory of psychoanalysis. Prior to becoming interested in emotional conditions, Freud was a neurologist. Unfortunately, he was unable to make the link between psychologic defenses against anxiety and the biologic processes of anxiety. Nonetheless, Freud made greatly significant contributions to the developing, although inexact, science of psychiatry, allowing for the unfolding of new ideas and a reexamination of old beliefs about mental disorders.

A major shift in contemporary Western psychiatry occurred during the 1930s and 1940s with the introduction of solely biologic therapies, e.g., shock treatment and various psychosurgeries. These treatments, with their subsequent successes and failures, kindled a strong interest in the biology of behavior. This trend led to biologic research and new treatments. An important step in the development of a biologic model in psychiatry was the introduction of psychotropic drugs, substances that had affected the brain and central nervous system to produce a desired change in behavior. This intervention was revolutionary. Psychotropic medications clearly refuted dualism and gave psychiatry objective evidence for a holistic view of the person. Although the effects of the drugs were clearly visible in the behavior of the people who took them, many mental health professionals continued to deny the existence of a biologic basis of mental disorders. Despite empirical evidence to the contrary, many today continue to explore solely psychologic explanations for behavior when physical explanations exist. The persistent denial of the physiologic aspects of mental illness possibly constitutes a nemesis. In the words of Illich (1976), a *nemesis* is "the inevitable punishment for attempts to be a hero rather than a human being" (p 35). It is dreadful to think that people bear the "punishment" of continued symptoms of mental disorders because a professional believes that "the harder the client works, the better the cure" (Lickey and Gordon 1983, p 9). Anyone who has ever tried to talk someone out of a hallucination, delusion, major depression, anorexia nervosa, or panic attack knows how ineffective this can be. However, because psychiatric illness is not unlike other forms of illness, it responds to varied interventions, depending on its severity. For some unbalanced states of emotion, behavioral intervention may be adequate. For clients with more severe states of disequilibrium, medications may be necessary for a full return to wellness. Psychobiology and its behavioral correlates are undeniable, and nurses need to foster an understanding of psychobiologic principles in practice. Such applied knowledge is likely to lend greater integrity to the practice of psychiatric-mental health nursing, while refuting the ancient tradition of dualism.

Dualism versus Holism in Nursing

An article in a recent nursing journal reported the outcomes of a conference on holistic nursing. According to the report, nurses from around the country had gathered to share their views on how nursing can be practiced more holistically, how holistic principles need to be more fully integrated into programs of nursing education, and finally, how to measure outcomes of care delivered in a holistic versus traditional fashion. Although the article was clear,

the need for such a conference seemed confusing. Nursing schools everywhere teach students to examine client problems from a biopsychosocial perspective, which was not addressed in the report. What the nurses at this conference were calling holistic included such practices as massage therapy, therapeutic touch, and other techniques that seemed more alternative or novel than holistic. The next questions in response to the report of the holistic conference were, "What, then, is holism and how does this influence nursing function?"

To appreciate holism more fully, we might explore its opposing perspective, dualism, from which the need for holism perhaps arose. Dualism maintains a view of the person as consisting of two irreducible elements: mind and body. From the dualistic perspective, the mind is separate from the body. In pure dualism, the interrelationships between mind and body are few or essentially nonexistent. Dualism receives support from many of the world's major religions, which accept the separateness of the body and soul and view the mind as sacred and the body as a banal dwelling spot of the mind and soul.

The holistic perspective views the person as an integrated whole whose parts share an organic and functional relationship. In the holistic view, the mind is not separate from the body, but it is a biochemical manifestation of the brain. A truly holistic approach in nursing allows for nothing but a biopsychosocial perspective in client care. In psychiatric nursing, holism means incorporating psychobiologic principles in assessment and intervention strategies in an innovative fashion.

BRAIN, MIND, AND BEHAVIOR

A Neuroanatomic Review

Volumes have been written about the anatomy of the nervous system. In this chapter it is impossible to even touch upon all of the major neuroanatomic structures. The points of interest here include the structures of the brain believed to be involved in the formation of thought and emotion. The first half of this section focuses on gross neuroanatomy, and the latter explores neuroanatomy and physiology from a cellular perspective.

The brain is defined in various ways. The definition that best suits the perspective of this chapter is that of Restak (1984), who states that the brain is that part of the central nervous system encapsulated by the skull. The brain is the core of our humanity. Intercommunications of different parts of the brain yield the experiences of love, hate, elation, joy, or madness. The brain provides the underlying biology for will, determination, hopes, and dreams. Without the brain to integrate experience, people would neither enjoy the wonder nor fear the horror of life.

This review explores the following six anatomic structures of the brain: cerebrum, diencephalon, cerebellum, medulla oblongata, pons, and midbrain; the last three comprise the brain stem.

The Cerebrum

The **cerebrum** is the largest part of the human brain. It is divided into two seemingly equal components, the *cerebral hemispheres.* The deep furrow that divides the hemispheres is known as the *longitudinal sulcus.* A small but important piece of tissue, the *corpus callosum,* connects the two hemispheres medially and allows communication between them. In the past, scientists believed that each hemisphere had separate functions such as logic or creativity and spatial accommodation. With the advent of new technologies such as positive emission tomography, it is now possible to assess metabolic activity in the brain as it occurs. Scientists are able to observe brain activity and have realized that creative as well as logical activities require input from both cerebral hemispheres.

The brain in general, and the cerebral hemispheres in particular, are well protected not only by the skull but also by a protective fluid (cerebrospinal fluid) that circulates around and within the brain. Deep within the brain are three spaces or *ventricles* that aid in the circulation of cerebrospinal fluid.

The cerebral hemispheres are divided into lobes, which are named after the parts of the skull under which they lie, i.e., frontal, temporal, occipital, and parietal (see Box 9–1 and Figure 9–1). All of the lobes contain many *gyri* (ridges) and *sulci* (grooves) that maximize brain surface area.

The cerebral hemispheres consist of both white and gray matter. Gray matter consists of myelinated fibers that are referred to as *nerves;* bundles of nerves are called *tracts.* The cerebral cortex consists solely of gray matter with underlying white matter. The cerebral cortex works much as the processing unit of a computer does. The cortex is the part of the brain that makes sense out of the volumes of input. It synthesizes thought, reasoning, will, and choice and is the seat of dreams.

As essential as the cerebral hemispheres are to emotional, intellectual, and biologic functioning, they are only as good as the quality of other interdependent structures in the brain. For example, people need various input and clear communication between different brain structures to produce efficient and purposeful behavior. An example of

---

Box 9–1
GROSS FUNCTIONS OF THE CEREBRAL LOBES

Frontal Lobes

- Responsible for any movements; the right frontal lobe controls left side body movement and vice versa
- Contain the *premotor cortex,* which organizes complicated movement
- Contain *prefrontal fibers,* which produce a "social conscience," inhibiting unacceptable behaviors

Parietal Lobes

- Contain the *sensory cortex,* which interprets contact sensations such as touch
- Facilitate spatial orientation

Temporal Lobes

- Involved in hearing and memory
- Connect with the limbic system (the "emotional brain") to allow for memory and expression of emotions such as anger, fright, and possibly love

Occipital Lobes

- Contain centers responsible for the complete experience of vision
- Are involved in language formation
- Collaborate with other brain structures in the formation of memory

---

the intercommunication between brain structures is the activity of the **limbic system.** This system, often referred to as "the emotional brain," is believed to be responsible for the modulation of emotions, memory, and possibly some aspects of attention (Andreasen 1984). The limbic system consists of neuroanatomic structures from the cerebral hemispheres and the **diencephalon,** a part of the brain located between the cerebrum and midbrain (Figure 9–2).

Two limbic structures play an especially important role in the enactment of emotion: the *amygdala* and the *hippocampus.* Begley et al. (1983, p 42) define the amygdala as a "bulbous waystation . . . [that] seems to process sensations wrapped in an aura of happiness or sadness and, perhaps, index the memory under the headings such as 'joy' or 'grief.' " Restak (1984) discusses the amygdala in relation to the hippocampus for the purpose of understanding the role both structures play in the formation of memories. Do you remember what you were doing on January

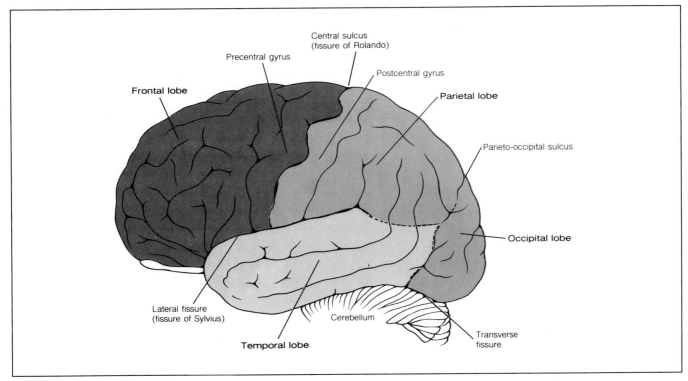

Figure 9–1
Delineation of the cerebral lobes.
Source: Spence AP, Mason EB: Human Anatomy and Physiology, *ed 3. Benjamin/Cummings, 1987, p 341.*

20, 1986? Unless that day had some major significance for you, chances are that you don't remember that day or remember it only vaguely. If, however, you won a million dollars on that day or attended a close friend's wedding or funeral, you are likely to remember it clearly. Emotion and memory are closely linked and are mediated through the structures of the limbic system. Of course, the view presented here is brief and oversimplified. All of the psychobiologic components of emotion, memory, and cognition are not known. What is known is that expression of thought or emotion involves the coordination of many different areas of the brain. An important assumption is that the neuroanatomy and physiology underlying thought and emotion must be relatively intact for an individual to think clearly and experience emotion fully. What is not clearly known is the degree of neurophysiologic variability among normal people. The behavioral correlates of neurophysiologic activity are seen in the behaviors of familiar persons and strangers. A busdriver making change for a rider, a police officer directing traffic, a mentally ill person on the street mumbling and yelling to seemingly nobody—all of these behaviors are the result of some form of activity in the brain. Surely a huge variance exists between illness and wellness behavior, but the finer points of how these differences manifest themselves in the realm of neurobiologic activity are not yet completely known.

Thalamus and Hypothalamus

Other limbic structures are in the diencephalon and include the thalamus and the hypothalamus. The *thalamus* functions as a relay station, receiving many impulses from the spinal cord, brain stem, and cerebellum. With the aid of many connections in the cerebral hemispheres and cortex, the thalamus regulates activity and movement, sensory experience, and emotional behavior.

The *hypothalamus* is a neuroanatomic marketplace of sorts, consisting of many structures such as the *supraoptic nuclei,* parts of the *pituitary gland,* and the *mamillary bodies.* The hypothalamus weighs approximately four grams and is less than 1 percent of the total brain volume (Restak 1984). However, its size is not a good indication of its importance. The hypothalamus is responsible for appetite control, fluid balance within the body, sexual impulse regulation, endocrine function, and temperature modulation. Within the hypothalamus lies the motivation of humankind and an awesome coordination of behaviors accom-

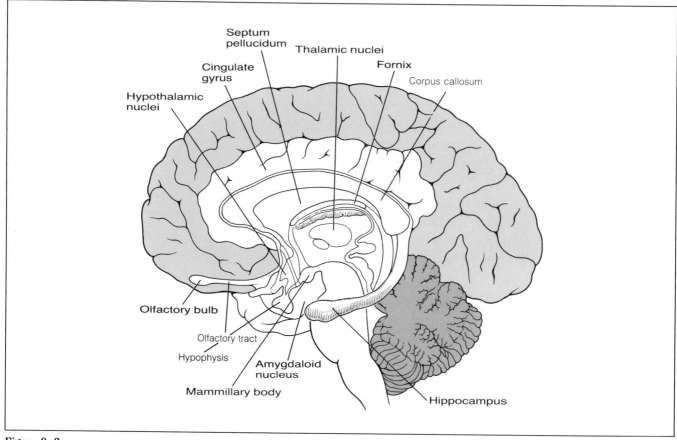

Figure 9–2
Structures of the limbic system.
Source: Spence AP, Mason EB: Human Anatomy and Physiology, *ed 3. Benjamin/Cummings, 1987, p 350.*

panying emotional expression. Mahler's frenzy, Frankenstein's monster's rage, and Lady MacBeth's woeful fears are most likely complements of hypothalamic activity. Students may be very aware of their hypothalamic activity when they experience fatigue after final examinations, middle-of-the-night munchies, and irritation at an inconsiderate roommate. Currently, some psychobiologists believe that the roots of such disorders as bulimia and anorexia nervosa lie in the hypothalamus.

Cerebellum

The **cerebellum** is that part of the brain that lies below the posterior section of the cerebrum. It is the second-largest structure within the brain (Figure 9–3). Like the cerebral hemispheres, the cerebellum has an outer layer of gray matter and is mainly composed of underlying white matter. The main function of this highly specialized part of the brain is movement and coordination. The hand-eye coor-

dination of a diamond cutter, the fluid movements of a ballerina, and the success of a quarterback's moves all depend on cerebellar functions. As you read this page, you are depending on your cerebellum to send messages to your eyes that allow you to follow the print as you read from one line to the next.

Brain Stem

The final section of this review involves an examination of the brain stem. The brain stem consists of three smaller structures: the medulla oblongata, the pons, and the midbrain (Figure 9–4). The **medulla oblongata** (Latin for oblong marrow) is the connecting piece of tissue between the brain stem and the spinal cord. It is less than two inches long but is responsible for many vital functions including respiration, regulation of blood pressure, and partial regulation of heart rate. It also controls vomiting, swallowing, and some aspects of talking. Incoming fibers from the spinal

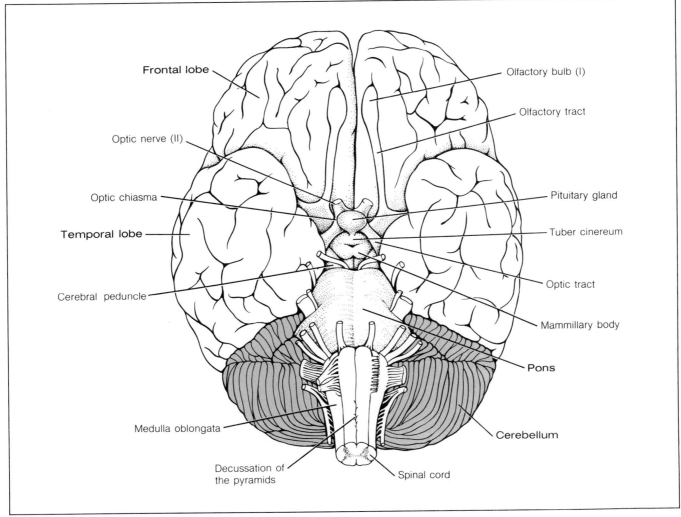

Figure 9–3
The cerebrum and cerebellum.
Source: Spence AP, Mason EB: Human Anatomy and Physiology, *ed 3. Benjamin/Cummings, 1987, p 346.*

cord cross over in the medulla, yielding left cerebral hemispheric control of the right side of the body and vice versa.

Pons means *bridge,* and bridging is its function. The pons contains conduction paths between the spinal cord and the brain. It also contains reflex centers that mediate sensations of the face, chewing, abduction of the eyes, facial expressions, balance, and regulation of respiration. Connections with the limbic system allow the pons to modulate expressions that indicate states such as tenderness, anger, fear, or happiness.

The **midbrain** is above the pons and below the cerebral hemispheres. Not unlike the pons, the midbrain (or mesencephalon) is a reflex center for the regulation of eye movement, visual accommodation, and regulation of pupil size. Additionally, the midbrain is essential for relaying

impulses to the cerebral cortex and sending behavior-producing messages back to the periphery.

Certain portions of the brain function in concert with other parts to create a system with a given function; the limbic system is a good example. Other systems that are of special interest to psychiatric nurses include the reticular activating system and the extrapyramidal system.

The **reticular activating system (RAS)** consists of nerve pathways that originate in the spinal cord and connect in the reticular formation, a system of neurons that modulates awareness and states of consciousness. The RAS screens stimulation from the environment and allows people to concentrate. Imagine what it would be like to have to pay attention to all sounds, smells, and sights in the environment around you as you read this page. Reading would be impossible and concentration would suffer greatly. The RAS also permits routine inattention, allowing for sleep. In states of mental illness, there is obviously some biologic disequilibrium of the RAS. However, the details of this imbalance are complex and not well understood at this time.

The **extrapyramidal system** consists of tracts of motor neurons from the brain to parts of the spinal cord. This system has complex relays and connections to areas of the cortex, cerebellum, brain stem, and thalamus. These tracts play an important role in gross movements and responses of emotional tone, e.g., smiling and frowning.

Antipsychotic drugs create side effects that affect the extrapyramidal system, hence extrapyramidal side effects

or EPS. The four general classes of extrapyramidal side effects include (a) parkinsonism, (b) dyskinesias and dystonias, (c) akathisias, and (d) tardive dyskinesia.

Central Nervous System Cells

The anatomic structure of the brain is incredibly complex on gross examination; things become even more complex as one looks at the biochemical processes that occur with every thought, emotion, inspiration, dream, or hope. Thought and feeling are made possible by complex interplays and communications between cells in the central nervous system in relation to the environment. The specialized cells of the nervous system are called **neurons**. Like other cells in the body, each neuron has a cell body that contains the cytoplasm and the nucleus. Unlike other cells, a neuron has at least two other processes: an axon and one or more dendrites (Figure 9–5). An **axon** is that portion of

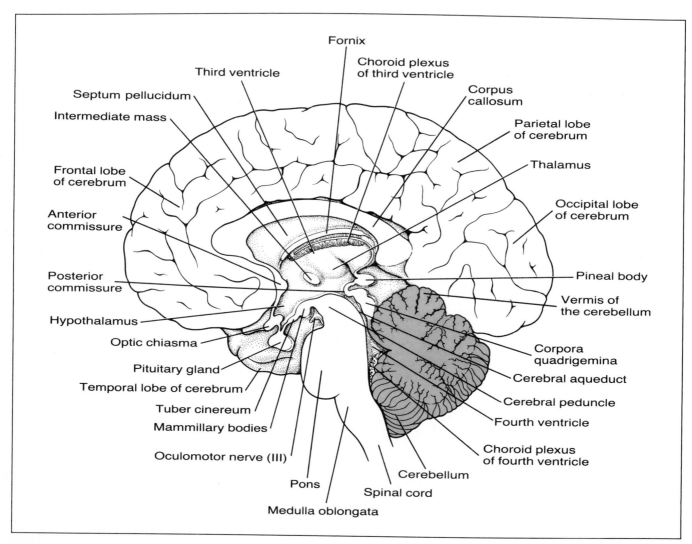

Figure 9–4
Structures of the cerebrum and cerebellum.
Source: Spence AP, Mason EB: Human Anatomy and Physiology, *ed 3. Benjamin/Cummings, 1987, p 348.*

the neuron that conveys electric impulses *from* the cell body to other neurons. Axons are covered with a white myelin sheath and compose the white matter in the brain and spinal cord. **Dendrites** are *not* myelinated but allow for the conduction of electric messages *to* the cell body. There are approximately one hundred billion neurons in the brain with nearly an equal number of supporting (glia) cells (Hubel 1979).

Neurons are classified according to the direction in which they conduct impulses. *Sensory neurons,* also known as afferent neurons, send messages from the periphery to the brain. For example, if someone puts a foot into a tub of scalding water, the message that the water is too hot is sent to the brain on sensory neuron pathways. *Motor* or

efferent *neurons* carry messages that originate in the brain and yield a behavioral change in the periphery. In the example of the foot in the hot water, the message from the brain is to remove the foot (quickly!) from the hot water; this message travels on motor neuron paths. Sometimes, specialized neurons that communicate between sensory and motor neurons help to produce a given, desirable behavior.

Communication among and between neurons is complex and specific. This communication is believed to be the

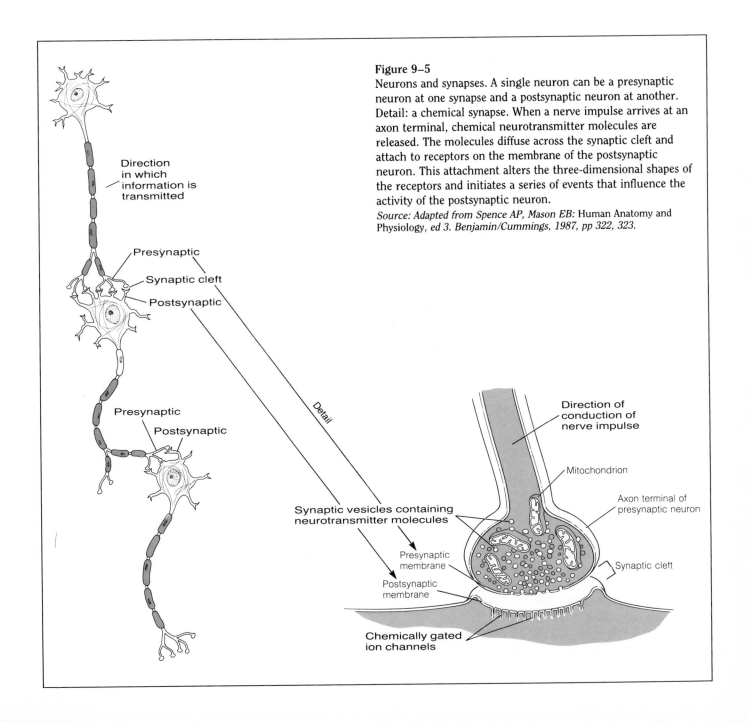

Figure 9–5
Neurons and synapses. A single neuron can be a presynaptic neuron at one synapse and a postsynaptic neuron at another. Detail: a chemical synapse. When a nerve impulse arrives at an axon terminal, chemical neurotransmitter molecules are released. The molecules diffuse across the synaptic cleft and attach to receptors on the membrane of the postsynaptic neuron. This attachment alters the three-dimensional shapes of the receptors and initiates a series of events that influence the activity of the postsynaptic neuron.
Source: Adapted from Spence AP, Mason EB: Human Anatomy and Physiology, *ed 3. Benjamin/Cummings, 1987, pp 322, 323.*

Direction in which information is transmitted

Presynaptic

Synaptic cleft

Postsynaptic

Presynaptic

Postsynaptic

Detail

Synaptic vesicles containing neurotransmitter molecules

Presynaptic membrane

Postsynaptic membrane

Chemically gated ion channels

Direction of conduction of nerve impulse

Mitochondrion

Axon terminal of presynaptic neuron

Synaptic cleft

basis of behavior. Any given neuron is likely to have contact with hundreds or thousands of other neurons, and the actual number of synaptic contacts in the brain alone may number 100 trillion (Hubel 1979). Interneuron communication is electric and chemical and occurs at the synapses, or points of contact between neurons, as well as along the neuron itself. The **synapse** is a microscopic gap on the cleft between neurons. Disordered activity can occur in this space, perhaps causing affective and schizophrenic illnesses.

Neurotransmitters

A closer look at the synapse reveals some fascinating information (Figure 9–5). The membrane of the end point or axon terminal of one neuron contains many saclike projections known as **synaptic vesicles**. The vesicles contain the chemicals that allow the transmission of electric impulses across the synapse. These chemicals are known as **neurotransmitters**. As an impulse travels down an axon toward the synapse, it stimulates a change in the cell membrane and commands the vesicles to release the neurotransmitter into the synaptic cleft. The results in the neurotransmitter chemicals binding to specific receptors on the dendrites of the adjacent neuron, allowing the electric impulse to cross the synapse and continue its course to the next neuron. It takes less than 0.0005 second for the impulse to move from the presynaptic terminal to the postsynaptic receptors (Lickey and Gordon 1983). What happens to the neurotransmitter substance that was released into the synapse *after* the impulse has passed? One of two things can occur: The neurotransmitter can be dissolved by enzymes in the synapse, or the chemical can be reabsorbed for recycling by the presynaptic neuron (re-uptake). In either case, the synapse and its pre- and postneurons are reset for the next impulse, at which time the process is repeated.

At this time, nobody actually knows how many neurotransmitters exist in the human brain. Box 9–2 lists those neurotransmitters that are currently known. Current estimates of the number of possible neurotransmitters exceeds forty (Iversen 1982). Part of the problem has been in deciding specific criteria to determine what chemicals in the brain can actually be called neurotransmitters. Several other neurochemical substances, known as neuromodulators, neurohormones, and neuroregulators, modify the actions of neurotransmitters but are not neurotransmitters themselves (Lander 1983). The following section examines the neurotransmitters and their functions.

Biogenic Amine (Monoamine) Neurotransmitters

This group of neurotransmitters includes dopamine, norepinephrine, serotonin, and histamine; the first three are implicated in mood disorders and schizophrenia (Brown and Mann 1985). Dopamine is a plentiful neurotransmitter synthesized from the dietary amino acid tyrosine and found in three parts of the brain: the brain's substantia nigra motor center (which affects movement and coordination), midbrain (involving emotion and memory), and the hypothalamus/pituitary connection (involving emotional responses and stress-coping patterns). Norepinephrine receptors are found in the cerebral cortex (affecting cognitive functions), the limbic system (yielding emotional responses), and hippocampus and thalamus (contributing to emotion, pleasure, and memory), the cerebellum (influencing movement), and the hypothalamus (influencing thirst, body temperature, and appetite). Serotonin pathways are somewhat similar to norepinephrine pathways and have similar effects and influences. Histamine, while of extreme importance in the peripheral nervous system, has not received great attention as a central neurotransmitter (Lander 1983).

Acetylcholine

Acetylcholine is the "grandparent" of neurotransmitters as it was the first neurochemical to be identified as a true

---

Box 9–2
KNOWN NEUROTRANSMITTERS IN THE BRAIN

Amine Neurotransmitters

- Serotonin
- Dopamine
- Norepinephrine
- Histamine

Cholinergic Neurotransmitters

- Acetylcholine

Amino Acid Neurotransmitters

- Glycine
- Gamma Aminobutyric Acid
- Glutamate

Source: Andreasen NC: The Broken Brain. Harper & Row, 1984, p 133.

neurotransmitter. It is available practically everywhere in the brain and spinal cord but is especially abundant in the neurons involved with some form of movement (motor neurons). It is considered to be highly significant in neuromuscular transmission (Iversen 1982).

Amino Acids

This group of neurotransmitters is of special interest to many, including the psychiatric nurse, because they are readily available in the form of proteins in the diet. As ingested proteins, these substances are precursors to neurotransmitters; brain cells convert these proteins into neurotransmitters. For example, there is truth in the folk wisdom that warmed milk with honey helps people sleep. Milk contains the amino acid *tryptophan.* In the presence of a carbohydrate such as honey, the tryptophan molecule binds with the glucose (carbohydrate) from the honey. Since the brain runs on glucose, the glucose/tryptophan combination can cross the blood/brain barrier. Once inside the brain, tryptophan is converted to serotonin and aids in the induction of sleep. Other examples of dietary amino acids include glutamate (also known as monosodium glutamate), choline (available from soybeans), and tyrosine. These amino acids are discussed later in this chapter. Amino acids in the central nervous system seem to be used for fast transmission of impulses in all regions of the brain. Chains of amino acids are believed to have a regulatory effect on central nervous system activity, especially in the area of pain regulation.

Neurotransmitter activity cannot be underestimated in states of both health and illness. If synaptic activity controls events such as thought, emotion, movement, and overall biologic functions, then one can anticipate that attention and research will expand knowledge in this area, eventually offering greater options for intervention in psychiatry and psychiatric nursing.

Psychoendocrinology and Psychoimmunology

Earlier in this chapter the notion of holism versus dualism was explored; this section further refutes the concept of dualism by examining the interaction of the brain and two subsystems: the endocrine and immune systems.

Grebb and Reus (1984) describe psychoendocrinology as a subspecialty of endocrinology that explores the relationship between behavior, biology, and endocrine function. Endocrine action is mediated through chemical substances such as hormones. Three classes of hormones exist: steroids, peptides, and amino acids. The peptides are of special interest to those in psychiatry because these hormones coexist with certain neurotransmitters (monoamines) and affect actions in the synapse. The peptides function as neuroregulators, i.e., they assist in neurotransmission but are not solely responsible for the entire bio-

chemical synaptic sequence. The peptides are also involved in the regulation of hormonal axes; recently, the cortisol axis has received significant attention in conjunction with the dexamethasone suppression test for depression. Box 9–3 shows the main hormonal axes and conditions that result from disordered peptide functioning. It is important to remember that neuroregulators are influenced by input from the limbic system (the "emotional" brain), the cerebral cortex (the "thinking" brain), and the hypothalamus and pineal gland (involved in hormonal secretion).

In the last few years there has been an upsurge of interest by psychiatrists and psychiatric nurses in the behavioral manifestations of thyroid dysfunction. As Vogel (1986, p 9) points out, clients with thyroid dysfunction present a "mixed bag" of symptoms including those that suggest mood disorders, heart disease, organic brain syndrome, and lithium toxicity.

A psychiatric nurse, for instance, might encounter the following scenario. The nurse walks into the room of Rose, a 44-year-old depressed woman.

Nurse: Hello, Rose.
Rose: (Rose is initially silent but rolls over in her bed and looks at the nurse.) Leave me alone . . .
Nurse: It's clear to me that you'd like to be left alone, but it's 8:30 in the morning, and you're expected at breakfast.
Rose: Take a hike, nurse! I'm exhausted, I've got aches and pains. If I eat, I'll just get more constipated. And besides, it's freezing in this place! Don't you people believe in using heat? What day is this anyway? And who *are* you? Did I work with you yesterday? I can't remember your name . . .

Rose's behaviors match the DSM-IIIR criteria for major depressive disorder. But what other behaviors is she demonstrating? She complains of fatigue, constipation, and vague pains and aches. She reports feeling cold, and her memory is poor. She is not oriented to the day. One of a thousand things might be going on with Rose, right? Not necessarily. Rose is perhaps demonstrating early signs of hypothyroidism. A quick review of her laboratory tests show normal thyroid function. Reviewing her admission physical exam, the nurse notices that her thyroid was basically normal, although slightly larger on the left than the right. At this point the nurse might abandon the idea that Rose's behaviors may be linked to thyroid dysfunction. But did the physician check Rose's thyroglobulin and thyroid microsomal antibodies? Gordin and Lamberg (1976), endocrine researchers from the University of Helsinki, report that some clients who show no clinical signs of thyroid dysfunction actually suffer from *autoimmune thryoiditis.* This condition produces an autoimmune process within the thyroid that eventually leads to atrophy of the gland and subsequent hypothyroidism. The early clinical indices used are those aforementioned thyroid antibody tests.

The nurse's expert clinical skills proved to be correct in Rose's case. It was not just depression that caused Rose to behave as she did. She was suffering from a treatable psychobiologic condition, autoimmune thyroiditis. Because of the nurse's keen assessment and interdisciplinary col-

laboration, Rose can receive the appropriate treatment and care.

Psychoimmunology explores the relationships among the central nervous system, the immune system, and behavior. Nurses, physicians, and others working in the health sciences have long been aware of the relationship between stress and illness. Arthritis, colitis, thyrotoxicosis, asthma, and cancer are a few of the conditions believed to be influenced by inordinate stress and its effect on immune system mediation. McKegney (1982) points out that within the last decade the relationship between stress and illness has been documented in numerous instances in the scientific literature and is not solely limited to "physical" illness. Of course, to a holistic practitioner, to speak of physical illness as different from mental illness makes little sense other than describing the qualities of the presenting symptoms.

The ways in which stress influences illness and disease are mostly unknown at this time. Most researchers who

---

Box 9–3
BEHAVIORAL CONDITIONS RELATED TO HORMONAL DISRUPTION

Cortisol

Hypercortisolism may lead to:

- Depression
- Mania
- Psychosis
- Confusion

Hypocortisolism may lead to:

- Apathy
- Fatigue
- Depression

Thyroid

Hyperthyroidism may lead to:

- Anxiety
- Restlessness
- Irritability

Hypothyroidism may lead to:

- Depression
- Cognitive impairment
- Confusion
- Psychosis

Autoimmune thyroiditis may produce a variety of concurrent behaviors, including:

- Anxiety
- Depression
- Somatic complaints (common)

Growth Hormone

- May be involved peripherally in the mechanism of Alzheimer's disease
- Causes acromegaly or dwarfism

Prolactin

Hyperactivity of the prolactin regulatory system may lead to:

- Lethargy
- Irritability
- Increased thirst

Other hormones of behavioral interest include endorphins, enkephalins, and cholecystokinin.

Source: From Table 11-3, p 134, "Neurobehavioral Chemistry and Physiology" by JA Grebb, VI Reus. Reproduced with permission from Review of General Psychiatry *by HH Goldman (ed). Copyright © 1984 by Lange Medical Publications. Reprinted by permission of Appleton-Lange Publishing Co., Los Altos, CA.*

have examined the effects of stress on disease states conducted animal studies that are difficult to generalize to a human population. However, as McKegney (1984) points out, the hypothalamic-pituitary-adrenal cortex axis is likely to be involved.

Circadian Rhythms

Life on this planet has evolved by the rhythm of the day-and-night cycle, and humans are no exception. Human life and biology demonstrate cycles of approximately 24 hours. Moore-Ede and his colleagues (1983) at Harvard Medical School have a special interest in circadian rhythms as they affect health and disease. They believe that one of the major functions of the circadian timing system is the sequencing of metabolic/physiologic events and compatible coordination of the same. Additionally, they believe that certain sleep disorders, endocrine disorders, and bipolar disorders may have circadian bases.

What underlies the human propensity for maintaining this approximate 24-hour cycle? Circadian rhythms within the body are believed to be *endogenous*, i.e., diurnal changes are likely to occur even when people are not in the natural environment. In other words, if a person were placed in a room that had a constant amount of light and sound over 24 hours but was not exposed to natural events such as sunlight and darkness, there would still be predictable shifts in cortisol, body temperature, sleep, and other circadian-dependent variables. The cyclic pattern is likely a response to the environment that evolved over time.

Currently, two circadian pacemakers are believed to exist: One is connected to the eyes and vision, and the location of the other is uncertain (Moore-Ede et al 1983). Because at least one of the pacemakers is located in a light-sensitive area, it makes great sense to hypothesize that the body learns its rhythms from light-dark cycles. Disorders of rhythmicity are observed in insomnia and affective disorders; some clinicians report seeing clients whose symptoms seem to be seasonally related. The belief is that these clients are very sensitive to changes in the number of hours of exposure to light each day. Also, early morning awakening is a common complaint of depressed people. High serum cortisol levels are common in depressed people. Is the sleep disturbance a part of the depression, a result of high serum cortisol, or an independently disturbed rhythm? Determination and resolution of such a question require accurate assessment and appropriate intervention.

Research at the National Institute of Mental Health (NIMH) suggests that defective circadian mechanisms may cause depressed or manic symptoms in vulnerable people. Such people who have affective illnesses demonstrate behavior indicative of faulty circadian pacemaker systems (Alper 1983). Additionally, follow-up studies at NIMH showed that people who respond to antidepressants do so in a fraction of the usual time if they are deprived of sleep for one

night. Other people with *bipolar disorder* are demonstrating a keen sensitivity to changes in the length of day due to seasonal changes; they experience seasonal depression in the autumn that terminates in hypomania in the spring (Alper 1983).

Some disturbances of circadian rhythm are amenable to nursing intervention. For instance, the nurse can help to "reset" a client's circadian clock by regulating that person's sleep pattern. Plumlee (1986), a nurse who has written on the subject of biologic rhythms, offers several helpful suggestions to psychiatric nurses who need to assess client rhythms. Other interventions, prescribed by physicians, include circadian rhythm–altering substances such as lithium, some steroids, and possibly tricyclic antidepressants (Moore-Ede et al 1983).

Stress and Biology

In the last thirty years, since Hans Selye introduced the concept of stress in his *general adaptation syndrome,* the topic of stress-induced illness has been the subject of much discussion and research. The last section presented some recent advances in psychoimmunology and psychoendocrinology, two areas in a growing body of psychobiologic knowledge.

Zegans (1982) discusses possibilities for a theory of stress and illness. He states: "Certain environmental, maturational, and intrapsychic events can initiate the stress response. Each state of this response has associated cognitive, affective, and physiological components. . . . Critical to any theory that claims that stress of a psychosocial nature can alter body function is the demonstration that brain structures exist that can mediate between cognitive-affective representations in higher cortical centers, and those lower nuclei systems that regulate hormonal and autonomic activity" (p 147).

Although no *unified* theory of how stress interacts with the body subsystems to produce illness and disease currently exists, many new possibilities are currently being developed. Some investigators choose to look at specific variables that predispose people to stress-related illnesses. Farber (1982) is interested in genetic diversity and differing reactions to stress. She points out that people respond differently to stressors because of endogenous factors. Farber states that delineating the interaction between genetic constitution and the environment is difficult but not impossible. Researchers have demonstrated a connection between genetic predisposition and coronary heart disease, alcohol consumption, asthma, ulcers, colitis, menstrual complaints, enuresis, and psychosis.

PSYCHOBIOLOGY AND MENTAL DISORDERS

This section examines current theories of the causes of schizophrenia, mood disorders (bipolar disorder, mania, depression), anxiety disorders, dementia, seizure disorders, and disorders of clinical ecology and environmental illness.

Schizophrenia

Schizophrenia continues to be the subject of heated debate among psychiatric professionals. Some maintain that schizophrenia is a single disorder, but others argue that the condition is a complex of disorders that produce symptoms labeled as schizophrenia. Some scientists believe that *if* schizophrenia is a single entity, then a single cause for the condition will be found. As of this writing, no cause is known for schizophrenia, but several psychobiologic hypotheses exist.

The *dopamine hypothesis* is the most probable explanation of schizophrenia to date. Schwartz and Africa (1984) note that this psychobiologic explanation has an established relationship to schizophrenia. Dopamine is a plentiful neurotransmitter within the brain. The dopamine hypothesis is that the amount of dopamine available at certain synapses is significantly altered in persons demonstrating schizophrenic symptoms. A clinical observation that contributed information to the development of this hypothesis was that antipsychotic drugs decrease dopamine at the synapse and lessen schizophrenic symptoms. When *neuroleptics* (substances that act on the autonomic nervous system) are given to clients with Parkinson's disease, a condition of dopamine deficiency, their symptoms become markedly worse. The correlation between dopamine, antipsychotic drugs, and schizophrenic symptoms does not establish a causal relationship. Some psychobiologists suggest that the reason why schizophrenic symptoms improve with dopamine blocking agents is that the synaptic biochemistry of schizophrenics is dysfunctional.

The *monoamine oxidase* (MAO) hypothesis of schizophrenia is that a certain type of MAO is lower in chronic schizophrenic clients than in the normal population (Schwartz and Africa 1984). This MAO abnormality may be indicative of an abnormality of neurotransmitter metabolism, especially that of dopamine. As with the dopamine hypothesis, there is no way of knowing the significance of this finding on the source or clinical course of schizophrenia.

The *transmethylation hypothesis* of schizophrenia is interesting but of uncertain clinical significance. The hypothesis is that certain catecholamines (specific neurotransmitters) undergo an abnormal chemical transformation process known as o-methylation. The end result of this chemical transformation is a substance that is very close in chemical structure to mescaline. This substance produces illusions, hallucinations, and other symptoms common to the experience of psychosis. Discussion continues regarding whether the transmethylation process is the result of an endogenous substance or something externally induced, perhaps by diet.

In recent years there has been significant discussion about whether the "human-made" morphines—the enkephalins and endorphins—play a part in the emergence of schizophrenic symptoms. To date, however, there is no empirical basis for such a claim. Several researchers have tagged certain proteins (e.g., immunoglobulins) or electrolytes (e.g., calcium) in an effort to find the cause of schizophrenic symptoms; none of these attempts have met with success. As more psychobiologic research is done to examine the causes of schizophrenia, answers may be found. The findings to date suggest that either the condition has multiple causes or one complex and multifaceted cause.

Mood Disorders

The term *mood disorders* covers a lot of psychiatric turf. Much research is being conducted on mood disorders. There are several schools of thought about the cause of mood disorders. Some psychobiologists believe that most psychiatric conditions, including anorexia nervosa and bulimia, are simply variants of affectively disordered states, while others maintain more traditional psychiatric nomenclature and classification.

Of great interest is a new classification that delineates the finer differences between unipolar and bipolar affective subtypes. Akiskal (1984, p 274) proposes the following subtypes:

- Recurrent mania: no evidence of clinical depression
- Bipolar I: depression and mania
- Bipolar II: depression and spontaneous hypomania
- Unipolar I: infrequent episodes of depression and no bipolar history
- Unipolar II: recurrent depressions with bipolar family history; many switch to hypomania with pharmacologic challenge.

This classification system presents a challenge to other, more established diagnostic systems such as the DSM-IIIR. This is not to say that one system is better than the other, but rather that the science is in such a flux at present that stability in nomenclature is difficult.

Psychobiologists are gaining a more refined understanding of the neurochemical correlates of such behaviors as mania, depression, and bipolarity. Disorders such as cyclothymia, dysthymia, and atypical affective states are apparently variants of the major conditions listed above.

Since little is known about the specific psychobiology of mania, our discussion focuses on the psychobiologic processes hypothesized in bipolar disorder and in depression. In the past, the psychobiologic focus for affective disorders was the catecholamine hypothesis. This theory holds that manic states are marked by an excess of a catecholamine neurotransmitter in certain synapses and that depression is characterized by the opposite. This hypothesis has essentially been refuted by recent research.

According to Reus (1984), the major focus of affective disorder research concerns one of the metabolites of norepinephrine, a catecholamine neurotransmitter. The metabolite is referred to as MHPG. When researchers measured MHPG in clients with the diagnosis of bipolar disorder, depression, two groups emerged: those who secreted more than normal and those who secreted less than normal amounts of MHPG. The clinical implications of this finding are unclear. However, an abnormal level of MHPG is a specific marker for a biochemical process involving neurotransmitters in people diagnosed with bipolar disorder. Other markers for bipolar disordered clients include electrolyte and serotonin disturbances as well as alterations in monoamine oxidase, an enzyme involved in breaking down certain neurochemicals.

The endocrine model of depression continues to attract adherents. The theory is that changes in the endocrine system occur after a given period of exposure to stress. These changes bring about biophysical changes known as *vegetative signs of depression*. They include psychomotor retardation, anorexia, constipation, lethargy, diminished libido, poor concentration, and insomnia.

While cortisol has received substantial attention from psychobiologists as possibly contributing to depression, other hormones, too, have been of interest. Growth hormone, thyroid-stimulating hormone, thyroid-releasing hormone, luteinizing hormone, and prolactin all have been found in abnormal levels in depressed clients, bolstering the case for psychoendocrinologic mechanisms in depression.

Anxiety Disorders

The clinical arena for conditions termed as anxiety disorders is bustling with activity, especially since 1977 when

---

RESEARCH NOTE

Citation

Nasrallah AH, Coryell WH: Dexamethasone nonsuppression predicts the antidepressant effects of sleep deprivation. Psychiatry Res 1982; 6: 61–64.

Study Problem/Purpose

Dexamethasone nonsuppression has been linked to disrupted circadian rhythms in depressed persons. Sleep deprivation allegedly exerts a transient antidepressant effect. This study aims to examine dexamethasone nonsuppression as a predictor of antidepressant response to sleep deprivation with clients who are diagnosed as having major depression.

Methods

Twenty-two depressed (by DSM-IIIR diagnostic criteria) adults received the dexamethasone suppression test (DST) upon admission to the hospital. Two to three days after the DST, the participating clients were deprived of sleep for 36 hours. Baseline depression severity was rated by a psychiatrist (blind to the DST results) on a valid/reliable scale (Hamilton Depression Scale). Clients also rated their own depression using a visual analog scale. At 8:00 A.M. on the day following sleep deprivation, a psychiatrist and nurse rated the clients' global improvement, and the clients simultaneously rated their own improvement. Improve-

ment was defined as receiving a higher rating from at least one staff member in addition to a higher self-rating by the client or "improved" ratings from both staff members without improved self-rating.

Findings

Four of the dexamethasone nonsuppressors and one suppressor improved with sleep deprivation. Three dexamethasone nonsuppressors and fourteen suppressors remained unimproved after sleep deprivation. The difference between the suppressor/nonsuppressor improvement is significant ($p = 0.02$, Fisher Exact Test).

Implications

This study documents a psychobiologic index of circadian rhythmicity in conjunction with sleep/wake cycles of depressed clients. The authors of the study point out that the antidepressant effects of sleep deprivation are possibly related to a correction of an abnormal diurnal biorhythm in depression. Although few nurses have studied circadian rhythmicity in depressed clients, the opportunity exists for an explanation of such rhythms through a nursing perspective. Such knowledge might allow for the evaluation of specific nursing assessment measures to examine circadian rhythms and to prescribe nursing interventions aimed specifically at correcting imbalance in biorhythm.

an actual mammalian neuron cell surface was found to have specific receptors for benzodiazepine drugs (e.g., diazepam) (Breier et al 1985). The clinical significance of that finding is that neurotransmitters are involved in the mediation of anxiety, making anxiety a psychobiologic condition with identifiable biologic markers. Braestrup (1982, p 1030) states: "All we can now say is that anxiety occurs when, in the brain, there is a certain activity pattern in certain neurons that are firing in a certain spatial and temporal pattern, and that this structurally complex activity is anxiety." Braestrup believes that anxiety probably involves neurotransmitters from the brain such as GABA, serotonin, norepinephrine, and dopamine. Psychobiologists believe that at least serotonin and norepinephrine are implicated in depression. How then, can one determine with any certainty that anxiety disorders that can be mediated by serotonin and norepinephrine are not simply variants of depression? At this time, it is impossible to make such a distinction in a reasonable fashion. But the question opens the door to an ongoing discussion among psychobiologists: Since some anxiety disorders respond to antidepressant medications, are they not, in fact, depressions? Relationships exist among panic disorder, generalized anxiety disorder, and major depressive disorder; these relationships need further exploration if we are to discover more specific and effective interventions.

Nurses, especially those working with psychiatric clients, constantly deal with anxious clients. How do nurses differ in their approaches to mildly anxious clients versus clients with moderate, high, or crisis levels of anxiety? Providing that nurses assess the client's anxiety accurately, how *prescriptive* are the interventions, and what *objective* evaluative measures of anxiety control do nurses use? Anxiety is a psychobiologic condition that responds to both behavioral and pharmacologic interventions; it is recognized as amenable to nursing care. Although many nurses have written about or researched anxiety and its related behaviors in clients, there remains a need to use this knowledge in the clinical arena more fully, allowing for more consistent assessment and more prescriptive interventions for anxiety.

Dementia

There are many causes of dementia. The most common is Alzheimer's disease, a psychobiologic process of slow onset and uneven progression leading to death. What happens to the brain of someone with Alzheimer's disease? The destruction of neurons begins in the memory centers in the brain. The destroyed nerves are replaced with non-functional fibers, preventing smooth transmission of impulses from neuron to neuron. As memory deteriorates, so does overall brain functioning. The resulting behaviors include disorientation, rambling speech, unstable emotions, and a poor understanding of the environment. Eventually, the affected individual seems to lose personality features and over time seems to become a totally different person. Unfortunately, no cure for Alzheimer's disease exists at this time.

Seizure Disorders

Recent advances in neurophysiology and psychoneurobiology have greatly contributed to the understanding of seizures from a cellular perspective. Niedermeyer (1984, p 100) discusses "epileptic neurons" and points out that these neurons are characterized by "autonomous and sustained abnormal firing as well as increased electrical excitability." Niedermeyer goes on to say that the cause of the abnormal behavior of the epileptic neurons is likely to be related to ionic changes in the neuron, especially involving calcium.

Of the many types of seizures, the ones of greatest interest to people working in psychiatry are probably those involving the temporal lobe. Psychomotor or complex partial seizures fit into the category of temporal lobe seizures. They involve limbic structures, particularly the amygdala. This type of seizure activity is characterized by movements such as chewing, swallowing, and lip smacking (Niedermeyer 1984). Such seizure-related behaviors can be easily overlooked because they occur normally. However, close assessment allows nurses to delineate seizure-related behaviors from normal behaviors.

What emotional changes can be anticipated in someone who suffers from temporal lobe seizures? According to Bear et al. (1984), among the possible behavioral changes are hyposexuality, anger, irritability, aggression, deepened emotions, religiosity, hypergraphia, psychosis, and dissociative states. Consideration must be given to the individual manifestations of the seizure disorder, as no one particular client is likely to develop all of these symptoms.

Clinical Ecology and Environmental Illness

Iris Bell (1982), an expert in the field of clinical ecology (CE) describes CE as an interdisciplinary subgroup of environmental medicine. The CE group proposes that chronic exposure to chemicals and inhalants in the environment and in ordinary foods may lead to psychobiologic disorders in people who are susceptible to this form of illness (see Box 9–4). Clinical ecologists emphasize that to understand environmental illness, one must consider the total load of low-dose environmental stressors a person encounters and the frequency of, as well as time between, exposures to substances.

Clinical ecologists observe for reactions in the behavior of the environmentally ill person. Common reactions include psychiatric, central nervous system, and psychophysiologic symptoms. Bell points out that the mechanisms involved in environmental illness are likely to be both immune and nonimmune. No particular abnormality is consistently noted among environmentally ill persons, but trends among this population point to a variety of immune and central nervous system changes.

There are three approaches to the treatment of environmentally ill clients (Bell 1982, p 47):

- Avoidance of offending substances
- Rotation diet of tolerated foods
- Neutralization or prevention of adverse reactions by subcutaneous injections or sublingual drops

Clinical ecology is in its early stages of development. Although many of the assumptions that underlie this science are not yet tested, clinical ecology does illuminate issues that need attention in the arena of psychoneuroimmunology and its related fields.

PSYCHOBIOLOGY AND NURSING

The idea of applying psychobiologic principles to psychiatric nursing practice seems reasonable, even though they are not commonly applied today. It is an idea whose time has come. The advances in the understanding of the brain and its functions give nurses an opportunity for advancements in the areas of nursing assessment, planning, implementation, and evaluation.

There are many unanswered questions about the connections between the brain and behavior. For example, nurses may be able to do psychobiologic assessments of diet, sleep, anxiety, and their effects on other behaviors but may not yet have any interventions *specific to nursing* that address such behaviors.

Nursing science is at a stage in its development that invites exploration of nursing approaches, models, and theories that help nurses to function more from a theoretical/empirical base rather than from intuition. In medical-surgical nursing, many interventions have been researched, refined, and used in practice with empirical backing. For example, a nurse who works in a cardiac intensive care unit has knowledge relevant to cardiac symptomatology and bases nursing intervention on that knowledge. At present, psychiatric nurses have the opportunity to help eliminate a dualistic approach to their work by incorporating psychobiologic principles into their care of clients, thus truly making psychiatric nursing practice a holistic science and art that is theoretically based.

Box 9–4
POTENTIAL MECHANISMS IN ENVIRONMENTAL ILLNESS

Hypotheses Derived from Clinical Observations

1. Specific foods in a susceptible individual can cause multisystem symptoms.

2. Symptoms can include emotional, cognitive, behavioral, somatic features—e.g., anxiety, irritability, depression, fatigue, impaired memory, difficulty concentrating, poor coordination, hyperactivity, sleepiness, grand mal seizures—in individual patterns in a given person.

3. Different foods can cause the same symptoms in different individuals, i.e., no single food triggers a particular disorder in all individuals with that disorder.

4. Multiple foods can provoke the same symptoms in a given individual.

5. Increased frequency of ingestion leads to increased sensitivity and vice versa.

6. Frequent ingestion can mask the presence of sensitivity; therefore, diagnosis depends on unmasking (avoiding the food) for four or more days before challenging with the food.

7. Adverse food reactions often have delayed onset from 1 to 24 hours after the meal and can last up to three to four days.

8. Mechanisms for such reactions are unknown, but classical IgE-mediated allergy is unlikely. Postulated mechanisms include IgG, immune complexes, complement, mediators such as neuro/gut peptides, prostaglandins, kinins.

9. Behavioral reactions can be biphasic in course, with stimulatory and depressed phases.

Source: Iris R. Bell, MD PhD: Personal communication, 25 March 1986.

The following case study and nursing care plan in this chapter incorporate psychobiologic principles into a nursing perspective. Many of the psychobiologically oriented concepts discussed in this chapter are novel, and applying psychobiologic principles to nursing care is new to many nurses. As nurses learn more about how their interventions affect the psychobiology of clients and subsequent client behaviors, psychiatric nursing intervention can become truly

Text continued on p. 193

CASE STUDY: Client with Recurrent Major Depression and Psychoactive Substance Dependence

Identifying Information

J.R. is a 28-year-old, single male who works as a technician in a medical intensive care unit. He lives alone in a single-bedroom apartment. He is enrolled in courses at the local junior college, taking night courses to get academic prerequisites completed so that he may apply to nursing school for the fall. Aside from the hospitalization discussed in this case presentation, J.R. has never been hospitalized for psychiatric difficulties.

Client's Definition of Present Problem, Precipitatory Stress, Coping Strategies, and Goals for Care

J.R. recognized his current problem as a mood difficulty, not dissimilar from the problems he experienced after the deaths of his family members. Although not fully aware of all of the potential precipitating factors, J.R. sees two major stressors, loneliness and academic pressure, as partially responsible for his current condition.

While J.R. has tried to remain active to ward off worsening of his depressive symptoms, he is aware that his functional abilities are rapidly deteriorating. He decides that he needs help and seeks out his therapist. His goals for reentering psychotherapy are to decrease his depression and suicidal thoughts and to learn better coping skills to prevent a recurrence of his illness.

Psychiatric History/Family History/Social History

J.R. had been under the care of a psychiatrist for six months, nearly five years ago. When J.R. was 23, both of his parents and his only sister died when their house burned as a result of an oil burner explosion. J.R. and his two older brothers lived away from home at the time of the fire and were spared. Shortly after the fire, J.R. reported symptoms of sleep disturbance, intermittent agitation, and disinterest in his usual activities. J.R. remembered his psychotherapy as "very helpful" in his emotional resolution of the tragic deaths of his family. While he received no psychopharmacologic intervention during his first psychotherapy experience, J.R. reported abatement of symptoms at the time he ended psychotherapy.

Health History

J.R. returned to therapy four weeks ago with complaints of inordinate fatigue, sleeplessness, anxiety, loss of interest in work, social withdrawal, and diminished libido. According to J.R., each day was comparable: After a fitful sleep, J.R. got out of bed and had two cups of coffee and several cigarettes before getting dressed and heading off to work. During the work day he had difficulty concentrating on his work. He found himself making errors more frequently than in the past. He reported his mood during the morning as "terribly grim" with occasional periods of uncontrollable tearfulness, seemingly precipitated by no specific event. By 2:00 P.M., J.R. noted his mood to have improved; by 10:00 P.M. he felt "somewhere near average." The cycle repeated itself daily, except on days of unusual stress, at which time his mood remained low throughout the day. In the last week, J.R.'s supervisor suggested that he take some time off from work, as his performance continued to deteriorate. J.R. accepted the supervisor's suggestion and planned to take the following week off from work. During that week, J.R. became suicidal, stating that he planned to asphyxiate himself with carbon monoxide exhaust from his car. As he sat in his closed garage with the car motor running, J.R. became frightened and called his therapist. J.R.'s therapist placed him in the hospital for treatment of depression with suicidal ideation.

continued

Current Mental Status

On examination, J.R. presented himself as a casually dressed man who appeared his stated age. His affect was grossly anxious, and his mood was depressed. Speech was slow and in soft tones (Figure 9–6). J.R.'s thought content focused on his present state of incapacity and desire to be dead; process was markedly blocked at times, but generally logical. He denied hallucinations and failed to demonstrate any formal thought disorder. He was oriented to person, time, and place, but his immediate memory was impaired, evidenced by an inability to recall two of four objects at five minutes. Short- and long-term memory were intact. J.R. was unable to do calculations, stating that he "needed a calculator" for serial sevens. Insight and judgment were fair. In response to questions about suicidal thoughts or plans, J.R. reported that he still planned to suffocate himself by inhaling automobile exhaust.

Diagnostic Impressions

Nursing Diagnoses (PND-I/ NANDA)

07.06.02.02	Altered systemic processes: less than body requirements /Alteration in nutrition: less than body requirements /Knowledge deficit, nutrition
07.99	Potential for altered physiologic processes /Alteration in nutrition: more than body requirements
01.04.03	Insomnia /Sleep pattern disturbance
04.02.02	Anxiety /Anxiety
05.99.01	Potential for violence (self-directed) /Potential for violence: self-directed

DSM-IIIR Multiaxial Diagnosis

Axis I: 296.30 Major depression, recurrent
          304.90 Psychoactive substance dependence, not otherwise specified
Axis II: Deferred
Axis III: None
Axis IV: 2 Mild (school pressure: acute; loneliness: enduring)
Axis V: 50—Severe symptoms

Collaborating with the Client to Reach Goals

J.R. developed the following goals for hospitalization:

1. To feel like my old self again—energetic, interested in life, cheerful
2. To get a handle on my nervousness
3. To sleep better
4. To completely get rid of these thoughts about killing myself
5. To get a new job because I'm too embarrassed to return to my old one.

Nursing staff met with J.R. after he wrote up his goals to discuss what could be accomplished in the hospital, given the constraints of length of stay. Staff believed that *direct* nursing intervention could be of help with goals 2 and 3. Most likely, goals 1 and 4 would be partially met during the hospital stay but would require ongoing attention after discharge from the hospital. Nursing staff referred J.R.'s goal 5 to a vocational rehabilitation therapist. In addition to J.R.'s goals, nursing staff negotiated with J.R. to add three more goals.

continued

LANGLEY PORTER PSYCHIATRIC INSTITUTE
HOSPITAL AND CLINICS
University of California, San Francisco

NURSING DATA BASE
ADULT ADMISSION INFORMATION

PATIENT'S NAME

BIRTHDATE

SERVICE

LPPI#

ADDRESSOGRAPH PLATE IMPRINT

HOW ARRIVED: Ambulatory X W/C __ Crutches __ Guerney __ Restraints __

Accompanied By _____ Alone X

Reason for Admission

Patient's: ___ "I can't function ... I want to have my life over."

Referral Source's: ___ Depression with suicidal ideation; S/P suicide attempt.

Current Psychiatric Treatment (include Meds):
    Individual psychotherapy weekly; currently on no medications
Current Medical Treatment (Include Meds):
    As above
Drug Sensitivities: ___ sulfa

Other Allergies: ___ Morphine sulfate, pollens, molds

No Known Allergies: ___
Health Problems/Physical LImitations/Special Needs:
    Allergies as listed above. S/P carbon monoxide inhalation.
Current Use of Alcohol, Street Drugs and/or Over the Counter Drugs:
    Occasional 1-2 beers. No drugs (illicit) in present/past. No OTC drugs.
    Takes 1 ounce of brandy for sleep 1-3 times weekly.
Previous Hospitalizations:

	WHERE	WHEN	RESPONSE/REACTION(Patient's Self Report)
1.	None		
2.			

Significant Others:

	NAME	RELATIONSHIP	PHONE
1.	MLR	brother	(415) 555-1954
2.	BG	friend	(415) 555-1862

Is the patient oriented to:

Person: Yes X No __ Time: Yes X No __ Present Situation: Yes X No __

Memory: Recent: Good X Fair __ Poor __
          Remote: Good X Fair __ Poor __
Speech: Quality _____ Slow _____ Quantity: ___ Sparse
          Organization: ___ logical

Affect: Anxious

Response to Admission Procedure:

Cooperative? Yes X No __ Angry? Yes __ No X Suspicious? Yes __ No X Fearful? Yes X No __

Patient Participation (specify): ___ Full Participant in interview

Figure 9–6
Psychiatric nursing data base: Adult admission information.
Source: Langley-Porter Hospital Nursing Service, University of California, San Francisco.

Case Study (continued)

6. To limit coffee intake to two cups per day (J.R. ingested about 750 mg caffeine daily; caffeine toxicity may occur with as little as 250 mg per day).

7. To regain 2 pounds per week during each week of hospitalization.

8. Not to harm himself during hospitalization but to seek out assistance from staff when needed, especially during periods of suicidal thinking.

J.R. agreed to work with nursing staff on these additional goals. The following nursing care plan is the direct result of collaboration between staff and client.

During the course of a 22-day hospitalization, J.R. demonstrated marked improvement and substantial lessening of depressive symptoms. He worked hard with the nursing staff to meet the goals that he and his primary care nurse developed. By discharge, he had made some psychobiologic alterations in his daily routine. Specifically, he eliminated caffeine from his diet and continued to use tryptophan dietary loading with specific relaxation interventions to control anxiety and sometimes to go to sleep. J.R. reset his circadian clock by adjusting his rest/activity schedule and eliminating his exposure to light after retiring each night. Affectively, he demonstrated abatement of depressive symptoms and suicidal ideation.

Of course, determining the *specific* effects of the antidepressant medication and anxiolytic medication versus the *specifics* of nursing intervention is difficult at best. Future nursing research will help to develop means to measure these differences and outcomes in client care.

Nursing Care Plan

Nursing Diagnosis (PND-I/NANDA)	Client Care Goals	Nursing Planning/ Intervention	Evaluation

07.06.02.02 Altered systemic processes (less than body requirements)* /Nutrition, altered; less than body requirements /Knowledge deficit	J.R. agrees to attend all meals and will gain 2 lbs per week while hospitalized.	1. Weigh client in the morning (bathrobe only) on Monday and Friday.
		2. Assist client weekly with menu selection for the following week. Include in the teaching:
		  a. Information on caloric requirements for weight gain
		  b. Basic food groups
		  c. Effects of anxiety/ depression on appetite and metabolism
			Document in progress notes on Mon-Wed-Fri J.R.'s compliance/progress with above plan. Primary care nurse to evaluate effectiveness of this plan each week by monitoring client's weight gain and assimilation of nutrition teachings.

07.99 Potential for altered physiologic processes (associated with excessive caffeine intake 7–10 cups/ day; risk for caffeine withdrawal) /Nutrition, altered: more than body requirements
 	
*PND-1 diagnosis also in NANDA list.
	J.R. agrees to limit coffee intake to 2 cups per day and will report psychobiologic symptoms of caffeine withdrawal to staff.	1. Teach client to report the following symptoms of caffeine withdrawal:
		  a. Listlessness
		  b. Headache
		  c. Irritability
		2. Teach J.R. the reasons for reducing his caffeine intake:
			1. Observe for noncompliance with caffeine restriction by assessing symptoms of moderate to high caffeine intake:
			  a. Restlessness
			  b. Agitation
			  c. Rapid heart rate,

continued

Case Study (continued)

Nursing Diagnosis (PND-I/NANDA)	Client Care Goals	Nursing Planning/ Intervention	Evaluation
		a. Caffeine toxicity mimics anxiety. b. Clear assessment of anxiety and/or sleep disturbance is impossible in presence of caffeine toxicity. c. Caffeine exerts an antagonistic effect on select medications (especially benzodiazepines). d. Caffeine affects neurotransmitters such as norepinephrine, leading to changes in usual patterns of thought.	possibly arrhythmia d. Demonstrations of high energy 2. Document J.R.'s compliance with above plan in the nursing notes; the primary care nurse will formally evaluate the effectiveness of this plan each week.
01.04.03 Insomnia* /Sleep pattern disturbance	Balanced sleep/activity cycles	1. Since disturbed sleep is potentially worsened by disturbed activity patterns, J.R. is to remain out of bed after 7:30 A.M. 2. J.R. will take one 15-minute walk with staff accompaniment each shift and perform scheduled activities. 3. Instruct the client in the importance of a high-tryptophan diet and suggest tryptophan loading before bedtime (physician can prescribe high-dose (2 g) tryptophan tablets). The tryptophan must be given with carbohydrate to be effective. 4. J.R. is to retire at 10:00 P.M. Since circadian patterns are light sensitive, make certain that the room is adequately darkened. Keep interruptions to a minimum.	Document effectiveness of plan each day, including an evaluation of the client's quantity and quality of sleep.
04.02.02 Anxiety* /Anxiety	1. J.R. will report a subjective reduction in	1. J.R. will write out a list of behaviors that he	With each episode of anxious behavior, evaluate

continued

Case Study (continued)

Nursing Diagnosis (PND-I/NANDA)	Client Care Goals	Nursing Planning/ Intervention	Evaluation
	his level of anxiety. 2. J.R. will learn early signs of anxiety and will learn to intervene before the symptoms become uncontrollable. 3. J.R. will demonstrate a decrease in the frequency and intensity of psychobiologic indices of anxiety (e.g., rapid heart rate, tremor, insomnia).	identifies as anxious. 2. When J.R. is *initially* aware of anxious feelings, he agrees to contact staff. 3. Staff will consistently intervene by: a. Assessing the degree of anxiety as mild (e.g., minimal subjective discomfort, hyper-attentiveness), moderate to severe (e.g., heart pounding, dry mouth, perspiration, wandering thought). Symptom severity increases directly with level of anxiety. b. For mild anxiety, spend 5–10 minutes with the client to discuss antecedents to anxious feelings. Then, redirect client to guided imagery relaxation work. c. For anxiety that is between moderate and severe, bring the client to a quiet place. Remain with the client but do not engage in discussion of the anxiety-producing event. Assist with deep breathing relaxation. Assess need for medication. d. For severe anxiety, assess for anxiolytic medication and administer the same, if appropriate. Do not engage in discussion but give direct, brief commands (e.g., to remain in a quiet area, to regulate breathing to prevent hyperventilation, etc.).	the effectiveness of the intervention using subjective and objective data. Document findings in a progress note.

continued

Case Study (continued)

Nursing Diagnosis (PND-I/NANDA)	Client Care Goals	Nursing Planning/ Intervention	Evaluation
		e. When the client demonstrates learning readiness (ability to concentrate and retain information reliably), embark upon medication teaching. Include information about drug name, dose, time of administration, purpose, side-effects, self-care measures to counteract side-effects, and toxic signs.	
05.99.01 Potential for violence* /Violence, potential for: self-directed	The client will not act on suicidal thoughts during hospitalization and will remain safe during this hospital stay.	1. Nursing staff is to do a formal suicide assessment each shift and document findings in a progress note. 2. If the client reports suicidal thoughts, inquire about the existence of a specific plan for suicide or self-harm. 3. If the client reports a specific plan, place the client on 1:1 contact with nursing staff and assess need for p.r.n. medication. 4. During the 1:1, follow assessment and intervention procedure outlined above for anxiety abatement. 5. Reassess suicidal thoughts following anxiety-reduction evaluation. 6. When client demonstrates adequate impulse control, evidenced by an ability to contract *not* to harm self in a suicide gesture/ attempt, discontinue 1:1 nursing contacts.	1. If the client demonstrates a worsening of suicidal thoughts and diminished impulse control, assess need for seclusion. 2. Document course of assessment/ interventions/evaluations in progress notes.

more prescriptive. This shift in nursing approach, of course, will take time. Nurses and other health team members need time to learn more about the psychobiology of behavior. The profession must slowly adjust educational and clinical approaches to accommodate the psychobiologic perspective. This is an exciting time in nursing in general and especially in psychiatric nursing as objective data are uncovered that yield explanations for the complexity of human behavior.

- Certain forms of seizures can produce behavioral alterations that appear like other forms of mental illness. These require close nursing assessment.

- Nurses have an ongoing opportunity to apply psychobiologic principles to psychiatric nursing practice.

Chapter Highlights

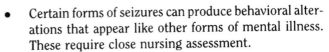

- Psychobiology is not a new concept, but we are gaining knowledge about the underlying biologic bases of human behavior.

- From a psychobiologic perspective, the human brain is the source of creativity, logic, thought, and emotion.

- Ancient Greeks who influenced early psychobiologic thought included Hippocrates, Plato, and Aristotle.

- Throughout history, dualism has been a common approach to illness; psychobiology closes the dualistic gap and approaches behavior holistically.

- Behavior is the result of a complex interplay of chemical and electric processes within the brain; intercommunication among the various parts of the brain produce behavior.

- The limbic system is commonly referred to as "the emotional brain" and consists of structures from the cerebral hemispheres, the diencephalon, and the midbrain.

- The reticular activating system is a complex of neurons that modulates states of consciousness and awareness.

- The extrapyramidal system consists of tracts of motor neurons from the brain to parts of the spinal cord; this system coordinates coarse automatic movements.

- Psychoendocrinology and psychoimmunology are two subspecialties that explore the relationships between behavior, biology, and endocrine/immunologic functions.

- Thyroid dysfunction is often masked as depression and when due to autoimmune thyroid processes is difficult to assess.

- Human functions demonstrate a 24-hour cycle; these cycles are commonly referred to as circadian rhythms.

- Several biologic explanations of schizophrenia exist, but the most probable is the dopamine hypothesis.

- Several hypotheses explore the psychobiologic basis of mood disorders, anxiety disorders, and dementia.

- Clinical ecology is a subgroup of environmental medicine that proposes that chronic exposure to chemicals, inhalants, and foods may cause psychobiologic disorders in susceptible individuals.

References

Akiskal HS: The bipolar spectrum: New concepts in classification and diagnosis, in Grinspoon L (ed): *Psychiatry Update.* American Psychiatric Press, 1984.

Alper J: Biology and mental illness. *The Atlantic Monthly,* December, 70–76, 1983.

Andreasen NC: *The Broken Brain.* Harper & Row, 1984.

Bear D, Freeman R, Greenberg M: Behavioral alterations in patients with temporal lobe epilepsy, in Blumer D (ed): *Psychiatric Aspects of Epilepsy.* American Psychiatric Press, 1984.

Begley S, Carey J, Sawhill K: *Newsweek,* February 7, 40–47, 1983.

Bell IR: *Clinical Ecology.* Common Knowledge Press, 1982.

Binder RL: Organic mental disorders, in Goldman HH (ed): *Review of General Psychiatry.* Lange Medical Publications, 1984.

Braestrup C: Anxiety. *Lancet* 1982; 2(November 6): 1030–1034.

Breier A, Charney DS, Heninger GR: *Am J Psychiatry* 1985; 142(7):787–797.

Brown RP, Mann JJ: A clinical perspective on the role of neurotransmitters in mental disorders. *Hosp Community Psychiatry* 1985; 36(2):141–150.

Farber SL: Genetic diversity and differing reactions to stress, in Goldberger L, Breznitz S (eds): *Handbook of Stress— Theoretical and Clinical Aspects.* The Free Press, 1982.

Gordin A, Lamberg BA: Natural course of symptomless autoimmune thyroiditis. *Lancet* 1976; 2(December 20): 1234–1237.

Grebb JA, Reus VI: Neurobehavioral chemistry and physiology, in Goldman HH (ed): *Review of General Psychiatry.* Lange Medical Publications, 1984, pp 125–138.

Harris E: The dexamethasone suppression test. *Am J Nurs* 1982; 82(5):784–785.

Hubel DH: The brain. *Sci Am* 1979; 241(3):45–53.

Illich I: *Medical Nemesis.* Random House, 1976.

Iversen LI: Neurotransmitters and CNS disease. *Lancet* 1982; 2(October 23):914–918.

Kaplan HI, Saddock BJ: *Modern Synopsis of Comprehensive Textbook of Psychiatry,* ed 4. Williams & Wilkins, 1985.

Lander M: *Introduction to Psychopharmacology.* The Upjohn Company, 1983.

Lickey ME, Gordon B: *Drugs for Mental Illness—A Revolution in Psychiatry.* Freeman, 1983.

McKegney FP: Psychoimmunology: What lies ahead. *Drug Ther* 1982; August, 61–72.

Moore-Ede MC, Czeisler CA, Richardson GS: Circadian timekeeping in health and disease. *N Engl J Med* 1983; 309(8):469–476.

Nasrallah HA, Coryell WH: Dexamethasone nonsuppression predicts the antidepressant effects of sleep deprivation. *Psychiatry Res* 1982; 6:61–64.

Niedermeyer E: Neurologic aspects of the epilepsies, in Blumer D (ed): *Psychiatric Aspects of Epilepsy.* American Psychiatric Press, 1984.

Pincus JH, Tucker GJ: *Behavioral Neurology,* ed. 2. Oxford University Press, 1978.

Plumlee AA: Biological rhythms and affective illness. *J Psychosoc Nurs Mental Health Serv* 1986; 24(3):12–17.

Restak R: *The Brain.* Bantam Books, 1984.

Reus VI: Affective disorders, in Goldman HH (ed): *Review of General Psychiatry.* Lange Medical Publications, 1984.

Schwartz SR, Africa B: Schizophrenic disorders, in Goldman HH (ed): *Review of General Psychiatry.* Lange Medical Publications, 1984.

Vogel P: Lithium and the thyroid. *J Psychosoc Nurs Mental Health Serv* 1986; 24(3):9–14.

Zegans LS: Stress and the development of somatic disorders, in Goldberger L and Breznitz S (eds): *Handbook of Stress—Theoretical and Clinical Aspects.* The Free Press, 1982.

PART TWO

Processes for Psychiatric Nursing Clinical Practice

TEN

Ethical Reflectiveness

Holly Skodol Wilson

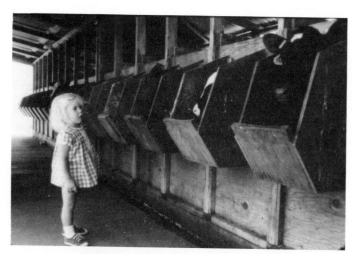

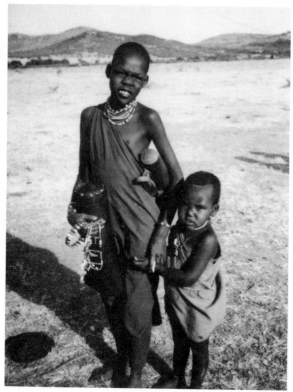

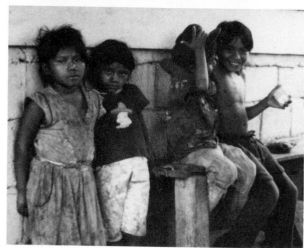

Learning Objectives

After reading this chapter, students should be able to

- Discuss the process of ethical reflection used in analyzing an ethical issue
- Compare and contrast dominant ethical perspectives
- Define the six major principles of bioethics
- Identify and discuss ethical dilemmas in psychiatric nursing
- Formulate a personal stand on the ethics and politics of psychiatric nursing practice

Cross References

Other topics relevant to this content are: Conceptual frameworks, Chapter 5; Cultural considerations, Chapter 38; Elder abuse, Chapter 35; Ethics in milieu therapy, Chapter 30; History, Chapter 2; Legal issues, Chapter 39; Management strategies for violence, Chapter 25; Philosophy, Chapter 1.

This book is dedicated to personal and professional ideals.

Key Terms

deontology
egoism
euthanasia, active
euthanasia, passive
ideal observer

justice
obligation
universality
utilitarianism
V-code

THE PROCESS OF ETHICAL REFLECTION

A young teacher of nursing bioethics and philosophy once said, "Reasoning in ethics means bringing all one's faculties in a balanced way to bear on the sincere concern for human well-being in general and the meaning of human experience. Being reasonable in ethics is more like having integrity than like being smart." This chapter describes a process of ethical reflection to be used as a framework for analyzing ethical issues and resolving ethical dilemmas in psychiatric nursing. Reason and reflection have always held an important place in the study of ethics, for ethics is more than a personal or inspirational enterprise used to answer moral questions. Moral judgments are most highly developed when the *process of arriving at them* and the *reasons for believing in them* are clear and convincing. At the heart of ethical judgments are the reasons for them. The process of applying ethical reflection to concerns in psychiatric nursing can:

- Improve the quality of our professional decisions
- Raise the level of our ability to communicate with others
- Increase our sensitivity to others
- Offer a sense of moral clarity and enlightenment about our work

Throughout the history of nursing education, teachers and students alike have been concerned with ethical matters. A closer look, however, reveals that the concern has been less with moral principles and ethical dilemmas and more with legal aspects of practice and what psychiatric nurse–bioethicist Anne Davis refers to as "the etiquette of the profession" (Davis and Aroskar 1978). Nursing has made notable advances toward professional autonomy in recent years. Greater autonomy, however, has created a greater need and responsibility to account for and accept the consequences of professional decisions and actions. Autonomy, according to Aroskar (1980) has to do with the right of self-determination, governance without outside control, and the capability to exist independently. Professionals do this by:

- Developing codes of ethics, which provide guidelines for defining professional responsibility
- Setting rigorous qualifications for entry into the profession
- Establishing peer review procedures
- Setting standards for practice, such as the *ANA Standards of Psychiatric and Mental Health Nursing Practice*

Professionals need to balance the goal of more autonomy in nursing with efforts to achieve what providers and consumers determine is the common and the individual "good" in health care.

On a personal level, however, each reader begins a chapter on ethical concerns with the hope of finding an uplifting code or credo of beliefs that can provide a standard against which to judge the rightness or wrongness of thinking and practice. Such a hope—easy and comforting though it may be—is somewhat short-sighted. In the words of Alfred North Whitehead, "The single-minded use of the notions of right or wrong is one of the chief obstacles to the progress of understanding." The goal of this chapter is not to preach right and wrong but to help students develop a way of thinking about complex ethical issues and dilemmas in psychiatric nursing.

Analyzing Ethical Issues

One of the major difficulties in ethical analysis is that there are no definite, clear-cut solutions to ethical dilemmas. For centuries moral philosophers—beginning with Socrates, Plato, and Aristotle—have struggled with two main ethical questions: (a) What is the meaning of right or good? and (b) What should I do? To identify, clarify, define, and defend a stand on an ethical issue, we must engage in a process of reflective thinking about data that can be gathered by using the framework of six critical questions set out in Box 10–1.

Psychiatric nurses must often identify alternative courses of action and decide what to do when there is a conflict of rights and obligations between clients and families, between themselves and other mental health workers, or between the clients' good and the community or social good. For example, if a woman's disturbed functioning or distress is in part a reaction to aspects of her social context, a therapist can alleviate the disturbance either by helping the person adjust to her situation as it is or by helping her

---

> ## Box 10–1
> # FRAMEWORK OF QUESTIONS FOR ANALYZING AN ETHICAL ISSUE
>
> 1. Who are the relevant actors in the situation?
> 2. What is the required action?
> 3. What are the probable and possible consequences of the action?
> 4. What is the range of alternative actions or choices?
> 5. What is the intent or purpose of the action?
> 6. What is the context of the action?

to change her situation. In a sense a psychiatric nurse becomes both an ethicist and a political agent in resolving this choice.

Dominant Ethical Perspectives

Various ethical perspectives provide different ways of structuring the answers to the questions in Box 10–1, thus leading to different decisions about what is the right action. The dominant ethical perspectives include the following traditions.*

- **Egoism.** The egoist answers questions about the morally right thing to do by saying that something is good because "I desire it." The right act, then, is the one that maximizes the pleasure of the person asking the question.
- **Deontology.** The deontologic or formalist approach suggests that rightness or wrongness depends on the nature or form of the action for moral significance. In this tradition there are both *act deontologists* and *rule deontologists*—i.e., rightness may be based on performing certain morally significant acts properly or adhering to certain preestablished rules or principles. This position requires a commitment to the principle of universality—i.e., one will make the same moral judgment in any similar situation regardless of time, place, or persons involved. Many rule deontologists believe in the divine command theory—an act is wrong because it is forbidden by God. The difficulty for both

*Adapted from Davis AJ, Aroskar MA: *Ethical Dilemmas and Nursing Practice.* Appleton-Century-Crofts, 1978.

believers and nonbelievers in this theory is that sometimes the rules conflict. In an attempt to get out of the problem of conflicting rules, Immanuel Kant, writing in the late eighteenth century, stated that you should act only on a maxim that you can simultaneously will to be a universal law. Unfortunately, Kant's position doesn't help with moral *conflict*. For example, if returning the institutionalized mentally disturbed to the community was identified as a morally good action, Kant would have us ignore any specifics of a particular situation, even though an individual might end up living in a dingy stairwell and stealing food.

- **Utilitarianism.** In the theory of utility, good is "happiness or pleasure," and right is "the greatest good for the greatest number of people." Implicit in this position is the assumption that one can weigh and measure harm and benefit and come out with the best possible balance of good over evil. Among the questions raised by this position is what happens to individual justice when the general welfare is emphasized.

- **Theory of obligation.** The basic principles of the theory of obligation are: (a) the principle of beneficence, which requires that we not just *want* good but *do* good rather than evil, and (b) the principle of justice, which requires that we distribute benefits and burdens equally through society. A problem with this position is what to do when the two principles conflict at the public and individual levels.

- **Ideal observer theory.** This perspective outlines the characteristics of ethical reason as consistency, disinterest, dispassion, omnipresence, and omniscience. These are the qualities of an *ideal observer* or *moral judge*. The ideal observer has only general interests, such as the welfare of all, and does not make decisions on practical or emotional grounds. Needless to say, the questions of who should be the moral judge and where the development of this moral consciousness will occur are left unanswered.

- **Justice as fairness.** The principles of justice as fairness are: (a) each person is to have an equal right to the most extensive liberty for all, and (b) social and economic injustices are to be addressed so that the least advantaged receive the greatest benefit. In this system, the first principle of maximizing liberty for all has absolute priority. Five criteria emerge from this tradition for judging the rightness of any ethical principles:

  1. Universality. The same principles hold for everyone.
  2. Generality. They must not be geared to specific people or situations.
  3. Publicity. They must be known and recognized by all.
  4. Ordering. They must order conflicting claims.
  5. Finality. They may override the demands of law or custom.

Principles of Bioethics

The preceding ethical traditions or a combination of them operate when nurses reflect on ethical dilemmas. Bioethics is a field that applies ethical reasoning to issues and dilemmas in the area of health care.

Taking a stand on an ethical issue involves much more than merely accepting the moral position or personal values of another. Bioethicists (Davis 1981) offer the six principles in Box 10–2 as important guidelines.

ETHICAL DILEMMAS IN PSYCHIATRIC NURSING

Contemporary psychiatric nursing is in the process of being redefined to emphasize enhancing the quality of life for clients, who are seen in a holistic view. Nurses no longer view people as totally propelled by instinctual drives and partially restrained by defense mechanisms such as repression. Rather they take the view that people construct their actions based on the meanings that their particular circumstances hold for them. People who are labeled psychiatric clients are no longer excused for their actions by virtue of having an illness over which they have no control. It is thus no longer easy to justify restrictive interventions such as seclusion, involuntary intramuscular medication,

---

Box 10–2
PRINCIPLES OF BIOETHICS

1. Autonomy—the right to make one's own decisions
2. Nonmaleficence—the intention to do no wrong
3. Beneficence—the principle of attempting to do things that benefit others
4. Justice—the distribution, as fairly as possible, of benefits and burdens
5. Veracity—the intention to tell the truth
6. Confidentiality—the social contact guaranteeing another's privacy

Source: Davis AJ: Ethical dilemmas in nursing. Recorded at JONA and Nurse Educator's 1981 Joint Leadership Conference. Available from Teach'em Inc., 160 East Illinois St., Chicago, Ill. 60611.

and restraint on the ground that the client's behavior is always crying out for others to control it.

The nurse must protect the rights of the individual client yet mediate between these rights and the interests of the social group. Sometimes the two are in conflict. To complicate the situation, Kai Erikson (1962) and Thomas Szasz (1974) argue that deviance can sometimes help stabilize society and therefore actually makes a valuable contribution to social life. According to these authors, only by public displays of rule-breaking behavior can the group learn its tolerance ranges for acceptable behavior. This position is a far cry from a view of the psychiatric client as a dangerous enemy of society—an actual or potential aggressor to be controlled by society's designated keepers. Ultimately nurses must reconcile a number of crucial ethical dilemmas with their personal and professional values. Among these issues are:

- The potential stigma of psychiatric diagnostic labels
- Psychiatry's right to control individual freedom
- The justification for involuntary confinement
- The use of restrictive treatment interventions
- The client's right to suicide
- The client's right to privacy
- The politics and ethics of women's mental health
- Psychiatry's responsibility in defending society's dominant life-style
- The psychiatric professional's role in social and political reform

To practice psychiatric nursing requires ethical responsibility. The quality of a nurse's moral commitment is a measure of professional excellence. However, problems arise when there is conflict about the ground rules for behavior, whether the conflict is between client and social group, nurse and profession, or nurse and agency. These problems are phrased in the ethical language of right and wrong. Circumstances likely to give rise to such problems include the following:

- The professional and the client are from different social classes and have different statuses or cultural values
- The voluntary nature of the client's participation is compromised
- The client's competence to enter into an agreement about intervention is questionable, or the client is subjected to interventions that he or she does not realize are in effect

Every nursing relationship begins with an unusual burden of ethical responsibility. The following pages explore some of these moral issues.

The Stigma of Psychiatric Diagnoses

The list of stereotypes associated with diagnostic categories is well known to most nurses. Equally familiar are the consequences to people with these diagnoses. Psychiatric diagnoses may have fateful consequences for clients and their families. For this reason, psychiatric professionals need to encourage research on this topic.

Diagnostic labels can come to have a life of their own. People labeled as drug addicts, alcoholics, homosexuals, convicts, paranoids, etc. acquire a discredited social identity because of the character flaws often associated with these categories. To much of society, the labels used in psychiatry suggest decadence, immorality, and wanton disregard for society's values. Sociologist Erving Goffman subtitles his monograph on stigma *Notes on the Management of Spoiled Identity* (1963). It is important to consider how and when psychiatric nurses, while advocating humane treatment for clients, indirectly contribute to their spoiled identities by participating in the arbitrary use of oppressive labels.

The Need to Label

Diagnosis has considerable value in psychiatric practice. Putting clients into diagnostic categories makes it easy for health professionals to communicate with each other about the client. Occasionally the diagnosis dictates a particular course of treatment and enables the health team to prognosticate about a client's recovery. Diagnostic categories enable nurses to plan comprehensively for client care and to conduct research.

Before the publication of the third edition of American Psychiatric Association's *Diagnostic and Statistical Manual of Mental Disorders* (DSM-III) and its recent revised edition, diagnostic categories such as schizophrenia, paranoia, or sociopathy were not sufficiently precise to give a clear idea of desirable treatment. A person labeled schizophrenic can be treated with phenothiazines, milieu therapy, or behavior modification techniques. All of these could be justified by one theoretical orientation or another. Nonetheless, the diagnostic label was felt to be the key to subsequent decisions about a client, especially the choice of medication. In some cases when clients failed to respond favorably to the medication indicated by their diagnosis, the diagnosis was changed.

We missed the diagnosis initially. We focused on the paranoid schizophrenic elements and missed the cycles. We need to take him off the Prolixin and consider Lithium for his manic depression.

Advocates for the criteria-based DSM-IIIR believe that its use will greatly improve diagnostic practices.

The Labeling Process

A substantial proportion of "treatment time" in any modern in-patient setting is devoted to piecing together stories about the clients in order to assign diagnostic or legal labels. Intelligence-gathering tactics consume staff attention and energy during the early days of a client's confinement, if not longer. Staff members trying to uncover information about a client interact with clients trying to hide what they believe are damaging data about themselves. One staff member comments to another, "Have you picked up a little paranoia in David or is it only guardedness?" Clients often sense that they are being evaluated for fateful decisions. They try to learn the scripts that will produce the most positive fates for them. One client asked the nurse, "Does it go against you to be lying down two hours in a row?"

A highly ritualized example of the process of piecing together a story occurs in group intake interviews in most in-patient settings.

Bianca, a newly admitted client, is confronted by a group of eight staff members in an interview room and questioned in a mildly interrogative style. Because of the need to "get to know the client as quickly as possible," her story does not just unfold. Instead she is frequently faced with a barrage of questions. She is standing, barefoot, in a robe, in front of eight strangers. At one point, she pleads: "I just want to go home. I feel like I'm going to be put away for the rest of my life. I don't like it here. I'm sorry, I'm trying to cooperate. I just don't feel I can be close to any of you." She starts to cry. "I'm confused because you ask so many questions. I just don't trust a group of strangers. I'm sorry, but I just need time to think."

Based on this interview and data in the client's chart, the staff pieces together her "story." One staff member summarizes: "I think we've observed a depressed gal with a history of inadequacy and dependency. The pathology is first and foremost depression with her hysterical personality disorder coming out to cover up."

The Self-Fulfilling Label

One of the most common characteristics of psychiatric labeling might be called a *correctness assumption*. Fre-

quently, staff members have already decided that a client will be given medication, even though the client has refused it. Before the start of the precertification observation period, staff members may have decided that the client will be certified for fourteen days. Contacts with the client are then used more to justify the decision than to make a decision in the first place.

Another major characteristic of psychiatric diagnosis is the *invalidation of the client's point of view*. A client's statement that he or she does not want psychiatric help is used as evidence that the person needs it. A client's tears

RESEARCH NOTE

Citation

Akerlund BM, Norberg A: An ethical analysis of double-bind conflicts as experienced by care workers feeding severely demented patients. Int J Nurse Stud 1985;22: 207–216.

Study Problem/Purpose

What is the nature of care workers' experiences when they must feed clients with incurable dementia who no longer take food or fluid voluntarily?

Methods

Thirty-nine care workers were interviewed about their thoughts, feelings, and attitudes toward feeding severely demented clients. Sample members were chosen using a stratified random procedure with number of years in the profession as the stratified variable. The interviews were semistructured and covered nine topics that were raised in no consistent sequence. Tape recordings of the interviews were analyzed using phenomenologic strategies, including text interpretation.

Findings

Feeding clients presented ethical conflicts between two principles: "Keep the client alive" and "Don't cause the client suffering." Care workers fell into four categories according to which ethical rule they gave priority to and how they felt about it. Feeding was a source of conflict for most workers. Workers' attitudes about autonomy and paternalism and time in the profession were not sources of significant differences.

Implications

According to this study, the source of anxiety for care workers feeding demented clients was a lack of discussion about ethics. A theory of ethics applicable to urgent nursing problems is needed.

The Homosexual

Acts of physical love with a member of the same sex often provoke harsh responses and attitudes in the United States. Society's aversion to homosexuality is demonstrated by the fact that it has been considered both a crime and a disease. Oppression of the homosexual today is maintained primarily by the fear that homosexuality threatens the stability of the society, by the irrational belief that homosexuality implies weakness, and by widespread concern about catching AIDS from homosexuals. Even though the label of homosexuality has been replaced in the psychiatric nomenclature by the more limited *ego-dystonic homosexuality* (meaning that the pattern of homosexual arousal causes distress to the client and is unwanted), some psychiatric professionals continue to view this particular lifestyle as reflecting immaturity, deep-seated psychologic problems, emotional disturbances, and severe conflicts.

The Schizophrenic

On the basis of a rather vague concept, thousands of Americans have been labeled and hospitalized as schizophrenics. An individual designated schizophrenic becomes an outcast who is approached with a mixture of distrust and fear. The labeled schizophrenic may be denied employment, particularly in sensitive or important jobs. The pride and self-confidence of diagnosed schizophrenics are often shattered, and they may come to view themselves as incapable of controlling their impulses. Some clients living in agony find reassurance in being told that at least they are not schizophrenic. This diagnosis has become psychiatry's equivalent of cancer in its connotation of hopelessness. Again, DSM-IIIR considerable narrows the concept of schizophrenia.

The Paranoid

The diagnostic term *paranoid* has taken on an almost totally negative meaning. The term is not restricted to those who behave strangely, are overtly suspicious, or tend to blame their failings on others. Professionals apply it to many who take deviant positions on social issues. To accuse an adversary of being paranoid has become a kind of trump card for discrediting any opponent's position.

The Addict

A person who uses alcohol or other drugs to excess may be overwhelmed with all sorts of personal and social difficulties and still maintain a respectable role in society. However, once labeled an alcoholic or addict, the person is often viewed as disgraced rather than as having a disease. Programs like Alcoholics Anonymous work to educate others about addictive disease and enhance the addict's self-esteem.

---

in an interview are viewed as a psychiatric symptom rather than a result of the immediate social context of interrogation, locked ward, involuntary confinement, fatigue, or other stressful circumstances.

Setups—contrived situations—often characterize the information-gathering operations prerequisite to diagnosis. Because diagnostic decisions usually must be made on the basis of limited contacts with clients, setting a situation up to "see how the client reacts" is sometimes used to help establish one diagnosis over another. The client's response to the setup is considered evidence of illness.

A client's diary had been brought to the hospital by a friend. Some discussion ensued among the psychiatric team members about whether "she knows we have this." The staff members decided to leave the diary on the desk in front of the interviewee to "see how she reacts." Any sign of outrage and anger would be viewed as an indicator of her emotional disorder rather than as a justified response to the circumstances.

Sociocultural Influences on Diagnosis

The diagnostic labels used in Western psychiatry have been of limited value in cross-cultural comparisons. Observations indicate that the behavior called *schizophrenia* differs from one culture to another. Even in Western society, the diagnostic label given to a particular behavior under DSM-III's predecessors was related to the client's position in the class structure. "Neurotic" disorders predominated among the upper classes and psychoses characterized the lower classes. Repressive attitudes toward women, blacks, and homosexuals influenced diagnoses. In sum, more often than we would like, conventional psychiatric diagnoses may be affected by characteristics of the social situation in which the deviant and the labelers interact. Factors that influence the outcome of deviant acts include (a) whether the act is labeled as symptomatic by a professional outsider, (b) how serious the act itself is, (c) how frequently the act has occurred, and (d) the social context. Most of the time families develop elaborate accommodation mechanisms to keep a deviant member within the home setting. These accommodation patterns are disrupted only when the public visibility of deviant behavior is highlighted by a diagnosis. The "V-codes" of DSM-IIIR are intended to improve this situation. The V-codes refer to problems in living that are a focus of attention but *do not reflect a mental disorder*.

Addicts elicit pity from some, scorn from others. Under some circumstances they can be imprisoned, even though the substances they use are harmful only to themselves. Mandatory drug screening is an emerging social trend.

The Nurses's Moral Stance on Diagnoses

Does labeling with psychiatric diagnoses merely provide psychiatric professionals with some additional sense of control in their dealings with clients? It is true that a diagnosis gives staff members an increased sense of being able to predict client behavior and a way of viewing calmly what might otherwise be upsetting behavior: "That's just her hysterical personality coming out," or "Those complaints are just paranoid delusions." The consequences of psychiatric labels for clients and their families, however, raise moral questions about the legitimacy of their arbitrary use. Consider the following, adapted from a letter to a newspaper advice columnist.

I am a 12-year-old girl who is left out of all social activities because my father is an alcoholic. I try to be nice and friendly to everyone, but it's no use. The girls at school have told me that their mothers don't want them to associate with me because my father might be dangerous. Is there anything I can do? I am very lonesome because it's no fun to be alone all the time. My mother tries to take me places with her, but I want to be with people my own age. Please give me some advice.

Sincerely,
An Outcast

Nurses have a moral responsibility to question practices that exact a price from clients far in excess of the benefits. Only through involvement in such issues can nurses create a moral environment for health care in which practices truly respond to clients' needs. Every moment of moral injustice takes its toll on nurses as well as clients. Every moment of moral responsibility strengthens their sense of personal integrity.

Control of Individual Freedom

Psychiatric professionals limit and control the freedom of clients through the subtle process of assigning labels to their behavior. These labels can have fateful consequences. Professionals also control individual freedom in more straightforward ways. The most frequent examples of direct controlling interventions are involuntary hospitalization,

and use of restrictive treatments, usually when a person is judged to constitute a danger to self or others.

Involuntary hospitalization and treatment of psychiatric clients are usually considered humanitarian efforts to help "the mentally ill." Yet any practice that directly and coercively deprives a person of freedom has political implications. In most states a client who is involuntarily committed to a mental hospital has few of the legal protections that even a criminal offender has. In addition, in some states clients have no guarantee that they will ever be released from this hospital unless they alter their behavior sufficiently to please their keepers.

Violence and Social Control

Violence Against Others

Psychiatric nurses are faced with the dilemma of trying to be both healer-helpers and agents of social control. In dealing with violently destructive clients, and some others, the value of life is being balanced against the value of liberty. Thomas Szasz (1974) argues that there is never adequate justification for involuntary commitment under the guise of medical help. He believes that violence toward others is a crime and should be treated as such, not as a mental disease. Szasz argues that contemporary psychiatrists confuse deviance with disease and control with cure and make decisions and policies that constitute grave threats to personal freedom and dignity. Seymour Halleck (1971), another politically oriented psychiatrist-writer, suggests that society needs to make distinctions among the kinds of violence to decide which kinds might legitimately be controlled by civil procedures. His intent is to limit severely the instances that justify psychiatric intervention. Like Halleck, psychiatrists Andrew Skodol and T. B. Karasu (1978) contend that psychiatric professionals can do little to help prevent spontaneous violence. So many variables contribute to such behavior that it is practically impossible for anyone to predict its occurrence. Because it is so difficult to know precisely who will be violent, it is an unjustifiable violation of civil liberties to lock up someone who behaves peaceably most of the time and has not committed a crime but is only suspected of being prone to impulsive outbursts. In contrast, Halleck identifies a group of people who plan violence and act in irrational, strange, or self-defeating ways even with members of their own subculture. It is reasonable to assume that these people are experiencing emotional difficulty, he feels. In this group would be a woman who talks of killing her children because she is commanded to do so by God, or a person who feels driven to obtain sexual pleasure by mutilating and molesting strangers. These individuals are justifiable candidates for involuntary detention on psychiatric grounds, in Halleck's view. Szasz, on the other hand, prefers the application of legal-criminal controls to this category of people.

Suicide

Suicide is a form of violence to oneself. As such, it raises for psychiatric nurses the moral issue of balancing liberty and life. The extent to which homicide and suicide are equivalent is another basic ethical question that bears on society's right to control suicide. Szasz believes that homicide and suicide bear the same relation to each other as rape and masturbation do. Homicide, according to Szasz, is the gravest crime, while suicide in his opinion is a basic human right.

Traditionally, nurses have felt that they should do everything possible to preserve life. They have relied on this imperative to justify coercive intervention in suicide attempts as well as heroic technical measures to avert impending deaths. Recent reconsideration of euthanasia, however, seems to raise questions about a client's right to suicide. *Euthanasia* has been defined as the intentional termination of a life of such poor quality that it is not worth living. The concept of allowing a person to die without the use of life-prolonging treatment is called **passive euthanasia**. **Active euthanasia**, by contrast, is defined as an act that results in the death of a person. The treatment given to dying clients is often in conflict with the treatment they desire. For example, a physician may disregard a client's protests against treatment. The doctor may assert that the client's medical condition is causing the client to behave irrationally. It is no great logical jump from clients dying of physical deterioration to clients dying of emotional or mental deterioration. Many of the same ethical questions emerge about the suicidal client:

- How is *quality of life* defined?
- Is the definition limited to physical factors?
- Who should have the right to make the definition?
- How is rationality to be measured?
- Are people always in conscious control of their choices?

An individual's right to choose when and how to die is a complex biomedical issue currently receiving more attention that ever before. The thoughtful professional nurse needs to clarify the issues, give them careful consideration, and search for a personal position. There are many ways in which people can deliberately shorten their own lives. They can destroy themselves quickly with a gun, or slowly through the chronic use of drugs such as tobacco or alcohol. When is coercive intervention by psychiatric practitioners justified? Do professionals have the right to restrain people against their will if those people have not committed an illegal act?

Use of Restrictive Treatments

At some time in their lives, all people experience the kind of excessive stress that makes them feel miserable or even desperate. Some people, however, communicate these feelings in ways that are inappropriate, troublesome, unreasonable, or frightening to others. A young woman who in times of stress mutilates her body by burning it repeatedly with cigarettes; a teenager who breaks everything in sight during violent, destructive outbursts; and a belligerent male who initiates physical fights with anyone and everyone without provocation all usually become candidates for *symptomatic treatments*—behavioral control measures often used against the person's will.

Psychosurgery

The most dramatic of restrictive measures is *psychosurgery*, the surgical removal or destruction of brain tissue with the intent of altering behavior even though there may be no direct evidence of structural disease or damage in the brain. Psychosurgery has become the subject of marked controversy on ethical grounds. Advocates claim that it is done to restore rather than destroy individual freedom. They argue that before psychosurgery, the client is crippled by mental illness. Individual autonomy is compromised by the client's bizarre behavior or internal psychologic state. After the surgery, clients supposedly are more autonomous than before, by their own and others' criteria. Advocates of selective use of psychosurgery, even when it is against the client's will, outline three conditions that must be met to justify it:

1. The illness being treated is seriously disabling and untreatable by nonsurgical means such as medication or therapy.
2. The treatment is undertaken with some sort of systematic investigative protocol—in short, it is accompanied by evaluation research.
3. The treatment occurs in settings with as many safeguards as possible to arrive at informed consent, if possible, perhaps using a client advocate during the procedure.

Psychotropic Drugs

The discovery that certain drugs can radically alter human emotions has had an enormous impact on psychiatry. The mental hospital is no longer seen as a warehouse for storing society's deviants; it is now a clearinghouse where clients are sorted, renovated, and dispatched back into their communities with symptomatic behavior under control through one or another of the current psychiatric medications.

Psychiatric professionals have associated the advent of psychotropic medications with a new optimism and less fear about working with persons labeled mentally ill. Conceivably, the impact of the drugs on attitudes of nurses may increase the amount of humane contact clients are given while in the hospital. Furthermore it might be argued that the drugs have helped keep people out of the hospital and have decreased the need for other more dramatic treatments, such as electroshock treatment.

Drugs that make people feel better, however, can lessen their motivation to confront an oppressive situation. This can have serious implications for the political and moral climate of society. Consider, for example, a common clinical problem:

A woman is married to a domineering and insensitive man. She becomes increasingly unhappy, then intensely anxious. When she is on the verge of fighting back to try to alter her oppressed situation, she becomes more agitated and visits a psychiatric clinic. Her therapist prescribes a medicine that alleviates her tension. As a consequence the client has less awareness of her plight and is less inclined to confront her problems. She ultimately continues to submit to her husband's oppressiveness.

It is conceivable that pills could be developed to keep such a woman quietly enslaved throughout her married life. Suppose drugs were coercively given to anyone whose unhappiness was rooted in social oppression. We can even contemplate the possibility that the government might become repressive enough to force all dissidents to take medicine.

Drugs cautiously and judiciously used with the consent of clients can be helpful to people. Used unreflectively, they can close off moral and political confrontations. Decisions about the use of drugs must be made in the context of the social situation and environment.

In the in-patient setting, medications are regularly used to reduce symptoms and make client behavior more manageable. Most staff members legitimize their use of chemical controls by defining violent or bizarre behavior as an indirect request for limits. When this kind of meaning is assigned to the use of drugs, practitioners can feel that their actions to suppress symptoms are based on the needs of the client rather than on the staff's management motives.

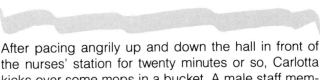

After pacing angrily up and down the hall in front of the nurses' station for twenty minutes or so, Carlotta kicks over some mops in a bucket. A male staff member shouts to the nurse to get her p.r.n. medication ready and strides into the hall telling the client to stop it. She cries and shouts, and they begin struggling. Several other staff members rush over to assist. They drag and carry her into her room, where she gets Haldol (10 mg). She continues fighting and screaming. The staff members decide to put her in "soft" restraints and continue to wrestle with her in her room. Finally they decide to transfer her to the ward downstairs, where she can be put into a seclusion room. In a report, a staff member describes the incident as, "Carlotta blew up and needed controls." In further discussion of the case, it became apparent that the decision to put her into seclusion was made because restrained clients have to be checked and released every ten minutes, which is a lot of work for the staff.

It is possible that all these controls would not have been necessary had a nurse behind the glass windows of the nurses' station responded to the nonverbal cues of mounting tension that the client communicated before kicking over the mops.

Structural Controls

Even the physical characteristics of psychiatric in-patient settings convey the notion that clients are not expected to be capable of self-control and that staff members have the responsibility for providing it. Many clients view these interventions as forms of abuse, while the staff sees them as "helping people who can't take care of themselves." Consider the following directions on use of restraints:

> The acutely psychotic client who is delusional, the angry individual who is testing limits, and the intoxicated client are the types of individuals to whom restraints may be applied for their own protection and that of others. These individuals are nonverbally asking for help to control their potentially inappropriate behavior. When all other techniques have failed and it is quite obvious that the client is out of control, the staff must take action and forcibly apply restraints.

All the judgments that must be made about restraints involve moral decisions. What other techniques have been tried?

Box 10–3

MENTAL PATIENT'S BILL OF RIGHTS

We are ex-mental patients. We have been subjected to brutalization in mental hospitals and by the psychiatric profession. In almost every state of the union, a mental patient has fewer de facto rights than a murderer condemned to die or to life imprisonment. As a human being, you are entitled to basic human rights that are taken for granted by the general population. You are entitled to protection by and recourse to the law. The purpose of the Mental Patients' Liberation Project is to help those who are still institutionalized. This Bill of Rights was prepared by those at the first meeting of MPLP held on June 13, 1971, at the Washington Square Methodist Church. If you know someone in a mental hospital, give him/her a copy of these rights. If you are in a hospital and need legal help, try to find someone to call the number listed below.

1. You are a human being and are entitled to be treated as such with as much decency and respect as is accorded to any other human being.

2. You are an American citizen and are entitled to every right established by the Declaration of Independence and guaranteed by the Constitution of the United States of America.

3. You have the right to the integrity of your own mind and the integrity of your own body.

4. Treatment and medication can be administered only with your consent and, in the event you give your consent, you have the right to demand to know all relevant information regarding said treatment and/or medication.

5. You have the right to have access to your own legal and medical counsel.

6. You have the right to refuse to work in a mental hospital and/or to choose what work you shall do and you have the right to receive the minimum wage for such work as is set by the state labor laws.

7. You have the right to decent medical attention when you feel you need it just as any other human being has that right.

8. You have the right to uncensored communication by phone, letter, and in person with whomever you wish and at any time you wish.

9. You have the right not to be treated like a criminal; not to be locked up against your will; not to be committed involuntarily; not to be fingerprinted or "mugged" (photographed).

10. You have the right to decent living conditions. You're paying for it and the taxpayers are paying for it.

11. You have the right to retain your own personal property. No one has the right to confiscate what is legally yours, no matter what reason is given. That is commonly known as theft.

12. You have the right to bring grievance against those who have mistreated you and the right to counsel and a court hearing. You are entitled to protection by the law against retaliation.

13. You have the right to refuse to be a guinea pig for experimental drugs and treatments and to refuse to be used as learning material for students. You have the right to demand reimbursement if you are so used.

14. You have the right not to have your character questioned or defamed.

15. You have the right to request an alternative to legal commitment or incarceration in a mental hospital.

The Mental Patients' Liberation Project plans to set up neighborhood crisis centers as alternatives to incarceration and voluntary and involuntary commitment to hospitals. We plan to set up a legal aid society for those whose rights are taken away and/or abused. Although our immediate aim is to help those currently in hospitals, we are also interested in helping those who are suffering from job discrimination, discriminatory school admissions policies and discrimination and abuse at the hands of the psychiatric professions. Call the number listed below if you are interested in our group or if you need assistance.

Mental Patients Alliance of Central New York
P.O. Box 158
Syracuse, N.Y. 13201
(315) 947-5822

Source: Mental Patients Alliance of Central New York Inc.

Is the client obviously out of control? How does the nurse decide? What will be the effects on the client of such a dramatic intervention? What are the effects on others in the milieu? In weighing decisions, nurses must keep in mind that any intervention that removes symptoms without simultaneously increasing the client's awareness of the underlying experience is potentially repressive. Clients themselves have begun to guard against repressiveness by issuing a bill of rights (Box 10–3).

Client Privacy and Confidentiality

When people seek psychiatric help, they must usually reveal highly personal, possibly embarrassing, and potentially damaging information about themselves. Almost all modes of therapeutic intervention rely on the client's willingness to talk openly and honestly about personal concerns, feelings, or problems. The solo therapist in private practice with voluntary clients is usually able to avoid compromising the clients' rights to confidentiality. In fact, many private therapists view themselves as vigilant protectors of their clients' privacy. Nurses, however, may encounter a serious ethical conflict in being at the same time the confidant of the client and an employee of the organization. These nurses have dual allegiances—to the client and to the agency. Clients usually assume that health professionals have no other purpose than to help them. They lose sight of the fact that nurses often are asked to collect data about them that might be highly influential in determining their medications, their disposition, and even their civil rights. While it is often the psychiatrist who makes final pronouncements about a client's mental health status, diagnosis, prognosis, and the like, such pronouncements rest on information collected and communicated to the doctor by nurses. This information-gathering process merits serious scrutiny.

It is not unusual for a kind of fiction to develop about a hospitalized client, in the staff's eagerness to gather juicy tidbits of information. Data are passed from one nursing shift to another and written on the chart without thought to their validity or reliability. These are then used to make generalizations about the client. The following are typical entries about clients in nurses' notes:

Little socialization

Somewhat seclusive

Superficially appropriate

Looks flat

Very poor insight

High as a kite

May be hallucinating

Often the requirement that nurses exchange tidbits such as these with each other becomes the motivation for getting out to talk to the clients so that the nurse will have something to report. Yet it is considered sufficient simply to have a comment to make. Little concern is shown about how representative that comment may be.

The information garnered in this way may be confirmed by repetition in shift reports and daily charting, without additional exploration. This arouses another reaction in some nurses—reluctance to report any observations.

On one occasion a few staff members in an in-patient facility expressed concern about the things people choose to put in reports, because of "the way things get latched onto around here." For example, a client may acquire a reputation as a homosexual or heroin addict because of revealing one experimental experience to a nurse in what the client believed to be a confidential exchange. One nurse said, "Somehow it seems more ethical to write 'I didn't talk to the client today' or 'I don't know what's going on with this person' than to select out of an eight-hour period one or two phrases or behaviors, often expressed in clichés."

Information gathering and sharing are part of the psychiatric nurse's role. When the employer is a federal- or state-supported agency that might have some investment in quelling deviants, however, the nurse is put in a double-agent role. The client's rights to privacy and confidentiality are increasingly threatened by computerized data banks for information storage, certain medical and other insurance procedures, and even the professional standards review organization (PSRO) system in clinical agencies. Thoughtful handling of this dilemma is facilitated by two safeguards:

1. Nurses must convey to clients the limit of confidentiality in their exchanges—that is, what the nurses do with the information a client shares.
2. Nurses must attempt to portray accurately to others how reliable, valid, and representative are the data they communicate about a client.

The Ethics and Politics of Women's Mental Health

In the past two decades, nurses have become aware of the impact of feminism on the institution of psychotherapy and the sensibilities of those professionals who concern themselves with a special subsection of the client population—women. Brodsky's (1973) review of a decade of feminist influence on psychotherapy cited changes in theories, treatment techniques, and assessment approaches, all reflecting more enlightened attitudes toward women as therapists and clients. Yet in 1978, a special populations subpanel on the mental health of women submitted a report to the President's Commission on Mental Health that began (Task Force, 1978):

> American women rank with the racial and ethnic minorities as a segment of the population who are overrepresented among the mentally ill, and underserved by the mental health system. While the numbers place women clearly in a majority position, other data suggest that women continue to be accorded disadvantaged status in all areas of American society. Despite the 1974 amendments to the Civil Rights Act of 1964, discrimination against women continues in all major institutions of this society.

The report further describes the documented social, economic, and psychologic status of women as follows:

- More than half the women in the United States are now employed outside the home, but they are clustered in the lowest-paying occupations and at the bottom of the achievement ladder.

- Equal opportunity programs and affirmative action notwithstanding, qualified women employed full-time in 1976 earned less than 56 percent of what men earn.

- One woman in four but one man in eighteen lives on an annual income of less than $4,000.

- Increasing numbers of families are comprised of a mother and her children, and there are few social supports for her outside the immediate family.

- Whether or not women are employed outside the home, housework remains largely women's work. Thus many American women have two full workdays every twenty-four hours.

- Fifty percent more women than men report having used barbiturates.

- Estimates of the proportion of alcoholic women in the population range from 20 percent to 50 percent, but the numbers are increasing.

- Twice as many women as men use the two most popular tranquilizers, Valium and Librium.

- Although exact numbers are not yet available, increasing numbers of women are reporting that they have been beaten, raped, or abused, often in their own homes.

- There are 175 women to every 100 men admitted to hospitals for the treatment of depression.

- There are 283 women to every 100 men treated for depression in outpatient services.

- More women than men in the general population report that they experience symptoms of depression.

- The highest rate for treatment in public facilities is for nonwhite women and women between twenty-five and forty-four who are separated or divorced.

- Among married women in the general population, symptoms of depression are more common among women whose children are living with them.

- Older women whose children have left home and women who have never married show fewer symptoms of depression.

- The conflict between self-esteem and incongruent role is reported as a source of stress for women.

- Since no evidence suggests that women are innately more vulnerable to mental illness, it must be assumed that social institutions have a different, more stressful impact on women than on men.

- Most mental health professionals are men, and most clients are women.

- Women in therapy comment that many therapists: foster traditional sex roles; have biases and expectations that devalue women; use traditional psychoanalytic concepts in a sexist way; and often respond to women as sex objects.

This rather disconcerting and thought-provoking summary underscores the necessity of viewing women's mental health as a clinical or research area requiring our most responsible and expert ethical and political reflectiveness.

Phyllis Chesler (1972), the outspoken author of *Women and Madness,* analyzes the status of women in our culture in her own unique, rhetorical style.

> Women are submissive. We're altruistic. And especially we're self-sacrificing. Usually our altruism comes from very low self-esteem. We're always guilty. We're losers— trained to be losers in life. We're also mothers or can be mothers and that's another reason why we might be altruistic.

Chesler goes on to identify four premises that run through all the theories of psychiatry and apply to most clinical practices. These premises, in Chesler's view, reflect how the mental health professions see women and how women have been taught to see themselves.

1. Everybody is crazy.
2. While everybody is crazy, women are crazier. To be mentally healthy is to be male.
3. Male homosexuality is sick, and lesbians don't exist.
4. In order for a woman to be a real woman, she's got to become a mother, and once you've become a mother, everything that goes wrong with your family's mental health is your fault.

The End of Neutrality

For a long time nursing has hidden behind the cloak of political neutrality, arguing that the role of caretakers and healers permits, even demands, a detachment from political, economic, and social issues. Psychiatric nursing services have been defined as client-oriented activities designed to reduce pain and discomfort and to increase the capacity of the individual to adjust satisfactorily. As long as nurses saw their psychiatric work as simply treating illnesses of the mind in the same way they treated illnesses of the body, they could accept the notion that psychologic illness, like physical illness, indicated a defect in the individual, not in the social milieu. Practitioners tended to search for the causes of emotional suffering exclusively in anomalies of the client's biologic or psychologic past. They did not consider the interaction of factors in the client's environment that might account for strange, troublesome, or irrational behavior. This view of the human condition and the nurse's role avoided any critical examination of society and the nurse's relationship to it.

New conceptual frameworks and nursing theories take into consideration not only internal individual perceptions of stress but also the immediate and broader social contexts that contribute to an individual's experience of stress. Nurses are beginning to realize that a person identified as a client may be miserable and not coping at any given moment not only because of personal perceptions of oppression, but also because they are actually being oppressed. As the saying goes, "Even paranoids have real enemies."

Combating Environmental Stress

In the complex superstructure of global society, environmental stresses may be generated both directly by the selfishness, apathy, or malice of those in power and indirectly by subtly imposed prejudices, outmoded and inflexible rules, the threat of nuclear war, and an economic system that deprives certain citizens (often the poor and members of minority groups) of basic human needs. Black people directly exposed to humiliation by bigoted whites have a clear idea who their oppressors are. They are aware of their anger and know toward whom it is directed. Black people living in a society where racism is institutionalized but not openly expressed may be exposed to repeated indirect aggressions that leave them frustrated and angry, but they have difficulty identifying the source of their sense of oppression. Halleck (1971) asserts that any citizens who believe in the basic benevolence of their society but do not partake of its benefits have similar reactions. It is not unusual for people in these circumstances to express their frustration and anger in alcoholism, drug use, violence, or suicide.

Environmental stress is also generated in immediate families or groups of significant others. A parent may abuse a child. An employer may harass or insult an employee. These are direct sources of stress.

Stress generated in immediate social systems also may be indirect, leaving the individual totally or partially unaware of its source. For example, a domineering husband may send day-to-day demeaning messages that chip away his wife's self-esteem in disguised ways. She may find herself feeling chronically depressed or anxious without knowing why. A domineering wife may do the same to her husband.

The Social Psychiatric Model

A psychiatric nurse who is willing to try to help clients to change the stresses in their environment rather than adapt to them is engaging in an aspect of social psychiatric practice. Halleck (1971), describing a social psychiatric model for practice, urges psychiatric professionals to abandon the hoax of a politically neutral profession and make their personal political positions explicit. He feels that it is illogical to believe that professional activities designed to change the status quo are political, while those designed to strengthen the status quo are neutral. Halleck emphasizes the important role of psychiatric professionals in social reform. All therapists base their efforts to help clients and society on some idea of the optimum human condition. Therefore, psychiatric professionals must think through the meaning of *optimum human condition* to gain insight into their own ideologies and to sharpen their ethical criteria for intervening in social systems or sustaining the status quo.

Acting to sustain and preserve a desirable social order is by no means immoral or unethical. Society relies on psychiatric professionals as agents of social control to bring a humane and caring perspective to their often difficult and uncertain work with clients. Many of these clients have engaged in behavior patterns believed to be evil, destructive, and burdensome to others. As one somewhat hardened nurse put it:

We are the junk pickers of society—picking up society's casualties and trying to rework them into some useful form.

Balancing the Individual and the Social Good

The judgments that label someone's experience as paranoid rather than simply unpopular are frequently based on arbitrary and shifting criteria. Behavior that is considered bizarre or unreasonable in one cultural context may be considered desirable in another. The definitions of those who need psychiatric help are constantly changing. Nurses are necessarily guided in therapeutic work by a belief system—by some vision of what kinds of changes would improve a client's life. Nurses are further guided by some moral principles that limit the extent to which they will help a client obtain happiness at the expense of others and the extent to which they will participate in the oppression of an individual in the interests of societal control. Laws represent yet another source of limits.

Nursing is frequently faced with two goals:

- To respond to the therapeutic needs of individuals.

- To serve society by preserving some degree of social order.

Often these two goals are in conflict, and nurses must face the dilemma of placing one above the other. The only way to resolve the conflict is for them to clarify their own goals and values through a process of ethical reflection.

Chapter Highlights

- Ethical reflection is a process for achieving clear and convincing reasons for making moral decisions rather than discovering a singular right or wrong solution for ethical dilemmas.

- An ethical dilemma is a conflict between two obligations.

- Nurses move toward professional autonomy through development of codes of ethics, setting qualifications for practitioners, participating in peer review, setting standards, and accepting consequences for professional decisions.

- Known dominant ethical perspectives include egoism, deontology, utilitarianism, theory of obligation, ideal observer theory, and justice as fairness.

- The egoistic perspective is that the right act is the one that maximizes the pleasure of the person asking the question, "How do I act?"

- In the deontologic view, rightness or wrongness depends on the form of the action for moral significance.

- Adherents of the theory of utilitarianism define good as happiness and right as maximizing good and minimizing harm for the greatest number of persons.

- Adherents of the theory of obligation suggest that individuals ought to do good, not just want good, and that benefits and burdens ought to be distributed equally throughout society.

- According to the ideal observer theory, the characteristics of ethical reason are consistency, disinterest, dispassion, omnipresence, and omniscience.

- The justice-as-fairness perspective is that each person is to have maximum liberty, and social and economic injustices are to be addressed so that the greatest benefit goes to the least advantaged.

- Principles of bioethics include autonomy, nonmaleficence, beneficence, justice, veracity, and confidentiality.

- Contemporary health-related ethical dilemmas include the effects of psychiatric labeling, control of personal freedom, use of restrictive treatments, the rights of the client, and the ethics and politics of women's mental health.

- The nurse must protect the rights of the individual yet mediate between these rights and the interests of the social group.

References

American Association of Colleges of Nursing: *Essentials of College and University Education for Professional Nursing; Final Report.* 1986, pp. 6–7.

American Psychological Association. Task Force on Sex Bias and Sex Role Stereotyping in Psychotherapeutic Practice: Guidelines for therapy with women. *Am Psychol* 1978; 33:1122–1123.

Aroskar MA: Establishing limits to professional autonomy: Whose responsibility? *Nurs Law Ethics* 1980; 1.

Brodsky A: The consciousness-raising group as a model for therapy with women. *Psychother Theory Re Prac* 1973; 10:24–29.

Chesler P: *Women and Madness.* Doubleday, 1972.

Davis AJ: Ethical dilemmas in nursing. Recorded at JONA and Nurse Educator's 1981 Joint Leadership Conference, available from Teach'em Inc., 160 East Illinois Street, Chicago, Illinois.

Davis AJ, Aroskar MA: *Ethical Dilemmas and Nursing Practice.* Appleton-Century-Crofts, 1978.

Erikson K: Notes on the sociology of deviance. *Soc Probl* 1962; 9:308.

Goffman E: *Stigma: Notes on the Management of Spoiled Identity.* Prentice-Hall, 1963.

Halleck SL: *The Politics of Therapy.* Harper and Row, 1971.

Skodol A, Karasu TB: Emergency psychiatry and the assaultive patient. *Am J Psychiatry* 1978; 135:202–205.

Szasz T: *The Myth of Mental Illness,* rev ed. Harper and Row, 1974.

Task Force on Mental Health of Women. *Report to the President's Commission on Mental Health.* U.S. Government Printing Office, 1978.

ELEVEN

Communication

Carol Ren Kneisl

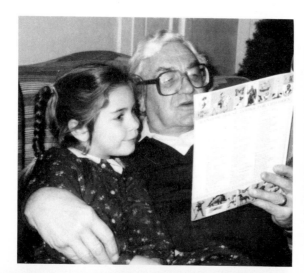

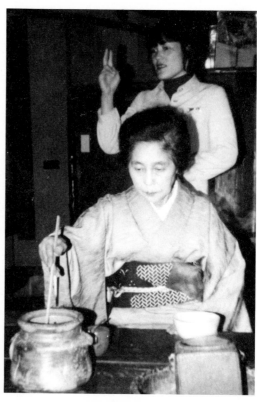

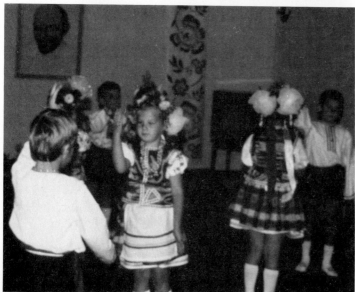

After reading this chapter, students should be able to

- Describe the process of human communication
- Compare linear, interactional, and transactional models of communication
- Identify the major concepts in a humanistic interactionist approach to communication
- Discuss verbal and nonverbal modes of communication
- Relate three major theories of communication to humanistic psychiatric nursing practice
- Identify concepts of facilitative communication that are essential ingredients of interpersonal relationships
- Apply skills that foster effective communication throughout the nursing process

Cross-References

Other topics related to this content are: Culture, Chapter 38; Empathy, Chapter 3; Influence of territoriality and personal space on communication, Chapter 13; and Role of human values in the communication of the nurse, Chapter 3.

Imagine a world beyond war.

Key Terms

Adult ego state
Child ego state
checking perceptions
clarifying
complementary relationship
complementary transaction
confronting
crossed transaction
feedback
game
illusion
imparting information
informational confrontation
interpersonal communication
interpretive confrontation
intrapersonal communication
kinesics
linking
mirroring
mixed message
neologism
neurolinguistic programming (NLP)
nonverbal communication
overload
paralanguage
paraphrasing
Parent ego state
perception
pinpointing
processing
proxemics
questioning
reflecting
structuring
summarizing
symmetrical relationship
tangential reply
transactional analysis (TA)
ulterior transaction
underload

When John Bowlby (1951) discovered that infants in foundling homes were literally dying for lack of contact and affection, the scientific community began to attach new importance to the old dictum that *people need people.* It is recognized today that the mechanism for establishing, maintaining, and improving human contacts is interpersonal communication. Communication is a very special process and the most significant of human behaviors. Moreover, it is the main method for implementing the nursing process.

The therapeutic interpersonal relationship in humanistic psychiatric nursing practice often develops through a storytelling experience. Telling stories is as natural and human as breathing. When they tell "their story," clients explain themselves, the events of their lives, and the circumstances they face.

The major role of the psychiatric nurse is to help clients tell their stories, explore the circumstances of their lives, and resolve the things that have gone wrong. However, the process of communication is so complex and multidimensional that it cannot be reduced to a few simple steps that nurses can memorize and perform.

THE PROCESS OF HUMAN COMMUNICATION

Communication is an ongoing, dynamic, and ever-changing series of events, each of which affects and is affected by all the others. The essence of effective communication is *responding with meaning* to the series. Unfortunately, some persons define communication simply as the transfer of information or meaning from one human being to another. However, meaning cannot be transferred from one human being to another but must be mutually negotiated, because meaning is influenced by a number of significant variables.

Variables That Influence Communication

Perception

A person's image or perception of the world is an essential element in communicating. The term **perception** refers to the experience of sensing, interpreting, and comprehending the world in which the person lives. This makes perception a highly personal and internal act.

The information that people have of the world around them is processed through their senses. However, seeing is not always believing. Contemporary communication specialists have discovered that because of human physiologic limitations, the eye and brain are constantly being tricked into seeing things that are not really what they seem (**illusions**). Figure 11–1 shows an illusion that reflects physiologic constraints. Before continuing to read, stare at Figure 11–1 for 20 seconds. The illustration will appear to swing back and forth. Verify that the movement is an illusion by checking the visual perception against tactile sensations.

What people "see" or sense is influenced very strongly by a number of factors. Stop reading here and look at Figure 11–2. Past experiences have prepared us to see things, persons, and events in particular ways. When we read the sayings in Figure 11–2, past experience encourages us to see them inaccurately as the familiar sayings "Snake in the grass," "Quick as a flash," and "Paris in the spring." The words actually are "Snake in *the the* grass," "Quick as *a a* flash," and "Paris in *the the* spring."

People tend to observe more carefully when a purpose guides the observation. The purposes or reasons for engaging in an observation also determine what is observed. The nurse in an intensive care unit observes a cardiac surgery client differently than a family member does.

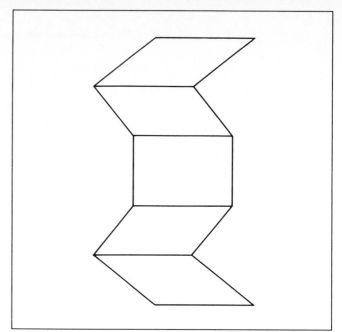

Figure 11–1
A perceptual illusion.

Finally, when understandings differ, people can look at the same object and see different things. Mental set helps determine how and what a person perceives. Before you read any further, look at the picture of the young woman in Figure 11–3. Do you see the silhouette of a young woman? Do you also see the face of an elderly woman? Our use of the phrase *the picture of the young woman in Figure 11–3* encouraged you to perceive the illustration in a particular way. Now you should also be able to see the elderly woman in the illustration.

As the illustrations demonstrate, the old axiom might be better stated: "Believing is seeing." Because people tend to perceive in terms of past experiences, expectations, and goals, perceptions may be a prime obstacle to communication. No two individuals perceive the world in exactly the same way, and the meanings of events differ because people's perceptions of them differ. Perceptions of other human beings are of particular importance since human com-

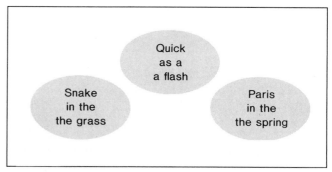

Figure 11–2
The influence of past experience on perception.

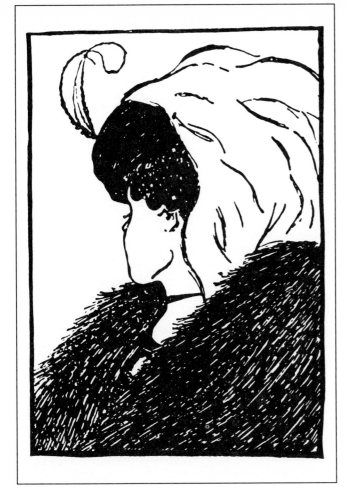

Figure 11–3
The influence of mental set on perception.

The parents of a 15-year-old girl were upset to find a small plastic bag of marijuana in her dresser drawer. She had been playing hooky from school and wore jeans that her parents considered sloppy. After a series of lengthy, angry discussions with her parents, she was confined to her room. During this period she refused to eat or drink.

When the girl was seen by a mental health treatment team, the members' opinions were divided. Some said that her behavior signaled an emotional disturbance and labeled her antisocial, depressed, and anxious. Others believed her parents were too rigid in attempting to force her to accept their values.

In another instance, a 35-year-old man was firmly committed to prayer. Most of his spare time was connected in some way to church-related activities. Staff members at a mental health clinic where he sought counseling told him that he was resorting to an early infantile attitude about God as the magic worker.

Clearly, these staff members were influenced by their own values.

The daily roles people take also influence their values. In any one day a man may be a student, husband, father, nurse, citizen, speaker, artist, son, and teacher.

munication is inevitably affected by participants' perceptions of one another. To see others at all as they are, people need to know themselves and to know how the self affects the perception of others.

Values

Values are concepts of the desirable. People value what is of worth to them. Values influence the process of communication, because people's values, like their perceptions, differ.

Value systems differ for a number of reasons. Age is one. Children's values shift when they become teenagers. The college or work experience generally influences values in yet other directions. Marrying or being a parent or grandparent may cause other value changes or shifts.

Psychiatric nurses must ultimately come to terms with the problem of values, because conflicting value systems among mental health professionals expose clients to uncertainty and confusion. Consider the following examples:

Culture

Each culture provides its members with notions about how the world is structured and what it means. These preconceptions, learned at an early age, are so subtle that they often go unrecognized. They nonetheless set limits on communication and interaction with others. Relying on culturally determined generalizations or stereotypes can have profound effects on people's relationships with others.

Communication is culture-bound in a wide variety of ways. The culture and the subculture (the culture within the culture) teach people how to communicate through language, hand gestures, clothing, and even in the ways they use the space around them.

The nurse who does not know that "run it by me" means to explain something, that a "close-knuckle drill" is a fistfight, or that "hit on a broad" means to sweet-talk a female may be confused by conversations with members of certain subcultures—adolescents and street people, for example. The nurse who overhears two clients talking about "angel dust" is likely to come to erroneous conclusions if unaware that the term refers not to a Christmas decoration but to PCP—an animal tranquilizer. In some cultures, belching after dinner is a compliment to the host and is considered proper etiquette. In other cultures, belching may be thought uncouth or an insult. When Americans make a circle with thumb and forefinger and extend the other fingers, they mean "OK." To Brazilians, the same gesture is an obscene sign of contempt. These examples make it obvious that communicating with meaning requires that the participants take culture well into account. How people communicate with others who do not share similar histories, heritages, or cultures is of critical importance in humanistic psychiatric nursing practice.

Levels of Communication

Communication takes place on at least three different levels—intrapersonal, interpersonal, and public. **Intrapersonal communication** occurs when people communicate within themselves. When a nurse walks into a client's room and thinks, "The first pint of blood is almost finished. I'd better get the next one ready for infusion," the nurse is communicating intrapersonally.

Interpersonal communication, which this chapter discusses in depth, takes place between dyads (groups of two persons) and in small groups. This level of person-to-person communication is at the heart of humanistic psychiatric nursing.

Public communication is communication between a person and several other people. Its most common form is the presentation of a public speech. Communications through the mass media are other forms of public communication.

MODELS OF HUMAN COMMUNICATION

One of the easiest ways to illustrate the nature of human communication and the elements or components that make up the process is through a model, or visual representation.

People use models frequently for many purposes. They might use a map, which is a visual representation of a territory, to find their way to the community mental health center they plan to visit. Health professionals use EEGs to see a visual representation of the electrical activity in the brain. However, models provide incomplete views—a map does not show all the trees, buildings, or park statues in the territory, and the EEG tracing does not show the color,

size, or blood supply of the brain. It is important to keep this in mind when looking at models. They sometimes make a process look simpler than it is.

Communication As an Act

Viewing human communication as an act is a linear concept of communication. Communication is seen as a one-way phenomenon: A talks to B. Communicators who follow this concept attempt to transfer the thoughts or ideas in their heads into someone else's head. Communication then becomes something that is done *to* another person. The process is illustrated in Figure 11–4.

Two major assumptions behind this view are that skill is all important, and that meaning is transferable. Such a model fails to take into account the variables discussed earlier—perception, values, and culture. It suggests that the receiver plays a passive role and does not affect the communicator. It places primary emphasis on the selection of "correct" messages. When misunderstandings occur, either the communicator is faulted for failing to send the correct message or the receiver is faulted for having allowed something to interfere with the transmission of a correct message. Both persons become preoccupied with laying blame and the need to construct "perfect messages." These implications and assumptions are evidence that the model of communication as an act is inadequate.

Communication As an Interaction

The interactional perspective takes into account the process of mutual or reciprocal influence in communication. In this view, when two people interact, they put themselves into each other's shoes. Each tries to perceive the world as the other perceives it, in order to predict how the other will respond. In other words, communication is not a one-way process. It is a circular process in which the participants take turns at being communicator and receiver: A (communicator) talks to B (receiver), and B (communicator) talks to A (receiver). Figure 11–5 illustrates communication as interaction.

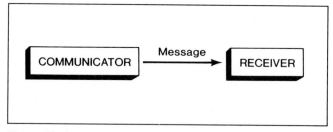

Figure 11–4

A linear model of communication (communication as an act).

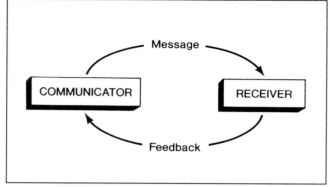

Figure 11–5
A circular model of communication (communication as an interaction).

Clearly, the model is not as reductionistic as the previous model. However, it still oversimplifies human communication, because it treats it as a series of causes and effects, stimuli and responses.

Communication As a Transaction

Mutual Influence between Communicators

In a transaction, the participants are both communicators. No one is labeled either as communicator or receiver. Communication is viewed as a process of simultaneous mutual influence rather than as a turn-taking event.

In a transactional perspective, participants are who they are in relationship to the other person with whom they are communicating. For example, in each dyadic communication event there are at least *six* persons involved: A's A, A's B, A's impression of the way B sees A, B's B, B's A, and B's impression of the way A sees B. Therefore, in addition to the content message, a relationship message also exists. Suppose A passes B in the corridor, and A says "Hi, how are you." B answers, "Just fine, thanks," moving down the corridor and away from A as quickly as possible. B's behavior is a comment on the relationship between A and B. Their subsequent communication will be affected by how A perceives B's response. If A thinks B walked away because B wanted to get home before the thunderstorm that was predicted, A is likely to respond one way to B the next time they meet. If A believes B is angry with A, A is likely to respond quite differently at the next encounter. The symbolic interactionist model described below helps explain what takes place between A and B.

A Symbolic Interactionist Model of Communication

A symbolic interactionist model is based on a transactional perspective. It views human communication on the social, interpersonal level and accounts for the whole persons involved in the process. The participants are products of their social system and integral parts of it. In the communication, some events take place *within* the participants (they are intrapersonal), and some take place *between* the participants (they are interpersonal).

A model constructed by Hulett (1966, p 14) according to symbolic interactionist principles, and adapted for this text, is shown in Figure 11–6. It shows five phases in each person's communication sequence: input, covert rehearsal, message generation, environmental event, and goal response.

The phase of *input* is one in which the person is motivated through some stimulus, either external or internal, toward some goal that requires engaging in a social relationship with another. Let us say that Jeff is attracted to Sarah and would like to get to know her better.

In the *covert rehearsal* phase, the person moves to make sense of the input received and develops and organizes a message *before* generating it. Figure 11–7 represents the symbolic interactionist model of the covert rehearsal. The individual first scans the information about self and others (Jeff enjoys theater and remembers hearing Sarah tell a friend that she'd really like to see the new musical comedy in town) and then rehearses, within his or her own head, possible actions to take (role playing) and possible reactions of the other (role taking). Successive readings of the map of the social structure and the resulting refinements give the person the opportunity to organize the eventual message as closely as possible to that desired. (Jeff thinks of four different ways to approach Sarah.) This process is represented by the intrapersonal feedback loop.

The covert rehearsal phase is really the core of the communication process. In it, Jeff decides what to say, how to say it, and even whether to send the message to Sarah at all.

Message generation, the third phase, is one in which the instrumental act of giving a message is performed. (Jeff asks Sarah to the theater.) A message generated by one person serves as the input or the stimulus for another person. (Sarah thinks about Jeff's invitation, decides whether she wants to go to the theater with him, and considers what response to make to Jeff.) Once the second person has completed his or her covert rehearsal and generates a message, this message becomes an *environmental event* for the first person. In our example, the environmental event is the fourth stage in the sequence of Jeff, whose *goal response* serves as another environmental event for Sarah, and so on.

A second, or interpersonal, feedback loop connects the person's environmental event phase to the covert rehearsal stage. It allows the person an opportunity to determine whether he or she has made an error in the approach to the other and to make appropriate corrections by repeating

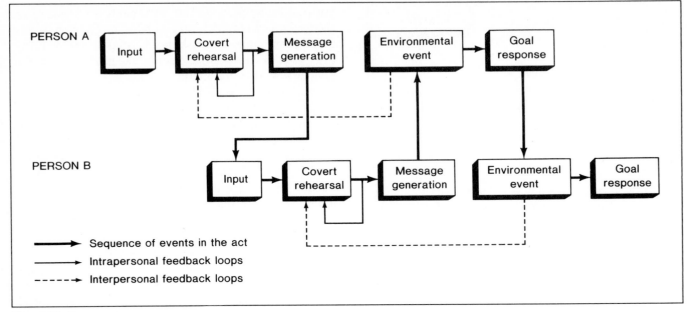

Figure 11–6
Symbolic interactionist model of communication.
Source: Adapted from Hulett JE Jr: A symbolic interactionist model of human communication. AV
Communication Review *1966;14:14.*

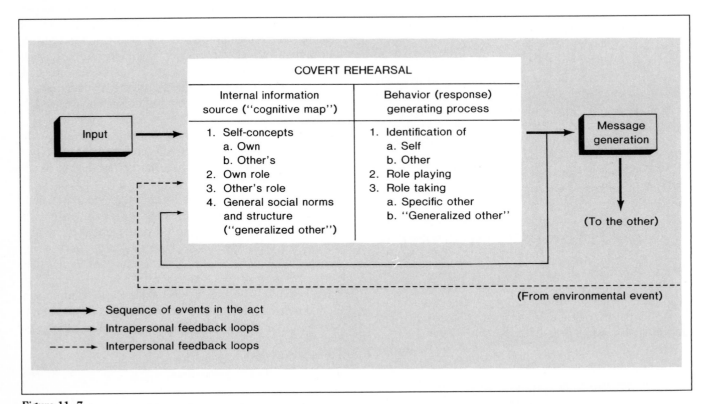

Figure 11–7
Symbolic interactionist model of the covert rehearsal phrase.
Source: Adapted from Hulett JE Jr: A symbolic interactionist model of human communication. AV
Communication Review *1966;14:18.*

the covert rehearsal and devising an altered message. (Jeff carefully considers Sarah's response. He listens to what she says and watches her behavior toward him. If her response is less than enthusiastic, he will try to determine what went wrong and how it can be corrected.)

In summary, the symbolic interactionist view of communication includes the following concepts:

- People run through a series of internal trials in the process of organizing a message.
- People select and transmit the message that will, in their view, have the highest probability of success.
- Success depends on the accuracy and completeness of the cognitive map of the environment and the accuracy and efficiency of the intrapersonal and interpersonal feedback loops.
- Communication is a dynamic (ever-changing) process that is unrepeatable and irreversible.
- Communication is complex.
- The meaning of messages is not transferred, it is mutually negotiated.

Communication is, at the very least, a very complicated process.

MODES OF COMMUNICATION

The Spoken Word

Verbal language, the ability to utter the spoken word, makes people human and distinguishes them from other animals. Yet problems arise as humans discover that words mean different things to different people. That is, *words* do not "mean" something, *people* do.

If communication between nurse and client is to be mutually negotiated, the nurse at least must understand the four concepts discussed next.

Denotation and Connotation

A *denotative meaning* is one that is in general use by most persons who share a common language. A *connotative meaning* usually arises from a person's personal experience. While all Americans are likely to share the same general denotative meaning of the word *pig*, the word may have completely different connotations for a farmer, a butcher, a consumer of meat, a person of the Moslem faith, an orthodox Jew, a college student, a prisoner, and a police officer. These positive and negative connotative meanings can arouse powerful emotions.

Private and Shared Meanings

In order for communication to take place, meaning must be shared. What happens when meaning is not shared is illustrated in a bewildering conversation between Alice and Humpty Dumpty:

> ". . . There's glory for you!"
> "I don't know what you mean by 'glory.' " Alice said.
> Humpty Dumpty smiled contemptuously. "Of course you don't—till I tell you. I meant 'there's a nice knock-down argument for you!' "
> "But 'glory' doesn't mean 'a nice knock-down argument,' " Alice objected.
> "When I use a word," Humpty Dumpty said, in rather a scornful tone, "it means just what I choose it to mean—neither more nor less."
>
> (Carroll 1965, p 93)

By assigning meanings to a word without agreement, Humpty Dumpty essentially created a private language.

Private meanings can be used to communicate with others only when the parties agree about what the word means. The private meaning then becomes a shared meaning. It is common for families, two friends, or members of larger social groups (military personnel, drug users, adolescents, etc.) to use language in highly personal and private ways. Problems arise when assumptions are made that persons outside of the group share these meanings.

People labeled schizophrenic may use language in an idiosyncratic way or may use a private, unshared language referred to as **neologisms**. Such people are unaware that this use of language is not shared with others. They expect to be understood and may become upset when they are not.

A young man who was hospitalized on a psychiatric unit complained to other clients and staff that he had been *odenated,* and he became increasingly frustrated and anxious when it became apparent that he wasn't being understood. With some help he was able to explain that he was upset about having been moved to a private room. The room was, he said, so dark and dingy that it looked like a cave. Animals live in caves that are called *dens.* In his view he had been o-*den*-ated—put in a cave.

In trying to make private meanings shared, the nurse should make an effort to reach mutual understanding of the client's message. It is insufficient, and quite possibly inaccurate, to attach meaning based solely on the nurse's (or the client's) interpretation of an event, a word or phrase, or a nonverbal gesture.

Nonverbal Messages

Most researchers agree that nonverbal communication channels carry more social meaning than verbal channels. Nonverbal cues help us judge the reliability of verbal messages more readily, especially in the presence of a mixed message (inconsistency between the verbal and nonverbal components).

There is a wide variety in nonverbal channels—facial expressions; hand gestures; body movements; use of space; pitch, rate, and volume of the voice; touch; body aromas; and so on. The following categories will be considered here: kinesic behavior (body movement), paralanguage (voice quality and nonlanguage sounds), proxemics (use of personal and social space), touch, and use of cultural artifacts (such as clothing and cosmetics).

Kinesics

The study of body movement as a form of nonverbal communication is called **kinesics**. Facial expressions, gestures, and eye movements are the most commonly used categories.

Facial expressions are the single most important source of nonverbal communication. They generally communicate emotions. The silent film comedians—blank-faced Buster Keaton and comic, endearing Charlie Chaplin—and the great mime Marcel Marceau communicate not only isolated acts but complete sequences of behavior with kinesics alone.

An infinite range of body movements and gestures provide clues about persons and about how they feel toward others. Hand gestures can communicate anxiety, indifference, and impatience, among other things. Foot shuffling and fidgeting may express the desire to escape. Body position gives cues about how open a person is to another person, or how interesting and attractive one person is to another. People tend to position their bodies according to their feelings about the person with whom they are communicating.

Eye contact is another very important cue in communicating. For example, proper sidewalk behavior among Americans is for passers-by to look at each other until they are about eight feet apart. At this distance, both parties look downward or away so they will not appear to be staring. Erving Goffman (1963, p 84) refers to this phenome-

non as a "dimming of our lights." Michael Argyle (1967, pp 105–116) points out several of the unstated rules about eye contact.

- Interaction is invited by staring at another person on the other side of a room. If the other person returns the gaze, the invitation to interact has been accepted. Averting the eyes signals a rejection of the looker's request.
- A looker's frank gaze is widely interpreted as positive regard.
- Greater mutual eye contact occurs among friends.
- Persons who seek eye contact while speaking are usually perceived as believable and earnest.
- If the usual short, intermittent gazes during a conversation are replaced by gazes of longer duration, the person looked at is likely to believe that the person gazing considers the relationship between the two persons as more important than the content of the conversation.

Paralanguage

Paralinguistics or **paralanguage** refers to something beyond or in addition to language itself. The two principal components are *voice quality,* such as pitch and range, and *nonlanguage vocalizations,* such as sobbing, laughing, or grunting—noises without linguistic structure.

Vocal cues can differentiate emotions. Who hasn't heard the injunction: "Don't speak to me in that tone of voice!" Sometimes vocal cues are used to make inferences about personality traits. For example, persons who increase the loudness, pitch, timbre (overtones), and rate of their speech are often thought to be active and dynamic. Those who use greater intonation and volume and are fluent are thought to be persuasive. Status cues in speech are based on a combination of word choice, pronunciation, grammatical structure, speech fluency, and articulation, among other features.

Proxemics

Proxemics is the study of space relationships maintained by persons in social interaction. It includes the dimensions of *territoriality* (fixed and permanent territory that is somehow marked off and defended from intrusion) and *personal space* (a portable territory surrounding the self that others are expected not to invade).

Knowing something about proxemics is useful, for example, in planning the physical space in which communication is to occur. Furniture can be arranged to increase or decrease interpersonal distance. Nurses should be especially sensitive to the constraints imposed on communication by physical objects. Nurses can use proxemics to decipher verbal communication by paying attention to how others use interpersonal space.

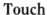
Touch

Touching behaviors, because they tend to personalize communication, are extremely important in emotional situations. In American society, the use of touch is governed by strong social norms. Who, when, why, and where people touch are all controlled by unwritten guidelines.

Most of the taboos against touching seem to stem from the sexual implications of touching behavior. However, although touching is a physical act, it may or may not be sexual in nature. A realization of the importance of touch and an understanding that touching is not necessarily a sexual behavior may make this channel of communication available to more people. It is equally important to be sensitive to the other person's disposition toward touching, so as not to alienate another by infringing on the person's right not to be touched.

Cultural Artifacts

Artifacts are items in contact with interacting persons that may act as nonverbal stimuli: clothes, cosmetics, perfume, deodorants, jewelry, eyeglasses, wigs and hairpieces, beards and mustaches, and so on.

Think about what information is communicated through artifacts such as a full-length mink coat, hair that has been dyed purple, a gold band on the third finger of the left hand, a military uniform, or a Phi Beta Kappa key.

Relationships between Verbal and Nonverbal Systems

The verbal and nonverbal elements of human communication are inextricably linked. Six different ways in which verbal and nonverbal systems interrelate are discussed below.

Repeating

A nonverbal cue may say the same thing as a verbal cue but in a different way. The deep-sea fisherman who tells verbally how big the sailfish that he caught was may also extend both hands to indicate its length. The gesture serves to repeat the idea.

Contradicting

Nonverbal behavior may also contradict verbal behavior. Consider the woman who meets a college roommate she hasn't seen for quite some time. She says, "You haven't changed a bit," but her tone of voice and facial expression convey sarcasm. When verbal and nonverbal cues contradict one another, it is usually safer to put more faith in the nonverbal cues.

Complementing

Nonverbal messages that add to or modify verbal messages are said to be complementary. When a man says he is a "little" irritated about being kept waiting, his tone of voice and body actions may indicate a more profound anger.

Accenting

Certain nonverbal cues accent or emphasize verbal cues. A woman shrugs her shoulders when she says she doesn't really care which movie she and her companion see. A master of ceremonies holds up his hand when he asks for quiet. These gestures and body movements emphasize the words.

Relating and Regulating

Cues that tell people when to start talking or when to stop talking are usually nonverbal. A woman who keeps opening and closing her mouth briefly while others are talking is indicating that she wants a turn too.

Substituting

Sometimes nonverbal cues are used in place of words. A wave from a friend at a distance says "hello." Applause at the end of a play tells the actors that they have pleased the audience.

COMMUNICATION IN HUMANISTIC PSYCHIATRIC NURSING

Ruesch's Theory of Therapeutic Communication

A theory of therapeutic communication has been developed by the psychiatrist Jurgen Ruesch (1961). In his view, communication includes all the processes by which one human being influences another human being. Ruesch's theory applies to the humanistic interactionist view because it takes into account the perceptions and interpretations that influence one person's view of the other. Further, Ruesch assumes that in order to survive, the individual must communicate successfully.

Basic Concepts

The basic concepts of this theory are:

- Communication occurs in four different settings—intrapersonal, interpersonal, group, and societal.

- The ability to receive, evaluate, and transmit messages is influenced by perception, evaluation (which involves memory, past experiences, and value systems), and transmission quality of messages (amount, speed, efficacy, and distinctiveness).

- Communication occurs in five systems of codification:

  1. Somatic language—statements mediated through the autonomic nervous system

  2. Sign language—gestures

  3. Action language—movements as statements mediated primarily through the central nervous system

  4. Object language—intentional and nonintentional display of material things, such as clothing and jewelry, art objects, and footprints

  5. Digital language—verbal or discursive language, spoken words

- Messages achieve meaning when they are mutually validated or verified between the two parties. (In Ruesch's view, however, it is the psychiatric therapist's reality that verifies a message. The definition is not mutually agreed on by client and therapist.)

- Metacommunicative messages (messages about the message) contain instructions on interpretation of messages by both sender and receiver on the levels of denotation and connotation.

- Correction through feedback is basic to adaptive, healthy behavior and successful communication.

Growth and Development in Communication

According to Ruesch, communication is one of the hardest human functions to master. It takes a long time to learn because it occurs in a series of steps, each built from the previous one. Effective communication requires decades of continuous practice. It is believed that interference hampers development and leaves an indelible mark.

Characteristics of Successful and Disturbed Communication

The four formal criteria for successful communication are efficiency, appropriateness, flexibility, and feedback. When these criteria are not met, communication is disturbed.

Efficiency

Simplicity, clarity, and timing are all components of efficient messages. Psychiatric nurses and other mental health professionals may find themselves using complex and scientific words or professional mental health jargon to convey messages. Obscure or clumsy language and introduction of irrelevant or useless information may also prevent others from understanding a message.

Clear messages have a sense of order or structure and reduce ambiguity by narrowing the number of possible interpretations or meanings. Emphasizing the important ideas helps.

Proper timing also is important. It is best to give messages when the other person is able to "hear" them, when there are no intervening noises or inputs, and when the others person can interpret them without undue haste. Problems occur if the time interval between the messages of two people is either too short or too long.

Appropriateness

Messages are appropriate when they are relevant to the situation at hand and when there is mutual fit of overall patterns and constituent parts. Communication that does not fit the circumstance, is irrelevant, or is misconstrued is inappropriate.

Communication can also be inappropriate in amount. Since every individual has both high and low tolerance levels for stimulation, a person's ability to cope with ideas, make decisions, and act is affected by the amount and rate of sensory input received. Exceeding a tolerance level is called overload. A person who is overloaded by too many messages or by messages too closely spaced cannot handle incoming messages. Underload occurs when delay or lack of information interferes with the person's ability to comprehend the message of another. The infants in foundling homes that John Bowlby (1951) studied were subjected to underload both verbally and emotionally.

The tangential reply is another example of inappropriateness. A tangential reply to a statement disregards the content of the message and is directed toward either an incidental aspect of the initial statement, the type of language used, the emotions of the sender, or another facet of the same topic.

People cannot always be sure how a message will be received, because each person with whom they communicate is unique and changing. Since they cannot expect constancy from others, people need to be flexible. In communication, lack of flexibility manifests itself as either exaggerated control or exaggerated permissiveness. Both extremes increase the likelihood of frustrating, ungratifying, or disturbed communication.

It is occasionally difficult to maintain flexibility when it requires a person to desert or temporarily lay aside a carefully planned goal. To be flexible, a person must have the ability to set new priorities and to move to meet immediate goals. People who practice humanistic psychiatric nursing work to achieve flexibility in their relationships with clients and colleagues.

Feedback

Feedback is the process by which performance is checked and malfunctions corrected. It performs a regulatory function in the communication process. Feedback enables people to decide which messages have been understood as intended. It requires the cooperation of two persons—one to give it, and one to receive it.

Under certain circumstances of disturbed communication, feedback either fails to function or functions poorly. When messages do not get through or are distorted, appropriate replies cannot be obtained and corrective feedback does not occur. If content elicits anxiety, fear, shame, or any of several other strong emotions, feedback is likely to be hampered. Feedback is discussed in greater depth later in this chapter.

The Theory of Pragmatics of Human Communication

Another theory of human communication was developed by Watzlawick, Beavin, and Jackson (1967), based on the assumption that communication is synonymous with interaction. These authors maintain that, in the presence of another, all behavior is communicative. This theory is concerned with the pragmatics, or the behavioral effects, of human interaction. Here, the term *pragmatics* refers to the interpersonal relation between communicators. What makes this theory particularly useful for this book is its conception of human communication as a reciprocal process.

Some Axioms of the Theory

According to this theory, one cannot *not* communicate. Message value is found in both activity and inactivity, verbalizations and silences. This communication occurs on two levels. The *content level* of a communication is the report aspect, in which information is conveyed. The *relationship level* is communication about a communication, a *metacommunication,* which says something about the relationship between the participants.

RESEARCH NOTE

Citation

Hurley PM: Communication variables and voice analysis of marital conflict stress. Nurs Res 1983;32;164–169.

Study Problem/Purpose

This study was based on the idea that the ability of the marital dyad to resolve power conflicts in a mutually satisfying way is one factor that distinguishes functional from dysfunctional families. The purpose of this study was to determine whether communication variables such as pauses, laughter, interruptions, and questions are inversely related to marital conflict stress.

Methods

The sample for this study consisted of sixty-eight middle-class couples married for five years or less. Subjects were asked to read and discuss eighteen vignettes that portray common marital disagreements (The Inventory of Marital Conflicts, intended to stimulate conflict between spouses). The couples' discussions of each vignette were tape recorded, and their physiologic responses during the discussions were measured using the Psychological Stress Evaluator (PSE), an instrument that measures changes in voice under stress by registering fluctuations in the microtremors of the muscles of the voice mechanism.

Findings

The data did not support the study hypothesis that pauses, laughter, interruptions, and questions are inversely related to marital conflict stress. However, the communication variables appeared to be significantly correlated, suggesting (a) that in functional marital dyads these variables constitute a pattern of speed and (b) that the presence or absence of this pattern may have value in family system assessment.

Implications

The presence or absence of pauses, laughter, interruptions, and questions in the communication of marital couples may have value in family system assessment. Becoming better able to identify characteristics common to functional and dysfunctional families will enhance the nurse's ability to tailor interventions to couples and their families.

All interchanges can be viewed as either **symmetrical** (based on equality) or **complementary** (based on difference). In symmetrical relationships, the partners usually mirror each other's behavior, thus minimizing difference. Complementary relationships, in contrast, are characterized by the maximization of difference.

Disturbances in Human Communication

Communication can be disturbed when a person attempts *not* to communicate. In this framework, the basic dilemma in schizophrenia is considered the schizophrenic person's attempt not to communicate. However, since it is impossible not to communicate, the person is faced with the need to deny that he or she is communicating while denying that this denial is a communication.

Another disturbance occurs when a person communicates in a way that invalidates the messages sent to or received from the other person. Such communications, called *disqualifications,* include a wide range of behavior: self-contradictions, inconsistencies, subject switches, incomplete sentences, misunderstandings, obscurities in style, literal interpretations of metaphors, and metaphorical interpretations of literal statements.

A person may communicate in a way that confirms, rejects, or disconfirms the other person's view of self. Confirmation of one person's self-view by another is thought to be the greatest single factor ensuring mental development and stability. Rejection of the other's definition of self essentially conveys this message: "You're wrong." Disconfirmation, by contrast, conveys this message: "You don't exist." Disconfirmation questions the other's authenticity. Disconfirmation leads to alienation and has been found to occur with some regularity in interactions between persons labeled schizophrenic and the members of their families.

Although all relationships are necessarily either symmetrical or complementary, *runaways* (exaggerations to the point of disturbance) may occur in either of the patterns. For example, the danger of competitiveness is ever present in symmetrical relationships. Symmetrical interactions that lose their stability may enter a spiral in which each individual attempts to be just a little bit "more equal" than the other. Runaways are seen in quarrels between people or wars between nations, behaviors that are relatively open. Rejection of the other's self is generally observed when a symmetrical relationship breaks down.

Breakdowns in complementary relationships, however, are generally characterized by disconfirmations of the other. For this reason, they are usually viewed as more serious.

Eric Berne's (1960) **transactional analysis** is a model of communication analysis proposing that a person may display the self from different psychologic positions. Transactional analysis (TA) is a method of therapy as well as a method of communication analysis. Transactional analysis theory is appropriate to this chapter because it is concerned with the changes in a person's posture, verbalization, voice, attitude, and feeling. Transactional analysis is both quick and easily understood. It is useful in brief contacts with clients or colleagues when there is little time to establish a rewarding relationship. Nurses can use TA concepts in understanding their own behavior as well.

Structural Analysis

Each person has three main sources of behavior, or ego states—the Parent, the Adult, and the Child. The **Child** is manifested through archaic modes of communication and relationship as well as by childlike behavior similar to that of an actual child less than seven years old. Giggling, coyness, naïveté, charm, boisterousness, and whining are characteristics of the Child ego state. So are "I want"; "gosh"; "golly"; "me"; "mine"; "I dunno."

By the time children become adults they learn that the spontaneous and free expression of feelings in their natural state, the Natural Child ego state, must be adapted to meet the demands and expectations of parents and the culture in which they live. Their adaptive behavior results in the Adapted Child ego state, which has two common manifestations: compliance with parents or other authority figures or rebellion and refusal to follow orders. Most people's Child falls somewhere between the two extremes.

Objective appraisal of reality and the capacity to process data are the domain of the **Adult.** The Adult is manifested in accomplishments beyond those of children, such as accurate analysis of complex realities and realistic manipulation of concepts. Perceptive skill, data processing, sociability, and communicativeness are attributed to the Adult. So are "it appears"; "I think"; "why"; "what"; "where"; "when"; "how."

The **Parent** incorporates the feelings and behaviors learned from parents or authority figures. A Parent ego state can be identified when the person's behavior includes the language, intonations, attitudes, postures, and mannerisms of one or both parents. All-wise, all-knowing, benevolent, prim, critical, or righteous attitudes are some examples. So are "if I were you"; "how many times have I told you"; "poor dear"; "disgusting"; "now what"; "do it this way." The Nurturing Parent ego state cuddles, protects, and cares for, while the Critical Parent ego state corrects or condemns.

Berne postulated that an individual exhibits a Parent or an Adult or a Child ego state, and that shifts can occur from one ego state to another. A nursing student, new to an in-patient unit of a community mental health center, reported her ego state switches in the following situation.

When I walked into the TV room to pick up the pen that I had left there, I saw a man pacing the floor; he was angrily muttering a string of obscenities. (Adult ego state) I don't mind telling you that I was plenty scared. I was afraid that he might hurt me. (Child ego state) I told myself that I should do something about reducing his anxiety and distress. (Parent ego state) But, I felt so helpless and dumb. (Child ego state) Then I decided that I really didn't know how to handle this situation and remembered something you said in class—that it's OK to ask for help—and I didn't feel scared or dumb any more. This has really turned into a good learning situation for me. (Adult ego state)

In TA theory, structural analysis includes the determination of which ego state controls the executive power at a particular time. Spontaneity, charm, creativity, and enjoyment reside in the Child. The Adult not only is necessary for survival in dealing effectively with the outside world but also regulates and mediates the activities of the Parent and the Child. The Parent enables an individual to act effectively as a parent and makes many automatic responses that free the Adult from routine, trivial decisions. Each of the three ego states serves vital functions.

Ego States in Wellness/Illness

Most of the time, persons who are ill or hospitalized are in a Child ego state. In the general hospital setting, one may hear of the "problem client" who is demanding, extremely dependent, or refusing to follow a prescribed medical regimen. That problem client is using his or her Adapted Child in unfamiliar or frightening situations. The overly cheerful, overly friendly, or overly helpful client is less often identified as a problem but is also using the Adapted Child ego state to cope with the stress of hospitalization. The Child ego state may also be seen in the client who is confused, disoriented, screaming, enraged, striking out at others, or withholding information because of fear of retaliation.

Sick people in their Parent ego state may be critical of hospital staff or suspicious of their intentions. Sometimes they nurture and protect other clients or even the staff. A person in a Parent ego state is critical of himself for being ill or for being unable to cope with the stresses of life. Such people berate themselves for bothering staff, family, and friends. Some persons even hallucinate figures

or voices that criticize them for their real or imagined transgressions.

The client who is able to decide when to sleep or rest, whether to visit with friends or family, and what steps to take to decrease stress contributes to wellness in the Adult ego state. People in this ego state are able to accept the temporary limitations imposed by illness or stress, to care for themselves within the confines of the limitations imposed, and to seek partnership in decisions about the directions of health care.

Obviously, the sick person in the Adult ego state is in the best possible situation under the circumstances. However, other ego states can also contribute to both illness and wellness. For example, persons in the Nurturing Parent ego state can allow themselves to be taken care of by others and may give themselves "permission" to be sick or to feel depressed. A quicker return to a state of well-being is more likely for these people than for those who are constantly berating themselves for being ill or succumbing to life's stresses. The Child ego state is helpful in achieving wellness, because it allows for the natural expression of feelings that can then be handled. These ego states in a wellness/illness relationship are illustrated in Figure 11–8.

Transactional Analysis

While structural analysis is directed more toward the analysis of the individual's personality, transactional analysis is broadened to focus on what occurs between two or more persons.

Complementary Transactions

Complementary transactions are those in which the transactional stimulus and the transactional response occur on identical ego levels. Transactions are complementary when a message sent to an ego state is responded to from that ego state. Complementary transactions can go on uninterrupted until one or the other of the participants changes ego state. Most of the time, productive communication occurs in complementary transactions, because the participants behave according to the perceived and predicted ego states of one another. However, continuing, or locked, complementary transactions—as from Critical Parent to Adapted Child—result in uninterrupted but uncomfortable, nonfacilitative communication. The Parent-Child transaction of nurse and client in Figure 11–9 limits the client's growth. It encourages dependency and discourages responsibility.

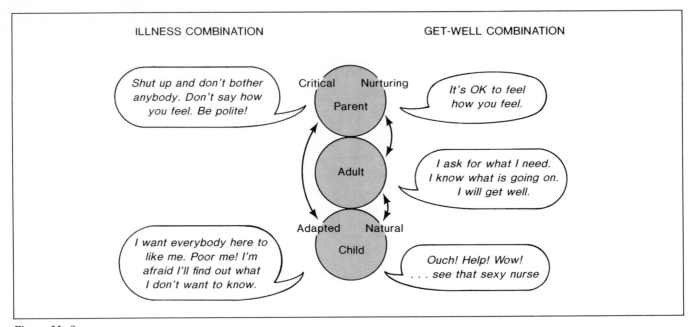

Figure 11–8
The wellness/illness relationship.
Source: Elder J: Transactional Analysis in Health Care. *Addison-Wesley, 1978, p 19.*

Crossed Transactions

Crossed transactions result from changes in ego states that terminate the complementary relationship. A crossed transaction occurs if the client tries to relate to the nurse on an Adult to Adult level but the nurse responds on a Parent to Child level, such as in Figure 11–10. In instances of crossed transactions, communication is usually not smooth or satisfactory and is soon terminated. When complementary transactions have become locked (and interpersonally uncomfortable), it may be useful to cross ego states to move the communication forward. For example, if a nurse is aware of having behaved like a Critical Parent to a client who responds from the Adapted Child state, the nurse can alter communication behavior by switching to Adult ego state. The client will probably follow this lead, leaving client and nurse better able to work together effectively.

Ulterior Transactions and Games

Ulterior transactions are complex phenomena that occur on two levels—social (the surface, or overt one) and psychologic (the hidden, or covert one). **Games** are series of ulterior transactions with concealed motivations. Figure 11–11 shows an ulterior transaction as it occurs in the "Why don't you . . . Yes, but . . ." game. In this game, one

person presents a problem to another person or to members of a group, who offer solutions to the problem. All solutions, however, are rejected by the first player. The gimmick, or concealed motivation, is that, although this is supposedly an Adult request for information, the psychologic level is Child to Parent. The Child always wins, as the supposedly "wise" Parents are confounded and confused one by one.

Since the interactions are complementary at both social and psychologic levels, the game can be played indefinitely until the Parents give up or a more sophisticated person who recognizes what is happening breaks it up. "Why don't you . . . Yes, but . . ." can also take place in one-to-one relationships, particularly when it is a behavioral pattern of the client and the nurse is unaware of the psychologic level. The following interaction is a typical of such a client-nurse situation. The client has been discussing her view of the problems she has experienced since her mother-in-law moved in.

Nurse: The problem seems to be that you give in to your mother-in-law all the time. How about trying to talk to her?

Client: If I talk to her, it won't do any good. She'll just continue to act the same way.

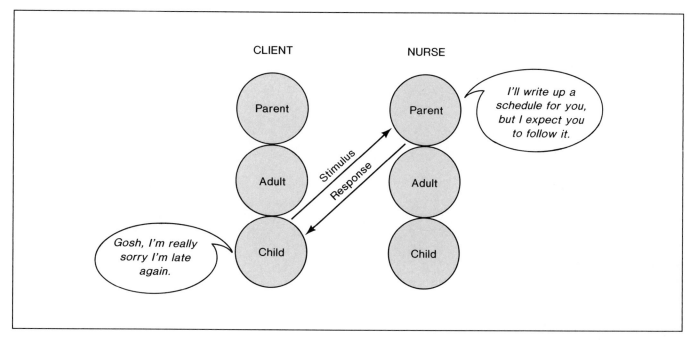

Figure 11–9
Complementary transaction.

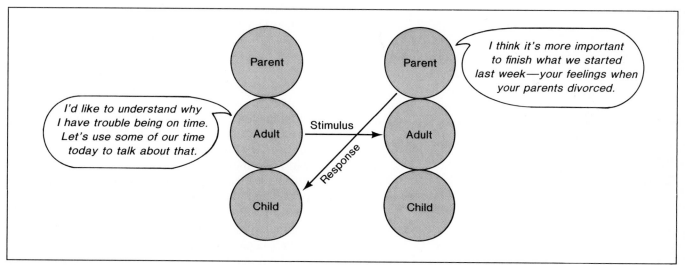

Figure 11–10
Crossed transactions.

Nurse: How about getting your husband to help?

Client: I'd ask him to talk to her, but he says that it's my house, so I should give the orders and there should be no problem.

Nurse: You mentioned that she has another son. Do you think that you could talk to him and work out some plan to have her live by herself?

Client: No. We haven't talked to him in a long while, and anyway she doesn't have enough money to live on her own.

Nurse: How about a nursing home?

Client: We can't afford to send her to a nursing home.

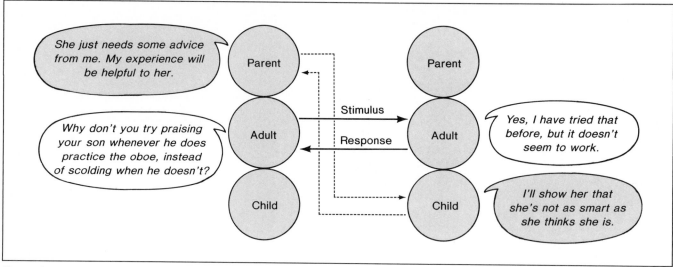

Figure 11–11
Ulterior transaction in "Why don't you . . . Yes, but . . ." game.

Apparently giving up on finding a solution for the client's "mother-in-law problem," the nurse begins to work on other tangentially related household problems.

Nurse: You said that taking care of six children is quite a job. Do you think you could hire a baby-sitter to watch them in the afternoon?

Client: There's nobody in the neighborhood who I can get to sit. Either they're too young or they don't want to.

Nurse: Do you think you could hire someone to clean the house one day a week?

Client: Well, we could afford it, but my husband says that I don't need anyone to help me and that I could do everything by myself.

The game was broken up, and the participants moved on to more productive communication after the nurse assessed her own and her client's ego states. She was able to do so by moving into her Adult ego state, figuring out the dynamics and her contributions to them, and then changing her responses.

Analysis of Ego States in Clinical Practice

The transactional analysis of ego states helps nurses gain a better understanding of the processes and behaviors that take place in an interpersonal relationship. It is a way of viewing the self-in-process—i.e., the self changing in response to interaction with another self—a way of understanding a person in the process of becoming. It can be used to understand how ego states of participants—nurses as well as clients—help or hinder communication efforts.

Neurolinguistic Programming Theory

Neurolinguistic programming (NLP) is a communication model developed in the early 1970s by Richard Bandler and John Grinder (1975, 1976). The model is derived from theory in linguistics, neurophysiology, psychology, cybernetics, and psychiatry. Relatively new to nursing, NLP first appeared in the nursing literature in 1983 (Brockopp 1983, Knowles 1983).

Bandler and Grinder first observed psychotherapists who were known as expert communicators to discover what made them so effective as therapists. They concluded that people take in, or *access* information in three sensory modalities—the auditory, the visual, or the kinesthetic modalities. Further, each person prefers one mode over the others. Sounds may facilitate communication with one person, while touch or sight may be more effective with another person. In addition, people also *process* information, or make sense out of it, according to the representational system (the NLP phrase for sensory modality) through which they receive it.

They also found that the expert communicators they observed were able to adapt themselves to match the client's representational system and to imitate the client in a natural and respectful way. Bandler and Grinder theorized that by tuning in to and then using the other person's preferred sensory mode, one could greatly enhance the ability to establish rapport. The most effective communicators, according to NLP theory, are those who can use all three modalities and can easily move from one representational system to another.

Determining the Representational System

To determine whether a client's representational system is auditory, visual, or kinesthetic, one identifies the client's:

- Preferred predicates (verbs, adjectives, adverbs that tell something about the subject)
- Eye-accessing cues
- Gross hand movements
- Breathing pattern
- Speech pattern and voice tones

Preferred Predicates

The predicates in Table 11–1 are categorized according to the auditory, visual, and kinesthetic modes. Observing the client to see which is the preferred set of predicates is a necessary first step before attempting to link words with nonverbal behavior.

Eye-Accessing Cues

Eye-accessing cues correlate with an individual's thinking process. Persons who are visualizing generally have their eyes turned upward or defocused straight ahead. The eyes usually move from side to side when someone is processing auditory information. When a person engages in intrapersonal communication, the eyes are usually focused down in the direction of the nondominant hand. A person in the kinesthetic mode looks down toward the dominant hand when experiencing sensations or emotions.

Gross Hand Movements

Gross hand movements also give clues to the client's sensory mode. People have a tendency to point toward or touch the sense organ that matches their current sensory mode. The person in a visual mode often points toward the eye, and the person in an auditory mode often points toward or touches the ear.

Breathing Pattern

Assessing the breathing pattern helps the observer understand the client's representational model. Shallow, thoracic breathing is often associated with visual accessing. Even breathing or prolonged expiration is associated with

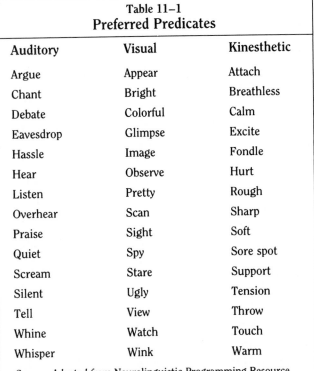

Table 11–1
Preferred Predicates

Auditory	Visual	Kinesthetic
Argue	Appear	Attach
Chant	Bright	Breathless
Debate	Colorful	Calm
Eavesdrop	Glimpse	Excite
Hassle	Image	Fondle
Hear	Observe	Hurt
Listen	Pretty	Rough
Overhear	Scan	Sharp
Praise	Sight	Soft
Quiet	Spy	Sore spot
Scream	Stare	Support
Silent	Ugly	Tension
Tell	View	Throw
Whine	Watch	Touch
Whisper	Wink	Warm

Source: Adapted from Neurolinguistic Programming Resource Manual. *American Society for Training and Development, 1986.*

auditory accessing, and deep abdominal breathing is associated with kinesthetic accessing.

Speech Pattern and Voice Tones

Visual accessing often correlates with quick bursts of words that are high pitched, strained, or nasal. Auditory accessing is often associated with a clear, midrange voice tone or with a rhythmic tempo and clearly enunciated words. Kinesthetic accessing is associated with a slow voice and a low volume or deep tone, or with a breathy tone and long pauses.

Therapeutic Use of NLP

Using NLP theory in psychiatric nursing practice gives us yet another way to empathize with clients by "trying on" their style. People tend to be less anxious with the familiar. Nurses who mirror the client's sensory mode are likely to be experienced as more comfortable and safer to be with, conditions that facilitate rapport.

Knowles (1983) suggests that nurses can use **mirroring** to help the client follow the nurse's lead. For example, with an anxious client, the nurse might being by mirroring the behaviors that indicate the client's anxiety and then shift into a more relaxed posture and less anxious behaviors. According to Knowles, the nurse can lead the client from a more anxious state to a less anxious state by employing the NLP principles discussed here.

An important benefit of the NLP approach is that it allows nurses to assess the client's style and preferred sensory mode and to communicate more effectively with clients by using both verbal and nonverbal communication in the client's preferred mode. Brockopp gives these examples of how the same nursing intervention can be expressed with different predicates, depending on the client's preferred mode (Brockopp 1983, p 1014):

- Visual—"Yes, I can *see* that you are much better. You *look* good, your eyes are *clear,* your *appearance* has certainly changed."

- Auditory—"Yes, I can *hear* from the *sound* of your *voice* that you are better. *Talking* with you today is quite different from yesterday."

- Kinesthetic—"Yes, you do seem to be *feeling* much better today, you're *holding* your head up, and your *grasp* is certainly *firmer* than yesterday."

By expanding their abilities to communicate with clients in all three modes, nurses can become more effective communicators. This section is a brief introduction to some of the basic uses of NLP; see the references at the end of this chapter for further information.

FACILITATIVE COMMUNICATION

Facilitative communication aims at initiating, building, and maintaining fulfilling and trusting relationships with other people. Communicating ideas and feelings with clarity, efficiency, and appropriateness helps a person be interpersonally effective. In reading the rest of this chapter, try to relate the therapeutic communication principles and practices discussed earlier to these ideas about facilitative communication.

Social Superficiality versus Facilitative Intimacy

Most relationships between people begin at the level of social superficiality. In a client-nurse relationship, we try to develop facilitative intimacy, which differs from social

intimacy. For example, the interdependence that characterizes the social relationship is greatly reduced. In social relationships participants may "tell their stories" to one another. In facilitative relationships that have therapeutic goals, only the client is engaged in storytelling with the nurse. The process is specifically focused. Clients not only explain themselves, the events of their lives, and the circumstances they face but also do so with a purpose in mind—understanding the circumstances through exploring them and moving to improve the circumstances of their lives.

The movement toward therapeutic intimacy may be difficult at first. For one thing, such intimacy violates certain social taboos. For example, at a cocktail party it may be socially incorrect to comment on a person's anxiety, stuttering, or facial tic. During facilitative and therapeutic communication, all messages, including these nonverbal ones, are heeded and may be discussed.

Therapeutic intimacy also requires that the participants move beyond social chitchat into meaningful areas of concern for the client. Therapeutic intimacy requires high involvement and commitment.

Essential Ingredients

Several interpersonal principles and practices are essential to the achievement of facilitative intimacy.

Responding with Empathy

Most theorists believe that empathy is the most important dimension in the helping process. Without a high level of empathic understanding, there is no real basis for helping. Empathy facilitates interpersonal exploration.

Responding with Respect

Responding with respect demonstrates that the nurse values the integrity of the client and has faith in the client's ability to solve his or her problems, given appropriate help. By encouraging the client to put forward possible plans of action, the nurse conveys respect for the client's ability to take charge of his or her destiny. On the other hand, giving advice conveys a directly opposite message.

Responding with Genuineness

Genuineness refers to the ability to be real or honest with another. To be effective, genuineness must be timed properly and based on a solid relationship. Honesty is not always the best policy, especially if it is brutal or if the client is not capable of dealing with it.

To the extent the client can experience the authenticity of the nurse, the client can risk greater genuineness and authenticity herself or himself. The nurse who is genuine is more likely to deal with and eventually help the client resolve real problems rather than just those that are safe or socially acceptable.

Responding with Immediacy

Responding with immediacy means responding to what is happening between the client and the nurse in the here-and-now. Because this dimension may involve the feelings of the client toward the nurse, it can be one of the most difficult to achieve. For example, the client may confront the nurse with overt or implied criticism of the nurse's role or competence. If the nurse responds in a defensive or evasive way, the relationship may be threatened. If the nurse is open, reasonable, and concerned, the relationship may be strengthened. However, if the nurse focuses attention on the relationship too early, the formation of an adequate base may be impaired.

Responding with Warmth

Warmth is so closely linked with empathy and respect that it is seldom communicated as an independent dimension. It is important, however, to note some additional points about the expression of warmth. Effusive, chatty, "buddy-buddy" behavior should not be confused with warmth. Warmth is most often conveyed in communications of respect and empathy.

The nurse should be aware of and accept the client's right to maintain distance. Warmth and intimacy cannot be forced. Initially high levels of warmth can be counterproductive for clients who have received little warmth from others in their lives or have been taken advantage of by others. Warmth alone is insufficient for building a relationship and solving problems.

Facilitative Communication Skills

To present a how-to manual or cookbook of communication skills goes against the thrust of this book. A set of communication skills employed rigidly as a sort of relationship "magic" is antihumanistic in many ways. Relationships, and the people in them, are unique and much too complex for the nurse to rely on a formula for facilitative communication. The following skills are therefore presented with many misgivings. It is important to remember that a holistic approach essentially precludes the rigid, inflexible application of communication techniques. Those presented here should be viewed as having the potential to

foster effective communication. They must be adapted individually for each human encounter.

Reflecting Context

Reflecting is repeating the client's verbal or nonverbal message for the client's benefit. In reflecting the *content* of the message, the nurse basically repeats the client's statement. This gives the client the opportunity to hear and mull over what he or she has said:

- "You believe things will be better soon."
- "You think it would be better to take a part-time job."

Content reflection is perhaps one of the most misused and overused methods in mental health counseling. It loses its effectiveness when used for lack of other choices.

Reflecting Feelings

Reflecting *feelings* consists of verbalizing what seems to be implied about feelings in the client's comment.

- "Sounds like you're really angry at your brother."
- "You're feeling uncomfortable about being discharged from the hospital."

In reflecting feelings, the nurse attempts to identify latent and connotative meanings that may either clarify or distort the content. Reflection is useful because it encourages the client to make additional clarifying comments.

Imparting Information

Imparting information is helping the client by supplying additional data. This therefore encourages further clarification based on new or additional input.

- "Group therapy will be held on Tuesday evening from 6:30 until 8:00."
- "I am a psychiatric nurse."

It is not constructive to withhold helpful or useful information from the client or to reply "What do you think?" to a straightforward information-seeking question. However, the nurse must be careful not to distort the giving of information into advice or use it to avoid an area of interpersonal difficulty. If the nurse gives personal social information, the conversation may move out of the realm of therapeutic intervention.

Clarifying

Clarifying is an attempt to understand the basic nature of a client's statement.

- "I'm confused about . . . Could you go over that again, please."
- "You say you're feeling anxious now. What's that like for you?"

Asking the client to give an example to clarify a meaning helps the nurse understand the client's intended message better. A person who describes a concrete incident is more likely to be able to see the connections between it and similar occurrences. Illustrations are very useful qualifiers.

Paraphrasing

In paraphrasing, the nurse assimilates and restates what she or he has heard the client communicating.

- "In other words, you're fed up with being treated like a child."
- "I hear you saying that when people compliment you, you feel embarrassed. If they knew the real you, they'd stay away."

Paraphrasing offers the opportunity to test the nurse's understanding of what the client is attempting to communicate. It is reflective in nature, in that it lets the client know how another person is understanding the message.

Checking Perceptions

The nurse who shares how she or he perceives and hears the client is engaged in the process of checking perceptions. After sharing perceptions of the client's behaviors, thoughts, and feelings, the nurse asks the client to verify the perception.

- "Let me know if this is how you see it too."
- "I get the feeling that you're uncomfortable when we're silent. Does that seem to fit?"

A perception check is used to make sure that the nurse understands the client. An effective perception check con-

veys the message "I want to understand. . . ." It allows the other person the opportunity to correct inaccurate perceptions. It also allows the nurse to avoid actions based on false assumptions about the client.

Questioning

Questioning is a very direct way of speaking with clients. But when used to excess, questioning controls the nature and range of the client's responses. Questions can be useful when the nurse is seeking specific information. When the nurse's intent is to engage the client in meaningful dialogue, however, questions should be limited.

When the nurse is using questions, it is best to make them open-ended rather than closed. An *open-ended question* focuses the topic but allows freedom of response.

- "How were you feeling when your mother said that to you?"
- "What's your opinion about . . . ?"

The *closed question* limits the client's choice of responses, generally to "yes" or "no" ("Were you feeling angry when your mother said that?"). Closed questions limit therapeutic exploration.

"Why" questions usually have the same effect. They often are impossible to answer and rarely lead to a clearer understanding of the situation. However, "who," "what," "when," and "how" questions may be helpful when used judiciously.

Structuring

Structuring is an attempt to create order or evolve guidelines. The nurse helps the client to become aware of problems and the order in which they might be dealt with.

- "You've mentioned that you want to improve your relationships with your wife, your sister, and your boss. Let's put them in order of priority."
- "No, I won't be giving you advice, but we can discuss the possible solutions together."

Structuring is particularly useful when clients introduce a number of concerns in a brief period of time with little idea of which to begin work on. In addition to structuring content, nurses use structuring to delimit the parameters of the nurse-client relationship and identify how the nurse will participate with the client in the problem-solving process.

Pinpointing

Pinpointing calls attention to certain kinds of statements and relationships. For example, the nurse may point to inconsistencies among statements or to similarities and differences in the points of view, feelings, or actions of two or more persons, or between what one says and what one does.

- "So, you and your wife don't agree about how many children you want."
- "You say you're sad, but you're smiling."

Linking

In **linking**, the nurse responds to the client in a way that ties together two events, experiences, feelings, or persons. Linking may be used to connect past experiences with current behaviors. Another example is linking the tension between two persons with current life stress.

- "You felt depressed after the birth of both your children."
- "So the arguments didn't really begin until after you got your promotion."

Giving Feedback

Feedback helps others become aware of how their behavior affects us and how we perceive their actions. Responding with feedback can be therapeutic self-disclosure. It allows the nurse to offer clients constructive information to help them become more aware of their impact on others. Total self-disclosure by the nurse is inappropriate in the nurse-client relationship. It would place a burden of interdependence on the client and limit the time and energy available to work on the client's concerns. Reciprocal self-disclosure is more appropriate in friend and colleague relationships.

- "When you wring your hands I feel anxious."
- "Sometimes when you turn your head away from me I think you're angry."

It is important to give feedback in a way that will not be threatening to the client and increase defensiveness. The more defensive the client, the less likely it is that she or he will hear and understand the feedback. Some characteristics of helpful, nonthreatening feedback are listed in Table 11–2.

Confronting

Productive change often results from constructive confrontations. **Confronting** is a deliberate invitation to another to examine some aspect of personal behavior in which there is a discrepancy between what the person says and what he or she does. Confrontation requires careful attention to nonverbal communication and the discrepancies between nonverbal and verbal messages.

Confrontations may be informational or interpretive, and they may be directed toward both the resources and the limitations of the client. An **informational confrontation** describes the visible behavior of another person. An **interpretive confrontation** expresses thoughts and feelings about the other's behavior and includes drawing inferences about the meaning of the behavior.

- "You characterize yourself as 'the dummy in the family,' yet none of your brothers or sisters made the honor roll like you did."
- "Ever since Sally and Joe criticized the way you conducted the meeting, you haven't spoken to them. It looks like you're feeling angry."

Six skills to be incorporated in constructive confrontations are:

1. Use of personal statements with the words *I, my,* and *me*
2. Use of relationship statements in which the nurse expresses what she or he thinks or feels about the client in the interaction
3. Use of behavior descriptions (statements describing the visible behavior of the client)
4. Use of description of personal feelings, specifying the feeling by name
5. Use of responses aimed at understanding, such as paraphrasing and perception checking
6. Use of constructive feedback skills (see Table 11–2)

Summarizing

Summarizing is a way of highlighting the main ideas that have been discussed. It reviews for the client and the nurse what the main themes of the conversation were. Summarizing is also useful in focusing the client's thinking and aiding conscious learning.

- "The last time we were together you were concerned about. . . ."
- "You had three main concerns today. . . ."

This technique can be used appropriately at different times in the client-nurse interaction. For example, summarizing the previous interaction is useful in the first few minutes of the time the nurse and the client spend together. When summarizing occurs early, it helps the client recall the areas discussed and also provides the client with the opportunity to see how the nurse has synthesized the con-

Table 11–2
Characteristics of Helpful, Nonthreatening Feedback

Strategy	Rationale	Strategy	Rationale
Focus feedback on behavior rather than on client.	Refer to what client actually does rather than how nurse imagines client to be.	Focus feedback on exploration of alternatives rather than answers or solutions.	Focusing on variety of alternatives for accomplishing a particular goal prevents premature acceptance of answers or solutions that may not be appropriate.
Focus feedback on observations rather than inferences.	Refer to what nurse actually sees or hears client do; inferences refer to conclusions or assumptions nurse makes about client.	Focus feedback on its value to client rather than on catharsis it provides nurse.	Feedback should serve needs of client, not needs of nurse.
Focus feedback on description rather than judgment.	Report what occurred rather than evaluating it in terms of good or bad, right or wrong.	Limit feedback to amount of information client is able to use rather than amount nurse has available to give.	Overloading will decrease effectiveness of feedback.
Focus feedback on "more or less" rather than "either/or" descriptions of behavior.	"More or less" descriptions stress quantity rather than quality (which may be value laden).	Limit feedback to appropriate time and place.	Excellent feedback presented at an inappropriate time may be ineffective or harmful.
Focus feedback on here-and-now behavior rather than there-and-then behavior.	The most meaningful feedback is given as soon as it is appropriate to do so.	Focus feedback on what is said rather than why it is said.	Focusing on why things are said or done moves away from observations and toward motive or intent (which can only be assumed, unless verified).
Focus feedback on sharing of information and ideas rather than advice.	Sharing ideas and information helps client make decisions about own well-being; giving advice takes away client's freedom to be self-determining.		

tent of a previous session. Summarizing is useful because it keeps the participants directed toward a goal.

The most frequent error with this technique is injudicious use. A nurse may rush to summarize despite other, more pressing and immediate concerns of the client. In this instance, summarizing is likely to meet the nurse's need for structure while disregarding the client's here-and-now concerns.

Processing

Processing is the most complex and sophisticated technique used by the nurse. Process comments are those that direct attention to the interpersonal dynamics of the nurse-client experience. These dynamics are illustrated in the content, feelings, and behavior expressed.

- "It seems that important things that need to be taken care of come up in the last five minutes we have together in our session."

- "Today is the first day our session has started out with silence. Last week it seemed there wouldn't be enough time."

Processing is most useful when therapeutic intimacy has been achieved.

Ineffective Communication Styles

Three clinical situations are presented below to give examples of some ways of responding to clients that are generally not helpful and may even be harmful (adapted from

Gazda 1973, pp 62–65). They illustrate a few of the common response styles that are not facilitative. An example of a helpful response is given at the end of each of the situations.

Situation 1

Client: "They wouldn't let me join their pinochle game!"

Responses that are not helpful:

Detective: Who wouldn't?

Detectives are eager to track down the facts of the case. They grill the client about the details of what happened and respond to this factual content instead of giving attention to feelings. Detectives control the flow of the conversation, and this often puts the client on the defensive.

Magician: It's time to eat dinner, so it doesn't matter now, does it?

Magicians try to make the problem disappear by telling the client it isn't there. This illusion is not lasting. Denying the existence of a problem denies the validity of the client's own experience and perception.

Manager: Would you help me get everyone together for the picnic?

Managers believe that if the client can be kept too busy to think about the problem, there will be no problem. Doing this has the effect of saying that the task assigned to the client by the manager is more important than the client's problem. An effective nurse communicates awareness of the magnitude of any particular problem to the client.

Judge: Remember yesterday when you didn't play fair? Of course they wouldn't want to play with you today!

Judges give rational explanations to show that the client's past actions have caused the present situation—that the client is the guilty party. Although such responses may be accurate, they are rarely helpful, because they are premature—they are being given before the client is ready to accept and use them.

Responses that are helpful:

"It hurts to be turned down!" or "That hurt!"

Situation 2

Client: "You asked me to chair the community meeting next week, but I can't do that. Please get somebody else. Anybody would be better than me."

Responses that are not helpful:

Drill sergeant: Later tonight figure out what each person should do. Give them assignments and make sure they work on it some each day. Get organized now and it will come out fine.

Drill sergeants give orders and expect them to be obeyed. Because they know just what the client should do, they see no need to give explanations, listen to the client's feelings, or explain their commands to the client.

Guru: You won't find out what you can do if you don't try new things. It's better to try and fail than not to try at all.

Gurus dispense proverbs and clichés on every occasion, as though they were the sole possessors of the accumulated wisdom of the ages. Unfortunately, their words are too impersonal and general to apply to any individual's situation with force or accuracy, and often the sayings are too trite to be noticed at all.

Magician: You don't *really* mean that do you?

Responses that are helpful:

"You're sort of afraid to accept this responsibility. It looks like more than you can handle."

Situation 3

Client: "I don't know what to do with my kids! They won't listen!"

Responses that are not helpful:

Detective: What's causing the problem?

Florist: With all your ability? I can't believe that! Why, you're such a good parent.

Florists are uncomfortable talking about anything unpleasant, so they gush flowery phrases to keep the client's problem at a safe distance. Florists mistakenly think that the way to be helpful is to hide the problem under bouquets of optimism.

Judge: You know, you got off to a bad start with your kids. You are going to have a hard time changing them.

Sign painter: You're a born pessimist!

Sign painters think a problem can be solved by being named. They have an unlimited inventory of labels to affix to persons and their problems.

Drill sergeant: First get them all tested psychologically. Then write up some behavior contracts. Keep your kids busy with simple projects. Then . . .

Guru: Things always look the worst before they get better.

Prophet: If you don't get some results with them pretty soon there will be trouble!

Prophets know and predict exactly what is going to happen. By declaring the forecast, prophets relieve themselves of responsibility. They sit back to let the prophecy come true.

Magician: You're imagining things. They're good kids, and you know it. They're a lot better than you give them credit for!"

Responses that are helpful:

"I guess it gets you down when you do all you know how to do and then don't get results."

Chapter Highlights

- Communication is an ongoing, dynamic, and ever-changing series of events, each of which affects all others; it is the mechanism by which people establish, maintain, and improve their human contacts.

- Meaning cannot be transferred from one human being to another but must be mutually negotiated between persons. Words and gestures do not "mean" something, people do.

- Communication takes place on intrapersonal, interpersonal, and public levels and includes nonverbal messages that are interrelated with the spoken word.

- Relationships with clients are initiated, built, and maintained through the vehicle of interpersonal communication.

- To help clients deal with problems, nurses need to be aware of how their own perceptions, values, and culture influence the way they process information about the world.

- The symbolic interactionist view of human communication posits that (a) after a series of internal trials people reflect and transmit the message they believe has the highest chance of success; (b) success depends upon the accuracy and completeness of the person's "cognitive map" of the environment and of the intrapersonal and interpersonal feedback loops; (c) communication is a complex, dynamic process in which the meaning of messages is mutually negotiated, not merely transferred.

- Nonverbal communication channels that help us judge the reliability of a message include facial expressions; hand gestures; body movements; use of space, voice, touch; and body aroma.

- In the development of the client-nurse relationship, a major focus is the development of facilitative intimacy.

- Facilitative intimacy is enhanced when nurses respond with empathy, respect, genuineness, immediacy, and warmth.

- Relationships are unique and too complex for a set of rigid, inflexible communication techniques to be consistent with humanistic psychiatric nursing practice.

- Communication skills that may foster facilitative communication include reflecting content, reflecting feelings, imparting information, clarifying, paraphrasing, checking perceptions, questioning, structuring, pinpointing, linking, giving feedback, confronting, summarizing, and processing.

References

American Society for Training and Development: *Neurolinguistic Programming Resource Manual.* The Society, 1986.

Argyle M: *The Psychology of Interpersonal Behavior.* Penguin, 1967.

Bandler R, Grinder J: *The Structure of Magic.* Science and Behavior Books, 1975, vol 1.

Bandler R, Grinder J: *The Structure of Magic.* Science and Behavior Books, 1976, vol 2.

Bashor P: A nursing communication assessment guide. *Rehab Nurs* 1983;8(1):20+.

Berne E: *Games People Play.* Grove Press, 1964.

Berne E: *Transactional Analysis in Psychotherapy.* Grove Press, 1960.

Black K: *Short-Term Counseling.* Addison-Wesley, 1983.

Bowlby J: *Maternal Care and Mental Health,* ed. 2, World Health Organization, 1951.

Bradley E, Biedermann H: Bandler and Grinder's neurolinguistic programming: Its historical context and contribution. *Psychother* 1985;22(1):59–62.

Bradley J, Edinberg M: *Communication in the Nursing Context.* Appleton-Century-Crofts, 1982.

Brockopp D: What is NLP? *Am J Nurs* 1983;83:1012–1014.

Carroll L: *Through the Looking Glass and What Alice Found There.* Random House, 1965.

Collins M: *Communication in Health Care: The Human Connection in the Life Cycle,* ed 2. Mosby, 1983.

Davis AJ: *Listening and Responding.* Mosby, 1984.

Duldt B, Griffin K, Patton B: *Interpersonal Communication in Nursing.* F.A. Davis, 1984.

Elder J: *Transactional Analysis in Health Care.* Addison-Wesley, 1978.

Faules DP, Alexander DC: *Communication and Social Behavior: A Symbolic Interaction Perspective.* Addison-Wesley, 1978.

Fritz PA et al: *Interpersonal Communication in Nursing: An Interactionist Approach.* Appleton-Century-Crofts, 1984.

Gazda GM: *Human Relations Development.* Allyn and Bacon, 1973.

Gazda G, Childers W, Walters R: *Interpersonal Communication: A Handbook for Health Professionals.* Aspen, 1982.

Goffman E: *Behavior in Public Places.* Free Press, 1963.

Hardin SB, Halaris AL: Nonverbal communication of patients and high- and low-empathy nurses. *J Psychosoc Nurs* 1983;21:15–20.

Heidt P: Effect of therapeutic touch on anxiety level of hospitalized patients. *Nurs Res* 1981;30:32–37.

Heineken J: Disconfirmation in dysfunctional communication. *Nurs Res* 1982;31:4–9.

Heineken J: Treating the disconfirmed psychiatric client. *J Psychosoc Nurs* 1983;21(1):21–25.

Hulett JE Jr: A symbolic interactionist model of human communication. *A V Communication Review* 1966;14:5–33.

Kalisch B: What is empathy? *Am J Nurs* 1983;83:1548–1552.

Kasch C: Interpersonal competence and communication in the delivery of nursing care. *Adv Nurs Sci* 1984;6(2):71–88.

Knapp M: *Nonverbal Communication in Human Interaction,* ed. 2, Holt, Rinehart & Winston, 1978.

Knowles RD: Building rapport: Through neuro-linguistic programming. *Am J Nurs* 1983;83:1011–1014.

Lasagna L: Three Christs. *Psychol Today* 1983;17(3):64–66.

Leininger M (ed): *Caring: An Essential Human Need.* Slack, 1981.

Leonard R: Speak for yourself. *Nurs 85* 1985;15:30–31.

Long L, Prophet P: *Understanding/Responding: A Communication Manual for Nurses.* Wadsworth, 1981.

Mehrabian A: *Silent Messages: Implicit Communication of Emotion and Attitude,* ed 2. Wadsworth, 1981.

Nelson M, Paluck R: Territorial markings, self concept, and mental status of the institutionalized elderly. *Gerontol* 1980;20(1):96–104.

Pelletier LR: Interpersonal communications task group. *J Psychosoc Nurs* 1983;21(9):33–36.

Ricci M: An experiment with personal space invasion in the nurse-patient relationship and its effect of anxiety. *Issues Ment Health Nurs* 1981;3(3):203–218.

Ruesch J: *Disturbed Communication.* W.W. Norton, 1957.

Ruesch J: *Therapeutic Communication.* W.W. Norton, 1961.

Ruesch J, Bateson G: *Communication: The Social Matrix of Psychiatry.* W. W. Norton, 1968.

Sommer R: *Personal Space: The Behavioral Basis of Design.* Prentice-Hall, 1969.

Stewart CJ, Cash WB: *Interviewing Principles and Practices,* ed 4. William C. Brown, 1985.

Taylor S: Rights and responsibilities: Nurse-patient relationships. *Image* 1985;17(1):9–14.

Watzlawick, P, Beavin, J, Jackson, D: *The Pragmatics of Human Communication.* New York: W. W. Norton, 1967.

TWELVE

Assessment

Holly Skodol Wilson
Carol Ren Kneisl

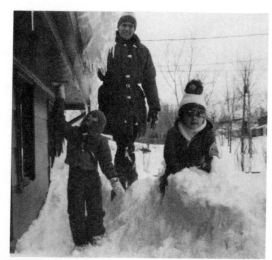

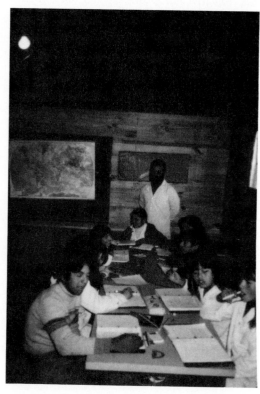

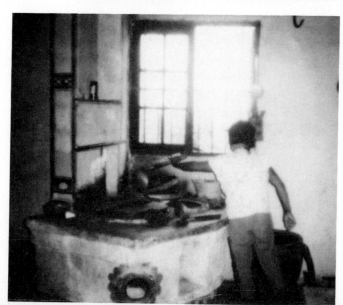

After reading this chapter, students should be able to

- Describe the processes of psychiatric history taking, mental status examination, neurologic assessment, and physiologic and psychologic testing

- Discuss the DSM-IIIR's multiaxial system for making a psychiatric diagnosis

- Evaluate the DSM-IIIR's congruence with psychiatric nursing diagnoses

- Describe the process of individual psychosocial assessment

- Discuss the differences between processes of source-oriented and problem-oriented systems of recording

- Identify methods for recording verbatim nurse-client interactions

- Comprehend the organization and function of the Interaction Process Analysis (IPA)

Cross References

Other topics relevant to this content are: Assessing clients with mood disorders, Chapter 18; Assessing clients with organic mental disorders, Chapter 15; Assessing clients with psychoactive substance use disorders, Chapter 16; Assessing clients with schizophrenic disorders, Chapter 17; Family characteristics and dynamics, Chapter 33; Group process, Chapter 13; Nursing process and nursing theory, Chapter 4; Small group assessment, Chapter 30; and Suicide assessment, Chapter 29.

Imagine an end to nuclear weapons—a time when they rust in peace

Key Terms

algorithms
Bender-Gestalt test
Diagnostic and Statistical Manual of Mental Disorders third edition revised (DSM-IIIR)
Global Assessment of Function (GAF) scale
intelligence tests
interaction process analysis (IPA)
mental disorder
mental status examination
Minnesota Multiphasic Personality Inventory (MMPI)
multiaxial system
neurologic assessment
Nursing Adaptation Evaluation (NSGAE)
projective (personality) tests
psychiatric audit
psychiatric history
Rorschach test
Stanford-Binet Test
Thematic Apperception Test (TAT)
Wechsler scales

COLLECTING, ASSESSING, AND RECORDING CLIENT DATA

The systematic scientific approach known among nurses as the *nursing process* has evolved as the cornerstone of clinical practice. The nursing process begins with assessment designed to collect and analyze objective and subjective data about the clients with whom nurses work. The primary sources for client data in most instances are the clients themselves. Other sources, such as psychologic tests, nurses' notes, and physicians' orders, are secondary data sources that can enlarge, clarify, and substantiate data obtained directly from the client.

The Psychiatric Examination

Systems of collection and assessment vary among mental health agencies. The psychiatric examination consists of two parts: psychiatric history and mental status exam. It is most often done during initial or early interactions with a client. It is often seen as a function of the psychiatrist, because a major goal of the examination is making a psychiatric diagnosis, although in some agencies it has become the responsibility of the intake worker. The traditional psychiatric examination is discussed in this chapter because it is still used in settings in which psychiatric nurses work and is considered the counterpart of the physical examination and history.

In less traditional settings, the psychiatric history and the mental status examination have given way to the *psychosocial assessment*—an assessment of the social and psychologic data gathered from interaction with the client. The primary goals of a psychosocial assessment are a psychiatric diagnosis and an assessment of the client's difficulties in living. A psychosocial assessment form is given in Appendix A.

Initial Contact Form

The following initial contact form (Figure 12–1) is filled in before the history and mental status exam are done. It provides basic demographic and problem information at the time the client requests service or is referred by another person or agency. This information should provide the clinician with enough data to make some early key decisions:

- How urgent is the situation (Box 12–1)?
- Who is to be assigned responsibility for proceeding with the next step?
- What type of response is indicated as "the next step"?

This form is used chiefly by the member of the mental health team designated to handle all incoming calls and requests for service during a specified period of time.

The Psychiatric History

Data Sources

The information gathered during psychiatric history-taking can be obtained from multiple sources. Family, friends, police, mental health personnel, and others may contribute data to the psychiatric history. Not all data are provided by the client. When the sources are varied, the psychiatric history focuses on the perceptions of others, how they see the client and the circumstances of the client's life. It is necessary to include the perceptions of the client if the data are to be meaningful from that person's viewpoint. The sources of the psychiatric history and their relationship to the client should always be clearly indicated. Information given by these sources should be reviewed and understood in terms of their relationship.

Categories of Data

The psychiatric history generally includes the following information:

- *Complaint*—the main reason the client is having a psychiatric examination. The client may have personally initiated the psychiatric examination, or it may

have been initiated by others (courts, hospital staff, family, referral from school or industry). The "chief complaint" should be recorded verbatim and indicated as such with quotation marks in the write-up ("I just don't want to live any longer" or "My drug use has become unmanageable").

- *Present symptoms*—the nature of the onset and the development of symptoms. These data are usually traced from the present to the last period of adaptive functioning.
- *Previous hospitalizations and mental health treatment.*
- *Family history*—generally, whether any family members have ever sought or received mental health treatment.
- *Personal history*—the person's birth and development; past and recent illnesses; schooling and educational problems; occupation; sexual development, interests, and practices; marital history; use of alcohol, drugs, and tobacco; and religious practices.
- *Personality*—the client's relationships with others, moods, feelings, interests, and leisure-time activities.

The main purpose of history-taking is to gather information, although it is often effective in establishing rapport with a client. Rapport is more likely to occur if the client's story is allowed to unfold naturally and the interviewer avoids an interrogative approach.

Box 12–1
CRISIS RATING: HOW URGENT IS YOUR NEED FOR HELP?

- *Very urgent:* Service request requires an immediate response within minutes; e.g., crisis outreach; medical emergency—requiring an ambulance to be called (overdoses); severe drug reaction; police contacted if situation involves extreme danger or weapons.
- *Urgent:* Response requires rapid but not necessarily immediate response, within a few hours. Example: low/moderate risk of suicide, mild drug reaction.
- *Somewhat urgent:* Response should be made within a day (approximately 24 hours). Example: planning conference in which key persons are not available until the following evening.
- *Slightly urgent:* A response is required within a few days. Example: client's funding runs out within a week and needs public assistance.
- *Not urgent:* When a situation has existed for a long time and does not warrant immediate intervention, a week or two is unlikely to cause any significant difference. Example: child with a learning disability, certain types of marital counseling.

INITIAL CONTACT SHEET

Today's Date _12-4-88_
Time _9_ AM
            PM

Walk-in _____
Phone ✓ _____
Outreach _____
Written _____

ID # _____
SS # _123-45-6789_
Welfare /
Medicaid # _____

SERVICE REQUESTED FOR
Client's NAME _Mary_ _Jane_ _Smith_
First   Middle   Last

Permanent ✓ _____
Temporary _____

Address _1 Success Drive_ _West Egg, N.Y. 10101_ _____
        Street   City / Town   Zip   County

Catchment Area _____

Phone # _666-1234_ Means of Transportation _Auto_ _____
Directions to home _____
(if outreach)
Sex __ Male _____ Date of Birth _1-14-43_ Age _45 yrs_ _____
Female ✓

SERVICE REQUESTED BY
☐ AGENCY   Name _____   Phone # _____
☐ OTHER   Address _____   Time(s) seen by
☑ SELF   If Agency-Contact Person _____   the agency _____

PRESENTING SITUATION / PROBLEM - What made you decide to seek help today?
(use other side if needed)

Feeling depressed about relationship with husband and life in general. Difficulty sleeping, low energy level, "I need to get help."

Have you talked with anyone about this?   Yes _____ Who? _____
Address _____   No ✓
                                            Date of last contact _____   Phone # _____
Are you taking ANY medication now?   Yes ✓   What? 1. _Valium_
(If more than 3 begin list on MH-2) No _____   2. _Dalamane_
                                                           3. _Aspirin_

CRISIS RATING How urgent is your need for help?
☐ Immediate (within minutes)
☐ Within a few hours
☐ Within 24 hours
☐ Within a few days
☑ Within a week or two

Comments
Intelligent housewife with marital problems — would probably benefit from counseling and perhaps couples group later

DISPOSITION (Check all that apply)
☐ Crisis
☐ Medical Emergency
☐ Assessment (specify) _____
☐ Discharge Planning
☐ Expediting / Advocacy
☐ Other (explain) _____
☑ Referral made to _Individual Counseling_ _____ Confirmed—Yes ✓ No _____ Date _12-14-88_
Date of Next Contact _12-15-88_ _____ Assigned to _____
Date of Assignment _____ Request taken by _____

MH-1

Figure 12–1
Initial contact sheet.
Source: Reproduced by permission of the Erie County Department of Mental Health; Mental Health Services, Erie County, Corporation IV, South East Corporation V, and Lakeshore Corporation VI.

The Mental Status Examination*

The mental status examination is usually a standardized procedure in agencies that use it. Its primary purpose is to gather more objective data to be used in determining etiology, diagnosis, prognosis, and treatment. The sections of the mental status examination that deal with *sensorium* and *intellect* are particularly important in sorting out the existence of organic brain disease. The purpose of this examination differs from that of psychiatric history in that it is used to identify the person's *present* mental status.

The mental status examiner generally seeks the following categories of information, not necessarily in the sequence presented here.

1. *General behavior, appearance, and attitude*—a complete and accurate description of the client's physical characteristics, apparent age, manner of dress, use of cosmetics, personal hygiene, and responses to the examiner. Postures, gait, gestures, facial expression, and mannerisms are included in the description. The examiner also notes the client's general activity level.

A 35-year-old white male, dressed in torn, disheveled jeans. Presented a blank facial expression, slouched posture, shuffling gait, generally low activity level, and sullen behavior.

Other descriptors that may be used include "frank," "friendly," "irritable," "dramatic," "evasive," "indifferent," and so forth. Details should be sufficient to identify and characterize the client.

2. *Characteristics of talk*—the form, rather than the content, of the client's speech. The speech is described in terms of loudness, flow, speed, quantity, level of coherence, and logic. A sample of the client's conversation with the examiner may be included in quotation marks. The goal is to describe the quantity and quality of speech to discern difficulties in thought processes. The following patterns, if present, should be particularly noted.

   a. *Mutism*—no verbal response from the client despite indications that he or she is aware of the examiner's questions.

   b. *Circumstantiality*—cumbersome and convoluted detail volunteered by the client but unnecessary to answer the interviewer's questions.

   c. *Perseveration*—a pattern of repeating the same words or movements despite apparent efforts to make a new response.

   d. *Flight of ideas*—rapid, overly productive responses to questions that seem related only by chance associations between one sentence fragment and another. Associated with flight of ideas might be rhyming, clang associations, punning, and evidence of distractibility.

   e. *Blocking*—a pattern of sudden silence in the stream of conversation for no obvious reason but often thought to be associated with intrusion of delusional thoughts or hallucinations.

3. *Emotional state*—the person's pervasive or dominant mood or affective reaction. Both subjective and objective data are included. Subjective data are obtained through the use of nonleading questions such as: "How are you feeling?" If the client replies by using such general terms as "nervous," he or she should be asked to describe how the nervousness shows itself and its effect, since such words may mean different things to different individuals. Objectively, the examiner should observe facial expression, motor behavior, the presence of tears, flushing, sweating, tachycardia, tremors, respiratory irregularities, states of excitement, fear, and depression. Much valuable information may be obtained by noting the relationship between the client and the examiner. Attitudes of hostility, suspiciousness, or flirtatiousness, a desire for bodily contact, or outspoken criticisms should be noted.

The psychiatric client is apt to have a persistent emotional trend based on a particular emotional disorder, such as depression. If this is true, further inquiry should attempt to reveal the intensity and persistence of this reaction.

It is desirable to record a verbatim reply to questions concerning the client's mood. The relationship between mood and the content of thought is particularly significant. There may be a wide divergence between what clients say or do and their emotional state as expressed by attitudes or facial expressions.

Note whether intense emotional responses accompany discussion of specific topics. *Shallowness* or *flattening of the affect* is indicated by an insufficiently intense emotional display in association with ideas or situations that ordinarily would call for a more adequate response.

Dissociation or *disharmony* is often indicated by an inappropriate emotional response, such as smiling or silly behavior, when the attitude should be one of concern, anxiety, or sadness.

Evaluation of emotional reactions may be even more difficult because some clients may use *simulation* or play-acting. Clients who are trying to cover up a deep depression may feign cheerfulness and good spirits. The reverse may also be true.

The client's emotional reactions may be constant

*Reprinted with permission of Sandoz Pharmaceuticals, Division of Sandoz, Inc. From Small SM: *Outline for Psychiatric Examination,* 1980.

or may fluctuate during the examination. Try to specify the ease or readiness with which such changes occur in response to pleasant or unpleasant stimuli. Use such terms as the following to indicate intensity of response:

- Composed, complacent, frank, friendly, playful, teasing, silly, cheerful, boastful, elated, grandiose, ecstatic

- Tense, worried, anxious, pessimistic, sad, perplexed, bewildered, gloomy, depressed, frightened

- Aloof, superior, disdainful, distant, defensive, suspicious

- Irritable, resentful, hostile, sarcastic, angry, furious

- Indifferent, resigned, apathetic, dull, affectless

The relationship of affect to content should be noted in terms of the influence of content on affect and disharmony between affect and content or thought. Constancy and change in the emotional state should be noted.

4. *Content of thought: special preoccupations and experiences*—delusions, illusions, or hallucinations, depersonalizations, obsessions or compulsions, phobias, fantasies, and daydreams. (These terms are defined in the glossary.) These data may be elicited by asking the client questions, such as "Do you have any difficulties?" or "Have you been troubled or ill in any way?"

If the client has delusions of being the object of environmental attention, some of the following questions might reveal them: "Do people like you?" "Have you ever been watched or spied upon or singled out for special attention?" "Do others have it in for you?"

Delusions of *alien control* (passivity) are feelings of being controlled or guided by external forces. If these delusions are suspected, ask the client such questions as "Do you ever feel your thoughts or actions are under any outside influences or control?" "Are you able to influence others, to read their minds, or to put thoughts in their minds?"

Nihilistic delusions are those in which the client more or less completely denies reality and existence. The client states that nothing exists, or everything is lost. He or she may say such things as "I have no head, no stomach," "I cannot die," or "I will live to eternity."

Delusions of *self-deprecation* are often seen in connection with severe depressions. The client describes feelings of unworthiness, sinfulness, ugliness, or emitting obnoxious odors.

Delusions of *grandeur* are associated with elated states, such as great wealth, strength, power, sexual potency, or identification with a famous person or even God.

Somatic delusions are focused on having cancer, obstructed bowels, leprosy, or some horrible disease. These are to be distinguished from a preoccupation with normal, visceral, or peripheral sensations.

Hallucinations are false sensory impressions with no external basis in fact. Try to elicit the clearness of the projection to the outside world (e.g., whether the client hears voices from outside or inside his or her head, the clarity and distinctness of the perception, and the intensity). Be tactful in approaching the client for evidence of hallucinatory phenomena, unless he or she is obviously hallucinating.

Obsessions are insistent thoughts recognized as arising from the self usually regarded by the client as absurd and relatively meaningless, yet they persist despite endeavors to get rid of them.

Compulsions are repetitive acts performed through some inner need or drive and supposedly against the subject's wishes. Yet they produce feelings of tension and anxiety if omitted.

Fantasies and *daydreams* are preoccupations that are often difficult to elicit from the client. The difficulty may be due to a lack of understanding on the part of the client of what the examiner wants, but he or she is often ashamed to talk about them because of their content.

5. *Sensorium or orientation*—orientation in terms of time, place, person, and self to determine the presence of confusion or clouding of consciousness. One may introduce such questions by asking "Have you kept track of the time?" If so, "What is today's date?" If the client says he or she does not know, he or she should be asked to estimate approximately or to guess at an answer. Many clinicians begin the mental status exam with these questions since the validity and reliability of subsequent data require that the client be reasonably oriented.

6. *Memory*—the person's attention span and ability to retain or recall past experiences in both the recent and the remote past. If memory loss exists, the examiner should determine whether it is constant or variable and whether the loss is limited to a certain time period. The examiner should be alert to the client's *confabulations*—attempts to devise memories to take the place of those he or she cannot recall. It is useful to introduce questions relating to memory by some general statement such as "Has your memory been good?" or "Have you had difficulty remembering telephone numbers or appointments?"

a. *Recall of remote past experiences.* The person can be asked to review the important chronological facts of his or her life. The information given can be compared with information obtained from other sources during the history-taking.

b. *Recall of recent past experiences,* such as the events leading to the present seeking of treatment.

c. *Retention and recall of immediate impressions.* The examiner might ask the client to repeat a name, address, or name of a set of objects, e.g., car, coin, and telephone, immediately and again after three to five minutes, or to repeat three-digit numbers at a rate of one per second, or to repeat a complicated sentence.

  d. *General grasp and recall.* The person might be asked to read a story and then repeat the gist of it with as many details as possible. "The Cowboy Story" is an example suggested for this purpose in a concise guide for conducting a psychiatric examination developed by S. M. Small (1980).

The Cowboy Story

A cowboy from Arizona went to San Francisco with his dog, which he left at a friend's while he purchased a new suit of clothes. Dressed in the new suit, he went back to the dog, whistled to him, called him by name, and patted him. The dog would have nothing to do with him in his new hat and coat, but gave a mournful howl. Coaxing had no effect, so the cowboy went away and donned his old garments. Then the dog immediately showed his wild joy on seeing his master as he thought he ought to be.

7. *General intellectual level*—a nonstandardized evaluation of intelligence. The examiner looks for the person's ability to use factual knowledge in a comprehensive way.

  a. *General grasp of information.* The person may be asked to name the five largest cities of the United States, the last four presidents, or the governor of the state.

  b. *Ability to calculate.* Tests of simple multiplication and addition may be given. Another test consists of subtracting from one hundred by sevens until the person can go no further (serial sevens test).

  c. *Reasoning and judgment.* Clients are commonly asked what they might do with $10,000 if it were given to them. Examiners must be particularly careful to correct for their own biases and values in assessing each client's answer.

8. *Abstract thinking*—the distinctions between such abstractions as poverty and misery or idleness and laziness. It is common to ask the client to interpret simple fables or proverbs, e.g., "Don't cry over spilled milk."

9. *Insight evaluation*—whether the client recognizes the significance of the present situation, whether the client feels the need of treatment, and how the client explains the symptoms. Often it is helpful to ask the client for suggestions for his or her own treatment.

10. *Summary*—the important psychopathologic findings and a tentative diagnosis. Any pertinent facts from the medical history and/or physical examination should be added to the summary.

Table 12–1 differentiates some of the mental status examination findings in organic brain syndromes, psychosis, and mood disorders.

Physiologic Assessment

As the summary of the mental status examination and Table 12–1 suggest, nurses must carefully consider the possibility that a client's symptoms may have a physiologic, particularly neurologic, basis. In some reported instances, clients with brain tumors or bromide intoxication have been hospitalized on psychiatric units and treated exclusively for their seemingly psychiatric symptoms. Such a critical oversight obviously delays and seriously hampers appropriate treatment of an organic or neurologic problem. The value of careful screening for physiologic disorders cannot be overemphasized in the assessment of an individual client. In many community settings in which psychiatric nurses practice, these nurses are the only mental health care providers prepared to undertake a physiologic and neurologic assessment and interpret the results.

Objectives of Neurologic Assessment

1. Detection of underlying and perhaps unsuspected organic disease that may be responsible for psychiatric symptoms

2. Understanding of disease as a factor in the overall psychiatric disability

3. Appreciation of somatic symptoms that reflect primarily psychologic rather than organic problems

Physiologic History-Taking

Of several procedures that enlighten the nurse who is attempting to rule out organic causes of psychiatric symptoms, the client's history is certainly a major one. The nurse should inquire into two primary aspects of physiologic history: (a) facts about known physical diseases and dysfunction, and (b) information about specific physical complaints. Information about previous illnesses may provide essential clues. If the presenting symptoms include paranoid delusions and the client has a history of similar episodes, each of which responded to diverse forms of treatment and left no residual symptoms, there is a strong possibility of amphetamine- or other drug-related psychosis, and a drug screen laboratory test may be indicated. An occupational history may provide information about exposure to inorganic mercury that has led to symptoms of psychosis or exposure to lead that has produced an organic mental disorder.

Table 12–1
Differentiation of Mental Status Examination Findings

| | Organic Brain Syndrome | | Psychotic Disorders | | Mood Disorders |
	Delirium	Dementia	Manic Episode	Schizophrenic Disorder	Depressive Disorder
Appearance and behavior	Fluctuating impairment of consciousness, restlessness	May show deterioration of personal habits but state of consciousness not clouded	Hyperactive, elated, assertive, boisterous, with rapid emphatic speech; may become suddenly angry or argumentative	Variable	Dejected, slowed, slumped, troubled
Mood	Anxiety, fear, lability	Irritability, lability	Elation, sometimes anger and irritability	Blandness, impoverishment or inappropriateness of affect	Depression, hopelessness
Thought processes and perceptions					
Coherence and relevance	May be confused, incoherent	May become confused	Rapid association of ideas that may seem illogical	Often incoherent, disorganized	
Thought content	May have delusions		May have delusions and feelings of persecution	May have feelings of unreality, depersonalization, persecution, influence and reference; delusions that are bizarre and symbolic	May have delusions, often involving guilt, self-depreciation, somatic complaints
Perceptions	May have illusions, hallucinations		May have illusions, rarely hallucinations	May have hallucinations and illusions, often bizarre and symbolic	May have illusions, rarely hallucinations
Cognitive functions					
Orientation	May be disoriented	May be disoriented	Well-oriented	Usually but not always well-oriented	Well-oriented
Attention and concentration	Poor	Poor	Distractable		
Recent memory	Poor	Poor		Usually well-preserved but may be difficult	

continued

Table 12–1 (Continued)
Differentiation of Mental Status Examination Findings

| | Organic Brain Syndrome | | Psychotic Disorders | | Mood Disorders |
	Delirium	Dementia	Manic Episode	Schizophrenic Disorder	Depressive Disorder
				to test because of inattentiveness and indifference	
Remote memory	May become poor	May become poor		Usually well-preserved but may be difficult to test because of inattentiveness and indifference	
Information	Preserved until late	Preserved until late			
Vocabulary	Preserved until late	Preserved until late			
Abstract reasoning	Concrete	Concrete		Concrete, may be bizarre	
Judgment	Poor	Poor			
Perception and coordination	May be poor	May be poor			

Source: Adapted from Bates B: A Guide to Physical Examination. *ed 3. Lippincott, 1983, pp 312–313. Reprinted by permission of Lippincott/Harper & Row.*

The second emphasis in history-taking is eliciting information from the client about specific physical complaints. Again, it is crucial that the nurse be aware of symptoms in terms of not only assessing psychiatric conditions but also detecting physical diseases. Symptoms that are atypical of psychiatric disorders are particularly effective clues. For example, if a client with hallucinations and delusions also complains of a severe headache at the onset of the symptoms, the symptoms together suggest possible brain disease and call for careful and repeated neurologic assessment. History-taking should also include information about medications currently being taken. Digitalis intoxication may result in impairment. Reserpine may produce symptoms generally considered psychiatric in nature.

Observation

The nurse's powers of observation also yield important data bearing on the possible presence of organic disorders:

- An unsteady gait may suggest diffuse brain disease or alcohol or drug intoxication

- Asymmetry—dragging a leg or not swinging one arm—might be a sign of a focal brain lesion
- Although inattention to proper dress and hygiene is common in people with emotional disorders, it is also a hallmark of organic brain disease, particularly lapses such as mismatching socks or shoes
- Frequent, quick, purposeless movements are characteristic of anxiety, but they are equally characteristic of chorea or hyperthyroidism
- Tremors accompanied by anxiety may point to Parkinson's disease
- Recent weight loss, although often encountered in depression and schizophrenia, may be due to gastrointestinal disease, carcinomatosis, Addison's disease, and many other physical disorders

The nurse should observe the skin color, pupillary changes, alertness and responsiveness, and quality of speech and word production, keeping in mind the possibility of organic brain dysfunction, substance intoxication, or other diseases.

Neurologic Assessment

A careful **neurologic assessment** is mandatory for each client suspected of having organic brain dysfunction. Its goal is to discover signs pointing to circumscribed, focal cerebral dysfunction or diffuse, bilateral cerebral disease. A guide for evaluating the presence of signs of central nervous system disorders or "neurologic soft signs" is presented in Figure 12–2.

Authorities in mental health practice consistently remind clinicians of the need for thorough physiologic assessment of clients seen in psychiatric settings. The psychiatric literature abounds with stories of clients whose symptoms were initially considered exclusively psychiatric but ultimately were proved to be organic, especially neurologic. Assessment errors occurred not because there were no features to suggest organic disease but because such features were accorded too little weight or were misinterpreted by the evaluator.

Psychologic Testing

Clinical psychologists administer and interpret a wide variety of psychologic tests. There are two types of psychologic tests: (a) those concerned with intelligence, and (b) those concerned with personality. Both kinds are included in a comprehensive psychologic evaluation.

Intelligence Tests

Intelligence tests may be useful particularly in evaluating the presence and degree of mental retardation. Commonly used intelligence tests are the **Stanford-Binet Test**, the **Wechsler Adult Intelligence Scale**, the **Wechsler Intelligence Scale for Children**, the Gesell Developmental Schedules, and the Vineland Social Maturity Scale.

Personality Tests

Personality tests are also called **projective tests** because they evoke projection in the responses of the person being tested.

The Rorschach Test

Hermann Rorschach, a Swiss psychiatrist, developed the **Rorschach Test** in 1921. It consists of ten standardized inkblots in black and white or color on separate cards, displayed one by one, to which clients are asked to respond in terms of their associations, thoughts, and impressions. Since each card contains only inkblots, clients' responses are *projected,* that is, they come from within the clients

themselves. People may see persons, animals, insects, objects, anatomic parts, or other things. The examiner scores the response using a system of symbols in relation to the following:

- *Location.* Where on the blot area was the response seen?
- *Content.* What did the client see?
- *Determinant.* What characteristic of the blot prompted the response?
- *Form–level.* How closely did the response correspond to the contour of the blot area used?
- *Originality.* How common a response is it?

Interpretation is based on a complicated system of scoring symbols and analyzing content. The Rorschach is the most highly developed of all the projective tests used to evaluate the personality.

The Thematic Apperception Test (TAT)

The TAT also consists of a series of cards shown one by one. However, TAT cards are pictures of people in various emotional situations (see Figure 12–3). Clients are asked to describe what seems to be happening in the picture or to tell a story about it. The pictures themselves are quite ambiguous, so that what clients choose to say reveals aspects of their own emotional lives. The psychologist who interprets and scores the TAT looks for themes, threads, and patterns in the responses to the cards. Some adaptations of the TAT for use with children are available.

The Minnesota Multiphasic Personality Inventory (MMPI)

The MMPI is a complex and lengthy test consisting of 550 questions asked of the client. Scoring is done in relation to nine areas: preoccupation about body diseases; depression; hysteria; antisocial personality; masculine or feminine features; paranoid qualities; anxiety, phobias, and psychogenic fatigue states; schizophrenic features; and manic features. A clinical profile of personality structure is drawn from the client's responses in these areas.

Since the MMPI is largely self-administered and can be scored quickly on computers, it has been advocated as a screening measure for colleges and universities, industry and business, and government agencies, among others. The large-scale collection and use of such information is alarming because of the negative labeling that such psychologic testing may lead to.

| TIME & DATE | PUPILS | | | L.O.C. | S-R | T.R. | MOTOR | | | | TOTAL |
	R	 = >	L				RUE	RLE	LUE	LLE	MAX. 25

Explanation of Codes

Pupils

Reaction time, right (R) and left (L)

(2) Reacts briskly

(1) Reacts slowly

(0) No reaction

Size

(=) Equal

(<) Right lesser than left

(>) Right greater than left

Level of Consciousness (L.O.C.)

(5) Alert and oriented x 3 = awakens easily; oriented to person, place, time

(4) Alert and partially oriented = awakens easily but oriented in only one or two of the three spheres

(3) Lethargic but oriented = slow to arouse, possibly slurred speech, but oriented x 3

(2) Lethargic and disoriented = slow to arouse, oriented in only one or two spheres or completely disoriented

Chart continues on next page

Figure 12–2
Neurologic Assessment Guide.
Source: Copyright © 1977. American Journal of Nursing Company. From American Journal of Nursing, *September, Vol. 77, No. 9.*

The Draw-a-Person Test

In the Draw-a-Person test, clients are asked first to draw a human figure and then, usually, to draw a figure of a member of the opposite sex (see Figure 12–4). The drawings may be interpreted to give information about clients' concepts of their own bodies and personality structures; their relationships with persons of the opposite sex, the same sex, and parents; and their views of the roles of men and women.

OR

(2) **Restless/combative (confused)** = spontaneously thrashing about in bed; striking out at others; inattentive to commands

(1) **Responds to stimulation only** = exhibits only some type of withdrawal or posturing in response to stimulation

(0) **Unresponsive** = gives no response of any kind

Stimulus-Response (S-R)

(5) **Responds to commands** = gives appropriate responses to orientation questions, complies with instructions on hand grasp, toe wiggling, etc.

(4) **Responds to name** = opens eyes to name or gives some indication that he or she hears (nods, moves, etc.), but does not follow all commands

(3) **Responds to shaking** = responds only to vigorous physical stimulation

(2) **Responds to pinprick** = responds to light pain applied with pin to trunk or extremities to elicit either withdrawal or posturing

(1) **Responds to deep pain** = responds only to mandibular pressure, periorbital rub, sternal rub, or pinch

(0) **Unresponsive** = gives no response to any stimulus

Type of Response (T.R.)

(3) **Complex withdrawal** = withdrawal and attempt to remove stimulus

(2) **Simple withdrawal** = withdrawal from stimulus alone

(1) **Posturing** = decorticate—head, arms, and hands flexed; decerebrate—head extended, arms extended and pronated, back arched

(0) **Flaccid** = no response

Motor

Right Upper Extremity (RUE)
Right Lower Extremity (RLE)
Left Upper Extremity (LUE)
Left Lower Extremity (LLE)

(2) **Full spontaneous use** = moves designated extremity or extremities with or *without* any stimulus

(1) **Moves to stimulus only** = responds only to touch, pin, or deep pain

(0) **No movement** = does not respond to any stimulus

Weakness of an extremity is indicated by writing "weaker" under the appropriate column.

Figure 12–2 (continued)

The Sentence Completion Test

The Sentence Completion test presents an extensive series of incomplete sentences to clients, who are asked to complete the sentences with the first thoughts that come to mind. The sentences are designed to elicit responses concerning fantasies, fears, daydreams, and aspirations, among other things.

The Bender-Gestalt Test

The Bender-Gestalt test asks clients to reproduce, as best they can, nine geometric designs that are printed on sep-

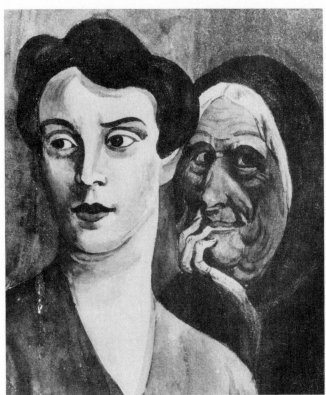

Figure 12–3
Card 12 GF of the Thematic Apperception Test.

Source: Reprinted from Murray HA: Thematic Apperception Test.
Harvard University Press, 1943. Copyright © 1943 by the President and
Fellows of Harvard College; 1971 by Henry A. Murray. Reprinted by
permission.

arate cards. Because this test can be used to evaluate memory, it is believed to be particularly helpful in identifying organic brain damage. It is also used to evaluate the maturation level of children in the coordination of visual, motor, and intellectual functions. For an example of a Bender-Gestalt design series, see Figure 12–5.

These and other instruments commonly used by clinical psychologists are briefly discussed in Table 12–2.

Psychiatric Diagnostic Practice According to APA's Criteria (DSM-IIIR)

The American Psychiatric Association (APA) published a revised third edition of the **Diagnostic and Statistical Manual of Mental Disorders** in 1987. (See Appendix B for an outline of categories for diagnosis and numeric codes.) Important features distinguish DSM-IIIR from its predecessors, DSM-II and DSM-III. It uses specified diagnostic criteria to improve the reliability of diagnostic judgments and offers a multiaxial or multidimensional approach to clinical assessment of psychiatric clients in which five different classes of data are collected and assessed.

The first edition of the DSM was published by the APA in 1952. In 1968 the main achievement of the second edition was to move into compatibility with the International Classification of Diseases, Injuries, and Causes of Death (ICD-9) published by the World Health Organization. The DSM-II was widely criticized for its low reliability and tendency to reflect an individual psychiatrist's philosophy or such client characteristics as social class rather than actual clinical data. In the first edition of this text, we charged that most psychiatric diagnostic practice had been subject to speculation about unconscious dynamics, was limited

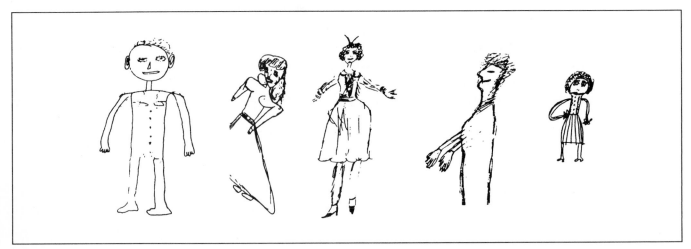

Figure 12–4
Examples of the Draw-a-Person test done by five women who had been hospitalized for two years.

Source: Spire RH: An experimental study of the use of photographic self-image confrontation as a
nursing procedure in the care of chronically ill schizophrenic female patients. (Project in partial
fulfillment of MS degree, State University of New York at Buffalo), 1967, pp 243, 248, 249, 251, 256.

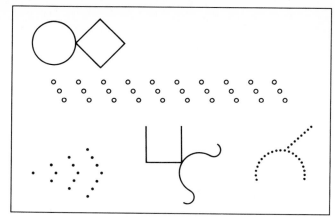

Figure 12–5
Examples of figures to be copied on Bender-Gestalt test. Subjects are asked to copy the figures on a single sheet of paper and then to draw them from memory. The clinician looks for distortion of the figures in terms of incompleteness, rotation, oversimplification, perseveration (giving more than is present in the stimulus). The interpreter also looks at the use of space on the page. The recall drawings also test for memory deficits.
Source: Bender L: A Visual-Motor Gestalt Test and its Clinical Use, Research Monograph no. 3. American Orthopsychiatric Association, 1938.

to intrapsychic variables, and represented a reductionistic and dualistic approach to human beings.

The DSM-IIIR represents the current state of knowledge about diagnosing **mental disorders**. It is composed of a list of all the official numeric codes and terms for all recognized mental disorders, along with a comprehensive description of each and specified diagnostic criteria that must be present in order to make each diagnosis.

Nurses have historically avoided instruments and tools for client assessment that ignore stressors in a person's social context and emphasize symptoms or illness to the exclusion of strengths, capabilities, and areas of adaptive functioning. In short, nurses have avoided exclusively "medical model approaches." Many of our colleagues believe that the new DSM-IIIR, while not entirely free of controversy, represents the state-of-the-art in the field of psychiatric diagnosis. According to Spitzer, Williams, and Skodol (1980), the DSM-III had been adopted for use in most facilities throughout the United States.

Basic Principles of the Multiaxial System

The multiaxial framework for client assessment provided by DSM-IIIR is congruent with holistic views of people, recognizes the role of environmental stress in influencing behavior, and requires that the clinician collect data about client adaptive strengths as well as about symptoms or problems. One of the most important features of DSM-IIIR is its increased interclinician reliability due to the use of specified observable criteria rather than diverse theories of etiology for mental disorders (Spitzer and Forman 1979).

Its multiaxial approach is undoubtedly of equal significance to psychiatric nursing (Williams and Wilson 1982).

The principle behind a multiaxial system is illustrated in the following example.

A 35-year-old man came to an out-patient mental health clinic for evaluation. This young man came in for treatment of a severe fear and avoidance of flying that amounted to a phobia. However, he also had a long-term personality disturbance, and suffered from eczema. If three different clinicians were asked to evaluate this man, a clinician who was particularly biologically oriented would certainly diagnose the eczema but might fail to notice the personality disturbance and make little of the phobia. A more psychodynamically oriented clinician would be sure to diagnose the personality disorder but might overlook the eczema and the phobia, considering them to be merely manifestations of the underlying personality disturbance. Finally, a clinician who was more behaviorally oriented would notice the phobia, but might fail to diagnose the personality disturbance and the eczema. It is clear, then, that due to their differing theoretical orientations these clinicians have a rather high likelihood of diagnostic disagreement.

This same man was presented to the same three colleagues, and this time each of the clinicians was required to evaluate him in each of three different areas of functioning: (a) behavioral or psychologic, (b) personality, and (c) physical functioning. In this case, all three clinicians would be much more likely to diagnose all three conditions and thus agree on the total evaluation of the individual.

In the DSM-IIIR **multiaxial system**, each individual is evaluated on five axes, each dealing with a different class of information about the client. A multiaxial evaluation system provides a much more comprehensive evaluation of an individual and increases the likelihood that clinicians will agree among themselves about the condition of the individual being evaluated.

The DSM-IIIR multiaxial system includes the five axes presented in Box 12–2. Axes I and II include all the mental disorders in DSM-IIIR and so might be said to represent the intrapersonal or *psychologic* area of functioning. Axis III is for recording physical disorders and conditions that are related to the understanding or management of the individual, and thus represents the area of *physical* functioning. Axes IV and V, for psychosocial stressors and a global assessment of functioning, includes an evaluation

Table 12–2
Common Psychologic Tests in Clinical Use

Name of Test	Description	Method
Bender-Gestalt test	A test of visual-motor coordination that is most useful with adults as a screening device to detect the presence of organic impairment. It may also be used to evaluate the level of maturation in the coordination of intellectual, muscular, and visual functions in children.	The client is asked to copy nine separate geometric designs onto plain white paper, one at a time. Sometimes the client is asked to draw the design from memory after an interval of forty-five to sixty seconds.
Blacky test	A projective test used most frequently with children (although it is also designed for adults) to determine the level of psychosexual development.	The client is shown various cartoons about a dog (who may be identified as male or female) and the dog's family and is asked to make up a story about each cartoon.
Draw-a-Person test	A projective test used with both adults and children to elicit information on the client's body image or perception of self and the client's relationship to the environment. It is also used as a screening device to detect the presence of organic impairment. With children it may be used to compare the age level of expression with the child's chronological age for a rough approximation of intelligence.	The client is asked first to draw a human figure and later to draw a person of the opposite sex. The test may be expanded by asking the client to draw a picture of a house and a tree as well (called the House–Tree–Person Test), an animal, or a family.
Minnesota Multiphasic Personality Inventory (MMPI)	A self-administered objective (as opposed to projective) personality test designed to yield a broad examination of personality functioning that is amenable to statistical interpretation—such as self-attitudes, certain aspects of ego functioning, and profiles of symptoms or psychopathology.	The client responds to 550 statements, by indicating either "true," "false," or "cannot say." The client's personality profile is sketched in terms of: • Preoccupation with body diseases • Depression • Hysteria • Antisocial personality • Masculine or feminine features • Paranoid qualities • Anxiety, phobias, and psychogenic fatigue • Schizophrenic features • Manic features
Rorschach test	A projective test that is the most highly developed of the personality tests. It reveals personality features and symptoms and is commonly used as a diagnostic tool.	The client responds to ten cards, one at a time, consisting of black-and-white or colored standardized inkblots. Responses include the impressions, thoughts, and associations that come to mind while the client looks at the inkblot.
Sentence Completion test	A projective test designed to elicit conscious associations to specific areas of functioning to illustrate the fears, preoccupations, ambitions, and idiosyncrasies of the client.	The client is asked to complete spontaneously sentences such as: "I feel guilty about. . . ," "Sex is. . . ," "My mother. . . ," "Sometimes I wish. . . ," Both mood and content are noted.
Stanford-Binet Intelligence Test	A general intelligence test based on an age-level concept from two years to about fifteen years. It is particularly useful to test children and to evaluate mental retardation.	The client is asked to do a graded series of tasks designed to correlate with the abilities of children of a particular age group. Each set is more difficult than the one before it.

continued

	Table 12–2 (Continued) Common Psychologic Tests in Clinical Use	
Name of Test	Description	Method
Thematic Apperception Test (TAT)	A projective test offering a standardized set of stimuli for exploring the client's emotional life. Themes and interpersonal problems emerge in the client's responses.	The client is shown a series of ambiguous pictures of people in various emotionally significant situations and is asked to respond by describing what is happening in the picture and telling a story about it. Adaptations have been designed for use with children. In these, the central figure is a child or the pictures are cartoons of animals.
Wechsler Adult Intelligence Scale (WAIS)	A general intelligence test for persons sixteen years of age and older. It is the most widely used and best standardized intelligence test.	The client completes eleven subtests, which yield both verbal and performance scores as well as full-scale IQs. Subtest raw scores may also be compared to reveal variability in functioning. The subtests are: information, comprehension, arithmetic, similarities, memory for digits, vocabulary, digit symbol, picture completion, block design, picture arrangement, and object assembly.
Wechsler Intelligence Scale for Children (WISC)	A general intelligence test for children from five through fifteen years of age.	Similar to the Wechsler test for adults, this test asks the client to complete ten subtests, which yield separate verbal, performance, and full-scale scores.
Wechsler Memory Scale	A psychologic test for immediate, short-term, and long-term memory.	The client is asked to do seven memory tests, including current information, orientation, mental control, logical memory, digits forward and backward, visual reproduction, and associate learning. A memory quotient (MQ) score is useful in the determination of organic mental syndrome.
Word Association test	A projective test similar in form and organization to the Sentence Completion test. It is designed to elicit associations to areas of conflict.	The client is asked to respond spontaneously to a series of fifty or more words, presented one at a time. Words presumed to be related to the conflicts of the specific client are mixed with words that generally produce an emotional reaction.

of the individual's *social* functioning. In this sense, the multiaxial system provides a more comprehensive bio-psychosocial approach to assessment.

Description of the Axes

It is essential that nurses understand the components of the multiaxial system thoroughly to use it effectively.

Axes I and II: Clinical Syndromes, V-Codes, Personality and Developmental Disorders

Axes I and II comprise all the "mental disorders and conditions not attributable to a mental disorder that are a focus of attention or treatment" (called V-codes). The easiest way to differentiate between these first two axes is to deal first with Axis II. On Axis II are personality disorders, usually diagnosed in adults, and developmental disorders

---

Box 12-2
DSM-IIIR AXES

Axis I: Clinical syndromes

Conditions not attributable to a mental disorder that are a focus of attention or treatment (V-codes)

Additional codes

Axis II: Personality disorders

Developmental disorders

Axis III: Physical disorders

Axis IV: Severity of psychosocial stressors

Axis V: Global assessment of functioning (GAF)

---

including mental retardation, diagnosed in children and adolescents. The remaining mental disorders and associated conditions are recorded on Axis I. The classes of disorders on Axis II were given their own axis because their usually mild and chronic symptomatology is often overshadowed by a more florid Axis I condition. DSM-IIIR clarifies the conceptual distinction between Axis I and Axis II by noting that Axis II conditions

- Have an early onset
- Have a stable, not episodic, course

V-Codes

In addition to the other mental disorders, Axis I includes the V-codes. The V-codes include such conditions as marital problems, occupational problems, and parent-child problems, in which the problem being evaluated or for which clinical care is sought is not due to a mental disorder. *A mental disorder is differentiated from other problems in living as a clinically significant behavioral pattern that occurs and is associated with either a painful symptom (distress) or impairment in functioning (disability).* Further, the distress or disability does not primarily reflect a conflict between an individual and society.

If a person with bipolar disorder, a mental disorder that has been in remission for many years, now develops marital difficulties for reasons unrelated to that person's psychiatric history or condition (perhaps, for example, a conflict has arisen because that person's wife wants

to resume a career), both "Marital problem" and "Bipolar disorder in remission" could be recorded on Axis I. If, however, the bipolar disorder is not in complete remission, and marital conflict develops as a result of the person's changeable moods and other symptoms associated with the mental disorder, the marital problem would not be recorded in addition to the bipolar disorder, since the marital problem in this case is due to the person's mental disorder.

Axis I also includes a code for "Unspecified mental disorder (nonpsychotic)," which indicates that the clinician has determined that there is some (nonpsychotic) Axis I mental disorder but, perhaps due to lack of information, cannot yet be more specific. Finally, there are codes for indicating that a diagnosis or condition is deferred on either Axis I or Axis II, or that there is no mental disorder. Examples of evaluations of individuals using only Axes I and II are presented in Box 12-3.

Axis III: Physical Disorders and Conditions

Axis III is for recording physical disorders and conditions that are important to take into account in planning treatment or are relevant to understanding the etiology or worsening of the mental disorder. A clinician might also want to record other significant physical findings, such as "soft" neurologic signs or even a single symptom (e.g., vomiting). An example of an evaluation done through Axis III is presented in Box 12-4.

In this example, in addition to the fact that diabetes is a major physical disorder and should always be noted, the child will probably not be very compliant with treatment, due in large part to his psychologic problems (conduct disorder, as the mental disorder, being noted on Axis II).

If there is lack of information on Axis III, that fact should be stated: "No information" or "Diagnosis deferred—not evaluated" or "Referred to Dr. Smith for evaluation."

Box 12-3
EXAMPLES OF DSM-IIIR MULTI-AXIAL EVALUATION ON AXES I AND II

Example 1

Axis I: 303.93   Alcohol dependence, in remission

Axis II: 301.70   Antisocial personality disorder

Example 2

Axis I: V71.09   No diagnosis

Axis II: 301.22   Schizotypal personality disorder

In any event, *something* should be noted on this axis, omitting it for lack of information undermines the purpose of a holistic multaxial system.

Axis IV: Severity of Psychosocial Stressors

Axis IV provides the rating scale shown in Table 12–3. This scale rates the severity of the psychosocial stressors that in the nurse's judgment helped to bring about, worsened, or account for a recurrence of a mental disorder. In making this judgment, the nurse should generally take into account only stressors that occurred in the year preceding the mental disorder.

To standardize the severity ratings across stressors, and to avoid rating an individual's idiosyncratic vulnerabilities, the evaluator should rate the severity of the stressors with an "average" person in mind. The nurse should take into account the individual client's circumstances and sociocultural background, and rate the severity of the stressors as experienced by the "average" person under these circumstances. In this way, an abortion would probably be more stressful for a Catholic than for an atheist.

The nurse should also take into account: (a) the total number of stressors the client recently experienced, (b) how desirable they were; to what extent they were under the client's control (e.g., whether the individual quit a job or was fired), and (c) the amount of change they caused in the individual's life (e.g., the development of a serious chronic physical illness could be expected to cause a great deal of change in the "average" person's life).

In addition to rating the severity of the stressors, evaluators should also note in their own words the specific stressors that they consider pertinent. Thus a multiaxial evaluation, up through Axis IV, might look like the example in Box 12–5. Changes in DSM-IIIR required stating if stressors were enduring or discrete events. In this example, the client developed panic disorder (a condition in which there are recurrent panic attacks) as she began classes in college.

Axis V: Global Assessment of Functioning

This axis in DSM-III provided the rating scale shown in Table 12–4. One of the most accurate indicators of clinical outcome is the level of premorbid functioning that an indi-

---

Box 12–4
EXAMPLE OF DSM-IIIR MULTI-AXIAL EVALUATION ON AXES I, II, AND III

Axis I:	V71.09	No diagnosis
Axis II:	312.23	Conduct disorder, socialized, aggressive
Axis III:		Diabetes

Box 12–5
EXAMPLE OF A DSM-IIIR MULTI-AXIAL EVALUATION ON AXES I, II, III, AND IV

Axis I:	300.01	Panic disorder
Axis II:	301.83	Borderline personality disorder
Axis III:		No diagnosis
Axis IV:		3–Mild (began college)

---

vidual sustained. For this reason, Axis V provides a **Global Assessment of Function Scale (GAF)** to rate the highest level of psychologic, social, and occupational functioning that an individual was able to sustain for at least a few months during the past year as well as at the time of evaluation.

Overall adaptive functioning was defined in DSM-III (1980) by three areas of functioning: (a) social relations, (b) occupational functioning, and (c) use of leisure time. The quality of the client's functioning in each of these three areas should be considered, with the breadth and quality of social relationships being given the greatest weight because of their high prognostic value. Use of leisure time is a serious consideration only in those individuals who have been functioning on a very high level.

Summary of Changes from DSM-III to DSM-IIIR*

With the widespread use of DSM-III and the publication of a revised form in spring of 1987, psychiatry has moved beyond an inclination to engage in lengthy justifications for classification and nosology (the science of naming) to the simple position that the ability to name and describe something is crucial to our ability to think meaningfully about it. Although it took five years to plan DSM-III, within three years of its publication efforts to revise it were underway. Yet, this fact was not a reflection of DSM-III's failure. It sold over 700,000 copies and came in behind the *Fanny Farmer Cookbook* on the nonfiction best-seller list. Its publication made an impressive impact on the field if only in view of the amount of research it stimulated. The architect of its development, Dr. Robert Spitzer, chair of the APA's DSM-III Task Force, described it as "one still-frame" in a process of increasing our understanding of mental

---

*For a complete discussion of changes from DSM-III to DSM-IIIR, see Wilson and Skodol (in press).

Table 12–3 Axis IV: Severity of Psychosocial Stressors Scale			
Code	Term	Examples of Stressors	
Adults		Acute Events	Enduring Circumstances
1	None	No acute events that may be relevant to the disorder	No enduring circumstances that may be relevant to the disorder
2	Mild	Broke up with boyfriend or girlfriend; started or graduated from school; child left home	Family arguments; job dissatisfaction; residence in high-crime neighborhood
3	Moderate	Marriage; marital separation; loss of job; retirement; miscarriage	Marital discord; serious financial problems; trouble with boss; being a single parent
4	Severe	Divorce; birth of first child	Unemployment; poverty
5	Extreme	Death of spouse; serious physical illness diagnosed; victim of rape	Serious chronic illness in self or child; ongoing physical or sexual abuse
6	Catastrophic	Death of child; suicide of spouse; devastating natural disaster	Captivity as hostage; concentration camp experience
0	Inadequate information, or no change in condition		
Children and Adolescents			
1	None	No acute events that may be relevant to the disorder	No enduring circumstances that may be relevant to the disorder
2	Mild	Broke up with boyfriend or girlfriend; change of school	Overcrowded living quarters; family arguments
3	Moderate	Expelled from school; birth of sibling	Chronic disabling illness in parent; chronic parental discord
4	Severe	Divorce of parents; unwanted pregnancy; arrest	Harsh or rejecting parents; chronic life-threatening illness in parent; multiple foster home placements
5	Extreme	Sexual or physical abuse; death of a parent	Recurrent sexual or physical abuse
6	Catastrophic	Death of both parents	Chronic life-threatening illness
0	Inadequate information, or no change in condition		

Source: American Psychiatric Association: Diagnostic and Statistical Manual of Mental Disorders, *ed 3, revised. APA, 1987.*

disorders. This statement captures the spirit in which it was so quickly revised.

The goals for DSM-IIIR were to address three problems identified with DSM-III: (a) ambiguities in terminology, (b) inconsistencies in the manual, and (c) need to incorporate research findings published since 1980. The process of revision was as elaborate as the process of generating DSM-III. A group of fifteen senior nosologists from across the United States worked with twenty-five advisory committees representing 230 expert consultants. The revision went through two preliminary drafts before its final publication in May 1987.

Table 12–4
Axis V: Global Assessment of Functioning Scale (GAF Scale)*

Code

90 | 81	Absent or minimal symptoms (e.g., mild anxiety before an exam), good functioning in all areas, interested and involved in a wide range of activities, socially effective, generally satisfied with life, no more than everyday problems or concerns (e.g., an occasional argument with family members).
80 | 71	If symptoms are present, they are transient and expectable reactions to psychosocial stressors (e.g., difficulty concentrating after family argument); no more than slight impairment in social, occupational, or school functioning (e.g., temporarily falling behind in school work).
70 | 61	Some mild symptoms (e.g., depressed mood and mild insomnia) *or* some difficulty in social, occupational, or school functioning (e.g., occasional truancy, or theft within the household), but generally functioning pretty well, has some meaningful interpersonal relationships.
60 | 51	Moderate symptoms (e.g., flat affect and circumstantial speech, occasional panic attacks) *or* moderate difficulty in social, occupational, or school functioning (e.g., few friends, conflicts with co-workers).
50 | 41	Serious symptoms (e.g., suicidal ideation, severe obsessional rituals, frequent shoplifting) *or* any serious impairment in social, occupational, or school functioning (e.g., no friends, unable to keep a job).
40 | 31	Some impairment in reality testing or communication (e.g., speech is at times illogical, obscure, or irrelevant) *or* major impairment in several areas, such as work or school, family relations, judgment, thinking, or mood (e.g., depressed man avoids friends, neglects family, and is unable to work; child frequently beats up younger children, is defiant at home, and is failing at school).
30 | 21	Behavior is considerably influenced by delusions or hallucinations *or* serious impairment in communication or judgment (e.g., sometimes incoherent, acts grossly inappropriately, suicidal preoccupation) *or* inability to function in almost all areas (e.g., stays in bed all day; no job, home, or friends).
20 | 11	Some danger of hurting self or others (e.g., suicide attempts without clear expectation of death, frequently violent, manic excitement) *or* occasionally fails to maintain minimal personal hygiene (e.g., smears feces) *or* gross impairment in communication (e.g., largely incoherent or mute).
10 | 1	Persistent danger of severely hurting self or others (e.g., recurrent violence) *or* persistent inability to maintain minimal personal hygiene *or* serious suicidal act with clear expectation of death.

Consider psychological, social, and occupational functioning on a hypothetical continuum of mental health-illness. Do not include impairment in functioning due to physical (or environmental) limitations.

Note: Use intermediate codes when appropriate, e.g., 45, 68, 72.

Source: American Psychiatric Association: Diagnostic and Statistical Manual of Mental Disorders, ed 3, revised. APA, 1987.

A comparison of DSM-III and DSM-IIIR reveals five types of changes:

1. Changes in the concepts underlying the axes of the multiaxial system
2. A shift in classification approach from "classical categories" to "prototype categories"
3. Less emphasis in diagnostic hierarchies
4. Revisions of some diagnostic criteria
5. Revisions of some textual descriptions

Changes in Concepts Underlying Axes

1. *Axes I and II.* The conceptual distinction between Axis I clinical syndromes and Axis II disorders was clarified by adding two characteristics to distinguish Axis II disorders: They all have early onsets, and they have a stable rather than episodic course. Consequently Axis II now includes:

   Personality disorders

   Developmental disorders (including)

Mental retardation
Pervasive developmental disorders
Specific developmental disorders

2. *Axis III.* Axis III was virtually unchanged and remains physical illness important to understanding or managing a psychiatric disorder. This axis is widely used, but there has been little research on the relationship of physical conditions and psychiatric disorders.

3. *Axis IV.* Axis IV presented a number of problems in DSM-III:

- Grouping stressors under one global rating was not very meaningful.

- Enduring rather than single, acute stressful life events seem more important in putting people at risk for developing mental disorders.

- It was difficult to sort out stresses that are etiologically significant from stresses that are not.

- Some research suggested that stressful life events in some clients do not make as much difference as the individual's vulnerability.

In the absence of any conclusive evidence, the belief persists that noting stress is important to planning treatment. Axis IV has been revised to include a six- rather than seven-point scale. The clinician is asked to note whether the stress listed and rated is acute or enduring in nature.

4. *Axis V.* Axis V has been revised to a ninety-point scale. It now includes a measure of psychologic function as well as social and occupational function. It resembles a well-established test called the Global Assessment of Function Scale in its present form. Ratings on Axis V should be made over two time periods: current and past year. Some critics, however, suggest that inclusion of a psychologic rating confuses the intent of separate multiaxial evaluations since psychologic functioning is obviously reflected in the criteria of other axes.

5. *Additional axes.* Many believe that a sixth axis should be added to the multiaxial system. Family therapists, psychodynamic psychiatrists, and psychiatric nurses proposing the **Nursing Adaptation Evaluation (NSGAE)** (Morrison 1985) have been among them. (See Boxes 12–6 and 12–7.) But the majority opinion was that it would be premature to make such a change in the DSM-IIIR. A compromise solution for the need for more psychodynamic material was to (a) include a glossary of defense mechanisms and (b) urge clinicians to list defensive functions among Axis II disorders.

Box 12–6
RATING SCALE FOR PATIENT'S CURRENT OVERALL LEVEL OF FUNCTIONING ON NSGAE

Level 1. The patient demonstrates self-care abilities in meeting all the basic biological needs and consistently uses appropriate resources when difficulties become manifest.

Level 2. The patient demonstrates the ability to independently accomplish specific self-care activities, but limited ability to utilize available resources.

Level 3. The patient is limited in the ability to accomplish self-care and requires either physical assistance or consistent verbal direction to ensure needs being met.

Level 4. The patient is severely limited in the ability to accomplish self-care and requires either physical assistance or consistent verbal direction to ensure needs being met.

Source: Morrison E, et al: NSGAE: a proposed Axis VI of DSM-III. J Psychosocial Nurs 1985;23(8):11.

Shift from Classical Categories to Prototype Categories

Mental disorders are rarely discrete entities, and conditions such as anxiety and depression cannot be separated into neat categories. For this reason, the basis for classification has shifted. A client no longer has to manifest all attributes listed (the classifical classification approach) to fit into a certain category. Under the prototype approach, the client can be included in a category if he or she displays some but not all of the symptoms associated with that category. This new approach to classification, which acknowledges overlap, obviously has implications for future reliability. Validity, however, has been enhanced through this change.

Move Away from Diagnostic Hierarchies

In DSM-III, the principle of diagnostic parsimony applied. If one made a diagnosis inclusive of another, only the inclusive diagnosis was made. For example, if anxiety was present in a depressed person, one diagnosed only depression because anxiety is part of depression. Because tracking heterogeneity is important to treatment response and long-term outcome, DSM-IIIR encourages making multiple independent diagnoses rather than ruling out something because it is "due to" something else.

Changes in Categories and Descriptions

1. *Psychoactive substance dependence.* The distinction between dependence, with its cornerstones of toler-

ance and physical withdrawal symptoms, and abuse has been deleted in DSM-IIIR. The new conception of psychoactive substance dependence disorders is consistent both with commonsense notions that compulsive, out-of-control drug use is troublesome and with the World Health Organization's current definition of substance dependence. The DSM-IIIR lists nine symptoms. In the presence of any three, a client meets the criteria for a diagnosis of "psychoactive substance dependence disorder." Substance abuse is now a residual category referring to hazardous use when three of the criteria are not met.

2. *Schizophrenic disorders.* Other psychotic disorders differ from core or true schizophrenia because of the latter's deteriorating downhill course. For this reason, attempts to differentiate other psychotic disorders from schizophrenia have intensified in DSM-IIIR. "Paranoid dis-

orders" have been renamed "delusional disorders" so as to include other nonbizarre delusions that tend to cluster. Schizophreniform subtypes have been included, and schizoaffective disorder, which had been a residual category with no diagnostic criteria, has been redefined with diagnostic criteria that delineate a syndrome in which the individual experiences either a major depressive or a manic syndrome concurrent with symptoms of the "A" criterion for schizophrenia.

3. *Mood disorders* (previously Affect disorders). The name of the category has been changed from affective to mood disorders. A number of clarifications, particu-

---

Box 12–7
DEFINITIONS AND BEHAVIORAL CRITERIA FOR NSGAE

Nutrition Level (N)

1. Is able to maintain nutrition and hydration independently.

2. Needs assistance with culturally accepted table manners.

3. Needs assistance selecting food or staying with meal.

4. Cannot report hunger or thirst.
   Inadequate/excessive intake due to fear of food, inability to be with others, medications or physical handicap.

Solitude and Social Interaction Level (S)

1. Is able to constructively use non-hospital support system to meet basic needs.

2. Is able to use nurse-patient relationship to problem-solve and validate feelings and perceptions of self and others.

3. Is preoccupied with internal stimuli, but responds when approached.
   Verbally provocative with peers or staff.

4. Is withdrawn or mute.
   Unable to control excitement, intrusiveness, or abusiveness.

Grooming and Personal Hygiene Level (G)

1. Is able to dress and groom self at own initiative according to environmental demands and cultural norms.

2. Is able to use hospital structure to care for own clothes, personal space, and grooming.

3. Needs assistance to prepare and complete hygiene tasks. Has no belongings and needs interventions to obtain basic articles of clothing or grooming tools.

4. Cannot dress self according to environmental demands or cultural norms.
   Cannot perform basic hygiene tasks.

Activity and Rest Level (A)

1. Is able to select and participate in activities, able to sleep restfully.

2. May still have sleeping difficulties but able to verbalize and problem-solve solutions.

3. Is over or underactive, but has some control over behavior and responds to direction.

4. Cannot sleep for restful periods or sleeps continuously. Is unable to control harmful activity without locked seclusion, restraints, and medications.

Elimination Level (E)

1. Able to regulate elimination pattern independently.

2. Able to ask for help to maintain elimination pattern.

3. Cannot maintain elimination without medication or other active treatment.

4. Cannot report bowel/bladder function.
   Antisocially urinates, defecates, or smears feces.

Source: Adapted from Morrison E, et al: NSGAE: A proposed Axis VI of DSM-III. J. Psychosocial Nurs 1985;23(8):13. Adapted from Smith S: In Underwood P: Self-Concepts Manual. University of California, Department of Mental Health and Community Nursing, 1981.

larly with respect to panic attacks and their distinction from generalized anxiety disorders, appear in DSM-IIIR.

Controversial Categories

Some arguments for including several additional diagnoses in DSM-IIIR met with resistance. These controversial categories included:

- Late luteal phase dysphoric disorder (formerly called premenstrual tension syndrome or PMS)
- Self-defeating personality disorder (listed as masochistic personality under the "Other" category in DSM-III)
- Sadistic personality disorder

Critics objected to these proposed diagnoses on a number of fronts:

- Their use as an insanity defense in a court of law would be counterproductive.
- They discriminate against women.
- Insufficient evidence exists to justify their inclusion.
- Some of the diagnostic criteria are ambiguous.
- "Self-defeating personality" concept is rooted in Freudian theory and its inclusion violates the atheoretical goal of DSM-IIIR.

The compromise conclusion was that such controversial categories would appear in an appendix with the indication that they deserve further study before becoming part of the official nomenclature. The impact on psychiatric practice and research of this decision and all other changes in DSM-IIIR is already being felt.

DSM's Usefulness to Psychiatric-Mental Health Nursing

From the perspective of psychiatric nursing, the DSM-IIIR represents some progress toward values that mental health nurses have espoused for decades. For example, as Williams and Wilson have stated (1982), DSM-III (and DSM-IIIR):

- Provides a framework for interdisciplinary communication
- Based revisions on a series of formative evaluations
- Represents a collaborative achievement
- Represents progress toward a more holistic view of mind-body relations

- Provides for diagnostic uncertainty
- Incorporates, at least in part, biologic, psychologic, and social variables
- Has achieved positive results of extensive field testing for validity and reliability
- Considers adaptive strength as well as problems
- Reflects a descriptive, phenomenologic perspective rather than any psychiatric theoretical orientation

Of all the axes represented in DSM-IIIR, Axes IV and V, Psychosocial Stressors and Functioning, are the areas in which nursing can make the greatest contribution. The Nursing Adaptation Evaluation (NSGAE) represents one proposed refinement of Axis V useful in planning and determining resources for nursing care (Morrison et al. 1985). The rating format appears in Box 12–6. The NSGAE could also become a sixth axis on its own.

Psychosocial Assessment

The psychosocial assessment is a dynamic process. While it is begun in the initial contact with the client, it continues throughout the nurse-client experience. Psychosocial assessments may be made of an individual, a family, or a group. In any case, they begin with the identifying characteristics, such as name, sex, age, marital status, and ethnic and cultural origins. Problem identification and definition are also necessary phases in the assessment process. The method for assessment described below has been adapted from the problem-solving model of Compton and Galaway (1979, pp 250–251).

Individual Assessment

During the individual assessment, the following factors should be considered:

1. *Physical and intellectual*
   a. Presence of physical illness and/or disability
   b. Appearance and energy level
   c. Current and potential levels of intellectual functioning
   d. How client sees personal world, translates events around self; client's perceptual abilities
   e. Cause and effect reasoning, ability to focus
2. *Socioeconomic factors*
   a. Economic factors—level of income, adequacy of subsistence: their effect on life-style, sense of adequacy, and self-worth
   b. Employment and attitudes about it
   c. Racial, cultural, and ethnic identification; sense of identity and belonging

d. Religious identification and link to significant value systems, norms, and practices

3. *Personal values and goals*

   a. Presence or absence of congruence between values and their expression in action; meaning of values to individual

   b. Congruence between individual's values and goals and the immediate systems with which client interacts

   c. Congruence between individual's values and assessor's values; meaning of this for intervention process

4. *Adaptive functioning and response to present involvement*

   a. Manner in which individual presents self to others—grooming, appearance, posture

   b. Emotional tone and change or constancy of levels

   c. Style of communication—verbal and nonverbal; ability to express appropriate emotion, follow train of thought; factors of dissonance, confusion, uncertainty

   d. Symptoms or symptomatic behavior

   e. Quality of relationships individual seeks to establish—direction, purposes, and uses of such relationships for individual

   f. Perception of self

   g. Social roles that are assumed or ascribed; competence in fulfilling these roles

   h. Relational behavior

      (1) Capacity for intimacy

      (2) Dependence-independence balance

      (3) Power and control conflicts

      (4) Exploitiveness

      (5) Openness

5. *Developmental factors*

   a. How role performance is equated with life stage

   b. How developmental experiences have been interpreted and used

   c. How individual has dealt with past conflicts, tasks, and problems

   d. Whether present problem is unique in life experience

The Place of Assessment in Practice

Assessment is essential in clinical practice and serves several purposes:

- Identifying problems
- Identifying client motivations, strengths, and resources

- Identifying forces that may hinder the therapeutic plan (forces both internal and external to the client)
- Setting reasonable goals
- Determining appropriate intervention strategies
- Providing continuous evaluation of the process and indicating when the therapeutic plan should be changed

Although the individual assessment has been presented in linear form, it would be a mistake for nurses to make assessments in this structured way. Assessment is an ongoing, continually changing, dynamic process that Compton and Galaway (1979, p 287) describe as a "squirming, wriggling, alive business." It provides an opportunity for nurse and client to engage in a partnership based on mutual definition of problems and goals.

SYSTEMS OF RECORDING

It is necessary to communicate adequately in writing to inform mental health team members of the client's patterns of interaction. Recording is an important process; it often provides the basis for:

- Altering a treatment plan
- Determining appropriate intervention strategies
- Allowing communication among members of the mental health team or mental health agencies
- Providing around-the-clock data on hospitalized clients
- Evidence in court
- Research

An often unrecognized or disregarded purpose of recording is to provide quality accountability of psychiatric nursing practice. Recorded data can be used to give nurses feedback about their practice, through processes such as the *psychiatric audit* (discussed later in this chapter). Exactly what system of recording is used depends on the agency.

What to Record

The most significant events the nurse records are the behavior patterns and interpersonal interactions of the client. It may also be important to record other significant happenings—the client's sleeping, eating, and elimination patterns; physical appearance; somatic treatments and medications; and so on.

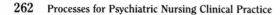

The following types of notes should be made:

- *Progress over time.* Mental health agencies may require that notes be entered at specific times, e.g., at the end of each eight-hour shift or at the end of each 24-hour period. When events of special significance occur, they should be recorded as soon after the event as possible, not held until the 8 or 24 hours have elapsed.

- *Nurse-client relationship.* Notes are often made after each session with the client in individual, group, or family therapy. These notes summarize what occurred during the experience.

- *Summary report.* Summary reports are usually made at the termination of contact with the client—i.e., when individual, group, or family therapy has ended. The summary report presents a clear and concise picture of the highlights of the experience.

Behavior and interaction notes should include examples rather than interpretations. Instead of writing "Ms W. is hallucinating," it is preferable to write "Ms W. states she hears Moses telling her not to get dressed today or leave her room."

Psychiatric Jargon: What to Avoid

The mental health field is rich in terms that nurses must learn if they are to speak the language in which mental health professionals converse. However, too much jargon may cloud meaning. The language of mental health, which relies heavily on words and phrases from psychology, has also borrowed from public health, sociology, anthropology, philosophy, and the federal bureaucracy. As Morgan and Moreno put it (1973, p 2): "In staff meetings of some centers, English is hardly spoken at all."

Nurses should use jargon sparingly. The glossary at the end of this book may be particularly useful not only in defining the terms that mental health professionals use but also in identifying the point of view or perspective from which the terms have come into popular use.

Source-Oriented Recording

Source-oriented records are becoming less common as more agencies institute problem-oriented methods of recording. Source-oriented recording usually consists of a clinical record or chart that includes unassembled chronological notations made by individual health team members. Phy-

sicians write orders and progress notes in one place, and nurses chart their notes in another. Other members of the team may not contribute in writing at all. Laboratory findings are kept in a third isolated section of the chart. Close communication among mental health team members is hindered by source-oriented recording. Such systems often duplicate efforts and fail to pull information about the client into a logical whole.

Problem-Oriented Recording

The problem-oriented system of recording is a major improvement over the source-oriented form. It is a way of organizing the same raw data into a comprehensive whole that can be used for assessment, planning, evaluation, research, and health care audits. The process stimulates mental health team members to gather, document, and describe data.

There are four necessary elements in problem-oriented recording systems:

1. *Data base.* The data base consists of all the information gathered at the initial contact with the client. It includes psychiatric history, psychosocial assessment, laboratory and physical findings, and the results of mental status examinations and psychologic tests. The mental health supplement to the standard defined data base that is used in one mental health facility is presented in Figure 12–6.

2. *Problem list.* The problem list emerges from the data base and summarizes the problems of the client. It should also include the client's assets. It is continually updated to present an accurate picture of the client's current situation.

3. *Initial plans.* A section of the record delineates the therapeutic plans for the client. Plans are formulated in terms of the problems to which they relate.

4. *Progress notes.* Progress notes parallel items in the problem list. They are used to monitor the plans, identify the need for modification, and provide a follow-up. The progress notes include narrative notes, flow sheets, and a discharge summary.

    a. Narrative notes are written in SOAP style, an acronym for *subjective* (the problem as perceived by the client), *objective* (clinical findings or observations), *assessment* (what is suggested by an analysis and synthesis of the subjective and objective data), and *plan* (proposed solutions for the identified problems).

    b. Flow sheets are used to tabulate information in graphic form. They are useful when some factor must be monitored frequently.

    c. The discharge summary is a summary of each problem area and the level of resolution reached.

It provides the essential data for community follow-up services.

Figure 12–7 demonstrates how one mental health facility uses problem-oriented progress notes.

Nursing Care Plans

Nursing care plans are a means of providing nursing personnel with information about the needs and therapeutic plans for each client. They are of major importance when an agency uses source-oriented recording methods, because they provide an ongoing, up-to-date record of goal-directed, individualized nursing care. When problem-oriented recording methods are used, nursing care plans may be an outgrowth of the record.

Algorithms

Algorithms are behavioral steps, or step-by-step procedures, for the management of common problems. Algorithms have proved useful protocols, particularly in settings that employ large numbers of paraprofessionals. At intake points in community mental health settings, such as walk-in neighborhood clinics, mental health workers often make the initial psychosocial assessment and may plan and implement treatment strategies. Clinical algorithms for common mental health problems would provide the nonprofessional with structured, standardized guidelines for decision-making.

Professional nurses in nonpsychiatric settings find clinical algorithms particularly useful. Algorithms for depression and suicidal lethality have been found to be reliable and valid in these circumstances.

Psychiatric Audits

The psychiatric audit is one way to evaluate the quality of mental health services received by consumers. The client's chart is reviewed to compare criteria for quality care with actual practice. Problem-oriented recording systems provide the descriptive documentation necessary for such a program. Although documentation may not always accurately indicate the quality of the care given, it is an important part of the process of keeping mental health workers accountable to consumers of their services.

The Interaction Process Analysis (IPA)

The interaction process analysis is a verbatim and progressive recording of the verbal and nonverbal interactions that ensue between client and nurse within a given time. It is an important means of communication between nurses or nursing students and their clinical supervisors, consul-

tants, or instructors about their client relationships. If nurses are to learn the function of therapeutic intervention, they must be able to study and review with objectivity the verbal and nonverbal components of the interaction to learn their potential significance. These components may express the existence of problems or attempts at resolution of these problems.

Purposes

The IPA serves a number of purposes:

- It helps nurses sharpen their skills of observation and listening by providing an opportunity to find clues that were not recognized during the face-to-face encounter.

Text continues on p. 267.

RESEARCH NOTE

Citation

Cox C: The health self-determinism index. Nurs Res 1985;34:177–183.

Study Problem/Purpose

To conduct a psychometric evaluation of a new measure of motivation in health behavior titled the Health Determinism Index.

Methods

The Health Determinism Index was completed by 202 randomly selected adults via a mail survey. The multidimensionality of the construct basic to this index was examined through factorial isolation for four subscales: self-determined health judgments, self-determined health behaviors, perceived competency in health matters, and internal-external cue responsiveness.

Findings

The four factors accounted for 56 percent of the total variance in the measure. The reliability coefficient for the total scale was 84, the internal consistency of the four subscales was supported by similar alpha reliability coefficients.

Implications

This instrument offers a means of examining nursing's ability to alter clients' motivation in relation to specific health behaviors. It also offers a basis for beginning a study of the role of motivation in health outcomes.

MEDICAL RECORD	SUPPLEMENT DEFINED DATA BASE

SUPPLEMENT TO (Check only one) PART ☑ I ☐ II ☐ III ☐ IV ☐ V ☐ VI

PREPARED BY (Signature & Title)	SERVICE	DATE
T. Knight, R.N. Clinical Specialist	*Emergency*	*12-23-88*

CHIEF COMPLAINT: In patient's own words and your impressions.

Gaunt, disheveled man in mid-thirties complains, "I have no purpose in life".

HISTORY AND DEVELOPMENT OF COMPLAINT

A. Date of onset and circumstances under which complaint developed.

Since resigning responsible position as electronics engineer 10 years ago, client has been drifting aimlessly, living at minimal level of subsistence. Brought in by police who found him living in his car in a school parking lot.

B. Previous hospitalizations and treatment-response to psychotropic drugs.

Unkown

C. Previous history of violent behavior, suicidal behavior, alcohol and drug abuse, previous arrests, and treatment by alcohol, drug and forensic program.

Experimentation with LSD and marijuana for 10 years at least 3x per week ... often once per day, with related impairment of social & occupational function. (No job, no dating relationships or social life)

MENTAL STATUS EXAMINATION

A. Overall general appearance. *Thin, unshaven dirty man in mid-thirties with poor nutrition, hygiene and tearful expression.*

B. Attitude and degree of cooperativeness.

Generally despondent but passively cooperative

C. Thought content and process—what patient thinks about—how patient thinks over and underproductive, spontaneous, circumstantial.

Thought content focuses on discovering solution to life's mysteries ... finding the key or answer.

Thought processes are vague and disconnected. Long periods of silence between verbalizations.

SUPPLEMENT

DEFINED

DATA BASE

VA FORM 10-7978g

Figure 12–6

Example of supplement to data base.

Source: Veterans Administration Hospital, Buffalo, NY.

D. Motoric behavior—overactive, underactive, inappropriate.

*Slow, underactive bordering on catatonic
low energy level*

AFFECT

A. How the patient feels—shallow, anxious, depressed appropriate, inappropriate.

Depressed and discouraged — feelings of inadequacy

SENSORIUM MENTAL GRASP AND CAPACITY

A. Orientation/memory

Oriented to time, place + person

B. Abstract thinking

Can interpret proverbs but ponderously

C. Judgment/insight, adequate, complete, incomplete, distorted

Questionable

D. Cognitive disorder—hallucinations and delusions

No data available at this time

E. Estimate of intelligence

Average or above

DIAGNOSTIC IMPRESSION

*Substance use disorder, Dysthymic Disorder (or
Depressive Neurosis), Possible Avoidant Personality*

TREATMENT PLAN

PROBLEMS	GOALS	TREATMENT
Poor nutritional status	*Improve status*	*Offer balanced, high cal diet suited to his vegetarian preference.*
Poor hygiene status	*Improve status*	*Encourage daily bathing. Refer to Dentist*
Dependence on Cannabis	*Decrease usage*	*Refer to Group Therapy*
Depression	*Control Sx*	*Prescribe anti-depress. medication. Refer to Psych. Therapist for individual counseling*

Figure 12–6 (continued)

MEDICAL RECORD		PROBLEM-ORIENTED PROGRESS NOTES

PROBLEM

DATE | **NO.**

Format—Problem title (Do not abbreviate) S-Subjective O-Objective A-Assessment P-Plans. (All notes must have signature and title of person making entry.) Continue on reverse.

12-4-88 | 3 | Problem Title: Angry and agitated.

Subjective: "I can't take anymore of this — I have to get out!"

Objective: Client is pacing, crying, waving his hands, yelling at nursing staff and other patients. Looks very upset.

Assessment: Client has just completed interview with his private therapist, who told him his wife has filed for divorce, and won't talk to him about it.

Plan: 1. Give client time and space to decrease agitation
2. Offer him use of quiet room
3. Keep him in eye contact but do not engage him at this time
4. If he is not quieter in 1 hr offer PRN medication.

J. Knight, RN
Clinical Specialist

PROBLEM-ORIENTED
PROGRESS NOTES

EXISTING STOCK OF VA FORM 10-7978i,
OCT 1974, WILL BE USED.

VA FORM 10-7978i

Figure 12–7
Sample form for problem-oriented progress notes.
Source: Veterans Administration Hospital, Buffalo, NY.

- It improves the communication skills of nurses. When nurses examine their words, gestures, and nonverbal communication, they can reduce their use of clichés, double messages, and stereotyped, automatic comments.
- It gives the nurse a tool for assessing nurse-client interactions and gives the instructor, clinical supervisor, or consultant a tool for assessing and guiding the nurse in clinical work. It supplements memory, facilitates evaluation, and acquaints the student with rudimentary applied research skills. It also asks the nurse to produce written comments grounded in theory.
- It provides data from which nurses can assess their own behavior in interactions with clients. By encouraging nurses to examine their personal reactions to client behavior, the IPA enriches their self-understanding and experience. An added advantage of the IPA is that it allows nurses to look at the dynamics of nurse-client behavior when they are away from the interpersonal situation. They can often gain some objectivity through distance.
- It helps nurses plan nursing interventions. By evaluating the effectiveness of therapeutic strategies in actual clinical situations and linking their observations to theory, nurses can identify additional or alternative nursing interventions.

Methods

There are several ways to structure IPAs. Two-, three-, or four-column styles may be used. Regardless of the organizational style, however, the IPA should include these components:

- The verbal and nonverbal communication of the client
- The verbal and nonverbal communication of the nurse
- Analysis or interpretation of the possible significance of the communication
- Identification of the nurse's own feelings
- Identification of the possible intent of the nurse's communication
- Identification of the nurse's perception of the client's emotions and the intent of the client's communication
- Evaluation of the effectiveness of the approach, based on the above data
- The nursing alternatives used and the rationale for their use

The raw data or verbatim recording can be obtained in a number of ways.

On-the-Spot Recording

The nurse may make brief notes on the spot, often using some type of shorthand code consisting of symbols and

abbreviations, in a stenographer's notebook. There are several advantages to this form of recording. Notes on verbal communication can be made easily, it is a more accurate technique than attempting to recall after the experience, and it prevents the nurse from unwittingly omitting important material. It also demonstrates that the nurse is paying close attention to what the client says and does. However, the nurse usually interacts less freely and becomes less spontaneous when recording on the spot, because of the need to attend to the note-taking task. It may also limit observation of the nonverbal components of the client's communication.

After-the-Fact Recording

When gathering data by recall, it is important to record them as soon as possible after the interaction with the client. The most successful method is for nurses to structure their time so that they can begin writing in a quiet area immediately. The longer the time between interaction and recording, the less able nurses are to remember words and actions and their sequence. If it is difficult to set aside enough time, raw data alone should be recorded at once, and analysis of the data may be delayed. A delay may actually improve analysis. It may allow a more objective interpretation, as time and distance make nurses less protective of their original behavior.

This method of recording is advantageous in that it does not require the nurse to take notes while paying close attention to the client. It thus does not curtail the nurse's spontaneity. The major disadvantage is that the nurse may not remember completely and thus distort the interaction. Nurses using this method of recording tend to omit or shorten important details.

Tape Recording

The most common form of mechanical recording is by audiotape. Tape recorders are now smaller, less expensive, and less obtrusive than earlier models were. Videotape recordings may also be used. Although now available in portable form, they are costly and are less commonly used.

Tape-recorded data can be transcribed at the nurse's leisure and provide a more accurate record of verbal interactions than notes do. The recording avoids unintentional editing or condensation of important content. Nurses who use a tape recorder can reexperience tones of voice, pauses, silences, speaking rates, actual words, and sequences of responses. Because tapes force nurses to listen to themselves as they actually are rather than as they would like to be, using a tape recorder may cause anxiety. Clients may fear being "on tape" and refuse to give the nurse permission to tape the session. Other disadvantages to tape-recording are that it does not pick up visual cues, and transcribing the tape can be costly and/or time-consuming.

Confidentiality and Comprehensiveness of IPAs

The nurse who records client data has the responsibility to protect the client from unwarranted exposure. The client's name should not appear on the IPA, and the record should not be treated carelessly or left lying about. The nurse's respect for the client's self-disclosures is one way for the client to gauge the nurse's trustworthiness.

Cutting corners in preparing an IPA is inadvisable, because meaningful exchanges may be bypassed. In order to be an effective learning tool, the IPA should be comprehensive.

Chapter Highlights

- The nursing process begins with assessment, and the primary source of client data in most instances is the client.

- Correct problem identification and intervention strategies often depend on the quality of information sharing.

- Psychiatric client information is gathered and assessed through psychiatric history-taking, mental status examination, physiologic assessment, psychologic testing, psychosocial assessments, and interaction process analysis.

- Traditionally, history-taking has followed a medical model and is most concerned with gathering information about a client's psychiatric problem.

- The mental status examination is used to identify a person's general behavior and appearance, characteristics of talk, emotional state, special preoccupations and experiences, sensorium or orientation, memory, general intelligence, abstract thinking, and insight; its primary purpose is to gather data to formulate a psychiatric diagnosis, prognosis, and treatment plan.

- Psychologic tests are tests concerned with measuring intelligence or personality.

- It is particularly important for the nurse to rule out a physiologic or neurologic basis for mental symptoms by conducting a thorough history, directly observing the client, and completing a neurologic assessment.

- The DSM-IIIR is the APA's most recent system for diagnosing and classifying mental disorders and is more congruent with holistic views of people than were DSM-II or DSM-I.

- Axes IV (Severity of Psychosocial Stressors) and V (Global Assessment of Functioning in the past year) of DSM-IIIR best represent the practice domain of nursing and are the areas in which nursing's greatest contribution may lie.

- In conducting a psychosocial assessment to determine a client's problems, the nurse should include physical, intellectual, socioeconomic and developmental factors, personal values and goals, adaptive functioning, and response to present involvements.

- Recording provides the basis for altering treatment plan, determining intervention, linking health team members, gaining around-the-clock data on hospitalized clients, evidence in court, and research.

- The most significant events the psychiatric nurse records are the behavior patterns and interpersonal interactions of the client.

- The psychosocial nurse uses psychiatric jargon sparingly, recognizing its inadequacies for understanding the depth and variety of human problems.

- Problem-oriented systems of recording are comprehensive and logically structured; they can be used in the psychiatric audit, to develop nursing care plans, and to devise algorithms.

References

Carpenito L: *Nursing Diagnoses: Applications to Clinical Practice.* Lippincott, 1983.

Compton BR, Galaway B: *Social Work Processes,* ed 2. Dorsey Press, 1979.

Diagnostic and Statistical Manual of Mental Disorders, IIIR. American Psychiatric Association, 1987.

Hagerty B: *Psychiatric-Mental Health Assessment.* Mosby, 1984.

Kaplan HI, Sadock BJ: *Modern Synopsis of Comprehensive Textbook of Psychiatry,* ed 4. Williams & Wilkins, 1985.

McFarland GK, Wasli EL: *Nursing Diagnosis and Process in Psychiatric Mental Health Nursing.* Lippincott, 1986.

Morgan AJ, Moreno JW: *The Practice of Mental Health Nursing: A Community Approach.* Lippincott, 1973.

Morrison E, et al: The NSGAE. *J Psychosocial Nurs* 1985;23(8):10–13.

Patient assessment: Neurological examination. (Programmed instruction.) *Am J Nurs* 1975;75 (Part I, September): PI, pp 1–24. 1975;75 (Part II, November): PI, pp 1–24. 1976;76 (Part III, April): PI, pp 1–25.

Small SM: *Outline for Psychiatric Examination.* Sandoz, 1980.

Spitzer RL, Forman JBW: DSM-III field trials: II. Initial experience with the multiaxial system. *Am J Psychiatry* 1979;136:818–820.

Spitzer RL, Williams JBW, Skodol AE: DSM-III: The major achievements and an overview. *Am J Psychiatry* 1980;137:151–164.

Williams JBW: DSM-IIIR preview: Psychotic and mood disorders. *Hosp Community Psychiatry* 1987;38(1):13–14.

Williams JBW, Wilson HS: A psychiatric nursing perspective on DSM-III. *J Psychosocial Nurs* 1982;20:14–20.

Wilson HS, Skodol AE: Introduction and overview of changes in DSM-III-R. *Arch Psychiatric Nurs* (in press.)

THIRTEEN

Group Process

Carol Ren Kneisl

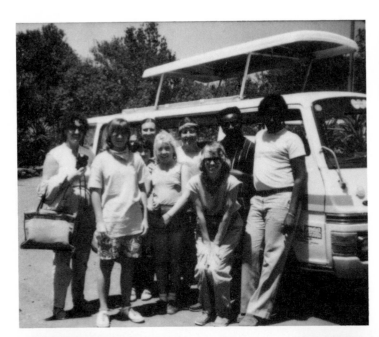

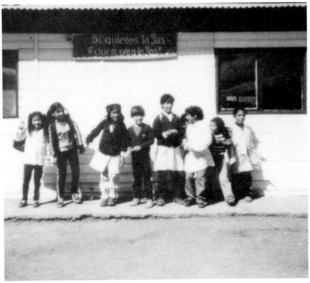

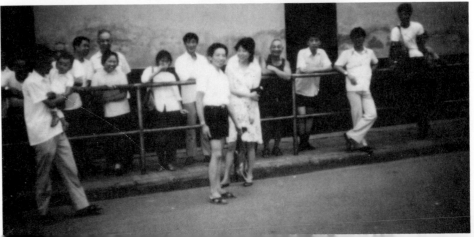

After reading this chapter, students should be able to

- Develop an appreciation for the influence of group dynamics in the lives of people

- Recognize the influence of the physical environment on a group

- Discuss the influence of the leadership approach on a group

- Identify the process of decision making and the various decision-making methods in groups

- Discuss the importance of trust in group functioning

- Explain the importance of cohesion to effective group functioning

- Describe how power influences the nature, operation, and interpersonal patterns in groups

- Apply knowledge of group process in work with groups of clients and groups of colleagues

Cross References

Other topics related to this content are: Client government groups, Chapter 31; Groups as a means of social support, Chapter 8; Group therapy with adolescents, Chapter 35; Group therapy with children, Chapter 34; Techniques of group therapy, Chapter 30; and Theories and models for understanding group therapy, Chapter 30.

Imagine teaching people to think and relate in mature productive ways in the international arena.

Key Terms

cohesion	norms
group dynamics	personal space
groupthink	task roles
hidden agenda	territoriality
maintenance roles	trust

People live most of their lives in groups. They depend on others for much of their sense of personal fulfillment and achievement. The activities they undertake toward personal fulfillment are, more often than not, activities that are carried out in the company of others.

Why are groups so important? Human beings are born into a group—the family—and their survival from the moment of birth depends on relationships formed with other human beings. The sense of self, of being, of personal identity derives from the ways in which people are perceived and responded to by the other members of the groups to which they belong. The self, according to the symbolic interactionist George Herbert Mead (1934), is essentially a social structure that arises from social experience. People interact with others at all stages of their lives in various groups—family groups, peer groups, work groups, play groups, worship groups.

Many of the goals people set for themselves cannot be achieved without membership in groups. Other people are important to each of us, just as we are important to others. Through cooperation and coordination in groups, we are able to achieve objectives and reach goals that would be unreachable through individual effort alone. In this way groups help us improve the quality of our lives.

Much of the nurse's professional life is spent in groups—groups of clients and groups of colleagues with whom the nurse plans and implements the delivery of health care services. To use groups rationally and effectively, nurses must understand the forces that underlie small group interactional processes and recognize their own patterns of participation. The goal of this chapter is to help the nurse understand group process and to lay the foundation for understanding Chapter 30, which deals with group therapy.

HISTORICAL AND THEORETICAL PERSPECTIVES

Although small groups have been around for as long as history itself, scientific interest in the operation and dynamics of small groups can be traced to the work of sociologists and social psychologists in the 1940s and 1950s. Notable among these early theorists was Kurt Lewin, who introduced the notion that a group was different from the simple sum of its parts. Lewin theorized that the behavior of an individual in a group cannot be based on an understanding of the psychodynamics of that individual alone but must be understood in relation to the group itself.

The small-group theories that resulted from these early studies form the base for understanding **group dynamics,** Lewin's term for the total of all the interactions among members of a group. Although there is as yet no one theory that adequately explains why people behave the way they do when in groups, several theoretical constructs help to explain the forces that modify and shape groups. Among these are decision-making processes, leadership, and power. These explanations are discussed later in this chapter.

Since World War II there has been a tremendous growth in the group movement and a corresponding increase in the variety of group methods and group approaches in existence. In addition to the recreational groups, educational groups, and even therapy groups that gained acceptance after the war, growth groups have become popular. These are oriented to understanding the self and the experience of membership by analyzing interactions with others in groups. Sadock (1985) proposes that an important factor that accounts for this growth is the waning influence of such natural groupings as the family and organized religion. Because human beings are gregarious animals with a strong desire to belong, small groups can provide the social network to help satisfy our strong desires to belong.

There are similarities and differences among the characteristics of various types of groups, e.g., task groups, self-awareness/growth groups, therapy groups, and social groups. Their characteristics are compared in Table 13–1.

IMPORTANCE OF GROUP DYNAMICS

A Study in Contrast

The Health Science Student Council at Anomie University held its monthly meeting yesterday. The council is composed of six members, four men and two women, who represent the health science schools on campus. The women represent nursing and occupational therapy; the men, medicine, dentistry, pharmacy, and physical therapy. The members arrived out of breath and in disarray. The meeting had been called only one hour before by the council president, the representative from the medical school. One member arrived in damp and sweaty clothes directly from the racquetball court; another had been taking a nap and arrived without changing his clothes or washing his face; a third arrived in uniform and breathless, after dashing from the hospital unit to which she was assigned. The meeting was held in the health science library in a cramped and dusty room that stored little-used books from the early 1900s. The vice-president of the council chose to sit at the head of the rectangular table, forcing the president to take a seat on one side.

The meeting, to decide joint projects to be undertaken during the current academic year, got off to a rocky start. The vice-president attempted to open the meeting, until the president reminded him of his subordinate status. The president then reminded the members at length that, of all the health science schools on campus, the medical school could provide the largest money grants to the council, because of that school's large alumni contributions and research grants. Most members expressed their unhappiness with the president's lecture. Members then began to debate which school was "better," had greater university and national recognition, had more money, and represented the most prestigious health science profession. Within ten minutes, the vice-president, the secretary, and two members had walked out. The question of which joint projects the council would undertake had not even been raised.

At the same time a group meeting was taking place at Connection College. Six women elected by their classmates represented the freshman, sophomore, junior, senior, first-year graduate, and second-year graduate nursing classes. The members arrived at the meeting ahead of the scheduled time. The chairperson had reserved one of the conference rooms at the Student Union, which are made available to student organizations, clubs, and committees for meetings. It was a comfortable room with bright windows, lounge chairs, and coffee service. The members sat around the circular table to discuss the items on the agenda—the choice of a place, date, and speaker for the commencement banquet.

The hour-long meeting proceeded smoothly. It was opened by the chairperson, who identified the group task and reviewed the experiences of the previous year's committee. She requested the opinions and ideas of each member and paid careful attention to any ideas or suggestions offered. Each suggestion was discussed and evaluated by the entire group before being either accepted or rejected. Unanimous decisions were reached. After adjournment most members stayed behind to chat about matters unrelated to the commencement banquet.

These two group meetings were clearly different experiences for their members. The Health Science Student

Table 13–1
Differences in Characteristics of Types of Groups

Characteristic	Task Groups	Self-Awareness/ Growth Groups	Therapy Groups	Social Groups
Purpose, goals	Performance of specific job or task explicitly agreed on by all members at initiation of group. Member participation is determined by task.	Development or use of interpersonal strengths. Broad objectives, such as to study group process, communication patterns, or problem solving are usually apparent at initiation of group.	Clearly defined: to do the work of therapy. Individual works toward self-understanding, more satisfactory ways of relating, handling stress, and so on.	Recreation, relaxation, and comfort promoted through mutual pleasure and enjoyment among friends and acquaintances in a social situation such as a party at someone's home.
Shared aim	To achieve group's task goal.	To improve functioning of group one returns to (job, family, community) through translation of one's own interpersonal strengths or to improve perception of members.	To improve perception of members and to improve individual health.	To experience fun, companionship, and satisfying relationships with friends.
Format	Defined at outset by leader and/or members. Method is specific to task to be performed.	Specific format, if any, and methods defined throughout group process by all members and leader/ trainer. Lack of agenda and structure may produce some difficulty.	Defined by therapist within context of some psychotherapeutic orientation. Definition is apparent through implementation of therapeutic principles.	Usually spontaneous. May be defined by members in case of planned recreational activities.
Focus	Completion of specific task.	Interpersonal concerns around current situations.	Member-centered. Past experiences may be just as relevant as current concerns depending on therapist's orientation.	Member-centered toward enjoyment and mutual meeting of needs.
Role of leader	To establish exchange of information among members and direct group toward task accomplishment, adhering to agenda.	To establish group interaction at emotional level among group members, and to serve as resource person guiding group by calling attention to certain events or processes and facilitating problem solving, mutual understanding, communication.	To establish group interaction between self and individual members and among group members. To facilitate members' interactions in work of therapy.	To meet basic requirements for social companionship, providing place, planning activity, preparing food, drink, etc.
Title of leader	Usually called chairperson.	Usually called trainer.	Usually called therapist.	Usually called host or hostess.

continued

Table 13–1 (continued)
Differences in Characteristics of Types of Groups

Characteristic	Task Groups	Self-Awareness/ Growth Groups	Therapy Groups	Social Groups
How leader differs from members	Chairperson identifies specific task, clarifies communication, and assists in expressing opinions and offering solutions.	Trainer differs from members by having superior skills in specialized area (understanding and facilitating group process). Trainer's superiority diminishes as group continues and members learn and implement similar skills.	Therapist differs from members by having superior skills in specialized area (group psychotherapy). Therapist never truly becomes member but may at times take on members' roles.	Host or hostess is member of group and works toward own as well as others' pleasure and enjoyment.
Requirements of leader	Qualified background and expertise in area of task emphasis. Must be accepted by members as an appropriate leader.	Sufficient preparation, experience, and skill to maintain effective control of interpersonal tensions.	Sufficient preparation and skill to undertake psychotherapy within context of situation.	Willingness to take steps to initiate social interaction.
Orientation of group work	Reality oriented in terms of adhering to explicit work goal. If group deviates into interpersonal realm, task is not accomplished most efficiently.	Reality testing with here-and-now emphasis. Assumption is that members can correct inefficient patterns of relating and communicating with each other. Members learn group process experientially through participation and involvement.	Oriented toward having members gain insight as basis for changing patterns of behavior toward health.	Oriented toward having fun, seeking pleasure and relaxation, releasing tension.
Selection of members	Selection made possibly in terms of individual's functional role, not usually in terms of personal characteristics, often in terms of employment status.	Selection criteria range from simply expressed desire to become more self-aware to mixture of criteria based on personality characteristics.	Selection usually based on extensive consideration of constellation of personalities, behaviors, and needs and identification of group therapy as treatment of choice.	Selection based on considerations of friendship or social obligation. Host or hostess chooses whom to invite.
Title of members	Known as committee members.	May be called trainees.	Known as clients or, in some settings, patients.	Known as guests.
Interviewing of prospective members	Usually not interviewed before entry into group.	May or may not be interviewed and/or requested to complete questionnaires on personal data and personality characteristics before entry into group.	Extensive selection interview(s) required before entry into group.	Not interviewed. Usually known through prior social acquaintance.
Length of group life	Target date usually set in advance.	Tends to be short term, with target date set in advance.	Usually not set. Termination date usually determined mutually by therapist and members.	May be set in advance or spontaneously determined.

Council meeting at Anomie University was characterized by dissension, unilateral activity on the part of members, interpersonal conflict, and ineffectiveness. The Commencement Banquet Committee at Connection College was friendly, organized, thorough, and effective. This chapter will demonstrate that the factors that influence the behavior of the members of the Health Science Student Council and the Commencement Banquet Committee are factors that influence all groups in action—nursing teams, therapy groups, governing boards, and so on. These are the factors that make the difference between effective and ineffective groups.

Characteristics of an Effective Group

To be effective, any group must accomplish three main functions:

1. Accomplishing its designated goals
2. Maintaining its own cohesion
3. Developing and modifying its structure to improve its effectiveness

Some factors that influence these functions and can be used to evaluate the effectiveness of a given group are detailed in Table 13–2. They constitute the major characteristics generally observable in effective and ineffective groups and illustrate different ways of dealing with the dynamic forces in every group.

FORCES THAT MODIFY AND SHAPE GROUPS

Several forces shape the structure and functioning of groups. The following sections elaborate on factors such as: space and seating arrangements; color, noise level, and decor; leadership styles and roles; methods of decision making; member trust; risk-taking behavior; cohesion and conformity; interpersonal attraction; and power and influence.

Physical Environment

Groups exist in complex environmental settings that strongly influence the group process. The building, room, and chair and table arrangements are aspects of the environmental setting that influence the operation of the group. Super-

---

RESEARCH NOTE

Citation

Selander JM, Miller WC: Prolixin group: Can nursing intervention groups lower recidivism rates? J Psychosoc Nurs Ment Health Serv *1985;23:16–20.*

Study Problem/Purpose

The purpose of this study was to answer the research question: Does receiving fluphenazine (Prolixin) in a nursing intervention group versus receiving neuroleptics in a variety of settings reduce the relapse rate of the group members?

Methods

The number of psychiatric admissions and the duration of hospitalizations of clients after they became members of a Prolixin group were compared to the number of admissions and the duration of hospitalizations before they entered the group. During each meeting, members had fifty minutes of group discussion; ten minutes were spent on fluphenazine injection. For each subject, the ratio of the total time spent in the hospital divided by the total number of admissions to the hospital was computed both over the total number of months in the Prolixin group and over a matching number of months prior to membership in the Prolixin group. Correlated *t*-tests were then computed.

Findings

The mean number of admissions was reduced from 2.6 before treatment to 1.0 after treatment. The mean of the total duration of hospitalizations in days was 133.7 before treatment compared to 30.8 after treatment. The mean average duration of each hospitalization was 71.4 days before treatment compared to 13.2 days after treatment.

Implications

A Prolixin group can reduce the relapse rate of its members as evidenced by fewer and shorter hospitalizations. In these days of decreased funding and increased accountability, this method offers nursing an opportunity to demonstrate that it can cost effectively combine nursing intervention though the group process with medication surveillance and medication administration. The group is also a way to teach clients group process, the target symptoms of schizophrenia, and the effects and side-effects of medications.

Table 13–2
Comparative Features of Effective and Ineffective Groups

Factor	Effective Groups	Ineffective Groups
Atmosphere	Informal, comfortable, and relaxed. It is a working atmosphere in which people demonstrate their interest and involvement.	Obviously tense. Signs of boredom may appear.
Goal setting	Goals, tasks, and objectives are clarified, understood, and modified so that members of the group can commit themselves to cooperatively structured goals.	Unclear, misunderstood, or imposed goals may be accepted by members. The goals are competitively structured.
Leadership and member participation	Shift from time to time, depending on the circumstances. Different members assume leadership at various times, because of their knowledge or experience.	Delegated and based on authority. The chairperson may dominate the group, or the members may defer unduly. Member participation is unequal, with high-authority members dominating.
Goal emphasis	All three functions of groups—goal accomplishment, internal maintenance, and developmental change—are emphasized.	One or more functions may not be emphasized.
Communication	Open and two-way. Ideas and feelings are encouraged, both about the problem and about the group's operation.	Closed or one-way. Only the production of ideas is encouraged. Feelings are ignored or taboo. Members may be tentative or reluctant to be open and have "hidden agendas" (personal goals at cross-purposes with group goals).
Decision making	By consensus, although various decision-making procedures appropriate to the situation may be instituted.	By the highest authority in the group with minimal involvement by members, or an inflexible style is imposed.
Cohesion	Facilitated through high levels of inclusion, trust, liking, and support.	Either ignored or used as a means of controlling members, thus promoting rigid conformity.
Conflict tolerance	The reason for disagreements or conflicts are carefully examined and the group seeks to resolve them. The group accepts basic disagreements that cannot be resolved and lives with them.	Attempts may be made to ignore, deny, avoid, suppress, or override controversy by premature group action.
Power	Determined by the members' abilities and the information they possess. Power is shared. The issue is how to get the job done.	Determined by position in the group. Obedience to authority is strong. The issue is who controls.
Problem-solving ability	High. Constructive criticism is frequent, frank, relatively comfortable, and oriented toward removing obstacles to problem solving.	Low. Criticism may be destructive, taking the form of either overt or covert personal attacks. It prevents the group from getting the job done.
Self-evaluation as a group	Frequent. All members participate in evaluation and decisions about how to improve the group's functioning.	Minimal. What little evaluation there is may be done by the highest authority in the group, rather than by the membership as a whole.
Creativity	Encouraged. There is room within the group for members to become self-actualized and interpersonally effective.	Discouraged. People are afraid of appearing foolish if they put forth a creative thought.

imposed on the physical structure are the influences of territoriality, personal space, and cultural background. As you read about these influences, try to visualize the specific and peculiar features of hospital units, nurses' stations, and ward versus private accommodations for hospitalized clients.

Territoriality

Most people at some time have experienced violating an unspoken and unwritten rule by sitting in someone else's chosen seat. The violator may be treated to some form of protest—a direct one in which the "proprietor" of the seat points out the transgression, or a less direct one in which the proprietor may complain of the behavior to others and/or send darting glances of hostility in the violator's direction.

This assumption of proprietary rights to space is but one example of the notion of territoriality. **Territoriality** can be defined as the assumption of a proprietary attitude toward a geographic area by a person or a group. People defend their right to the designated territory against invasion by others despite the lack of legal sanction. People do not really "own" their territory but rather occupy it, permanently or intermittently, and act as if the property belonged to them.

Avoidance of intragroup conflict depends in part on the degree to which group members respect one another's territorial rights. Intergroup conflict may result when one group fails to respect the territorial rights of another group; in fact, this is how most wars between nations begin. In addition, territoriality provides a modicum of privacy for the individual or the group. It may also serve as a method of dominance by an individual or a group over others. The head nurse's chair, or the unit chief's chair at the head of the conference table, are concrete examples.

Personal Space

Personal space is an invisible bubble of territory around a person's body into which intruders may not come. It differs from territoriality in that it is space maintained and carried around with the person, rather than a specific geographic location. Robert Sommer (1969), a psychologist who studied the effects of physical setting on attitudes and behavior, has stated that the best way to learn the location of the invisible boundary of personal space is to keep walking toward a person until he or she complains.

A common defensive response to unwanted intrusion is selecting a position that is as inaccessible as possible. Another common response is flight. The need to defend personal space may also interfere with group functioning. Unwanted intrusion of one member into another's personal space creates discomfort, unease, and other negative feelings. These feelings are revealed in the group dynamics and interfere with group progress.

Cultural Background

The anthropologist Edward T. Hall (1969) identifies cultural background as a strong influence on territoriality and personal space. An American who wants to be alone goes into a room and shuts the door, relying on architectural features for screening. English people have never developed the habit of using space to protect themselves from others. They use other barriers, such as "the silent treatment," which they expect others to recognize and respect. When an Englishman becomes silent in the company of an American man, the American is likely to expend extra effort to break through the barrier to assure himself that all is well.

Americans believe that propinquity (geographic nearness) is an acceptable basis for interaction. Living next door to a family entitles a neighbor family to socialize with the members, borrow a cup of flour from them, and have its children play with theirs. To others, propinquity is not enough, especially when relationships are patterned around social status rather than space.

Most Europeans perceive Americans as loud. They believe this to be an intrusive trait, for being overheard interferes with the privacy of others. Americans perceive their "loudness" as an expression of openness or having nothing to hide. They perceive the quiet or hushed conversations of others as sly or secretive.

Conditions that people in the United States perceive as crowded, others (Latin Americans and those from Mediterranean cultures) may perceive as spacious. A North American in Latin America or the Middle East is likely to feel crowded and hemmed in. In this person's view, people come too close and touch too much. The Middle Eastern or Latin American may experience the North American as cold. But, in English and Scandinavian cultures, it is the North American who perceives the others as aloof.

Influences from the various cultures carry over from generation to generation. For satisfactory functioning, a group must pay attention to the cultural factors that influence the individual member. In the large hospital or metropolitan mental health center where members of many cultures come together, these differences may promote misunderstandings and thwart effective group functioning.

Material Aspects of the Setting

The material aspects of the physical environment influence the functioning of groups in interesting ways. Students in social science courses are generally told of the well-known studies of worker productivity conducted at Western Electric Company (Roethlisberger and Dickson 1939). The investigators found that workers at first were more productive when the intensity of lighting was increased. However, after a period of weeks, production fell. This time the researchers decreased the lighting intensity and found the same effect—productivity increased again—even though this environmental change was directly opposite to the first one. This phenomenon, called the *Hawthorne effect,* spurred a host of other studies. Similar results were reported in studies that introduced music, coffee breaks, and so on. The primary variable seemed to be the workers' perception of the situation; if they believed that someone cared enough about them to be concerned about the conditions under which they worked, they responded by working harder and/ or more effectively than when they believed no one cared about them.

Color and noise have been found to influence people's perceptions and performance. In one work situation, women workers complained of feeling uncomfortably cold with the thermostat at seventy-five degrees when the room was painted a cool blue (Seghers 1948). The same women complained of feeling too warm at the same temperature, when the room was painted in warm yellows and restful greens. Recent research indicates that a specific shade of pink initially decreases aggressive behavior. In response, some prisons have painted their jail cells pink. Unpredictable noise has been found to evoke feelings of frustration and lead to a decrease in performance. Sound conditioning of work areas has been found to reduce worker discomfort and annoyance.

Other studies have been done on the effects of "beautiful" rooms versus "ugly" rooms. The beautiful room was an attractively decorated, comfortable study. The ugly room was a cluttered, messy, and unsightly storeroom. Participants in the ugly room reported more headaches, monot-

ony, fatigue, hostility, discontent, and room avoidance than did participants in the beautiful room (Mintz 1956).

These studies about the material aspects of a setting indicate that elements of the environment are important in determining group and individual behavior (Figure 13–1). Productivity, interpersonal behavior, and intrapsychic experiences are all affected.

Spatial Arrangements

Seating arrangements have been methodically studied since Bernard Steinzor first wrote about the face-to-face discussion groups he was conducting in 1950. His interest was piqued by the behavior of one of his group members—a man who changed his seat in order to sit directly opposite another man with whom he had previously had an argument. Since that time, researchers have found that adults prefer a side-by-side arrangement for cooperation and a direct face-to-face arrangement for competition. This knowledge can be helpful in understanding the interaction among members of a psychotherapy group, a nursing team conference, or an interdisciplinary clinical conference at a community mental health agency.

People also select positions according to their perceived status in the group. Studies of twelve-person jury tables have demonstrated that jurors holding managerial or professional status frequently select the chair at the head of the table. Jurors seated at the end positions of the rectangular jury table tended to be more influential and to participate more than persons who chose side positions (Strodtbeck and Hook 1961).

There is also a relationship between spatial arrangement and leadership. Since the person who sits at the head of the table is usually perceived as the leader, the spatial position a person occupies in a group has important consequences for that person's chances of emerging as a group leader or for undertaking significant leadership responsibilities. Round tables tend to enhance the development of leadership traits among the membership rather than to invest certain members with authority because of their spatial position.

There are many other fascinating facets to the influence of space and environment on groups and individuals. This presentation provides only a starting point for further study by interested readers.

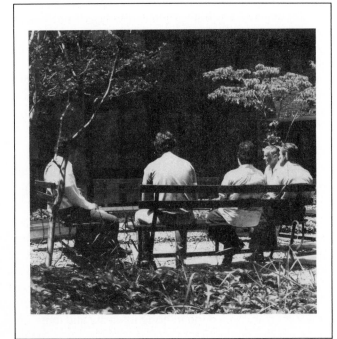

Figure 13–1
An attractive setting helps to enhance a group's ability to work effectively. A flexible seating arrangement is even better.

Leadership

Leadership functions within a group are executed under two general conditions: (a) by the person designated as the leader, and (b) by members who engage in leadership behavior. This distinction is an important one for understanding the emergence of leadership within groups.

The process of leadership is an influence relationship that occurs among mutually dependent group members in their attempts to achieve the group's goals. Because all group members influence other members, at times, each member will exert leadership at some time in the group's life. This approach to understanding leadership behavior is called the *distributed functions approach*. Other approaches are also considered in this section.

Distributed Functions Approach

The functional approach to group leadership is based on two major beliefs:

1. Any member of a group may become a leader by taking actions that serve group functions.
2. Different members may fulfill various functions.

Each member may enact more than one role during a meeting of the group and a wide range of roles in successive participations. Any or all of the roles may be played by any member. The various functional roles may be grouped in two categories:

1. **Task roles** are related to the task of the group. Their purpose is to facilitate and coordinate group efforts in the selection, definition, and solution of a group problem. Examples of task roles are *information seeker, information giver, elaborator, procedural technician, coordinator, opinion seeker,* and *opinion giver* among others.
2. **Maintenance roles** are oriented toward building group-centered attitudes among the members and maintaining and perpetuating group-centered behavior. Members who function as *encourager, compromiser, standard setter, follower, group observer,* or *harmonizer* carry out some of the maintenance roles possible in groups.

Sometimes members of a group behave in ways designed to satisfy individual needs that are irrelevant to the group task. These *self-serving roles* (the *recognition seeker, blocker, aggressor, dominator, self-confessor,* and *playboy* for example) may also be negatively oriented to group maintenance functions. If a group is to function effectively, it must perform a self-diagnosis to determine what the needs of the group are, and how they can be met, so that the self-serving roles no longer present obstacles to effective functioning.

The functional theory of group leadership emphasizes the importance of distributing leadership functions among the group members. Distributed leadership is believed to be the most effective approach, because it teaches people the diagnostic skills and behaviors needed to accomplish the group task and maintain good interpersonal relationships. The distributed functions approach can be best described through its main assumption: *Responsible mem-*

bership is the same thing as responsible leadership. Of course, in psychotherapy groups, there may be some functions or activities that are largely, or even solely, the province of the therapist.

Trait Approach

The trait approach is essentially a "great person" theory. It is based on the belief that a leader is a charismatic person who possesses unique, inborn leadership traits. Its central thesis is that leaders are born, not made; discovered, not trained.

However, researchers have found similar traits both in leaders and in followers, so this theory does not explain what makes one person assume a leadership role while another does not. The assumption can be made, however, that people who are energetic, self-confident, determined, and motivated to succeed will become leaders, because they work hard to reach positions of leadership.

Position Approach

The position approach defines leadership as a position of authority in the formal role system that defines the authority hierarchy. Although this approach can certainly explain who has the designated title of leader at a drug-abuse outreach center, for example, it does not take into account the fact that other members beside the designated leader influence the group's activities.

Style Approach

This classic theory of leadership behavior developed in 1939 by Lewin, Lippitt, and White identified three leadership styles: democratic, autocratic, and laissez faire. In the *democratic* style, the leader functions as a facilitator who encourages group discussion in decision making. The *autocratic* leader is one who determines policies unilaterally and gives orders and directions to the group members. The *laissez faire* condition is characterized by a hands-off style in which the leader participates at a minimal level.

The democratic style has proved the most effective. However, there are conditions under which each of the other two styles seems to be the most effective. For example, when an urgent decision is necessary, the autocratic style may be the most effective. A laissez faire style facilitates group functioning best when a group has made an effective decision, is committed to it, and is able to implement it.

Popularity of the style approach has waned in favor of the more comprehensive distributed functions theory of leadership.

Decision Making

A group that makes sound decisions is a group that functions effectively. The purpose of group decision making is to construct well-conceived, well-understood, and well-accepted realistic actions toward the goals agreed on by the group.

Effective Decisions

Five major characteristics of effective decisions are:

1. The resources of the group members are well used. The group listens to all members who have ideas or input helpful to the decision-making process.
2. The group's time is well used. The group concentrates on the task at hand and keeps interruptions and side-tracks to a minimum.
3. The decision is correct or of high quality. The alternative the group picks to execute is appropriate, reasonable, and error free.
4. The decision is put into effect fully by group members. Members feel committed to the decision and responsible for its implementation.
5. The problem-solving ability of the group is enhanced. Members feel satisfied with their participation, and the positive group atmosphere increases the members' perception of themselves as adequate problem solvers.

Decision Methods

There are several ways in which decisions can be made by a group.

- Decisions by *consensus* are reached when a group arrives at a collective opinion after each member has had a fair chance to exert influence. Unanimity is not always present in consensus decisions. However, members support the decision and are willing to give it a try.
- Sometimes group decisions are made by the person selected as the *group expert.*
- *Averaging members' opinions* is another method for arriving at decisions. It means that the most popular

opinion becomes the group decision. It may nonetheless be held by fewer than half the members.

- *Decision by majority vote,* 51 percent or more of the members, is the most common method used.
- Decisions can be made through *minority control* of a group. Executive committees of groups with many members exercise minority control of the whole group. A small minority may also quickly and forcefully "railroad" decisions (force the group to accept them by exerting intense pressure).
- In decision making by an *authority after discussion* with the members, the designated leader makes the final decision but first discusses the issue with the members to get their ideas and views.
- In decisions by *authority rule without discussion,* the designated leader makes decisions without consulting the group.

Each of these decision-making methods is appropriate at certain times. In psychotherapy groups, certain decisions (such as whether to add a new member, for example) should be made by the group expert—in this instance the group therapist—who has the clinical expertise. A group that has to make a decision must take several factors into account before selecting a method. Questions such as these should be raised: What type of decision has to be made? How much time can be spent in the decision-making process? What resources are available to the group? What is the past history of the group? What is the task to be worked on? How does the setting influence the method that should be chosen? What are the consequences of the particular method for the group's future operation? These questions are answered for each of the seven decision-making methods in Table 13–3.

Risk Taking in Group Decisions

An interesting phenomenon, the *risky shift,* occurs in the decision-making process of groups. Social psychologists Kogan and Wallach (1964) observed individuals who had previously made private decisions and then engaged in group discussion. The decisions made by the group were riskier than the members' private decisions. A risky shift has profound implications, particularly when the decision of a group may involve a large number of people.

Three major explanations for the risky shift have been given. The first is that high risk takers are more influential and persuasive than low risk takers. Thus, in a group decision the high risk takers' position will tend to win out over less risky alternatives. The second hypothesis is that in group decision-making, responsibility is diffused. Any cost or imagined loss that might result from a risky decision is borne by all rather than just one individual. The final explanation is that information about peer norms is received by group members through decision making. They learn the

Table 13–3
Strengths and Limitations of Decision-Making Methods

Method	Strengths	Limitations
Consensus	Produces innovative, creative, and high-quality decision; elicits commitment by all members to implement decision; uses the resources of all members; enhances future decision-making ability of group; is useful in making serious, important, and complex decisions requiring commitment from all members	Takes great deal of time and psychologic energy and high level of member skill; can be used only when time pressure is minimal and no emergency is in progress
Expert	Is useful when expertise of one person is so far superior to that of all other group members that little is to be gained by discussion; should be used when need for membership action in implementing decision is slight	Can be ineffective when it is difficult to determine who is expert; does not build commitment for implementing decision; loses advantages of group interaction; may result in resentment and disagreement that can sabotage group effectiveness; does not use resources of other members
Average of members' opinions	Is useful when it is difficult to get group members together to talk, when decision is so urgent that there is no time for group discussion, when member commitment is not necessary for implementing decision, and when group members lack skills and information to make decision any other way; is applicable to simple, routine decisions	Does not allow enough interaction among group members for them to gain from each other's resources and to get benefits of group discussion; does not build commitment for implementing decision; leaves unresolved conflict and controversy that may damage future group effectiveness
Majority vote	Can be used when sufficient time is lacking for decision by consensus or when decision is not so important that consensus needs to be used, and when complete member commitment is not necessary for implementing decision; closes discussion on issues that are not highly important for group	Usually leaves an alienated minority, which damages future group effectiveness; may lose relevant resources of many group members; does not build total commitment for implementing decision; does not obtain full benefit of group interaction
Minority control	Can be used when everyone cannot meet to make decision, when group is under such time pressure that it must delegate responsibility to committee, when only few members have any relevant resources, when broad member commitment is not needed to implement decision; is useful for simple, routine decisions	Does not use resources of many group members; does not establish widespread commitment for implementing decision; can leave unresolved conflict and controversy that may damage future group effectiveness; does not obtain much benefit from group interaction
Authority rule after discussion	Like consensus, uses resources of group members more than other methods; gains some benefits of group discussion	Does not develop commitment for implementing decision; does not resolve controversies and conflicts among group members; tends to create situations in which group members either compete to impress designated leader or tell leader what they think leader wants to hear
Authority rule without discussion	Applies more to administrative needs than to member needs; is useful for simple, routine decisions; should be used when very little time is available to make decision, when group members expect designated leader to make decision, and when group members lack skills and information to make decision any other way	Uses only one person as resource for every decision; loses advantages of group interaction; develops no commitment among other group members for implementing decision; can produce resentment and disagreement that may sabotage and reduce group effectiveness; does not use resources of other members

Source: Johnson DW, Johnson FP: Joining Together: Group Theory and Group Skills, 3/E, © 1987, pp 104–105. Adapted by permission of Prentice-Hall, Inc., Englewood Cliffs, New Jersey.

value attached to being risky in the process. Members then attempt to meet the group norm in relation to both risk and caution.

Indecisiveness

Sometimes a group has a hard time making decisions. Members find themselves unable to agree what the decision should be. Some reasons for indecisiveness are:

- Fear of the consequences of the decision

- Conflicts among members that make cooperative activity difficult

- Choice of a decision-making method inappropriate to the immediate situation

- Member loyalty to other groups that makes it difficult to commit themselves to making good decisions in this group

Once the reasons for indecisiveness have been identified and put on the table, a group can work to remove the obstacles in its way. It may be necessary for the group to rearrange its membership, redefine its task, select another decision-making method, or work at resolving the conflicts among its members before continuing its work on the identified task.

Trust

The complex phenomenon of **trust** has been studied by a variety of theorists and researchers. Some of the better-known work has been done by Morton Deutsch (1949, 1958). In this view, trusting behavior consists of the following four steps:

1. A person is in a situation where the decision to trust another may result in either positive or negative consequences for the self. The person realizes the risk involved in trusting another.

2. The person realizes that the future behavior of the other determines whether trusting will bring positive or negative consequences for the self.

3. The person will suffer more if the trust is violated than the person will gain if the trust is fulfilled.

4. The person feels reasonably confident that the other will behave in ways that will bring the beneficial consequences.

The person who decides to have minor elective surgery of little consequence is engaging in the four steps of trusting

behavior. The client: (a) recognizes that the choice could lead to either beneficial or harmful consequences, (b) realizes that the consequences of the choice depend on the behavior of the surgeon, (c) would suffer much more if the trust is violated and the surgeon does a bad job, and (d) feels relatively confident that the surgeon will make sure that beneficial consequences result.

Trust within relationships is built when people disclose more and more of their thoughts, perceptions, attitudes, and reactions to one another. The group member who makes a suggestion; discloses an attitude, feeling, experience, or perception; gives feedback; or confronts another also engages in trusting behavior and assumes the risks inherent in trusting. Trusting and being trusted are intimately linked to risk taking. The level of trust among the members of a group determines the extent of risk-taking behavior in the group.

Cohesion

"Hanging together" is the aspect of group life generally referred to as group **cohesion**. Groups that hang together or cohere possess a certain spirit of common purpose. The members have a yen for each other, for mutual association. Groups in which cohesion is minimal are those that seem always on the verge of breaking up or falling apart. Cohesion is the primary factor keeping a group in existence and working effectively.

The Need for Attraction

A group is cohesive when its members are attracted to it. People are attracted to a group for a wide variety of reasons. The group may meet their needs for affiliation, interpersonal security, or financial security. It may have admired members who not only are available for human interaction but also have important shared attitudes, values, interests, and beliefs. An attractive group has explicit, mutual, and attainable group goals with clear paths to goal attainment. Its members engage in a sort of interdependence that is cooperative rather than competitive. The activities the group undertakes are satisfying and successful, and there is a high degree of member participation in a democratic structure. Communication networks are open, central, and flexible in a warm and friendly atmosphere (Figure 13–2).

This implies that cohesive groups are not born but developed. While some features of attraction may account for a "love-at-first-sight" phenomenon, others do not become evident until the group has come together long enough to have shared experiences that provide the basis for attraction.

Evaluating Cohesion

What indicates that the spirit of cohesion exists in a given group? How do groups with sufficient cohesion differ from groups with minimal cohesion? At the beginning of this section on group dynamics we introduced two groups whose characteristics were radically different. The Health Science Student Council at Anomie University was only minimally cohesive. The more effective group, the Commencement Banquet Committee at Connection College, was "groupier." Table 13–4 identifies the characteristics of highly cohesive groups and compares them to those of minimally cohesive groups.

Building Cohesion

How can a group's tendency to cohere be enhanced? Some methods are increasing: the trusting and trustworthy behavior of members; the affection expressed among members; the expressions of inclusion and acceptance among members; and the influence that members have on one another. Two other methods for building cohesion are promoting group norms and structuring cooperative relationships among group members.

Promoting Group Norms

Norms are the set of unwritten rules of conduct or prescriptions of behavior established by members of a group. They derive from the common beliefs of the group about appropriate behavior. In other words, they tell how members are expected to behave. Norms prevent chaos because they lay out the expectations of members. They help members predict the behavior of others and anticipate the actions that they should take themselves.

Norms are evaluative. They tell members what ought and ought not be done. They represent value judgments that establish accepted standards for behavior. Some of the characteristics of norms that influence group behavior are:

- Norms are developed around situations that are important to the group. Groups do not establish norms for every conceivable situation.

- Norms may apply to every member of a group, or to certain members in specific roles only. For example, skiers are expected to wait their turn in the chair lift line, but a member of the National Ski Patrol may cut in at the head of the line without challenge.

- Norms vary in the degree to which they are accepted by group members. Most persons accept the norm that the driver of a vehicle should not pass a stopped school bus, but many violate the norm that drivers of slow-moving vehicles should stay in the right lane.

- Norms vary in the extent to which people can permissibly deviate from them. Violating a norm that members arrive for meetings on time is a more acceptable transgression than violating the norm against killing another person.

- Norms differ in the sanctions applied for their violation. Members who arrive late may be subjected to mild disapproval, but the member who kills another may be punished with life imprisonment or the death penalty.

The importance of norms in the power, influence, and conformity aspects of group life is discussed more completely later in this chapter.

Structuring Cooperative Relationships

All task groups have group goals. Anomie University's Health Science Student Council had the goal of deciding the joint projects to be undertaken during the current academic year. Connection College's Commencement Banquet Committee's goal was to decide the place, date, and speaker for the banquet. It takes cooperative action on the part of members to meet group goals.

In addition to group goals, members have individual goals. When the personal or individual goals of group members differ from the group goals, competitive relationships may develop that destroy the effectiveness of group relationships. For example, it is common for members who are in disagreement with the group goals to acquire hidden agendas that interfere with group functioning. A **hidden agenda** may be defined as a personal goal, unknown to the other group members, which is at cross-purposes with the dominant group goals. The vice-president of the Health Science Student Council at Anomie University may have

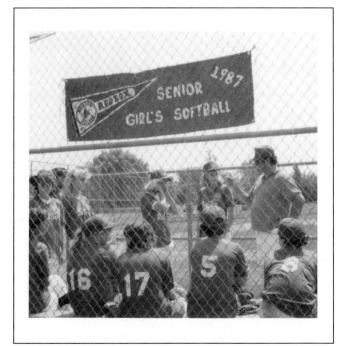

Figure 13–2
A high level of cohesion in this girl's softball team turned it into a championship team with a strong feeling of "we-ness."

	Table 13–4 Group Cohesion Assessment		
Characteristics of High-Cohesion Groups	**Characteristics of Low-Cohesion Groups**	**Characteristics of High-Cohesion Groups**	**Characteristics of Low-Cohesion Groups**
Members like one another	Members seem uncaring or may actively dislike one another	Group goals are consistent with goals of individuals	Group goals and individual goals are not consistent
Members are friendly and willing to interact	Members seem unfriendly and unwilling to become involved	Group goals can best be handled by group action	Goals can best be handled by individual action
Members enjoy interacting with one another and interact readily	Members get little pleasure from interaction and interact reluctantly	Group goals difficult to achieve are met by persistent efforts	Group goals difficult to achieve are given up
Members receive support on issues from one another	Members do not give one another active support	Attendance is high, and members arrive on time	Attendance is low or uneven, and members may arrive late or leave early
Members praise one another for accomplishments	Members do not acknowledge one another's accomplishments or belittle them	Efforts are directed toward maintaining, strengthening, and regulating group	Efforts are not directed toward maintaining, strengthening, and regulating group
Members share similar opinions and attitudes	Members have dissimilar or mutually exclusive opinions and attitudes	Risk taking is high	Risk taking is low
		Participation is high	Participation is low
Members are likely to influence one another and are willing to be influenced by other members	Members make few influence attempts and are unwilling to be influenced by other members	Commitment to group goals increases	Commitment to group goals is minimal
		Communication is high	Communication is low
		"We" is frequently heard in discussions	"I" is frequently heard in discussions
Members accept assigned tasks and roles readily	Members are reluctant or refuse to accept assigned tasks and roles	Leadership is democratic	Leadership is autocratic
		Group action is interdependent and cooperative	Group action is independent and competitive
Members trust one another	Members do not trust one another	Group output and productivity are high	Group output and productivity are low
Members are loyal to group and defend it against external criticism and attack	Members do not defend group and may criticize it to others	Group norms are adhered to and protected	Group norms are violated
		Members experience increase in security and self-esteem and reduction in anxiety	Members experience decrease in security and self-esteem and increase in anxiety
Members stay in group	Members drop out		
Group goals are valued	Group goals are not valued	Satisfaction with members and work of group is high	Satisfaction with members and work of group is low

had a hidden agenda (deposing the president, for example) that influenced his selection of a seat at the traditional "head of the table" position and his usurping of the president's privilege of opening the meeting.

To structure cooperative relationships around group and individual goals, members need to review and discuss group goals thoroughly when the group is formed even though goals may have been prescribed for the group by others. Member understanding of the goals and the tasks necessary to reach them will be clarified or corrected through discussion. The group goals should be recognized and rephrased during the discussion, encouraging members to feel a sense of "ownership" toward the goals. Table 13–5 provides suggestions for dealing with hidden agendas.

Cooperative relationships to meet goals are extremely important for group effectiveness. When hidden agendas structure a group competitively, members will strive for individual goal accomplishment in a way that blocks others from obtaining the group goal.

Groupthink: A Special Case of Cohesion

The Bay of Pigs incident during the administration of President John F. Kennedy was based on the beliefs of the in-group that the Cuban air force was ineffectual and the army weak, that a small group of Cuban exiles could establish a beachhead, and that Fidel Castro would be unable to suppress an uprising in support of the exiles. All these beliefs proved false, and the invasion of Cuba based on them was a fiasco. Similarly, the in-group around Admiral H. E. Kimmel failed to prepare for the Japanese assault on Pearl Harbor during World War II despite repeated warnings that such an attack was imminent.

Groups that "hang together" can sometimes be more easily hanged. Irving Janis (1971a, 1971b) has coined the term **groupthink**, a word reminiscent of George Orwell's *1984* society, as a way to refer to the mode of thinking engaged in by members of a highly cohesive in-group in which uniformity and agreement are given such high priority that critical thinking is impossible or unacceptable. Groups infected with groupthink have developed group norms around the maintenance of unity and loyalty, no matter what the cost.

How can one tell if a group is obsessed with the need for concurrence that characterizes groupthink? Janis (1971a, p 44) lists the following main symptoms of groupthink:

- *Invulnerability.* Most or all members of the in-group share an *illusion* of invulnerability that gives them some degree of reassurance about obvious dangers. It makes them overoptimistic and willing to take extraordinary risks. It also makes them ignore clear warnings of danger.

- *Rationalization.* Victims of groupthink collectively construct rationalizations to discount warnings and other forms of negative feedback that, taken seriously, might lead the group members to reconsider their assumptions each time they recommit themselves to past decisions.

- *Morality.* Victims of groupthink believe unquestioningly in the inherent morality of their group. This belief inclines the members to ignore the ethical or moral consequences of their decisions.

- *Stereotypes.* Victims of groupthink hold stereotyped views of outsiders. These stereotyped views are usually negative ones.

- *Pressure.* Victims of groupthink apply direct pressure to any individual who momentarily expresses doubts about any of the group's shared illusions or questions the validity of the arguments supporting an alternative

Table 13–5
Steps for Dealing with Hidden Agendas

Suggestion	Rationale
Look for the presence of hidden agendas.	The group cannot diagnose or solve a problem until its presence is recognized.
Once the presence of hidden agendas has been pinpointed, judge whether or not they should be brought to the surface and rectified.	Sometimes hidden agendas should be left undisturbed, if the consequences of bringing them to the attention of the entire group may be negative, rather than facilitating the work of the group.
Determine whether group members are willing and able to deal with hidden agendas. Suggest that perhaps not all there is to say has been said, but do not force members to disclose their hidden agendas.	Disclosing hidden agendas may be harmful to group attempts to reach cohesion and may result in the premature ouster of the member with the hidden agenda.
Accept members whose hidden agendas have been revealed, without rejecting or criticizing them.	Hidden agendas are common and legitimate group occurrences. They should be worked on in the same way that group tasks are.
Devote group time to working on the hidden agendas of members.	Hidden agendas impede group progress. The attention given to hidden agendas should be determined by the extent of the effect on group effectiveness.
As a group, evaluate the group's ability to deal with hidden agendas.	Learning better ways of handling agendas more openly will result from evaluation and reduce the need for keeping agendas hidden.

favored by the majority. This gambit reinforces the concurrence-seeking norm that loyal members are expected to maintain.

- *Self-censorship.* Victims of groupthink avoid deviating from what appears to be a group consensus. They keep silent about their misgivings and minimize even to themselves the importance of their doubts.

- *Unanimity.* Victims of groupthink share an *illusion* of unanimity within the group about almost all judgments. This is expressed by members who speak in favor of the majority vote.

- *Mindguards.* Victims of groupthink sometimes appoint themselves as mindguards to protect the leader and fellow members from adverse information that might break the confidence they share in the effectiveness and morality of past decisions.

Members afflicted with groupthink behave in characteristic ways, according to Janis (1971a, p 75):

- They limit group discussions to a few alternative courses of action (often only two) without an initial survey of all worthwhile alternatives.

- Members fail to reexamine the course of action initially preferred by the majority after they learn of risks and drawbacks they had not considered originally.

- Members spend little or no time discussing whether there are gains they may have overlooked in a rejected alternative or ways of reducing the seemingly prohibitive costs that made a rejected alternative appear undesirable to them.

- Members make little or no attempt to obtain information from experts within their own organizations who might be able to supply more precise estimates of potential losses and gains.

- Members show positive interest in facts and opinions that support their preferred policy. They tend to ignore facts and opinions that do not.

- The group spends little time deliberating about how the chosen decision might be hindered by bureaucratic inertia, sabotaged by opponents, or temporarily derailed by common accidents. It fails to work out contingency plans to cope with foreseeable setbacks that could endanger the overall success of the chosen course.

How can groupthink be prevented? Table 13–6 identifies goals that prevent or remedy groupthink and suggests constructive behaviors a group may undertake to correct its functioning.

Groupthink has a negative influence on the quality of the decisions made by a group. The groupthink decision is less reliable than decisions by consensus. Too much cohesiveness leads members to pat each other on the back even while headed toward disaster.

Power is a potent force that explains a good deal about the nature, operation, and patterns of interpersonal behavior. It is impossible to discuss group dynamics without discussing power because it is impossible to interact without influencing, and being influenced by, others. This process constantly occurs within groups, forcing members to adjust to one another and modify their behavior. In some instances, attitudes and beliefs are modified as well. *Power* can be defined as the ability to do or act, to have possession of command or control over others, to achieve the desired result (Ferguson 1985). The terms *power* and *influence* are used interchangeably in this chapter.

There is a definite process by which power is mobilized to help in accomplishing goals. Powerful people:

- Determine and clarify their personal goals
- Affirm the resources or informational level they bring to the group (what they can contribute toward the accomplishment of their goals and the goals of group members)
- Determine what coalitions are necessary to secure the information and resources needed to accomplish the goals
- Develop the necessary coalitions so that the resources can be applied (i.e., find out what they want from the others, what the others want from them, and what they can exchange so that everyone can accomplish the goals)
- Carry out the necessary activities for reaching the goals.

Some people perceive power and influence as negative forces. These people are frequently unaware of the influence they themselves exert on others, or they confuse the judicious use of power in building effective groups with the use of power to control, manage, and manipulate others. Nurses are only now becoming aware of how they might employ power and influence in the service of their clients and their profession.

Power Sources

According to power theorists, there are six possible sources of a person's power:

1. Reward power
2. Coercive power
3. Legitimate power
4. Referent power
5. Expert power
6. Informational power

Table 13–6 Preventing Groupthink			
Goal	**Preventive and Remedial Behaviors**	**Goal**	**Preventive and Remedial Behaviors**
Discouraging members from soft-pedaling their disagreements; not allowing their striving for agreement to inhibit critical thinking.	Each member should be assigned the role of critical evaluator to encourage the group to assign high priority to open airing of objections and doubts. This practice needs to be reinforced by the leader's acceptance of criticism.	Challenging the majority position.	Whenever the agenda of the group calls for an evaluation of policy alternatives, at least one member should take on the "devil's advocate" role, functioning as a good lawyer would in challenging the testimony of those who favor the majority position.
Encouraging open inquiry and impartial probing of a wide range of alternatives.	An impartial stance, rather than a statement of preferences and expectations at the beginning, should be adopted by the key members of a hierarchy when they assign a policy-planning task to any group within their organization.	Discouraging stereotyped views of other groups.	When the issue involves relations with a rival group, the group should devote a sizable block of time to surveying the signals and cues from the other group and writing alternative scenarios on the rivals' intentions.
Preventing the insulation of an in-group.	Several outside policy-planning and evaluation groups with different leaders should be set up to work on the same policy question.	Encouraging alternative plans.	The group should, from time to time, break up into two or more subgroups that meet separately, with different leaders, develop separate plans, and then come back together to negotiate differences.
Preventing the establishment of desire for "unity at all costs."	Each member should be asked at intervals to check out group conclusions with trusted associates and to report their reactions back to the group.	Rethinking the entire issue.	After reaching a preliminary consensus, the group should hold a "second chance" meeting, encouraging each member to express residual doubts before making a final choice.
Discouraging members from accepting unchallenged the views of core members.	One or more outside experts should be invited to each meeting, on a staggered basis, and encouraged to challenge the views of core members.		

Source: Compiled from Janis IL: Groupthink. Psychology Today, *November 1971, p 76. By permission of Ziff Davis Publishing Company.*

People have *reward power* if they can deliver positive consequences or remove negative ones in response to the behavior of group members. They have *coercive power* if they can deliver negative consequences or remove positive ones in response to the behavior of group members. When group members believe a person ought to have influence over them because of the person's position in the group or organization, that person can be said to have *legitimate power*. A person has *referent power* when group members identify with or want to be like that person. Members do what that person wants out of liking, respect, and the desire to be liked themselves. The person with *expert power* is seen by the group as trustworthy and having some special knowledge or skill. When a person has *informational power,* group members believe that this person has access to information not available elsewhere that will be useful in accomplishing their goal.

The Problem of Unequal Power

A group in which certain members have much power and others have little power is likely to be in trouble. The unequal distribution of power affects both the task and the maintenance functions of a group. Members who believe they have little influence within the group are unlikely to feel committed to group goals and to implementation of group decisions. Their dissatisfaction with the group decreases its attractiveness and reduces its cohesion.

High-power people often are the most popular or have the most authority. Neither circumstance is satisfactory for high-quality decision making. High-quality decision making results when power is based on expertise, competence, and relevant information, not on popularity or authority.

Destructive Obedience to Authority

Stanley Milgram (1963, 1964) conducted an absorbing and rather frightening series of social science experiments on obedience to authority. Milgram became interested in the obedience phenomenon that occurred during World War II, which formed the defense of many accused war criminals during the Nuremberg trials. He set up experiments in which subjects were to administer increasingly high doses of electric shocks to others who failed to memorize a given sequence of words. Subjects believed they were administering mild to severe (up to 300-volt) shocks that could have damaging physical consequences. Despite the possible severe consequences, 62 percent of the subjects administered the most extreme level of electrical shock under no compulsion other than the repeated verbal requests of the experimenter. Such unquestioning obedience to authority may prevent rational and humane decision-making behavior. Group members should assess and critique suggestions from the authority to avoid the consequences of uncritical obedience.

Because much of the role socialization of the nurse emphasizes "following orders," nurses must be especially critical of an unquestioning tendency to behave in concert with the wishes of persons in authority. Psychiatric nurses need to find a balance between a submissive role and an autocratic role, seeking instead to temper autonomy with reason and sensitivity. The autocratic and powerful personas of such motion picture nurse figures as the icily dictatorial Miss Davis in *The Snake Pit* and the ruthlessly punitive Nurse Ratched in *One Flew Over the Cuckoo's Nest* are examples of misdirected autonomy.

arises through membership in groups that help achieve goals they set for themselves.

- Nurses interact with groups of clients and colleagues in a wide variety of settings. To use groups rationally and effectively, nurses must understand the forces that underlie small group interactional processes and recognize their own patterns of participation.

- Varieties of groups, developed since World War II, include recreational groups, educational groups, therapy groups, and growth groups.

- Effective groups accomplish their goals, maintain cohesion, and develop and modify their structure in ways that improve effectiveness.

- Regardless of setting or composition, several forces shape and modify the structure and functioning of groups. They include space and seating arrangements, material aspects of the physical environment, leadership styles and roles, methods of decision making, trust, risk-taking, cohesion and conformity, interpersonal attraction, and power and influence.

- The most effective group leadership is one based on the assumption that responsible membership is the same thing as responsible leadership. In this distributed-functions approach, both the leader and the members engage in leadership behavior.

- Groups make decisions by consensus, selection of a group of experts, averaging members' opinions, majority vote, minority control, authority rule after discussion, and authority rule without discussion. Each method is appropriate at certain times.

- Sound decision making that leads to well-conceived, well-understood, and well-accepted realistic actions toward the goals agreed on by the group is the hallmark of a group that functions effectively.

- The existence of trust in groups allows members to make suggestions; disclose attitudes, feelings, experiences, and perceptions; give feedback; and confront one another.

- Cohesion in groups is the spirit of "we-ness" that develops when a group has had shared experiences that provide a basis for attraction—the primary factor keeping a group in existence and working effectively.

- Power and influence in groups operates constantly and forces members to adjust to one another and modify their behavior.

- Too much cohesiveness (groupthink) may have a negative influence on the quality of a group's decisions.

Chapter Highlights

- Most people's lives are spent interacting with other human beings in groups. An individual's sense of being

References

Aldag RJ, Brief AP: *Managing Organizational Behavior.* West, 1981.

Beck CT: The conceptualization of power. *Adv Nurs Sci* 1982;4:1–2.

Benne KB, Sheats P: Functional roles of group members. *J Soc Issues* 1948;4:41–49.

Booth RZ: Conflict and conflict management, in Mason DJ, Talbott SW: *Political Action Handbook for Nurses.* Addison-Wesley, 1985, pp 115–127.

Browne SE: Group leadership experiences for students. *Nurs Outlook* 1980;28:166–169.

Cartwright D, Zander A: *Group Dynamics: Research and Theory.* Harper and Row, 1968.

Davis JH: *Group Performance.* Addison-Wesley, 1969.

Deutsch M: The effects of cooperation and competition upon group process. *Hum Relations* 1949;2:129–152, 199–231.

Deutsch M: Trust and suspicion. *J Conflict Resolution* 1958;2:265–279.

Deutsch M: Conflicts: Productive and destructive. *J Soc Issues* 1969;25:7–41.

Ferguson VD: Power in nursing, in Mason DJ, Talbott SW: *Political Action Handbook for Nurses.* Addison-Wesley, 1985, pp 88–94.

Fisher DW: Guidelines to effective group functioning. *Point View* 1985;22:6–8.

Francis D, Young D: *Improving Work Groups: A Practical Manual for Team Building.* University Associates, 1979.

Hall ET: *The Hidden Dimension.* Doubleday, 1969.

Heineken J, McCloskey J: Teaching power concepts. *J Nurs Educ* 1985;24:40–41.

Hersey P, Blanchard K, Natemeyer W: Situational leadership: Perception and impact of power. *Group Org Stud* 1979;4:418–428.

Janis I: Groupthink. *Psychology Today,* November 1971a, p 43.

Janis I: Groupthink among policy makers, in Sanford N (ed): *Sanctions for Evil.* Jossey-Bass, 1971b, pp 71–89.

Johnson DW, Johnson FP: *Joining Together: Group Theory and Group Skills.* Prentice-Hall, 1975.

Kogan N, Wallach MS: *Risk-Taking: A Study in Cognition and Personality.* Holt, Rinehart and Winston, 1964.

Larson ML, Williams RA: How to become a better group leader? Learn to recognize the strange things that happen to some people in groups. *Nurs 78* 1978;8:65–72.

Lewin K, Lippitt R, White RK: Patterns of aggressive behavior in experimentally created social climates." *J Soc Psychol* 1939;10:271–299.

Luthans F: *Organizational Behavior.* McGraw-Hill, 1981.

May R: The meaning of power, in *Power and Innocence.* W.W. Norton, 1972, pp 99–119.

Mead GH: *Mind, Self, and Society.* University of Chicago Press, 1934.

Milgram S: Behavioral study of obedience. *J Abnorm Soc Psychol* 1963;67:371–378.

Milgram S: Group pressure and action against a person. *J Abnorm Soc Psychol* 1964;69:137–143.

Mintz N: Effects of esthetic surroundings: II. Prolonged and repeated experience in a "beautiful" and an "ugly" room. *J Psychol* 1956;41:459–466.

Roethlisberger FJ, Dickson WJ: *Management and the Worker.* Harvard University Press, 1939.

Sadock BJ: Group psychotherapy, combined individual and group psychotherapy, and psychodrama, in Kaplan HI, Sadock BJ: *Comprehensive Textbook of Psychiatry,* ed 4. Williams & Wilkins, 1985, pp 1403–1427.

Sampson EE, Marthas MS: *Group Process for the Health Professions.* Wiley, 1981.

Seghers CE: Color in the office. *Management Rev* 1948;37:452–453.

Shotman L: *The Skills of Helping Individuals and Groups,* ed 2. Peacock, 1984.

Small LL: Finding your leadership style in groups. *Amer J Nurs* 1980;80:1301–1303.

Sommer R: *Personal Space: The Behavioral Basis of Design.* Prentice-Hall, 1969.

Steinzor B: The spatial factor in face-to-face discussion groups. *J Abnorm Soc Psychol* 1950;45:552–555.

Strodtbeck FL, Hook LH: The social dimensions of a twelve man jury table. *Sociometry* 1961;24:397–415.

FOURTEEN

Research in Psychiatric Nursing

Anita Werner O'Toole
Susan L. Jones
Holly Skodol Wilson

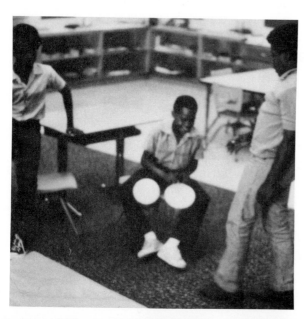

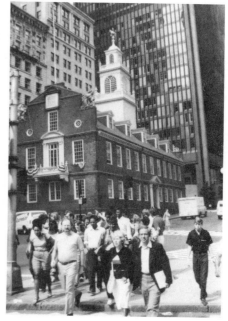

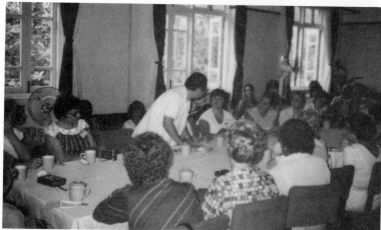

After reading this chapter, students should be able to

- Appreciate the usefulness of scientific research in psychiatric nursing practice

- Specify the assumptions, characteristics, and aims of the scientific way of knowing

- Explain the typical steps in the research process

- Discuss considerations crucial to evaluating the credibility of research findings

- Advocate the protection of human rights and the principles of ethical scientific work

- Summarize the current state of published research in psychiatric-mental health nursing

- Formulate fruitful directions for future research in the discipline

- Summarize important strategies for evaluating research for clinical utility and merit

Cross References

Other topics relevant to this content are the Nursing process and nursing theory, Chapter 4.

Key Terms

concept	inductive
conceptual framework	null hypothesis
confounding variable	mean
construct	median
construct validity	mode
data	population
deductive	random sample
dependent variable (DV)	reliability
elements	sample
extraneous variable	theory
hypotheses	uncontrolled variable
independent variable (IV)	validity

Psychiatric nursing is in the midst of an information revolution. Every psychiatric nurse needs to respond knowledgeably about such diverse issues as the influence of neurotransmitters on adolescents with eating disorders, dietary restrictions for depressed adults taking antidepressant medications, the most effective strategies for providing social support to family caregivers of the demented elderly, or the projected trends in the needs of the homeless chronically mentally ill. Information on these issues comes from research. Regardless of the nurse's educational preparation, all nurses in the future will require an ability to read, understand, and judge the usefulness of studies conducted by others and the motivation and skill to participate in clinical nursing research as well. Psychiatric nursing has been in the vanguard of the discipline throughout its history. Building a body of knowledge based on research findings and applying research knowledge to clinical decisions should be no exception.

This chapter is about research in psychiatric nursing both as a process for discovering knowledge and as a body of scientific findings that have accumulated as a consequence of studying human responses. The first section of the chapter is an overview of selected ideas about research as a process for acquiring knowledge. The second section summarizes the current state of research in psychiatric nursing and suggests fruitful directions for future research. This chapter cannot substitute for a good introductory research text (see Wilson 1985, Wilson 1987). Instead, it is intended to make readers intelligent and informed consumers of research and sensitive to worthwhile problems for future clinical research.

Imagine a future when economic prosperity and social programs become alternatives to military spending.

Portions of this chapter appeared in Wilson HS: Research in nursing, in Kozier B, Erb G: *Fundamentals of Nursing*, ed 3. Addison-Wesley, 1987.

WHAT IS NURSING RESEARCH?

The history of nursing research encompasses only about three decades, since its beginnings are usually traced to the early 1950s. Certain historians may point out that although nursing research had a rebirth in the 1950s and 1960s, Florence Nightingale changed health care with her carefully researched case studies and detailed statistical accounts in the Crimea (Chenitz 1985).

Nursing research is more than just scientific investigations conducted by a person educated and credentialed as a nurse. It refers instead to research directed toward building a body of nursing knowledge about "human responses to actual or potential health problems" (ANA 1980, p 9) and about the effects of nursing action on such human responses. The human responses of people may be (a) reactions of individuals, groups, or families to actual health problems, e.g., the burden a family experiences when they must care for an elderly relative with senile dementia; and (b) concerns of individuals and groups about potential health problems, e.g., stress management in an industrial setting. The purpose of nursing research is to improve health care.

Nursing research also reflects the traditional nursing perspective. In this perspective, the client is seen as a whole person, with physiologic, psychologic, social, cultural, and economic components. In addition to reflecting concern for the whole person, a nursing perspective implies 24-hour-a-day responsibility. Thus, this perspective encompasses all of the factors in a client's environment, such as fatigue, noise, sensory deprivation, nutrition, and positioning, that might influence coping patterns. Diers (1979) lists three distinguishing properties of nursing research:

1. The goal of nursing research is to improve client care in a way that matters.
2. Nursing research has the potential for contributing to theory development and the body of scientific nursing knowledge.
3. A research problem is a nursing research problem when nurses have access to and control over phenomena being studied.

WHAT IS RESEARCH IN NURSING?

Some authors make a distinction between nursing research (i.e., research that focuses on human responses, clinical problems, and processes of care encountered in the practice of nursing) and research in nursing (the broader study of the nursing profession including historical, ethical, and political studies). However, the American Nurses' Association (ANA) Cabinet on Nursing Research (1985) identifies the following as priorities for nursing research.

- Promote health, well-being, and ability to care for oneself among all age, social, and cultural groups
- Minimize or prevent behaviorally and environmentally induced health problems that compromise the quality of life and reduce productivity
- Minimize the negative effects of new health technologies on the adaptive abilities of individuals and families experiencing acute or chronic health problems
- Ensure that the care needs of particularly vulnerable groups—e.g., the elderly, children with congenital health problems, individuals from diverse cultures, the mentally ill, and the poor—are met in effective and acceptable ways
- Classify nursing practice phenomena
- Ensure that principles of ethics guide nursing research
- Develop instruments to measure nursing outcomes
- Develop integrative methodologies for the holistic study of human beings as they relate to their families and life-styles
- Design and evaluate alternative models for delivering health care and for administering health care systems so that nurses will be able to balance high quality and cost-effectiveness in meeting the nursing needs of identified populations
- Evaluate the effectiveness of alternative approaches to nursing education for the kind of practice that requires broad knowledge and a wide repertoire of skills, and for the kind of practice that requires specialized knowledge and a focused set of skills
- Identify and analyze historical and contemporary factors that influence the shaping of nursing professionals' involvement in national health policy development

Nursing research is both basic and applied. A variety of methodologies are used to accomplish its purposes.

WHY IS RESEARCH IN PSYCHIATRIC NURSING IMPORTANT?

In the information revolution transforming the present and shaping the future, reading and understanding nursing research is as fundamental to professional practice as knowledge of the nursing process and communication. The ability to access, evaluate, and interpret findings from nursing studies is a source of power in clinical decision making and a strategy for achieving excellence in the delivery of care.

Research in psychiatric nursing is not only a tool for discovering solutions to clinical practice problems but also a political tool. "Research provides knowledge necessary to improve practice and achieve professional status. Through research, nursing can improve the care of persons in need of health service and affect policy that directs the way health services are provided. Political wisdom is an integral part of the research act" (Chenitz 1985, p 314).

Ways of Knowing

Nurses rely on diverse ways of knowing when they confront day-to-day clinical questions. Some may:

- Retreat to established tradition and authority as reflected in a procedure book or established protocol
- Use trial and error combined with their own common sense or past experience
- Consult an expert
- Attempt to arrive at a logically reasoned decision

The Scientific Way of Knowing

The way of knowing that is the focus of this chapter is scientific inquiry as evidenced in nursing research. The scientific approach is a process of learning about truth by systematically collecting and comparing observable, verifiable data through the senses to describe, explain, and/or predict events and phenomena. The scientific approach as reflected in nursing research has two characteristics that other usual ways of knowing in nursing do not: (a) It has a built-in system of checks to ensure objectivity and the potential for self-correction and (b) it relies on sensory evidence or empirical data that are collected in a systematic, carefully prescribed manner (Wilson 1985, Wilson and Hutchinson 1986).

A system of checks and balances to minimize bias is applied to knowledge generated through the research process. Nurse scientists who find that one particular hypothesis is supported also check whether alternative hypotheses are supported as well, perhaps more strongly. The research methods and conclusions drawn from a study's findings must always be open to the criticism of others. Following the steps in the research process is one way of determining whether a study complies with accepted conventions for conducting credible research studies.

Steps in the Research Process

The truly important discoveries made in the health care field have not been made by scientists who think in dog-matic, mechanical fashion, who focus on knowledge of irrefutable facts without interpretation, or who forget that research is most often a process that moves back and forth between ideas, hunches, existing knowledge, and carefully made observations. Yet, for the sake of clarity, the research process is generally conceptualized as a series of steps or phases. Although these phases are dynamic, flexible, and expandable, they can be formalized as follows:

Step 1. Stating a Research Question or Problem

An investigator's initial task is narrowing a broad area of interest to a delimited problem that specifies exactly what she or he intends to study. Most investigators try to define a research problem as precisely as possible. A problem is often stated in the form of a question.

If a study problem is too broad or vague, proceeding to subsequent stages of the process becomes confusing. A research question, according to Brink and Wood (1983, p 2), "is an explicit query about a problem or issue that can be challenged, examined, analyzed, and will yield useful new information."

Step 2. Defining the Purpose of a Study

The second step is sometimes called defining the rationale of the study. It is the researcher's statement of why the question is important and what use the answer will serve. It lets the reader or funding agency know what to expect from the study.

Step 3. Reviewing Related Literature

If researchers want their study to build on, confirm, or even transcend the existing knowledge in a discipline and thereby qualify as a real contribution to science, they must know what has already been done. A review of the literature provides the researcher with a framework of background ideas. In a theoretical framework the investigator relates the existing concepts, theories, research methods, and findings to her or his study question and purpose (Brink and Wood 1983). At the least, constructing such a framework provides relevant concepts for the research; at best, it gives the researcher a full awareness of facts, issues, prior findings, theories, and instruments that might be related to the study question.

Step 4. Formulating Hypotheses and Defining Variables

Hypotheses are statements of the relationship between two or more concepts, or variables. Some studies are intended to develop hypotheses (exploratory, descriptive, and grounded theory designs), and others are intended to test hypotheses using statistical procedures. Stating hypotheses requires not only sufficient knowledge about a topic to predict the outcome of the study but also definitions that specify the variables under investigation in measurable terms. Finally, the investigator must articulate the relationships among the variables.

Hypotheses (H) may be stated as **null hypotheses** (H$_0$), which essentially test the premise that there are no significant differences in the outcome or dependent variable other than those that can be attributed to chance. To formulate hypotheses, the investigator must specify the concepts being studied; thus, it is important at this point to determine how to define these variables for the purpose of measuring them. For example, social support might be defined as a score on a written self-report scale, or inventory. This step is called operationally defining the variables. If one does a convincing job, the study is said to have **construct** (or concept) **validity**.

Step 5. Selecting the Research Design

A research design is a well-formulated, systematic, and controlled plan for finding answers to study questions. The design is a road map or blueprint for organizing a study. Everything from methods of data collection through methods of data analysis should be spelled out in the research design.

Step 6. Selecting the Population, Sample, and Setting

After narrowing a general area of interest to a specific study question, reviewing the literature, and deciding on a research design, the researcher must choose a study population, select a sample, and decide on a setting where the sample can be located. The **population** is the group to be studied. To whom do the findings apply? Some recent studies, for instance, have focused on these populations: divorced fathers, older persons, hospitalized children, disadvantaged minorities, depressed women, people with AIDS, clients who have had disfiguring surgery, and psychiatric nurses. The **sample** is that segment of a population from whom data will be collected. Findings from the sample are generalized to

the population. Subjects who comprise the sample are called **elements**.

Step 7. Conducting a Pilot Study

A pilot study helps the researcher discover the strengths and weaknesses of the intended design, sample size, and data-collection instrument of the larger project. Pilot studies strengthen nursing studies by weeding out problems in advance; many funding agencies do not approve study proposals unless a pilot study has been conducted.

Step 8. Collecting the Data

The scientific method is characterized by a reliance on empirical data: information collected from the observable world. These data are used to make statements about what is true. Any study that goes beyond armchair speculation eventually requires the researcher to collect data. Data sources may be people, documents, or laboratory materials. Data-collection instruments include interviews, questionnaires, and biologic and psychologic tests. The basic point, however, is that by moving either from observation to idea (an **inductive** process) or from idea to observation (a **deductive** process), the scientist relies on empirical data to discover or test knowledge. The researcher uses the senses and measurement tools to collect data relevant to the variables being studied. The time and energy required for this step vary according to the research design. Field studies, historic research, surveys, and most experiments are time-consuming and intellectually demanding.

Step 9. Analyzing the Data

The next step in the research process is reorganizing the collected data to relate them to the study question, research objectives, or stated hypotheses. The most important part of this step is to have a procedural plan in mind, have the requisite skills for analysis (such as knowledge of statistics), and realize that analysis provides the answers to the original research questions.

Step 10. Communicating Conclusions and Implications

The researcher's challenge at the final stage is to explain the results of the investigation and link them to the existing body of knowledge in the discipline. Whether results are published or reported verbally, the study's contribution cannot be judged unless the conclusions are communicated to colleagues and critics. Communicating the conclusions, interpreting the meaning and implications of the findings, recognizing the study's limitations, and suggesting directions for future study culminate the research process.

The steps of the research process provide the tools with which scientists achieve their major aims or goals. These basic aims are: (a) to develop theories, or explanations of the world, and (b) to find solutions to practical problems.

THE INVESTIGATIVE ROLES OF ALL NURSES

The majority of career scientists in nursing are prepared at the doctoral and postdoctoral level, although an increasing number of clinicians with master's degrees are beginning to participate in research activity as part of their nursing role. However, "if nursing is to emerge in society as a socially significant, credible, scientific, and learned profession with a commitment to high-quality patient care, then research (for all nurses) is a necessity" (Starzomski 1983). It may be unrealistic to expect each nurse to conduct a study in the clinical setting. Many constraints in clinical settings must be reckoned with before research can become a legitimate and comfortable activity. However, if nursing is to develop as a research-based practice, it is not unreasonable to expect the nurse in the clinical area to:

- Have some awareness of the process and language of research
- Be sensitive to issues related to protecting the rights of human subjects
- Participate in the identification of significant researchable problems
- Be an informed consumer of research findings

The nursing student must learn these investigative functions early in her or his career to establish the connection that "knowing how we know is fundamental to doing what we do" (Wilson 1985, p viii). Bridging the research-practice gap, i.e., bringing research into the clinical practice arena, is a key strategy in uniting the scholarly, scientific, and caring aspects of nursing in the future. Box 14–1 summarizes this position in the ANA's "Guidelines for the Investigative Function of Nurses" (1981), which specify the generally expected research competencies of nurses with associate, bachelor's, master's, and doctoral degrees.

THE RESEARCH-PRACTICE GAP

It is apparent that nurse leaders want to make nursing practice a more frequent focus of nursing research and increase the application of valid research findings in clinical work. Yet progress toward achieving these goals is often slowed by several barriers.

Lack of Cumulative Order in the Literature

A scientist from another discipline, according to Gortner, would probably characterize most nursing research as "discrete, nonaggregated studies of isolated empirical phenomena for which the explanatory theory is not yet well known or defined" (Gortner 1980). It would be much easier for nurse generalists and clinicians with no specialized research training to apply research findings to their practice if nursing research were organized into well-defined programs that would yield cumulative discoveries. In selected instances, this pattern has been more successfully attained than in others.

Insufficient Preparation by Nurses

Building a cumulative, organized, scientific knowledge base to replace traditions, habits, and trial and error as the basis for practice decisions is not enough. Nurses must be motivated and competent to read, understand, evaluate, and interpret this body of work. Reports of research findings are not always easy to locate through the professional media or in the most widely read journals. Once reports are located, nurses may find their traditional scientific format and specialized language difficult or intimidating. To read and interpret them, nurses need to become wise and proactive consumers of research findings.

Service Organization Structure

Until recently, most service settings rarely encouraged clinical nurses to make changes in interventions based on systematic appraisals or participation in nursing research. Here are some successful strategies for introducing a research orientation into an institution whose focus is the delivery of client care:

- Legitimize the research activities of clinical nurses by granting release time for research and recognizing nursing research through the institution's formal reward system.
- Form a research reference group for clinical nurses. Such a group would bring together nurses who value research, raise research consciousness among nurses, and allow members to exchange formal and informal knowledge about research.
- Help clinical nurse investigators explore the researcher role. In particular, give nurses access to clients for

---

Box 14–1
INVESTIGATIVE FUNCTIONS OF A NURSE
AT VARIOUS EDUCATIONAL LEVELS

Associate Degree in Nursing

1. Demonstrates awareness of the value or relevance of research in nursing
2. Assists in identifying problem areas in nursing practice
3. Assists in collecting data within an established, structured format

Baccalaureate in Nursing

1. Reads, interprets, and evaluates research for applicability to nursing practice
2. Identifies nursing problems that need to be investigated and participates in the implementation of scientific studies
3. Uses nursing practice as a means of gathering data to refine and extend practice
4. Applies established findings of nursing and other health-related research to nursing practice
5. Shares research findings with colleagues

Master's Degree in Nursing

1. Analyzes and reformulates nursing practice problems so that scientific knowledge and scientific methods can be used to find solutions
2. Enhances the quality and clinical relevance of nursing research by providing expertise in clinical problems and by providing knowledge about the way in which these clinical services are delivered
3. Facilitates investigations of problems in clinical settings through such activities as contributing to a climate supportive of investigative activities, collaborating

with others in investigations, and enhancing nursing's access to clients and data

4. Conducts investigations for the purpose of monitoring the quality of the practice of nursing in a clinical setting
5. Assists others to apply scientific knowledge in nursing practice

Doctoral Degree in Nursing or a Related Discipline

1. Provides leadership for the integration of scientific knowledge with other sources of knowledge for the advancement of practice
2. Conducts investigations to evaluate the contribution of nursing activities to the well-being of clients
3. Develops methods to monitor the quality of the practice of nursing in a clinical setting and to evaluate contributions of nursing activities to the well-being of clients

Graduate of a Research-Oriented Doctoral Program

1. Develops theoretical explanations of phenomena relevant to nursing by empirical research and analytic processes
2. Uses analytic and empirical methods to discover ways to modify or extend existing scientific knowledge so that it is relevant to nursing
3. Develops methods for scientific inquiry of phenomena relevant to nursing

Source: From Guidelines for the investigative function of nurses. *Published by ANA and reprinted by permission of the American Nurses' Association.*

---

research purposes and help nurses discover differences in the rhythm of research work and clinical work. Clinical nurses are accustomed to a large volume of work that must be accomplished in a short time. Learning how much scholarly and research work to expect from oneself in a specific time represents a major shift for most clinical nurses, who must learn to spend more time in the sedentary activities of prolonged reading and thinking (Davis 1981).

Nurses must overcome these obstacles if they are to incorporate nursing research into the practice arena and make research an important area of nursing skill and

expertise. The following sections address the nurse generalist's investigative roles in more detail.

PROTECTING THE RIGHTS OF HUMAN SUBJECTS

Because nursing research usually focuses on humans, a major nursing responsibility is to be aware of and advocate clients' rights. All clients must be informed about the consequences of consenting to serve as research subjects. The client needs to be able to assess whether an appropriate balance exists between the risks of participating in a study and the potential benefits, either to the client or to the development of knowledge.

Research ethics not only protect the rights of human subjects but also encompass a broader list of characteristics. Most of these characteristics are reflected in the ANA's "Human Rights Guidelines for Nursing in Clinical and Other Research." These guidelines are based on historical documents, such as the Nuremberg Code, the Declaration of Helsinki, and United States federal regulations, all of which set standards governing the conduct of research involving human subjects. The ANA Guidelines are presented in Box 14–2.

The Nurse's Role

All nurses who practice in settings where research is being conducted with human subjects or who participate in such research as data collectors or collaborators play an important role in safeguarding the following rights:

Right Not to Be Harmed

The Department of Health and Human Services defines risk of harm to a research subject as exposure to the possibility of injury going beyond everyday situations. The risk can be physical, emotional, legal, financial, or social. For instance, withholding standard care from a client with delirium tremens (DTs) so as to study its natural course clearly poses a potential physical danger. Risks can be less overt and involve psychologic factors (e.g., exposure to stress or anxiety) or social factors (e.g., loss of confidentiality or loss of privacy).

Right to Full Disclosure

Even though it may be possible to collect data about a client as part of everyday care without the client's particular knowledge or consent, to do so is considered unethical. Full disclosure is a basic right. It means that deception, either by withholding information about a client's participation in a study, or by giving the client false or misleading information about what participating in the study will involve, will not occur. Full disclosure involves informing study subjects about the following aspects of any study:

- The nature, duration, and purposes of the study
- The methods, procedures, and processes by which data will be collected, expressed in lay language rather than technical terms (for example, teaspoons of blood to be drawn, rather than milliliters)
- The use to which the findings will be put and any benefits that could be derived

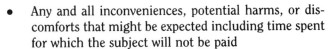

- Any and all inconveniences, potential harms, or discomforts that might be expected including time spent for which the subject will not be paid
- Any possible results or side-effects that might follow, including being sent more questionnaires
- The client's alternatives to participating in the study
- The right to refuse to participate or to withdraw at any point
- The identities of the investigators and how to contact them

Right of Self-Determination

Many clients in dependent positions, such as people in nursing homes, feel pressured to participate in studies. They feel that they must please those doctors and nurses who are responsible for their treatment and care. The right of self-determination means that subjects should feel free from constraints, coercion, or any undue influence to participate in a study. Masked inducements, for instance, suggesting that they might become famous by making an important contribution to science or get special attention by taking part in the study, must be strictly avoided. Nurses must be assertive in advocating this essential right as well.

Right of Privacy, Anonymity, and Confidentiality

Privacy enables a client to participate without worrying about later embarrassment. Anonymity in a study is ensured if even the investigator cannot link a specific subject to the information reported. Confidentiality means that any information a subject relates will not be made public or available to others. Investigators must inform research subjects about the measures that provide for these rights. Such measures may include using pseudonyms, code numbers, or reporting only aggregate or group data in published research.

Nurses who participate in scientific investigations that involve human subjects are in a key position to serve as advocates for research subjects. All of the study topics in Box 14–3 could put human subjects at risk.

Vulnerable Subjects

Certain subjects, including children, fetuses, the mentally disabled, the elderly, captives, the dying, and the sedated or unconscious, are considered particularly vulnerable subjects. The guiding principle in these cases is that the less a subject is able to give informed consent, the greater the nurse's responsibility to protect the client's rights.

The desire for scientific knowledge must be compatible with the need to preserve the dignity and rights of individuals and social groups. The following principles of ethical research (Wilson 1985) are worth remembering:

1. (S) Scientific objectivity. Objectivity ensures that the research is conducted without bias, misconduct, or fraud.

Box 14–2
ANA GUIDELINES FOR NURSING RESEARCH

The following guidelines attempt to specify several important entities: (1) the type of activities that are involved, (2) the rights that are to be protected, (3) the persons to be safeguarded, and (4) the mechanisms necessary to ensure that protection is adequate.

Guideline 1: Employment in Settings Where Research Is Conducted

Conditions of employment in settings in which clinical or other research is in progress need to be spelled out in detail for all potential workers. . . . Anyone employed in work that carries the potential of risk to others needs to be advised as to the types of risks involved, the ways of recognizing when risk is present, and the proper actions to take to counteract harmful effects and unnecessary danger.

Guideline 2: Nurses' Responsibilities for Vigilant Protection of Human Subjects' Rights

In all instances the prospective subject must be given all relevant information prior to participation in activities that go beyond established and accepted procedures necessary to meet his personal needs. . . . Nurses must be increasingly vigilant in their concern for subjects and patients who by reason of their situation and/or illness are not able to protect themselves effectively from externally imposed threat or injury. They must be sensitive to the tendency toward exploitation of "captive" populations such as students, patients, and inmates in institutions and prisons. All proposals to be used need to be discussed with the prospective subject and with any worker who is expected to participate as a subject or data collector or both. Special mechanisms must be developed to safeguard the confidentiality of information and protect human dignity.

Guideline 3: Scope of Application

The persons to whom these human rights guidelines apply include all individuals involved in research activities and include the following groups: patients, donors of organs and tissue, informants, normal volunteers including students, and vulnerable populations that are "captive" audi-

ences, such as the mentally disordered, mentally retarded, and prisoners.

Guideline 4: Nurses' Responsibility to Support the Accrual of Knowledge

Just as nurses have an obligation to protect the human rights of patients, so do they also have an obligation to support the accrual of knowledge that broadens the scientific underpinnings of nursing practice and the delivery of nursing services.

Guideline 5: Informed Consent

To safeguard the basic rights of self-determination, nurses must obtain consent from the prospective subject or his legal representative to participate in research or unusual clinical activities. The subject needs to receive:

- A description of any benefit to the subject or the development of new knowledge that might be expected

- An offer to discuss or answer any questions about the study

- A clear statement to the subject that he is free to discontinue participation at any time he wishes to do so

- Full freedom from direct or indirect coercion and deception

Guideline 6: Representation on Human Subjects Committee

There is increasing public support for systematic accountability to ensure that individual rights are not denied to human subjects who participate in research studies. In most instances, the protective mechanism takes place through a committee judged competent to review studies and other investigative activities that involve human subjects. The profession of nursing has an obligation to publicly support the inclusion of nurses as regular members of institutional review committees of this kind.

Source: Adapted and summarized from Human rights guidelines for nurses in clinical and other research. *Published by ANA and reprinted by permission of the American Nurses' Association.*

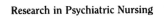

2. (C) Cooperation with duly authorized review groups, agencies, and institutional review boards (IRB). These committees are charged with reviewing provisions for protecting the rights of human subjects and interpreting law and ethics.

3. (I) Integrity in representing the research study. Integrity means that the researchers do not deceive subjects about the risks, discomforts, or potential benefits of participating as a research subject.

4. (E) Equitability in acknowledging the contributions of others. The researcher should acknowledge coauthors, research associates, and clinical nurses who provided access to clients and participated in data collection.

5. (N) Nobility in the application or processes and procedures to protect the rights of human subjects. Subjects' rights should never be compromised to facilitate the research.

6. (T) Truthfulness about a study's purpose, methods, and findings. "Undercover research" is no longer considered ethical.

7. (I) Impeccability in the use of privileges associated with the researcher's role. Researchers often have access to privileged, private information. This information must be kept confidential and anonymous. All nurse researchers must be as discrete about clients as nurse clinicians are.

8. (F) Forthrightness about a study's funding sources and sponsorship. Any published research must disclose all sources of financial support and any special sponsorship.

9. (I) Illumination of knowledge through contributions to publications and presentations of research findings.

Nurse clinicians need to be assured that efforts by nurse researchers will be available to them.

10. (C) Courage to clarify publicly any distortions or misinterpretations of research findings.

As the list acronym (SCIENTIFIC) suggests, following these principles of ethical research makes the scientific ethical (Wilson 1985). See Figure 14–1.

FINDING RESEARCHABLE PROBLEMS

Protecting the rights of human research subjects and advocating ethical research are crucial investigative roles for all nurses. Another important role is to identify, in the course of giving nursing care, problems and questions that call for research-based explanations. Identifying problem areas in nursing practice is an investigative skill that all nurses need to master if the interplay between research and practice urged by the ANA is to be achieved (ANA 1981). A clinician with a research orientation can turn a nursing problem into a nursing research problem.

Box 14–3
RESEARCH STUDIES WITH ETHICAL ISSUES AT STAKE

1. A nurse who had worked for 6 years in a setting for demented elderly clients was concerned about the tendency for nurses to avoid certain clients. She decided to conduct a study of how nurses care for the demented elderly.

2. In a study of impaired nurses, several nurse informants revealed some very personal and damaging information about themselves, but this was only a pilot study and they had not signed a consent form.

3. In a study of care of mentally retarded children, the researcher found that there were some glaring deficiencies in the care of these children. For example, children were often left in uncomfortable positions for hours at a time, were rarely offered fluids, and received diaper changes infrequently.

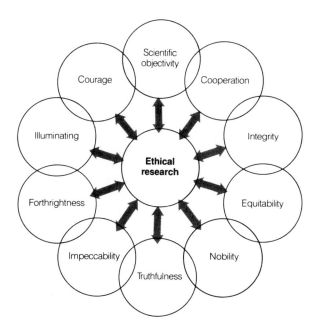

Figure 14–1
Making the scientific ethical.
Source: Wilson HS: Research in nursing, in Kozier B, Erb G: Fundamentals of Nursing, *ed 3. Addison-Wesley, 1987, p. 125. Copyright © 1987 Addison-Wesley Publishing Company, Inc.*

Sources of Research Problems

For the nurse with observation skills and an inquiring mind, each interaction is not only a way to meet the client's needs for comfort and support but also an opportunity to recognize discrepancies between what is (existing nursing practice or client status) and what is desirable. Every discrepancy is a potential source of research problems. Valid sources of researchable topics include one's own clinical experience, patterns or trends in someone else's observations or research, and one's own intellectual and scientific interests. Consider these examples:

A staff nurse on an in-patient psychiatric unit reads about the hypnotic effects of a dietary amino acid, L-tryptophan, on clients who have recently experienced a major stress. The nurse wonders if the effects of the amino acid could be approximated by serving certain amounts of dairy products and some meats to these clients.

An out-patient clinic nurse who does psychosocial assessments on elderly clients wonders if a program of daily hydration would improve their orientation and decrease their confusion.

From Clinical Nursing Problem to Research Problem

Research questions usually begin with *who, what, when, where,* or *why.* Some researchers have sorted questions into different levels, suggesting that some questions are most appropriate when the existing knowledge is at a certain level. For example, if very little is known about a certain topic, it makes sense to ask a *what, who,* or *where* question to acquire descriptive information:

> What are the unmet mental health needs of the frail elderly?
>
> Where would people prefer to die?
>
> Who should assume responsibility for teaching self-care to the chronically mentally ill?

When more is known about a topic, it is appropriate to ask *how* or *why* questions:

> How do nurses decide when to initiate suicide precautions?
>
> Why do clients fail to comply with drug therapy?

Research problems come from a variety of sources. In one's own clinical practice they may come from gripes, wishes, observed patterns of needs, conventions or traditions in nursing care, and the like. Changing a clinical nursing problem into a researchable one can involve four straightforward steps.

1. State the wish, gripe, etc.
2. Identity the constraints that contribute to the discrepancy between what is going on and what should occur.
3. From the brain-stormed list generated in step 2, select the most likely explanation for the discrepancy.
4. Rephrase the problem in conceptual terms so that solutions are not applicable to one case alone, but rather can be generalized to clients with similar characteristics and in similar circumstances.

A researchable problem is stated clearly and unambiguously as either a question or a statement, for example:

> What are the predictive factors in repeated adolescent suicide attempts?

Probably the most important point to keep in mind when developing the skills to recognize researchable nursing problems is that much of the tradition of nursing practice is based on just that—tradition—rather than on carefully controlled research. Many conventional nursing interventions are open to investigation through nursing research.

In the near future, nursing research will focus on the interaction of psychologic and psychosocial mechanisms in human experiences of coping with health and illness, the evaluation of nursing interventions, the application of research findings in practice, and underserved and high-risk groups, such as the elderly and minority groups. The nurse of tomorrow will be directly involved in the conduct and application of research. Examples of areas for research in psychiatric nursing appear in Box 14–4.

BECOMING AN INTELLIGENT RESEARCH CONSUMER

Clinical nursing research is the answer to the dilemmas that routinely face the practicing nurse, even when the questions begin with "how do I," "what if," and "what is the best way?" Before clinical nurses can evaluate the worth of a research report, however, they have to understand it. This goal is an ongoing one throughout one's nursing education, but beginning steps include: (a) understanding the format of a research journal article, (b) translating the vocabulary of scientific research, and (c) evaluating the credibility of a scientific presentation of findings.

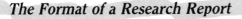

The Format of a Research Report

Almost all reports of research findings in research journals have a standardized format. The nursing student who becomes familiar with it gets the most out of time spent reading the report. It is easier to grasp the meaning of unfamiliar terminology if one understands the context in which the information is being presented. The typical research article is organized in the following way:

1. Abstract
2. Introduction
    a. Review of related literature (including theoretical framework)
    b. Statement of the purpose or specific goals of the study (including hypotheses)
3. Methodology
    a. Procedure for selecting the study sample
    b. Study design
    c. Data collection tools or strategies
    d. Data analysis procedures
4. Results or findings
5. Discussion and implications
6. References

Once the nurse has a general idea of how a research report is organized, she or he must read it with understanding. This involves developing the skill to "come to terms with research terminology" (Wilson 1985, p 98).

Research Terminology

Concepts, Constructs, Conceptual Frameworks, and Theory

Nurses work with **concepts** all the time. *Bonding, self-care level, loss, stress, burnout, decentralization,* and *deinstitutionalization* are all terms for categories of phenomena that share certain characteristics. Some phenomena, such as the presence of mood-altering chemicals, can be measured directly with blood or urine screening. Others, because they are more abstract, call for proxy measures. For example, anxiety may be measured by a score on an anxiety scale alone or by the combination of an anxiety scale score and some physiologic measures, such as respiration and pulse

> ### Box 14–4
> # EXAMPLES OF AREAS FOR RESEARCH IN PSYCHIATRIC–MENTAL HEALTH NURSING
>
> 1. Identification of determinants (personal and environmental, including social support networks) of wellness and health functioning in individuals and families, e.g., avoiding abusive behavior such as alcoholism and drug use, successfully adapting to chronic illness, and coping with the last days of life
>
> 2. Identification of phenomena that negatively influence the course of recovery and that may be alleviated by nursing practice, e.g., anorexia, diarrhea, sleep deprivation, deficiencies in nutrients, electrolyte imbalances, and infections
>
> 3. Development and testing of care strategies to do the following:
>
>   - Facilitate individuals' ability to adopt and maintain health-enhancing behaviors (e.g., exercise and alterations in diet)
>
>   - Enhance clients' ability to manage acute and chronic illness so as to minimize or eliminate the necessity for institutionalization and to maximize well-being
>
>   - Reduce stressful responses associated with the medical management of clients (e.g., surgical procedures, intrusive examination procedures, or extensive use of monitoring devices)
>
> 4. Enhance the care of clients culturally different from the majority (e.g., black Americans, Mexican Americans, native Americans) and clients with special problems (e.g., teenagers, prisoners, mentally ill), and the underserved (the elderly, poor, and the rural)
>
> 5. Design and assess, in terms of effectiveness and cost, the models for delivering nursing care strategies found to be effective in clinical studies
>
> 6. Provide more effective care to high-risk populations (e.g., maternal and child care service to vulnerable mothers and infants, family planning services to young teenagers, services designed to enhance self-care in the chronically ill and the very old)

rate. Certain abstract concepts are often called **constructs.** Examples of constructs from various theories are *social class* from sociology, *locus of control* from psychology, and *leadership style* from management theory. Science is concerned with identifying, refining, and explaining relationships among concepts by comparing them to empirical observations. For this reason, deciding whether a study uses appropriate, valid, and believable measures for concepts and constructs is an important step in judging the credibility of a nursing research study. Conceptual or theoretical frameworks (sometimes simply called theories) are systems that interrelate concepts and constructs. Most nursing students are familiar with the theories of relativity, gravity, and evolution as well as psychoanalytic theory and learning theory.

Independent and Dependent Variables

The term *variable* refers to anything that varies. The **dependent variables** (DV) in a study may also be called the output, outcome, or criterion variables. Change or the lack of it presumably depends on causes or conditions that the investigator can manipulate. In most cases, the dependent variable is what the researcher is trying to study. The **independent variables** (IV) are *existing* conditions that the researcher manipulates to affect the dependent variable. It is possible to have multiple independent and dependent variables. Most research is designed to clarify the relationships among them. The ability to recognize the dependent and independent variables in a study is an important step in grasping a study's potential meaning and significance.

Uncontrolled Variables

Determining the dependent and independent variables in a research study is usually straightforward. Interpreting the study's findings, however, is more complicated. The researcher must take into consideration all the other relevant variables, other than the identified IV, that might affect the DV. Sometimes these other variables relate to how standardized and unbiased the data-collection procedures are. Sometimes they relate to characteristics of the subjects in the sample or how they were chosen. Sometimes, unwanted variables may be introduced through the passage of time or through unforeseen events in the course of conducting the study. A well-designed study specifies the precise steps the researcher must take to be as certain as possible that the results or findings are not a result of **uncontrolled (extraneous or confounding) variables.** If such variables cannot be controlled through sampling procedures or analysis procedures, the researcher should report their possible influence on the findings and list them as a limitation of the study. When one reads the results of a study, it is important to ask what else could have accounted for the study findings or have influenced them in one way

or another. A good practice when one is in doubt about the credibility of a research study's findings is to refer to a research critique (see, for example, Wilson 1985, Chapters 6 and 7).

Data

Data is a plural noun meaning information, in this case the information that a nurse researcher collects from the subjects of a research study. Data may be physiologic measurements (e.g., blood pressure readings or pulse readings), psychologic measures (e.g., scores on intelligence, personality, or other mental measurement scales), or sociologic measures (e.g., social class reflected by such factors as educational preparation, occupation, income, and the like). Data are obtained from subjects through instruments (or tools). Many instruments are used in nursing studies, including interviews, questionnaires, intelligence tests, rating scales, and such biologic measures as blood pressure or pulse rate.

Validity and Reliability

Among the most important concerns of the reader evaluating the worth of instruments used to measure variables in a nursing study are their **validity** and **reliability.** A valid instrument measures what it is supposed to measure. A reliable measure produces consistent results or data on repeated use because the researcher has established a carefully standardized procedure for administering it. If blood pressure readings are taken several times on the same subject under unchanging conditions, and the results are consistent, the measure (the procedure for taking the reading) is reliable.

Populations and Samples

The population for a study (N) is the total possible membership of the group being studied. Because it is not always possible or feasible to study everybody in a population, a representative part of the population, called a **sample** (n) of participants or respondents, is usually used. When reading a study, the research consumer must attempt to determine if the findings were obtained from a sample that is representative of the study population. A **random sample** is one in which all members of a population have an equal chance of being included in the study sample.

Tables and Graphs

It is beyond the scope of this text to teach the reader how to evaluate whether qualitative or statistical analysis procedures in a nursing study were appropriate. However, a research consumer must learn to read and comprehend findings that customarily are presented in tables and graphs. The following guidelines should prove helpful:

- Try to spot trends.

- Decide if the researcher has picked the correct measure of central tendency. It can be the **mean** (the total divided by the number of cases); the **median** (the midpoint between the upper and lower halves); or the **mode** (the case that is most common). The consumer must determine which is the best way to describe the central tendency for any particular study question.

- Pay attention to the range of numbers in charts and graphs. The range can reveal how typical the dominant response was.

- Look for exceptions. Sometimes these are missing data or "outlyers": instances, observations, or scores that don't fall into the typical pattern.

- Compare findings presented in the text of a research article against data presented in tables, charts, and their captions, keeping alert for any inconsistencies.

- Look up unfamiliar statistical procedures in a good basic statistics book.

The word *criticism,* in everyday language, has negative connotations. When the nurse is analyzing, reviewing, carefully dissecting, evaluating, and even judging the merits of a research report, criticism becomes a professional responsibility. In fact, the word as Aristotle used it meant a standard for "judging well." A thoughtful research critique requires more than just following the steps of a process that begins with the question, "Is the problem clearly stated?" The student must learn the standards against which to judge research reports. What are the qualities of good problem statements? How does one judge the credibility of evidence, the adequacy of explanations, the reliability and validity of a study's instruments and design? These investigative skills will be required of all nurses in the future.

RESEARCH IN PSYCHIATRIC NURSING: THE CURRENT STATE

Two of the authors (O'Toole and Jones) undertook a qualitative and quantitative analysis of psychiatric nursing research articles to summarize the characteristics of research in psychiatric mental health nursing. O'Toole (1981) had previously analyzed the literature to determine the adequacy of theory development. Between the years of 1970 and 1985, twenty-four journals were reviewed. There were 153 psychiatric nursing research articles in fifteen journals. Nine journals contained no psychiatric nursing research articles. Although the authors may have inadvertently failed to locate certain articles, the survey is essentially a population survey rather than a sampling of articles. (See Jones and Jones [1987] for additional discussion of this survey.)

Methodology

Each article was subjected to an intensive critical reading independently by the authors. The article was then discussed and evaluated according to specified criteria. An analysis of the 153 studies evaluated the methodology and statistical procedures used. Each study was classified by journal type, time trends, author characteristics, kinds of statistics, number of subjects, number of variables, methodologic characteristics, type of design, age of subjects, specification of variables, and reported differences in groups (if any) further identified by kind of differences.

A subset (N = 136) of the studies was analyzed further to determine characteristics of the content of each article. These articles were selected because of their focus on psychiatric nursing practice, including the liaison role of the psychiatric nurse. Thus, 17 articles were eliminated because they were studies of staff or student attitudes. The analysis classified articles by type of design, developmental age of subjects, and content of independent and dependent variables.

Findings

Type of Journal

Table 14–1 shows the number and percentage of psychiatric nursing research articles classified by type of journal. There are four types of journals: research (32 percent), theoretical/clinical/research (8 percent), clinical-psychiatric (51 percent), and clinical-nonpsychiatric (9 percent). It is interesting to note that most research articles appeared in clinical-psychiatric journals.

Table 14–2 shows time trends in number of articles published in the various types of nursing journals. In the period from 1970–1974, 54 percent of the articles were in research journals. This declined to 22 percent in the most recent period (1980–1985). In contrast, clinical-psychiatric journals increased their share from 41 percent to 60 percent in the corresponding time periods. Clinical-nonpsychiatric journals increased their share from 0 percent to 10 percent during this time.

Author Characteristics

A comparison of author characteristics by year of publication is presented in Table 14–3. Of primary importance is that the percentage of authors with doctorates is constant across the three time periods (45 percent overall).

Table 14–1
Articles Classified by Journal Type

Journal	Number of Articles	Percent
Research	(48)	(32%)
International Journal of Nursing Studies	9	6%
Nursing Research	30	20%
Research in Nursing and Health	5	3%
Western Journal of Nursing Research	4	3%
Theoretical/Clinical/Research	(13)	(8%)
Advances in Nursing Science	2	1%
Image	1	<1%
Journal of Advanced Nursing	10	6%
Clinical-Psychiatric	(78)	(51%)
Issues in Mental Health Nursing	26	17%
Journal of Psychosocial Nursing	46	30%
Perspectives in Psychiatric Care	6	4%
Clinical-Nonpsychiatric	(14)	(9%)
Heart and Lung	9	6%
Issues in Pediatric Nursing	1	<1%
Journal of Gerontological Nursing	1	<1%
Journal of Obstetrics and Gynecology	1	<1%
Maternal Child Nursing	1	<1%
Public Health Nursing	1	<1%
Total	153	100%

Source: Jones SL, Jones PK: Research in psychiatric and mental health nursing: The emergence of scientific rigor. Arch Psych Nurs 1987;1(3):157. © 1987 by Grune & Stratton, Inc.

However, the percentage of authors with a master's degree has steadily increased from 27 percent to 45 percent, whereas the percent of authors with a baccalaureate degree has decreased over time from 20 percent to 5 percent. The percent of M.D.'s has decreased from 7 percent to 2 percent.

Kinds of Statistics

Table 14–4 shows the kinds of statistics reported by year of publication. The percentage of articles presenting descriptive statistics only has declined from 59 percent to 39 percent over the time span, reflecting an increase in sophistication of the psychiatric nursing research. In contrast, the percentage of articles presenting descriptive plus more complex parametric inferential statistics has increased from 23 percent to 35 percent.

Number of Subjects

Table 14–5 shows the number of subjects by journal classification. Research and theoretical/clinical/research journals report studies with large sample sizes, i.e., more than 75 subjects. Clinical journals tend to report studies with smaller sample sizes.

Table 14–2
Time Trends in Journal Articles

Nursing Journal Type	Number of Articles	Year of Publication			
		1970–1974 N = 22	1975–1979 N = 44	1980–1985 N = 87	Total N = 153
Research	48	54%	39%	22%	32%
Theoretical/Clinical/Research	13	5%	11%	8%	8%
Clinical-Psychiatric	78	41%	39%	60%	51%
Clinical-Nonpsychiatric	14	0%	11%	10%	9%
Total	153	100%	100%	100%	100%

Source: Jones SL, Jones PK: Research in psychiatric and mental health nursing: The emergence of scientific rigor. Arch Psych Nurs 1987;1(3):157. © by Grune & Stratton, Inc.

Table 14–3
Comparison of Author Characteristics by Year of Publication

Percent of Authors	Year of Publication			
	1970–1974 N = 22	1975–1979 N = 44	1980–1985 N = 87	Total N = 153
With doctoral degree	46%	40%	47%	45%
With master's degree	27%	45%	45%	42%
With baccalaureate degree	20%	12%	5%	10%
Who are nurses	59%	65%	75%	69%
Who are M.D.'s	7%	6%	2%	4%

Source: Jones SL, Jones PK: Research in psychiatric and mental health nursing: The emergence of scientific rigor. Arch Psych Nurs 1987;1(3):158. © by Grune & Stratton, Inc.

Table 14–4
Kinds of Statistics Reported by Year of Publication

Kinds of Statistics Reported	Year of Publication			
	1970–1974 N = 22	1975–1979 N = 44	1980–1985 N = 87	Total N = 153
Descriptive only	59%	41%	39%	42%
Descriptive plus parametric inferential	23%	27%	35%	31%
Descriptive plus nonparametric inferential	18%	14%	21%	18%
Descriptive plus combination	0%	16%	3%	7%
Unspecified	0%	2%	2%	2%

Table 14–5
Number of Subjects by Journal Classification

Number of Subjects	Research N = 49	Theoretical/ Clinical-Research N = 13	Clinical-Psychiatric N = 78	Clinical-Nonpsychiatric N = 13	Total N = 153
None	8%	0%	8%	0%	6%
1–25	22%	23%	28%	54%	28%
26–75	33%	23%	37%	46%	36%
>75	37%	54%	27%	0%	30%
Total	100%	100%	100%	100%	100%

Table 14–6
Number of Variables Analyzed by Year of Publication

Number of Variables Analyzed	Year of Publication			
	1970–1974 N = 22	1975–1979 N = 44	1980–1985 N = 87	Total N = 153
One (univariate)	77%	48%	44%	50%
Two (bivariate)	23%	34%	47%	40%
Three (multivariate)	0%	18%	9%	10%
Total	100%	100%	100%	100%

Number of Variables

Table 14–6 shows the number of variables analyzed by year of publication. There has been a decline in the percentage of articles reporting univariate analysis only, from 77 percent in 1970–1974 to 44 percent in 1980–1985. In contrast, there has been an increase in the use of bivariate and multivariate procedures. This trend reflects psychiatric nursing's concern with clients as biopsychosocial in nature and with the complexities of interaction.

Methodologic Characteristics

Table 14–7 shows the methodologic characteristics of journal articles. Most articles (82 percent) contain a clear statement of the problems, and two-thirds (66 percent) include a review of the literature. In contrast, only about one-third (32 percent) include a theoretical/conceptual framework. About half of the articles contain conceptual and opera-

Table 14–7
Methodologic Characteristics of Journal Articles

Methodologic Characteristic	Percent N = 153
Clear statement of problem	82%
Review of literature	66%
Theoretical/conceptual framework	32%
Conceptual *and* operational definitions of variables	50%
Sample criteria outlined	56%
Sample description given in results	49%
Data-collection procedures outlined	61%

Source: Jones SL, Jones PK: Research in psychiatric and mental health nursing: The emergence of scientific rigor. Arch Psych Nurs 1987;1(3):158. © by Grune & Stratton, Inc.

Table 14–8
Type of Design by Year of Publication

Type of Design	Number of Articles	Year of Publication		
		1970–1974 N = 16	1975–1979 N = 44	1980–1985 N = 76
Descriptive	50	38%	34%	38%
Associational	48	25%	36%	37%
Experimental (nonnursing)	4	0%	2%	4%
Experimental (nursing intervention)	34	38%	27%	21%
Total	136	101%*	99%*	100%

*Total percents do not equal 100 because of rounding errors.

tional definitions of variables, sample criteria for inclusion of subjects, and a sample description given in the results. Less than two-thirds (61 percent) include a description of data-collection procedures.

Type of Design by Year of Publication

An analysis of type of design by year of publication is presented in Table 14–8. There has been a decline in the percentage of studies using an experimental design that tested a nursing intervention as the experimental variable: 38 percent in the first time period compared with 21 percent in the last time period. Associational designs increased from 25 percent in the first time period to 37 percent in the last time period. Studies using descriptive designs remained constant over the time period studied.

Age of Subjects

Table 14–9 gives a frequency analysis of the developmental age of the subjects. The majority (89 percent) of the studies used adults as subjects. Only 7 percent investigated children, and 3 percent investigated the elderly. These data illustrate the paucity of research in psychiatric mental health nursing on the underserved populations of children and the elderly.

Specification of Variables

As shown in Table 14–10, the majority of studies specified or defined an independent variable (86 percent) as well as a dependent variable (84 percent). Further analysis of the

subset of studies in which an independent variable was specified (N = 86) is shown in Table 14–11. Almost half (47 percent) of the 86 studies investigated the effects of the therapy process, counseling, or the nurse-client relationship on the dependent variable. Illness/hospitalization was the independent variable in only 12 percent of the articles, social role/social support in 10 percent, and social demographics in 9 percent. It is interesting to note that milieu intervention was investigated as an independent variable in only 6 studies (7 percent).

PND-I Response Class

Table 14–12 presents an analysis of the sample of studies categorized by response class. The response class categorization was taken from the early drafts of the *Classification*

Table 14–9
Developmental Age of Subjects
(N = 136)

Age of Subjects	Number of Articles	Percent
Infants	0	0%
Children	10	7%
Adult	121	89%
Elderly	4	3%
Multiple age groups	1	1%
Total	136	100%

Table 14–10
Variables Specified as Independent and Dependent
(N = 136)

	Number of Articles	Percent
Independent Variable Specified		
Yes	86	63%
No	50	37%
Total	136	100%
Dependent Variable Specified		
Yes	84	62%
No	52	38%
Total	136	100%

of *Individual Human Responses of Concern for Psychiatric/Mental Health Nursing Practice* (Loomis et al. 1987). All dependent variables from studies in which a dependent variable was specified plus the single variable in descriptive studies were combined and subjected to a content analysis according to the major response classes. Over one-third (38 percent) of the studies were classified in the sociobehavioral response class, 18 percent in the emotional response class, and 17 percent in the perceptual/cognitive response

Table 14–11
Categorization of Independent Variable
(N = 86)

Category	Number of Articles	Percent
Illness/hospitalization	10	12%
Therapy/nurse-client relationship	40	47%
Milieu intervention	6	7%
Social demographics	8	9%
Social role/social support	9	10%
Life events/stress/disaster	5	6%
Other	8	9%
Total	86	100%

Table 14–12
Categorization of Dependent and Descriptive Variable by PND-I Category
(N = 136)

Response Class*	Number of Articles	Percent
Physiologic	4	3%
Sociobehavioral†	52	38%
Emotional	25	18%
Defensive	1	1%
Perceptual/cognitive	23	17%
Value/belief	0	0%
Other	31	23%
Total	136	100%

*This analysis was based on on an early draft of PND-I. In subsequent drafts some categories have been added and others deleted.

†Currently termed interpersonal class.

class. In contrast, only 3 percent were physiologic variables, and less than 1 percent were classified in the defensive response class. The defensive class has been eliminated from PND-I. Of interest is that almost one-fourth (23 percent) could not be classified in one of the major response classes. These were usually studies that evaluated a single program and failed to identify what was to be changed or influenced by the program.

Breakdown by Sociobehavioral Class

Table 14–13 gives a frequency distribution of a subset (N = 52) of the studies that related to the sociobehavioral response class, currently termed the interpersonal class. A third of these articles were about conduct/impulse control, 29 percent focused on role performance, 19 percent on self-care, and 17 percent on communication. In contrast, there were no articles on sexuality or motor behavior and only one on sleep/arousal.

FUTURE RESEARCH DIRECTIONS

The current state of research in psychiatric nursing suggests some important future directions for clinicians who wish to advance the scientific knowledge base in the field. Research of importance could address any of the following areas or client groups.

- Studies advancing the psychobiology knowledge base for nursing interventions regarding nutrition, exer-

Table 14–13
Sociobehavioral* Response Class
(N = 52)

Sociobehavioral Response Class	Number of Articles	Percent
Communication	9	17%
Conduct/impulse control	17	33%
Motor behavior	0	0%
Role performance	15	29%
Self-care	10	19%
Sleep/arousal	1	1%
Sexuality	0	0%
Total	52	99%†

*Currently termed interpersonal class.

†Total percent does not equal 100 because of rounding errors.

cise, and sleep. For example: What nutrients affect brain function? How do caffeine and chocolate consumption influence drug withdrawal? What is the relationship of dehydration to confusion among elderly clients?

- Studies advancing knowledge about the effectiveness of psychiatric nursing interventions. For example: What are the most effective strategies for using restraints with a violent client? What are the effects of "white noise" on sleep in anxious clients?

- Studies on target populations such as the elderly, the chronically mentally ill, AIDS clients, and children, who represent a rapidly growing segment of clients in need of psychiatric services.

THE MERIT AND UTILITY OF RESEARCH FOR PSYCHIATRIC NURSING PRACTICE

Building a scientific basis for clinical practice is the most important priority for research in psychiatric nursing. Applying research findings in practice requires that all nurses be competent in judging the merit and utility of the research findings they read.

Guidelines for Judging the Merit and Utility of Clinical Studies

1. Has the original study been replicated?
2. If replicated, do findings support original findings?
3. Was the study conducted in real-world clinical conditions?
4. What was the risk/benefit of the nursing intervention tested?
5. Does the study address a significant clinical practice problem?

RESEARCH NOTE

Citation

Dennis KE, Strickland OL: The clinical nurse researcher: Institutionalizing the role. Int J Nurs Stud 1987;24:25–33.

Study Problem/Purpose

The purpose of this study was to examine the implementation of the nurse researcher role within the clinical setting.

Methods

Data were collected through interviews with ten nurse researchers from six agencies in the eastern United States. All of the researchers interviewed were associated with large medical centers, and all had been in their positions less than five years. Eight had doctoral degrees or were doctoral candidates. Two who had master's degrees worked with nurses holding doctorates. Interviews were unstructured, and categories emerged through content analysis of the hand-recorded interview notes. Categories were identified independently and then validated by a second reader and follow-up interviews.

Findings

Implementation of the clinical nurse researcher role occurred under four major nursing models: nursing research unit, dual roles, collaborative roles, and functional role division. Organizational and colleague support were crucial to the visibility and viability of the clinical nurse researcher role.

Implications

If the clinical researcher role is to be fully institutionalized in clinical settings, administrators and clinicians must clearly understand its potential benefits and contributions. Establishment of the clinical nurse researcher role within the clinical setting can benefit the client, the institution, and the discipline of nursing. The survival of the role will be contingent on its demonstrated benefits and cost-effectiveness in providing direction for the delivery of nursing care.

6. Do psychiatric nurses have control over the study variables?

7. Is it realistically feasible to implement the nursing intervention?

8. What is the cost of implementing the intervention?

9. What contribution to the client's human responses does the nursing intervention make?

10. What overall contribution to psychiatric nursing knowledge does the study make?

Chapter Highlights

- In the information revolution transforming the present and shaping the future, reading and understanding nursing research are as fundamental to professional practice as knowledge of the nursing process and communication skills are.

- The ability to access, evaluate, and interpret findings from nursing studies is a source of power in clinical decision making and a strategy for achieving excellence in the delivery of care.

- The scientific approach is a process of learning about truth by systematically collecting and comparing observable, verifiable data through the senses to describe, explain, and/or predict events and phenomena.

- The scientific approach as reflected in nursing research has two characteristics that the major ways of knowing in nursing do not: (a) It has a built-in system of checks to ensure objectivity and the potential for self-correction and (b) it relies on sensory evidence or empirical data that are collected in a systematic, carefully prescribed manner.

- The research process is generally conceptualized as a series of steps or phases, which, however, are dynamic, flexible, and expandable.

- The steps of the research process provide the tools with which scientists achieve their major aims or goals. These basic aims are to develop explanations of the world called theories and to find solutions to practical problems.

- If nursing is to emerge as a socially significant, credible, scientific, and learned profession with a commitment to high-quality client care, then research (for all nurses) is a necessity.

- If nursing is to develop as a research-based practice, the clinical nurse must know the process and language of research, be sensitive to protecting the rights of human subjects, participate in the identification of significant researchable problems, and be a discriminating consumer of research findings.

- Bridging the research-practice gap, that is, bringing research into the clinical practice arena, is a key strategy in uniting the scholarly, scientific, and caring aspects of nursing in the future.

- All nurses who practice in settings where research is being conducted with human subjects or who participate in such research as data collectors or collaborators play an important role in safeguarding the rights of human subjects.

- Certain subjects, including children, the mentally disabled, the elderly, captives, the dying, and the sedated or unconscious, are considered particularly vulnerable.

- Identifying problem areas in nursing practice is an investigative skill that all nurses need to master if the interplay between research and practice urged by the ANA is to be achieved.

- A researchable problem is one that can be investigated using the steps of the research process.

- Judging the merit and quality of clinical studies is a professional responsibility of readers of nursing research.

- Most research in psychiatric nursing between 1970 and 1985 has been published in clinical journals and reveals major gaps and future needs for focused directions.

References

American Nurses' Association: *Human Rights Guidelines for Nurses in Clinical and Other Research.* The Association, 1975.

American Nurses' Association: *Nursing: A Social Policy Statement.* The Association, 1980.

American Nurses' Association, Commission on Nursing Research: *ANA Guidelines for Investigative Functions of Nurses.* The Association, 1981.

American Nurses' Association, Cabinet on Nursing Research: *Directions for Nursing Research: Toward the Twenty-First Century.* The Association, 1985.

Brink P, Wood M: *Basic Steps in Planning Nursing Research, from Question to Proposal.* Wadsworth, 1983.

Chenitz C: The politics of nursing research, in Mason DJ, Talbott SW: *Political Action Handbook for Nurses.* Addison-Wesley, 1985.

Davis M: Promoting nursing research in the clinical setting. *J Nurs Admin* 1981;March:122–127.

Diers D: *Research in Nursing Practice.* Lippincott, 1979.

Gortner S: Out of the past and into the future. *Nurs Res* 1980;29:204–207.

Jones SL, Jones PK: Research in psychiatric and mental health nursing: The emergence of scientific rigor. *Arch Psych Nurs* 1987;1(3):155–162.

Loomis M, O'Toole AW, Brown ML, West PP, Wilson HS: Development of a classification system for psychiatric/mental health nursing. *Arch Psych Nurs* 1987;1:16–24.

O'Toole AW: When the practical becomes theoretical. *J Psychosoc Nurs* 1981;19(12):11–19.

Starzomski R: The place of research in nursing. *Can Nurse* 1983;October:34–35.

Wilson HS: *Research in Nursing.* Addison-Wesley, 1985.

Wilson HS: *Introducing Research in Nursing.* Addison-Wesley, 1987.

Wilson HS, Hutchinson SA: *Applying Research in Nursing.* Addison-Wesley, 1986.

PART THREE

Human Responses to Distress and Disorder

FIFTEEN

Applying the Nursing Process for

Clients with Organic Mental Syndromes and Disorders

Gail DeBoer
Holly Skodol Wilson

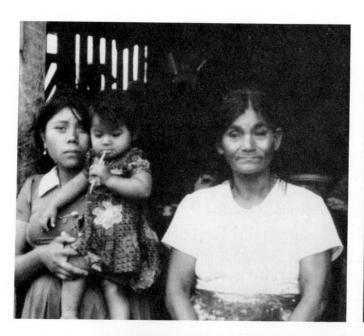

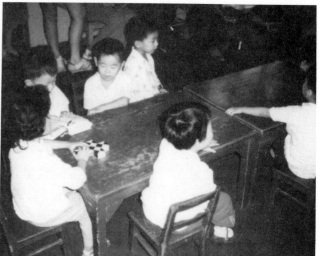

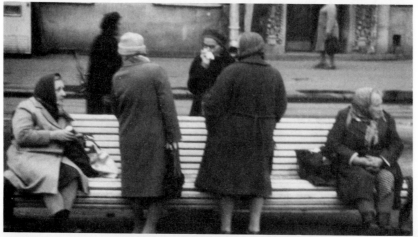

After reading this chapter, students should be able to

- Understand theories that explain the psychopathology of organic mental syndromes and organic brain disease

- Differentiate among types of dementias and delirium

- Specify diagnostic criteria for dementia and delirium

- Apply the nursing process with clients who have organic mental syndromes and organic brain disease

- Assess relevant subjective and objective data for clients with organic mental syndromes and organic brain disease

- Formulate psychiatric nursing diagnoses for clients who have organic mental syndromes and organic brain disease

- Plan and implement nursing interventions for clients who have organic mental syndromes and organic brain disease

- Identify outcome criteria to evaluate nursing interventions for clients with organic mental syndromes and organic brain disease

Cross References

Other topics relevant to this content are: Dying clients and their families, Chapter 37; Elderly, Chapter 36; Families, Chapter 33; Neuropsychiatric complications of AIDS, Chapter 26; Older adults, Chapter 6; Social support, Chapter 8; Substance abuse–related organic brain syndrome and organic mental disorder, Chapter 15.

Imagine a future when nations renounce war as a way to settle disputes.

Key Terms

agnosia
Alzheimer's disease
amnestic syndrome
aphasia
apraxia
Creutzfeldt-Jakob disease
delirium
dementia
Huntington's chorea
Kluver-Bucy-like syndrome
mnemonic disturbance
multi-infarct dementia (MID)
neurofibrillary tangles
neurosyphilis
normal pressure
   hydrocephalus
organic anxiety syndrome
organic brain syndrome
   (OBS)

organic delusional syndrome
organic hallucinosis
organic mental disorder
   (OMD)
organic mental syndrome
   (OMS)
organic mood syndrome
organic personality
   syndrome
organic hallucinosis
Parkinson's disease
Pick's disease
progressive supranuclear
   palsy
pseudodementia
pseudodelirium
senile plaques
tetrahydroaminoacridine
   (THA)

Ms L was a 57-year-old widowed schoolteacher who had begun experiencing difficulties with her memory for the past year. She complained that she was having problems selecting the words she wanted to use and putting her thoughts on paper. She began to miss appointments and scheduled workdays. Gradually, handling her own financial affairs became impossible.

Over three years, Ms L was forced to quit her job and become more and more dependent on her family. Her eldest daughter moved into her home, and other friends and family took turns sitting with her. Ms L became incontinent as she wandered confusedly about the house, unable to find the bathroom. Increasingly anxious and paranoid, she began to see things crawling on the walls and mistook her own reflection in a mirror for a painting. When agitated she was just as likely to walk out into the street as to become belligerent with her daughter.

Ms L was finally admitted to a long-term care facility when she became increasingly belligerent and aggressive with her daughter, wandering the house at night, sleeping sporadically. After two years, Ms L was bedridden and unable to speak. She had to be tube fed. Ms L finally succumbed to pneumonia.

Until very recently psychiatric nursing has for the most part ignored mental disorders due to cerebral dysfunction. Recent developments have changed the focus, however, and interest is growing in the organic mental syndromes and disorders. Lipowski (1980) identifies the factors behind this shift:

- The ever-increasing number of people over age 65 who have a high prevalence of organic mental disorders
- A growing awareness of the psychiatric manifestations of cerebral disorders resulting from acute systemic and chronic metabolic disturbances
- Advances in the neurosciences, especially in our knowledge of neurotransmitters
- Improvements in the classification of organic mental disorders through the DSM-III and DSM-IIIR

HISTORICAL AND THEORETICAL FOUNDATIONS

Before the twentieth century, all organic brain disorders of the aged were categorized as *senile dementia*. Beginning at the turn of the century, neuropathologists doing autopsy work distinguished senile dementia from arteriosclerotic conditions and neurosyphilis (Butler and Lewis 1982). Arteriosclerotic brain disease was then considered the primary cause of confusional states in the elderly. It was believed to be the result of diseased cerebral vessels (Wolanin and Fraelich-Philips 1981). By the middle of this century, a new category, *organic brain disease (OBD)* was added. This category was broader, allowing for both a defect in the vessels and in the brain itself. The category **organic brain syndrome (OBS)** then followed, which recognized the need for a diagnosis that included symptoms without a known cause. Today, the term **organic mental syndrome (OMS)** refers to a group of psychologic or behavioral signs of no specific etiology. **Organic mental disorder (OMD)** refers to a particular syndrome whose etiology is known or presumed. In an effort to connect cause and effect more clearly and to avoid the negative connotation of the word *senile,* psychiatric professionals are proposing terms such as *brain failure, cognitive decrement,* and *poor cerebral support.*

PSYCHOPATHOLOGY

Dementia

In the United States today, approximately 5 percent of people over age 65 suffer from dementia to the extent that they cannot care for themselves, and 10 percent suffer from a milder form (Gershon and Herman 1982). Over 60 percent of people in nursing homes have been diagnosed with

dementia (Brody et al. 1984). A now common clinical syndrome, **dementia** is marked by alterations in the cognitive areas of

- Orientation
- Memory
- Intellectual function
- Judgment
- Affect

In its broadest sense, dementia is defined as an altered mental state secondary to cerebral disease (Hamill and Buell 1982). Symptoms related to specific areas of brain damage are shown in Figure 15–1. The DMS-IIIR further differentiates *dementia* as "a disturbance severe enough to interfere significantly with work or usual social activities or relationships with others" (DSM-IIIR, p 103). (See Box 15–1 for the DSM-IIIR diagnostic criteria.)

Dementias are classified according to causal agent (Box 15–2) or area of neurologic damage. The latter scheme distinguishes between cortical and subcortical dementias. Alzheimer's disease is the classic cortical dementia, while Huntington's chorea and Parkinson's disease are common subcortical types. These categories are quite similar. People with subcortical dementias, however, have a higher order of functioning. That is, insight is retained and signs of aphasia, apraxia, or agnosia are not present (Huber and Paulson 1985).

Alzheimer's Disease

Alzheimer's disease, an OMD, is the form of dementia most commonly seen in the elderly. It accounts for over 50 percent of the dementias of old age (Small et al. 1981). Louis Alzheimer first recognized it in 1907 while conducting an autopsy on a 55-year-old woman with a history of dementia. **Senile plaques** and other pathologic lesions that he then called **neurofibrillary tangles** were discovered. These are now referred to as Alzheimer-type changes. This disease may also destroy those neurons that secrete the neurotransmitter acetylcholine, which plays a role in memory and learning (Wells, 1962).

Alzheimer's disease is defined as a progressive, age-related chronic cognitive dysfunction (Schneck et al. 1982). The usual age of onset for the presenile type is from 40 to 54; for the senile type, 70 to 84. Death usually follows in six to seven years after the diagnosis is confirmed.

Signs of Alzheimer's Disease

Wolanin and Fraelich-Philips (1981) describe four signs of this disease:

1. Aphasia (loss of language ability). Initially, the person experiences difficulty in searching for words, becoming mute as the disease progresses.

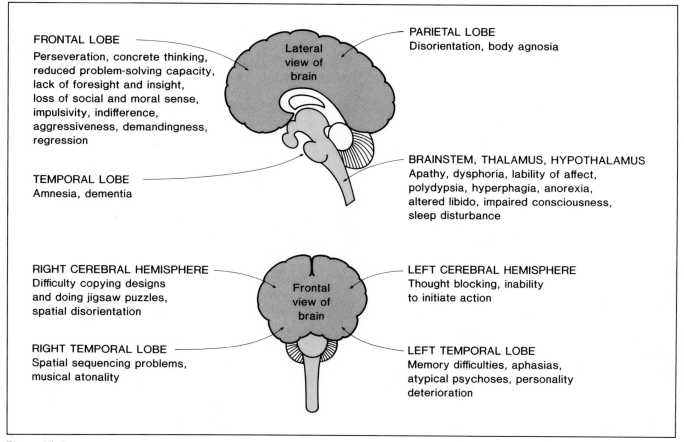

Figure 15–1
Behavior changes related to specific areas of brain damage.

2. **Apraxia** (loss of purposeful movement without loss of muscle power or coordination in general). In the early stages, the individual has difficulty reproducing a picture in perspective. In time, the person is no longer able to perform previously mastered purposeful and skilled activities, such as dressing himself or herself.

3. **Agnosia** (loss of sensory ability to recognize objects). Initially, the person will have difficulty recognizing everyday objects. In the later stages, he will recognize neither loved ones nor his or her own body parts.

4. **Mnemonic disturbances** (memory loss). The inability to remember recent events extends to profound memory loss of both recent and past events.

The Progression of Alzheimer's Disease

Stages of the progression of Alzheimer's disease have been variously described in the literature. In the early stages, called "the forgetfulness phase" (Schneck et al 1982), the person has difficulty remembering names, appointments, and where things were placed. The person may also have problems with spatial orientation, show affect changes, and seem emotionally unstable at times. Epileptiform seizures may occur, along with muscle twitching. (See Table 15–1.)

More advanced stages present with apparent cognitive deficits. Memory for past events may still exist, but the person has no recall of recent ones. Orientation and concentration are now affected, and the person has increasing difficulty comprehending everyday events. Restlessness at night and increased aphasia, agnosia, and apraxia are seen. Activities of daily living must be supervised, and former social habits are forgotten. Hypertonia and an unsteady gait are seen, along with perseveration phenomena, hyperorality, and an insatiable appetite without weight gain.

The final stage is the terminal phase, usually not lasting for more than one year. Severe disorientation, psychotic symptoms (e.g., delusions, hallucinations, and paranoid ideation), and severe agitation are present. A Kluver-Bucy-like syndrome occurs, which includes hyperorality, blunting of emotions, bulimia, and attempts to touch every object in sight. The individual eventually becomes bedridden, emaciated, and helpless. Death usually results from

---

Box 15–1
DSM-IIIR DIAGNOSTIC CRITERIA FOR DEMENTIA

1. Demonstrable evidence of impairment in short- and long-term memory. Impairment in short-term memory (inability to learn new information) may be indicated by inability to remember three objects after five minutes. Long-term memory impairment (inability to remember information that was known in the past) may be indicated by inability to remember past personal information (e.g., what happened yesterday, birthplace, occupation) or facts of common knowledge (e.g., past Presidents, well-known dates).

2. At least one of the following:

   a. Impairment in abstract thinking, as indicated by inability to find similarities and differences between related words, difficulty in defining words and concepts, and other similar tasks

   b. Impaired judgment, as indicated by inability to make reasonable plans to deal with interpersonal, family, and job-related problems and issues

   c. Other disturbances of higher cortical function, such as aphasia (disorder of language), apraxia (inability to carry out motor activities despite intact comprehension and motor function), agnosia (failure to recognize or identify objects despite intact sensory function), and "constructional difficulty" (e.g., inability to copy three-dimensional figures, assemble blocks, or arrange sticks in specific designs)

   d. Personality change, i.e., alteration or accentuation of premorbid traits

3. The disturbance in A and B significantly interferes with work or usual social activities or relationships with others.

4. Not occurring exclusively during the course of delirium.

5. Either a or b:

   a. There is evidence from the history, physical examination, or laboratory tests of a specific organic factor (or factors) judged to be etiologically related to the disturbance

   b. In the absence of such evidence, an etiologic organic factor can be presumed if the disturbance cannot be accounted for by any nonorganic mental disorder, e.g., Major Depression accounting for cognitive impairment

Criteria for Severity of Dementia

Mild: Although work or social activities are significantly impaired, the capacity for independent living remains, with adequate personal hygiene and relatively intact judgment.

Moderate: Independent living is hazardous, and some degree of supervision is necessary.

Severe: Activities of daily living are so impaired that continual supervision is required, e.g., unable to maintain minimal personal hygiene; largely incoherent or mute.

Source: American Psychiatric Association: Diagnostic and Statistical Manual of Mental Disorders, ed 3, revised. *APA, 1987, p 107.*

---

pneumonia or other infection, malnutrition, and dehydration.

Cause of Alzheimer's Disease

The actual cause of Alzheimer's remains unknown, but several factors are believed to play a role. Genetics, especially in the presenile type, may play a role; as evidenced by the occurrence in members of the same family (Wright and Whaley 1984). Work is also being done to discover a slow-acting viruslike causal agent. This work has been prompted by the findings of just such an agent in Creutzfeldt-Jakob disease (Schneck et al. 1982). Aluminum has also been implicated, since it can cause dementia in animals and has been found in significantly higher than normal concentration on autopsy in people with Alzheimer's disease (Wells 1982). Alzheimer's disease may also be related to a specific chromosome or genotype. People with Down's syndrome who survive to adulthood eventually develop Alzheimer lesions in the brain. Last, a possible defect in the immune system, as evidenced by detected brain antibodies in people with Alzheimer's disease, is under investigation (Schneck et al. 1982).

Multi-Infarct Dementia

Multi-infarct dementia (MID), an OMD, accounts for about 15 percent of the dementias. Unlike Alzheimer's disease, which is slowly progressive, MID is usually abrupt in onset and episodic, with multiple remissions (Gershon and Herman 1982). The client also demonstrates focal neurologic signs, such as one-sided weakness, emotional outbursts when frustrated, a stepwise rather than progressive decline in intellectual functioning, and a history of hypertension (Small et al. 1981).

Box 15–2
CLASSIFICATION OF DEMENTIAS (ORGANIC MENTAL DISORDERS)

	Rate of Occurrence
Primary dementia	
Alzheimer's disease	50%
Pick's disease	—
Huntington's chorea	—
Progressive supranuclear palsy	—
Creutzfeldt-Jakob disease	—
Vascular	
Multi-infarct dementia	15%
Secondary causes	
Normal pressure hydrocephalus	5%–6%
Korsakoff's psychosis	—
Trauma (chronic subdural hematoma)	—
Central nervous system masses	—
Metabolic (thyroid, pernicious anemia, renal, or hepatic disease)	—
Central nervous system infections (viral encephalitis, tertiary neurosyphilis, tuberculous and fungal meningitis, acquired immune deficiency syndrome, AIDS-related complex)	—
Drugs	—
Pseudodementia of depression	10%

Source: Adapted from Gershon S, Herman S: The differential diagnosis of dementia. J Am Geriatr Soc 1982;30:558–566.

In MID, brain tissue is destroyed by intermittent emboli. The result is widely distributed areas of microinfarction with diffuse, asymmetrical regions of cerebral softening (Gershon and Herman 1982). Factors contributing to MID include:

- Myocardial infarction
- Hypertension
- Diabetes mellitus
- Transient ischemic attacks
- Peripheral vascular disease
- Obesity
- Smoking

Parkinson's Disease

Only recently has the OMD, **Parkinson's disease**, been associated with dementia. Historically, this disease was believed to involve only tremors, rigidity, and *bradykinesia* (slow movement) without cognitive involvement (Huber and Paulson 1985). It is now estimated that about one in three people with Parkinson's disease will become demented over time (Wells 1982). It has also been suggested that there may be two separate disorders: Parkinson's disease without dementia, and Parkinson's with dementia. The former is

Table 15–1
The Progression of Alzheimer's Disease*

Early Stages	Advanced Stages	Later and Terminal Stages
Memory loss (recent)	Memory loss (recent and remote)	Irritability and severe agitation
Spatial disorientation	Difficulty comprehending	Seizure
Time disorientation	Disorientation	Apraxia
Mistakes in judgment	Restlessness at night; wandering	Loss of appetite with emaciation
Mood changes	Aphasia	Bedridden and helpless
Decreased concentration	Agnosia	Kluver-Bucy-like syndrome
Carelessness in actions and appearance	Apraxia	Delusions
Epileptiform seizures	Perseveration	Hallucinations
Muscular twitchings	Hyperorality	Paranoid ideation
Difficulty focusing attention	Unsteady gait	Unresponsive coma
Decreased interest in environment	Hypertonia	Susceptibility to infection and injury
Increased indifference to social courtesies	Socially unacceptable behavior	Incontinence
	Increased appetite without weight gain	Ataxia
		Little or no response to stimuli

*Behaviors observed in the progression of the disease are categorized variously in the literature into three or four stages.

seen more often in younger clients who experience a longer and more benign course and respond well to levodopa therapy. The dementia is seen in the older group who experience cognitive dysfunction following motor dysfunction and do not respond well to the drug levodopa (Huber and Paulson 1985).

These clients also show, on autopsy, the characteristic brain changes associated with Alzheimer's disease (Wells 1982), indicating a relationship between these two diseases. Work is also being done with L-dopa as a possible causal agent; however, this work remains speculative.

Huntington's Chorea

A hereditary disease, **Huntington's chorea** involves both motor and cognitive changes. This OMD usually begins between the ages of 30 to 50 years. Subtle changes in memory function are believed to precede physical changes by several years (Huber and Paulson 1985). The motor dysfunction is characterized by chorea: quick, jerky, purposeless, involuntary movements. Subcortical dementia is seen, with personality and cognitive changes ranging from apathy to violent emotional outbursts, inability to solve problems and process information quickly, and poor concept formation (Wolanin and Fraelich-Philips 1981). Average life span after an initial diagnosis is fifteen years.

Pick's Disease

Pick's disease is a presenile dementia with age of onset in the mid-fifties. This OMD resembles Alzheimer's disease clinically, but senile plaques and neurofibrillary tangles are not found on autopsy. Cerebral atrophy is confined to the frontal and temporal cortex (Small et al. 1981).

Early signs of Pick's disease include emotional blunting, lack of inhibitions, and lack of insight and social awareness. As the disease progresses, the deterioration becomes more global, affecting memory and language. The expected life span after the original diagnosis is seven years. A higher incidence is seen in some families, pointing toward a genetic predisposition (Wolanin and Fraelich-Philips 1981).

Creutzfeldt-Jakob Disease

Creutzfeldt-Jakob disease is a presenile dementia that usually begins at age 50 to 60. This OMD affects the cerebral cortex through cell destruction and overgrowth. It is marked clinically by a very rapid onset. The first symptoms noted are motor or sensory disturbances, which may include visual and hearing disturbances, loss of muscle strength, and

problems with coordinated movements. With rapid progression, the person may suffer from blindness, deafness, severe ataxia, *myoclonus* (muscle spasm), and tremors. Cognitive decline includes deterioration in language, memory, and intellectual functions. Life expectancy after diagnosis is approximately one year. In the final stage, the person is confined to bed with brain failure (Wells 1978, Wolanin and Fraelich-Philips 1981).

This is the only dementia of aging for which there is documented evidence of a slow-acting virus being the cause. The disease has been reproduced in 70 percent of primates inoculated with affected brain tissue. Researchers are trying to isolate the virus, and there is speculation about the possibility of human-to-human transmission, especially through blood transfusions.

Normal Pressure Hydrocephalus

First recognized in 1965, **normal pressure hydrocephalus** is a presenile dementia affecting about 5 percent of those diagnosed with dementia. Gait disturbance is often the earliest sign of this OMD. This symptom may lead to incorrect diagnosis as Parkinson's disease. Urinary incontinence and mild dementia are later stage symptoms. Clients are usually slow and withdrawn, and depression is frequently present (Hamill and Buell 1982).

The syndrome is believed to occur when the flow of cerebrospinal fluid over the cerebral hemispheres is blocked and absorption at the superior sagittal sinus is impaired, with resulting ventricle enlargement and decreased cerebral bloodflow. Neurosurgical shunting is the usual treatment, although results are mixed. The syndrome has various causes; two-thirds of clients have an identified cranial disease (e.g., cerebral trauma, tumors, or infections) (Wells 1978).

Neurosyphilis

Neurosyphilis or *dementia paralytica* is the direct result of untreated primary syphilis. The infecting organism (*Treponema pallidum,* a spirochete) produces cerebral atrophy in the frontal and anterior temporal lobes. Symptoms of this OMD may appear two to thirty years following the primary lesion (Wolanin and Fraelich-Philips 1981). The usual symptoms are paranoia, poor memory, faulty judgment, and disturbed emotional displays. Neurologic signs include fine and coarse tremors, abnormal reflexes, *dysarthria* (difficulty in speaking), and convulsions. Untreated, the disease is usually fatal within three years of onset.

Progressive Supranuclear Palsy

Progressive supranuclear palsy is a presenile subcortical dementia resulting from cell atrophy in the midbrain. Gait disturbances, flat affect, impaired ocular movement, forced laughter or crying, recent memory loss, and a general slowing of cognitive processes are all present in this OMD. There is no known cause or treatment (Huber and Paulson 1985).

Pseudodementia

The syndrome of pseudodementia has been the subject of increasing attention. This OMD is particularly common in the elderly and most difficult to assess among elderly clients (McAllister 1983). **Pseudodementia** is a syndrome in which dementia is mimicked by a psychiatric illness (Wells 1978). The course of the illness is influenced by the underlying psychiatric disorder (Table 15–2). The mood disorders are the most common cause of pseudodementia, which can be appropriately viewed as a depression-induced organic mental disorder (McAllister 1983).

This syndrome is significant because of the great number of depressed elderly people. It is estimated that about 15 percent of the elderly living in the community experience some form of depression and that 4 percent have

major symptoms of depression (Reifler, Larson, and Hanley 1982). Failure to recognize the syndrome may lead to inappropriate treatment. The person may be labeled as senile, and the stigma attached to the label deepens the person's depression. The prognosis, if the syndrome is recognized, is excellent (McAllister 1983).

Delirium

Mr. R, an 80-year-old bachelor with bilateral cataracts, lived alone in a small midwestern town with his pet cat, Suzy. With help from family and friends, he lived a full, active life. He walked a mile daily, did his own cooking, and attended church services regularly.

RESEARCH NOTE

Citation

Monsour N, Robb S: Wandering behavior in old age: A psychosocial study. Soc Work 1982;September:411–416.

Study Problem/Purpose

Why do some elderly people wander while others do not despite their similar ages, mobility levels, and degrees of confusion?

Methods

This was a retrospective study of differences in the psychosocial life-styles between groups of male wanderers and nonwanderers. Twenty-two matched pairs of wanderers and nonwanderers were selected from a population of approximately 400 residents in the long-term care division of a Veterans Administration medical center.

Procedures

A personal structured interview was conducted with each subject's closest significant other to collect data related to the life-style of each subject during the period after age 40. Interview schedules were derived from scales selected to measure variables such as preferred social and leisure activities, experiences of stressful life events, and responses to stress. Background demographic data were also obtained from records and in the interviews with significant others.

Findings

Paired *t*-test statistics were used to evaluate four major hypotheses. The findings were as follows:

1. Wanderers engaged in more social and leisure activities than nonwanderers did before their illness.

2. Before their illness, wanderers experienced more stressful life events than nonwanderers did.

3. Wanderers, in contrast to nonwanderers, had motor reactions to stress in their earlier years.

4. Wanderers demonstrated more physically active behavior styles in their earlier years than did nonwanderers.

Implications

Wanderers may have had the need not only to participate in physical activity but also to be productively absorbed during their leisure time. Thus, previous life-style deserves more attention as a possible explanatory variable than it has received from researchers and clinicians endeavoring to understand wandering behavior in elderly people. Management implications include: (a) It is important to record the history of wandering clients' life-styles rather than accepting too readily the organic dysfunctions of old age. (b) Such interventions as physical restraints or drugs ought to give way to alternatives that have the potential to achieve the same goal of stopping or managing wandering behavior. For instance, the environment can be structured so that wandering behavior is more appropriate and safer. A retrieval program, such as that used at the Ebenezer Society in Minneapolis, can be instituted. Another intervention is to decrease the individual's desire or need to wander by encouraging physical exercise or decreasing environmental stressors that may lead wanderers to react with increased motor activity.

	Table 15–2 Impaired Cognitive Function		
	Dementia	**Delirium**	**Depression**
Essential Features	Demonstrable evidence of impairment in short- and long-term memory. Multifaceted deficit: loss of intellectual abilities of sufficient severity to interfere with social or occupational function, judgment, impulse control, abstract thought, and a variety of other higher cortical functioning. Changes in personality and behavior.	Reduced ability to maintain attention and shift attention. Manifestations: reduced level of consciousness, sensory misinterpretation, disordered stream of thought. Disturbances of sleep-wakefulness and psychomotor activity.	Dysphoric mood, loss of interest or pleasure in usual activities and pastimes, appetite disturbance, change in weight, sleep disturbance, psychomotor agitation or retardation, decreased energy, feelings of worthlessness or guilt, difficulty concentrating or thinking, thoughts of death or suicide or suicide attempts.
Associated Features	Mild dementia: awareness of deteriorating faculty leading to anxiety, depression. May conceal or compensate for deficit. Paranoid ideation. Vulnerable to physical and psychologic stressors.	Emotional disturbance: fear, anxiety, irritability, anger, euphoria, apathy. Neurologic signs: presence of abnormal movements, e.g., tremors, asterixis (flapping movement of hyperextended hands). Autonomic signs: tachycardia, flushed face, increased blood pressure. Disorders of higher cortical function: dysnomia (inability to name objects), dysgraphia (impaired ability to write).	Depressed appearance, tearfulness, feelings of anxiety, irritability, fear, brooding, excessive concern with physical health, panic attacks, phobias. Delusion or hallucinations may be present. In elderly, see symptoms suggesting dementia (e.g., disorientation, memory loss, distractibility, apathy, difficulty in concentration, inattentiveness).
Onset	Depends on underlying etiology. May be rather sudden (e.g., head trauma) or insidious in onset and slow, but progress is relentless over several years (e.g., primary degenerative dementia).	May begin abruptly. Relatively rapid—over hours. Short period of time—few days. Especially common in children and after the age of 60.	Usually able to date onset with some precision. Onset is variable; symptoms usually developing over a period of days to weeks but may be sudden. In some instances, prodromal symptoms may occur over several months.
Course	Depends on underlying etiology. May be progressive, static, or remitting.	Fluctuates; symptoms usually worse at night; lucid intervals usually in the morning.	Often not recognized or misdiagnosed in the elderly. Need to differentiate from dementia.
Duration	May progress to death over several years. May be arrested or reversed.	Brief—usually one week, rarely over a month.	Self-limiting. Median time period is eight months; may last up to two years.
Outcome	Reversibility depends on underlying pathology, timely diagnosis, and treatment. The more widespread the structural damage to the brain, the less likely the clinical improvement.	Recovery if underlying disease is corrected or self-limiting. If disorder persists, shift to another more stable organic brain syndrome. May cause death.	Can be successfully treated. Spontaneous recovery is expected. Severe depression may end in suicide.
Etiologic Factors	Primary degenerative dementia, Alzheimer type. Infections of central nervous system. Brain	Systemic infections. Metabolic disorders (hepatic or renal disease, hypoxia, hypercapnia,	Situational—bereavement, loss of health, major catastrophic event in person's life.

continued

Table 15–2 *(Continued)* **Impaired Cognitive Function**		
Dementia	**Delirium**	**Depression**
trauma. Virus (e.g., acquired immune deficiency syndrome, Creutzfeldt-Jakob disease). Toxic metabolic disturbance. Vascular disease (e.g., multi-infarct dementia). Normal pressure hydrocephalus. Neurologic diseases such as Huntington's chorea, multiple sclerosis, Parkinson's disease. Postanoxic or posthypoglycemic states.	hypoglycemia, ionic imbalances, thiamine deficiency). Postoperative states. Substance intoxication and withdrawal. Head trauma. Lesions of the right parietal lobe and occipital lobe.	

Sources: American Psychiatric Association: Diagnostic and Statistical Manual of Mental Disorders, *ed 3, rev. APA, 1987. Blazer DG: Epidemiology of late life depression.* J Am Geriatr Soc *1982;30:587–592. Raskind MA, Storrie MC: The organic mental disorders, in Busse EW, Blazer DG (eds):* Handbook of Geriatric Psychiatry. *Van Houten, 1980, pp 305–328.*

Mr. R was admitted to the community hospital for a hernia repair that he had been putting off for several months. Never hospitalized before, he was extremely anxious on admission and became more so with each preoperative procedure that day. By ten o'clock that evening, Mr. R was found wandering in the hallway looking and calling for Suzy. The nurse gave him a barbiturate sleeping preparation and returned him to his room. Three hours later he was again found wandering, this time nude and more disoriented than before. He was again sedated and confined to bed with a vest and soft wrist restraints. By morning, Mr. R was so disoriented and agitated that the surgery was canceled. Mr. R's physician then ordered Valium for sedation and the client remained confined to bed. Within one week, Mr. R's behavior had deteriorated to the extent that he was felt to need institutionalization. He was transferred to a local nursing home for permanent care.

The elderly, especially the demented, are prone to transient cognitive disorders, usually referred to as either *delirium* or *acute confusional states*. It is estimated that 30 to 50 percent of elderly medical/surgical clients will experience a life-threatening acute confusional state. One-fourth of these delirious elderly die within one month of admission (Foreman 1986). In spite of these and other compelling statistics, research in this area continues to be grossly neglected (Lipowski 1983).

Delirium has been called senile delirium, acute confusional states, acute brain syndrome, acute brain failure, pseudosenility, and clouded states. Delirium is defined as an "organic brain syndrome, characterized by global cognitive impairment of abrupt onset and relatively brief duration (usually less than 1 month) and by concurrent disturbances of attention, sleep-wake cycle, and psychomotor behavior" (Lipowski 1983, p 1427). (See Box 15–3 for DSM-IIIR diagnostic criteria.)

Signs of Delirium

Cognition

The three components of cognition—perception, thinking, and memory—are all disrupted in delirium:

- *Perception.* The person shows reduced ability to distinguish and integrate sensory information and to discriminate it from hallucinations, dreams, illusions, and imagery.
- *Thinking.* This process is fragmented and disorganized to the extent that the elderly person is unable to reason, judge, abstract, or solve problems.
- *Memory.* Memory is impaired in all three spheres; the elderly person is unable to register, retain, or recall information.

Attention and Wakefulness

Attention is impaired in all three spheres. The person has difficulty with:

- Alertness or the maintaining of vigilance

- Selectiveness, or the ability to focus on and selectively attend to stimuli at will

- Directiveness, or the ability to direct and focus one's mental processes

Wakefulness is usually reduced during the day, and the person experiences sleeplessness, restlessness, and agitation at night. Interestingly, delirium and dreaming are characterized by the same electroencephalographic (EEG) changes. The elderly person is then caught between dreaming and hallucinating, sleep and wakefulness.

Psychomotor Behavior

The delirious client is either hyperactive or hypoactive, often alternating between. Approximately 10 percent of clients display violence toward others (Lipowski 1983). Speech may be slurred and disjointed, with aimless vocalizations and repetitions. Tremors and irregular spasmodic (*choreiform*) movements may be present.

Miscellaneous Features

The delirious person may manifest rage, depression, fear, and apathy. Incontinence of urine and feces is not uncommon.

Causes of Delirium

Delirium in the elderly usually has multiple causes. Often several organic agents are responsible, along with environmental stressors, poor sensory input, and any of a wide variety of psychosocial problems. Due to the aging process, impairments in hearing and vision, and the possible presence of dementia, the elderly have great difficulty in maintaining homeostasis when faced with stress. The following are suggested causes of delirium secondary to aging (Lipowski 1983):

- Changes in the hypothalamic nuclei, which operate to maintain body homeostasis and are vulnerable to high levels of corticosteroids present during periods of stress

- Loss of cells in the cerebral cortex, frontal cortex, and hippocampus, the centers of cognition

- Dysfunction of the locus ceruleus, a structure in the fourth ventricle of the brain that has been associated with nocturnal delirium

- Reduction in acetylcholine synthesis, which directly affects normal memory, learning, attention, wakefulness and the sleep-wake cycle

---

Box 15–3
DSM-IIIR DIAGNOSTIC CRITERIA FOR DELIRIUM

1. Reduced ability to maintain attention to external stimuli (e.g., questions must be repeated because attention wanders) and to appropriately shift attention to new external stimuli (e.g., perseverates answer to a previous question).

2. Disorganized thinking, as indicated by rambling, irrelevant, or incoherent speech.

3. At least two of the following:

   a. Reduced level of consciousness, e.g., difficulty keeping awake during examination

   b. Perceptual disturbances: misinterpretations, illusions, or hallucinations

   c. Disturbance of sleep-wake cycle with insomnia or daytime sleepiness

   d. Increased or decreased psychomotor activity

   e. Disorientation to time, place, or person

   f. Memory impairment, e.g., inability to learn new material, such as the names of several unrelated objects after five minutes, or to remember past events, such as history of current episodes of illness

4. Clinical features develop over a short period of time (usually hours to days) and tend to fluctuate over the course of a day.

5. Either a or b.

   a. Evidence from the history, physical examination, or laboratory tests of a specific organic factor (or factors) judged to be etiologically related to the disturbance

   b. In the absence of such evidence, an etiologic organic factor can be presumed if the disturbance cannot be accounted for by any nonorganic mental disorder, e.g., Manic Episode accounting for agitation and sleep disturbance

Source: American Psychiatric Association: Diagnostic and Statistical Manual of Mental Disorders, *ed 3, revised. APA, 1987, p 103.*

- Reduction of cerebral blood flow and metabolism, producing hypoxia

Compounding the normal aging process, chronic or acute physical illnesses are usually associated with delirium. (See Box 15–4.) Systemic diseases are the most frequently implicated, and intoxication with prescription drugs is the most common cause of delirium. High consumption of many different drugs, including prescription and over-the-counter drugs, is common among these clients. With the age-related changes in metabolism, renal clearance,

Box 15–4
PHYSIOLOGIC, PSYCHOLOGIC, AND ENVIRONMENTAL ETIOLOGIES OF ACUTE CONFUSIONAL STATES IN THE HOSPITALIZED ELDERLY

I. Physiologic

  A. Primary cerebral disease

    1. Nonstructural factors

      a. Vascular insufficiency—transient ischemic attacks, cerebral vascular accidents, thrombosis

      b. Central nervous system infection—acute and chronic meningitis, neurosyphilis, brain abscess

    2. Structural factors

      a. Trauma—subdural hematoma, concussion, contusion, intracranial hemorrhage

      b. Tumors—primary and metastatic

      c. Normal pressure hydrocephalus

  B. Extracranial disease

    1. Cardiovascular abnormalities

      a. Decreased cardiac output states—myocardial infarction, arrhythmias, congestive heart failure, cardiogenic shock

      b. Alterations in peripheral vascular resistance—increased and decreased states

      c. Vascular occlusion—disseminated intravascular coagulopathy, emboli

    2. Pulmonary abnormalities

      a. Inadequate gas exchange states—pulmonary disease, alveolar hypoventilation

      b. Infection—pneumonias

    3. Systemic infective processes—acute and chronic

      a. Viral

      b. Bacterial—endocarditis, pyelonephritis, cystitis

    4. Metabolic disturbances

      a. Electrolyte abnormalities—hypercalcemia, hyponatremia and hypernatremia, hypokalemia and hyperkalemia, hypochloremia and hyperchloremia, hyperphosphatemia

      b. Acidosis/alkalosis

      c. Hypoglycemia and hyperglycemia

      d. Acute and chronic renal failure

      e. Volume depletion—hemorrhage, inadequate fluid intake, diuretics

      f. Hepatic failure

      g. Porphyria

    5. Drug intoxication—therapeutic and substance abuse

      a. Misuse of prescribed medications

      b. Side-effects of therapeutic medications

      c. Drug-drug interactions

      d. Improper use of over-the-counter medications

      e. Ingestion of heavy metals and industrial poisons

    6. Endocrine disturbance

      a. Hypothyroidism and hyperthyroidism

      b. Diabetes mellitus

      c. Hypopituitarism

      d. Hypoparathyroidism and hyperparathyroidism

    7. Nutritional deficiencies

      a. B vitamins

      b. Vitamin C

      c. Hypoproteinemia

    8. Physiologic stress—pain, surgery

    9. Alterations in temperature regulation—hypothermia and hyperthermia

    10. Unknown physiologic abnormality—sometimes defined as pseudodelirium

II. Psychologic

  A. Severe emotional stress—postoperative states, relocation, hospitalization

  B. Depression

  C. Anxiety

  D. Pain—acute and chronic

  E. Fatigue

  F. Grief

continued

Box 15–4 (continued)

G. Sensory/perceptual deficits—noise, alteration in functioning of senses

H. Mania

I. Paranoia

J. Situational disturbances

III. Environmental

A. Unfamilar environment creating a lack of meaning in the environment

B. Sensory deprivation/environmental monotony creating a lack of meaning in the environment

C. Sensory overload

D. Immobilization—therapeutic, physical, pharmacologic

E. Sleep deprivation

F. Lack of temperospatial reference points

Source: Foreman MD: Acute confusional states in hospital elderly: a research dilemma. Nursing Research *1986;35:37–38. Copyright © 1986 The American Journal of Nursing Company.*

and overall body composition, the elderly are as a group critically susceptible to drug intoxication. Drugs with anticholinergic effects are frequently prescribed and probably are the most common cause of delirium.

Differentiating Delirium from Dementia

Although it is extremely important to distinguish delirium from dementia, the task is difficult. The difficulty is compounded by the fact that about one-third of hospitalized demented clients also experience delirium. In the client who is already demented, the delirium is usually modified to include apathy and periods of noisy restlessness, as well as periods of acute and fluctuating diminished cognitive functioning.

Pseudodelirium

In 5 to 20 percent of the cases of delirium, no organic cause can be identified. As in pseudodementia, the presence of inconsistencies in cognitive functioning (e.g., the client does not know where he or she is but can find the bathroom, bed, etc.) should raise the suspicion of a **pseudodelirium**. If the client also has a history of psychiatric illnesses, is grossly and consistently delusional, has marked manic or depressive features, or is unmotivated during cognitive testing, the diagnosis of this OMS may be appropriate (Lipowski 1983).

Amnestic Syndrome

Amnestic syndrome, an OMS, is characterized by memory deficits, both *anterograde* (of events after the episode precipitating the disorder) and *retrograde* (of events prior to the episode precipitating the disorder). The syndrome results from lesions involving bilateral temporal structures, or the diencephalon, or both (Lipowski 1980).

Organic Hallucinosis

In **organic hallucinosis**, persistent hallucinations are due to an organic factor. The type of hallucination depends on the organic factors (e.g., alcohol usually produces auditory hallucinations and cataracts may stimulate visual hallucinations). Use of hallucinogens and prolonged use of alcohol are the most common causes of this disorder.

Organic Anxiety Syndrome

The essential feature of **organic anxiety syndrome** is recurrent panic attacks or overwhelming anxiety that has organic bases. The attacks range from mild to severe, with cognitive impairment especially in the ability to sustain attention. Etiology is usually related to psychoactive substances (caffeine, cocaine, amphetamines) or endocrine disorders such as hyperthyroidism and hypothyroidism. Full recovery can be expected when the cause is removed.

Organic Delusional Syndrome

In **organic delusional syndrome**, both paranoid and schizophrenia-like symptoms are present. Although delusions are the dominant symptom, hallucinations, catatonia, and other typical schizophrenia-like patterns may be present. Intellectual functioning is intact. The OMS is believed to be a result of cerebral disorders that involve the temporal lobe, e.g., epilepsy, encephalitis, or cocaine and amphetamine intoxication (Lipowski 1980).

Organic Mood Syndrome

Organic mood syndrome is characterized by an abnormal mood (depressive or manic) that is the result of a cerebral disorder only. Clinically, the person appears to be acutely manic or in a major depressive episode. Possible causal agents of this OMS include acute viral infections, Cushing's syndrome, pernicious anemia, hyperthyroidism or hypothyroidism, Parkinson's disease, and hallucinogens and reserpine (DSM-IIIR 1987).

Organic Personality Syndrome

The distinguishing symptoms of **organic personality syndrome** involve disturbances of motivation and of emotion and impulse control, with resulting lability and impulsiveness. Cognitive functions are intact, even though social judgment is not. The causes are usually structural damage to the brain. Endocrine diseases and certain toxic substances can also be involved.

THE NURSING PROCESS AND CLIENTS WITH OMS AND OMD

Assessment

Gathering data about clients with organic mental syndromes and disorders is often made difficult by the clients' anxiety and defensiveness, their questionable reliability as historians when confusion is present, and the frequent lack of a reliable secondary source of information. All data should be gathered in a milieu that is free of distraction. The questions should be paced slowly to allow the client time to answer comfortably. Aging people can normally process information once it is received but may have difficulty taking in information. Placing the client in a situation that interferes with an already compromised sensory apparatus only heightens the client's anxiety and seriously compromises the nurse's attempts to evaluate effectively.

Subjective Data

Confusion

Confusion is the most common complaint of the elderly seeking assistance. The complaint may come from the client, family, or friends. Wolanin and Fraelich-Philips (1981) define *confusion* as a condition characterized by disorientation to time and place, memory deficits, poor conceptual boundaries, and inappropriate verbal statements. When assessing for confusion, the nurse can keep the following questions in mind:

- How long has the confusion been present? Acute and chronic episodes may suggest delirium versus dementia. More precisely, they may point to an acute organic cause versus a progressive degenerative process.

- When does the confusion seem most apparent? Nighttime confusion can be a sign of intoxication from sedatives or age-related changes in sleeping habits. Daytime confusion may indicate a bilateral cerebral vascular accident or lingering effects of hypnotics (Wolanin and Fraelich-Philips 1981).

- Does the family report client behaviors that they call confusion? The client may minimize problems as an ego-protection reaction.

Health History

When completing the client's health history, the nurse must include all past and present medical conditions. Special attention should be given to chronic conditions for which the client is being treated, along with any recent changes in health status. Box 15–4 indicates the significant number of medical syndromes that may result in cognitive changes. The client should be asked, "Are you seeing a physician at this time?" "Why did you seek medical help?" "What does the doctor say is the problem?"

Sensory Impairment

The elderly are particularly sensitive to the confusion associated with sensory deprivation. Physiologic changes in their sensory apparatus may be directly related to aging or to pathologic processes. Both diminish sensory receptive ability. The sensory changes, however, are not clear-cut. The person may have difficulty hearing high-frequency sounds, such as consonants. Turning up the volume on the radio may help the person hear one range of sounds but produce sensory overload because the rest of the sounds are too loud. The result is deprivation and distortion.

The nurse should try to ascertain any possible sensory problems, especially in hearing and vision. To test hearing, stand directly in front of the client so that he or she can see your face and ask a question in a normal tone of voice. The question should require more than a yes/no answer. Vision can be tested with pictures that the client will easily recognize.

Dietary History

When possible, the nurse should obtain an estimate of the client's food intake. "What do you eat for breakfast? lunch? dinner?" Special note should be made of protein and vitamin intake. Avitaminosis, pellagra, anemia, and hypoglycemia have all been associated with reversible brain syndromes (Butler and Lewis 1982). Hydration is also an important factor, easily noted in the client's physical state (e.g., saliva pool below the tongue). Dehydration can also cause confusion.

Head Trauma

Falls are common among the elderly. Cerebral contusions, midbrain hemorrhage, and subdural hematoma should all be considered. Confusion may be the primary result of such trauma.

Medication

The elderly are prone to adverse drug reactions as a result of age-related bodily changes. These factors are compounded by high consumption of many different drugs: 45 percent of all prescriptions are written for elderly clients. Medications are thus a common cause of delirium. The aged are particularly susceptible to drugs with anticholinergic properties (major tranquilizers, antidepressants, barbiturates, adrenal steroids, atropine, alcohol, antihypertensives, and diuretics). The client needs to be questioned about both prescription and over-the-counter drugs: "Are you now taking any medicines that your doctor prescribed?" "Do you take laxatives, cold pills, or other medicines that you buy at your drug store without a prescription?"

The client should also be questioned about alcohol consumption. Alcohol is a central nervous system depressant, and intoxication may mimic symptoms of OMD. Alcohol also compromises nutritional status and may cause withdrawal effects. Ask questions such as "How much alcohol do you drink in one day/week?" and "Have you ever had periods of not remembering after drinking?"

Cognitive functioning includes memory, reasoning, abstraction, calculations, and judgment. For the client to respond effectively, the nurse must be sure that the information requested is relevant to the client, that the client sees some purpose in the interview, and that the client is interested in the material. Testing materials should be chosen carefully, and the endurance of the client should be kept in mind at all times.

Appearance   Clients who appear disheveled, dirty, or sloppy may be experiencing problems with poor memory or a shortened attention span. This deficit may not be apparent if the client has a caretaker who helps with grooming.

Manner   Some clients may exaggerate mannerisms to compensate for a perceived decline in functioning. For example, a compulsive person may become more set in his or her ways.

Attitude   An attitude of defensiveness, withdrawal, or paranoia may be a response to increasing anxiety about diminished abilities.

Communication   Communication is assessed in the areas of speech, gestures, facial expression, and writing (Ninos and Makohon 1985). The client's ability to find words and name objects is assessed. Difficulty may suggest expressive aphasia. Difficulty grasping complex concepts (receptive aphasia) is also evaluated by the use of object and pictures rather than just words. The client's ability to use gestures and facial expressions to compensate for verbal aphasia is also noted. Not using facial expressions and gestures and speaking in a monotone may indicate depression. Written communication and reading ability are also tested.

The nurse can ask the client to follow verbal instructions, increasing the number of sequential commands. ("Please pick up the paper, fold it in half lengthwise, and place it on the other side of the table.") A knowledge of the client's ability to follow instructions helps the nurse intervene appropriately. Overly difficult communications confuse the client, but infantile communications rob the client of dignity.

Perception   Perception is the client's ability to recognize and integrate sensory information. It also includes the conscious recognition of oneself in relation to the environment. Clients with asymmetrical brain involvement of Alzheimer's disease may neglect one side of their body. These clients may also have difficulty recognizing objects (*agnosia*).

Clients with perceptual difficulty may distort sensory information, with resulting hallucinations and delusions. Auditory hallucinations are the most common; visual hallucinations usually indicate an acute toxic state. When listening to a client describe a delusional system, the nurse notes the underlying feelings and theme, e.g., fear, sorrow. Also keep in mind that the isolation and fear that are the usual causative agents may be as much a product of hearing loss as of the imagination.

Attention and Wakefulness Attention refers to alertness and the ability to attend selectively to stimuli and to direct one's focus. Can the client sustain or pay attention to the interview process, or is he or she easily distracted by the environment? Wakeful states range from hyperalertness to stupor. Stupor can be the result of medication intoxication or an acute systemic disease, e.g., a brain abscess or pneumonia.

Motor Activity Lethargy often is a symptom of depression but can also be the result of such medications as tranquilizers, antihypertensives, antidepressants, and antihistamines. Lethargy can also be caused by a number of disease processes, e.g., urinary tract infection, anemia, and meningitis. A shift between hypermotor and hypomotor activity is a sign of delirium. Agitation and physical striking out are occasionally demonstrated.

Mood and Affect Depression may accompany the earlier stages of dementia. The more demented the client, however, the less depressed he or she is. Clients with organic disease of the cerebral area are emotionally labile. The client should be asked about any changes in eating or sleeping habits. The nurse should also inquire about a recent loss of energy and interest in usual activities. If depression is suspected, the client needs to be evaluated for risk of suicide. "Have you felt like life is not worth living?" "Do you think you would take your own life?" All questioning in the area of suicide must be done matter of factly and without hesitation.

Orientation Disorientation to time, place, and person must be measured in an environment where the client has easy access to the information. Days in a hospital are all the same to many of us. Acute disorientation in all spheres is commonly found in toxic states and traumatic brain disease. Disorientation to place and person usually indicates a degenerative disorder.

Memory At present there is no set of tests that can adequately measure the memory capacity of demented clients (Tariot et al. 1985). (See Table 15–3.) Most tests measure *episodic memory*—the processing and storage of information, e.g., recalling the events of the day. This type of memory is impaired in most clients with OMD, depression, and drug or alcohol intoxication. *Semantic memory,* or knowledge memory, allows people to synthesize and think about events. It is used in language, abstraction, and logical operations. People with Alzheimer's disease have difficulty with semantic memory; however, depressed clients do not. Episodic memory can be quickly tested by asking

the client to repeat a series of words or to recall a recent event, such as a meal. Semantic memory can be tested by asking the client to develop a scenario, such as describing what he or she did from dinner until bedtime in the evening.

Episodic memory is also tested in relation to time and usually divided into three spheres—recent, remote, and past. It was previously believed that recent memory is lost before remote, and remote before past. No research validates this theory. Rather, past memory is now believed to be memory that cannot be refuted. The accuracy of past memory is not readily assessed. People with dementias have difficulty in recent memory acquisition or learning; this symptom may be a key to early detection of dementia. Unfortunately, most testing is done in past and remote memory (Whelihan et al. 1984).

Abstract Reasoning Proverbs are the most common way of testing abstract reasoning. "What does it mean when we say, 'People who live in glass houses shouldn't throw stones'?" "What does 'A stitch in time saves nine' mean to you?" Clients with Alzheimer's disease often interpret these proverbs quite literally.

Calculations The most common test of calculation ability is the serial sevens test: The person counts back from 100 in decrements of 7. This is a difficult process for the demented or delirious client. The test measures the client's ability to concentrate and focus thought. Unfortunately, it may also be a measure of educational level.

Judgment The test for judgment should predict whether a person will behave in a socially accepted manner, including the planning and carrying out of activities that call for the client to discriminate reality from unrealistic situations. You might ask the client, "If you needed help during the night, how would you get it?" "If you had lost your wallet while on errands, what would you do?"

Psychosocial History

The psychosocial history should include an assessment of the client, his or her family, and their joint coping styles and level of intimacy. Some assessment of the client's function in the community should be included. Unlike cognitive testing, this assessment shows what the client is doing rather than what he or she might possibly do.

Family History

The families of impaired older persons can be a major source of information and support. In the United States, almost

90 percent of the elderly have seen one or more relatives the previous week, and more than 75 percent live within 30 minutes of their nearest child. Common living arrangements for the elderly include living with a spouse, child, or sibling (Reifler and Eiserdorfer 1980). The family assessment includes:

- Living arrangements
- Care arrangements for the elderly, e.g., shopping assistance, daily visits, telephone calls
- Family knowledge of the current illness
- Family expectations for the future
- Special family concerns about client care
- Family style of coping with stress, e.g., death of a relative, illness
- The identified spokesperson for the family
- The family's perception of the client's coping abilities

Throughout the interview, the nurse should note the interactions between the family and the client. Do they support the client and respect what he or she has to say? Do people listen to one another? What is the atmosphere in the group? What is the level of intimacy between members?

Activities of Daily Living

The client must be carefully assessed for level of self-care. What can the client do without help? What can't he or she do without help? What type of help is needed? As cognitive deficits increase, the client will be more dependent on others for assistance.

Community Functioning

The Comprehensive Functional Assessment (CFA) tool measures the client's ability to sustain himself or herself in the community (Besdine 1983). The nurse needs to assess not only the client's ability to live independently in the community but also his or her degree of social involvement. Does the client belong to any clubs or groups? Do friends visit in his or her home? Does he or she belong to a particular church or temple?

Objective Data

Larson et al. (1984) have developed a three-step process for evaluating the elderly with mental impairment.

Step 1: Physical assessment. The client is given a thorough medical workup, including a complete neurologic exam and a psychiatric consultation for possible functional illness. Because elderly people with organic illness frequently manifest confusion and depression, one works from the assumption that reversible organic illness is present. Chest x-ray films and an electrocardiogram are taken.

Step 2: Laboratory assessment. The following tests are routinely ordered for the elderly:

- Complete blood count, including folic acid and vitamin B_{12} levels to detect anemia
- Erythrocyte sedimentation rate to detect infection
- SMA-12 to detect electrolyte imbalances
- Syphilis tests (VDRL)
- Thyroid function studies
- Serum levels of barbiturates, bromides, and digitalis

Step 3: Computed axial tomographic brain scan (CT scan). This test is ordered for those clients at high risk, e.g., those having acute deterioration in cognitive functioning of recent onset.

A number of elective procedures can also be used. Their use should be limited unless indicated, due to their cost to the family and client. These are:

- Skull x-ray films
- Lumbar puncture
- Electroencephalography
- Positron emission tomography (PET)
- Cerebral angiography
- Isotope cisternography

There are a number of brief rating scales for testing cognitive impairment (see Table 15–3). None of these is perfect, and most need to be augmented by another test. The SET test, developed in Scotland, is a tool for effective and quick nursing assessment (Hays and Borger 1985). The test measures mental function as a whole rather than its individual components. The test requires the person to count, name, and remember items, demonstrating motivation, alertness, concentration, short-term memory, and problem-solving ability.

The test takes less than five minutes to administer. The client is asked to list ten items from each of four groups: fruits, animals, colors, and towns/cities (FACT). The maximum is 40; a score of 15 or below is positively correlated with dementia. Scores between 15 and 24 may not indicate dementia but may indicate some early mental changes due to other factors. The mood disorders do not affect the results of this test as much as they do those of so many others.

Nursing Diagnosis

Psychiatric nursing diagnoses (PND-I) common to clients with organic mental syndromes and disorders are listed in

Table 15–4, as are NANDA diagnoses. A brief discussion of each of the PND-I diagnostic categories follows.

Human Response Patterns in Activity Processes

01.01 Altered Motor Behavior Gait changes due to neurologic involvement are seen in a number of the dementias. These include Alzheimer's disease, Huntington's chorea, Parkinson's disease, Creutzfeldt-Jakob disease, normal pressure hydrocephalus, and progressive supranuclear palsy. Restlessness in the delirious client is reflected in hyperactive behavior. The client usually alternates between hyperactivity and hypoactivity.

01.03 Altered Self-Care The delirious client is unable to perceive, organize, or carry out the activities of daily living. He or she is far too distracted by stimuli and unable to focus. The Alzheimer's client has a distinct problem: *apraxia,* or the loss of ability to perform formerly known skills. In the late stages of all the dementias, total care is a necessity as the client moves toward brain failure.

01.04 Altered Sleep/Arousal Patterns *Sundowning*—confused behavior at night when environmental simulation is low—is commonly seen in delirious clients. The client catnaps during the day and wanders at night. Poor sensory processing can also be seen in demented clients who also wander at night. The client with Alzheimer's disease may not sleep for several days, moving about in a confused state.

Human Response Patterns in Cognition Processes

02.03 Altered Knowledge Processes *Agnosia,* the failure to recognize familiar objects, is a progressive problem that eventually renders the person without knowledge of loved ones. Overall, in both delirium and dementia, the client's ability to utilize information to make judgments may be seriously impaired.

02.05 Altered Memory Episodic short-term memory is affected by delirium, dementia, and the affective illnesses. Long-term memory is diminished in the later stages of Alzheimer's disease and acute delirium.

02.06 Altered Orientation Disorientation is seen in both the dementias and delirious clients. In the former it is related to progressive cerebral changes and in the latter to an acute, usually identifiable causal agent.

02.07 Altered Thought Content Delusions may be present in delirium and dementia. The client is sensitive to these cognitive processes as a result of the client's reduced ability to distinguish and integrate sensory information. The problem is compounded by short- and long-term memory loss.

Human Response Patterns in Interpersonal Processes

05.01.02 Altered Verbal Communication Aphasia, both receptive and expressive, is one of the hallmarks of Alzheimer's disease. In the late stage of this illness, the client is completely mute. Confabulation is a common defense

---

Table 15–3
Brief Rating Scales for Assessing Organic Mental Impairment

Title	Items Measured
Cognitive Capacity Screening Examination (CCSE)	Orientation, memory, recall Calculation, language
Mental Status Questionnaire (MSQ)	Orientation, memory, general knowledge
Short Portable Mental Status Questionnaire (SPMSQ)	Orientation, memory, general knowledge, subtraction
Mini-Mental State (MMS)	Orientation, registration, recall, calculation, language, graphomotor function
Cognitive Assessment Scale (CAS)	Orientation, general knowledge, mental ability, psychomotor function
Global Deterioration Scale (GDS)	Assessment of primary degenerative dementia and its stages, including orientation, memory, neurologic exams
Functional Dementia Scale (FDS)	Activities of daily living, orientation, affect
SET Test	Alertness, concentration, short-term memory, problem solving
Nurse's Mental Status Exam (NMSE)	Consciousness, mood, orientation, memory, language, judgment
Extended Mental Status Questionnaire (EMSQ)	Orientation, remote memory, lower/higher levels of cognitive functioning
Philadelphia Geriatric Center (PGC)	Recent memory (story recall)

Source: Adapted from Cooper B, Bickel H: Population screening and the early detection of dementing disorders in old age: A review. Psychol Med 1984;14:81–95. Cambridge University Press, England.

Table 15–4

Comparison of DSM-IIIR and Nursing Diagnoses Commonly Related to OMD and OMS

DSM-IIIR		PND-I Diagnoses		NANDA Diagnoses
290.00	Primary degenerative dementia of the Alzheimer's type, senile onset, uncomplicated	01.01	Altered motor behavior	Mobility impaired, physical
		01.01.03	Impaired Coordination	
		01.03	Altered self-care	Self-care deficit: feeding, toileting, dressing, grooming
		01.04	Altered sleep/arousal patterns	
290.43	Multi-infarct dementia, uncomplicated	02.03	Altered knowledge processes	
		02.03.01	Agnosia	
293.00	Delirium	02.03.02	Altered intellectual functioning	
293.81	Organic delusional disorder	02.05	Altered memory	
		02.05.03	Long-term memory loss	
		02.05.04	Short-term memory loss	
293.82	Organic hallucinosis	02.06	Altered orientation	
293.83	Organic mood disorder	02.06.01	Confusion	
		02.06.02	Delirium	
294.00	Amnestic disorder	02.06.03	Disoriented	
294.10	Dementia	02.07	Altered thought content	Thought process, altered
294.80	Organic anxiety disorder	02.07.01	Delusions	
294.80	Organic mental disorder NOS	05.01	Altered communication processes	
		05.01.02	Altered verbal communication (associated with aphasia, confabulation)	Communication, impaired: verbal
		05.02	Altered conduct/impulse processes	Violence, potential for: self-directed or directed at others
		05.02.01	Dysfunctional behaviors	
		05.02.02.05	Unpredictable behavior	
		05.03	Altered role performance	Role performance, altered
		05.03.01	Altered family role	
		06.01	Altered attention	
		06.01.01	Distractibility	
		06.01.02	Hyperalertness	
		06.03	Altered self-concept	Self-concept, disturbance in: self-esteem
		06.03.04	Altered self-esteem	
		06.04	Altered sensory perception	Sensory/perceptual alterations
		06.04.03	Hallucinations	
		07.02	Altered elimination processes	
		07.02.01	Altered bowel elimination	Bowel elimination, altered patterns
		07.02.01.03	Incontinence	
		07.02.02	Altered urinary elimination	Urinary elimination, altered patterns
		07.02.02.01	Incontinence	
		07.06	Altered nutrition processes	Nutrition, altered: less than body requirements
		07.06.03	Altered eating processes	

used by clients who cannot remember required information and therefore use fantasy to fill in the memory gaps.

05.02 Altered Conduct/Impulse Processes In clients with Alzheimer's disease and the majority of the other dementias, there is a gradual decline in social acceptability of behavior. Hyperorality and touching all objects seen are a few of these impulsive and unpredictable behaviors. The client may also strike out at others while hallucinating or in a hyperactive phase. These behaviors are also seen in clients with delirium who are similarly unpredictable.

05.03 Altered Role Performance As the result of decreasing intellectual competence, the demented client moves from role of spouse, parent, employee, and community member to that of a dependent, regressed family member. The role loss and role change is anxiety-provoking and at times overwhelming for the client and family. Characteristically the family members experience a period of acute grief after receiving the diagnosis. Their level of depression should be assessed. Feelings of isolation and being overwhelmed are common (Kuale 1986).

Human Response Patterns in Perception Processes

06.01 Altered Attention The inability to attend and focus concentration is a hallmark of delirium. Decreased attention is also seen in the later stages of the dementias when the client loses the ability to encode.

06.03 Altered Self-Concept During the first stage of Alzheimer's disease and other dementias, the client is acutely aware of cognitive failure. This awareness and the resulting anxiety can be damaging to the self-esteem of a person living in a culture that does not tolerate or provide for dependence.

06.04 Altered Sensory Perception Delirium alters perception by reducing the client's ability to distinguish and integrate sensory information. As a result, the client has difficulty in discriminating reality from hallucinations, dreams, illusions, and imagery. In the later stages of dementia, clients also experience hallucinations and delusions, which complicate delivery of care.

Human Response Patterns in Physiologic Processes

07.02 Altered Elimination Processes Incontinence of urine or feces is usually the result of confusion and failure to use the facilities. In the later stages of dementia, clients lose cortical control but physiologic function remains. Incontinence of urine may also be an indication of normal pressure hydrocephalus.

07.06 Alterations in Nutrition/Metabolism Poor nutrition and some metabolic disorders can be the direct cause of confusion in the elderly. The reverse can also be true; confusion and cerebral change can cause nutritional deficits. Without supervision, many clients will not be able to provide for or ingest adequate amounts of food. In the later stages of Alzheimer's disease, the client has symptoms of bulimia followed by total loss of appetite.

Planning and Implementing Interventions

Nursing interventions for clients with organic mental syndromes and disorders can be divided into two broad groups: interventions for demented clients and those for delirious clients. Sample nursing care plans for these are presented on pages 334–339. With few exceptions, the interventions are similar, although the overall goals are different. The goal with the demented client is to minimize the loss of self-care capacity. Although functional loss is progressive,

at every stage of the illness the client's self-care capacity needs to be assessed and supported. With the delirious client the overall goal for nursing intervention is to support existing sensory perception until the client's cognition state can return to previous levels of functioning.

Promote Normal Motor Behavior With the demented client's impaired coordination, falls become a safety concern. Living areas need to be well lit and furniture left in one consistent place. The client needs to be evaluated for visual and balance disturbances. Safety bars should be installed near toilets, showers, and tubs. Clients who need assistance should be taught the safe use of walkers and wheelchairs (Burnside 1981). All clients using tranquilizers and antidepressants need to be evaluated for postural hypotension. Blood pressure taken supine and standing will be an indication. Restlessness and wandering can be dealt with by allowing the demented client to wander in a closed milieu. Avoid crowds or large open spaces without boundaries.

With the delirious client, hyperactivity can be decreased by controlling environmental stimuli. If this does not help, medications can be used judiciously. A low dose of haloperidol (Haldol) may be prescribed. Taking vital signs one hour before and after the administration of any medication is necessary, and the client must be observed carefully for signs of stupor. Restraint in both the demented and delirious client should be avoided if at all possible, since most people respond by becoming extremely agitated and disoriented. Prolonged periods of hypoactivity need to be interrupted with range-of-motion exercises, frequent turning, and having the client stand up at bedside, as tolerated. During periods of fluctuating motor behavior, there is always concern for the client's safety. Staff should be present at all times, and side rails of the bed should be up and the bed lowered.

Maintain Self-Care Allow the client to do as much as possible unassisted. The more the client can effectively control his or her daily routine, the less anxiety the client will experience. Remind the client about daily grooming and personal hygiene and repeat instructions. If the client is resistive to oral hygiene, mouth swabs with dilute hydrogen peroxide can be used. If the client resists this as well, having the client eat an apple may help to clean the mouth. For all routine procedures, if the client resists, wait a few moments and try again. The client often forgets what he or she was resisting. As discussed earlier, the "leading" technique may help encourage clients who are experiencing apraxia to complete these routines. Clients who are acutely delirious or who are in the last stages of dementia will need total bed care.

Text continues on p. 336.

Nursing Care Plan: The Client with Dementia

Nursing Diagnosis (PND-I/NANDA)	Client Care Goals	Nursing Planning/ Intervention	Evaluation
01.01 Altered motor behavior* /Mobility, impaired: physical	Promote normal motor behavior.	Evaluate the environment for hazards that may cause falls, e.g., throw rugs, poorly lit rooms; lack of safety bars in bathroom; teach client use of walkers and wheelchairs. Client using tranquilizers needs standing and supine blood pressures taken to check for hypotension. Allow wandering in a prescribed area.	Maintaining full physical activity.
01.03 Altered self-care* /Self-care deficit	Maintain self-care.	Encourage independence in self-care; use verbal and nonverbal communication when making requests; repeat requests as needed. Use clothing with elastic, eliminating buttons and zippers if possible. Label clothing items and important rooms. Provide mouth swabs and fresh fruit if refusing oral hygiene. Repeat self-care requests at a later time if client is resistant, total physical care during last stages.	Functioning at highest possible level for self-care.
01.04 Altered sleep/ arousal patterns /Sleep pattern disturbances	Promote adequate sleep.	Offer beer or wine at bedtime; allow client to wander in a prescribed area till tired; if restraints used, remove them when client has fallen asleep. Active daily schedule.	Able to sleep at regular intervals in amount necessary to maintain health.
02.03.01 Agnosia	Support optimal cognitive functioning.	Use the same interventions prescribed for altered memory. Enhance with labels to objects, supervising client when warranted. Support family as they care for a loved one who no longer recognizes them as individuals.	Participates in self-care and family environment at optimal level.
02.05 Altered memory	Support optimal memory function.	Structure ward environment to enhance memory, e.g., clocks, calendars, orientation board. Use verbal and nonverbal communication to emphasize requests, repeating as necessary. Have client attend music therapy and other "reminiscing" groups; place familiar objects in room; allow open visiting with family.	Participating in self care and groups at optimal level.
02.06 Altered orientation	Promote optimal orientation.	Provide easily read clocks and orientation boards, consistent daily	Oriented to time, place, and person if possible.

*PND-I diagnoses also in NANDA list.

continued

Nursing Care Plan: The Client with Dementia *(Continued)*

Nursing Diagnosis (PND-I/NANDA)	Client Care Goals	Nursing Planning/ Intervention	Evaluation
		routine, socialization that does not produce sensory overload. Maintain physical activity; avoid use of tranquilizers. Client should be wearing aids (hearing/vision) as needed.	
02.07 Altered thought content* /Thought process, altered	Support clear thought processes.	Structure ward environment to enhance memory and orientation. Do not argue with validity of delusions, rather try to understand the feelings being indirectly expressed. Low-dose haloperidol may be prescribed.	Does not verbally express delusional material.
05.01.02 Altered verbal communication* /Communication, impaired: verbal	Support optimal verbal expression.	Call client by name, approach in clear view, and give simple commands. Substitute pictures if client experiencing aphasia. Attempt to attach meaning to nonverbal communications, checking interpretations with client or family.	Able to communicate needs.
05.02 Altered conduct/ impulse processes /Violence, potential for	Support appropriate conduct/impulse control.	Decrease environmental stimuli; make all changes slowly; make nondemanding requests; refrain from touching. Always approach in full view calling client by name. Distract as necessary; low dose of antipsychotic p.r.n.	Participating in daily living situation without striking out at self or others.
05.03 Altered role performance* /Role performance, altered	Support optimal role performance.	Use community resources to support family and client in home, e.g., day care, home visits, respite care, family support groups. Encourage family to participate in client's daily activities once institutionalized and include client in family functions. Support family through their own grieving as their loved one becomes more confused and withdrawn.	Functioning at highest possible level within the community and family.
06.01 Altered attention	Maintain optimal attention span.	Decrease environmental stimuli that agitate client. Repeat requests in a clear, simple manner, using gestures to supplement.	Able to focus long enough to participate in simple tasks.
06.03 Altered self-concept* /Self-concept, disturbance in: self-esteem	Promote optimal self-concept/self-esteem.	Encourage client to express feelings in a nonjudgmental environment; allow for expression of anger and sadness. Encourage	Participating in self-care as much as possible; able to express both positive and negative comments about

continued

Nursing Care Plan: The Client with Dementia *(Continued)*

Nursing Diagnosis (PND-I/NANDA)	Client Care Goals	Nursing Planning/ Intervention	Evaluation
		family to include client in social activities. Gently remind client of forgotten events. Organize the environment to enhance memory, e.g., label rooms and contents of drawers, write notes to remind to do some things.	personal level of functioning.
06.04 Altered sensory perception* /Sensory/perceptual alterations	Support optimal perceptual functioning.	Decrease environmental stimuli; provide soft music, slower-paced unit, eyeglasses and hearing aids as needed. Restrain client if combative; distract if agitated; reassure client that he or she is safe and will not be harmed; postpone procedures if client is agitated.	Able to perceive environment with a minimum of distortion.
07.02.01.03 Altered bowel elimination*, incontinence /Bowel elimination, altered 07.02.02.01 Altered urinary elimination,* incontinence /Urinary elimination, altered	Promote optimal patterns of elimination.	Establish regular toileting schedule; use disposable diapers/ pants if client will not participate willingly in toileting; do not use catheters or condoms if possible.	Continent of urine and feces; elimination controlled by other safe means.
07.06.03 Altered eating processes* /Nutrition, altered: less than body requirements	Maintain optimal nutritional status.	Monitor food and fluid intake, 24-hour intake; output documented as necessary. Supervise at mealtimes and assist as necessary. Give diet high in protein and carbohydrates in finger-food form with double portions. Weigh client frequently; increase caloric intake p.r.n.; if client refuses to eat, administer nasogastric, gastrostomy, or IV feedings.	Adequate daily intake of food and fluids; no weight loss; able to assist self as much as possible.

Promote Adequate Sleep Clients with dementia and delirium respond poorly to hypnotics, which increase confusion and aggravate sundowning in the elderly. Beer or wine at bedtime may produce enough relaxation without side-effects. If the client is having problems sleeping, allowing the client to wander in a confined area until he or she is tired may be the most helpful. If the client is disorganized at night, make sure the room is light and without shadows. Possibly leave a radio on to provide more stimulation. Low doses of haloperidol or an antianxiety agent may be prescribed. A Posey vest and soft restraints may have to be used if a staff member cannot sit with the delirious client or if the client attempts to remove IV tubing or bandages. Reassure the client that he or she is safe and that the

Text continues on p. 340.

Nursing Care Plan: The Client with Delirium

Nursing Diagnosis (PND-I/NANDA)	Client Care Goals	Nursing Planning/ Intervention	Evaluation
01.01 Altered motor behavior* /Mobility, impaired physical	Promote normal motor behavior.	Decrease environmental stimuli if client is hyperactive, a low dose of antipsychotic medication (haloperidol) may be necessary; check vital signs one hour before and after administration. If client is hypoactive, use range-of-motion exercises, up at bedside. Fluctuating hypoactivity to hyperactivity: staff should be present to ensure safety; side rails up, bed lowered.	Normal motor behavior in response to stimuli.
01.03 Altered self-care* /Self-care deficit	Maintain self-care.	Encourage client to do as much for self as possible; assist as necessary. Explain all procedures simply and clearly.	Able to perform activities of daily living (ADL) without assistance.
01.04 Altered sleep/ arousal patterns* /Sleep pattern disturbance	Promote adequate sleep.	Prevent nighttime confusion by increasing stimulation, e.g., light in room, radio; give low dose of antipsychotics or antianxiety agents. Restrain only if absolutely necessary. Reassure client that the environment is safe. Discourage daytime napping.	Able to sleep at regular intervals in the pattern normal to the client prior to delirium.
02.03.02 Altered intellectual functioning	Support optimal cognitive functioning.	Present new information as client is able to accept without confusion; keep requests that require judgment to a minimum. Support the orientation and memory of the client.	Able to participate in daily decision making.
02.05 Altered memory	Optimal memory function.	Speak to client about mutual areas of interest. Do not dispute memory discrepancies, this will only increase anxiety.	Able to remember recent and remote experiences.

*PND-I diagnoses also in NANDA list.

continued

Nursing Care Plan: The Client with Delirium *(Continued)*

Nursing Diagnosis (PND-I/NANDA)	Client Care Goals	Nursing Planning/ Intervention	Evaluation
02.06 Altered orientation	Promote optimal orientation.	Gently orient the client. Surround client with familiar objects from home, clocks, calendars, etc. Client should be wearing aids (visual/hearing) as needed. Familiar objects from home along with clocks, calendars, etc. Orient client during conversation; do not quiz.	Oriented to time, place, and person.
02.07 Altered thought content* /Thought processes, altered	Support clear thought processes.	Structure ward/ environment to enhance memory and orientation. Do not agree with delusional material; however, do not argue. Respond to feelings being indirectly expressed.	No longer verbally expresses delusional material.
05.02.02.05 Un-predictable behavior* /Violence, potential for	Support appropriate conduct/ impulse control.	Use the measures to support orientation and perception. Medicate with a low dose of an antipsychotic (e.g., haloperidol). Restrain to protect self/others only if an emergency or when staff presence is no longer effective. Move slowly in the room, speak clearly, and explain all procedures.	Socially appropriate behavior; able to verbalize fears/concerns without striking out.
05.03 Altered role performance* /Role performance, altered	Support optimal role performance.	Encourage family to participate in client's care. Support family emotionally as they work with a loved one whose behavior may be very bizarre.	Client's role within the family is not jeopardized by the period of delirium.
06.01 Altered attention 06.01.01 Dis-tractibility 06.01.02 Hyper-alertness	Maintain optimal attention span.	Reduce environmental stimuli; all procedures should be reduced to only those absolutely necessary. While working with client, move slowly, speak clearly, and	Able to sustain a normal attention span to participate in ADL.

continued

Nursing Care Plan: The Client with Delirium *(Continued)*

Nursing Diagnosis (PND-I/NANDA)	Client Care Goals	Nursing Planning/ Intervention	Evaluation
		provide information slowly; reduce the number of different people having contact with client.	
06.04.03 Hallucinations* /Sensory/perceptual alterations	Support perceptual functioning.	When speaking to the client, stand or sit so client can clearly see you, touch to hold his or her attention, and slowly explain all procedures. Respond to hallucinations by orienting without arguing; do not ask for elaboration. Reassure client that these perceptions will go away. Do not isolate; maintain stimulation, e.g., adequate lighting, another person present to speak to. Restrain only as a last resort.	Able to perceive environment as it is without distortion; not frightened by environmental changes.
07.02 Altered elimination processes* /Bowel elimination, altered patterns /Urinary elimination, altered patterns	Optimal patterns of elimination.	Maintain regular toileting schedule; check frequently for incontinence to prevent skin breakdown. Supervise food and fluid intake to prevent constipation; administer stool softeners p.r.n.	Continent of urine and feces; routine bowel functioning.
07.06.03 Altered eating processes /Nutrition altered: less than body requirements	Maintain optimal nutritional status.	Monitor food and fluid intake; document 24-hour intake-output as necessary; supervise at mealtimes, assisting as needed. Note condition of skin for hydration. Weigh frequently.	Adequate daily intake of food and fluids; no weight loss; able to feed self.

restraints are there to protect and help. If restraints are used, remove them as soon as the client has fallen asleep (Dietsche and Pollman 1982).

Support Knowledge Processes   The same interventions that are used to support memory and orientation are applied to the support of knowledge processes. Family education is imperative and can take the form of professional help or self-help groups.

Support Optimal Memory Function   Gently orient the client. To allay anxiety, do not argue with the client about verbal discrepancies. Rather, direct the client toward areas of interest that are familiar and pleasurable to him. The environment needs to support whatever memory functions are still intact. Do not test the client for episodic memory unless it is absolutely necessary. If the client uses confabulation, do not argue; rather note it as an ego-protective mechanism.

Because of his or her episodic memory loss, the Alzheimer's client does not respond well to reality orientation classes, although the ward environment can be structured to support what episodic memory is present (Hanley et al. 1981). The nurse, however, can positively trigger semantic memory by initiating a procedure that the client can then complete. In this leading technique, a combination of words and nonverbal cues are used. For instance, while handing the client a toothbrush and pointing toward his or her mouth with a brushing motion, the nurse says, "Brush your teeth." Constant repetition in a kind, firm manner is often necessary. Music therapy may also trigger past associations, aid the client's long-term memory, and help a normally aphasic client to participate in a group (Dietsche and Pollman 1982).

Drug therapy has also been proposed to assist the client in the early stages of Alzheimer's disease to maintain memory and orientation. **Tetrahydroaminoacridine (THA),** a potent anticholinesterase is currently being studied in human trials. Of the fifteen clients who were given the drug at the time of this report, twelve who took it for one year showed striking improvement in memory and participation in activities of daily living. Tetrahydroaminoacridine is not proposed as a cure but rather as an approach that may make early stages of Alzheimer's disease more bearable (Lancet 1987).

The family of clients experiencing advanced agnosia need support when their loved one no longer recognizes them.

Promote Optimal Orientation   The client's environment must be structured to support his or her cognitive functions. The client should be wearing whatever aids (hearing,

vision) are necessary to prevent sensory loss or distortion. Familiar objects from home, such as slippers, robe, and photographs, also help to orient the client. Easily read clocks, orientation boards, and a consistent daily routine that includes physical activity and socialization without sensory overload also helps to orient the client (Wolanin and Philips 1981). Verbally orient the client during conversation. Do not quiz the client. Avoid the use of drugs if at all possible.

Support Optimal Verbal Expression   As communication skills decrease, the client's nonverbal communications become more important. The client will respond physically to the environment, especially if he or she feels threatened. Call the client by name, approach in clear view, and give simple commands.

Support Appropriate Conduct/Impulse Control   All measures used to support perception and orientation are imperative here. The client may strike out in response to hallucinations or delusions. These clients function best in an environment where stimulation is controlled and sensory overload prevented. All changes, whether environmental or personal, need to be made slowly. Always approach the client in full view, calling his or her name, and refrain from touching the client. Requests should be simple and nondemanding. Clients who are agitated and striking out may need to be given a psychotropic medication, such as haloperidol. As low a dose as possible should be used, and the client should be carefully observed for the onset of **extrapyramidal symptoms.** Clients with short-term memory loss can often be distracted. As a last resort, restraints may be used to protect the client and others. They are, however, a last resort when the presence of staff members is no longer effective.

Support Optimal Role Performance   If the client is to keep functioning within the family, he or she must be viewed as an active member. Most demented clients remain at home with their families until the caregiver is exhausted and can no longer manage the client's round-the-clock needs. The family needs support throughout this time. Formal support includes home visits, day care, respite care, and family support groups. A four-year day-care program at the Cornell Medical Center was evaluated; 24 percent of participating families reported that without this program they would have had to institutionalize their loved one sooner and 40 percent would have had to hire more home help (Panella et al. 1984). There also appears to be a positive correlation between the amount of social support available to the family and their morale.

Regardless of the client's behavioral problems, the more support the family receives the better their morale (Zarit et al. 1980, Gilhooly 1984). After the client is institutionalized, the family should be made an integral part of the client's daily routine. The family needs extra emotional support as the client no longer recognizes them and the rewards for maintaining involvement diminish. Role maintenance with the delirious client involves supporting the ongoing need for the client to be oriented as well as assisting the family through the acute period.

Maintain Optimal Attention Span   Repeat requests as needed. Speak in simple phrases, loud enough to be heard, and reinforce meaning with nonverbal gestures. To decrease distractability and hyperalertness, keep environmental stimulation at a minimum. Every effort should be made to lower the client's anxiety level by moving slowly, speaking clearly, and providing new information slowly.

Promoting Optimal Self-Concept/Self-Esteem   During the early stages of dementia, every effort should be made to maintain the client's self-esteem as he or she struggles with the personal awareness of cognitive loss. Encourage the client to express fears and concerns and listen attentively. Allow for the expression of anger and sadness.

The environment can be manipulated to help the client with a failing memory. Helpful measures include labeling the bathroom and bedroom, posting notes to remind the client to turn off the stove and lock the door, and labeling the contents of drawers. Gently remind the client of forgotten events, and do not confront confabulations. Encourage the family to maintain the client as a productive member of this important group.

Support Optimal Perceptual Functioning   A quiet environment with soft music will prevent the client from experiencing sensory overload. When speaking with the client, stand or sit so that he or she faces you directly. With verbal warning, touch his or her shoulder or hand, and slowly and clearly explain all procedures. Touch should be used with caution. Sometimes a very soothing touch can overexcite the client, who may respond by striking out. Make sure that the client is wearing hearing aids and eyeglasses if necessary.

In responding to hallucinations, simply state that you understand that these thoughts are very real to him or her, but that you do not experience the same thoughts. Do not argue or ask the client to elaborate. Reassure him or her that these thoughts will go away and that he or she is in a safe place. Do not leave the client alone or in an isolated room without some stimulation to help the client block out the hallucinations and support reality testing. The room should be well lit without shadows or glare. If the client becomes combative, physically restrain him or her for as brief a period as possible. Then attempt to distract, reassuring the client that he or she is in a safe place. Restraints should not be used unless the client is a threat to others or self; restraints only frighten and aggravate perceptual problems further.

Promote Optimal Patterns of Elimination   A regular toileting schedule helps the delirious client control bowel and urine incontinence. Clients are often not able to let the nurse know when they have to use the toilet or have soiled themselves.

During the early stage of dementia, a toileting routine is essential. As the disease progresses and the client no longer recognizes a toilet or its purpose, he or she may resist sitting on the toilet. Forcing the client will only produce agitation and combativeness. Distract and try again. If all efforts at maintaining a routine fail, then disposable pants or diapers are recommended. The use of catheters and external drains are not recommended due to the possibility of infection and their certain removal by a confused client.

Promote Optimal Nutritional Status   The client's food and fluid intake needs to be monitored. Clients who experience motor hyperactivity should be fed a diet high in protein and carbohydrates, and in finger-food form. Double portions of food may also be necessary. Clients who chew constantly need to be reminded to swallow. Depending upon the client's level of perception and motor activity, he or she will need to be supervised at mealtimes and assisted as necessary. The phenomenon of bulimia, seen in later stages of Alzheimer's disease, results in weight loss regardless of increased feeding. Weigh the client routinely and increase caloric intake as needed. In the final stages of the disease, the client loses all interest in food and must receive nasogastric, gastrostomy, or intravenous feedings (Dietsche and Pollman 1982).

Evaluation

Specific outcomes for the clients experiencing the organic mental syndromes and disorders are listed in the care plans.

Dementia Evaluation Criteria

The process of dementia is one of progressive intellectual, behavioral, and physiologic deterioration. The goal of nursing care is not to effect a cure but rather to sustain the client at his or her optimal level of self-care. Focus is also turned toward the family to help them sustain a personally rewarding relationship with their loved one throughout this terminal process.

Text continues on p. 345.

CASE STUDY: Client with Organic Mental Disease*

Identifying Information

Rosie W is an 83-year-old white Jewish woman, living alone in an apartment in the city; she was widowed 2 years ago. She was referred by her brother who states, "She has been extremely forgetful recently." She lives off her husband's retirement and also receives social security. She completed 9 years of school and has no current therapist.

Client's Definition of Present Problem, Precipitative Stresses, Coping Strategies, Goals for Care

Rosie comes to the clinic this morning at the request of her brother, stating "I had nothing to do with it. My brother's daughter must have a friend here." She states that she has been feeling "confused" and cannot remember things "from one moment to the next." She cannot remember how long this has been going on. She attributes this to getting old.

History of Present Problem

Rosie states that nothing unusual has happened over the past year. She is able to provide limited information about her present problem. Her brother was contacted to provide the necessary details. According to Rosie's 72-year-old brother, she has become increasingly disoriented over the last six months. On his own initiative, he brought her to her doctor who was unable to find anything physically wrong. Her brother describes her as "forgetful and just not herself. She doesn't even remember my name sometimes." On occasion, when he has gone to visit her, he has found her door unlocked, and the burner on the stove left on. He says he now manages her finances, since she can no longer balance the household budget herself. She has become increasingly withdrawn and no longer spends time with her friends. When he does take her out, she will often act in an embarrassing manner and say inappropriate and rude things. She is easily distracted, and he finds her mumbling to herself frequently. He states, "She will often start to do something, and right in the middle of doing it, she will go and start something else." He feels she is not reliable enough to prepare her own meals and is concerned that if he or his daughter do not bring her food, she will not eat. He is concerned that something will happen to her living alone and feels that she should have somebody live with her. She has refused to live with her brother, and because it is becoming increasingly difficult for him to get around, he cannot visit her as frequently as he would like. He thinks that Rosie's memory has gotten even worse over the past two to three months, although he cannot recall precisely when it all started.

Rosie has lived in her apartment for thirty-five years with her husband and for the past two years alone following his death. She states that she likes being "left alone." Her daily routine consists of "cleaning the apartment and shopping." She says she keeps her apartment "very orderly," so that she knows exactly where everything is. Recently, she has found it helpful to write things down so that she does not forget anything. When asked what she had for breakfast, she responded, "I don't remember, exactly." She states that she has difficulty sleeping because of all the noise and awakens frequently during the night.

Rosie describes her brother as her "right hand." She states that she has "a few friends" who live in the apartment building where she lives, but she does not socialize with them anymore because "There just isn't enough time in the day."

This case study was provided by Kathleen Tomaselli, a graduate student in psychiatric nursing at University of California, San Francisco.

continued

Case Study (Continued)

She says that she has been surrounded by people all her life but now prefers to be left alone. She has a 52-year-old married daughter, who lives about 300 miles away and with whom she speaks once a week. When asked when she saw her daughter last, she responded "last Thanksgiving . . . she ruined my grandson; now he's into dope!"

Psychiatric History

No previous hospitalizations and no previous therapists or treatments.

Family History

According to Rosie, her husband of 60 years "dropped dead two years ago while watching TV." She was unable to recall exactly when her parents died. However, she says that it was "many years ago." Rosie has one brother, 72 years old who is married with one daughter and who also lives in the city, and a daughter, 52 years old, who is married with three children and lives "in another state." Her older sister died 10 years ago. Her son died "quite young" of a brain tumor. The client says that she is close to her brother. During the interview, she repeatedly interjects, "I love my brother, but I wish he'd get off my back! I am I, as I am, not who he wants me to be!"

Social History

Rosie appears to have had a normal adulthood, passing through developmental milestones—such as marriage, parenting, grandparenting, retirement, widowhood—without any problems. Rosie states that she was forced to quit high school because of a nose condition. Her brother states that she completed nine years of school, but was not aware of Rosie's being forced to quit school. Rosie has no formal occupational training. She reminisces at length and with great detail about her work at the theater as a dresser. She quit the theater when she was offered a job as business agent for the wardrobe union. She does not remember for how, long she worked at either job nor at what age she retired. She recalls that "It was a very happy time for me. I was very well received." Her recollection of the events that have taken place between the time she retired from the wardrobe union and the present is sketchy.

Rosie was married when she was 21-years old. When asked how long she had been married before her husband died, she replied, "too many years." Her brother was able to report that she had been married for sixty years before her husband's death. Rosie described their relationship as "not very good. He had no use for me and I never knew what he wanted from me." She continued, "Oh, he fooled around alright, but that never bothered me. I had gorgeous red hair that every man admired. All the attention I received made my husband jealous."

Rosie never smoked and denies any history of drugs and alcohol.

Rosie spends most of her days in her apartment. She leaves the apartment only to go to the YWHA for her lunch and dinner. "I know my way there because it's only a stone's throw from my apartment."

Significant Health History

No history of major illness or injuries. Has had cataract surgery on both eyes. According to her brother, surgery on her left eye was done three months ago and her right eye was operated on two weeks ago. Currently, her right eye is patched. She states that she has hypertension and takes medication for it, but is unable to recall when it was first diagnosed. According to Rosie's brother, she has no other medical problems. When asked if she has enough energy, she responded, "at my age, it's not too bad."

The client appears well nourished. She says her appetite is "so-so" but thinks

continued

Case Study (Continued)

she may have gained weight. When asked if she had any difficulty bathing, she responded defensively, "I don't smell! I don't need to bathe any more often than anybody else!" She states that she has no difficulty "getting around," except at night since her vision at night is poor and she cannot find her flashlight. Sometimes it is difficult for her to see objects clearly and she is unable to read most things. She states, "It doesn't matter, since I don't remember anything I read anyway."

Current Mental Status

Rosie is a cooperative, white-haired, elderly woman who appears somewhat unkempt with uncombed hair, wrinkled dress, and smelling of strong perfume. She sits learning forward, clutching her pocketbook in her lap. She is oriented to person and place, knows the year, but is unsure of the month and date. Her fund of general knowledge is poor and she is unable to name the last five presidents. When asked if she knew who the president of the United States is, she responded, "Do I *know* that so-and-so? I don't like him!" When asked if she knew who the current mayor is, she replied, "Of course I know who he is! Don't you?" Her memory and recall are poor, performs digit span $\times 4$ forward and $\times 2$ backward. She is unable to repeat the names of three objects after five minutes and unable to name objects (keys, quarter) on sight and feel.

Her calculations are poor (unable to perform simple addition and subtraction and serial 7's). Client states, "It's frustrating for me since I used to be a bookkeeper and I was very good at math." Her judgment is poor. When asked what she would do if she found a stamped, addressed letter on the street, she replied, "I would read it and then, of course, mail it."

Rosie is alert, labile, superficial; sporadically anxious and irritable. She appeared depressed when talking about her grandson but cheerful and elated when describing her work in the theater. She states that she has no thoughts or plans of suicide. Her voice is soft, speech fluent. She becomes slightly pressured when trying to remember.

She denies having illusions, hallucinations, or delusions. She shows loose associations but can be redirected easily. Her ability for abstract thought is impaired. She provides concrete interpretations of proverbs. Her thoughts are tangentially related and responses to questions are irrelevant and circumstantial at times. She seems distractible and appears to have difficulty concentrating. She answers "I just don't know" frequently.

Rosie becomes anxious and attempts to minimize cognitive defects. She tries to conceal them by circumstantiality, perseveration, and changing the topic. She has little insight into current situation. She states, "I wish people would just leave me alone and get off my back. I don't know why everyone is so excited. I'm just getting old."

Diagnostic Impression

Nursing Diagnoses (PND-I/NANDA)

01.02	Altered recreational patterns /Social isolation
01.04.03	Insomnia /Sleep pattern disturbance
02.03.02	Altered intellectual functioning /Coping, ineffective individual

continued

Case Study (Continued)

	02.05	Altered memory
	02.06.01	Confusion
	02.08.01	Altered abstract thinking /Thought processes, altered
	04.02.08	Sadness
	06.04.08	Visual, altered sensory perception

DSM-IIIR Multiaxial Diagnosis

Axis I: 290 Primary degenerative dementia of the Alzheimer's type, senile onset with depression

Axis II: V71.09 (No diagnosis or condition; obsessive compulsive traits)

Axis III: Poor vision, high blood pressure, Alzheimer's disease

Axis IV: 2 Mild (cognitive impairment: enduring)
4 High (psychosocial stressors resulting from severe loss of memory. These include inability to balance finances; isolation from community, family, and friends; inability to maintain independence and self-care functioning: acute)

Axis V: Current GAF: 50 Serious symptoms (social and cognitive impairment)
Highest GAF in past year: 60

Nursing Care Plan

See the nursing care plan for the client with dementia on pages 334–336.

Delirium Evaluation Criteria

The evaluation of nursing care in delirium is based on the premise that the client is capable of returning to his or her previous level of functioning. During that process the client will be able to maintain optimal levels of sensory perception, participate in activities of daily living, and maintain physiologic homeostasis.

Chapter Highlights

- Dementia is a condition marked by a loss of intellectual abilities of sufficient severity to interfere with social and/or occupational functioning.

- Dementias are classified as cortical and subcortical; clients with the latter retain higher levels of functioning than those with cortical dementias.

- Alzheimer's disease, the most common form of dementia seen among the elderly, is a progressive, age-related chronic dysfunction that progresses through phases: early phases of forgetfulness, more advanced phases of disorientation and diminished concentration, and later and terminal phases of severe agitation, disorientation, psychosis, and complete helplessness.

- Genetics, viruslike substances, aluminum intoxication, and immune dysfunctions are all under consideration as possible causes of Alzheimer's disease.

- Pseudodementia, progressive supranuclear palsy, neurosyphilis, normal pressure hydrocephalus, Creutzfeldt-Jakob disease, Pick's disease, Huntington's chorea, Parkinson's disease, and multi-infarct dementia are among the other dementias seen in psychiatric nursing practice.

- Delirium is an organic brain syndrome characterized by global cognitive impairment of abrupt onset and relatively brief duration in which perception, thinking, and memory are all disrupted.

- Delirium may be due to organic agents, environmental stressors, poor sensory input, and other causes.

- It is extremely important to differentiate delirium from dementia but difficult to do so because about one-third of clients hospitalized for OMS experience both dementia and delirium.

- Assessment for OMS and OBS is particularly challenging because confused clients are often poor historians; furthermore, the interview environment and procedure may increase the client's anxiety and seriously compromise the nurse's attempts to assess.

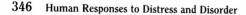

- Areas of subjective assessment include degree of confusion, health history (including psychosocial life-style patterns), sensory impairment, dietary history, possibility of head trauma, medication use, cognitive functioning, and overall mental status.

- Objective data are obtained from physical examination, laboratory assessment of routine tests, and objective rating scales of cognitive functioning.

- Psychiatric nursing diagnoses and interventions targeted toward them include those in the categories of: activity processes, perception and cognition processes, physiologic processes, and interpersonal processes.

- The overall goal of nursing interventions for clients with dementia is minimizing the loss of self-care capacity.

- The overall goal of nursing interventions for clients who have delirium is to support existing sensory perception until the client returns to previous levels of cognitive function.

- As knowledge in the field of psychobiology grows, psychiatric nurses will assume increasing responsibilities for designing intervention models for clients with OBS and OMS.

References

Besdine RW: The educational utility of comprehensive functional assessment in the elderly. *J Am Geriatr Soc* 1983;31:651–656.

Brody E, Lawton M, Liebowitz B: Senile dementia: Public policy and adequate institutional care. *Am J Public Health* 1984;74:1381–1383.

Burnside IM: Psychosocial issues in nursing care of the aged. *J Gerontol Nurs* 1981;7:689–694.

Butler RN, Lewis MI: *Aging and Mental Health,* ed 3. Mosby, 1982.

Cummings J: Multi-infarct dementia. *PSO* 1987;28(3): 117–125.

Dietsche LM, Pollman JN: Alzheimer's disease: Advances in clinical nursing. *J Gerontol Nurs* 1982;8:97–100.

Foreman MD: Acute confusional states in hospitalized elderly: A research dilemma. *Nurs Res* 1986;35:37–38.

Gershon S, Herman S: The differential diagnosis of dementia. *J Am Geriatr Soc* 1982;30:558–566.

Gilhooly ML: The impact of care-giving on caregivers: Factors associated with the psychological well-being of people supporting a dementing relative in the community. *Bri J Med Psychol* 1984;57:35–44.

Hamill RW, Buell SJ: Dementia: Clinical and basic science aspects. *J Am Geriatr Soc* 1982;30:781–787.

Hanley IG, McGuire RJ, Boyd WD: Reality orientation and dementia: A controlled trial of two approaches. *Br J Psychiatry* 1981;138:10–14.

Hays A, Borger F: A test in time. *Am J Nurs* 1985; 85:1107–1111.

Huber SJ, Paulson GW: The concept of subcortical dementia. *Am J Psychiatry* 1985;142:1312–1317.

Kuale JN: Alzheimer's disease. *Ann Fam Pract* 1986; 34:103–110.

Lancet: Cholinergic treatment in Alzheimer's disease: Encouraging results. *Lancet* 1987;1(8525):139–141.

Larson E, Reifler B, Canfield C, Cohen G: Evaluating elderly outpatients with symptoms of dementia. *Hosp Community Psychiatry* 1984;35:405–428.

Lipowski ZJ: A new look at organic brain syndromes. *Am J Psychiatry* 1980;137:674–678.

Lipowski ZJ: Transient cognitive disorders (delirium, acute confusional states) in the elderly. *Am J Psychiatry* 1983;140:1426–1436.

McAllister TW: Overview: Pseudodementia. *Am J Psychiatry* 1983;140:528–533.

Ninos M, Makohon R: Functional assessment of the patient. *Geriatr Nurs* 1985;6:139–142.

Panella J, Lilliston B, Brush D, McDowell F: Day care for dementia patients: An analysis of a four year program. *J Am Geriatr Soc* 1984;32:883–886.

Reifler B, Eisdorfer C: A clinic for the impaired elderly and their families. *Am J Psychiatry* 1980;137:1399–1403.

Reifler B, Larson E, Hanley R: Coexistence of cognitive impairment and depression in geriatric outpatients. *Am J Psychiatry* 1982;139:623–626.

Schneck M, Reisberg B, Ferris S: An overview of current concepts of Alzheimer's disease. *Am J Psychiatry* 1982;139:165–173.

Roca R: Bedside cognitive examination: Usefulness in detecting delirium and dementia. *PSO* 1987;28:2:71–76.

Small GW, Liston EH, Jarvik LF: Diagnosis and treatment of dementia in the aged. *West J Med* 1981;135:469–481.

Tariot P, Sunderland T, Murphy D, Cohen R, Weingartner H, Makohon R: How memory fails: A theoretical model. *Geriatr Nurs* 1985;6:144–147.

Task Force Sponsored by the National Institute on Aging. Senility reconsidered: Treatment possibilities for mental impairment in the elderly. *JAMA* 1980;244:259–263.

Wells CE: Pseudodementia. *Am J Psychiatry* 1978; 136:895–900.

Wells CE: Chronic brain disease: An update on alcoholism, Parkinson's disease, and dementia. *Hosp Community Psychiatry* 1982;33:111–126.

Whelihan WM, Lesher EL, Kleban MH, Granick S: Mental status and memory assessment as predictors of dementia. *J Gerontol* 1984;39:572–576.

Wolanin MO, Fraelich-Philips LR: *Confusion, Prevention and Care.* Mosby, 1981.

Wright AF, Whaley LJ: Genetics, aging and dementia. *Bri J Psychiatry* 1984;145:20–38.

Zarit S, Reever K, Bach-Peterson J: Relatives of the impaired elderly: Correlates of feelings of burden. *Gerontologist* 1980;20:649–655.

SIXTEEN

Applying the Nursing Process for
Clients with Psychoactive Substance Use Disorders

Sally A. Hutchinson

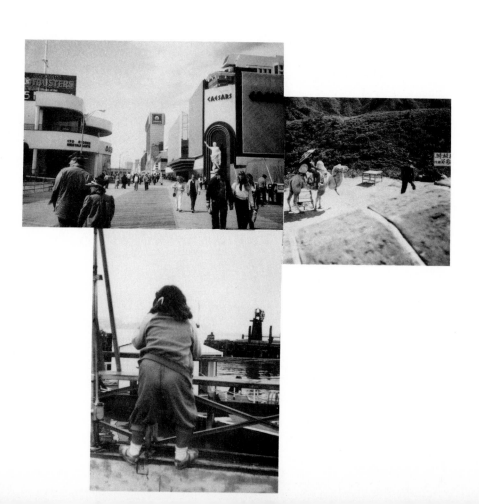

After reading this chapter, students should be able to

- Contrast the different definitions of substance abuse
- List key legislation in the history of substance abuse
- Analyze major theoretical explanations for substance abuse
- Compare and contrast the major categories of substance use
- Identify the groups at risk for substance abuse
- Assess the physical, psychologic, and withdrawal effects of the major categories of substance use
- Apply the nursing process with clients with psychoactive substance use disorders
- Identify questions that are integral to a nursing assessment of clients who are substance abusers
- Compare and contrast nursing diagnoses from NANDA and PND-I with diagnoses from DSM-IIIR
- Discuss a variety of nursing intervention strategies for clients demonstrating various types of substance abuse
- Identify evaluation/outcome criteria for clients who are substance abusers

Cross References

Other topics related to this chapter are: Adolescents, Chapter 35; Depression, Chapter 18; Organic mental disorders, Chapter 15; Polydrug use among the elderly, Chapter 36; Psychobiology, Chapter 9; Risk of AIDS for intravenous drug users, Chapter 26.

Key Terms

Al-Anon
Al-Ateen
Alcoholics Anonymous
Antabuse (disulfiram)
anterograde amnesia
blackouts
codependency
delirium tremens (DTs)
enabler
fetal alcohol syndrome (FAS)
psychoactive substance–induced organic mental disorders
psychoactive substance use disorders

Drug and alcohol abuse, already a widespread problem in most industrialized countries, is rapidly escalating in third world countries. Substance abuse is an international problem. In the United States and Europe, television and radio advertisements entice viewers with the hope of relief from pain and problems. The cultural values portrayed are clear: Discomfort should be erased; drinking is vital to a stress-free life; drugs are acceptable mediators of emotions. Note the following facts about substance abuse:

- Substance abuse strikes all ages, cultural groups, and socioeconomic classes.
- Drug abuse, excluding alcohol abuse, cost the United States $39 billion in 1985.
- Business loses an estimated $16 billion a year to drug and alcohol abuse on the job.
- One of ten American workers is a substance abuser.
- One of two families in the United States has a problem with chemicals.
- One of five nurses is a substance abuser.
- Americans spend $220 million a day on illegal drugs.
- Americans spend more than $6 billion a year on enforcement of drug laws.
- Sixty percent of the world's drugs are used in the United States.
- Alcohol is involved in:

  60 percent of fatal accidents

  70 percent of all murders

  41 percent of assaults

  53 percent of fire deaths

  50 percent of rapes

  60 percent of sex crimes against children

  90 percent of child abuse

  56 percent of fights and assaults in homes

  37 percent of suicides

  55 percent of arrests

Imagine a "no first strike" agreement.

36 percent of pedestrian accidents

22 percent of home accidents

45 percent of drownings

50 percent of skiing accidents

More admissions to mental hospitals than any other cause

More than 50% of traffic accidents

30 to 50 percent of all hospital admissions

- Alcohol is the number one killer of people under 25. More than 8000 young people are killed in alcohol-related highway accidents each year, and 40,000 suffer serious injury.

- Alcoholism costs the United States $25 billion in medical expenses, lost wages, and reduced productivity.

- 3,300,000 teenagers are alcoholics

- One of five children comes from a household with an alcoholic.

- Two-thirds of adolescent sexual encounters occur while teenagers are drinking at a family home, usually in a party situation.

- Nineteen percent of 12–17-year-olds have a serious drinking problem, which is defined as drinking at least once a week and consuming five to twelve drinks on a single occasion.

- Every five seconds, a teenager has a drug- or alcohol-related traffic accident.

- Sixty percent of American high school seniors have tried marijuana; one of fourteen is a daily user.

- Intellectually gifted adolescents are 400 times more likely to become chemically dependent than the general population.

- One of every five high school adolescents "does drugs" on a weekly basis.

- Twenty-five percent of 18–25-year-olds have tried cocaine and hallucinogens.

- Ten thousand cocaine users were treated in emergency rooms in 1985; the 1985 cocaine death rate was triple that in 1981.

- Four million people in the United States use cocaine.

Substance abuse is a major public health issue of grave ramifications. It increases the crime rate, auto accident deaths, number of teenage pregnancies, and the suicide rate. Individuals and families are destroyed. Every part of a substance abuser's life—social life, family life, work productivity and relationships, physical health—is affected.

Substance abuse in the work environment increases accidents, workers' compensation claims, absenteeism, and theft.

This chapter is an in-depth exploration of the substance abuse issues relevant to the practicing nurse.

HISTORICAL FOUNDATIONS

From the beginning of recorded history, humans have experimented with drugs and drink in an effort to feel good or to experience an altered state of consciousness. Drugs first touted for their healing effects, with time, often become problems to society. William James, a brilliant American psychologist, wrote of a "tremendously exciting sense of an intense metaphysical illumination" after using nitrous oxide (Klein 1985, p 40). Freud believed cocaine to be a new wonder drug because of its euphoric effects. William Halstead, a surgeon, used cocaine for regional anesthesia. Others found it useful for alcohol and morphine addiction, asthma, colds, corns, eczema, neuralgia, and even spiritual awakening (Rottenberg 1980). In the 1960s, Timothy Leary, a Harvard psychologist, was an avid supporter of the use of LSD for the purpose of achieving heightened awareness. Over time, each of these drugs has left a wake of horror in people's lives. Deaths, brain damage, violence, and ruined lives are the result of abuse.

New "wonder" drugs come on the market continuously. This pattern is not unusual: Scientists using animals experiment with drugs and notice their initial effects. The drug becomes available on the street, and people increase the dosage and adulterate it with various, often harmful substances. Consequently, the street version of the drug is far different from the original compound. Home chemists experiment in making similar drugs that are readily sold on the street. Side-effects appear, and the wonder drug is transformed into something unrecognizable. Because of this pattern and because a drug's total effects become evident only with time, new drugs must be subjected to controlled scientific tests. Such testing requires an experimental and control group, use of animal subjects before people, and timed trials, meaning that the drug is given under controlled conditions and its effects assessed over time. The research should then be reported in a reputable scientific journal.

Efforts at Controlling Substance Abuse

While one segment of the population experiments with drugs and alcohol, another segment attempts to set limits. By examining events over the last eighty years, we can trace changing perspectives on substance abuse and efforts to control it. This significant legislation mirrors changing trends:

- In 1914, the Harrison Narcotics Act became the first United States legislative act that attempted to control narcotics.
- In 1920, the Volstead Act prohibited alcohol.
- From 1919–1923, addicts were able to obtain heroin from clinics.
- In 1924, Congress passed the Narcotics Drugs Import and Export Act and the Marijuana Tax Act.
- In 1933, the Volstead Act was repealed.
- In 1946, the Mental Health Act brought increased attention to substance abuse.
- In 1946, the United Nations and World Health Organization became involved in the control of illicit drugs.
- In the 1960s, President Kennedy declared drug education a national priority, and federal monies were allocated to substance abuse programs.
- In 1968, the Bureau of Narcotics and Dangerous Drugs (formerly under the Food and Drug Administration) was transferred to the Department of Justice. Today, it is the Bureau of Narcotics and Dangerous Drugs and Customs.
- In 1970, the Harrison Narcotics Act was repealed. A new act, the Comprehensive Drug Abuse Prevention and Control Act (also known as the Controlled Substance Act) regulated the availability and use of controlled substances.
- In 1972, regulations for the handling and distribution of methadone were planned.
- In the 1980s, federal drug and alcohol funds were rechanneled into alcohol, drug abuse, and mental health block grants (ADAMH).
- In 1985, Congress pursued legislation attached to a foreign aid bill that required the Drug Enforcement Administration and the State Department to share information on international narcotics traffickers.
- By 1986, programs for nurses who are substance abusers were in effect in twenty-one states and were being developed in most other states.

Beliefs about Causes

Beliefs about the causes of substance abuse changed over the years. In the 1900s, alcoholics and drug addicts were considered morally weak people who yielded easily to temptation. In 1956, the American Medical Association declared alcoholism a disease; this relabeling had important ramifications for diagnosis and treatment. The following year, the American Hospital Association accepted alcoholism as an illness appropriate for treatment in general hospitals. At this time, insurance companies offered financial coverage.

Gradually, as substance abuse became redefined as a

psychiatric disorder, researchers found the topic worthy of study. Initial research was conducted in the 1950s at the Yale University Center of Alcohol Studies. The Controlled Substance Act of 1970 provided Department of Health, Education, and Welfare grants for treatment, rehabilitation, and education programs related to drug abuse. Today, substance abuse is a major public health issue and, con-

RESEARCH NOTE

Citation

Hutchinson S: Chemically dependent nurses: the trajectory toward self-annihilation Nurs Res *1986;35(4): 196–201.*

Study Problem/Purpose

Qualitative field research—interviewing and participant observation—was used to generate a substantive grounded theory that explains the process of nurses becoming chemically dependent.

Methods

Data collection methods included in-depth interviews with twenty chemically dependent nurses and a variety of participant-observation strategies, including attending a self-help group for impaired nurses for one year. Grounded theory methods were used for data analysis.

Findings

Findings reveal that as a result of physical and/or psychologic pain, nurses who became chemically dependent embarked on a trajectory of self-annihilation (Figure 16–3). The nurses began by experimenting with drugs or alcohol; over time they became committed to using chemicals as part of their life-style and soon they became possessed by their addiction, feeling a compulsion to "use." As they became addicted, they suffered the loss of family, friends, and work relationships. Often, they lost their jobs and were in trouble with the legal system and/or the Board of Nursing. Their attempt at self-care backfired, ultimately bringing more pain than ever.

Implications

An understanding of the processes nurses go through in becoming chemically dependent is useful for planning educational and administrative interventions. Hypotheses for experimental research may be derived from the theory.

sequently, research monies from federal and private agencies are plentiful.

As substance abuse was redefined, the writings about substance abuse gradually changed in quantity and quality. Initially confined to psychiatric nursing journals and medical journals, literature on alcoholism and drug addiction began to appear in the general nursing literature (Naegle 1983). At the present time, psychiatric nursing has yet to develop adequate theories to guide the care of clients who are substance abusers. Research is in the early phase of development: Theories are being generated and also borrowed from other disciplines and applied to nursing. Nursing research on the assessment, diagnosis, and intervention with the substance abusing client is increasing and should soon have some effects on nursing practice.

THEORETICAL FOUNDATIONS

Before examining the theories that attempt to account for the "why" of substance abuse we should define the term. According to the National Council on Alcoholism, a *substance abuser* is a person who experiences problems with health, work, family, and social relations as a result of drug or alcohol use.

According to Dr. G. Douglas Talbott, a pioneer in the study of addiction, *abuse* is the misuse of a drug that can be discontinued at will; addiction occurs when misuse is uncontrollable. Addiction, a disease, occurs when a person with a genetic predisposition to addiction abuses a drug (Gallagher 1986, pp 7–8).

In 1964, the World Health Organization (WHO) Expert Committee on Addiction-Producing Drugs voted to substitute the term *drug dependence* for *addiction* and *habituation*. In 1980, the American Psychiatric Association's *Diagnostic and Statistical Manual of Mental Disorders,* third edition (DSM-III), divided substance use disorders into two major categories: substance abuse and substance dependence. The DSM-IIIR proposes two major categories—**psychoactive substance–induced organic mental disorders** and **psychoactive substance use disorders** (American Psychiatric Association 1987). These various definitions and categories demonstrate the changing terminology of substance abuse.

In this chapter, *substance* refers to alcohol, prescription drugs, over-the-counter medications, and illicit drugs. Contemporary explanations of substance abuse derive from biologic, psychologic, sociocultural, and family systems theories.

The biologic explanation, especially of alcoholism, has assumed a greater importance in the last few years. Research to determine genetic predispositions to alcoholism continues. The following are examples of research that is gaining respect in the scientific community:

- Classic research by Jellinek in the 1940s and 1950s revealed that alcoholics proceed through phases, including the prealcoholic symptomatic phase, the prodromal phase, the crucial phase, and the chronic phase (Jellinek 1946). He recognized "loss of control" in addictive alcoholics and conjectured that it may have a biochemical basis.

- Cultural differences may affect alcoholism rates. For example, Oriental people frequently experience adverse reactions to alcohol, including palpitations and a flush of the skin. These responses are genetic and probably account for the lower rate of alcoholism in the Orient.

- Alcoholics have been noted to have a type of color blindness. A study of relatives of alcoholics indicates possible transmission by sex-linked recessive genes (Cruz-Coke and Varela 1966, Varela et al. 1969).

- In the late 1950s, researchers studied Scandinavian twins to determine if alcoholism was inherited. The scientists studied twins of alcoholic parents who were reared by (a) their own parents, (b) foster parents, and (c) different foster families. After twenty-five years, the records reveal that the degree of alcoholism in all three groups is almost identical. This finding suggests that a genetic factor predisposes to alcoholism (Mann 1983). A related direction for research is the effects of alcohol on the fetus.

- Some people are born with a faulty hepatic enzyme system that may predispose them to alcohol addiction.

- Researchers have found that alcoholics metabolize ethanol more efficiently than nonalcoholics through the creation of alternative pathways and in response to chronic high blood alcohol levels. This phenomenon suggests an explanation for the abnormal increase in ethanol tolerance noted in the alcoholic population (Lieber and DeCarli 1970, Ugarte et al. 1972).

- P-450, an enzyme with opiatelike characteristics, has been found to develop in alcoholics, possibly creating the craving and compulsion to drink addictively (Koop et al. 1982).

- In animals, alcohol is metabolized into tetrahydro-isoquinolones (TIQs), opiatelike compounds that affect nerve receptors much as morphine and endorphins (the body's naturally produced opiates) do. TIQ from alcohol has an opiate effect. In response, the body decreases or stops endorphin production. When the alcohol wears off, the endorphin levels remain low, and the alcoholic cannot feel good without drinking. Some researchers believe alcoholics may be born with an endorphin deficiency, creating a low tolerance to pain and stress (Franks 1985).

- Animal research advances the notion that alcoholics have a metabolic anomaly that causes them to derive more pleasure than other people do. When alcohol is absent from the body, the absence of this pleasure is felt as a deficiency (Franks 1985).

- Alcoholics may have neurophysiologic defects. They may be vulnerable to intense sensory input and use alcohol as a protection from this heightened sensitivity.

- Research demonstrates that children of alcoholics are at fourfold risk of becoming alcoholics. Even if they are adopted by different families at birth, identical twins of alcoholic parents have more than a 60 percent chance of becoming alcoholics; fraternal twins have less than a 30 percent chance. Children of nonalcoholics reared by alcoholics are not at increased risk of alcoholism (Schuckit 1985).

- When a control group of sons of nonalcoholics (a low-risk population) and an experimental group of sons of alcoholics (a high-risk population) were compared, three differences were found (Schuckit 1985):

  1. Sons of alcoholics appear to show less intense responses to modest ethanol dosages, demonstrate lower amplitudes of a brain wave that might measure selective attention, and may have different brain alpha rhythms.

  2. Subjective and objective tests showed that sons of alcoholics were less affected by ethanol than sons of nonalcoholics.

  3. When both groups were given the same dosage of ethanol, controls showed poorer performance on a number of cognitive and psychomotor tests and more intense changes in cortisol and prolactin, two hormones known to be affected by injection of ethanol.

Schuckit (1985) concludes "there is consistent evidence that those in the high-risk group demonstrate significantly less intense reactions to modest doses of ethanol than those in the low-risk group. It may be that they are feeling less ethanol effect at the blood alcohol concentrations at which most people make a decision to stop drinking" (p 2616).

Scientists now are working on computerized methods of analyzing blood chemistries. These techniques may help in diagnosing early alcoholism. Another blood test will detect liver changes that warn of cirrhosis (Franks 1985). When these tests are perfected, their use will raise difficult ethical and legal issues for employers, as the use of urinalysis to detect drug abuse does now. One such issue is the employee's right to privacy. A second is the possibility of error.

The error rate in urine tests is 50 to 100 percent (often due to technical errors and poor quality control), giving an unjustly accused employee a cause for legal action. Another problem with urine tests is that they cannot detect when a person used a drug or whether a person is an addict, a habitual user, or an occasional user. Also, test results do not indicate job performance. There remain the difficult questions of who to test, when to test, how to test, and what steps to take if the test is positive. In spite of these questions, one-third of the nation's largest companies are doing urinalysis on their employees.

Psychologic Perspectives

From the psychologic perspective, the substance abuser is viewed as regressed and fixated at pregenital, oral levels of psychosexual development. Some writers relate the pattern of drug taking to parental inconsistency, self-centeredness, and inner dishonesty. The following personality traits are often associated with disruptive drug use:

- Dominant and critical behavior with underlying self-doubts and passivity
- Tendency to describe own parents as self-reliant and efficient but not emotionally warm
- Personal insecurity
- Problems with sexual identification
- Rebellious attitudes toward authority
- Tendency to use defense mechanisms that are primarily escapist
- Difficulty with intimacy
- Absence of a strong and efficient superego
- Marked narcissistic trends

There is no real agreement about whether certain personality traits are sufficient to account for drug dependence, because the personality traits in question are studied after the diagnosis of substance abuse.

Presently, there is general agreement among the psychiatric community that people with certain personality traits are not substance abusers. Clients diagnosed with primary affective disorders, sociopathy, and certain personality disorders, however, often abuse alcohol and drugs. In such cases, initial assessment, after the client has undergone withdrawal, should focus on accurate diagnoses so that both conditions may be treated simultaneously.

Richard Marohn (1983), the president of the American Society for Adolescent Psychiatry, offers an interesting and plausible psychologic explanation for adolescent, and ultimately adult, substance abuse. Adopting a developmental perspective, Marohn views the alcohol or drugs as having a self-healing or self-medicating function. Adolescents who successfully separate from their parents do so by transferring their object attachment from their parents to idealized others, including peers. With time, adolescents learn how to master a variety of strong emotions—anger, guilt, joy, pain, sexual attraction, love—and recognize that these emotions emanate from themselves and are part of themselves. The adolescent can then care for himself or herself by living with and experiencing the powerful emotions that are part of being alive.

Adolescents who are substance abusers, Marohn believes, have severe problems with tension regulation. They have not been able to separate and individuate from significant others. They view their emotions as emanating from the other or from the external world, as children do. The expectation, then, is that the parents are responsible for the teenager's life and feelings. When this expectation is not met and when they experience strong emotions, adolescents resort to substance abuse to manage these emotions. Drugs and alcohol are an escape from powerful and often painful emotions, an attempt at self-soothing and self-care.

Sociocultural Perspectives

Life's harsh realities come in many forms: the hopelessness and defeat of urban slum dwellers, the academic and social pressures generated by upper middle class families, the adolescent's feeling of impotence and alienation, the peer group pressure to join in and share experiences, the social vacuum of unloving families, where meaningful attachments are dissolved or dissolving. All of these social conditions and contexts help create and sustain substance abuse. In addition, however, people who become addicts or alcoholics tend to live in environments where access to chemicals is easy and initiation into their use is widespread. Substance abusers describe in interviews how they learned to drink or use drugs at high school and college parties or at home by watching their families. They recognized chemicals as a remedy for psychic and physical pain.

Deviant subcultures encourage their members to adopt a drug-dependent life-style. The sociologist Howard Becker (1963) studied the process by which a person becomes a marijuana user. In this classic study, Becker emphasizes the role the subculture plays in teaching people to disengage from conventional social controls. The subculture also teaches them how to think about the experience and the techniques that ensure that they will enjoy using the

drug. Another sociologist, Alfred Lindesmith (1965), observes that people recognize that they are addicted at the moment when the appearance of withdrawal symptoms makes voluntary abstinence impossible. At this point, they are ready to be assimilated into a genuine drug-dependent life-style, because they must begin planning how to make sure they have a future supply. They must learn the sources, devices, and customs they will use to solve their problems.

Studies clearly show that substance abuse is present in all cultures; however, which substance people abuse is often culturally determined. In Western culture, alcohol is the drug of choice. Moslem countries have a problem with marijuana because Islam prohibits alcohol use. Opium is used in China and other Eastern countries, while people in India and Africa use native herbs and chemicals. Native Americans use peyote and alcohol more than other drugs.

Reasons for use are also different in different cultures. Many native Americans use peyote to communicate with the Great Spirit, and its use is culturally sanctioned. Some social scientists believe that alcohol abuse among native Americans is the result of white people's ignorant and harmful interference in native beliefs and traditions. The theory is that native Americans suffer from cultural dissonance because they still live between two cultures. The extreme poverty and political oppression of their lives make them susceptible to alcohol abuse, which was introduced at the time of contact with white people. In the native American culture, the problem of alcoholism has escalated over the years.

Family Systems Perspectives

A family systems explanation for substance abuse has gained increasing acceptance among health care professionals. Stanton and Todd's (1982) work is particularly useful because it proposes a theoretical framework, a treatment method, and evaluation methods based on family systems theory. Unlike social theorists who stress the power of the peer group, Stanton and Todd view adolescent drug abuse primarily as a family phenomenon. Adolescent drug addicts, they believe, are too close to their parents and consequently feel dependent, inadequate, and fearful of separation. The family is overly *enmeshed* or *entangled*.

Contrary to what one might expect, the adolescent drug abuser is striving to preserve the stability of the entangled family. He or she keeps the family in crisis and focused on the problems brought about by drug abuse. If the addict improves and begins to individuate and separate from the family, the underlying familial problems emerge. Thus, the entire family has a stake in keeping the addict on drugs. The drug use allows the addict to pseudoindividuate—to be both in and out of the family.

The family systems perspective also includes the phenomenon of **codependency**, an emotional dysfunction that is present in families with an alcoholic member (Friel et al. 1984). A codependent is the family member who alternately rescues and blames (persecutes) the alcoholic. Certain behaviors are characteristic of the codependent, also called the coalcoholic (see Box 16–1). Essentially, this person is a highly organized achiever who works continuously, attempting to maintain stability in the present situation. Usually, codependents are married to the alcoholic, and the children in the family are at high risk for becoming substance abusers and emotionally unstable. Survival patterns are usually different for each child. One may become a substance abuser, while another may become the family caretaker ("hero") at an early age. This young child actively "parents" the parents and siblings, covers up for them, and works to promote harmony (placator role) in a volatile, dysfunctional family. Another child may be a "scapegoat," behaving in negative ways so as to deflect blame from the alcoholic parent. Emotional and behavioral problems are common. This child is at high risk for becoming a substance abuser. "The lost child" escapes into fantasy and also is at high risk for addiction; the "mascot" plays the role of the clown, thereby diverting attention from the parents.

Families with alcoholic members suffer guilt, remorse, and alienation. Conflict is inevitable, and violence is common. The dysfunctional family patterns involve all family members and tend to be transmitted through the generations, making family systems intervention necessary for change.

Although **Alcoholics Anonymous (AA)**, a support group for alcoholics, does not openly endorse the family systems theory, they do recognize clearly that alcoholism is a family disease. **Al-Anon** and **Al-Ateen** are groups for spouses, parents, and teenagers who are involved with alcoholics. The focus is on helping these nonalcoholics learn to live and work effectively with alcoholics. The underlying belief is that family members often assume the role of **enablers**, or coalcoholics, perpetuating the alcoholic's drinking patterns. As the family attempts to adjust to the alcoholic's life-style, they develop behavioral and emotional problems (The Family Enablers, p 3).

A cycle begins when the enablers do what they think is best in the situation. They begin to cover for the alcoholic, e.g., by saying that he or she has a cold, is bruised because of stumbling in the dark, is asleep because of fatigue. Protected by the enabler, the alcoholic is spared the consequences of his or her behavior and continues drinking. The enabler, believing that the alcoholic is coping with family, marital, or work problems "the best way he can," denies the disease of alcoholism. The alcoholic blames the enabler; the enabler feels guilty and then attempts to control family life and the behaviors of the alcoholic, e.g., throwing out liquor, taking the car keys. Of course, this behavior does not work. The enabler has tried the roles of protector, rescuer, controller, and blamer, but none is effective in altering the course of the disease. Consequently, enablers feel worthless and helpless because they are unsuccessful in terminating the alcoholism. Intervention and confrontation are necessary to break the cycle.

All of these theories—biologic, psychologic, sociocul-

Box 16–1
CODEPENDENCY BEHAVIORS

- Highly organized
- Competent at a wide variety of tasks and able to learn new skills quickly
- Stable and not given to panic
- Skilled at diplomacy and emotional manipulation
- Resilient with a high tolerance for pain
- Energetic and not easily fatigued
- Good administrator
- Able to defer gratification indefinitely
- Skilled at crisis intervention
- Strongly moral; sense of right and wrong crucial to this person's thinking
- Loyal and willing to put the needs of an important group before own needs; out of touch with needs and feelings
- Very unlikely to ask "What's in this for me?"
- Able to do enormous amounts of work for a minimal payoff
- Excellent caretaker
- Overachiever and "workaholic"

Source: Adapted from Elkin M: Families under the Influence. W. W. Norton, 1984, pp 57–58.

---

tural, family systems—offer perspectives on the problem of substance abuse. Research that tests hypotheses derived from these theories is necessary to advance our knowledge and to contribute to further theory development.

CATEGORIES OF SUBSTANCE ABUSE

The DSM-III (American Psychiatric Association 1980, p 163) includes the diagnostic class "substance use disorders," which is concerned with

> . . . Behavioral changes associated with more or less regular use of substances that affect the central nervous system. Examples of such behavioral changes include impairment in social or occupational functioning as a consequence of substance use, inability to control use of or to stop taking the substance, and the development of serious withdrawal symptoms after cessation of or reduction in substance use.

orders result in dependence or abuse. (See Box 16–4 for the diagnostic criteria for dependence and abuse.)

The DSM-IIIR (American Psychiatric Association 1987) has two categories entitled psychoactive substance-induced organic mental disorders and psychoactive substance use disorders (see Boxes 16–2 and 16–3). Psychoactive substance-induced organic mental disorders result in intoxications, withdrawal, delirium, hallucinosis, and delusional disorders, among others. Psychoactive substance use dis-

ALCOHOL

Josie B, a 62-year-old woman, arrived at the hospital to be admitted for the fifth time. Her gait was unsteady and her speech slurred. Even though drunk, she avoided

---

Box 16–2
PSYCHOACTIVE SUBSTANCE–INDUCED ORGANIC MENTAL DISORDERS

Alcohol

303.00	Intoxication
291.40	Idiosyncratic intoxication
291.80	Uncomplicated alcohol withdrawal
291.00	Withdrawal delirium
291.30	Hallucinosis
291.10	Amnestic disorder
291.20	Dementia associated with alcoholism

Amphetamine or Similarly Acting Sympathomimetic

305.70	Intoxication
292.00	Withdrawal
292.81	Delirium
282.11	Delusional disorder

Caffeine

305.90	Intoxication

Cannabis

305.20	Intoxication
292.11	Delusional disorder

Cocaine

305.60	Intoxication
292.00	Withdrawal
292.81	Delirium
292.11	Delusional disorder

Hallucinogen

305.30	Hallucinosis
292.11	Delusional disorder
292.84	Mood disorder
292.89	Posthallucinogen perception disorder

Inhalant

305.90	Intoxication

Nicotine

292.00	Withdrawal

Opioid

305.50	Intoxication
292.00	Withdrawal

Phencyclidine (PCP) or Similarly Acting Arylcyclohexylamine

305.90	Intoxication
292.81	Delirium
292.11	Delusional disorder
292.84	Mood disorder
292.90	Organic mental disorder NOS

Sedative, Hypnotic, or Anxiolytic

305.40	Intoxication
292.00	Uncomplicated sedative, hypnotic, or anxiolytic withdrawal
292.00	Withdrawal delirium
292.83	Amnestic disorder

Other or Unspecified Psychoactive Substance

305.90	Intoxication
292.00	Withdrawal
292.81	Delirium
292.82	Dementia
292.83	Amnestic disorder
292.11	Delusional disorder
292.12	Hallucinosis
292.84	Mood disorder
292.89	Anxiety disorder
292.89	Personality disorder
292.90	Organic mental disorder NOS

Source: American Psychiatric Association: Diagnostic and Statistical Manual of Mental Disorders, *ed 3, revised. APA, 1987, p 51.*

eye contact, appeared embarrassed, and apologized profusely for "getting into this mess again." She said, "I really don't need to be here. I can handle this problem."

Box 16–5 presents the key facts about alcohol abuse. Several years ago alcoholism was considered a neglected disease. Recently, because of its increasing incidence and the highway carnage attributed to alcohol use, alcoholism has been the focus of magazine articles and radio and television programs. Perhaps this media blitz is in part a response to heightened awareness of the devastating effects of chronic alcoholism, e.g., depression; loss of self-respect; alienation from family, friends, and coworkers; malnutrition; infections; and damaging physiologic effects to most body systems (see Box 16–6). Although alcoholism historically was viewed as a moral problem, this increased awareness played a part in the redefinition of alcoholism as a disease. (The American Medical Association labeled alcoholism as a disease in 1956.) As research about its biochemical aspects became known, earlier beliefs were challenged. The social stigma attached to alcoholism is decreasing, and more people are seeking help. Professionals, laypeople, alcoholics, and nonalcoholics are attending workshops and seminars on alcoholism; college courses at the graduate and undergraduate levels are offered. Recovery programs are reported widely in the popular media.

Effects of Alcohol

A sedative anesthetic, alcohol is absorbed in the small intestine. Approximately 95 percent is broken down by the liver; the rest is excreted through the lungs, kidneys, and skin. Generally, a person can metabolize 10 mL of alcohol or 1 ounce of whiskey every ninety minutes. If taken in exceedingly high doses, alcohol can depress respiration and cause death. Intoxication occurs when a person's blood alcohol level is 0.10 percent or more. This blood alcohol level is the legal definition of inebriation in most states. Simple intoxication lasts less than twelve hours and is usually followed by a hangover. A *hangover* is the unpleasant

---

Box 16–3
PSYCHOACTIVE SUBSTANCE USE DISORDERS

Alcohol

303.90 Dependence
305.00 Abuse

Amphetamine or Similarly Acting Sympathomimetic

304.40 Dependence
305.70 Abuse

Cannabis

304.30 Dependence
305.70 Abuse

Cocaine

304.20 Dependence
305.60 Abuse

Hallucinogen

304.50 Dependence
305.30 Abuse

Inhalant

304.60 Dependence
305.90 Abuse

Nicotine

305.10 Dependence

Opioid

304.00 Dependence
305.50 Abuse

Phencyclidine (PCP) or Similarly Acting Arylcyclohexylamine

304.50 Dependence
305.90 Abuse

Sedative, Hypnotic, or Anxiolytic

304.10 Dependence
305.40 Abuse
304.90 Polysubstance dependence
304.90 Psychoactive substance dependence NOS
305.90 Psychoactive substance abuse NOS

Source: American Psychiatric Association: Diagnostic and Statistical Manual of Mental Disorders, *ed 3, revised. APA, 1987, p 6.*

symptoms occurring approximately four to six hours after alcohol ingestion. These symptoms include nausea and vomiting, gastritis, headache, fatigue, sweating, thirst, and vasomotor instability. The cause of the symptoms is uncer-

tain, but they are attributed to hypoglycemia and the accumulation of lactic acid and acetaldehyde in the blood.

Alcoholic hallucinosis refers to auditory hallucinations reported by clients with alcohol dependence. The hallucinations occur approximately forty-eight hours after heavy drinking.

Alcohol withdrawal syndrome refers to withdrawal symptoms unaccompanied by delirium. These include tremulousness and hallucinations. Tremulousness may

---

Box 16–4
DIAGNOSTIC CRITERIA FOR PSYCHOACTIVE SUBSTANCE DEPENDENCE

A. At least three of the following:

　1. Substance often taken in larger amounts or over a longer period than the person intended

　2. Persistent desire or one or more unsuccessful efforts to cut down or control substance use

　3. A great deal of time spent in activities necessary to get the substance (e.g., theft), taking the substance (e.g., chain smoking), or recovering from its effects

　4. Frequent intoxication or withdrawal symptoms when expected to fulfill major role obligations at work, school, or home (e.g., does not go to work because hung over, goes to school or work "high," intoxicated while taking care of his or her children), or when substance is physically hazardous (e.g., drives when intoxicated)

　5. Important social, occupational, or recreational activities given up or reduced because of substance use

　6. Continued substance use despite knowledge of having a persistent or recurrent social, psychologic, or physical problem that is caused or exacerbated by the use of the substance (e.g., keeps using heroin despite family arguments about it, cocaine-induced depression, or having an ulcer made worse by drinking)

　7. Marked tolerance: need for markedly increased amounts of the substance (i.e., at least a 50 percent increase) in order to achieve intoxication or desired effect, or markedly diminished effect with continued use of the same amount

Note: The following items may not apply to cannabis, hallucinogens, or phencyclidine (PCP):

　8. Characteristic withdrawal symptoms

　9. Substance often taken to relieve or avoid withdrawal symptoms

B. Some symptoms of the disturbance have persisted for at least 1 month, or have occurred repeatedly over a longer period of time.

Criteria for Severity of Psychoactive Substance Dependence

Mild: Few, if any, symptoms in excess of those required to make the diagnosis, and the symptoms result in no more than mild impairment in occupational functioning or in usual social activities or relationships with others.

Moderate: Symptoms or functional impairment between "mild" and "severe."

Severe: Many symptoms in excess of those required to make the diagnosis, and the symptoms markedly interfere with occupational functioning or with usual social activities or relationships with others.

In partial remission: During the past six months, some use of the substance and some symptoms of dependence.

In full remission: During the past six months, either no use of the substance, or use of the substance and no symptoms of dependence.

Diagnostic Criteria for Psychoactive Substance Abuse

A. A maladaptive pattern of psychoactive substance use indicated by at least one of the following:

　1. Continued use despite knowledge of having a persistent or recurrent social, occupational, psychologic, or physical problem that is caused or exacerbated by use of the psychoactive substance

　2. Recurrent use in situations in which use is physically hazardous (e.g., driving while intoxicated)

B. Some symptoms of the disturbance have persisted for at least 1 month or have occurred repeatedly over a longer period of time.

C. Never met the criteria for psychoactive substance dependence for this substance.

Source: Adapted from American Psychiatric Association:
Diagnostic and Statistical Manual of Mental Disorders, *ed 3, revised. 1987, pp 167–169.*

occur during the drinking period or up to two hours afterward, whereas hallucinations begin twelve to forty-eight hours after the person stops drinking. Grand mal seizures ("rum fits") may occur two to three days after the person stops drinking. **Delirium tremens** (DTs), a rare symptom of withdrawal, is a condition of severe memory disturbance, agitation, anorexia, and hallucinations. Generally, the DTs begin a few days after drinking stops and end within one to five days. Frequently, additional medical illnesses are present and may include pneumonia, pancreatitis, and hepatic decompensation (Kaplan and Sadock 1985). (See Boxes 16–5 and 16–6 for additional information.)

Medical Treatment

Various medical treatments for withdrawal exist. Many clients who are withdrawing from alcohol suffer from overhydration. Consequently, giving fluids intravenously may lead to seizures and delirium. One dose of furosemide (Lasix 40–80 mg) brings on safe, rapid diuresis and shortens the

detoxification period. Magnesium sulfate, given for central nervous system hyperirritability, helps prevent convulsions and decreases central nervous system edema. Phenobarbital provides useful and safe sedation. Because alcohol is cross tolerant with barbiturates, a larger than usual dose of phenobarbital may be required (e.g., 30 mg by mouth four times daily for two days and then in gradually decreasing doses for up to five days). Because alcohol interferes with absorption of B vitamins, clients often receive vitamins B_1, B_6, and B_{12}. After an initial dose given intramuscularly, daily doses of vitamin B complex and vitamin C are given orally. Diazepam (Valium) or chlordiazepoxide (Librium) may be given to help prevent DTs.

Disulfiram (**Antabuse**) may be prescribed for alcoholic clients. Disulfiram inhibits acetaldehyde dehydrogenase, which normally metabolizes acetaldehyde. As a result, acetaldehyde accumulates if alcohol is consumed. Acetalde-

---

Box 16–5
KEY FACTS ABOUT ALCOHOL

Examples

Liquor, wine, beer

Slang Terms

Hooch, booze, moonshine, sauce

Route of Administration

Oral (liquid)

Psychologic Symptoms

Irritability*
Mood swings*
Short attention span*
Talks a lot and loudly*
Decreased judgment
Decreased inhibitions
Interference with memory

Physical Symptoms

Slurred speech*
Lack of coordination*
Unsteady gait*
Blackouts
Decreased REM sleep
Nystagmus*
Flushed face*
Decreased psychomotor functions

Withdrawal Symptoms

Nausea or vomiting
Anxiety
Depressed mood or irritability
Malaise or weakness
Autonomic hyperactivity
Tachycardia
Sweating, elevated blood pressure
Orthostatic hypotension
Coarse tremor of hands, tongue, eyelids

Dangers

Car accidents
Physical injury
Malnutrition
Hepatitis
Cirrhosis
Gastritis
Suicide
FAS (fetal alcohol syndrome)

Typical Users

Teenagers
Adults

Symptoms of intoxication noted in DSM-IIIR.

hyde is highly toxic, producing nausea and hypotension. Hypotension leads to shock and may be fatal. The dosage of disulfiram is usually 250 mg daily. Often, clients stop taking the drug, and it may be useful to dispense the drug every four days during client visits to a clinic. If the client uses alcohol, a powerful disulfiram reaction may occur and last for up to two weeks. Reaction symptoms include nausea, vomiting, flushing, dizziness, and tachycardia.

Because of the potential danger of disulfiram, the client must be instructed orally and in writing not to use alcohol in any form, including alcohol-based cough syrups or cold remedies. Clients with myocardial disease or taking metronidazole (Flagyl) should not take Antabuse; in the latter case, a disulfiram reaction is possible.

Patterns of Use

According to the DSM-IIIR (p 173), alcoholics manifest one of three patterns of use: (a) regular daily intake of large amounts of alcohol, (b) regular heavy drinking limited to weekends, and (c) long periods of sobriety interspersed with binges of heavy drinking lasting for weeks or months. Regardless of the preferred pattern, people who drink excessively experience numerous negative physiologic and psychologic effects (see Boxes 16–5 and 16–6). For more information about the physical effects of alcoholism, see Bittle et al. (1986).

Blackouts

Having **blackouts** is frequently confused with passing out. In fact, passing out refers to unconsciousness, whereas a blackout is **anterograde amnesia**—loss of short-term memories with retention of remote memories. A person can function effectively for up to several days—talking on the telephone, working, and shopping—yet have absolutely no memory of what he or she has done. To others, the alcoholic may appear normal or "high." Interestingly, alcoholics appear unconcerned by the blackouts and eventually learn to cover them up. This appearance of unconcern may, in part, be due to *euphoric recall:* The alcoholic recalls only how good he or she felt but does not remember his or her behavior. Reality is distorted. Blackouts appearing later in the disease process may be indicative of physical dependence and are not related to the amount of alcohol consumed. They are unpredictable, and exactly how or why they occur is not clear. Some authorities believe blackouts are an acute brain syndrome due to dehydration of the brain tissue. When assessing an alcoholic client, psychi-

Box 16–6
PHYSICAL EFFECTS OF CHRONIC ALCOHOLISM

Hepatic System

Alcoholic fatty liver syndrome
Alcoholic hepatitis
Laënnec's cirrhosis

Neurologic System

Wernicke-Korsakoff syndrome (related to thiamine deficiency)
Peripheral neuropathy (related to vitamin B deficiency)
Marchiafava disease*
Central pontine myelinosis*
Cerebellar degeneration*
Alcoholic amblyopia*

Cardiovascular System

Alcoholic cardiomyopathy
Hypokalemia
Hypomagnesemia
Hyperlipidemia
Altered fluid balance
Beriberi heart disease (related to thiamine deficiency)
Hematologic abnormalities

Musculoskeletal System

Acute alcoholic myopathy
Subclinical alcoholic myopathy
Chronic alcoholic myopathy

Gastrointestinal System

Gastritis
Esophagitis
Mallory-Weiss syndrome
Boerhaave's syndrome
Pancreatitis
Nutritional deficiency diseases
Nausea
Abdominal pain
Erratic bowel function (constipation and diarrhea)
Gastrointestinal hemorrhage
Jaundice
High incidence of digestive tract cancers
Glucose intolerance

Reproductive System

Impotence
Sterility
Gynecomastia
Anorgasmic (women)
Fetal alcohol syndrome (FAS)

Very rare.
Source: Adapted from Kneisl CR, Ames SA: *Adult Health Nursing. Addison Wesley, 1986.*

atric nurses need to determine if blackouts are part of the symptoms.

Fetal Alcohol Syndrome

Nurses also need to be aware of the harmful effects of alcohol on pregnant women and unborn children. Fetal alcohol syndrome (FAS) is found in children of alcoholic women. Physical and mental defects include severe growth deficiency, heart defects, malformed facial features, mental retardation, low birth weight, learning problems, and hyperactivity. If a child has one or two of these characteristics, the condition is called *fetal alcohol effects.* FAS affects 1 of every 750 babies born in the United States. A baby born to an alcoholic mother may need to be gradually withdrawn from alcohol.

Suicide

Nurses must be alert to the possibility of suicide attempts by alcoholics. One percent of the general population attempt suicide, but 15 percent of alcoholics do so. The nurse should watch for self-destructive behavior and for events in a client's life that represent a loss, e.g., work, family, health, or legal problems. Such behavior and events put people in a high-risk category (Trenk 1986).

BARBITURATES OR SIMILARLY ACTING SEDATIVES OR HYPNOTICS

Elizabeth W, a 45-year-old housewife, has been depressed and irritable over an impending divorce. Her physician prescribed Valium (5 mg) for sleep and for anxiety (every six hours as needed). Because this dosage was not helping decrease her anxiety as much as she wanted, Ms W increased her dosage and began taking from 50–100 mg a day over a period of a few weeks. This evening Ms W's estranged husband found her mumbling incoherently. Her speech was slurred, she was bumping into furniture, and she was quite drowsy.

Box 16–7 presents the major facts about barbiturates. Barbiturates are highly addictive drugs that cause people to feel euphoric yet relaxed. They are frequently prescribed to relieve pain, reduce anxiety (sedative effects), and induce sleep (hypnotic effects). In party situations, teenagers and young adults take high doses, often in combination with alcohol, to get "high." The resultant CNS depression makes this practice especially dangerous. *"Speed freaks"* (amphetamine abusers) use barbiturates to "come down" from a high. Dependence, tolerance, and cross-tolerance to other depressant drugs develop rapidly.

Barbiturates are metabolized in phases by the liver. Initially they are absorbed if taken orally and are partially metabolized. However, the unmetabolized parts become active metabolites that are stored in the fatty tissues. Consequently taking these drugs over a period of time results in a cumulative effect, unsuspected dependence, and possible overdose.

More Americans die from barbiturate overdose than from opioid addiction. Many take alcohol and barbiturates together. While judgment is impaired, they take more pills, thereby unintentionally overdosing. Because alcohol and barbiturates are synergistic, an overdose can occur quickly. Barbiturates are often used in suicide attempts.

Barbiturate withdrawal is unpleasant and life threatening. A deep sleep is followed by respiratory depression, coma, and sometimes death. Babies born to mothers addicted to barbiturates are physically dependent and need to be helped through withdrawal.

OPIOIDS

Steven Y, a 20-year-old male, arrived at the hospital in an ambulance. He was unconscious. His respiration was slow, and his pupils were pinpoints. "Tracks" were visible on his arms and behind his knees. A source said Steven had just "shot up" heroin.

The opioids include heroin and morphine derived from the poppy plant and synthetic drugs, such as meperidine (Demerol), codeine, methadone, and others. Opioids have analgesic qualities and are prescribed after surgery. Depending on the person, the drugs may produce a euphoric high, as in drug addicts, but generally cause people to feel drowsy and out of touch with the world. Most opiate users are in their twenties or younger. See Box 16–8 for more facts about opioids.

In 1898 heroin became available and initially was not believed to be addictive. Within a short time, its addictive properties became known, and the government intervened (Harrison Narcotics Act of 1914). Addiction to opiates has increased through the years. Because most opioid abusers take the drugs intravenously, they are at high risk for acquired immune deficiency syndrome (AIDS) and hepatitis. Overdose, malnutrition, and infections spread by dirty drugs and needles are dangers. Dealers often add impurities to heroin (called "cutting" heroin), thus increasing the quantity and their own profit. The impurities may cause poisoning and other problems.

Because opioids are physically addicting, withdrawal is a threat. People who use high doses of a drug and who "shoot up" or "mainline" (use the drug intravenously) are at high risk for severe withdrawal symptoms. Withdrawal symptoms are usually evident within twelve hours after the last dose. The person experiences the most severe withdrawal within thirty-six to forty-eight hours, with the symptoms decreasing gradually over two weeks. During this stressful time, the person craves the drug. Babies born to addicted mothers must be treated for opioid withdrawal. The babies present with irritability, high-pitched crying, increased respirations, fever, sneezing, yawning, and tremors.

In 1964, Dole and Nyswander began to treat opiate addiction with methadone. By the late 1960s and early 1970s, when the federal government allocated money for treatment, methadone maintenance programs mushroomed all over the United States. Methadone, a synthetic narcotic, was dispensed daily at clinics to narcotic addicts. Although addictive, methadone does not produce the "rush" (ecstatic feeling) associated with heroin. Methadone alleviates the addicts' craving for narcotics and, therefore, was expected to decrease illicit drug trafficking, theft, prostitution, and crime necessary to obtain money for drugs, thereby allowing addicts to lead productive lives. Also, methadone therapy is far less expensive ($2000 annually) than residential programs ($5000) or jail ($23,000). Today, methadone maintenance programs remain a major treatment for opioid addicts.

Presently, clonidine hydrochloride (Catapres), a nonopiate hypotensive drug, is being investigated for use dur-

---

Box 16–7

KEY FACTS ABOUT BARBITURATES OR SIMILARLY ACTING SEDATIVE OR HYPNOTICS

Examples

Diazepam (Valium), chlordiazepoxide (Librium), chloral hydrate, methaqualone (Quaalude), secobarbital (Seconal), phenobarbital, pentobarbital (Nembutal)

Slang Terms

Downers, ludes, sopors, 714s, yellow jackets, reds, blues, rainbows, trenks

Route of Administration

Oral (pills or capsules), intravenous

Psychologic Symptoms

Euphoria
Mood lability*
Intoxication
Loquacity (talkativeness)*
Impaired attention and memory*
Irritability*
Anxiety
Sexual aggressiveness*

Physical Symptoms

Drowsiness
Slurred speech*
Long periods of sleep
Fever
Vomiting
Postural hypotension

Lack of coordination*
Unsteady gait

Withdrawal Symptoms

Nausea and vomiting
Malaise or weakness
Autonomic hyperactivity
Tachycardia
Sweating, elevated blood pressure
Anxiety
Depression or irritability
Orthostatic hypotension
Coarse tremor of hands, tongue, eyelids
Painful muscle contractions
Convulsions
Status epilepticus (major epileptic attacks succeeding each other with little or no intermission)
Hallucinations

Dangers

CNS depression
Possible overdose and death, especially if mixed with alcohol

Typical Users

Middle-class, middle-aged females
Teenagers
Young adults

*Symptoms of intoxication noted in DSM-IIIR.

ing the acute states of opiate withdrawal. If a client is assessed to be not at risk for complications of the drug, he or she is first stabilized on methadone (three to five days), the usual drug of choice for withdrawal. Within one to three days after the methadone is discontinued, opiate withdrawal symptoms often appear. At this time, clonidine is begun and is given in increasing doses, until withdrawal symptoms are alleviated (up to 14 days). Clonidine blocks the withdrawal symptoms, making the detoxification process less painful and more rapid than with methadone. Psychologically, the client feels less anxious and depressed. Side-effects of clonidine include insomnia, dry mouth, generalized weakness, and postural hypotension (Schloemer and Skidmore 1983).

Opioid intoxication is indicated by constricted pupils, euphoria, psychomotor retardation, slurred speech, and/or drowsiness. If a client has overdosed, naloxone (Narcan) (0.4 mg–0.8 mg IV repeated in five to fifteen minutes) is given. It is a fast-acting narcotic antagonist that counter-

acts respiratory depression. Abdominal cramps, rhinorrhea, and lacrimation may be treated with belladona alkaloids or with phenobarbital.

AMPHETAMINES OR SIMILARLY ACTING SYMPATHOMIMETICS

Laura S, a 16-year-old high school girl, was on a diet so she could get into a favorite bathing suit. Her friend's brother, a pharmacist, gave her some Dexedrine "just

---

Box 16–8
KEY FACTS ABOUT OPIOIDS

Examples

Heroin, morphine, hydromorphone (Dilaudid), codeine, methadone

Slang Terms

H, smack, junk, M, Miss Emma, Little D, School Boy, Horse

Route of Administration

Intravenous, oral, intramuscular, subcutaneous ("skin popping")

Psychologic Symptoms

Impaired attention/memory*
Euphoria*
Appears sedated ("nodding out")
Psychomotor retardation*
Insensitivity to pain
Agitation
Apathy*
Dysphoria*

Physical Symptoms

Pinpoint pupils
Drowsiness*
Slurred speech*
Nausea and vomiting
Hypothermia

Withdrawal Symptoms

(Presents much as influenza does)
Dilated pupils

Tearing
Runny nose
Piloerection
Sweating
Diarrhea
Fever
Yawning
Mild hypotension
Tachycardia
Insomnia
Restlessness and irritability
Muscle and joint pains
Increased respiration
Gastrointestinal symptoms
Loss of appetite

Dangers

Death (especially if combined with barbiturates)
Pulmonary edema
Opioid poisoning (coma, shock, respiratory depression)
Malnutrition
Hepatitis/infections
AIDS

Typical Users

Teenagers
Young adults

Symptoms of intoxication noted in DSM-IIIR.

until you lose the weight." Laura's mother initially noticed her rather unusual hyperactivity, her euphoria, and the fact that she refused dinner. Over a period of a few weeks Laura's behavior changed. She appeared suspicious and irritable and continued to speak and move rapidly.

The amphetamines/sympathomimetics include groups of synthetic drugs derived from ephedrine that stimulate the release of adrenaline. In small doses, they cause a person to feel energetic, euphoric, and "turned on" to life. Users take these central nervous system stimulants to feel good. A growing number of people, who do uppers and downers in a cyclic fashion, take amphetamines to coun-

teract the effects of barbiturates. Amphetamines are dangerous because they alter judgment and obscure feelings. Taken in high doses or intravenously, amphetamines can have dangerous side-effects (see Box 16–9).

In the 1950s and 1960s, amphetamines were heralded as wonder drugs for depression and lassitude. By the 1970s, their dangers became known, and physicians today prescribe them less frequently. Amphetamines are still used to control appetite and to treat depression, narcolepsy, minimal brain dysfunctions, and attention deficit disorders in children. Abusers are usually teenagers or people in their early twenties who are looking for a good time. Truck drivers may use amphetamines to stay awake on long trips, and students may use them to study for exams. Athletes, hoping to improve their performance, may use amphetamines. Tolerance develops rapidly, and chronic abusers may suffer a toxic psychosis presenting with the symptoms of paranoid schizophrenia. Delusions, hallucinations, stereotypical compulsive behavior, increased libido, panic, and violence may occur (Kneisl and Ames 1986). However, unlike

---

Box 16–9
KEY FACTS ABOUT AMPHETAMINES

Examples

Dexedrine, methamphetamine

Slang Terms

Bennies, dexies, uppers, black beauties, pep pills, crank, speed, diet pills

Route of Administration

Oral, intravenous

Psychologic Symptoms

Hypervigilance*
Irritability
Grandiosity*
Loquacity (talkativeness)*
Elation
Impaired judgment
Psychomotor agitation*
Aggressive, violent behavior
Paranoia
Hallucinations, delusions
Disorientation
Increased libido
Stereotypical compulsive behavior
Visual/auditory hallucinations

Physical Symptoms

Tachycardia*
Increased blood pressure*
Dilated pupils*

Perspiration or chills*
Nausea or vomiting*
Diarrhea
Headache
Dizziness
Cardiac arrhythmias
Hyperthermia
Decreased appetite
Delirium

Withdrawal Symptoms

Depression
Fatigue
Disturbed sleep
Dreaming
Restlessness
Disorientation

Dangers

Malnutrition
Cerebrovascular accident
Depression
Suicide
Hyperpyrexia
Convulsions

Typical Users

Teenagers
Young adults

Symptoms of intoxication noted in DSM-IIIR.

a chronic schizophrenic, a person who abuses amphetamines does not present with a thought disorder or a flat affect. Instead, these clients are agitated and extremely anxious. Clients who are chronic amphetamine abusers begin to crave the drugs and require higher and higher dosages. They are rowdy, paranoid, and irritable. A "crash" (depression), often with suicidal symptoms, may last for several weeks. Cyclical patterns of abuse and crashing may occur.

Chlorpromazine (Thorazine) may be ordered to combat the physiologic effects of amphetamines. Diazepam (Valium), given intravenously, decreases tachycardia and the chance of convulsions.

CANNABIS

Joe P, a 35-year-old captain of a rescue squad, was having trouble at his job. He paid less and less attention to the accuracy of his patient reports; he was often late for work; he forgot to repair and replace his equipment, causing his unit to be unsafe and ill equipped. Joe told an emergency room nurse that he felt all the marijuana he was smoking was beginning to affect him. He revealed he'd been a daily smoker for five years. At first, he felt there were no long-term effects, but lately he was concerned because "I never feel like doing anything."

Marijuana arrived in the United States in the early 1900s. Although it has been illegal in the United States since 1937, marijuana is used more than any other chemical except tobacco, alcohol, and caffeine (see Box 16–10). Derived from an Indian hemp plant (*Cannabis sativa*), marijuana contains the psychoactive substance delta 6-3,4-tetrahydrocannabinol (THC). THC is found in the sticky yellow resin secreted by the tops and leaves of the ripe plants (Kneisl and Ames 1986). Three grades of marijuana are available (Kaplan and Sadock 1985):

1. Bhang, the cheapest and least potent grade, is the cut tops of uncultivated plants; the resin content is low.

2. Ganja, made from the tops of cultivated plants, has a higher quantity and quality of resin.

3. Charas is made from resin from the tops of ripe plants. Also called hashish, this form is the most potent.

THC is transformed into metabolites in the body. Unlike alcohol, which is water soluble and leaves the body through urine, breath, and perspiration, THC is stored in the fatty tissues (especially the brain and reproductive system). Consequently, it can be detected in the body for up to six weeks. From 1984 to 1986, marijuana has increased in

---

Box 16–10
KEY FACTS ABOUT CANNABIS

Examples
Marijuana, hashish, THC

Slang Terms
Pot, grass, bhang, hashish, ganja, joint, reefer, weed, "shit"

Route of Administration
Smoked in a pipe or cigarette, oral (e.g., mixed in food)

Psychologic Symptoms
Initial anxiety, then euphoria
Altered perceptions
Sensation of slowed time
Decreased concentration
Lack of motivation
Loss of short-term memory
Passivity
Abrupt mood changes
Paranoid ideation
Impaired judgment

Physical Symptoms
Dry mouth
Increased heart rate
Conjunctival irritation
Dilated pupils
Decreased coordination
Increased appetite, thirst
Craving for sweets
Fatigue
Impaired ovulation, impaired sperm count and motility, increase in abnormal sperm cells

Dangers
Lung damage
Psychologic dependence
Panic reaction
Impaired driving ability

Typical Users
Teenagers
Young adults

---

potency ten times. Although marijuana contains over 400 chemicals, the THC content determines the potency. With an increase in potency comes an increase in health problems.

Researchers have found marijuana effective in treating epilepsy, glaucoma, asthma, hypertension, and the nausea and vomiting associated with chemotherapy. Researchers presently are studying the effects of marijuana smoking by the pregnant woman on her fetus. The cannabinoids of marijuana cross the placental barrier and are distributed to fetal tissues. The risk of fetal death and abnormalities—central nervous system disturbances, lower birth weight, decreased length, and smaller head circumference—increases when the mother uses marijuana. A suppressed prolactin level in the mother makes nursing impossible. If people with a history of schizophrenia or mood disorders use marijuana, they may have a relapse or their symptoms may worsen.

The National Federation of Drug Free Youth has published the following facts that clearly indicate the dangers of marijuana:

* Marijuana appears to lower testosterone levels in boys.
* In girls, hormone levels remain normal, but marijuana's chemicals possibly accumulate in the ovaries.
* Marijuana smoke has 50 percent more tar than regular cigarettes.
* Marijuana tar contains 70 percent more benzopyrene, a major cancer-causing chemical.
* Marijuana smoke produces greater cellular changes in the lungs than does tobacco smoke.
* Smoking two "joints" (marijuana cigarettes) can reduce lung capacity more than smoking one pack of tobacco cigarettes.
* Marijuana may cause emphysema twenty times faster than tobacco.
* Marijuana smoke increases airway resistance 25 percent under laboratory conditions in which a similar amount of tobacco smoke produces no significant increase in airway resistance.
* Brain wave tests show that teenagers who get high twice a week or more often have evidence of diffuse brain impairment for up to two months after the last time they use the drug.
* After a person smokes marijuana, THC can be found in the blood and urine for up to two weeks; if the THC is radioactively labeled, it can be detected for up to one month.

Because marijuana smoking is so prevalent among teenagers and because its dangers are becoming increasingly known, some health professionals advocate a urine screen when teenagers have a checkup by a family doctor. In 1985, the American Academy of Pediatrics was challenged to confront the problem of substance abuse among teenagers. A key point was that chemical dependency takes ten to fifteen years to develop in adults and only a few years to develop in a child. Only 25 percent of kids in drug rehabilitation succeed, compared with 75% of adults who succeed. Because substance abuse is a "neglected disease," pediatricians should initiate educational and treatment programs on drug and alcohol abuse (Cherskov 1985). Likewise, psychiatric nurses need to respond to this vital public health issue.

Marijuana use is endemic in the teenage culture. Therefore nurses who work with teenagers must be knowledgeable about marijuana and its effects. When admitting a teenager to a psychiatric unit or interviewing a teenager as an outpatient, be aware of a variety of indicators of marijuana use. Parents should know these facts about marijuana and indications of its use:

* Marijuana smells like hemp or burning rope.
* Teenagers often burn incense or use perfumed sprays to mask its pungent odor.
* Teenagers may use eye drops (e.g., Murine) so that their eyes will not be red, and they may cough a lot.
* A teenager who uses marijuana may have smoking paraphernalia, e.g., plastic baggies filled with dried leaves, rolling paper, and "roach" clips—a clip that holds the marijuana cigarette once it becomes too small to handle.

COCAINE

Will R, a 32-year-old male, was brought to the hospital by his father. Talkative and jumpy, his eyes darted around the examining room, and he repeatedly wiped his nose with his finger and rubbed the bottom of his face. He acted suspicious and kept saying someone was after him. His family stated he had a $400 a day cocaine habit.

Each year, 20 tons of cocaine enter the United States. After the cocaine is adulterated with sugar, quinine, amphetamine, ephedrine, or procaine, 80 to 160 tons are available on the streets (Cocaine: Some Questions and Answers 1983). Since cocaine abuse has been recognized as a widespread problem, government agencies have spent much money trying to block cocaine shipments from South America. Planes, boats, and "mules" (people who transport cocaine) have been seized, and tons of cocaine have been confiscated and destroyed. Yet it still is plentiful and is purer today than ever before. The cocaine industry is a multibillion dollar enterprise involving bribery, corruption, and murder (Cocaine: Some Questions and Answers 1983).

Cocaine is a stimulant derived from the coca plant found in Bolivia and Peru. It has long been known and used. For hundreds of years, South American Indians have chewed coca leaves, enjoying the effects of decreased appetite and increased ability to work at high altitudes. Slaves became more productive when given cocaine. Freud experimented with cocaine. It was an ingredient in Coca Cola before federal regulations prohibited it in 1903. Today, cocaine is used as a local anesthetic in ear, nose, and throat surgery.

Cocaine is the drug of the 1980s. It is no longer just the chic, expensive drug of choice (the champagne of drugs) of young upwardly mobile professionals and stars. Cocaine is now available to all cultural and socioeconomic groups; today, 50 percent of users are women. For some years cocaine was believed to produce euphoria without addictive potential and without negative side-effects. Lately the horrors of cocaine abuse have been described in both lay and professional literature. (See Box 16–11.)

That cocaine is physically addictive has not been proved, but its ability to cause psychologic dependency is clear.

Cocaine users crave the drug. After a brief postuse euphoria (lasting approximately five to ten minutes), they experience a strong desire to repeat the high. This high is followed by a "crashing," a terrible letdown called the "postcoke blues," or cocaine abstinence syndrome. Anxiety, depression, and fatigue are part of this syndrome (Rottenberg 1980). One addict described these postcoke blues as "pure hell, the most painful depression I have ever felt. I wanted to die from the pain." This painful depression, along with the memory of the cocaine high, causes people to want to use cocaine again and again to recapture the momentary ecstasy. The period of agitation, anxiety, and insomnia usually ceases within two weeks. Nurses need to assess clients carefully to differentiate cocaine use from manic-depression and chronic anxiety. The cocaine use cycle is depicted in Figure 16–1.

Box 16–11
KEY FACTS ABOUT COCAINE

Slang Terms

Coke, lady, blow, snow, rabbits, C, powder

Route of Administration

Intranasal (flakes or powder sniffed), subcutaneous or intravenous, smoked in a pipe (freebasing)

Psychologic Symptoms

Psychomotor agitation*
Anxiety
Elation
Talkativeness*
Grandiosity*
Hypervigilance*
Impaired judgment
Ideas of reference/paranoia
Hallucinations
Formication (sensation of insects crawling on the skin)
Euphoria followed by depression and let-down feeling
Violence
Insomnia
Anorexia

Physical Symptoms

Dilated pupils*
Tachycardia*
Elevated blood pressure*
Perspiration or chills*
Nausea or vomiting*

Anorexia
Dry mouth (characteristic bad breath)
Weight loss
Stuffy/runny nose
Burns and sores of nasal membranes
Tremors
Muscle cramping
Seizures

Withdrawal Symptoms

Severe craving

Dangers

Syncope
Fever
Chest pain
Depression
Death from convulsions
Cardiac/respiratory arrest

Typical Users

Teenagers
College students
Young urban professionals (yuppies)
Rock and movie stars
Executives

Symptoms of intoxication noted in DSM-IIIR.

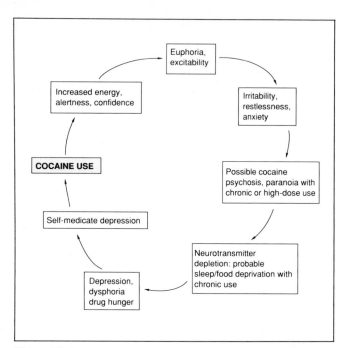

Figure 16–1
Cocaine use cycle.
Source: Landry M, Smith DE: Crack: Anatomy of addiction. Calif Nurs *1987;March/April:13.*

Detoxification for cocaine abusers is still in the experimental phase and may depend on the client's symptoms. Some hospitals use nothing; others administer diazepam (Valium) intravenously 1–20 mg at a slow rate (not more than 5 mg/minute). In some hospitals, cocaine abusers are treated with a Valium protocol that lasts approximately four days; Valium is decreased from 10 mg q 4 hours p.o./I.M. to 5 mg q 8 hours p.o./I.M. with additional doses as needed if the client has withdrawal symptoms. Other hospitals have p.r.n. Valium orders only. Another protocol involves the use of phenobarbital in decreasing doses and imipramine hydrochloride (Tofranil). Since the depression is so great, Tofranil or other tricyclic antidepressants may be given for several weeks after detoxification. Tricyclics build up existing levels of neurotransmitters and make them available for transmission.

Amino acids (tyrosine, phenylalanine, cysteine, glutamic acid) are often prescribed because they are converted by the body to neurotransmitters, which are depleted by cocaine abuse (see Chapter 9). With these additional amino acids, the body can replenish the depleted neurotransmitters, thereby alleviating the depression and fatigue common in withdrawal. Tryptophan is often prescribed to decrease depression and craving and promote sleep. A nat-

urally occurring amino acid, it is a precursor of a sleep hormone and the neurotransmitter serotonin.

Use of amino acid transmitter precursors to restore depleted neurotransmitters is called *presynaptic treatment* for cocaine withdrawal. Use of tricyclic antidepressants to increase the number of neurotransmitters in the synapse is called *synaptic treatment. Postsynaptic treatment* for cocaine withdrawal and dependence includes use of dopamine receptor antagonists, such as bromocriptine, that stimulate postsynaptic receptor actions of depleted neurotransmitters (see Figure 16–2).

Interestingly, low-level cocaine intoxication presents with symptoms similar to alcohol withdrawal—sweating, dilated pupils, psychomotor agitation, and increased blood pressure/heart rate. With higher doses of cocaine, a person becomes increasingly intoxicated. Symptoms include high fevers, cardiac arrhythmia, seizures, hallucinations, and a paranoid schizophrenic syndrome. Hallucinations typically involve "cocaine bugs," which feel like bugs under the skin. The client may scratch furiously in an attempt to get rid of them. Haloperidol (Haldol) is used to combat the psychotic symptoms; phenothiazines should not be used as they may decrease the seizure threshold.

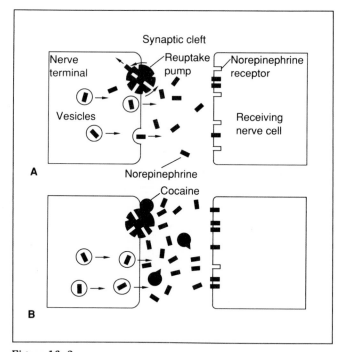

Figure 16–2
Neurotransmitter depletion in cocaine addiction. The action of cocaine results in part from blocking the reuptake of neurotransmitters such as dopamine and norepinephrine at nerve synapses. Treatment for withdrawal and dependence includes presynaptic, synaptic, and postsynaptic drugs that restore the available neurotransmitters that have been depleted because cocaine has blocked the reuptake system (A) and stimulated the postsynaptic neuron as the concentration builds up (B).
Source: Landry M, Smith DE: Crack: Anatomy of addiction. Calif Nurs *1987;March/April:35.*

The strength of the physiologic effects of cocaine are revealed by animal research. Monkeys work harder by pressing a bar to receive cocaine intravenously than to get any other drug. Even when starving to death or when confronted with a sexually receptive female, monkeys continue pressing the bar. Receiving an electric shock every time they touch the bar does not alter their behavior. Research with cocaine users indicates that the drug bromocriptine mesylate (Parlodel), a dopamine (DA) receptor agonist, eliminates the craving users feel after they stop using cocaine.

Cocaine initially increases DA neurotransmission. Over time, however, cocaine abuse depletes DA in the brain, and this depletion may be the basis for craving. In a preliminary study, bromocriptine proved successful in decreasing cocaine craving. The researchers suggest doing more studies that are placebo controlled and double-blind. They also suggest that doses of bromocriptine be varied for acute and long-term cocaine abstinence and craving (Bromocriptine as Treatment of Cocaine Abuse 1985, pp 1151–1152).

CRACK

"Crack" or "rock" cocaine, recently labeled "the most addictive drug known to man," is "a potent form of hydrochloride cocaine that is mixed with baking soda and water, heated, allowed to harden, and then broken or 'cracked' into little pieces and smoked in cigarettes or glass water pipes" (Gianelli 1986, p 2). Crack is more insidious, addictive, and toxic than cocaine. One user said, "I am worse in three weeks of using crack than in six years of using cocaine."

Crack is cheap and easily bought on the street or in special crack houses where people congregate to smoke. A crack high has a rapid onset and is intensely euphoric, followed by a dramatic crash. Within seconds after "coming down," users feel compelled to smoke more crack. Due to the rapid addiction, many people are "hooked" and seek help when they can no longer support their habit. In New York City in 1985, 55 percent of the cocaine arrests were due to crack. Crack users are flooding treatment centers, many of which have long waiting lists. Recidivism is estimated by some experts at 90 percent.

Symptoms of crack use (see Box 16–12) include irritability, paranoia, depression, and physical symptoms that go along with the smoking of a toxic chemical, e.g., wheezing and coughing blood and black phlegm. Cardiac arrhythmias caused by crack use may lead to death. There is an increase in the number of babies being born to mothers who use crack. These babies are more likely to be premature or have low birth weights. They present with irritability, tremors, and muscle rigidity. A related issue is the increasing number of children who are neglected or abused by crack-using parents. Drug needs seem to prevail over child care in many cases (Gianelli 1986, p 18).

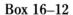

Box 16–12
KEY FACTS ABOUT CRACK (HYDROCHLORIDE COCAINE)

Slang Terms

Rock, crack

Route of Administration

Smoked

Psychologic Symptoms

Paranoia
Depression
Insomnia
Irritability
Deterioration of mental function
"Schizophrenic-like" psychosis
Appetite suppression

Physical Symptoms

Wheezing, shortness of breath
Black phlegm
Coughing blood
Parched throat and lips
Singed eyebrows and lashes
Increased heart rate and blood pressure
Weight loss

Dangers

Seizures
Cardiac arrhythmias
Respiratory paralysis
Paranoid psychoses
Pulmonary dysfunction

Typical Users

Teenagers
Young adults
All socioeconomic and cultural groups

PHENCYCLIDINE (PCP)

Pete O, an 18-year-old college student, was offered marijuana at a fraternity party. After smoking several joints he was driving home with a friend when he became severely agitated. He insisted his friend stop the car near a pay phone; he jumped out and attempted to call the police, believing someone was trying to kill him. When the police arrived because of the disturbance he was causing (by then he was shouting and hallucinating), he rushed them, kicking at passersby and shooting at them as if he had a gun. During an assessment interview, the friend confessed to putting PCP in the marijuana.

PCP was originally used as an anesthetic for humans and as a tranquilizer for animals. Because of its dangerous side-effects (see Box 16–13), it was removed from the market, except for veterinary use. However, by the mid-1960s, PCP was readily available as a street drug. PCP is inexpensive and easily synthesized by home chemists, making a supply always available.

People who use PCP frequently arrive at the emergency room in a psychotic, violent, and agitated state. Some fluctuate between coma and violence. Hallucinations are common. A differential diagnosis is important but difficult because the symptoms are similar to those of schizophrenia. It is believed that schizophrenics are particularly sensitive to PCP and that PCP may aggravate schizophrenic symptoms.

A PCP high appears about five minutes after a person takes the drug and lasts four to six hours. Effects may last up to forty-eight hours. PCP may be recovered from the blood and urine for seven to ten days. While using PCP, a person experiences a wide variety of feelings ranging from euphoria and utter peace to violence, confusion, and disorganization. Distorted sensory perceptions are common. In a bad "trip," anxiety, fear, and paranoia predominate.

Clients who have ingested PCP may be given diazepam for muscle spasms, seizures, and agitation. Haloperidol may be used for severe psychotic behavior, but phenothiazines are not used since PCP is anticholinergic. The dramatic physical and emotional effects of PCP may last for several weeks. Users may suffer from depression, fatigue, memory loss, difficulty in concentration, and poor impulse control.

A vital problem with PCP is the question of its purity and its concentration. Because it is generally manufactured illegally, users never really know what they are buying. Adulterants are often toxic to humans, causing a wide variety of responses, including death. Originally called the "peace pill," PCP is now recognized for its potential to cause violence, especially when the drug is taken in high dosages.

Box 16–13
KEY FACTS ABOUT PHENCYCLIDINE (PCP)

Slang Terms

PCP, angel dust, crystal, superjoint, hog, elephant tranquilizer, THC, rocket fuel, peace pill

Route of Administration

Oral, intravenous, smoked, inhaled

Psychologic Symptoms

Euphoria*
Psychomotor agitation*
Anxiety*
Grandiosity*
Disorientation swings
Emotional lability*
Sensation of slowed time*
Synesthesias (e.g., seeing colors when a loud sound occurs)*
Facial grimacing
Muscle rigidity
Hallucinations
Paranoid ideation
Violent or bizarre behavior
Hostility, apathy
Depersonalization, isolation

Physical Symptoms

Vertical and horizontal nystagmus*
Increased blood pressure/heart rate*
Insensitivity to pain*
Dysarthria*
Ataxia*
Perspiration
Salivation
Vomiting

Dangers

Violence
Hypertension
Respiratory depression/arrest
Stupor
Coma
Convulsions
Death
Suicide

Typical Users

Adolescents
Young adults

Symptoms of intoxication noted in DSM-IIIR.

HALLUCINOGENS

Two seniors in high school decided to take LSD. After eight hours, one student was enjoying music, describing the varied colors he saw as the music changed in tempo. The other student was sweating profusely. His pupils were dilated, and he was trembling. He saw brightly colored dogs with huge teeth and claws changing into cats, snakes, and lions. He said he felt his gallbladder working with his liver and stomach. He eventually became so out of control that the other student took him to the emergency room.

Hallucinogens are synthetic and natural drugs that cause hallucinations and unusual sensory experiences. Developed in 1938 for scientific research, LSD became popular in the 1960s when Timothy Leary, a Harvard psychologist, described how it stimulated great insight and increased awareness. In the 1960s and 1970s, the United States Army secretly experimented with LSD by giving it to unsuspecting army employees. One dramatic and much publicized event concerned the army officer who leapt to his death from a window after unknowingly ingesting LSD. At this time the danger of LSD became publicized, as did the unethical research. Physician researchers also were interested in experimenting with the uses of LSD in the treatment of a variety of diseases; however, in 1966, LSD became illegal and could no longer be used in human research. Peyote, however, is still an integral part of religious rituals of Indians in the Southwest and Mexico.

After a lull in use, LSD ("acid") is again being used by teenagers because it is cheap ($2.00–$5.00 a "hit") and causes an intense high that lasts six to twelve hours. Teenagers today are unacquainted with the horror stories of the 1960s. Today, people use LSD predominantly to get high rather than to expand consciousness. See Box 16–14 for additional information.

The dangers of hallucinogens include "bad trips" and flashbacks. Users who experience bad trips may appear psychotic and extremely fearful. Reassuring the person and pointing out reality are helpful; occasionally, tranquilizers or antipsychotics are given. The symptoms usually disappear within twelve hours but may persist for months. People who are mentally ill or emotionally conflicted are more likely to have bad trips and flashbacks and to require hospitalization than ordinary users are.

Flashbacks are a spontaneous reliving of the experiences the person felt while under the influence of the drug, although the person is drug free. The experience may involve perceptual distortions, a variety of physical feelings, and strong emotions, e.g., fear or pleasure. Flashbacks are generally brief, and they occur less frequently over time. Flash-

---

Box 16–14
KEY FACTS ABOUT HALLUCINOGENS

Examples
LSD, psilocybin, DMT, psilocin, Mescaline, peyote, MDA

Slang Terms
Acid

Route of Administration
Oral

Psychologic Symptoms
Intensification of perceptions
Depersonalization
Derealization
Illusions, pseudohallucinations
Synesthesias (e.g., seeing sound or hearing colors)
Anxiety
Depression
Intense emotions
Body image changes
Ideas of reference
Paranoid ideation
Impaired judgment
Mood swings

Physical Symptoms
Dilated pupils
Tachycardia
Sweating
Palpitations
Blurred vision
Tremors
Lack of coordination

Dangers
Unpredictable behavior, resulting in harm to self or others
"Flashback" hallucinations

Typical Users
Adolescents
Young adults

---

backs may be induced by stress, fatigue, and drug or alcohol ingestion.

Some authorities believe hallucinogens pose a particular danger to adolescents in that they may precipitate a psychosis. Because teenagers' egos and defenses are weak, they may be especially susceptible to the effects of hallucinogens.

Psychologic and physical dependence are unlikely because each experience with a hallucinogen is different. At the present time, researchers have demonstrated no relationship between hallucinogens and birth defects. Likewise, increased creativity and brilliant personality revelations, presumed effects of the drugs, are short-lived at best.

POLYDRUG USE

Most substance abusers today are polydrug users. This fact complicates diagnosis and treatment and increases the hazards associated with abuse. *Synergistic* or potentiating effects are possible. In other words, the effects of two or more drugs taken together are greater than the singular effects of each drug—the whole is greater than the sum of its parts, e.g., alcohol and barbiturates taken together. *Additive effects* occur when two drugs that have similar effects are used together. *Paradoxical effects* occur if a drug causes a reaction opposite to that expected. Paradoxical effects may occur when only one drug is taken or when several drugs are taken. A *pathologic reaction,* too, may result from ingestion of only one or several drugs: It is an unexpected and dramatic response to the drug. For example, the combination of alcohol and marijuana is especially dangerous because THC suppresses the nausea that results from an overdose of alcohol. Consequently, the person may continue to drink, risking respiratory depression, coma, and even death. Cocaine and alcohol are frequently used together; the cocaine gives the user a brief high, and the alcohol masks the ensuing depression. Prescription drugs and alcohol are also a common combination.

DESIGNER DRUGS

Designer drugs, a new threat on the drug scene, are chemical derivatives of controlled drugs. They are called analog drugs because they retain properties of controlled drugs, but one molecule is changed, making them initially not classifiable as controlled. According to the Controlled Substance Act of 1970, controlled substances (i.e., federally regulated substances) are classified from I (most regulated) through V, based on the potential for abuse and the current accepted medical use. As new information is made available, drugs may be reclassified.

Produced by underground chemists, analog drugs are initially legal until analyzed and researched by chemists. Once a dangerous pattern of use is determined (often three to six months after police discover the drug), the drug may be classified as a controlled substance. Fentanyl (Sublimaze), a synthetic anesthetic used in anesthesiology, is similar chemically to some designer drugs. Fentanyl is 100 times as strong as morphine and 20 to 40 times as strong as heroin. It provides a fast rush and an extraordinary high. A person can become addicted after one shot of fentanyl (Gallagher 1986, p 7). Ecstasy (MDMA, Adam) was a designer drug; it has recently been classified as a Schedule I narcotic because research demonstrates that ecstasy causes structural damage to the brain. MTPT (China white), an analog of meperidine (Demerol), has an adverse reaction similar to the rigidity caused by Parkinson's disease.

SUBSTANCE ABUSE AND GROUPS AT RISK

Teenagers

Drug abuse among teenagers is pervasive in our society. Although many adolescents experiment with drugs for only a brief time, many more who do so become addicted. Susceptibility to addiction seems to depend on several variables: the form and potency of the drug, the dosage, the frequency and the pattern of use, stress, the personality and genetic makeup of the user, and the family culture. Straight, Inc., views drug abuse as a primary disease—an incurable chronic disease that is progressive and terminal. Newton (1981) describes drug use as a disease of feelings. Newton believes that psychoactive drugs affect the "old brain," the limbic system and center of feeling, and not "the new brain" (neocortex), the center of conceptualization (p 33). Consequently, a teenager's moods are affected not only at the moment of use but also over time. People use drugs that initially produce good feelings to escape from the stress and strain of life. A teenager who relies on a quick "fix" (a drug) to ease mental pain does not learn healthy coping processes. If teenagers do not learn healthy coping mechanisms or work through the pains and mood swings associated with living, they never complete a necessary developmental stage. As a consequence, they remain fixated at a dependent level of development. A dangerous cycle is begun—a cycle that is unlikely to be interrupted without professional intervention. Drug use, regardless of what drug is used, inevitably affects all areas of a teenager's life—school, work, social and family relationships, and sense of self-worth (see Box 16–15).

Adolescent drug users manifest more psychopathologic conditions than nonusers do. Symptoms include feelings of depression, inadequacy, frustration, helplessness, and self-alienation. These teenagers also have ego structure deficiencies and poor impulse control (Pallikkathayil and Tweed 1983, p 314). Note the behavioral changes in Box 16–15. The earlier a child begins using a dependency-producing drug, the more likely that he or she will use other dependency-producing drugs. Alcohol and marijuana are "gateway" drugs; their use often leads to the use of narcotics, cocaine, or more dangerous drugs. There is a progression of drug use: alcohol, marijuana, tranquilizers, analgesics, hypnotics, cocaine, heroin, PCP (least commonly used). Teenagers who use alcohol and drugs are likely to continue to use them in adulthood.

Psychiatric Clients

Nurses need to be alert to possible substance abuse by psychiatric clients in a hospital setting. Problems may occur if clients take a combination of substances, and treatment is hindered if patients are under the influence of drugs or alcohol. Close observation of teenagers and their visitors is useful, and the nurse often needs to ask clients directly if they are taking drugs.

Women

Although alcoholism is a greater stigma for women than men, more women are drinking today. Many of these women are also using other drugs. Women respond to alcohol somewhat differently than men do. Finley (1982, pp 15–16) reviews the available literature on alcoholism and women and concludes:

- Most problem drinking in women occurs from 35–49 years of age.
- Depression often precedes alcoholism in women.
- Women are at greater risk of developing liver disease with a shorter duration of drinking at a lower level and at a younger age than men are.
- Women with acute liver disorders have a higher mortality than men with such disorders.
- Estrogen appears to effect alcohol intoxication and metabolism, e.g., a woman taking oral contraceptives of synthetic estrogens gets more intoxicated and remains intoxicated longer than a man who drinks the same amount.
- Women tend to drink in secret and drink continuously rather than binge.
- Women drink before stressful events and report increased drinking before their menstrual periods.
- Women describe personality changes from drinking.

Box 16–15
BEHAVIORAL CHANGES ASSOCIATED WITH TEENAGE DRUG ABUSE

- Unexplained periods or reactions of moodiness, depression, anxiety, irritability, oversensitivity, or hostility
- Strongly inappropriate overreaction to mild criticism or simple requests
- Lessening in accustomed family warmth—avoids interaction and communication with parents, withdraws from family activities
- Preoccupation with self, less concern for the feelings of others
- Loss of interest in previously important hobbies, sports, activities
- Loss of motivation and enthusiasm (amotivational syndrome)
- Lethargy, lack of energy and vitality
- Loss of ability for self-discipline and assuming responsibility
- Need for instant gratification
- Change in values, ideals, beliefs
- Changes in friends, unwillingness to introduce friends
- Secretive phone calls—callers refuse to identify themselves or hang up when you answer
- Unexplained absences from home
- Disappearance of money or items of value from home; handling of money becomes secretive
- Desire for increased sensory stimuli

Additional studies show:

- Premenstrual tension is related to alcohol abuse (Belfer 1971).
- When given the same dose of ethanol (adjusted for body weight), women have higher peak blood alcohol levels than men do (Jones and Jones 1976).
- Women have higher blood alcohol levels premenstrually than at other times in their menstrual cycle (Jones, Jones, and Paredes 1976).
- High alcohol intake can cause infertility, amenorrhea, and failure to ovulate (Pratt 1981).

- Women describe using alcohol and drugs in response to obstetric/gynecologic problems (Busch et al. 1986).

After reviewing existing research on women and alcohol, Blume (1986) suggests that treatment programs should be geared to women's needs. Such programs might include women-only groups, female therapists, meetings with recovered women alcoholics, and help for the clients' families.

General Hospital Clients

Nurses who work in the general hospital need to be alert to the possibility that clients presenting with other illnesses may be substance abusers and may be in danger of withdrawal. Chychula (1984, p 18) suggests that nurses be suspicious if physical assessment reveals:

- Debilitation out of proportion to the presenting health problem
- Physical findings that do not correlate to the chief complaint
- Unsteady gait, slurring of speech, dilated pupils, night sweats, chills, blackouts, tremors, skin tracks, abscesses, nasal septum perforation, jaundice
- Weight loss, poor hygiene, and poor nutrition

The nurse may want to alert the physician and suggest appropriate laboratory studies (e.g., liver function tests). A nursing assessment may include questions about a client's drinking habits. If alcoholism is suspected, the client needs to be confronted nonjudgmentally so that he or she can be treated for possible withdrawal symptoms.

The Elderly

Elderly clients who often are being treated for several chronic illnesses by different physicians are at risk for drug problems from drug interactions and/or for drug dependence. By being alert to this fact nurses can work towards getting a good history from the client, including a list of all the drugs taken, frequency of use, dosage, and length of time the client has been on the drug. Frequently the confusion seen in elderly clients is a direct consequence of drug interaction or malabsorption.

After reviewing the literature on drug abuse and the elderly, Caroselli-Karinja (1985, pp 25–27) presents the following critical facts:

- People 65 years old represent 11 percent of the United States population, yet they take 25 percent of all prescribed drugs.
- Older people often see a variety of physicians who prescribe medication without assessing the other drugs the client is taking.
- The physiologic and psychologic changes of aging may affect the way medication is metabolized. Adverse and toxic effects are more likely.
- The prescription drugs subject to abuse and misuse are anxiolytics, sedatives, hypnotics, and analgesics.
- Problems of the elderly—retirement, loss of independence, illness, loss of family/friends, decreased income—are likely to cause depression, anxiety, and loneliness. Such feeling states may cause clients to take over-the-counter drugs and physicians to prescribe drugs.
- The elderly often hoard unused drugs and share them with friends.

Adult Children of Alcoholics

Adult children of alcoholics are at great risk of becoming alcoholics. If both parents are alcoholics, a child has a 70 percent chance of becoming an alcoholic; if one parent is an alcoholic, a child has a 40 percent chance. This type of alcoholism has been labeled *familial.* Research on familial alcoholism has shown that (a) a family history of alcoholism is present, (b) alcoholism develops early, usually by the time the person is in his or her late twenties, (c) the alcoholism is generally severe and usually requires treatment, (d) the risk of alcoholism is increased but not the risk of other psychiatric disorders (Kaplan and Sadock 1985).

Nurses

The issue of chemically dependent nurses has received attention in professional journals and lay literature. Note the following facts:

- Chemical dependency is the number one health problem affecting nurses.
- Nurses have a 50 percent higher rate of dependency than nonnurses do.
- As early as 1973, 70 percent of all disciplinary hearings were related to chemical dependency. In 1981, 67 percent of 971 disciplinary cases were drug related (Green 1984).
- The majority of state nursing associations have passed resolutions about the problem.

Nurses generally work under a great deal of stress and have easy access to drugs. Every day, they give people medication to decrease pain. It is an easy leap to begin to self-

Box 16–16
WARNING SIGNS OF CHEMI-CALLY DEPENDENT NURSES

- Frequent absenteeism before and after days off; always working (for supply)
- Irritability
- Abrupt mood changes; inappropriate affect
- Sloppy charting and client care
- Problems with drugs (missing drugs, frequent "wasting" of drugs, inaccurate records)
- Frequent errors of judgment
- Alcohol (stale or fresh) on breath
- Frequent disappearance from the unit
- Offering to give medication to other nurses' clients
- Frequent night shift work
- Her or his patients complain of little or no pain relief

medicate (Figure 16–3). However, such behavior is a violation of the state nurse practice act and, depending on the drug and method of obtaining it, may be a criminal offense. Colleagues of chemically dependent nurses need to be alert to behavior that is suspicious (see Box 16–16) and to document and report such behavior to the head nurse or supervisor. It is very common to cover up such behavior. Shielding such a nurse puts the clients, the nurse, and the nursing profession at risk and violates the nurse practice act, the nurse code of ethics, and the law in many states.

It is most important that nurses view their chemically dependent colleagues as suffering from a disease rather than from moral problems. This understanding enables nurses to work together to help each other.

Only recently has nursing administration begun to confront the problem by writing policies and developing programs for the chemically dependent professional. Nurse self-help groups are springing up all over, and some hospitals are working closely with recovering nurses on intervention strategies and requirements for treatment. State boards of nursing are usually involved and in some cases hire a person to work with chemically dependent nurses all over the state. Depending on the circumstances, a chemically dependent nurse may need to be terminated or transferred. Voluntary surrender of the nursing license may be suggested. Each nurse is entitled to confidential medical treatment, freedom from stigma, and the opportunity to return to work upon recovering (Naegle 1985, p 24). Intervention with nurse substance abusers follows the pattern presented in the section, "Confrontation Strategies," later in this chapter. While in the process of recovery, chemically dependent nurses need regular drug screenings. Their work performance should be monitored, along with their attendance at a treatment program or group for a period of up to two years. With early intervention and continued support and treatment, chemically dependent nurses have a good prognosis.

Research in the area of chemically dependent nurses

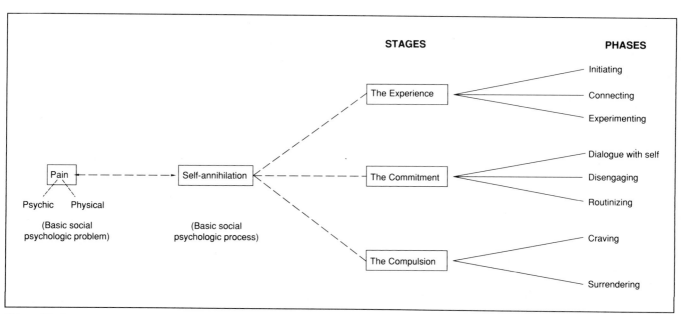

Figure 16–3
Chemically dependent nurses: the trajectory toward self-annihilation.
Source: Hutchinson S: Chemically dependent nurses: The trajectory toward self-annihilation.
Nursing Research *1986;34(4):196–201. Copyright © 1986 The American Journal of Nursing Company.*

is just beginning. Hutchinson's (1986) study describes the process of nurses becoming chemically dependent. Researchers need to continue studying substance abusers and specific groups at risk. Questions for research can address successful and unsuccessful intervention strategies, successful and unsuccessful treatment programs, the self-help group process, the relationships of environmental and/or personal factors to chemical dependency, and successful coping strategies of people at risk who are extremely stressed but do not use chemicals.

A HUMANIST-INTERACTIONIST PERSPECTIVE

Substance abuse needs to be viewed as a disease and not as a moral problem. A moralistic attitude always alienates the client. Recognizing and accepting that the disease is chronic, often with remissions and exacerbations, should keep the nurse from succumbing to the frustration felt by many who treat substance abusers. Even if the client regresses, there is hope if he or she learns something and alters behavior in some positive way. At certain stressful times in life, anyone may develop a dependency on drugs or alcohol; however, certain people seem to be predisposed to the illness. Nurses' expertise in the stages of the nursing process is vital to the care of the client with substance abuse problems. Chychula (1984) suggests that nurses focus on helping the client work toward self-awareness, good health, and good interpersonal relationships. With improvements in these areas and the development of alternative life-styles, these people can lead productive, fulfilling, happy lives.

THE NURSING PROCESS AND CLIENTS WHO ARE SUBSTANCE ABUSERS

As substance abuse becomes an increasing problem in society, more clients will be admitted to hospitals and clinics for help with intoxication and withdrawal. Drugs change rapidly, requiring that nurses keep up with "the drug scene" so that they can assess and treat clients. Along with the knowledge acquired from reading, continuing education programs, and seminars, nurses need self-knowledge to help them be good therapists with substance abusers. Ongoing critical self-analysis of feelings, attitudes, and behavior toward clients is useful. See Box 16–17 for a list of useful questions to guide this self-analysis.

Box 16–17
GUIDE TO ANALYZING PERSONAL RESPONSES TOWARD SUBSTANCE ABUSERS

Analyze your responses to the following questions:

1. What thoughts and feelings does the term *alcoholic* evoke in me?

2. What thoughts and feelings does the term *addict* evoke in me?

3. Do I believe that substance dependence occurs out of moral weakness?

4. Do I believe that substance dependence is an illness that can be treated?

5. Is the person who abuses substances deliberately destroying his or her life and the lives of significant others?

6. Who in my personal life has abused drugs, alcohol, or other chemicals?

7. How does my experience with relatives, friends, colleagues, or clients who have abused substances affect my attitude toward caring for a substance-abusing client?

8. Is substance abuse a social problem, an emotional-psychologic problem, or a physical abnormality?

9. How do I view the family, spouse, or friends of the substance abuser? Do they encourage the abuse, or otherwise "enable" the person to continue their abuse? Or are they victims?

10. How does my own personal use of nicotine, caffeine, drugs, or alcohol affect my attitude toward clients?

Source: Bittle S, Feignbaum JS, Kneisl CR: Substance abuse, in Adult Health Nursing: A Biopsychosocial Approach. *Addison-Wesley, 1986, p 254.*

Assessment

Substance Abuse Assessment Questions

Figure 16–4 presents Chychula's Substance Abuse Assessment Form. This form is comprehensive and can be modified if the nurse is under time constraints. In a rushed situation, as in an emergency room, a nurse need ask only a few key questions:

- What did you take?

- How much did you take?

- When did you take it?

Text continues on p. 380.

Substance Abuse Assessment Form

I. Admission profile
   A. Do you take any medications by prescription from a physician? If so, which do you take?
   B. For what physical conditions were these medications prescribed?
   C. How often and how long have you taken these medications?
   D. In what ways do these drugs help you?
   E. What medications or food are you allergic to?
   F. Have you ever used any drugs that were not prescribed by a physician?
   G. Types of drugs used

	Frequency of use		
	In last 30 days	In last 24–48 hours	Lifetime years/months
1. Heroin	⎯⎯	⎯⎯	⎯⎯
2. Non-RX methadone	⎯⎯	⎯⎯	⎯⎯
3. Other opiates, synthetics	⎯⎯	⎯⎯	⎯⎯
4. Barbiturates	⎯⎯	⎯⎯	⎯⎯
5. Other sedatives, hypnotics	⎯⎯	⎯⎯	⎯⎯
6. Amphetamines	⎯⎯	⎯⎯	⎯⎯
7. Cocaine	⎯⎯	⎯⎯	⎯⎯
8. Marijuana/hashish	⎯⎯	⎯⎯	⎯⎯
9. Hallucinogens	⎯⎯	⎯⎯	⎯⎯
10. Inhalants	⎯⎯	⎯⎯	⎯⎯
11. Tranquilizers	⎯⎯	⎯⎯	⎯⎯
12. Syrups with codeine	⎯⎯	⎯⎯	⎯⎯

   H. In which way have you used these drugs?
      Oral ⎯⎯
      Smoking ⎯⎯
      Inhalation ⎯⎯
      Intravenous ⎯⎯
      Intramuscular ⎯⎯
   I. What is the usual dose of each drug used?
   J. In what way do the drugs you use help you?

II. Severity of drug use
   A. What do you experience when you stop use of the drugs?
   B. Do you hoard any medication? Which ones?
   C. Did you ever have a blackout or any effects you didn't want to have while under the influence of drugs? How many times has this happened?
   D. Have you ever tried to hurt yourself? How many times?
   E. Have you ever overdosed on any drugs? How many times?
   F. Which drugs were the cause of the overdose?
   G. Have you ever missed work because of drug use?
   H. Does your family physician know you are using drugs?

Figure 16–4
Substance abuse assessment form.

continued

Source: Adapted from Chychula N: Screening for substance abuse in a primary care setting. The Nurse Practitioner *July 1984, 9:7, pp 15–24. Reprinted by permission of Vernon Publications, Inc.*

Substance Abuse Assessment Form (continued)

III. Treatment history and expectations of future use
    A. Have you had any drug-free periods during your drug use?
    B. How long did the drug-free periods last?
    C. Have you received treatment for drugs? How many times?
    D. What was your treatment experience(s)?
    E. Are you presently receiving drug treatment?
    F. What do you forecast about your future drug use?
    G. Can you see youself free of drugs?
    H. Do you want to stop using drugs?

IV. Licit drug history
    A. Alcohol
        1. Five-day alcohol use history

Days	Type of Alcohol Beverage	Amount of Alcohol Beverage
a. Today	_____	_____
b. Yesterday	_____	_____
c.	_____	_____
d.	_____	_____
e.	_____	_____
f.	_____	_____

        2. Date and time of last drink: _____ A.M./P.M.
        3. Last time sober for more than a week _____

Check one for reliability:
    ____ The client gave the information without any suggestion of inaccuracy.
    ____ The client was somewhat unsure of him/herself or was judged as such.
    ____ The client was unsure of him/herself or was not able to give any information or said he/she had forgotten.

        4. Frequency of alcohol use/seven days a week _____
        5. Duration of "heavy drinking" _____
        6. Duration of drinking _____
        7. Pattern:
           a. Typical drinking day
      ____ Starts in morning and drinks slowly and steadily throughout the day not becoming noticeably intoxicated.
      ____ Drinks and becomes noticeably intoxicated all day.
      ____ Drinks after work only.
      ____ Other—Describe: _____
           b. Typical drinking period:
      ____ drinks for ___ days, weeks, months, (circle one) and abstains for ___ days, weeks, months (circle one).
      ____ Drinks on weekends.
      ____ Drinks practically every day throughout the year.
      ____ Other—Describe: _____

Figure 16–4 (continued)

Substance Abuse Assessment Form (continued)

8. History of alcohol withdrawal syndrome (AWS):
   Have you experienced any of the following symptoms after drinking?
   ___ Shakes, sweating, restlessness, problems sleeping, decrease in appetite.
   ___ Hallucinations: visual, auditory, tactile.
   ___ Convulsions or seizures.
   ___ Delirium tremens (DTs or alcohol withdrawal delirium).

9. Treatment history (dates, location of program)
   Detoxifications: _____
   Rehabilitations: _____
   Antabuse treatments: _____

10. Have you ever been arrested for drunkeness or drunk driving? How many times?
11. Have you ever missed time from work due to drinking?
12. Have you ever lost a job due to drinking?
13. Has anyone in your family expressed concern over your drinking?

B. Over-the-counter products
   1. What types of over-the-counter preparations have you used?
      Vitamins _____
      Laxatives _____
      Antacids _____
      Cold remedies _____
      Aspirin _____
      Analgesics _____
      Weight-reduction products _____
      Sleeping aids _____
      Products to stay awake _____
      Caffeine _____
   2. How often do you use the over-the-counter product(s)?
   3. How long have you used the over-the-counter product(s)?

V. Significant others
   A. Of your family and friends, whom do you consider the most important person to you or someone you could confide in?
   B. Does this person know you take drugs?
   C. Does this person take drugs also?
   D. Does anyone in your family have drug problems?
   E. Does anyone in your family have alcohol problems?
   F. Do you conceal from others, including your family and friends, the kinds of drugs or the amount of drugs you take?
   G. What have been your usual living arrangements in the past year?
      1. With sexual partner and children _____
      2. With sexual partner _____
      3. With parents _____
      4. With friends _____
      5. Alone _____
      6. Controlled environment _____
      7. No stable living arrangements _____

Figure 16–4 (continued)

Substance Abuse Assessment Form (continued)

VI. Psychiatric conditions
   A. How many times in the last month have you experienced the following conditions that were not a direct effect of drug/alcohol use?
      1. Serious depression _____
      2. Serious anxiety or tensions _____
      3. Hallucinations _____
      4. Trouble with memory _____
      5. Trouble communicating _____
      6. Trouble following directions _____
      7. Difficulty completing work _____
      8. Difficulty controlling violent behavior _____
      9. Thoughts of suicide _____
      10. Thoughts of suspiciousness or paranoid feelings _____
      11. Trouble getting asleep _____

   B. Have you ever received treatment for a psychologic or emotional problem? What type of treatment?
   C. Have you ever received medications for a psychologic or emotional problem? What medications were prescribed?
   D. How did this treatment(s) help you?

Figure 16–4 (continued)

- What have you taken in the last twenty-four hours? the last week?

Of course, in an emergency situation, the client may be unable to give coherent answers and a friend may not have accurate information. In these cases, the presenting symptoms are treated, and the assessment is done when the client is alert and oriented. The kind and number of questions asked in a nursing assessment depend on the setting and the client's behavior.

Motivation for Treatment

Nurses need to consider some important psychosocial issues when clients come for treatment. Clients may enter a treatment program voluntarily. This situation is best, because they are internally motivated and therefore have a better chance of success. Clients, however, may be coerced by family, friends, physicians, or the police to undergo treatment. Coerced treatment inevitably causes anger and resentment. These clients may lash out at people, blame them (including the nurse), and demonstrate resistant or arrogant behavior. In these difficult situations, the nurse must remain detached and nonjudgmental to avoid both power struggles and taking the role of persecutor or rescuer. At this time, the nurse functions as a data gatherer: "I know you are (uncomfortable, anxious, afraid, angry) now. To help you feel better, I need to ask you some ques-

tions about your drug use." In contrast, a judgmental question is, "Don't you know that if you don't get help now you will only get worse?" Such questions prevent rapport and alienate the client from the therapeutic process.

The Importance of Language

Knowing the language of the drug world is important in obtaining an accurate nursing assessment of a substance abuser. Drug users have a language all their own; to understand them and the extent and nature of their habit, a nurse needs to "get hip." For example, "basing and balling" refers to freebasing (using ether to purify cocaine and make it more potent), and speedballing (combining heroin and cocaine); "copping an eight-ball" means acquiring one-eighth ounce of cocaine; "drug of choice" is the client's favorite drug. Often the clients themselves or a recovering addict can teach the nurse.

Rationale for Assessment

An accurate assessment of the substances used and abused is necessary to anticipate potential toxic and withdrawal effects and to make nursing care plans as specific and relevant as possible. For example, a chronic alcoholic who is malnourished, exhausted, and depressed needs immediate diet regulation, rest, and gradual involvement in a treatment program. Cocaine or crack abusers are likely to be resistant to treatment and need active staff intervention and a structured program immediately to involve them in treatment. They should not be left alone or purposefully isolated, as might be done with an alcoholic.

Common Defense Mechanisms

Denial and projection are two defense mechanisms common to substance abusers. These mechanisms along with other behaviors—conning, bargaining, feigning—complicate all phases of the nursing process. Alcoholics and other drug abusers tend to deny they have a problem or minimize the problem: "I drink/use every day but it rarely interferes with my work." Rationalization is common: "I know I shouldn't drink, and I'll stop as soon as I get through this problem. Drinking keeps me calm enough to function." A detailed assessment, along with family/coworker interviews, reveals that the problem is generally worse than the client says. Cocaine users tend to project and blame their difficulties on others, often a spouse. For instance, a man may bring up the issue of his wife's drinking and give a million reasons why he does not need treatment.

Substance abusers "con" (manipulate) people to get drugs. *DSB,* a term used in some treatment centers, refers to *drug-seeking behaviors,* e.g., feigning illness or an injury to get a drug. These people also bargain with themselves and staff to get what they want. For example, an alcoholic/drug abuser is likely to think, "I know I shouldn't hang out with B and P since we all get loaded together, but I like them. I'll just be with them, but I won't drink/use." Later on, he or she may think, "I'll only use a gram of cocaine"; later, "I'll just do an eight-ball." He or she might tell the nurse, "I'll be glad to go to group therapy next week; just let me rest for a few days. I'm really tired." Of course, substance abusers always con themselves first.

Useful Nursing Responses

Recognizing common defense mechanisms and behaviors should help nurses in their client interviews and later in intervention. Coleman (1985, p 74) suggests what nurses can do to refuse to "play the game":

- Recognize and pay attention if you think something is not right.
- Recognize when your feelings of sympathy or compassion are excusing bad behavior and letting someone off the hook.
- Stop and think before you act; check with others for their reactions.
- Decide on a course of action and stick to it; do not argue or explain.
- Do not assume the client's responsibility.

- Talk to the involved staff and agree on a unified course of action. Avoid sending contradicting messages to the client.
- Insist the client follow the rules.
- Negotiate, but do not change agreements.
- Do not scold, blame, or preach. Remain objective.
- Control your temper through the use of humor or detachment.

Substance abusers are frequently demanding (they are used to immediate gratification), frightened, dependent, and grandiose. They need consistency and firmness. Savvy, not naiveté, is required for accurate client assessment and successful interventions.

Nursing assessment requires observation of subjective and objective behaviors. Examples of subjective comments are: "I have a $3000 a week coke habit and I have no more money." "I took all the pills in my medicine cabinet (Tylenol, Valium, Darvocet)." "I've drunk a quart a day for the last three weeks." Objective data relevant to each substance used are given in Boxes 16–5 through 16–14.

Nursing Diagnosis

DSM-IIIR, PND-I, and NANDA diagnoses are compared in Table 16–1.

Planning and Implementing Interventions

Program Interventions

Nurses may hold positions in any of the following settings. Their roles may be slightly different in each setting, depending on the client's stage of illness and presenting symptoms. Solari-Twadell (1983) describes five types of treatment programs:

General Hospital Care

Substance abusers who are suicidal or acutely ill with delirium tremens, hepatic coma, respiratory depression, or cardiac arrhythmias are often treated in a medical-surgical unit of a general hospital. Life-threatening physiologic symptoms are attended to first. When the client is out of danger, the alcoholism or drug addiction issues are addressed.

Table 16–1
Comparison of a DSM-IIIR Diagnosis and Psychiatric Nursing Diagnoses

DSM-IIIR Diagnosis	PND-I Diagnoses		NANDA Diagnoses
305.30 Hallucinogen abuse	01.01.03	Impaired coordination	
	01.03	Altered self-care*	Self-care deficits
	01.04.03	Insomnia*	Sleep pattern disturbance
	02.02	Altered judgment	
	02.07.01	Delusions	
	02.07.02	Ideas of reference	Sensory/perceptual alterations
	06.04.03	Hallucinations	Thought processes, altered
	06.04.04	Illusions	Thermoregulation, ineffective
	05.02.02.05	Unpredictable behaviors	Coping, ineffective individual
	05.02.01.02	Aggressive/violent behaviors toward others*	Violence, potential for: self-directed or directed at others

*PND-I diagnosis also in NANDA list.

In this setting, nurses monitor vital signs and respiratory and cardiovascular support and administer prescribed medications. Ice packs may be used for fever, e.g., fever caused by amphetamine intoxication. If the client is hallucinating and very fearful, as with delirium tremens, the nurse decreases stimulation by providing a darkened room in a quiet area. The nurse points out reality: "I know you are seeing things, and I know you are frightened. You are in the hospital, and we are caring for you. There are no bugs (monsters, etc.) here. You are safe and will feel better soon."

Frantic, angry, paranoid, or irrational behavior may be seen in clients who have taken overdoses of amphetamines, LSD, PCP, or cocaine. Reassuring the client may be ineffective; often, the symptoms subside only with time. Occasionally, restraints may be necessary. The nurse makes sure that clients get adequate nutrition and fluids; they are disoriented and generally forget to eat and drink. The nurse plays a critical role in assessing why the client took an overdose.

Specialty Hospital Care

Specialty hospital care is given in in-patient hospital units that are geared specifically for substance abusers. If the hospital is equipped with trained personnel and appropriate resources, acutely ill clients may be admitted. The physical environment is modified to handle problems with substance abusers. For example, padded seclusion rooms devoid of all but a mattress offer a quiet, unstimulating environment that prevents convulsions and decreases anxiety. A primary nurse may be assigned to decrease confusion and stimulation. The staff are experts in detoxification, education, and treatment. Clients also receive treatment for coexisting medical and psychiatric problems. Staff efforts are geared toward stabilization.

Residential Rehabilitation

Residential rehabilitation facilities offer in-patients expert care for substance abuse, but staff are not skilled in treating medical or psychiatric problems.

Extended Residential Care

Extended care facilities provide services for people with physical impairments and provide a home for recovering alcoholics or drug addicts who have been rejected by their families. Apartments for independent living, a relatively new concept, are useful for these clients.

Outpatient care may consist of daily, weekly, or monthly individual, group, or family treatment in a variety of treatment centers. Daily care is usually given only in intensive programs of limited duration, usually one month. Employee assistance programs (EAP) are now common in many industries and are one example of outpatient care given not in a clinic but in the workplace. Substance abuse outreach counselors work with chemically dependent employees.

Nurses who work with substance abusers in any of these settings need to recognize that addiction is a chronic, progressive disease. The nurse needs different skills depending on the work setting. For example, in general or specialty hospitals nurses need psychosocial skills along with technical skills to assess and monitor the physiologic components of abuse and withdrawal. In residential rehabilitation and extended residential care centers, the nurse may educate clients about the disease, help clients reenter the community as much as possible, and facilitate or lead support groups. In an outpatient treatment center, the nurse functions as a counselor/therapist. In all cases, the nurse needs psychosocial skills. Such skills may include interviewing, teaching clients about the disease process and alternative coping strategies, referring clients to appropriate sources and community support systems, and knowing how to conduct individual, group, or family therapy. In all situations, the nurse needs an in-depth understanding of the disease process, from the varying theoretical explanations to the varying methods of treatment at different stages, to give quality nursing care.

Alcoholics Anonymous and Narcotics Anonymous

In contrast to the previously described treatment programs, Alcoholics Anonymous (AA) and Narcotics Anonymous (NA) are not specifically treatment programs, but AA/NA community groups do hold meetings at various treatment facilities. Both are successful self-help groups that meet daily in different parts of large cities and weekly in smaller towns. Anyone who has a desire to stop drinking or taking drugs is welcome. This belief pervades both organizations: "Once an alcoholic/addict, always an alcoholic/addict." Members admit they are powerless over chemicals, live "one day at a time," pray the serenity prayer, and believe in "a power greater than man." The members learn to turn their problems over to "the God of my understanding." Their philosophy is revealed in part through their key slogans, "First things first," "Easy does it," and "Let go and let God." Alcoholics learn the "Twelve Steps of AA" (see Box 16–18). Through AA/NA, people learn to change negative attitudes and behaviors into positive ones. A key concept of AA/NA is that total abstinence is essential to recovery. As members become sober or drug-free, they begin "sponsoring" (helping) other substance abusers. This offering

---

Box 16–18
TWELVE STEPS OF ALCOHOLICS ANONYMOUS

1. We admitted we were powerless over alcohol—that our lives had become unmanageable.

2. Came to believe that a Power greater than ourselves could restore us to sanity.

3. Made a decision to turn our will and our lives over to the care of God, as we understood Him.

4. Made a searching and fearless moral inventory of ourselves.

5. Admitted to God, to ourselves, and to another human being the exact nature of our wrongs.

6. Were entirely ready to have God remove all these defects of character.

7. Humbly asked Him to remove our shortcomings.

8. Made a list of all persons we had harmed, and became willing to make amends to them all.

9. Made direct amends to such people wherever possible, except when to do so would injure them or others.

10. Continued to take personal inventory and when we were wrong promptly admitted it.

11. Sought through prayer and meditation to improve our conscious contact with God, as we understood Him, praying only for knowledge of His will for us and the power to carry that out.

12. Having had a spiritual awakening as the result of these steps, we tried to carry this message to alcoholics, and to practice these principles in all our affairs.

Source: "The Twelve Steps" from Twelve Steps and Twelve Traditions *reprinted with permission of Alcoholics Anonymous World Services, Inc.*

---

of support is believed to be vital to recovery, as is regular attendance at AA/NA meetings.

Women for Sobriety

Women for Sobriety (WFS) is another self-help group. Unlike AA/NA, WFS is not based on a spiritual philosophy; instead, the program is based on abstinence. WFS's thirteen acceptance statements focus members on new ways of thinking. The women learn to cope and, over time, to change their daily lives. The group recognizes the differences in male and female alcoholism.

Treatment Models

Presently, contradictory beliefs exist about the correct treatment of substance abusers. In the AA/NA model of treatment, alcoholism and drug addiction are viewed as a primary disease process. Other psychiatric symptoms are seen as resulting from addiction. Certain residential treatment centers and in-patient programs use the AA approach exclusively, to the dismay of many psychiatric professionals. This latter group believes that many alcoholics and drug abusers have fundamental psychiatric problems, such as depression, personality disorders (especially antisocial personality disorders or borderline personality disorders). Such disorders are viewed as primary and substance abuse as secondary. Treatment, they believe, should reflect this reality. Drugs and traditional psychotherapy are often prescribed for these clients. This difference in ideology and philosophy is manifested clearly in different mental health groups and in different care facilities. Nurses should be clear about their own beliefs and about the philosophy of a hospital or clinic before they accept a position.

Other treatment modalities include biofeedback, relaxation techniques, group and individual therapy, and education about the disease. Research has not yet shown which, if any, treatment or combination of treatments yields the best results. At the present time, a variety of theories and treatment modes should be used and studied. The client's particular problems and circumstances should guide the treatment plan.

Citizens' Responses

Because of the increasing number of deaths due to drunk driving, a group of concerned citizens and relatives of those people killed have banded together to combat the problem. Mothers against Drunk Driving (MADD) and Students against Drunk Driving (SADD) are two new aggressive organizations that fund research, educate the public via the media and special programs, and work to pass stricter laws against drunk driving. Anti–drunk driving publicity was at an all time high during the 1985 holiday season. Bar owners were to stop serving drunk customers, and "care" cabs were available all over the nation to drive intoxicated people home. Nurses have been useful participants in this group because of their specialized knowledge.

Nursing Interventions

Confrontation Strategies

For many years, it was believed that alcoholics and drug abusers needed to "hit bottom" before they could accept their problem and request help. Today, most people believe that intervention can occur as soon as the problem is identified. Group intervention/confrontation is one strategy that aims to break down the substance abuser's denial. Nurses are often "intervention specialists" and leaders in the process.

Several family members, friends, employers, co-workers, and an alcohol/drug intervention specialist confront the substance abuser in a private meeting. They list the evidence by going around the group, one by one. For example,

> "You had slurred speech and didn't even respond when I told you I had to be hospitalized for surgery."
>
> "You have not made your daughter's dinner all week. And you forgot to pick her up from school."
>
> "You missed work for three days, and you have been late eight days in the past month."
>
> "You have alcohol on your breath (or needle marks on your arms)."
>
> "I found two bottles (a syringe and empty vial) hidden in the bathroom."

The people, following the leader's cues, speak calmly and slowly with minimal emotion. They are presenting the facts, the objective evidence. Yelling, blaming, and haranguing are avoided because the alcoholic/drug abuser will inevitably respond by denying the behavior or making excuses. However, confrontation by several people who really care and who persistently present the facts serves to break through the denial. The next step requires the family/friends/employer to make clear and direct statements about consequences:

> "Either you get help now or you will have to leave your job."
>
> "Either you enter a treatment program now or I will move out with the kids."

If the client agrees to treatment, the caring people agree to remain involved.

Avoiding Nontherapeutic Intervention

Michael Elkin (1984, pp 81–84), a family therapist, reviews the typical moves in the relationship between an alcoholic and a nurse/therapist (see Figure 16–5). He draws on Eric Berne's belief that the alcoholic plays the part of a victim and the therapist moves from being a rescuer to a persecutor. An inexperienced nurse/therapist is likely to perpetuate this dysfunctional pattern in a long-term "therapeutic" relationship. The typical steps are:

1. The alcoholic (victim) deceives the nurse/therapist (rescuer) into believing that she or he is an unusually perceptive therapist and that the two of them have a close relationship.

2. The victim does not cut down on drinking, but the rescuer avoids mention of this (becomes a patsy) because such confrontation may endanger the relationship.

3. The victim gets drunk and calls the rescuer.

4. The rescuer becomes furious and moves to the position of persecutor.

5. The victim realizes the rescuer is like everyone else and never really cared. The victim feels rejected and abandoned.

6. The rescuer feels guilty about getting angry and engages in self-blame.

7. The victim, feeling guilty and repentant, returns to see the rescuer. A pattern has begun.

Treatment strategies are designed to help the nurse avoid "taking the bait." The nurse/therapist should avoid the role of rescuer, patsy, and persecutor and function in the role of a nonjudgmental problem solver who points out the consequences of behavior. A focus on reality (e.g., "when you drink you seem to have severe physical, emotional, and family problems") and on strategies to achieve realistic goals is useful. The nurse should avoid collusion with the alcoholic or the family but rather should focus on helping them restructure their relationships to avoid the roles of rescuer and persecutor. Successfully working with substance abusing families is a demanding task that requires education and skill, but it can be a wonderfully rewarding experience. As in all active therapeutic relationships, both the clients and the therapists learn and share and grow.

Education

Education is a useful nursing intervention. Videotapes and talks by recovered substance abusers or experts in the effects

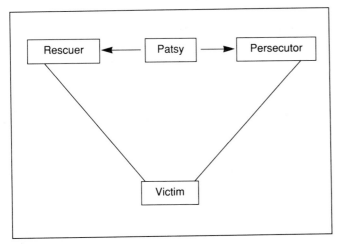

Figure 16–5
The rescue triangle. This diagram suggests that the victim (codependent or coalcoholic) often plays both the role of rescuer and of persecutor, depending on the situation. Whenever the victim plays these roles, she or he inevitably ends up being a patsy. Playing the role of rescuer or persecutor is not useful for the victim or the alcoholic client; it is a no-win situation.

Source: Reprinted from Families Under the Influence, Changing Alcoholic Patterns, *by Michael Elkin, by permission of W.W. Norton & Company, Inc. Copyright © 1984 by Michael Elkin.*

of substance abuse are helpful. Education may take place in or out of the hospital, in one comprehensive session or several sessions over a period of time. Nurse educators should focus on the types of abused substances and their physical, psychologic, and social effects. Families are often involved in these sessions because substance abuse is a family problem. The belief underlying such education is that knowledge and awareness may be useful in decreasing self-destructive behavior. Knowledge alone, however, is never enough.

Self-Help Groups

Support and self-help groups are extremely useful in helping clients to feel better about themselves and to acquire new attitudes and behaviors. Merely being with many people who are suffering in similar ways is beneficial. By observing people who have been sober or drug free for long periods, clients can begin to model similar behaviors. They can see that there is hope and that recovery is possible. Self-help groups also provide new friends, generally with healthy life-styles. Clients may choose to attend support groups for the rest of their lives. Some clients who experiment with drugs or alcohol during one period of their lives and who succeed in stopping may attend only during the crisis.

Support groups with cocaine abusers should initially (one to two weeks) be homogeneous and not include other substance abusers. Cocaine and crack are rapidly addicting and give an exhilarating high, and cocaine users are often aggressive, domineering people. For these reasons, some experts believe that initial group efforts should focus only on understanding cocaine addiction. After the two weeks, cocaine users are gradually incorporated into general chemical dependency education programs and AA/NA groups. Nurses often are facilitators in support groups.

Life-Style Change

An emphasis on the requirement for a total life-style change is necessary. Nurses can help clients discuss ways to alter their destructive habits by suggesting different coping strategies and by encouraging clients to discover new interests and capabilities within themselves. Nurses and clients can role play new responses to old situations. Recognizing that relapse is always a threat, nurses may set up contracts with clients. For example, clients may agree to contact the nurse or an AA/NA sponsor if and when they feel the urge to drink or do drugs. This agreement represents new behaviors that are necessary for a life-style change.

Clients must realize that spending time with friends who are substance abusers or hanging out at places where

Text continues on p. 393.

CASE STUDY: Client with Cocaine Intoxication

Identifying Information

Leigh S is a 25-year-old married woman who lives at 2205 Long Street. She was brought into the hospital by her husband. Leigh is an advertising executive with a large firm (Weeks, Bedde, and Law). She has a BA in business and an MBA in marketing. She is not and has never been under the care of a therapist.

Client's Definition of Present Problem, Precipitatory Stresses, Coping Strategies, Goals for Care

Leigh states she does not need to be in the hospital but rather needs to get back to work on her ideas for ads. She states that she is extremely creative and productive and needs "to get my ideas down on paper." She is incoherent occasionally during the interview. She does state that she is perspiring and "feels sick to my stomach." Leigh admits to "working very hard," but does not feel she needs care right now. She feels she can handle this herself.

History of Present Problem

Leigh states she has been using cocaine intranasally for one year. She admits to spending the majority of her salary on cocaine and states that she has used cocaine four to five times a day for the last five days. Prior to this, she generally used cocaine once or twice a week. She has increased her use because "it helps me work harder and faster. I feel more productive." She is having trouble sitting still and sleeping. Leigh thinks that she has not slept more than an hour or two for several days. Leigh's husband and one woman colleague are her main support system.

Psychiatric History

No prior psychiatric history

Family History

Leigh's parents are living and work in their own business, a shoe store. Leigh has one brother, 21 years old, a senior in college. She feels emotionally close to her family and brother, but because they live 2000 miles away, sees them only on holidays. Leigh's father has a history of alcoholism, which has been under control for five years.

Social History

Leigh has always excelled, both in her academic work and in her job. She is competitive and likes "being number one." She has a few close friends and socializes with numerous "acquaintances from work." She has smoked since age 17, drinks "moderately," but occasionally gets drunk on weekends. She has experimented with a variety of drugs but finds cocaine to be "what works for me." She describes herself as a "workaholic" but enjoys reading and tennis when time permits.

Significant Health History

Leigh has no current or past medical problems. She states that she is in good health, but "feels horrible now." Assessment reveals a blood pressure reading of 140/90 and pulse rate of 110.

Current Mental Status

Leigh is attractive, yet disheveled, agitated, hyperalert, alternately compliant and hostile, and occasionally incoherent. Her sensorium is impaired. She is oriented to time, place, and person; judgment is impaired. Her affect is labile (alternately hostile and compliant); mood swings are evident. She moves rapidly and frequently. Her thought content is grandiose. Delusions and illusions are present. She states that she wants to open her own advertising company very soon and

continued

Case Study (Continued)

	says she is more efficient, intelligent, and productive than her boss. She reports seeing "signs" at work that are messages to her that she should "move onward and upward." Her thought processes reveal a thought disorder; she is occasionally incoherent and tangential. She is easily distracted and has difficulty concentrating. Presently she denies her problem and has little insight, stating, "I can take care of myself. I know what I'm doing."
Other Subjective or Objective Clinical Data	Not on any medications; suicide/violence potential minimal
Diagnostic Impression	
Nursing Diagnosis (PND-I/ NANDA)	05.02 Altered conduct/impulse processes /Coping, ineffective individual 01.04.03 Insomnia* /Sleep pattern disturbance 05.05 Altered social interaction* /Social interaction, impaired 07.01.02 Altered cardiac circulation* /Cardiac output, altered 07.04 Altered gastrointestinal processes /Nutrition, altered: less than body requirements 05.01.02 Altered verbal communication* /Communication, impaired, verbal 02.02 Altered judgment 02.07.01 Delusions 04.02 Altered feeling patterns

DSM-IIIR Multiaxial Diagnosis	Axis I: 305.60 Cocaine intoxication (primary diagnosis)
	         304.20 Cocaine dependence
	Axis II: V71.09 (no diagnosis; denial and rationalization)
	Axis III: Hypertension
	Axis IV: 3 Moderate (unable to function at work: acute)
	Axis V: Current GAF: 40 Serious impairment in judgment
	        Highest GAF in past year: 60

PND-I diagnosis also in the NANDA list.

Nursing Care Plan

Nursing Diagnosis (PND-I/NANDA)	Client Care Goals	Nursing Planning/ Intervention	Evaluation
05.02 Altered conduct/ impulse processes /Coping, ineffective individual	Leigh agrees to become free from cocaine within 48 hours. Leigh will complete detox program.	1. Meet individually with client to discuss consequences of drug-using behavior, e.g., "You are having trouble at work, at home, and with friends. We will work with you on these problems."	Urine "clean" 2 days after admission.

continued

Case Study (Continued)

Nursing Diagnosis (PND-I/NANDA)	Client Care Goals	Nursing Planning/ Intervention	Evaluation
		2. Assign client to daily group therapy and to an individual counselor.	Meets with counselor and attends group according to schedule.
		3. Observe client every half hour; expect drug-seeking behavior. When you notice this, talk about client's feelings, explaining the anxiety and craving will, over time, disappear.	Talks about her feelings, including her anxiety and craving for cocaine. Discusses the problems cocaine has created for her.
01.04.03 Insomnia* /Sleep pattern disturbance	Leigh will sleep 5–6 hours a night after 1 week.	Record sleep activity every 24 hours. Administer medication (often tryptophan) as ordered.	Sleeps 5–6 hours a night. Takes tryptophan (or other medications).
05.05 Altered social interaction* /Social interaction, impaired	Leigh will attend group without leaving the room after 1 week.	Record group attendance and behavior.	Attends group therapy as scheduled and remains seated throughout. If agitated, discusses her feelings.
07.01.02 Altered cardiac circulation* /Cardiac output altered		Monitor and record vital signs q 1 hr × 4 or until stable, then q 4 hr.	
07.04 Altered gastrointestinal processes /Nutrition, altered: less than body requirements	Leigh will become physiologically stable and have no evidence of gastrointestinal upset.		Is physiologically stable. No GI upset.
		Encourage diet as tolerated; monitor food intake.	Eats three meals a day.
		Weigh each week.	Maintains stable weight or gains weight.
05.01.02 Altered verbal communication /Communication, impaired verbal	Leigh will speak clearly and sensibly within 72 hours. She will not mention how wonderful she is, how she will start her own company, or other signs of grandiosity. She will not evidence extreme anger or euphoria when in group or individual treatment or in conversations with others on the unit.	When client is incoherent, ask her to slow down and to repeat again what she was saying. Ask her to discuss some of the problems in her life that she feels are a result of cocaine. When she blames others, get her to focus on herself. When she is angry and agitated, you may say, "I know you have an idea that cocaine could help you now and I know you are suffering, but with hard work on your part, you will get better."	Repeats her statements when requested to do so by nurse. Makes sense. Discusses her own feelings and anxieties and fears.
02.07.01 Delusions			
02.02 Altered judgment /Coping, ineffective individual			
04.02 Altered feeling patterns			

*PND-I diagnosis also in NANDA list.

CASE STUDY: Client with Chronic Alcoholism

Identifying Information

John Mills of 6950 Warden Road is a 54-year-old married civil servant. He is Catholic; has a high school education; and was referred from the Care Unit (a specialty hospital), where he has been for the last thirty days. His therapist's name is J. P. Allen, Ph.D.

Client's Definition of Present Problem, Precipitatory Stresses, Coping Strategies, Goals for Care

"I've had a drinking problem for 15 years. My wife and boss told me if I don't shape up, they'll kick me out of my home and my job. I want to feel better. It's been a living hell. But, I'm not sure I can stop drinking. I've tried before." John describes drinking "to cope with my problems for most of my life." Wants to "stay dry."

History of Present Problem

Fifteen years ago, John's social drinking escalated, and he began binging on the weekends and, later, drinking throughout the week. He drank daily for most of the last three years. He drank "enough to keep a buzz on" and occasionally enough "to pass out." John has long-term problems with work (showing up late, absenteeism, errors on the job). He also has long-term problems with his wife, who "either yells at me or takes care of me." John describes years of her pouring out his hidden liquor and her calling his boss to say John had the flu when he really was "hung over."

Psychiatric History

John has been in and out of AA groups and has seen three different psychiatrists. He has been hospitalized three times for car accidents and injuries due to drinking (a broken leg, ribs, contusions, and a concussion). After the last general hospital admission, he was admitted to the Care Unit for a thirty-day alcohol treatment program.

Family History

Both of John's parents are deceased, and both were alcoholics. One female sibling, age 58, is a recovering alcoholic (has been "dry" for ten years). The family has never been close. John feels he was never really "allowed to be a normal, active child." He reports that his sister cared for him when he was young and was "like my mother."

Social History

John developed normally but always "felt different." He worked every summer and took a full-time job after high school graduation. He enjoyed "drinking buddies" from work, but has never had a close friend he could depend upon. John smokes one pack of cigarettes daily and uses no other drugs. He spends his leisure time watching TV and at bars with friends.

Significant Health History

Cirrhosis of the liver. Malnourished from history of chronic alcoholism. Long history of insomnia.

Current Mental Status

John is well-groomed, clean, and alert. Sensorium is within normal limits. Affect is appropriate, yet apathetic. He appears depressed, and he expresses feelings of self-reproach and guilt for his years of drinking and their effect on others. He speaks slowly yet spontaneously. Motor behavior, thought content, and thought

continued

Case Study (Continued)

processes are within normal limits. Defenses are down in that client recognizes his alcoholism and expresses his fear of not being able to stop drinking. Insight is questionable. He recognizes his problem but is only beginning to be knowledgeable about alcoholism as a disease and about the stresses that cause him to drink.

Other Significant Subjective or Objective Clinical Data

Client is on multivitamins qd and Antabuse qd; no indication of suicide or violence potential.

Nursing Diagnosis (PND-I/ NANDA)

07.06 Altered nutrition processes*
/Nutrition, altered: less than body requirements
01.04.03 Insomnia*
/Sleep pattern disturbance
02.08.03 Altered problem solving
/Thought processes, altered
04.02.05 Fear*
/Fear
04.02.02 Anxiety*
/Anxiety
04.02.07 Guilt
/Spiritual distress
05.05.02 Social isolation/Withdrawal*
/Social isolation
05.03.01 Altered family role
/Coping, ineffective family: disabled

DSM-IIIR Multiaxial Diagnosis

Axis I: 303.90 Alcohol dependence
Axis II: No diagnosis
Axis III: Malnourished, chronic insomnia, alcoholic cirrhosis of liver
Axis IV: Psychosocial stressors: attempting to combat alcoholism
Conjugal: severe marital discord
Occupational: threats of losing job
Financial: threat of losing job
Interpersonal: social isolation
Severity: 5 extreme (a combination of predominately enduring and acute circumstances)
Axis V: Current GAF: 50
Highest GAF past year: 30

Nursing Diagnosis (PND-I/NANDA)	Client Care Goals	Nursing Planning/ Intervention	Evaluation
07.06 Altered nutrition processes* /Nutrition, altered: less than body requirements	John will eat three meals a day, plus snacks, and take vitamins as ordered.	1. Monitor intake of meals and snacks. 2. Offer food/drink q 2 hours; initiate dietary consult to learn food preferences.	Gains 1 or more pounds a week; discusses relationship of alcoholism and malnutrition; discusses a well-balanced diet.

*PND-I diagnosis also in NANDA list.

continued

Case Study (Continued)

Nursing Diagnosis (PND-I/NANDA)	Client Care Goals	Nursing Planning/ Intervention	Evaluation
		3. During individual sessions, offer food or drink.	
		4. In individual meetings and in orientation seminar, discuss the relationship between alcoholism and malnutrition; discuss resultant problems; discuss a well-balanced diet.	
01.04.03 Insomnia* /Sleep pattern disturbance	John will sleep a total of 6 hours a night.	Assess client's typical sleep pattern and what strategies aid sleep, e.g., if client awakens after 2–3 hours of sleep, does reading or warm milk help client return to sleep? Once useful strategies are determined, have client put them into effect.	Sleeps 6 hours per night; uses sleep-inducing strategies nightly.

02.08.03 Altered problem solving /Thought processes, altered	John will not use alcohol. He will attend individual counseling sessions and take Antabuse as ordered. He will attend daily AA meetings. He will call counselor whenever he is anxious, fearful, depressed, or craving a drink.	1. Draw up a contract with the client and have client agree to it and sign it. In the contract, client should agree to:
		  a. Attend AA meetings every night.
		  b. See individual counselor from inpatient unit every week for the first month.
		  c. Take Antabuse and return to physician as scheduled for refill.
		2. Discuss with client that ambivalent feelings are normal but to counteract them he must call assigned counselor and/ or sponsor from AA *whenever* he feels the urge to drink. Client may also write down feelings and experiences
			Remains alcohol and drug free; attends treatment program as contracted; takes Antabuse as prescribed; feels proud for each day of sobriety; feels proud for sticking to contract. Repeats information learned about alcoholism as disease.

continued

Case Study (Continued)

Nursing Diagnosis (PND-I/NANDA)	Client Care Goals	Nursing Planning/ Intervention	Evaluation
		that increase the desire to drink.	
		3. Plan with client other stress-reducing activities, e.g., daily exercise, reading books from AA, etc.	
		4. Help condition client to call counselor and to execute planned strategies when feeling stressed.	
		5. Teach client about alcoholism as a disease with a biochemical basis.	
04.02.05 Fear* /Fear 04.02.02 Anxiety* /Anxiety 04.02.07 Guilt /Spiritual distress	John will discuss feelings at AA meeting and with counselor or sponsor.	1. Explain to client that all alcoholics experience these feelings and that they are worked on at the AA meetings, where clients learn to surrender their problems to "a God of my understanding" and to confess their guilt and pray for help. They also learn to make amends to people after a rigorous moral inventory. 2. Go over the 12-step AA program with client; encourage client to participate in AA and to read AA books. If necessary, help client obtain copies of books. 3. Each week, ask client if and how guilt and self-reproach have changed.	Works the 12-step program of AA; guilt and self-reproach decrease over time; client takes moral inventory and makes amends to selected people.
05.05.02 Social isolation/ withdrawal* /Social isolation	John will go to work. At work, he will eat lunch with one or more people. He will call a friend or acquaintance who does not drink at least once a week.	1. Discuss with client that it is important to stay away from people, places, and things that are associated with drinking: New friends can come from AA, and alcohol should not be available at new activities.	Makes new friends who are in the AA program; feels better about socializing with people at work; begins to attend social events with nondrinkers and enjoys them.

continued

Case Study (Continued)

Nursing Diagnosis (PND-I/NANDA)	Client Care Goals	Nursing Planning/ Intervention	Evaluation
		2. Make it clear to the client that he must develop an entirely new life-style and that this will be difficult and will take time. Encourage client to attend AA activities and educational programs. Church is another useful outlet.	
05.03.01 Altered family role /Coping, ineffective family: disabled	Understand alcoholism as a family disease.	1. Refer to family therapist or, if educationally prepared, work with alcoholic and wife and educate them about the typical alcoholic game (victim, rescuer/ persecutor). 2. Help client and wife see what games they have played and how these games only serve to perpetuate a dysfunctional family system. 3. Teach client new coping strategies such as honesty about self and disease. Help client learn to accept that life is difficult and painful and there is no "quick fix." Help client and wife talk openly with each other about their games.	Wife attends Al-Anon; client attends family therapy if prescribed; correctly recalls information about alcoholism as a family disease; begins to change coping mechanisms (e.g., avoids role of victim, decreases conning and manipulating behaviors); accepts responsibility for self.

they used to do drugs/alcohol is not helpful. The mere sight or smell of paraphernalia or alcohol/drugs is often enough to trigger a relapse. Old ties must be broken; new friends and activities must be pursued.

The two case studies and nursing care plans were chosen because cocaine and alcohol are commonly abused drugs. Short- and long-term interventions are quite different, as evidenced by the nursing care plans. Nursing interventions with other types of substance abuse have differences and similarities. Differences in intervention tend to be medical (e.g., clonidine for opiates; haloperidol for PCP) and symp-

tomatic (e.g., if a client hallucinates, decrease stimulation and point out reality). Similarities in intervention include confrontation strategies, therapeutic strategies, education, long-term self-help groups and emphasis on a total life-style change.

Evaluation/Outcome Criteria

Outcome criteria for substance abusers include sobriety (abstinence from drugs and alcohol, "being clean") and improvement of work, family, and social relationships. Clients become more effective in using new attitudes and behaviors. Better feelings about themselves result. Although the fear of relapse is always present, over time the craving for chemicals diminishes and a new, healthy life-style is established. Chychula (1984, p 24) lists ten criteria that are useful in evaluating the recovery process:

1. Is the client beginning to take responsibility for his or her own actions?
2. Is the abuse pattern decreasing without a dependence on other substances?
3. Is there any indication of increased job stability?
4. Is there improvement in interpersonal relationships with others?
5. Are problem-solving techniques improving?
6. Is the client setting goals and following through?
7. Is the client less impulsive and compulsive?
8. Is the client able to delay gratification?
9. Are stress and anxiety decreasing without the use of chemicals?
10. Is there evidence of increased assertiveness?

Additional questions include:

11. Is the client using community support systems?
12. Is the client engaging in social activities with people who are not substance abusers?

Improvement in these areas is a good indication the client is well on the road to recovery.

Chapter Highlights

- Drug and alcohol abuse are endemic problems in most industrialized countries.
- One segment of the population experiments with drugs or alcohol while another segment attempts to set limits.
- Contemporary explanations of substance abuse derive from biologic, psychologic, sociocultural, and family systems theories.
- Major DSM-IIIR categories of substance use include psychoactive substance–induced organic mental disorders and psychoactive substance use disorders.
- Groups at risk for substance abuse include teenagers, psychiatric clients, women, the elderly, adult children of alcoholics, general hospital clients, and nurses.

- Substance abusers suffer from intoxication and physical and psychologic withdrawal effects.
- To arrive at an accurate nursing diagnosis and design effective nursing interventions, the nurse must make a comprehensive assessment of the substance abuser, focusing on types and amount of substances used and frequency of use.
- Nursing diagnoses for substance abusing clients are gradually being generated.
- After the client is detoxified, effective nursing intervention strategies include education, support groups, writing a contract, and ultimately a change in life-style.
- Evaluation/outcome criteria include improvement in the areas of work, family, and social relationships; increased ability to solve problems and delay gratification; abstinence from all chemicals; increased feeling of well-being; and the use of community services.

References

American Psychiatric Association: *Diagnostic and Statistical Manual of Mental Disorders,* ed 3. APA, 1980.

American Psychiatric Association: *Diagnostic and Statistical Manual of Mental Disorders,* ed 3, revised. APA, 1987.

Becker H: *The Outsiders.* Free Press, 1963.

Belfer M, Strader R, Carroll M et al: Alcoholism in women. *Arch Gen Psychiatry* 1971; 25:540–544.

Bittle S, Feiginbaum J, Kneisl CR: Substance abuse, in Kneisl CR, Ames SA: *Adult Health Nursing: A Biopsychosocial Approach.* Addison-Wesley, 1986, pp 231–268.

Blume S: Women and alcohol. *JAMA* 1986; 256, 11:1467–1470.

Bromocriptine as treatment of cocaine abuse. *Lancet* 1985; May 18: 1151–1152.

Busch D, McBride A, Benaventure L: Chemical dependency in women: The link to Ob/Gyn problems. *J Psychosoc Nurs* 1986; 24:26–30.

Caroselli-Karinja M: Drug abuse and the elderly. *J Psychosoc Nurs* 1985; 23:25–30.

Cherskov M: Chemical dependency a major problem for youths. *American Medical News* 1985; Nov. 8; 29–30.

Chychula N: Screening for substance abuse in a primary care setting. *Nurse Pract* 1984; 9:15–24.

Cocaine: Some questions and answers. The American Council for Drug Education, 1983.

Coleman N: Check . . . Checkmate, Countering the con-games of drug abusers. *Drug Abusers* 1985; 77(Feb. 1):68–74.

Cruz-Coke R, Varela A: Inheritance of alcoholism: Its association with color blindness. *Lancet* 1966; 2:1282–1284.

Elkin M: *Families under the Influence.* W. W. Norton, 1984.

The Family Enablers. Johnson Institute, 1982.

Finley B: Primary and secondary prevention of substance abuse in nurses. *Occup Health Nurs* 1982; 30:14–18.

Franks L: A new attack on alcoholism. *The New York Times Magazine* 1985; November: 47–69.

Friel J, Sebby R, Friel L: Co-dependency and the search for identity: A paradoxical crisis. Health Communications, 1984.

Gallagher W: Pandora's pharmacy. *This World.* August 31, 1986; 7–9.

Gianelli D: Very addictive, appealing to youth, crack poses major health worries. *Am Med News* 1986; September 12, 1986.

Green P: The impaired nurse: chemical dependency. *J Emergency Nursing* 1984; 10(1):23–26.

Hutchinson S: Chemically dependent nurses: The trajectory towards self-annihilation. *Nurs Res* 1986; 35:196–201.

Jellinek E: *Phases in the Drinking History of Alcoholics.* Hillhouse Press, 1946.

Jones B, Jones M: Male and female intoxication levels for three alcohol dosages, or do women really get higher than men? *Alcohol Technical Report* 1976; 5:11–14.

Jones B, Jones M, Paredes A: Oral contraceptives and ethanol metabolism. *Alcohol Technical Report* 1976; 5:28–32.

Kaplan H, Sadock B (eds): *Comprehensive Textbook of Psychiatry,* ed 4. Williams and Wilkins, 1985.

Klein J: The new drug they call "ecstasy." *New York* 1985; May 20:38–43.

Kneisl CR, Ames SA: *Adult Health Nursing.* Addison-Wesley, 1986.

Koop D, Morgan E, Taer G, Coon M: Purification and characterization of a unique isozyme of cytochrome P-450 from liver microsomes of ethanol-treated rabbits. *J Biol Chem* 1982; 257:8472–8480.

Landry M, Smith DE: Crack: Anatomy of an addiction. *California Nursing Review.* 1987; March/April: 8–36.

Lieber C, DeCarli L: Hepatic microsomal ethanol oxidizing system: In vitro characteristics and adaptive properties in vivo. *J Biol Chem* 1970; 245:2505–2512.

Lindesmith A: *Opiate Addiction.* University of Indiana Press, 1965.

Mann G: *The Dynamics of Addiction.* Johnson Institute, 1983.

Marohn R: Adolescent substance abuse: A problem of self-soothing. *Adolesc Psychiatry* 1983; 1:2–11.

Naegle M: The nurse and the alcoholic: Redefining a historically ambivalent relationship. *J Psychiatr Nurs* 1983; 21:17–24.

Naegle M: Creative management of impaired nursing practice. *Nurs Adm Q* 1985; 9:16–26.

National Federation of Drug Free Youth, 1982.

Newton M: *Gone Way Down.* American Studies Press, 1981.

Pallikkathayil L, Tweed S: Substance abuse: Alcohol and drugs during adolescence. *Nurs Clin North Am* 1983; 18:313–321.

Pratt O: Alcohol and the woman of childbearing age: A public health problem. *Br J Addict* 1981; 76:383–390.

Rottenberg R: Cocaine: chic, costly, and what else? *The Care Medic* 1980; 1–8.

Royce, JE: *Alcohol Problems and Alcoholism: A Comprehensive Survey.* Free Press, 1981.

Schloemer N, Skidmore J: Opiate withdrawal with clonidine. *J Psychiatr Nurs* 1983; 21:9–14.

Schuckit M: Genetics and the risk for alcoholism. *JAMA* 1985; 254:2614–2617.

Solari-Twadell P: *The Multiple Roles of a Nurse in a Comprehensive Level of Care System for Alcoholic Patients.* Gateway Community Services, 1983.

Stanton M, Todd T: *Family Therapy of Drug Abuse and Addiction.* Guilford Press, 1982.

Trenk B: Biochemical abnormalities can be linked to suicide. *American Medical News* 1986; Jan 17:11.

Ugarte G, Perida I, Pino M, Iturriaga: Influence of alcohol intake, length of abstinence and meprobomate on the rate of ethanol metabolism in men. *Q J Stud Alcohol* 1972; 33:698–705.

Varela A, Rivera L, Mardones J, Cruz-Coke R: Color vision defects in nonalcoholic relatives of alcoholic parents. *Br J Addict* 1969; 64:67.

What parents must learn about teens and alcohol. National Federation of Parents for Drug Free Youths.

SEVENTEEN

Applying the Nursing Process for
Clients with Schizophrenia and Other Psychotic Disorders

Catherine Chesla

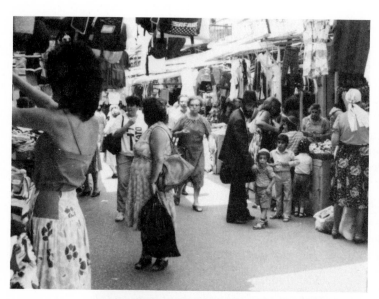

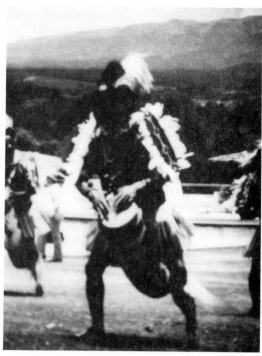

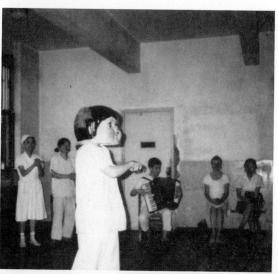

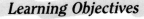

Learning Objectives

After reading this chapter, students should be able to

- Describe historical antecedents to the current treatment of schizophrenia

- Describe several competing theoretical explanations of schizophrenia

- Recognize the DSM-IIIR criteria for the diagnosis of schizophrenia

- Recognize key criteria that differentiate the schizophrenic disorders from other psychotic disorders

- Assess individual and family problems of clients diagnosed with schizophrenia

- Identify nursing diagnoses for clients who have schizophrenic disorders

- Construct nursing interventions appropriate for clients who have schizophrenic disorders and are treated in in-patient settings

- Evaluate the effectiveness of nursing interventions with the individual schizophrenic client and the family

Cross References

Other topics related to this chapter are: Biologic therapies, Chapter 32; Chronically mentally ill, Chapter 22; Communication, Chapter 11; Community mental health, Chapter 40; Family, Chapter 33; Psychobiology, Chapter 9; Social Support, Chapter 8.

Key Terms

ambivalence
anhedonia
apathy
bizarre delusion
blunted affect
brief reactive psychosis
catatonia
circumstantial communication
delusion
delusional disorder
dementia praecox
dopamine (DA) hypothesis
disengagement
enmeshment
expressed emotion

flat affect
hallucination
illusion
inappropriate affect
induced psychotic disorder
loose associations
magical thinking
schizoaffective disorder
schizophreniform disorder
tangential communication
thought blocking
thought broadcasting
thought insertion
thought withdrawal
type I schizophrenia
type II schizophrenia

HISTORICAL AND THEORETICAL FOUNDATIONS

Descriptive Psychiatry

The work of Kraepelin and Bleuler advanced the understanding of schizophrenia as a disease entity. Kraepelin began to describe the syndrome of schizophrenia, which he labeled dementia praecox, or early senility. He believed the syndrome was caused by an organic abnormality, was degenerative, and always ended in a state of disorganization that today would be called *psychosis*. Bleuler, who used the term *schizophrenia*, refined Kraepelin's descriptive picture of the illness. Bleuler attempted a psychologic explanation of schizophrenic symptoms but remained undecided whether the illness was organic or psychologic. Unlike Kraepelin, Bleuler believed that there were many possible courses and outcomes of the disease.

Psychoanalytic Therapies

Successful analytic work with schizophrenics by Sullivan and Fromm-Reichmann challenged earlier beliefs that schizophrenia could not be treated. By focusing on interpersonal relations, particularly from early childhood, these therapists attempted to understand and interpret the schizophrenic's symptoms. Their work represented a departure from Freud's belief that schizophrenics could not form a

Imagine a comprehensive test ban and antiballistic missile treaty.

therapeutic relationship and therefore could not be treated using analytic techniques. They claimed, as do their followers, that schizophrenic symptoms can be diminished through careful in-depth interpretive work. The effectiveness of insight-oriented therapies with schizophrenics continues to be debated today (Karon and Vandenbos 1981).

Somatic Therapies

Somatic treatments—e.g., insulin coma; drug or electrically induced shock treatments; and psychosurgery, including prefrontal lobotomies—were used in the 1930s. Many hoped these treatments were the long sought-after cure for schizophrenia because they were relatively quick and inexpensive treatments when compared with the analytic therapies. This hope was not realized.

Psychopharmacologic Treatments

The introduction of psychoactive drugs in the 1950s provided new alternatives for the treatment of schizophrenia. Psychotropic medications, which influence the thoughts, mood, and behavior of clients, made previously uncontrolled symptoms manageable. In the period following the introduction of psychotropic medications, the use of seclusion and restraints declined dramatically, as did the duration of hospital stays and numbers of clients in state hospitals.

A new optimism arose regarding the possible outcomes of mental illness. Because they controlled the most difficult symptoms of psychosis, psychotropic medications made psychosocial or behavioral treatments possible for a much greater percentage of psychiatric clients. Tranquilizing drugs did not live up to their promise of providing a cure for schizophrenia and other chronic psychiatric illnesses. However, these drugs relieved the most debilitating symptoms for many clients and were the beginning step toward recovery or a higher level of functioning.

Community Mental Health

Following the recommendations of the Joint Commission on Mental Health in 1961, Congress enacted legislation to establish a system of community-based mental health centers devoted to treating and preventing mental illness. New services established were community-based outpatient, day treatment, and crisis programs.

In the mid-1970s priority was given to the care of the chronically mentally ill in a federally funded Community Support Program. The aim of this program was to supplement natural helping networks in supporting the chronically mentally ill in the community. In addition to the traditional mental health services, psychosocial rehabilitation, residential services, assistance in securing medical and financial support, and backup support for families were called for.

Biologic Theories of Schizophrenia

It is unlikely that schizophrenia is caused by a specific biologic abnormality. Scientists have searched unsuccessfully for a unique biologic marker that is consistently found in schizophrenics and not found in healthy persons. At the same time, scientific evidence suggests that the disorder is not merely psychologic and that biologic alterations are present. Particularly convincing is the fact that the symptoms associated with schizophrenia, such as delusions or hallucinations, are found in normal persons only when they are in a state of metabolic imbalance or suffer from organic diseases. Persons with brain tumors, or who have ingested certain drugs, for example, may experience hallucinations (Liberman et al. 1984).

Genetic Theories

Schizophrenics inherit a genetic vulnerability for the disease rather than the disease itself. Evidence supporting this thesis is the fact that relatives of schizophrenics have a greater chance of developing the disease than the general population do. One percent of the population develops schizophrenia, while 10 percent of the first-degree relatives (parents, siblings, children) of schizophrenics are diagnosed with the disease during their lifetimes. The risk of developing schizophrenia increases with the closeness of relation with a diagnosed schizophrenic. Siblings of schizophrenics have a greater risk of developing the disease than do half-siblings or grandchildren, and these have a greater risk than more distant relatives, such as cousins.

Twin studies indicate that both environmental and genetic factors are important in schizophrenia. Concordance rates (both twins either express or do not express the trait) for schizophrenia are consistently higher for monozygotic twins than for dizygotic twins. This finding supports the hypothesis of genetic transmission. However, concordance rates for monozygotic twins is in the range of 35 to 58 percent, indicating that environment plays a large part in the expression of the illness. If the disease were solely genetically determined, the concordance rates in this group would be close to 100 percent (Liberman et al. 1984).

Biochemical Theories

Investigators believed that the biochemical basis of schizophrenia might be uncovered by studying the biochemical actions of drugs that reduce schizophrenic symptoms. The dopamine (DA) hypothesis is the most widely held and extensively studied biochemical mechanism thought to underlie schizophrenia.

In simplified form, the DA hypothesis is that schizophrenia may be related to overactive neuronal activity that is dependent on DA. The hypothesis is supported by pharmacologic research demonstrating that drugs that increase DA activity worsen schizophrenic symptoms and drugs that decrease DA activity alleviate symptoms. Two classes of drugs used most frequently in the treatment of schizophrenia, the phenothiazines (e.g., Thorazine) and the butyrophenones (e.g., Haldol), have been extensively studied. Although these drugs are chemically quite different, both block DA receptors. The extent to which they block DA is related to their clinical effectiveness. In addition, drugs within each of these classes of drugs that are chemically similar, yet do not block DA receptors, have little effect on schizophrenic symptoms (Shapiro 1981).

The cause of excessive DA activity in schizophrenics is not yet known, nor can we conclude that schizophrenia is caused by DA excesses. Biochemical states are influenced by the individual's genetic makeup and by such environmental factors as stress, nutrition, and exposure to viruses. There are many theories about the biologic mechanisms that lead to excessive DA, but none has been adequately tested to receive widespread approval.

Structural Alterations in Schizophrenia

Ventricular size has been found to be significantly larger in chronic schizophrenic clients than in control groups (Liberman et al. 1984). Computer tomography (CT), safer and less invasive than prior tests, has allowed researchers to study this abnormality. It is now believed that schizophrenics with enlarged ventricles may be a subgroup of all schizophrenics, who have similar biologic abnormalities and clinical pictures. For example, schizophrenics with enlarged ventricles have a poorer therapeutic response to antipsychotic drugs than those in a matched group of schizophrenics who do not show enlarged ventricles. Enlarged ventricles are also associated with poor performance on pyschologic tests.

Crow (1980) suggests that there are two types of schizophrenia, each with unique biologic abnormalities and clinical courses. **Type I schizophrenia** is characterized by *positive symptoms* of schizophrenia: hallucinations, delusions, and thought disorder. Type I schizophrenia is thought to be associated with the biologic abnormality of increased dopamine receptors. Its onset is acute, and it responds well to psychotropic medications. **Type II schizophrenia** is characterized by the *negative symptoms* of the disease: flattening of affect, loss of motivation, and poverty of speech. Type II schizophrenia shows little response to treatment with drugs.

Psychologic Theories of Schizophrenia

Information Processing

Many schizophrenic clients have information-processing deficits (Liberman et al. 1984). Two central types of information processing have been identified: (a) automatic and (b) controlled or effortful processing. Automatic processing is the taking in of information unintentionally. Automatic processing can occur without the individual's being aware of it, and it does not interfere with conscious thought processes occurring at the same time. Examples of automatic information processing are the initial awareness and coding of physical features of a new environment.

Schizophrenics are deficient in controlled information processing. Their ability to perform directed, conscious, sequential thinking—e.g., making comparisons between two stimuli or organizing a set of stimuli—is consistently inferior to that of nonschizophrenics.

We do not know whether the schizophrenic's inability to sustain conscious, directed thought is the primary problem or the result of a primary deficit in automatic thinking. If the primary deficit is in automatic processes, then the schizophrenic is forced to complete automatic tasks at the conscious level, inhibiting and slowing controlled information processing. Sufficient evidence to resolve this question is not yet available.

Attention and Arousal

Physiologic studies of attention and arousal in schizophrenics show promise of identifying clinically significant subgroups. Arousal and attention are measured by physiologic states and alterations, e.g., galvanic skin response, heart rate, blood pressure, skin temperature, or pupillary response. One subgroup of clients exhibits abnormally low response levels to novel stimuli. This finding suggests that these clients are less adept than normal persons at attending and responding to novel situations. Liberman et al. (1984) note that the 40 to 50 percent of schizophrenics who demonstrate this attention abnormality present clinical symptoms similar to those identified by Crow as type II schizophrenia.

A second subgroup of schizophrenics demonstrates a state of hyperarousal evidenced by elevated electrodermal activity, heart rate, and blood pressure. Hyperarousal has been noted in schizophrenics during both symptomatic and nonsymptomatic periods. Clinically, this subgroup has characteristics of Crow's type I schizophrenia. They demonstrate symptoms of irritability, excitement, and anxiety rather than apathy and withdrawal.

Family Theories of Schizophrenia

Numerous theories have been put forth implicating family interaction as a cause of schizophrenia. Terms that represent these theories include schizophrenogenic mothers, double-binds, and pseudomutuality. Research has failed to support the theory that dysfunctional family interaction causes the illness (Falloon et al. 1984).

Wynne (1981) suggests that disordered family communication causes schizophrenia only in the presence of a genetic vulnerability to the disease. A communication problem evident in some families of schizophrenics is the inability to focus on and clearly share an observation or thought. Living with this pattern of family communication during early development is thought to impair the schizophrenic's ability to perceive the environment and communicate with others about it.

A second theory is that the family's emotional tone can influence the course of schizophrenia over time (Falloon et al. 1984). Researchers found that schizophrenics who come from families who are highly critical, hostile, or overinvolved tend to relapse more often than those from families who do not demonstrate these characteristics. Families who demonstrate these characteristics have been described as having high **expressed emotion**. There is some evidence that family expressed emotion may be an influence on, rather than a response to, the illness, but this evidence is not definitive.

Humanist-Interactional Understandings of Schizophrenia

An interactional model of schizophrenia integrates many of the biologic and social theories already discussed. In this view, schizophrenia is due to the interaction of a biologic vulnerability, stress or change in the environment, and the individual's social skills and supports (Liberman et al. 1984). In an interactional model, the influences are multidirectional. Great biologic vulnerability may inhibit the individual's capacity to cope with even minor stressors. Loss of a primary source of support might trigger decreased

functioning in the schizophrenic. Similarly, the schizophrenic might grow worse upon entering an environment that demands coping skills he or she has not developed.

Figure 17–1 shows a schematic representation of an interactional model. This model depicts the biologic, behavioral, and environmental domains of variables that influence the disorder. Three time dimensions are also depicted: enduring vulnerability characteristics, more transient states, and outcomes for each domain.

Enduring vulnerability characteristics in the biologic realm include the genetic and biochemical defects already described. Enduring behavioral deficits include poor relationship skills, lack of motivation, and inability to perform productively at work or school. It is theorized that the environment of schizophrenics characteristically provides poor opportunities for learning. An example of a poor learning environment is the family milieu in which parents provide inaccurate or incomplete descriptors of the world, as described in the communication deviance theories.

According to the interactional theory, events in the schizophrenic's life are played out on this biologic, behavioral, and environmental stage. Disablement is the result of a balance or imbalance that develops as changes occur in each of the three domains. Stressors and life events constitute the changes in the schizophrenic's environment. Fluctuations in the schizophrenic's coping skills and problem-solving abilities comprise the behavioral changes. Neurotransmitter and neuroendocrine abnormalities as well as alterations in arousal and attention are the biologic changes thought to affect the schizophrenic's level of functioning.

The interactional theorists propose that disability may develop because of changes in any domain interacting with response or lack of response in any other domain. The two following examples illustrate this multidirectionality of causation.

Daryl, a 26-year-old with a diagnosis of paranoid schizophrenia, decided to stop taking his Haldol because it made him feel heavy and too tired to get up in the morning. Within a few days of stopping the medication, he was unable to leave the house for fear of someone harming him. Although he liked his unpaid job at the local cannery and knew that he had the chance to earn money in the near future, he refused to go to work for fear that he would be hit by a bus on his way there. He was eventually fired because of poor attendance. In this instance, a decrease in medication increased biologic vulnerability with marked behavioral and eventually environmental consequences.

Jean, 22, had lived with her divorced mother and younger sister Mary since her release from the hospital after her second psychotic episode. She found living alone too frightening and was more comfortable staying in her old room at home. When Mary began pre-

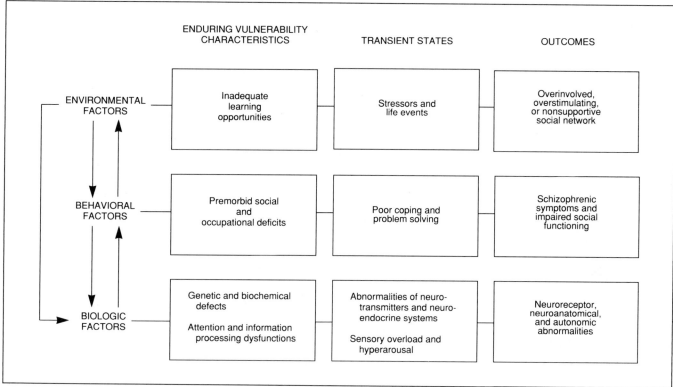

Figure 17–1

An interactional model for schizophrenia.

Source: Liberman RP, et al: The nature and problem of schizophrenia, in Bellack AS (ed): Schizophrenia, Treatment, Management and Rehabilitation. *Grune & Stratton, 1984, p 4.*

paring to leave home for college, Jean became increasingly anxious, demanding to sleep in Mary's room at night and hiding Mary's belongings. As Mary's departure drew near, Jean began actively hallucinating and withdrew to her room, refusing to talk to her mother or sister. In this case, the client did not have sufficient coping skills to deal with her sister's departure from the household, and the client retreated into psychosis.

PSYCHOPATHOLOGY

Diagnostic Criteria for Schizophrenia

In the most recent revision of the third edition of the *Diagnostic and Statistical Manual of Mental Disorders* (DSM-IIIR), the American Psychiatric Association (APA) made minor changes in the behavioral indicators that must be present to justify a diagnosis of schizophrenia. The criteria, including the changes, are specified in Box 17–1.

Five types of schizophrenia are specified in DSM-IIIR. Each type of schizophrenia is characterized by a set of predominant symptoms. The types of schizophrenia are labeled

- Paranoid
- Catatonic
- Disorganized
- Undifferentiated
- Residual

Clinical features of each subtype of the disorder are listed in Box 17–2.

The course of the illness varies from client to client, and thus the APA has specified five courses of the illness: chronic, subchronic, chronic with acute exacerbation, subchronic with acute exacerbation, or in remission. The DSM-IIIR indicators of the illness course are found in Box 17–3.

Box 17–1
DSM-IIIR DIAGNOSTIC CRITERIA
FOR SCHIZOPHRENIA

A. Presence of characteristic psychotic symptoms in the active phase: either (1), (2), or (3) for at least one week (unless the symptoms are successfully treated):

  1. Two of the following:

    a. Delusions

    b. Prominent hallucinations (throughout the day for several days or several times a week for several weeks, each hallucinatory experience not being limited to a few brief moments)

    c. Incoherence or marked loosening of associations

    d. Catatonic behavior

    e. Flat or grossly inappropriate affect

  2. Bizarre delusions (i.e., involving a phenomenon that the person's culture would regard as totally implausible, e.g., thought broadcasting, being controlled by a dead person)

  3. Prominent hallucinations [as defined in 1.b above] of a voice with content having no apparent relation to depression or elation, or a voice keeping up a running commentary on the person's behavior or thoughts, or two or more voices conversing with each other

B. During the course of the disturbance, functioning in such areas as work, social relations, and self-care is markedly below the highest level achieved before onset of the disturbance (or, when the onset is in childhood or adolescence, failure to achieve expected level of social development).

C. Schizoaffective disorder and mood disorder with psychotic features have been ruled out, i.e., if a major depressive or manic syndrome has ever been present during an active phase of the disturbance, the total duration of all episodes of a mood syndrome has been brief relative to the total duration of the active and residual phases of the disturbance.

D. Continuous signs of the disturbance for at least six months. The six-month period must include an active phase (of at least one week or less if symptoms have been successfully treated) during which there were psychotic symptoms characteristic of schizophrenia (symptoms in A), with or without a prodromal or residual phase, as defined below.

Prodromal phase: A clear deterioration in functioning before the active phase of the disturbance that is not due to a disturbance in mood or to a psychoactive substance use disorder and that involves at least two of the symptoms listed below.

Residual phase: Following the active phase of the disturbance, persistence of at least two of the symptoms noted below, these not being due to a disturbance in mood or to a psychoactive substance use disorder.

Prodromal or Residual Symptoms:

1. Marked social isolation or withdrawal

2. Marked impairment in role functioning as wage-earner, student, or homemaker

3. Markedly peculiar behavior (e.g., collecting garbage, talking to self in public, hoarding food)

4. Marked impairment in personal hygiene and grooming

5. Blunted or inappropriate affect

6. Digressive, vague, overelaborate, or circumstantial speech, or poverty of speech, or poverty of content of speech

7. Odd beliefs or magical thinking, influencing behavior and inconsistent with cultural norms, e.g., superstitiousness, belief in clairvoyance, telepathy, "sixth sense," "others can feel my feelings," overvalued ideas, ideas of reference

8. Unusual perceptual experiences, e.g., recurrent illusions, sensing the presence of a force or person not actually present

9. Marked lack of initiative, interests, or energy

Examples: Six months of prodromal symptoms with one week of symptoms from A; no prodromal symptoms with six months of symptoms from A; no prodromal symptoms with one week of symptoms from A and six months of residual symptoms.

E. It cannot be established that an organic factor initiated and maintained the disturbance.

F. If there is a history of autistic disorder, the additional diagnosis of schizophrenia is made only if prominent delusions or hallucinations are also present.

Source: American Psychiatric Association: Diagnostic and Statistical Manual of Mental Disorders, *ed 3, revised. APA, 1987.*

Planning care for individual clients requires diagnostic precision because interventions for clients with schizophrenic disorders differ from those for persons with other psychotic disorders. Two categories of psychotic disorders other than schizophrenia are specified in DSM-IIIR: delusional disorders, and psychotic disorders not elsewhere classified.

Delusional Disorders

Clients with **delusional disorders** are similar to schizophrenic clients because they hold unusual or bizarre beliefs and cannot be reasoned with regarding these beliefs. Unlike schizophrenic clients, delusional clients do not have persistent hallucinations and exhibit few or any of the other features of schizophrenia—e.g., flat or inappropriate affect, social withdrawal or isolation, and inability to care for themselves. The content of the delusions varies. For example, some delusional clients believe that they are being persecuted. Others may think they have special knowledge or powers, have a physical disorder, or are loved by a famous public figure.

Psychotic Disorders Not Elsewhere Classified

Psychotic disorders not elsewhere classified is a category of diagnoses for clients who present with psychotic features yet do not fully exhibit characteristics of the schizophrenic, delusional, or major mood disorders. Four disorders that fall in this category are:

1. Schizophreniform disorder
2. Schizoaffective disorder
3. Brief reactive psychosis
4. Induced psychotic disorder

General clinical features that differentiate delusional disorders and other psychotic disorders from schizophrenia

---

Box 17–2
DIAGNOSTIC CRITERIA FOR FIVE TYPES OF SCHIZOPHRENIA

Catatonic Type

1. Catatonic stupor (marked decrease in reactivity to the environment and/or reduction in spontaneous movements and activity) or mutism.
2. Catatonic negativism (an apparently motiveless resistance to all instructions or attempts to be moved).
3. Catatonic rigidity (maintenance of a rigid posture against efforts to be moved).
4. Catatonic excitement (excited motor activity, apparently purposeless and not influenced by external stimuli).
5. Catatonic posturing (voluntary assumption of inappropriate or bizarre postures).

Disorganized Type

1. Incoherence, marked loosening of associations, or grossly disorganized behavior.
2. Flat or grossly inappropriate affect.
3. Does not meet the criteria for catatonic type.

Paranoid Type

1. Preoccupation with one or more systematized delusions or with frequent auditory hallucinations related to a single theme.
2. None of the following: incoherence, marked loosening of associations, flat or grossly inappropriate affect, catatonic behavior, grossly disorganized behavior.

Undifferentiated Type

1. Prominent delusions, hallucinations, incoherence, or grossly disorganized behavior.
2. Does not meet the criteria for paranoid, catatonic, or disorganized type.

Residual Type

1. Absence of prominent delusions, hallucinations, incoherence, or grossly disorganized behavior.
2. Continuing evidence of the disturbance, as indicated by two or more of the residual symptoms listed in criterion D of schizophrenia (see Box 17–1).

Source: American Psychiatric Association: Diagnostic and Statistical Manual of Mental Disorders, *ed 3, revised. APA, 1987.*

Box 17–3
CRITERIA FOR CLASSIFICATION OF THE COURSE OF SCHIZOPHRENIA

1-Subchronic The time from the beginning of the disturbance, when the person first began to show signs of the disturbance (including prodromal, active, and residual phases) more or less continuously, is less than two years, but at least six months.

2-Chronic Same as above, but more than two years.

3-Subchronic with Acute Exacerbation Reemergence of prominent psychotic symptoms in a person with a subchronic course who has been in the residual phase of the disturbance.

4-Chronic with Acute Exacerbation Reemergence of prominent psychotic symptoms in a person with a chronic course who has been in the residual phase of the disturbance.

5-In Remission When a person with a history of schizophrenia is free of all signs of the disturbance (whether or not on medication), "in remission" should be coded. Differentiating "schizophrenia in remission" from no mental disorder requires consideration of overall level of functioning, length of time since the last episode of disturbance, total duration of the disturbance, and whether prophylactic treatment is being given.

0-Unspecified

Source: American Psychiatric Association: Diagnostic and Statistical Manual of Mental Disorders, *ed 3, revised. APA, 1987.*

are specified in Table 17–1. The nurse should consult DSM-IIIR for a complete description of criteria used to differentiate these disorders.

THE NURSING PROCESS AND CLIENTS WITH SCHIZOPHRENA

Assessment

Assessment of clients who have schizophrenia occurs at the individual, family, and environmental level. The nurse must be aware of the client's status and of changes in the client's personal life, family situation, and environment to plan care and intervene effectively. Additionally, care that

addresses multiple levels of the client's life is consistent with the interactional theory of schizophrenia because it is assumed that changes in any aspect of the schizophrenic's person or environment influence all other aspects of the personal environment balance.

Perceptual Changes

The perceptions of clients with schizophrenia may be either heightened or blunted. These changes may occur in all the senses, or in just one or two. For example, a client may see colors as brighter than normal or may be acutely sensitive to sounds. Another may have a heightened sense of touch and therefore be extremely sensitive to any physical contact.

Illusions occur when the client misperceives or exaggerates stimuli in the external environment. A schizophrenic client may mistake a chair for a person or perceive that the walls of a hallway are closing in. The perceptual changes are sufficient to cause the client to mistake the stimulus for something that it is not.

Hallucinations are the most extreme and yet the most common perceptual disturbance in schizophrenia. A **hallucination** is a subjective perception of something that does not exist in the external environment. Hallucinations can be visual, olfactory (smell), gustatory (taste), tactile (feel), or auditory. Auditory hallucinations are the most common. Although hallucinations are a hallmark of schizophrenia, their presence alone does not establish the presence of the disorder. Table 17–2 lists various types of hallucinations along with a disease process commonly associated with the symptom.

Nurses assess perceptual disturbances by asking the client about the experience and by observing for behaviors that indicate the client is frightened or attending to internal stimuli. The nurse asks the client to describe what he or she is experiencing and notes the degree to which this description differs from the nurse's perceptions of the environment.

Clients may be reluctant to discuss the extreme perceptual disturbance of hallucinations. A classic sign of auditory hallucinations is placing the hands over the ears. The client is frightened by the perception and tries to block it out. Less obvious signs of hallucinations are inappropriate laughing or smiling, difficulty following a conversation, or difficulty attending to what is happening at the moment. Fleeting, rapid changes of expression that are not precipitated by events in the real world can be a further sign. Finally, clients may talk to themselves, presumably in answer to the voices they hear.

Disturbances in Thought

Clients with schizophrenia find their thinking is muddled or unclear. Their thoughts are disconnected or disjointed, and the connections between one thought and another are vague, a characteristic called **loosening of associations**. When the associations between thoughts are based on the sounds of words rather than their meanings, the client is making *clang associations*, e.g., "I'm great (grate) like in the sewer (sue her), and I'll see you in court."

Schizophrenic clients also have difficulty thinking abstractly. Their responses may be inappropriate because they interpret words literally rather than abstractly. For example, when told to prepare to have his blood drawn, a young man readied some paper and marking pens. Abstract thinking can be assessed by asking clients the meaning of proverbs, a test requiring the client to abstract a general meaning from a specific or metaphysical statement, e.g., "People who live in glass houses shouldn't throw stones."

A disturbance in the content rather than the form of thought is a delusion. **Delusions** are fixed false beliefs about oneself, one's environment, or events occurring in it. A belief is delusional when it cannot be consensually validated. That is, persons who surround the delusional person cannot agree with or validate his or her belief.

Delusions vary in type and complexity. Table 17–3 describes several types of delusions frequently experienced by schizophrenics, including persecution, somatic, and control delusions. Delusions can be simple beliefs, relating to only a small part of the person's daily life, or highly complex systems of belief.

Changes in Communication

Clients with schizophrenia frequently have difficulty responding appropriately to events and people they encounter. The difficulties arise because of the schizophrenic's distorted perceptions, impaired ability to sort and assimilate these perceptions, and difficulty communicating his or her response clearly.

The clarity of the client's communication often reflects his or her level of thought disorganization. Client's responses may be simply inappropriate to the situation or conversation. They may have difficulties articulating a response or stop mid-sentence, as if they are stuck, a sign of **thought blocking**.

Nurses should note the rate and quality of client's speech. Is it unusually loud, insistent, and continuous? Does the client wander from topic to topic (**tangential communication**) or bring up details that are irrelevant to the topic at hand (**circumstantial communication**)? Are the client's responses slow and hesitant, reflecting difficulty in taking in stimuli and responding?

Disruptions in Emotional Responses

Tone of voice, rate of speech, content of speech, expressions, postures, and body movements indicate emotional tone. Disturbances in emotions commonly seen in schizophrenia are a restricted expression or inappropriate expression of emotions. Observe whether the client expresses

---

Table 17–1
Discriminating Criteria for Delusional and Other Psychotic Disorders

Delusional Disorders	Other Psychotic Disorders Not Elsewhere Classified
Clinically similar to schizophrenia only because of the presence of delusions. Differences include:	Clinical picture is very similar to schizophrenia, but one or more of the essential diagnostic criteria are not met. For example:
a. Delusions have a basis in reality.	a. Schizophreniform disorder: The duration of all symptoms (acute and residual) is less than six months and a return to normal functioning is possible.
b. Hallucinations are not a dominant feature.	b. Schizoaffective disorder: Dominant schizophrenic symptoms are accompanied at some, but not all times by a major depressive or manic syndrome.
c. Behavior is within normal range except in relation to the delusion.	c. Brief reactive psychosis: Psychotic symptoms appear shortly after a stressful event or series of events. Duration of symptoms is one month or less, with recovery to normal level of function.
d. Behavior does not meet the criteria for schizophrenia, i.e., catatonia, affective abnormalities, and loosening of associations are not present.	d. Induced psychotic disorder: A delusional system develops because of a close relationship with a person who already has a psychotic disorder with delusions. The second person to develop delusions receives this diagnosis.

Source: Adapted from American Psychiatric Association: Diagnostic and Statistical Manual of Mental Disorders, *ed 3, revised. APA, 1987.*

emotion that does not match what he or she is saying. For example, he or she may laugh when describing a frightening or sad incident. Additionally, lack of expressed emotion is often indicative of schizophrenia.

Motor Behavior Changes

Disruptions seen in schizophrenia include disorganized behavior and **catatonia**. Disorganized behavior lacks a coherent goal, is aimless, or is disruptive. Catatonic behavior is manifested by unusual body movement or lack of movement. This activity disturbance includes *catatonic excitement* (the client moves excitedly but not in response to environmental influences), *catatonic posturing* (the client holds bizarre postures for periods of time), and *stupor* (the client holds the body still and is unresponsive to the environment).

Changes in Role Functioning

An important factor in predicting the course of schizophrenia is the client's level of functioning before the symptoms of the disease became pronounced. Assessment should therefore include a complete history of the client's success at completing developmental tasks. The prognosis is best if the client functioned at a high level prior to the onset of schizophrenic disturbance. Nurses should assess how well the client fulfilled role responsibilities in the family, in school, in relation to peers, and in work. Nurses should obtain a history of the rate of decline in these various roles. The onset of schizophrenia may be relatively acute, or degeneration may be slow.

Drug Use

Clients with drug toxicity or withdrawal may present with behavior disturbances similar to those seen in schizophrenics. These clients may have auditory or visual hallucinations and may be confused, illogical, and highly anxious. For this reason, it is essential to obtain a detailed drug history. Both long-term and recent use of chemical substances must be assessed. If the client is not a reliable historian, family or friends should be interviewed. In addition, both blood and urine should be tested for drugs if reliable information cannot be obtained.

Family Health History

Part of assessment is noting any history of mental illness in the client's family. Of particular interest is a history of schizophrenia or any thought disorder, mood disorders (e.g., cyclical highs or depressions), or alcoholism in any family member. Any report that family members had "nervous breakdowns" or any other colloquial descriptions of mental or emotional disorders should be noted.

Family Cohesion and Emotion

A moderate level of family cohesion is optimal according to many family theorists (Olson et al. 1983). The two extremes—lack of cohesion (disengagement) and too much cohesion (enmeshment)—signify problems in family functioning. In families of schizophrenics, enmeshment, combined with a negative emotional tone, is thought to be detrimental to the ill member's well-being. Schizophrenics from overinvolved families who criticize the client have a high relapse rate (Falloon et al. 1984).

Much of the nursing assessment of families can be carried out unobtrusively. Levels of cohesion can be assessed by noting who accompanies the client when he or she is admitted. Is it the whole family or just one member? Does

Table 17–2 Disturbances in Perception		
Type of Hallucination	Commonly Associated Disease Process	Example
Auditory	Schizophrenia	Hearing voices of family members who aren't present
Visual	Acute organic brain syndrome	Seeing animals walking across the walls of the room
Tactile	Acute alcohol withdrawal	Feeling bugs crawl on the skin
Olfactory	Seizure disorders	Smelling foods that aren't present
Gustatory	Seizure disorders	Tasting a sharp sweet taste on the tongue, in the absence of food
Somatic	Schizophrenia	Sensing that one's head has a tunnel running through it

the client come in alone? Visits from family are a rich source of information. Who visits, how often, and for how long? How do family visitors behave with the client? Do the members spend time interacting and sharing activities, do they sit quietly together, or do they maintain physical and emotional distance from one another? Nurses document these patterns of family interactions and additionally monitor the effect of family visits on the client.

Formal family assessment interviews can be arranged by the nursing staff, in conjunction with the interdisciplinary team. In this forum, family history and current functioning can be completely assessed. Nurses should not overlook natural opportunities to assess families and their needs. During visits, the nurse can join the family for a few minutes to learn their understanding of the program, their concerns, and their questions. Establishing a trusting relationship with key members of the client's family is essential for establishing a flow of information and for planning care.

Family Communication Problems

Unclear or incomplete communication is frequently noted in families of schizophrenics. This area requires nursing assessment. Unclear communication may result from continual interaction with the ill member or may contribute to the illness. Although research on this issue is inconclusive, clinicians evaluate how effectively the family communicates to determine the potential need for intervention.

The nurse assesses these aspects of family communication: (a) ability to focus on a topic, (b) ability to discuss a topic in a meaningful way with other members, (c) ability to maintain the discussion without wandering from the subject or becoming distracted, and (d) use of language and explanations that are generally understandable, i.e., not peculiar to that family alone (Wynne 1981). In addition, nurses should note who in the family seems to do the

talking, who talks to whom, and whether members talk for or interrupt one another.

Family Burden

A majority of families of schizophrenics report that caring for the ill member places a burden on the family unit. Burdens reported most often are financial strains, disruption in family routines, worry about the future, and feeling overwhelmed or unable to cope. Additionally, families report these needs:

- Information about the disorder
- Information about how to manage day-to-day problems due to schizophrenic symptoms
- Support for family members in their roles as caregivers

Environmental Assessment

Nurses assess the availability of support and services beyond the bounds of the family, including extended family and friends, as well as community groups and organizations that support schizophrenic clients. Mental health programs that address the specific needs of schizophrenic clients should be sought.

Nursing Diagnosis

Nursing diagnoses with schizophrenic clients focus on alterations in the patterns of activity, cognition, emotion

Table 17–3 Disturbances in Thought		
Type	**Definition**	**Example**
Delusions of persecution	Belief that others are hostile or trying to harm the individual	A woman notices a man looking at her and believes that he is trying to follow her.
Delusions of reference	False belief that public events or people are directly related to the individual	A man hears a story on the evening news and believes it is about him.
Somatic delusions	Belief that one's body is altered from normal structure or function	An elderly woman believes that her bowel is filled with cement and refuses to eat.
Thought broadcasting	Belief that one's thoughts can be heard by people even though one has not spoken those thoughts	A young client believes that his attraction to a nurse is known to those around him although he has said nothing.
Delusions of control	Belief that one's actions or thoughts are controlled by an external person or force	A woman believes that her neighbor controls her thoughts by means of his home computer.

processes, interpersonal processes, and perception. Alterations in ecologic, physiologic, and valuation processes are assessed as well, but the central nursing problems relate to the former five processes. PND-I nursing diagnoses for schizophrenic clients are listed in Box 17–4.

Altered Communication

Altered Verbal Communication

Schizophrenic clients communicate in a disorganized, sometimes incomprehensible fashion. Clients with less severe disorganization skip from topic to topic, making few if any logical links. When more severe thought disorganization is present, the client's statements may be totally incoherent. Some clients manifest thought disorganization by speaking very little, a characteristic labeled *poverty of speech*.

Box 17–4

PSYCHIATRIC MENTAL HEALTH NURSING DIAGNOSES (PND-I) FOR CLIENTS WITH SCHIZOPHRENIC DISORDERS

05.01   Altered communication processes
        Altered verbal communication
        Altered nonverbal communication
05.02   Altered conduct/impulse processes
        Dysfunctional behaviors: Disorganized behaviors
01.03   Altered self-care
        Altered grooming
        Altered hygiene
01.02   Altered recreational patterns
        Inadequate diversional activity
05.03   Altered role performance
        Altered leisure role
02.02   Altered judgment
06.04   Altered sensory perception
        Hallucinations
        Illusions
06.03   Altered self-concept
        Altered body image
02.07   Altered thought content
        Delusions
        Magical thinking
04.98   Altered emotional processes (not otherwise specified)
        Inappropriate emotions
        Anhedonia

Nurses should also note poverty of content in speech, in which the client converses but says very little.

Often clients with schizophrenia communicate in ways that are overly concrete (a sign of an inability to think and communicate abstractly) or overly symbolic (a sign of preoccupation with unreal or delusional material). The symbols are usually difficult to decipher because their meanings are idiosyncratic.

Altered Nonverbal Communication

In schizophrenic clients, facial and body expressions that accompany verbal communication frequently do not match the content of the verbal message. This lack of congruence is primarily due to the blunting of emotions found in schizophrenia. Expected facial expressions—e.g., smiles, looks of concern or disgust—may not accompany the schizophrenic's statements. In addition, clients with motor or behavioral abnormalities—e.g., posturing, unusual movements, or grimacing—convey a confusing mix of verbal and nonverbal messages.

Altered Conduct/Impulse Processes

Disorganized Behavior

Thought disorganization can be manifested in disorganized behaviors as well as incoherent communication. Actions that appear random or lack coherent movement toward a goal are disorganized. Disorganized clients move quickly from one task to another, rarely completing or returning to the first. At times, such clients resist the nurse's attempts to help them focus on one activity at a time, but they sometimes welcome external structure and direction. Nurses should first document the pattern of activity observed. Nurses should attempt to understand the meaning of the behavior for the client and the meaning of the client's resistance or willingness to change the pattern.

Alterations in Self-Care

Altered Grooming and Hygiene

Persons with schizophrenia frequently appear indifferent to their personal appearance. They may neglect to bathe, change clothes, or attend to minor grooming tasks such as combing their hair. Some show little awareness of current fashion styles, wearing clothing that makes them look out of place. Of greater concern are those who wear clothing that is inappropriate to the current season and weather conditions.

Lack of attention to grooming might be a simple annoyance to those who must live in close proximity to the schizophrenic. Health risks related to prolonged poor hygiene also arise. The nurse should assess immediate problems, e.g., inadequate nutrition, fluid intake, and elimination, as well as long-term problems, e.g., dental caries and increased susceptibility to infections.

Disregard for appearance and hygiene may extend to the schizophrenic's environment. He or she may fail to maintain a clean and safe living space. The schizophrenic may not take good care of personal belongings and may misplace them. Self-care deficiencies may result from consistently disturbed thought and perceptual processes. For example, a young man whose chronic hallucinations are only partly relieved by medication has difficulty concentrating for long periods and therefore demonstrates variable attention to grooming.

Inactivity

The emotional disturbances of **ambivalence** and **apathy**, common in schizophrenic disorders, can result in lack of interest and inactivity. Inactivity induced by ambivalence is associated with higher levels of emotion. Anxious about choosing one course of action and rejecting another, the client is immobilized. Jim, for example, is ambivalent about taking a pass out alone for the first time. He is undecided about taking the risk of leaving the hospital ward without a staff member yet yearns for the freedom of walking the streets alone. Indecision leaves him standing, immobilized, by the doorway to the unit.

Extreme ambivalence can manifest itself in even the most automatic of behaviors. Mary cannot eat because of ambivalence about where to sit or what to eat. She stands in the center of the dining room, turning first to one chair and then another, unable to choose and thus begin eating.

Clients who are inactive because of apathy demonstrate little emotional tone. Such a client may spend long hours lying in bed staring into space or listening to music. Often, but not always, apathetic individuals prefer isolation. The nurse might find several clients sitting in the same room, engaged in no apparent activities and interacting with one another only when absolutely necessary.

Social Withdrawal

Extreme anxiety about relating to others often leads schizophrenics to withdraw from interaction and to isolate themselves. Some clients tolerate only a few moments of direct communication, whereas others can manage extended periods of contact. The nurse should assess the client's tolerance of brief periods of contact with nurses and other clients. The nurse should document patterns of relating and withdrawal, also noting which activities the client engages in when in contact with others and when alone.

Altered Judgment

Impaired judgment in schizophrenics is probably due to biochemical alterations in the brain that make it difficult for clients to take in, synthesize, and respond to information. Impaired judgment may be evident both in the

mundane activities of daily life (e.g., selecting one's diet) and in major life decisions. One example is Murray, who refuses to take medications, even though not taking them means that he will be evicted from the residential treatment program he likes.

Altered Perceptions

Hallucinations

Hallucinations are both a clinical diagnostic sign of schizophrenia and a focus for nursing care. Nurses need to know the extent and nature of clients' hallucinations. Monitoring a client's hallucinations over time provides information on stressors that precipitate hallucinations, the client's response to psychotropic medications, and nursing actions that may diminish this symptom.

If a client is willing to discuss his or her hallucinations, the nurse can begin to assess their content. Once trust has been established, the nurse can ask the client whether the hallucinations are sounds or actual voices. If the client hears voices, the nurse asks whether the voices are familiar and what they are saying. It is important to learn if the voices command the client to take any action. If so, the nurse must assess the client's ability to control behavior and ignore the command, and then the nurse must take action to prevent unsafe or dangerous behavior.

Events that precipitate hallucinations should be noted because these indicate factors in the client's environment that are particularly stressful. Precipitating events include participating in group activities, spending long periods of time in close contact with others, or being around objects, e.g., the television about which the client has delusional beliefs.

Illusions

Illusions—misperceptions of the environment—make the client vulnerable to emotional and physical injury. The level of misperception may vary from day to day and even throughout the day. Misperceptions of the social environment make the client vulnerable to inappropriate responses and therefore ridicule. Misperceptions of the physical environment, e.g., misjudging the speed of an oncoming car, may lead to physical harm.

Impaired Self-Awareness

An altered sense of self is common in schizophrenics. Clients may lose the sense of where their bodies leave off and where inanimate objects begin. They may become dissociated from various body parts and believe, for example, that their arms and legs belong to someone else. Schizophrenics may worry about the normalcy of their sexual organs. Clients often verbalize this altered sense of self straightforwardly, e.g., "I don't feel like myself" or "I feel like I am looking at my body from somewhere else in the room."

Altered Thought Content

Delusions

Clients express delusional thinking in direct interactions and, to a lesser extent, through behaviors. When asked, many clients willingly describe their delusional beliefs in detail. They seldom withhold this information because they believe firmly in the validity of the delusion, no matter how bizarre it seems to others. Clients' actions reflect the fixedness of their beliefs.

Jerry has the somatic delusion that her body is riddled with holes. She flatly refuses to drink, convinced that the fluid will flow directly out of the holes and soil her dress.

The content of delusions varies, e.g., delusions of persecution, reference, and so on. (Review Table 17–3.) Reality-based delusions may seem plausible because they could, under some circumstances, actually occur. **Bizarre delusions**, more common among schizophrenics, have no possible basis in reality. The false belief that one's husband is having an affair with a neighbor is a reality-based delusion. In contrast, the belief that one's thoughts are directed by a television announcer or that one's unspoken thoughts can be heard by others are bizarre delusions.

Delusions often reflect the client's fears, particularly about personal inadequacies (Barile 1984). For example, a man's grandiose delusion that he is the mayor of New York City is a defense against feelings of inferiority. Similarly, persecutory delusions defend against the person's own feelings of aggression. Aggressive feelings are projected onto a person or organization, e.g., the police, whom the client then fears.

Magical Thinking

Magical thinking is the belief that events can happen simply because one wishes them to. Some schizophrenics claim they can exert will to make people take certain actions or make specific events occur, e.g., winning the lottery.

Thought Insertion, Withdrawal, and Broadcasting

Hallmarks of schizophrenic thought are the beliefs that others can put ideas into one's head (**thought insertion**) or take thoughts out of one's head (**thought withdrawal**). In addition, some clients believe that their thoughts are trans-

mitted to others via radio, television, or other means but not directly by the client. This belief is known as **thought broadcasting**.

Altered Emotional Responses

Inappropriate Emotions

Many schizophrenics demonstrate **inappropriate affect**—emotional responses that are inappropriate to the situation. For example, a client may smile or laugh while relating a history of having been abused as a child. Or, the client may become angry and anxious when asked to join a group of other clients for dinner. The degree to which a client's emotions are inappropriate is a prognostic indicator. Clients whose emotional response is preserved and generally appropriate have a more favorable prognosis than clients who demonstrate inappropriate affect.

A marked decrease in the variation or intensity of emotional expression is called **blunted affect**. The client may express joy, sorrow, or anger, but with little intensity. **Flat affect** is a total lack of emotional expression in verbal and nonverbal behavior. The client's face is impassive, and voice rate and tone are regular and monotonous.

Anhedonia

Anhedonia is the inability to experience pleasure or to imagine a pleasurable emotion. This inability is very distressing to clients, who are aware of how they differ from other people. One young man lamented, "How can it be possible to feel so many awful things and *never* feel happy?"

Family Overinvolvement and Negativity

At present there are no clear-cut clinical markers of what constitutes overinvolvement and negative emotions in families. Research criteria, which are too complex to apply in clinical settings, have been developed to determine families at risk. Nurses should note families who seem excessively bonded emotionally. Family members' inability to maintain emotional, social, or physical separateness is a clear sign of this problem. A high level of criticism among family members should also be assessed. Families thought to be seriously enmeshed or hypercritical should be discussed with the treatment team.

Impaired Family Functioning

Families burdened with the long-term responsibility of caring for a schizophrenic relative may suffer disruptions in their household routine, work, social interactions, and physical well-being. The household may be disrupted by the client's insistence that the family act on and accommodate his or her delusional beliefs. The family may bend to the client's wish, fearing an increase in the client's anxiety and possible fighting or shouting if they do not comply. For example, one family built an extra bathroom rather than fight their schizophrenic son, who spends hours in the bath completing elaborate washing rituals. Another family must eat out several times each week because their schizophrenic daughter refuses to allow anyone in the dining room when she eats.

The family social life may be disrupted. For instance, the family may fear leaving the schizophrenic home alone or embarrassing the schizophrenic or visitors if friends are invited in. Some families are willing to be open about the adjustments they make in living with a schizophrenic, while others choose to live isolated lives.

Family members' work can suffer because of the emotional strain of living with a schizophrenic. Additionally, they must take time off to accompany the schizophrenic to doctors' appointments, make hospital visits, and help during interviews with social agencies or the police. Family health may suffer because of general inattention or because of prolonged stresses within the home.

Planning

When planning care for any client with a chronic illness, nurses must be careful to set realistic goals for client change. Particular care must be taken with schizophrenics because such clients are extremely sensitive to change and failure.

Deterioration in all aspects of functioning is characteristic of the disease. Nurses must focus upon the most troublesome areas of client functioning and set incremental, short-term goals that pave the way for successes in achieving long-term goals.

Jean May is a 50-year-old single woman diagnosed with schizophrenia, undifferentiated type. For the past seven years she has lived in a skilled nursing facility because of her extreme regression and inability to care for herself. The nursing home is changing acceptance criteria and will no longer care for clients with a primary psychiatric diagnosis. She is admitted for evaluation of her medications and for alternative placement.

Jean manages none of her own personal cares. Aides in the nursing home have bathed and dressed her, asking only that Jean brush her own teeth. She hasn't made her bed or cleaned up her own living space for years. She can, however, feed herself.

- Short-term goals: Jean participates in her own care by helping the nurse decide what Jean will wear and by helping the nurse draw the bath. Jean helps the nurse clean up the bedroom.

RESEARCH NOTE

Citation

Hartigan del Campo EJ, Carr CF, Correa E: Rehospitalized schizophrenics: What they report about illness, treatment and compliance. J Psychiatr Nurs 1983;21:29–33.

Study Problem/Purpose

Chronic schizophrenic clients relapse frequently and are highly noncompliant with medication regimens and programs designed to provide follow-up care. This noncompliance is associated with poor understanding of the illness, dissatisfaction with care, and the experience of side-effects of medications. An examination of clients' attitudes toward their illness and care is needed to intervene effectively in interrupting the cycle of relapse.

Methods

Twenty-five rehospitalized schizophrenics under the age of 35 were asked to complete questionnaires regarding: (a) demographic information, (b) personality inventories, (c) reason for current hospitalization, (d) participation in aftercare prior to readmission, and (e) understanding of their illness and medications prescribed.

Findings

Personality and demographic characteristics did not distinguish clients who did and did not accept their illness prior to rehospitalization. A full 80 percent of the relapsed clients admitted to noncompliance with out-patient treatment or taking medications, or both. A majority (76 percent) admitted they had a psychiatric condition, but only 52 percent believed the current hospitalization was for the treatment of that condition. Most clients (52 percent) felt they had an inadequate understanding of their medications and close to that number (44 percent) indicated a need for more information about their illness.

Implications

Client attitudes about their condition, and its treatment may be important influences on compliance with treatment prescribed. Since compliance with treatment affects relapse rates, understanding and influencing these attitudes are important nursing interventions. Educating clients about their illness and medications may be another important intervention in reducing relapse.

- Intermediate goal: Jean manages her personal care needs and cleans her room with only verbal direction from the nurse.
- Long-term goal: Jean independently manages her personal grooming and cleaning responsibilities on the ward.

Client goals are tailored to each person's specific needs and strengths. As the client's status changes during the course of treatment, nursing goals are altered to reflect these changes. Tables 17–4 through 17–6 list a sampling of nursing goals appropriate to specific problems of schizophrenic clients.

Implementing Interventions

Promoting Adequate Communication

Clients with schizophrenia try to communicate, even though their statements may be hard to understand. Close attention to what the client is saying and honest attempts to understand the real and symbolic aspects of the message are important. The client perceives nuances of the nurse's behavior. Therefore, one of the most direct and successful ways to demonstrate caring and respect is to attend seriously to what the client says.

Clients make valid observations about their environment, needs, and concerns. A client may make observations about events or situations that are beyond the nurse's awareness. For example, communications about another client's drug use or suicidal threats should be seriously considered. If a client complains of a physical symptom such as stomach distress, the nurse should consider the symptom as real until there is evidence otherwise. It is easy to dismiss a client's statements, particularly if he or she is delusional. Doing so, however, shows lack of respect for the client's intact capacities to see and respond to what is happening in the environment.

Promoting Compliance with Medical Regimen

Psychotropic medications play an important part in the treatment of schizophrenic disorders. Drugs that diminish focal symptoms (e.g., hallucinations and delusions) and yet produce relatively few untoward effects are now available. The nurse must recognize, however, that each individual responds to medications differently.

Table 17–4
Planning Care for Clients with Disorganized Behavior

Goals	Interventions
Participates in goal-directed activity	1. Approach client in a calm manner.
Completes tasks that are begun	2. Discuss basic behavioral expectations.
	3. Assess the client's preferred activities.
	4. Verbally guide clients step by step through essential activities.
	5. Provide prescribed psychotropic medication.
	6. Move client to a quiet environment.

Nursing interventions regarding medications are to:

- Administer prescribed medication
- Observe client behavior for therapeutic effects
- Monitor side-effects of the medications
- Teach the client about the therapeutic and possible untoward effects of the medications prescribed
- Help the client take action to prevent untoward effects, e.g., maintaining fluid intake to avoid postural hypotension
- Evaluate the client's subjective response to the medication and attitude toward continued use

Consistent compliance in taking medications as prescribed is not common among this client population. Researchers estimate that as few as 68 percent of psychiatric clients adhere to medication regimens while in the hospital. When these clients return to the community, 37 percent or fewer adhere to drug regimens. Clients may stop taking their medications because

- They don't understand the administration instructions.
- They are too disorganized to follow the instructions.
- The side-effects of major tranquilizers are too uncomfortable.
- They do not wish to be stigmatized as having schizophrenia and therefore reject treatment.

Schizophrenics who do not take medications are more vulnerable to stressors and risk more frequent relapse of symptoms than those who comply with medication regimens. Efforts to educate clients about their medications and to have them practice self-medication prior to dis-

Table 17–5
Planning Care for Clients with Hallucinations

Goals	Interventions
Demonstrates no signs of attending to internal stimuli Identifies stressors that precipitate hallucinations	1. Monitor client for signs of attending to internal stimuli and observe for precipitating stressors. 2. Discuss your observations with the client: "You appear to be listening to something." 3. Assess the nature of the hallucinations. 4. Encourage client to attend to stimuli in the environment, such as conversations, rather than to internal stimuli. 5. Make brief, frequent contacts with the client to interrupt hallucinatory cycle and to maintain trust. 6. Help the client to dismiss or ignore the hallucination by engaging in activities. 7. Assist the client to monitor events or interactions that precede an increase in hallucinations. 8. Protect the client and others who might be harmed by the client's acting on hallucinated commands.

Source: Adapted from Barile L: The client who is hallucinating, in Lego S (ed): American Handbook of Psychiatric Nursing. *Lippincott, 1984, p 446.*

Table 17–6
Planning Care for Clients with Delusions

Goals	Interventions
Statements and beliefs are reality based	1. Avoid arguing or attempting to disprove the delusion. 2. Observe for stressors that precipitate discussion of the delusion and help the client to avoid or eliminate these stressors. 3. Attempt to address the need that is met by the delusion, e.g., assure client of his or her safety. 4. Provide prescribed psychotropic medication. 5. Protect the client and others from delusional behaviors that might prove harmful.

Source: Adapted from Barile L: The client who is delusional, in Lego S (ed): American Handbook of Psychiatric Nursing. *Lippincott, 1984, p 446.*

charge have increased the rate of compliance only marginally (Battle et al. 1982). Clearly, such factors as the client's attitude toward the medications prescribed also influence his or her willingness to take medications. The nurse is an active participant in assessing compliance and fostering a positive attitude toward medications.

Nursing Interventions in the Milieu

Nurses often work with large numbers of clients in a physically limited space, e.g., a ward. More than any other members of the treatment team, nurses are responsible for monitoring and managing the treatment milieu. The tone of the milieu is set by the program structure, the regular group activities, and the expectations set out for clients, but this tone changes dramatically with various client groups.

When half the clients in a twenty-bed adult ward are diagnosed as having depression, for example, there is likely to be little energy or initiative in the milieu. In such a case, nurses must take much of the initiative to get groups started and help clients attend groups. In contrast, in a ward with many young, highly active schizophrenics, the milieu may be overly stimulating. In this case, nurses need to regulate the energy and activity of the milieu so that clients who are more fragile can tolerate it.

Nurses can regulate the milieu by:

- Varying the number and nature of structured activities
- Arranging for walks and activities in the community
- Consciously attempting to unite clients who might be helpful to one another
- Helping disruptive clients to learn more appropriate interactional skills
- Setting limits on disruptive behaviors

Assisting with Grooming and Hygiene

Helping clients to establish and maintain personal care habits is a complex process. If the client clearly lacks the skills, then the emphasis is on teaching these skills. If, however, the client has learned grooming skills but does not practice them, the nurse focuses on ways to motivate the client. Intervention begins by establishing clear expectations in regard to essential grooming habits. The frequency and timing of all aspects of grooming—including bathing, hair care, oral hygiene, and room care—should be specified in writing.

To help the client complete the plan, the nurse reminds him or her of the agreed time when tasks are to be completed. Power struggles regarding completion of tasks should be avoided. If initial prompts don't work, the client should be left alone for a period of time to see if he or she takes action. Any effort by the client to meet personal care needs should be noticed and praised. In addition, meaningful rewards—i.e., a walk outside alone with the staff member—can be used to encourage accomplishment of new and often challenging tasks.

Promoting Organized Behavior

Clients whose behavior is disorganized require direction and limits to make their actions more effective and goal directed. The first rule of working with a disorganized client is to go slowly and keep calm. The client's perception of the environment may be distorted, but the nurse's calmness can help to calm the client. The nurse tries to direct the client in simple, safe activities.

Examples of nursing goals and interventions for a disorganized client are given in Table 17–4. A case example of one such intervention follows.

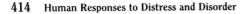

George is moving quickly yet aimlessly from the refrigerator to the cupboard. He pulls a box of cereal from the cupboard, opens it, and then wanders away. Next he goes to the refrigerator, opens the door, peers in, and closes the door. Rummaging through all his pockets, he locates a cigarette, lights it, places it in an ashtray, and wanders back to the cupboard. This effortful yet unproductive behavior continues for several minutes when the nurse enters.

Nurse: George, are you trying to get yourself some cereal?

George: Sort of. I was going to . . . smoke . . . no . . . eat something. Yeah, I wanted something to eat.

Nurse: Try to concentrate on one thing. First put out the cigarette. (He does so.) Now, come over here and get the cereal box. Here's a bowl. Here's a spoon. (She hands him the utensils.) Why don't you sit right here?

(She seats him so that he has his back to the rest of the activity in the room.) Can you sit still for a bit?

George: I think so.

Nurse: Pour yourself some cereal. I'll get the milk for you. (She does so.)

George begins to eat his cereal quietly. The nurse stays with him for a few minutes and directs him to continue eating when he becomes distracted by others who come into the room.

Promoting Social Interaction

The client's efforts to withdraw from social contact stem from past relationship failures and fear of rejection. Clients often find their internal world less risky and therefore more attractive than a world that requires interpersonal relating. When making efforts to help the client become less withdrawn, the nurse must respect the client's overwhelming anxiety about human contact.

After establishing a basic level of trust, the nurse can encourage the client to try out new behaviors within the relationship. The goal is to have the client experience success, and thus small increments of change should be encouraged. If, for example, the client has difficulty initiating conversation, the nurse could encourage the client to practice this skill once a day. Similarly, if the client avoids any activity in the milieu because of fear of relating to groups, the nurse might structure an activity involving the client, the nurse, and one other client.

Promoting Optimum Activity Levels

Immobility due to ambivalence is extremely uncomfortable. One of the ways to decrease immobilization is to limit the number of choices that the client has to make when he or she is suffering from indecision. For example, the nurse can help a man who is immobilized by his inability to decide whether to go out alone for the first time by telling him that it seems too soon for him to go out alone and that, for today, he must be accompanied. The nurse can remove extra chairs at the table in the dining room so that the young woman who is undecided about where to sit has only one choice.

Clients are often ambivalent about taking medications. Maintaining adequate blood levels of therapeutic medications is important for the schizophrenic. To help clients overcome ambivalence, the nurse gives them time to think about taking the medications. If the client is unable to act within a few minutes, setting a time limit may spur the client to decide to take it. If not, the nurse should leave and come back later to offer the medications. Two useful strategies are reminding clients of the positive effects of the medication and framing the action as a way for clients to help themselves get better.

Promoting Reality-Based Perceptions

Having illusions or hallucinations is often frightening for clients. Nurses can intervene by:

- Reassuring clients of their safety
- Protecting them from physical harm as they respond to their altered perceptions
- Validating reality
- Helping clients to distinguish reality from the hallucinatory experience

Some specific nursing actions to help clients who are actively hallucinating are listed in Table 17–5. General approaches to working with clients with altered perceptions are highlighted below.

Hallucinations are extremely frightening when the client has never experienced them before or when the content of the hallucination is threatening or angry. The nurse can begin to alleviate clients' anxiety by sharing her or his observation of the frightened behavior and asking clients to discuss what they are experiencing. It is helpful to make simple reassuring remarks, e.g., "I know the voices are real to you, but no one else can hear them. There is no one here that means to harm you."

The client should be protected from harm as well as reassured about safety. The client may take impulsive action to escape the frightening experience or to obey the voices he or she hears. The nurse must prevent this by:

- Closely observing client behavior during active hallucinations
- Intervening quickly by giving additional doses of psychotropic medications or placing the client in a quiet room
- If necessary, securing the unit so that the client cannot leave and take self-destructive or impulsive action

The nurse makes every effort to help the client attend to real rather than internal stimuli, orients the client to the real situation, and encourages the client to focus on the nurse rather than on the hallucination. For example: "George, listen to me rather than to the sounds you say you hear. Remember, you are in the hospital and I am your nurse. I will help you find your shoes. Come with me." Active involvement in some activity, e.g., finding shoes, helps the client to maintain a focus on real events and perceptions.

Some clients can diminish hallucinations by actively telling them to go away (Field 1985). This intervention should be attempted only when the hallucinations are threatening or negative. Work with the client to recognize when the hallucinations begin. Move the client to a private area, and have him or her tell the voices to go away. Auditory hallucinations can be decreased if the client verbally and vehemently demands that the voices go away each time they recur.

Intervening with Delusions

General guidelines for working with delusional individuals are not to argue with their false beliefs, to focus upon the reality-based aspects of their communications, and to protect them from acting on their delusions in a way that might harm themselves or others. Suggested nursing interventions with delusional clients are found in Table 17–6.

Promoting Congruent Emotional Responses

Working with clients who display blunted or flat affect can be confusing for nurses who are accustomed to reading emotional responses that fall within a more normal range. Nurses need to be aware that these clients have feelings about events around them, including their interaction with the nurse, yet have difficulty expressing these emotions.

Lack of congruence between the person's affect and the content of the message should be noted. If the relationship between the nurse and client is well established, then the nurse might comment on the incongruity and explore it with the client. (For example, "George, what you are telling me is sad but you are laughing. What shall I pay attention to?") Modeling clear, congruent communications is helpful. Little can be done to change the client's anhedonia, yet empathic listening might comfort the client.

Promoting Family Understanding and Involvement

When a schizophrenic is hospitalized, the family should be encouraged and helped to remain involved in his or her care. Information on the client's status, treatment program, and future treatment plans, including discharge plans, should be shared with the family except in unusual circumstances. Nurses need to comply with the client's wishes and with the laws governing disclosure of information, which vary by state and by institution.

Some mental health professionals have a bias against family involvement. This bias is a remnant of now-discredited theories that family interaction patterns cause schizophrenia. Nurses may need to be active advocates for families' rights to information about, and involvement in, the care of the schizophrenic member. This question is a useful way to check one's bias against the family's rights: Am I responding to this family any differently than I would to the family of a client with a medical condition?

If assessment suggests the family needs information about the disease and treatment, the nurse should refer the family to education programs, if they are available. Family psychoeducation programs are preferable to direct

Text continues on p. 420.

CASE STUDY: A Client With Schizophrenia, Paranoid Type

Identifying Information

Jim March is a 24-year-old single male who currently lives with his mother. He is unemployed and supports himself with SSI payments. Jim was brought up as a Catholic and attended Catholic schools through high school. He has sporadically attended the local community college, where he is attempting to complete an AA degree. He has not regularly attended school for two years. He currently attends a day treatment work program five times a week.

Dr. Taylor, Jim's private psychiatrist, referred Jim for admission. The evaluation is based upon the initial interview with Jim and his mother. Additional information is gained from a telephone call with Dr. Taylor and from a copy of Jim's day treatment record.

Client's Definition of Present Problem

The client states, "My mom and the cops said I had to come here. She's the crazy one. I just want her to leave me alone!"

History of Present Problem

Jim's mother reports that for the past three weeks Jim has been increasingly isolated at home, refusing to come out of his room, to eat, or to talk. She hears him mumbling to himself in his room and knows he runs into the kitchen to eat when she is not around.

Jim's behavior is quite erratic. He unexpectedly leaves the house any time, including the middle of the night, to go to the nearby community college computer center. There, he insists on using a computer terminal to work on his "plan." Lacking an access number, he cannot get the terminal to work, and the staff at the center call the security guard to have him removed. Jim has been unwilling to discuss the "plan" with anyone except to imply that it will protect him from someone who is trying to attack him. This episode of attempting to use the community college computer has been repeated six times in the last few weeks. The police are threatening to cite Jim if he does not agree to in-patient treatment at this time.

Two stressors probably precipitated this episode. First, Jim got a notice from his work program that he would be let go if he was late for work three additional times. He immediately stopped attending the work program. At first, he spent his free time walking the streets in the neighborhood and eventually went out less and less.

Prior to this episode, Jim had established a year-long pattern of fairly regular attendance at work program, which demanded six hours of work in a local restaurant, washing dishes for the breakfast and lunch trade. He worked from 10:00 A.M. to 4:30 P.M. five days a week. When not at work, he spent time in his room listening to rock music or watching television. He had few friends, although he did stay in contact with a few members of the bimonthly medication group conducted at the community mental health center.

A second stressor was Jim's father's announcement of his plan to remarry. When Jim first heard the news, he offered congratulations. He has subsequently refused to talk with his father.

continued

Psychiatric History

Hospitalizations

At age 20, Jim was hospitalized at Saint Mary's Hospital for six weeks for evaluation of extreme withdrawal and talking to himself. His diagnosis was schizophreniform disorder. Jim was treated with fluphenazine (Prolixin), which had a positive effect on symptoms. The precipitant of illness was probably his parents' separation.

At age 22, Jim was rehospitalized at Saint Mary's for evaluation of acting out behavior. Jim had failed all his course work in the community college and was making threatening statements toward his instructors. Hospitalization lasted four weeks. Jim was treated with thiothixene (Navane), with positive effects. He returned home and began attending the local day treatment program.

For the past two years, the client has been seeing a private psychiatrist for medication management and has attended programs at the community mental health center. He regularly attended day treatment for one year. Last year he began a job through the mental health center's work program. He was marginally successful in meeting the demands of the job, although he had problems with repeated tardiness.

Family History

Jim's parents are both living and well. They were separated four years ago and divorced within nine months of the separation. Jim's father is an attorney, and his mother works part time in a stationery store. There are no other children. Jim lives with his mother, and this arrangement is acceptable to both of them. He sees his father once a month and on holidays and special celebrations, such as birthdays.

Social History

Developmental History

Pregnancy, delivery, childhood, and early adolescence were unremarkable, with developmental tasks completed at the expected times. Jim's mother recalls that Jim was always physically active and skilled. Although he was never extremely popular, he always had one or two good friends, both male and female. He dated casually but never developed an intimate relationship with a woman.

Jim began to pull away from friends when he started community college. He claimed to have difficulty keeping up with course work and thus dropped out of most evening and weekend activities. Since his first hospitalization, he has vehemently refused to contact any of his old high school friends. The only people he sees socially are those whom he's met in day treatment or the work program.

Education

Jim performed at or above average through high school. He went on to community college, intending to get a degree in computer science. Beginning with his first quarter, he received barely passing grades and was asked to leave the program in his second year.

Habits

Jim smokes one pack of cigarettes per day and drinks occasionally, primarily beer. He denies any drug use, past or present, and his mother confirms this report.

Hobbies

Jim has always had a keen interest in computers. In high school, he took elective courses that introduced him to computer uses. Other hobbies in high school were co-rec basketball and track. He never tried out for a competitive team. As his interest in friends has waned, Jim has become increasingly intent on music and on increasing his music library. For the past two years, nearly all of his free time has been spent listening to records or watching television rock video programs.

continued

Case Study (Continued)

Health History	Jim has no notable medical problems. He has no known allergies, and he has never had a negative reaction to psychotropic medications.

Current Mental Status

General Appearance	Jim is a young-looking, 24-year-old white male who is quite anxious and guarded but cooperative during the interview. He is dressed in jeans and sweatshirt, and his hair is slightly unkempt. He sits kicking his right leg continuously throughout the interview. Jim gets up once during the interview to look out the window but does not explain this behavior.
Sensorium	Jim is alert and oriented to person, time, and place. He demonstrates an adequate fund of knowledge and can name past presidents through Kennedy. Memory and recall are good. He calculates serial sevens slowly but correctly to 58. His judgment is marginally impaired: He reports that if he found a signed blank check on the street he would put it in the church collection.
Feelings	Jim's affect is anxious, and his mood is angry.
Speech	Jim's speech is rapid, pressured, and tangential. He frequently interrupts the interviewer to ask questions about the hospital rules and treatment.
Motor Behavior	Jim sits holding himself rigidly in the chair, kicking his foot continuously throughout the interview. He gets up to examine things in the room and to ask about them as well as to peer suspiciously out the window.
Thought Content	Jim describes delusions of persecution and has a grandiose belief that his "plan" will ward off danger. He will not elaborate about the plan but insists that he needs access to a computer terminal while in the hospital. He admits to hearing voices for the past several weeks. It is through the hallucinations that he has become convinced that someone is trying to harm him. Occasionally he hears his father's voice, which is extremely frightening to him. He denies suicidal or homicidal ideation.
Thought Process	Some loosening of associations is evident. When asked about special eating habits, he relates a story about a religious sister he had run into recently. Abstractions are concrete and self-referential. When asked the meaning of "People who live in glass houses shouldn't throw stones," he responds, "If I threw a rock through that window, I'd get cut."
Insight	Jim believes that this hospitalization is a ruse by the police and his mother to keep him out of his room for a week. In this way, progress on his "plan" will be held up, and his mother will be able to clean his room. He is cooperative with admission but insists on a private room.

Diagnostic Impression

Nursing Diagnoses (PND-I/NANDA)	4.02.02	Anxiety* /Anxiety
	2.07.01	Delusions /Thought processes, altered
	5.02.02.05	Unpredictable behaviors (potential for elopement) /Noncompliance

PND-I diagnosis also in NANDA list.

continued

Case Study (Continued)

1.03.01	Altered eating (associated with suspiciousness)* /Self-care deficit: feeding	
5.01.02	Altered verbal communication (associated with social isolation) /Social interaction: impaired	
1.02.01	Inadequate diversional activity* /Diversional activity: deficit	

DSM-IIIR Multiaxial Diagnosis
Axis I: 295.34 Schizophrenia, paranoid type, chronic with acute exacerbation
Axis II: 799.90 Deferred
Axis III: No physical disorder at this time
Axis IV: Psychosocial stressors: 3, Moderate, acute (fired from part-time job that he held for the past year); 3, Moderate, enduring (father announced plans to remarry)
Axis V: Current GAF: 30
Highest GAF in the past year: 40

Nursing Care Plan

Nursing Diagnosis (PND-I/NANDA)	Client Care Goals	Nursing Planning/ Intervention	Evaluation
4.02.02 Anxiety* /Anxiety	Jim will be comfortable in the milieu.	1. Give Jim a private room. 2. Approach Jim with clear warning. 3. Make brief (ten-minute) contacts with Jim. 4. Provide private time in room to decrease anxiety.	Jim reports feeling safe in the milieu.
2.07.01 Delusions /Thought processes, altered	Jim will show less preoccupation with threats to his safety.	1. Reassure Jim of safety on the unit. 2. Avoid contradicting Jim's delusions. 3. Redirect Jim to discussion of other topics, e.g., music. 4. Give Jim prescribed medication.	Jim is able to carry on a conversation with the nurse without bringing up topic of threats.
5.02.02.05 Unpredictable behaviors (potential for elopement) /Noncompliance (with hospitalization)	Jim will not escape from the unit and will abide by unit rules regarding the use of passes.	1. Establish a contract to remain on unit with Jim. 2. Observe Jim closely during periods of increased stress. 3. Help Jim engage in quiet activity when he feels less in control of his impulse to leave.	Jim stays on unit except for planned outings with staff.

(continued)

Case Study (Continued)

Nursing Diagnosis (PND-I/NANDA)	Client Care Goals	Nursing Planning/ Intervention	Evaluation
		4. Use p.r.n. medications as needed.	
		5. Secure unit as needed.	
1.03.01 Altered eating (associated with suspiciousness) /Self-care deficit: feeding	Jim will maintain adequate intake of food and fluids.	1. Allow Jim maximum control over his choice of foods. 2. Have Jim eat in a private area to decrease anxiety. 3. Serve foods in their original containers to decrease Jim's fears of tampering. 4. Provide fluids frequently throughout the day.	Jim eats at least one-half of all meals and drinks a minimum of 2000 mL per day.
5.01.02 Altered verbal communication (social isolation) /Social interaction, impaired	Jim will participate in all unit activities.	1. Establish a schedule of daily activities. 2. Allow quiet time alone in room. 3. Prompt Jim to attend activities at scheduled times. 4. Praise Jim's attempts to follow through with schedule.	Jim participates in all daily activity included in his schedule.
1.02.01 Inadequate diversional activity* /Diversional activity: deficit	Jim will use free time constructively.	1. Explore Jim's preferred hobbies. 2. Help Jim gain access to materials needed, e.g., records. 3. Work with Jim during unstructured times to begin hobby or interaction. 4. Observe Jim's ability to pursue the activity and provide continued guidance if needed.	Jim works on hobbies or socializes with other clients during free time.

*PND-I diagnosis also in NANDA list.

teaching because they often combine education with mutual support. In such groups, families can meet others who share their life difficulties. These peers can provide informal support and information to help the family deal with the tasks that lie ahead. Nurses can reinforce the formal teaching that occurs in such programs when they meet with individual families.

Promoting Community Contacts

Awareness of clients' community supports and potential treatment programs guides nurses in preparing clients for discharge. For example, the client's most important peer support group might be the clientele at a local day treatment program. If so, several visits to the program prior to discharge will help the client make the transition back to the community.

Preparing the client for the type of residence he or she will enter after hospital discharge is a central nursing task. Often placement depends on how the client functions in the hospital. If the client is able to manage medications, participate in a variety of groups, and live cooperatively with other clients, then placement in a residential care facility that supports independent functioning is appropriate. In contrast, clients who need assistance with structuring free time, resist taking medications, or cannot take on responsibilities for self-care require a more structured environment.

Nurses work with clients to help them achieve their highest level of functioning. They document clients' abilities to perform various tasks and make recommendations to the treatment team about appropriate placements.

Evaluating

To complete the nursing process, nurses evaluate changes in client status and behavior in response to nursing interventions. Evaluation criteria are linked to nursing goals and reflect an understanding of the limitations of schizophrenic clients.

The focus of nursing evaluation should be on the behavioral, perceptual/cognitive, and emotional response systems. Improvements in the specific problem areas of communication, self-care, judgment, perceptions, thoughts, and emotions should be examined.

Evaluation of changes in the family and in the larger system of support is more difficult to accomplish. Family changes can be evaluated by the family's reports. Feedback to nurses from agencies in the community about the appropriateness of placements and the helpfulness of information contained in nursing discharge summaries comprise evaluations of community level interventions.

Chapter Highlights

- Persons with schizophrenia experience disturbances in perception, thought, affect, and activity.
- The biologic, psychologic, and family theories of schizophrenia can be largely incorporated into one interactional model of the disorder.
- Care of schizophrenic clients requires an awareness of the client's multiple functional deficits and of the nurse's personal response to working with this population.
- Nursing assessment of individual problems in schizophrenia focuses on the client's self-care and communication abilities, activity patterns, cognitive and perceptual functioning, and emotional expression.
- Nursing assessment of family problems in schizophre-

nia focuses on family communication, cohesiveness, emotions, and burdens.

- Nursing diagnoses for clients with schizophrenia identify the communication, conduct, judgment, perceptual, and emotional alterations commonly found in this disorder.
- Nursing interventions promote adequate communication, activity, social interaction, grooming, and perception in clients with schizophrenia.
- Nurses evaluate the effectiveness of their interventions with individual schizophrenic clients and their families.

References

Asaad G. Shapiro B: Hallucinations: Theoretical and clinical overview. *Am J Psychiatry* 1986; 143(9):1088–1097.

Barile L: The client who is hallucinating. The client who is delusional, in Lego S (ed): *American Handbook of Psychiatric Nursing.* Lippincott, 1984, p 446.

Battle EH, Halliburton A, Wallston KA: Self medication among psychiatric patients and adherence after discharge. *J Psychosoc Nurs* 1982;20:21–28.

Crow TJ: Regular review: Molecular pathology of schizophrenia: More than one disease process? *Brit Med J* 1980; 12 Jan:67.

Falloon IRH, Boyd JL, McGill CW: *Family Care of Schizophrenia.* Gilford Press, 1984.

Field WE: Hearing voices. *J Psychosoc Nurs* 1985;23:9–14.

Harding C, et al.: Chronicity in schizophrenia: Fact, partial fact, or artifact. *Hosp Community Psychiatry* 1987; 38(5):477–486.

Kane C: The outpatient comes home. The family's response to deinstitutionalization. *J Psychosoc Nurs* 1984;22:19–25.

Karon BP, Vandebos, GR: *Psychotherapy of Schizophrenia.* Jason Aronson, 1981.

Krauss JB, Slavinsky AT: *The Chronically Ill Psychiatric Patient and the Community.* Blackwell Scientific, 1982.

Liberman RP et al: The nature and problem of schizophrenia, in Bellack AS (ed): *Schizophrenia: Treatment, Management and Rehabilitation.* Grune & Stratton, 1984.

Olson DH, Russell CS, Sprenkle DH: Circumplex model of marital and family systems: IV. Theoretical update. *Fam Process* 1983;22:69–93.

Shapiro SA: *Contemporary Theories of Schizophrenia.* McGraw-Hill, 1981.

Wynne L: Current concepts about schizophrenia and family relationships. *J Nerv Ment Dis* 1981;169:82–89.

EIGHTEEN

Applying the Nursing Process for
Clients with Mood Disorders

Maxine E. Loomis

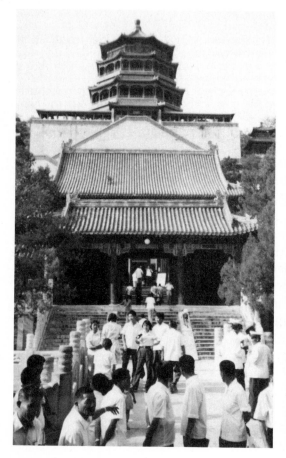

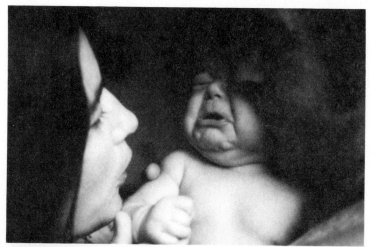

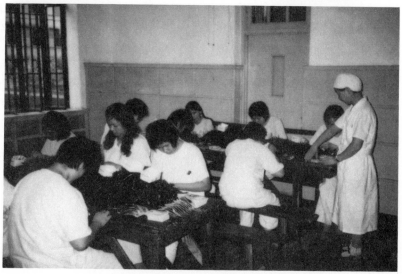

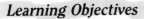

Learning Objectives

After reading this chapter, students should be able to

- Identify and discuss the early development and personality characteristics of persons with mood disorders

- Compare and contrast the behavioral manifestations of a manic episode, a major depressive episode, and dysthymia

- Describe and discuss application of the nursing process in working with persons with mood disorders

- Identify key elements in the human response patterns of persons with mood disorders

- Plan, implement, and evaluate nursing intervention designed specifically for persons with mood disorders

Cross References

Other topics related to this chapter are: Biologic therapies, Chapter 32; Growth and development, Chapter 6; Psychobiology, Chapter 9; Suicide, Chapter 25.

Key Terms

adrenocorticotropic hormone (ACTH)
Beck's Depression Inventory
bipolar disorder
cortisol
cyclothymia
depression
depressive disorder
dexamethasone suppression test (DST)
dysthymia
hypomanic
learned helplessness
limbic system
major depression
mania
"manic depressive"
manic episode
melancholia
object loss
pace and lead
seasonal affective disorder (SAD)
Zung's Self-Rating Depression Scale

Ron is a 47-year-old high school football coach whose wife brought him to the emergency room because he was unable to sleep, had not eaten in a week, and was keeping their family awake nights playing game films on their VCR at full volume. He had spent the previous day shouting obscenities from his bedroom window at passersby. He was combative and argumentative with the emergency room staff and had to be restrained prior to admission to the in-patient psychiatric unit.

Marcia is a very bright, poised, articulate, and engaging executive in the pharmaceutical industry whose mood has vacillated between excitement and total lack of energy since she was passed over for promotion six months ago. Marcia, age 32, decided to seek help from a private psychiatric outpatient clinic because she feared "losing control" of her behavior and emotions.

Ann, a 45-year-old secretary, asked for help at a community crisis clinic because she had been preoccupied with thoughts of killing herself. She said she had no friends and no time for fun because of the demands of her job.

What do these three people have in common? They are all suffering from mood disorders. The mood disorders (see Box 18–1) are a group of psychiatric diagnoses characterized by disturbances in emotional and behavioral response patterns. These patterns range from extreme elation and agitation to extreme depression and a serious potential for suicide. Accurate assessment, diagnosis, intervention, and evaluation by psychiatric nurses are essential in helping clients with mood disorders attain a more comfortable, safe, and productive life.

Imagine policy alternatives that yield a greater likelihood of global survival.

The author gratefully acknowledges the contributions of Sylvia Whiting, RN, MS, to the final revisions of this chapter.

Box 18–1
MOOD (AFFECTIVE) DISORDERS (DSM-IIIR)

Bipolar Disorders

296.6x   Bipolar disorder, mixed
296.4x   Bipolar disorder, manic
296.5x   Bipolar disorder, depressed
301.13   Cyclothymia
296.70   Bipolar disorder NOS (not otherwise specified)

Depressive Disorders

296.2x   Major depression, single episode
296.3x   Major depression, recurrent
300.40   Dysthymia
296.82   Depressive disorder NOS

HISTORICAL AND THEORETICAL FOUNDATIONS

Bipolar Disorders

The bipolar disorders are mood disorders characterized by episodes of mania and depression. Either mania or depression may be evident at any given time, elements of both may be present simultaneously, or symptoms of one may alternate with symptoms of the other. The manic phase is characterized by hyperactivity, excitement, agitation, euphoria, excessive energy, decreased need for sleep, and impaired ability to concentrate or complete a single train of thought. The depressive phase is characterized by underactivity, marked apathy, profound sadness, guilt, and lowered self-esteem. Bipolar disorders are referred to as manic-depressive disorders in some clinical settings.

Early Development

Arieti (1974) describes a common parenting experience that leads to one of three types of manic-depressive personality, depending on the young child's adaptation to this early situation. The home is one in which parents are willing to accept and care for the infant and the infant is receptive to parenting. Parent(s) and child are engaged with each other and available to interact and respond. To outsiders, the family appears normal and healthy, with parents and children doing all the happy, right, and healthy things one would expect of growing families.

The major problem, according to Arieti, is a sudden withdrawal of the previously available nurturing and attention. This withdrawal can be either physical—e.g., the sudden departure, illness, or death of a parent—or psychologic—e.g., preoccupation with a family problem, mother returning to work, or the birth of a sibling who draws attention away from the older child. Arieti makes no reference to the age at which this withdrawal of nurturance occurs, however, the trauma has been reported as occurring anywhere from 3 months to 5 years of age (Loomis and Landsman 1980).

Overadapted Response

Arieti (1974, p 465) describes the first type of manic-depressive adaptation to this type of parenting as that of "finding security by accepting parental expectations, no matter how onerous they are." The result is a well-behaved child and, later, a dedicated adult motivated by responsibility and with a high level of investment in doing things well. The important activities of life and the criteria for success are externally defined. The person later relives the experience of a withholding or depriving parent by attachment to a "dominant other" or by dedication to a profession, social cause, church, or some other social institution. The promise of nurturing and the disappointment of deprivation are repeatedly reenacted in these attachments.

Passive-Dependent Response

A second type of manic-depressive adaptation is more directly and obviously passive-dependent. Instead of adapting by doing things well, the youngster attempts to reengage parents and, later, parent figures by being a helpless baby. At times, these people present themselves as inept and incapable of managing their lives. They demand attention and expect to be taken care of by others. They often empower others as responsible for their happiness or unhappiness, success or failure.

Characterologic Response

Arieti's third manic-depressive personality type establishes characterologic defenses as a result of deciding not to incorporate or identify with the original parents. The youngster may attempt to identify with other adults or childhood heroes but forms no meaningful attachments. The result is an adult who has difficulty establishing permanent relationships and has few internalized values. This person is actively involved in doing things and may move from one successful, shady business to another. The purpose of all this activity is to escape from self-examination and to avoid closeness with others.

In clinical practice, the nurse also sees a fair number of manic-depressive people who have been exposed to inconsistent or abusive parenting. Inconsistent parenting often takes the form of alternating periods of nurturing and unpredictable periods of anger or neglect that seem unrelated to the child's behavior. The family presents an appropriate, loving appearance to the outside world but neglects or abuses the child within the privacy of the home. The person denies or represses memories of psychologic or physical abuse, which emerge only during the course of treatment. Because of these overwhelming inconsistencies and contradictions in parenting, the child often does not see adult logic as useful in establishing the cause-and-effect nature of early experiences. The youngster reacts to the unpredictable nurturing with elation and to the periodic abandonment and abuse with withdrawal and depression. In adult life, these extremes are repeated as the manic-depressive experiences "unexplainable" cyclic highs and lows.

Personality Structure

The personality structure of persons with bipolar disorders is built on a foundation of:

- Parenting from a competitive frame of reference
- An early emphasis on doing or not doing things
- A grandiose approach to thinking, feeling, and behaving
- Development of a fantasized nurturing parent

Regardless of the specific details of their early development, people with bipolar disorders appear to share a common set of personality characteristics.

Competitive Frame of Reference

A person with a competitive frame of reference believes that no two people can think, feel, or do the same thing at the same time. The competition can be over:

1. Sensations, e.g., the mother decides when the child is hungry, or the father maintains that his son's injury doesn't really hurt.
2. Affect, e.g., the mother is sad, the father is angry, one youngster is always scared, and the other child is not allowed to feel at all.
3. Cognition, e.g., a certain area of knowledge "belongs" to one family member, and the others are expected to know nothing about that information.
4. Behaviors, e.g., one child excels academically, another is athletic, and the third child is rebellious and won't do anything the others are doing.

Competition also sets up a polarity in which there are only winners and losers. These people feel they must compete about everything in life in order to survive.

Persons with bipolar disorders view the world from a competitive frame of reference. Many of them have inter-

nalized two conflicting messages: "You can do anything in the world you set your mind to, but you'll never do it well enough to please me." The conflict between these two messages is acted out in the manic belief that one can do anything and the depressive realization that one will never do well enough.

Doing or Not Doing

People with bipolar disorders and a competitive frame of reference wage war on the battleground of doing versus not doing. Some of these people appear very successful and experience difficulty only when that success is blocked in some way. Marcia came for treatment six months after being passed over for early promotion within the corporation in which she was a very successful executive. She was doing quite well professionally and had just been offered an excellent position with a competing company, but Marcia seemed unable to deal with the perceived rejection that had blocked her earlier advancement.

Other people with bipolar disorders appear comfortable with failure and seem to go out of their way not to succeed. One such client was a very bright lawyer who became depressed and unable to work every time the law firm he owned became involved in an important case that would enhance his reputation. Another young man wrecked his car during a manic episode following his graduation from college—a degree he achieved after ten years and numerous setbacks.

Regardless of their success or failure in doing things, these two types of people have a common problem. Their sense of themselves and their relationships are defined by what they do rather than who they are or what they feel. They have very little or no self-identity apart from what they do or do not accomplish. They are like small boats tossed about in a storm of opinions about the quality and quantity of their accomplishments, and they lack the internal definition of self that would provide a peaceful harbor.

Grandiosity

Grandiosity with respect to feeling, thinking, and behaving is a hallmark of the bipolar personality structure. Because of the competitive frame of reference and the emphasis on doing things within the parent-infant interaction, nurturing is not experienced as safe or comforting. Within the competitive frame of reference, the parent must win and do things right, resulting in a style of caretaking in which the parent sets the pace and discounts or defines the child's feelings and needs. Holding and feeding are the earliest parent-infant contacts, and here the competition begins about who will set the pace and win control. As a result, the infant experiences agitation or a lack of synchrony during nurturing as parent and child compete to get their needs met.

Parents in these families model inconsistency and agitation. The child experiences parenting that is alternately very good and very bad. Thus, the child must develop a structure that allows for drastic swings, and the self is experienced as either very good or very bad. Denial is the defense that allows the child to tolerate this discrepancy. The child uses denial to separate the experiences of being either very good or very bad and never integrates or realistically resolves the "good" and "bad" selves. A great deal of energy is needed to maintain the denial that keeps the two experiences separate. Denial allows a grandiose or exaggerated approach to feelings. For example, when these people are manic, they may deny ever having been depressed. When they are depressed, they report never having done anything worthwhile. Apparent inconsistencies or contradictions are not experienced as internal conflict.

Because feelings cause competition and agitation in the family, the child associates them with a grandiosity that leads the youngster to conclude that feelings are overwhelming. In families that demonstrate a high level of competition for specific feelings, the youngster may decide not to experience a feeling that "belongs" to the father (e.g., anger) or that "belongs" to the mother (e.g., fear). This system can be maintained only through extensive use of denial.

Within the competitive frame of reference, problems cannot be solved; instead, struggles can only be won or lost. In fact, the competition is more important than arriving at solutions. Because problems are perceived as overwhelming and insoluble, the youngster must learn to discount the significance of external stimuli or regard them as overwhelming. Either approach leads to a very grandiose approach to thinking.

Likewise, the grandiose parent message, "You can do anything," and the punitive parent message, "But you'll never do it well enough," are isolated as separate manic and depressive experiences. Manic persons evidence grandiosity about doing things as a need to be in constant motion. At times they may be involved in a dozen or more major projects at home and at work. The depressed person who claims that he or she can do nothing right or has no energy makes an equally unrealistic assessment of his or her capabilities.

Fantasized Nurturing Parent

The fantasized nurturing parent is an internal construct reported by many persons with bipolar disorders. The child develops this internal fantasy of the loving, kind, nurturing parent as a way to deal with the experience of inconsistent

or abusive parenting. "If I just work hard enough or do well enough, then they will love me" is the child's way of attempting to control an unpredictable environment. Since the child develops and maintains this construct internally and never tests it against reality, the construct can persist into adulthood. Adults then operate from the assumption that someday they will obtain the fantasized nurturing. They are not prepared for the realistic requirements of caring for themselves in a world that is at times hostile and at times benevolent. Their response to the normal successes and setbacks of life is either unrealistic elation or depression.

The expression of bipolar personality in adulthood varies a great deal. For example, some people are successful at working hard, doing things well, and finding a family and work environment that supports their success while not expecting intimacy. Many successful administrators and business executives find social and professional reinforcement for this personality structure. Others admire their success and constant energy. They may have infrequent episodes of physical illness or fatigue from overwork, but basically they thrive on doing things and are seldom or never depressed.

In contrast, some just cannot seem to get their lives together. They have difficulty focusing their energy or sustaining any goal-directed effort. They may alternate between periods of hypomanic activity and moderate depression, or they may just suffer from chronic fatigue and depression. It is important to realize that the basic personality structures of these people are similar, even though they are acted out differently. People with bipolar personality structures can be viewed on a continuum ranging from functional to dysfunctional. Their placement on this continuum is determined to a large extent by how comfortable or uncomfortable they are with themselves and how comfortable or accepting people around them are with this behavior.

Psychobiology

Considerable research has been conducted over the past twenty years to determine the physiologic correlates of bipolar disorders (Davis and Maas 1983). Most recent data indicate that the neurotransmitters norepinephrine and serotonin fluctuate during periods of mania and depression. Urinary levels of norepinephrine decrease as people become depressed and increase during manic episodes. Davison and Neal (1978) propose that a low level of serotonin may be a predisposing factor for mood disorders and that the manic or depressive direction of the disorder is determined by an increase or decrease of norepinephrine. Although these changes in the neurotransmitters are correlated with mood changes, there is not sufficient evidence to conclude that they cause the mood changes.

Genetic factors have also been linked to the development of mood disorders (Schuckit 1986). At least six longitudinal studies of twins show an extremely high concordance of mood disorders (70 percent for identical twins and 15 percent for fraternal twins). In addition, the risk of depressive disorder in close relatives of people with mood disorders is 20 percent, compared with 5 to 10 percent for the general population. Studies using genetic markers suggest that bipolar mood disorders are transmitted by an X-linked dominant gene (Weitkamp et al. 1980).

At this time, it is not possible to say exactly what causes bipolar mood disorders. There may very well be an inherited genetic factor that makes people more vulnerable to certain environmental stressor or parenting patterns. It is clear that certain neurotransmitters fluctuate with people's moods; however, the cause-and-effect relationship has not been determined. Regardless of the origins of bipolar disorders, both clients and psychiatric nurses must learn to deal with the human responses associated with these disorders.

Depressive Disorders

The depressive disorders are characterized by exaggerated feelings of sadness, melancholy, dejection, worthlessness, emptiness, and hopelessness that are not warranted by reality. Depressive disorders may be expressed in a wide range of biologic, emotional, cognitive, and motor human responses. They should be differentiated from the normal sadness and grief resulting from some personal loss or tragedy.

Early Development

There are several theories about the development of depressive disorders, some of which are similar to theories of the causes of bipolar disorders. Three theories specific to depression—anger turned inward, object loss, and learned helplessness—are discussed in this section.

Anger Turned Inward

Anger turned inward is central to the theory developed by Freud (1957) to explain the neurotic depression he observed in his patients. Freud believes that the loss of a significant object or person precipitates both a loving and an angry response in people, whether adults or children. Since the mixed reaction of love and anger is either emotionally confusing or socially unacceptable, the person deals with the lost object by loving and grieving its loss and turns the anger against the self. For example, a young husband may find it unacceptable to be angry with his wife who died in childbirth, leaving him alone to care for a baby. He therefore turns his anger inward and blames himself for not loving his spouse enough or perhaps even assumes that he was in some way responsible for her death. This man might remain depressed indefinitely, withdraw socially, and never

consider marriage again unless he received help in expressing his anger toward the wife who deserted him.

Object Loss

Object loss is the forced, often traumatic separation of a person from a significant object of attachment. Bowlby (1960) proposes that such a significant loss during infancy or childhood establishes a pattern of anxiety, grief, and helplessness/hopelessness that the person uses to deal with all subsequent losses. Since it is impossible to go through life without experiencing at least minor losses, separations, or blows to one's self-esteem, the person establishes a lifelong pattern of depression. The person feels helpless to cope with the ups and downs of life effectively and assumes a hopeless, depressed attitude toward existence.

Learned Helplessness

Learned helplessness is one of several theories that focus on depression as a learned response to life events that are or were originally outside one's control. Seligman (1975) proposes that depression is caused not by the trauma or loss alone but by the belief that one cannot control the important events in one's life. Similarly, Beck et al. (1979) propose that depression is caused by a cognitive mind set in which people have an extremely negative opinion of themselves. Learned in youth, this negative opinion is later converted into absolutes: "No one could ever love me" or "I can't do anything right."

Personality Structure

Regardless of the etiology or childhood antecedents of depression, Arieti and Bemporad (1980) describe three types of depressive personality structures. The *dominant other* type of depression is experienced by persons who rely on dominant or significant others for their self-esteem. Their sense of worth is determined externally, and rewards and values are offered by dominant persons or organizations. These people lack personal goals and direction, tend to focus on problems, and are seen as passive, manipulative, and clinging. They avoid anger and confrontation so as not to anger those in charge of determining rewards. The *dominant goal* type of depression occurs in people who invest all of their energies and self-worth in the attainment of some inflated goal. The goal may be attaining personal wealth or professional status, being elected to public office, or discovering the cure for cancer. Whether the goal is realistic or not, the problem is that the person's self-esteem is determined by goal attainment rather than an internal sense of worth. If the goal is blocked, the person becomes depressed, and his or her lack of self-esteem becomes evident.

The *depressive character* structure is exemplified by people who cannot form either dominant other or dominant goal attachments. Their lives are empty, their relationships are petty and shallow, and they have a harsh, critical attitude toward themselves and others. They generally have many physical complaints and are unpleasant companions. Depression is a way of life for these people.

Like persons with bipolar disorders, people with depressive disorders can be viewed on a continuum ranging from functional to dysfunctional. Their level of functioning is often determined by how comfortable they are with themselves and how accepting and comfortable people around them are with the behavior. It is also important to note that the nurse has no reliable way to determine the seriousness of the stressor that precipitates depression. Only the person whose self-esteem is affected can determine the significance of the loss or stress in relation to depression.

Psychobiology

As with the bipolar disorders, there has been a marked increase in research attempting to identify the biochemical correlates of depression. For example, recent research conducted at the National Institute of Mental Health and the National Institute of Child Health and Human Development in Bethesda, Maryland, have led researchers to postulate that the high levels of **cortisol**, a steroid hormone, seen in depressed persons reflect abnormally high levels of corticotropin-releasing hormone released by the hypothalamus (Science News 1986). Further, scientists have known for some time that urinary levels of the neurotransmitter, norepinephrine, are markedly decreased in people suffering from depression. While these biochemical correlates of depression exist, it is not known whether the biochemical changes cause depression or whether depression causes biochemical alterations.

One test used in the diagnosis of *endogenous depression* (chronic depression not caused by external factors such as grief or loss) is directly related to a psychobiologic theory of depression. The **dexamethasone suppression test (DST)** involves the administration of a single dose of dexamethasone followed by blood and/or urine monitoring of cortisol levels. In depressed people, the dexamethasone does not suppress adrenocortical functioning as it does in nondepressed people. Data indicate that there is a failure of the normal inhibitory influence of the brain on the release of **adrenocorticotropic hormone (ACTH)**, a hormone of the anterior pituitary gland, and cortisol in persons suffering from depression. This suggests that depressed people have a limbic system dysfunction that is not simply a response to stress and is associated with disturbances in mood, affect, appetite, sleep, and autonomic nervous system activity.

A related theory suggests that depressed people are suffering from a failure of the central nervous system circadian inhibitory mechanism. Data about the activity levels of depressed people indicate that many symptoms of the illness, previously thought to be random events, are actually abnormal biologic rhythms. Most recently, **seasonal affective disorders (SADs)** are being studied in people who live in the northern hemisphere and suffer increased depressions during the winter months when there is less sunlight. When these people are exposed to sunlight (even artificial sunlight) for at least eight hours per day, their depressive symptoms decrease markedly or disappear altogether. The mind-body-environment interactions implied by these theories offer exciting new treatment options for depressed people.

PSYCHOPATHOLOGY

The mood (affective) disorders are divided into two major categories in DSM-IIIR (see Appendix B).

1. Bipolar disorders
    a. Bipolar disorders (mixed, manic, depressed)
    b. Cyclothymia
2. Depressive disorders
    a. Major depression (single episode, recurrent)
    b. Dysthymia

With the exception of dysthymia, the diagnosis of bipolar disorders or depressive disorders is based on the past or present incidence of manic episodes and depressive episodes. These episodes and their symptoms are defined in Box 18–2, Manic Episode, and Box 18–3, Major Depressive Episode.

Bipolar Disorders

Bipolar disorders are of three different types: manic, mixed, and depressed. The episode that leads to hospitalization the first time is usually a manic episode. Both manic and depressive episodes occur more frequently than the depressive episodes falling under the category of major depressive episodes (described later). Often one type of episode under the bipolar category will be immediately followed by a short episode of another kind under the bipolar disorders. Thus, one might experience a manic episode and appear to recover, only to develop symptoms of bipolar disorder, depressed.

Bipolar Disorder, Manic

In bipolar disorder, manic, the most recent or current episode exhibits the full criteria for a manic episode. The full criteria need not be met, however, if there has been a previous manic episode.

Bipolar Disorder, Mixed

In bipolar disorder, mixed, the most recent or current episode is characterized by symptoms of both manic and major depressive episodes. There is rapid intermingling and alternation of symptoms. Depressive symptoms are prominent and last at least a full day.

Bipolar Disorder, Depressed

In bipolar disorder, depressed, the current or most recent episode is a major depressive episode. There will have been one or more manic episodes, and the full criteria need not be met if there has been a previous major depressive episode.

Cyclothymia

Cyclothymia is characterized by a period of two years in which there have been numerous periods with abnormally elevated, expansive, or irritable moods that did not meet the symptom criteria for a manic episode, and numerous periods with depressed mood or loss of interest or pleasure that did not meet the symptom criteria for a major depressive episode. During the previous two years, there will not have been a period without hypomanic or depressive symptoms for more than two months at a time. According to DSM-IIIR (1987) the following are seen in hypomanic episodes:

1. Moods for a distinct period of time that are abnormally and persistently elevated, expansive, or irritable.

2. During the period when mood changes occur, at least

Box 18–2
MANIC EPISODE

Note: A "manic syndrome" is defined as including criteria A, B, and C below. A "hypomanic syndrome" is defined as including criteria A and B, but not C, i.e., no marked impairment.

A. A distinct period of abnormally and persistently elevated, expansive, or irritable mood.

B. During the period of mood disturbance, at least three of the following symptoms have persisted (four if the mood is only irritable) and have been present to a significant degree:

1. Inflated self-esteem or grandiosity

2. Decreased need for sleep, e.g., feels rested after only three hours of sleep

3. More talkative than usual or pressure to keep talking

4. Flight of ideas or subjective experience that thoughts are racing

5. Distractability, i.e., attention too easily drawn to unimportant or irrelevant external stimuli

6. Increase in goal-directed activity (either socially, at work or school, or sexually) or psychomotor agitation

7. Excessive involvement in pleasurable activities that have a high potential for painful consequences,

e.g., the person engages in unrestrained buying sprees, sexual indiscretions, or foolish business investments

C. Mood disturbance sufficiently severe to cause marked impairment in occupational functioning or in usual social activities or relationships with others, or to necessitate hospitalization to prevent harm to self or others.

D. At no time during the disturbance have there been delusions or hallucinations for as long as two weeks in the absence of prominent mood symptoms (i.e., before the mood symptoms developed or after they have remitted).

E. Not superimposed on schizophrenia, schizophreniform disorder, delusional disorder, or psychotic disorder NOS.

F. It cannot be established that an organic factor initiated and maintained the disturbance. Note: Somatic antidepressant treatment (e.g., drugs, ECT) that apparently precipitates a mood disturbance should not be considered an etiologic organic factor.

Source: American Psychiatric Association. Diagnostic and Statistical Manual of Mental Disorders, *ed 3, revised. APA, 1987, p 217.*

Box 18–3
MAJOR DEPRESSIVE EPISODE

Note: A "major depressive syndrome" is defined as criterion A below.

A. At least five of the following symptoms have been present during the same two-week period and represent a change from previous functioning; at least one of the symptoms is either (1) depressed mood, or (2) loss of interest or pleasure. (Do not include symptoms that are clearly due to a physical condition, mood-incongruent delusions or hallucinations, incoherence, or marked loosening of associations.)

1. Depressed mood (or can be irritable mood in children and adolescents) most of the day, nearly every day, as indicated either by subjective account or observation by others

2. Markedly diminished interest or pleasure in all, or almost all, activities most of the day, nearly every day (as indicated either by subjective account or observation by others of apathy most of the time)

3. Significant weight loss or weight gain when not dieting (e.g., more than 5 percent of body weight in a month), or decrease or increase in appetite nearly every day (in children, consider failure to make expected weight gains)

4. Insomnia or hypersomnia nearly every day

5. Psychomotor agitation or retardation nearly every day (observable by others, not merely subjective feelings of restlessness or being slowed down)

6. Fatigue or loss of energy nearly every day

7. Feelings of worthlessness or excessive or inappropriate guilt (which may be delusional) nearly every

day (not merely self-reproach or guilt about being sick)

8. Diminished ability to think or concentrate, or indecisiveness, nearly every day (either by subjective account or as observed by others)

9. Recurrent thoughts of death (not just fear of dying), recurrent suicidal ideation without a specific plan, or a suicide attempt or a specific plan for committing suicide

B. 1. It cannot be established that an organic factor initiated and maintained the disturbance.

2. The disturbance is not a normal reaction to the death of a loved one (uncomplicated bereavement).

Note: Morbid preoccupation with worthlessness, suicidal ideation, marked functional impairment or psychomotor retardation, or prolonged duration suggest bereavement complicated by major depression.

C. At no time during the disturbance have there been delusions or hallucinations for as long as two weeks in the absence of prominent mood symptoms (i.e., before the mood symptoms developed or after they have remitted).

D. Not superimposed on schizophrenia, schizophreniform disorder, delusional disorder, or psychotic disorder NOS.

Source: American Psychiatric Association: Diagnostic and Statistical Manual of Mental Disorders, *ed 3, revised. APA, 1987, pp 222–223.*

---

three of the following symptoms have persisted to a significant degree. There will be four if the mood disturbance has been only irritable.

a. Inflated self-esteem or grandiosity

b. Decreased need for sleep, e.g., feels rested after only three hours of sleep

c. More talkative than usual or pressure to keep talking

d. Flight of ideas or subjective experience that thoughts are racing

e. Distractibility, i.e., attention too easily drawn to unimportant or irrelevant external stimuli

f. Increase in goal-directed activity (either socially,

at work or school, or sexually) or psychomotor agitation

g. Excessive involvement in pleasurable activities that have a high potential for painful consequences, e.g., the person engages in unrestrained buying sprees, sexual indiscretion, or foolish business investments

Major Depression

Major depression may occur as a single episode or as a recurrent episode, but the diagnosis is used when there is no history of a manic or hypomanic episode. The illness may be further classified according to the severity of the episode, which will be noted as mild, moderate, or severe and with or without psychotic symptoms. It is believed that over 50 percent of those experiencing major depression, single episode, will ultimately experience the illness again. Those with the diagnosis of major depression, recurrent, are at higher risk for developing a bipolar disorder.

Major Depression, Single Episode

Some individuals may experience only one episode of major depression in their lifetime. As opposed to bipolar disorder where the occurrence is equal for males and females, major depression, single episode occurs twice as often among females.

Major Depression, Recurrent

Major depression, recurrent, is diagnosed when there is no history of manic or hypomanic episodes. Recurrent depressive episodes may be separated by many years, may occur in clusters, or may increase as one grows older. Between episodes, functioning is generally at the premorbid level. There may be, however, some who experience a chronic condition with considerable impairment.

Dysthymia

Dysthymia, also known as depressive neurosis, is a condition essentially consisting of chronic depressive mood disturbances for extended periods of time. The diagnosis is made when the individual is never without symptoms for more than two months over a two-year period (one year for children and adolescents). The diagnosis is not made in the presence of a major depressive episode or when symptoms are superimposed on some chronic psychotic condition. Nor is the diagnosis made when the disturbance occurs during prolonged conditions wherein a specific organic factor exists. This includes periods when certain medications such as antihypertensives are in use. According to DSM-IIIR (p 232) the symptoms that characterize this condition are as follows:

- Poor appetite or overeating
- Insomnia or hypersomnia
- Low energy or fatigue
- Low self-esteem
- Poor concentration or difficulty making decisions
- Feelings of hopelessness

THE NURSING PROCESS AND CLIENTS WITH MOOD DISORDERS

"Nursing is the diagnosis and treatment of human responses to actual or potential health problems" (ANA 1980, p 9). This definition implies a linear, cause-and-effect relationship between health problems and human responses. This relationship may not always be so clearcut. For example, a client who is immobilized in traction with multiple fractures may become depressed as a response to the health problem. In contrast, a person might be depressed and preoccupied, thus precipitating an accident that results in multiple fractures as well as guilt and increased depression.

The cause-and-effect relationship between health problems and human responses is not always clear. Health problems and human responses may be interactive in many situations. In the practice of psychiatric nursing, health problems are defined by human responses. Human responses are behaviors—biologic, motor, emotional, and cognitive behaviors. A diagnosis is a predictable cluster or configuration of human responses. For example, medical/psychiatric diagnosis of the various bipolar disorders is based on behavioral criteria for a manic episode and a major depressive episode. The medical and nursing diagnoses are therefore very closely related, as the following sections demonstrate.

Nursing Assessment

Nursing assessment data relevant to all human response patterns listed in PND-I should be obtained from the client and significant others. Clients who are extremely upset or are using denial as a defense mechanism may not provide accurate information because they cannot remember details of past events. In these cases, a relative or close friend may be the primary source of assessment data. Relevant nursing assessment data includes:

- Identifying demographic information
- Client's definition of the problem
- Psychiatric history
- Family history
- Social history
- Health history
- Current mental status

A variety of assessment tools are available to assist the nurse with data collection. Beck's Depression Inventory

(Beck 1967) is a twenty-one-item multiple-choice questionnaire clients can use to rate themselves on variables related to depression, e.g., sadness, pessimism, guilt, suicidal ideas, social withdrawal, insomnia, weight loss, and fatigue. **Zung's Self-Rating Depression Scale** (Zung 1965) contains twenty descriptors of depression—e.g., "I feel downhearted and blue"—on which clients can rate themselves on a four-point scale ranging from "a little of the time" to "most of the time." This scale is helpful in determining the client's depth or intensity of depression. The dexamethasone suppression test is used in some interdisciplinary and in-patient settings to assess the presence of endogenous depression.

Another assessment tool useful for determining the presence and acuity of depression is the Algorithm for Depression (Orsolits and Morphy 1982). There are four sections consisting of yes-or-no response sets that yield a total score indicating the level of depression and risk factors involved (see Figure 18–1). The tool focuses on recent losses, behavioral and feeling states, suicidal ideation, lethality, social supports, and judgment of the clinician. It is simple to use and helpful in aiding the client and clinician in decision-making.

Nursing Diagnosis

Once the nurse has collected and analyzed data from the nursing assessment, multiple diagnoses can be formulated. The purpose of making a nursing diagnosis is to guide nursing interventions. The nursing diagnosis is a general label for a cluster of human responses. For example, the diagnosis "01.01 Altered motor behavior" may be based on observations of a client moving about the room, seemingly unable to sit still, and waving his arms rapidly in all directions. Table 18–1 contains a comprehensive listing of the general and specific human responses that are of concern for psychiatric-mental health nurses who work with clients who have mood disorders. Not all these nursing diagnoses will apply to every client, and the nurse will need to decide which diagnoses have priority with each client at a given point in time.

The case studies on pages 445 and 449 demonstrate how assessment data are used to arrive at nursing diagnoses with two very different clients.

Psychiatric nursing diagnosis for persons with mood disorders can be classified according to the eight human response patterns:

- Activity processes
- Cognition processes
- Ecologic processes
- Emotional processes
- Interpersonal processes
- Perception processes
- Physiologic processes
- Valuation processes

There is a great deal of similarity between the human responses of concern for psychiatric-mental health nursing practice and the diagnostic criteria for determining a DSM-IIIR diagnosis. Actually, human responses can be discussed using both systems simultaneously.

01. Human Response Patterns in Activity Processes

01.01 Altered Motor Behavior

Manic persons usually display gross levels of hyperactivity and are seemingly unable to sit still, agitating themselves and others around them. Depressed persons, in contrast, are hypoactive and do very little. Some may even sit and stare into space for hours to the point that those around them report feeling depressed. Both manic and depressed people, however, may report and display physical restlessness, especially if they are using activity as a way of avoiding their feelings.

01.01.01 Bizarre Motor Behavior   Any variety of behaviors may be seen in this category, ranging from sitting still but maintaining odd or even uncomfortable positions for a period of time. Positions may be assumed while standing or walking that appear very uncomfortable or almost impossible to achieve. Repetitive acts may be seen in which the client seems not to tire after lengthy periods of repetition.

01.01.03 Impaired Coordination   Coordination may be impaired for a variety of reasons, but one of the main reasons relates to medications to which the client may be adapting. If the client is suffering great anxiety as is usual in most psychiatric illnesses, there may be lack of coordination as well as interest or energy, which the client generally manages well.

01.01.04 Hyperactivity   Activity in this category is of such intensity that there is danger of the client's becoming fatigued to the point of collapse if untreated. Movement, consisting of walking, running, or dancing of the nonstop variety, is constant. Interest is constantly changing so that the client switches rapidly from one activity to another. Since judgment is also very poor, the client may proceed to do things that, if unchecked, would prove later to be very embarrassing.

01.01.05 Hypoactivity   Activity in this category is extremely limited, and because interest in anything is generally diminished, there is no impetus to engage in activity.

	Table 18–1		
	Nursing Diagnosis of Human Responses in Mood Disorders		
General Human Response Patterns	**Specific Human Responses**	**General Human Response Patterns**	**Specific Human Responses**
01. Human response patterns in activity processes		02.03 Altered knowledge processes*	02.03.02 Altered intellectual functioning 02.03.03 Knowledge deficit*
01.01 Altered motor behavior	01.01.01 Bizarre motor behavior 01.01.03 Impaired coordination 01.01.04 Hyperactivity 01.01.05 Hypoactivity 01.01.07 Psychomotor retardation	02.06 Altered orientation	02.06.01 Confusion 02.06.02 Delirium 02.06.03 Disorientation
		02.07 Altered thought content	02.07.01 Delusions 02.07.02 Ideas of reference 02.07.03 Magical thinking 02.07.04 Obsession
01.02 Altered recreation patterns	01.02.01 Inadequate diversional activity		
01.03 Altered self-care	01.03.01 Altered eating 01.03.02 Altered grooming* 01.03.03 Altered health maintenance 01.03.04 Altered hygiene* 01.03.05 Altered participation in health care 01.03.06 Altered toileting*	02.08 Altered thought processes*	02.08.01 Altered abstract thinking 02.08.02 Altered concentration 02.08.03 Altered problem solving
		03. Human response patterns in ecologic processes	
01.04 Altered sleep arousal patterns	01.04.01 Difficult transition to and from sleep 01.04.02 Hypersomnia 01.04.03 Insomnia 01.04.04 Nightmares 01.04.05 Somnolence	03.03 Altered home maintenance*	03.03.01 Home safety hazards 03.03.02 Home sanitation hazards
01.97 Undeveloped activity processes		**04. Human response patterns in emotional processes**	
01.98 Altered activity processes not otherwise specified		04.02 Altered feeling patterns	04.02.01 Anger 04.02.01 Anxiety* 04.02.03 Elation 04.02.07 Guilt 04.02.08 Sadness 04.02.09 Shame
01.99 Potential for altered activity processes			
02. Human response patterns in cognition processes		04.03 Undifferentiated feeling patterns	
02.01 Altered decision making		04.97 Undeveloped emotional responses	
02.02 Altered judgment		04.99 Potential for altered emotional responses	

PND-I diagnosis also in NANDA list.

continued

Table 18–1 (*Continued*)
Nursing Diagnosis of Human Responses in Mood Disorders

General Human Response Patterns	Specific Human Responses	General Human Response Patterns	Specific Human Responses
05. Human response patterns in interpersonal processes			05.05.02 Social isolation/ withdrawal*
		05.99 Potential for altered interpersonal processes	05.99.01 Potential for violence
05.01 Altered communication processes*	05.01.01 Altered nonverbal communication 05.01.02 Altered verbal communication*	**06. Human response patterns in perception processes**	
05.02 Altered conduct/impulse processes	05.02.01 Aggressive/ violent behaviors 05.02.01.01 Aggressive/ violent behaviors toward environment 05.02.01.02 Aggressive/ violent behaviors toward others 05.02.01.03 Aggressive/ violent behaviors toward self 05.02.02 Dysfunctional behaviors 05.02.02.01 Age-inappropriate behaviors 05.02.02.02 Bizarre behaviors 05.02.02.03 Compulsive behaviors 05.02.02.04 Disorganized behaviors 05.02.02.05 Unpredictable	06.01 Altered attention	06.01.01 Distractability 06.01.02 Hyperalertness 06.01.03 Inattention 06.01.04 Selective attention
		06.02 Altered comfort patterns*	06.01.01 Discomfort
		06.03 Altered self-concept	06.03.03 Altered personal identity* 06.03.04 Altered self-esteem*
		07. Human response patterns in physiologic processes	
		07.02 Altered elimination processes	07.02.01 Altered bowel elimination* 07.02.01.01 Constipation* 07.02.01.02 Diarrhea
05.03 Altered role performance	05.03.01 Altered family life 05.03.02 Altered leisure role 05.03.03 Altered parenting role* 05.03.04 Altered play role 05.03.05 Altered student role 05.03.06 Altered work role	07.06 Altered nutrition processes	07.06.02 Altered systemic processes 07.06.02.01 More than body requirements *07.06.02.02 Less than body requirements*
		08. Human response patterns in valuation processes	
05.04 Altered sexuality processes		08.01 Altered meaningfulness*	08.01.01 Hopelessness 08.01.02 Helplessness 08.01.03 Loneliness
05.05 Altered social interaction	05.05.01 Social intrusiveness		

Thus, the client just sits around and may even have to be urged to get out of bed or go to the bathroom.

01.01.07 Psychomotor Retardation In this condition the client is seen as extremely slowed down so that movement appears to take twice or three times as long to get done as is usual for the client. The client does not assume a negativistic attitude but just seems to have an inability to move at the rate necessary to get anything accomplished.

01.02 Altered Recreation Patterns

01.02.01 Inadequate Diversional Activity In order to maintain a healthy life-style, there must be a balance in the work and play aspects of life. Individuals who are uninterested or unwilling to participate in other than only certain specific activities would be seen as having problems in this area. Depressed clients are uninterested, unwilling, or unable to interest themselves in diversional activities.

01.03 Altered Self-Care

01.03.01 Altered Eating Persons in this category would have suffered either a loss of interest in normal food intake or would be ingesting larger than necessary or unusual amounts of food. In extreme cases there is danger to the individual who follows one or the other of these patterns. Manic clients tend to stay too busy to eat, although at times they may gorge themselves. Depressed patients are unwilling to eat because they feel so guilty and worthless.

01.03.02 Altered Grooming* This symptom may be seen in either manic or depressive conditions and indicates either disinterest, lack of awareness, and/or inability to attend to the problem. Manic patients tend to overdo their grooming as to appear grotesque and inappropriate.

01.03.03 Altered Health Maintenance This symptom occurs in situations similar to the previous one and may require the intervention of others to prevent serious illness or death. For the manic client, there is no time; for the depressed client, there is no interest.

01.03.04 Altered Hygiene* Again, this symptom is similar to those just preceding and may become serious enough as to cause further illness or at least to hamper relationships with others.

01.03.05 Altered Participation in Health Care Persons in this category may provide a threat to the community as well as to themselves. The manic client who falls within this category may have a contagious disease such as AIDS or tuberculosis, or may present problems of another kind (e.g., failure to take medications).

01.03.06 Altered Toileting* The client who is seriously depressed or clients in the geropsychiatric category are those who present problems of this nature. Sometimes there is a tendency to take this area for granted and to fail to pay sufficient attention to the needs of clients. The nurse needs to be aware of the physiologic manifestations that can arise when this situation exists.

01.04 Altered Sleep Arousal Patterns

01.04.01 Difficult Transition to and from Sleep Sleep is a healthy and necessary component of life, and many in the general population as well as the psychiatric population suffer in this area. There are significant measures, in addition to psychotherapy, that are useful in assisting clients to improve this area.

01.04.02 Hypersomnia The client with this problem requires an excessive amount of sleep and has confusion upon awakening. Depressed clients may fall into this category.

01.04.03 Insomnia This symptom is characterized by an inability to fall asleep, difficulty remaining asleep, and/or awakening early in the morning. This condition is seen in both manic and depressed clients.

01.04.04 Nightmares Though this is a common occurrence in the general population, it also represents a symptom in the psychopathology of many clients.

01.04.05 Somnolence The tendency toward drowsiness or sleepiness may be observed in depressed clients.

01.97 Undeveloped Activity Processes

This symptom indicates an individual who has either not had available or been able to utilize certain activity skills generally available to the population. Depressed clients are observed to exhibit this problem.

01.98 Altered Activity Processes Not Otherwise Specified

This category allows the clinician to identify symptoms related to activity processes that are not clearly addressed elsewhere.

Text continues on p. 439.

---

*PND-I diagnosis also in NANDA list.

---

*PND-I diagnosis also in NANDA list.

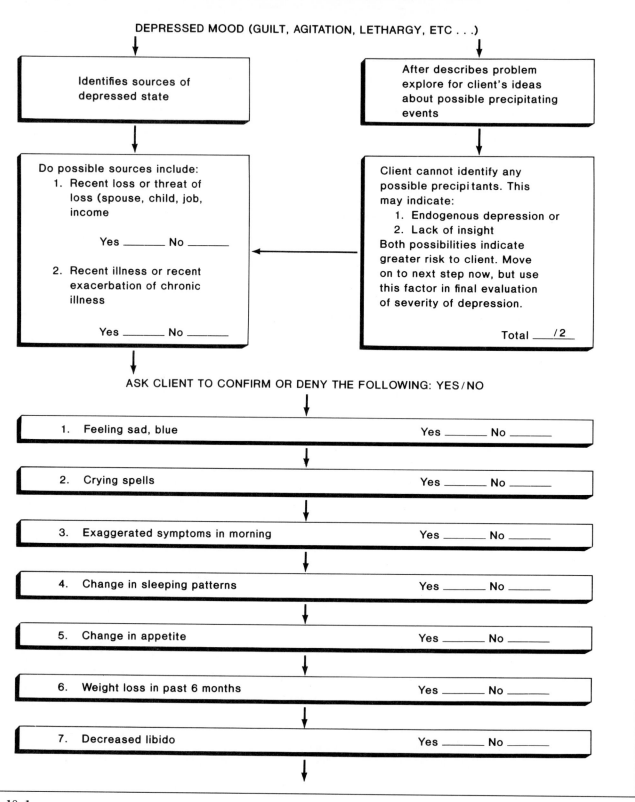

ALGORITHM FOR DEPRESSION

For use when client indicates problem related to depressed mood, feelings of guilt or shame, or when client exhibits agitation or lethargy not immediately attributable to organic cause.

DEPRESSED MOOD (GUILT, AGITATION, LETHARGY, ETC . . .)

Identifies sources of depressed state

After describes problem explore for client's ideas about possible precipitating events

Do possible sources include:
1. Recent loss or threat of loss (spouse, child, job, income

   Yes _____ No _____

2. Recent illness or recent exacerbation of chronic illness

   Yes _____ No _____

Client cannot identify any possible precipitants. This may indicate:
1. Endogenous depression or
2. Lack of insight
Both possibilities indicate greater risk to client. Move on to next step now, but use this factor in final evaluation of severity of depression.

Total ___/2___

ASK CLIENT TO CONFIRM OR DENY THE FOLLOWING: YES/NO

1. Feeling sad, blue   Yes _____ No _____

2. Crying spells   Yes _____ No _____

3. Exaggerated symptoms in morning   Yes _____ No _____

4. Change in sleeping patterns   Yes _____ No _____

5. Change in appetite   Yes _____ No _____

6. Weight loss in past 6 months   Yes _____ No _____

7. Decreased libido   Yes _____ No _____

Figure 18–1

Depression algorithm.

continued

Source: Orsolotis M, Morphy M: A Depression Algorithm for Psychiatric Emergencies. J Psychiatr Treatment Eval *1982;4:137–135. Reprinted with permission from* Journal of Psychiatric Treatment and Evaluation, *Pergamon Press, Ltd.*

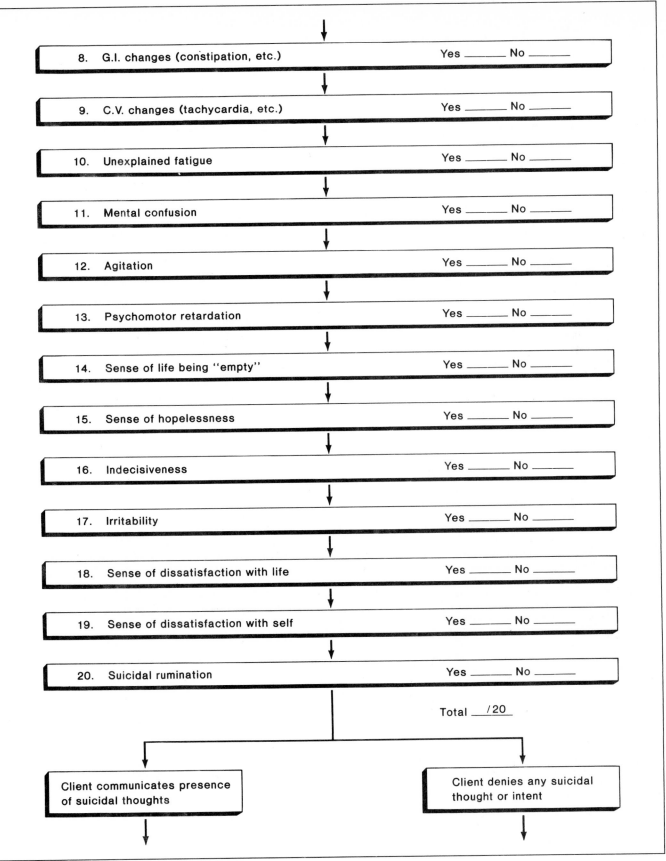

8. G.I. changes (constipation, etc.)   Yes _____ No _____

9. C.V. changes (tachycardia, etc.)   Yes _____ No _____

10. Unexplained fatigue   Yes _____ No _____

11. Mental confusion   Yes _____ No _____

12. Agitation   Yes _____ No _____

13. Psychomotor retardation   Yes _____ No _____

14. Sense of life being "empty"   Yes _____ No _____

15. Sense of hopelessness   Yes _____ No _____

16. Indecisiveness   Yes _____ No _____

17. Irritability   Yes _____ No _____

18. Sense of dissatisfaction with life   Yes _____ No _____

19. Sense of dissatisfaction with self   Yes _____ No _____

20. Suicidal rumination   Yes _____ No _____

Total ___/20___

Client communicates presence of suicidal thoughts

Client denies any suicidal thought or intent

continued

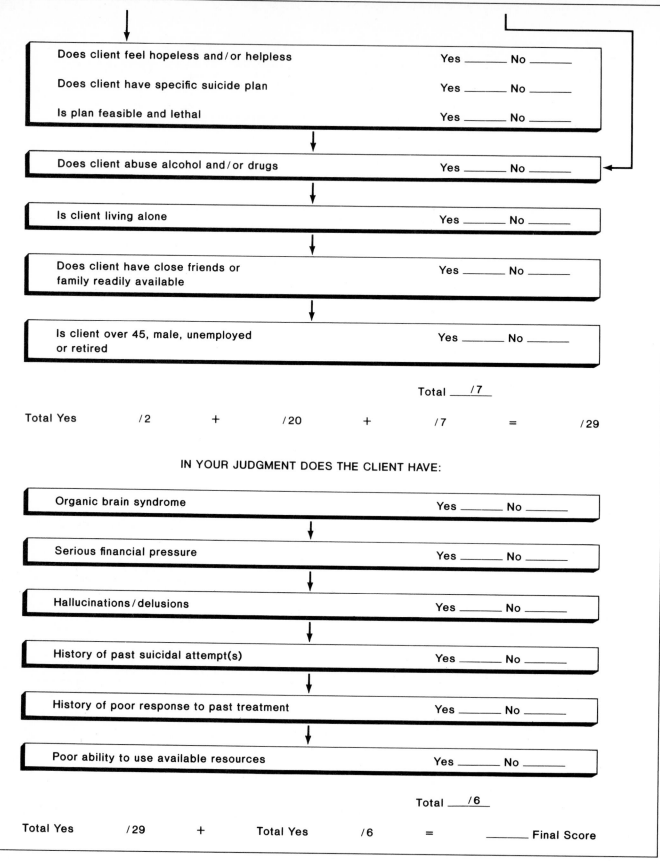

Does client feel hopeless and/or helpless   Yes _____ No _____

Does client have specific suicide plan   Yes _____ No _____

Is plan feasible and lethal   Yes _____ No _____

Does client abuse alcohol and/or drugs   Yes _____ No _____

Is client living alone   Yes _____ No _____

Does client have close friends or
family readily available   Yes _____ No _____

Is client over 45, male, unemployed
or retired   Yes _____ No _____

Total ___/7___

Total Yes   /2   +   /20   +   /7   =   /29

IN YOUR JUDGMENT DOES THE CLIENT HAVE:

Organic brain syndrome   Yes _____ No _____

Serious financial pressure   Yes _____ No _____

Hallucinations/delusions   Yes _____ No _____

History of past suicidal attempt(s)   Yes _____ No _____

History of poor response to past treatment   Yes _____ No _____

Poor ability to use available resources   Yes _____ No _____

Total ___/6___

Total Yes   /29   +   Total Yes   /6   =   _____ Final Score

continued

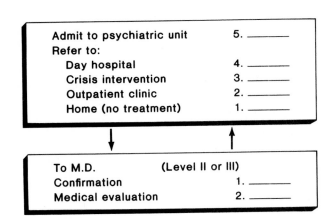

ALGORITHM SCORING

Add the number of ''Yes'' responses in each subsection to provide a final score. Scoring has been included in the algorithm's construction from the outset in order to facilitate future analysis of data. Correlations of disposition decisions, and possibly other outcome measures, with these subtotal and total scores can be completed.

01.99 Potential for Altered Activity Processes

In this category, the clinician has identified some signs indicating a client's potential for developing problems in a specific area of activity.

02. Human Response Patterns in Cognition Processes

02.01 Altered Decision-Making

The client demonstrates either an inability to decide or faulty decision-making processes. Both depressed and manic clients experience serious problems in this area.

02.02 Altered Judgment

The client's decision-making processes demonstrate poor judgment, which generally produces problems for the client or others.

02.03 Altered Knowledge Processes*

02.03.02 Altered Intellectual Functioning The client's intellectual ability falls far below the average levels in formal testing procedures.

02.03.03 Knowledge Deficit* The client does not possess certain information that one is generally expected to have at a particular point in time or experience.

02.06 Altered Orientation

02.06.01 Confusion Orientation to person, time, and place is disturbed.

02.06.02 Delirium Delirium is usually reversible, except when followed by dementia or death, when there is con-

---

*PND-I diagnosis also in NANDA list.

fusion and fluctuating consciousness due to an organic state. The condition may include delusions, illusions, and hallucinations. Outstanding symptoms are anxiety and agitation.

02.06.03 Disorientation   The client demonstrates lost awareness relative to the self in regard to space, time, or other persons.

02.07 Altered Thought Content

02.07.01 Delusions   The client holds ideas that are false and rigidly fixed so that he or she is unable to be convinced of the actual facts. This symptom may be observed in both manic and depressed clients.

02.07.02 Ideas of Reference   The client interprets casual and external events as having direct reference to the self when the contrary is true. This symptom is typical of depressed or manic clients.

02.07.03 Magical Thinking   The client has a belief that thinking is the same as doing. This condition occurs in dreams, in children, and in clients under a variety of conditions.

02.07.04 Obsession   The client holds a persistent idea that cannot be eliminated just by willing it so. Both depressed and manic clients may experience this phenomenon.

02.08 Altered Thought Processes*

02.08.01 Altered Abstract Thinking   Proverbs used to test thought processes are either interpreted in very concrete ways or out of the usual set of responses that logical persons would use.

02.08.02 Altered Concentration   The client has difficulty in reciting or recalling certain items just previously called out.

02.08.03 Altered Problem Solving   Difficulty performing a task that requires judgment and decision-making skills may be observed in both depressed and manic clients.

03. Human Response Patterns in Ecologic Processes

03.03 Altered Home Maintenance*

03.03.01 Home Safety Hazards   A situation in which this occurs may indicate the inability or disinterest of the client to manage in this area. It could relate to depressive or manic psychopathology of one or more persons in the home and may result in harm to the client as well as others.

03.03.02 Home Sanitation Hazards   These symptoms are similar to those in the previous diagnosis.

04. Human Response Patterns in Emotional Processes

04.02 Altered Feeling States

People experiencing mild, moderate, or severe depression invariably report a lack of joy, elation, or happiness. They do not necessarily report an accompanying excess of sadness, anger, distress, or guilt. In fact, they may report just feeling "empty" or "nothing." Further exploration and discussion of feelings over time may help such persons get in touch with anger or even rage, distress or anguish, or guilt or sadness accompanied by tearfulness or crying; however, these emotions may not be initially experienced or reported.

Incongruent emotions and their expression are characteristic of persons with manic and depressive disturbances. Depressed people are sad or guilty when others in their environment would normally experience pleasure or anger. Manic people are happy and elated and may even engage in inappropriate laughing, joking, or punning when the situation calls for some other emotional response. This incongruence makes other people uncomfortable or puzzles them.

04.02.01 Anger   Anger may manifest in a number of different ways. It may be explosive or of the "chip on the shoulder" variety. It may be passive-aggressive in nature so that it appears as complaining, pouting, or needling of others. Anger in the depressed person is often turned inward onto the self so that rather than showing outward manifestations of anger, the client appears sad and guilty.

04.02.02 Anxiety*   Anxiety is experienced as a sense of impending doom. It is different than fear in that the cause

---

*PND-I diagnosis also in NANDA list.

*PND-I diagnosis also in NANDA list.

is unknown; however, the uncomfortable feelings are the same. Depressed clients are prone to this symptom.

04.02.03 Elation Elation is the experience of extreme well-being and may occur in the manic period. It is unrelated to the situation at hand when it presents as a pathologic symptom.

04.02.07 Guilt Guilt is experienced from doing what is perceived as wrong, causing the individual to feel worthless and to desire punishment. This is a predominant symptom and underlying cause of depression and mania.

04.02.08 Sadness Feelings of gloom or low spirits are typically found in depressed individuals.

04.02.09 Shame Shame is an emotion that occurs when one has failed to live up to perceived expectations of self or others. This symptom may be a factor in depression and mania.

04.03 Undifferentiated Feeling Pattern

The client is unable to describe the feeling state and may appear very flat, a symptom found in depression.

04.97 Undeveloped Emotional Responses

For some individuals who are not encouraged to recognize or demonstrate feelings or who may not have such demonstrations modeled for them, there may be inability to express or demonstrate specific feeling states. This could be a prime cause of depression.

04.99 Potential for Altered Emotional Processes

Many clients who seek intervention prior to the development of a psychiatric condition may send signals relative to emotional processes indicating potential for future problems. Many others who are either not uncomfortable enough or who are unwilling to seek assistance for personal problems may also send signals indicating the potential for emotional problems.

05. Human Response Patterns in Interpersonal Processes

05.01 Altered Communication Processes*

In general, persons experiencing a manic episode are more talkative than usual and demonstrate a driven, pressured quality in their speech. People who are depressed are often

less talkative than usual; however, people attempting to avoid depression may also feel pressure to keep talking. Psychotic communication presents as difficult to understand because of the very personal and autistic needs of the client.

05.01.01 Altered Nonverbal Communication Nonverbal responses are not as usually displayed or as one would expect in a given situation.

05.01.02 Altered Verbal Communication* Verbal responses are not as usually displayed or as one would expect in a given situation. This is seen in clients whose psychopathology has become readily apparent. Speech may be retarded in the depressed client and rapid and disorganized in the manic client.

05.02 Altered Conduct/Impulse Processes

It is most important to assess a person's potential for harming himself or herself. Suicide attempts are the most obvious danger; however, there are numerous other ways of hurting oneself. Depressed people who are not actively suicidal may be accident-prone and report cutting or hurting themselves when not paying attention. Persons experiencing manic or hypomanic episodes often engage in potentially self-destructive activities, e.g., reckless driving, buying sprees, sexual indiscretions, and foolish business investments. In their manic excitement, these people simply do not stop long enough to consider their potentially harmful behaviors. Persons coming out of a severe depression are at a greater risk for suicide because they have increased energy to implement their self-destructive ideas.

05.02.01 Aggressive/Violent Behaviors

05.02.01.01 Aggressive/violent behaviors toward environment: Individuals with certain character disorders or clients experiencing organic or functional paranoid reactions may be prone toward violent behaviors.

05.02.01.02 Aggressive/violent behaviors toward others: Individuals designated above may act out their violence upon other people. Violent behavior may take the form of intermittent explosive acts or may occur as a single violent act with catastrophic impact on those around him.

---

*PND-I diagnosis also in NANDA list.

*PND-I diagnosis also in NANDA list.

05.02.01.03 Aggressive/violent behaviors toward self: Self-destructive behavior generally occurs when there is depression, although recent incidences of adolescent suicide appear to have been peer governed. Nurses need to recognize that suicide is highly possible among psychiatric clients, especially those who are depressed.

05.02.02 Dysfunctional Behaviors

05.02.02.01 Age-inappropriate behaviors: For a variety of reasons, certain individuals may fail to reach the appropriate level of maturity expected for their chronologic age, or there may be regression to earlier stages of development under periods of extreme stress. The behavior may appear as extremely dependent, even helpless, or the client may engage in temper tantrums or inappropriate sexual acting-out behaviors. This regression indicates a lack of resolution of earlier developmental tasks.

05.02.02.02 Bizarre behaviors: Maladaptive behavior that appears as bizarre is generally seen in clients with psychotic disorders, either of the functional or organic type but particularly prevalent in manic disorders.

05.02.02.03 Compulsive behaviors: Compulsive behaviors are seen in individuals with high levels of anxiety. Clients feel compelled to act in a certain way even when there is a preference not to do so (e.g., handwashing, repetitive phases, or other constant repetitious acts).

05.02.02.04 Disorganized behaviors: Clients in this category tend to behave in a manner that is incongruent with environmental expectations. Manic clients, especially, are apt to manifest such behavior (e.g., undressing in the day room).

05.02.02.05 Unpredictable behaviors: Clients in this category are difficult to assess and manage. They tend not to be goal directed or to be able to accomplish tasks. Clients who are manic tend to display unpredictability.

05.03 Altered Role Performance

05.03.01 Altered Family Life   This category indicates a discrepancy in usual family functions. This problem is certainly typical for depressed or manic clients who become so disorganized as to pose a serious threat to family stability.

05.03.02 Altered Leisure Roles   The client is unable to perform activities that might have been available in the past. Manic clients are totally unable to relax and enjoy leisure activities while depressed clients are just uninterested.

05.03.03 Altered Parenting Role*   Something has occurred to effect a change or deviation in the usual or expected role of parenting, and this is typical of both depressed and manic clients.

05.03.04 Altered Play Role   The ability to play has been hampered by some circumstance that prevents the usual experience of play. Both depressed and manic clients have problems in this area.

05.03.05 Altered Student Role   Some circumstance has occurred that causes an inability to meet student role expectations. The same problems exist for both depressed and manic clients.

05.03.06 Altered Work Role   Certain individuals may develop a condition that hampers their usual work functions. Again, this is another role affected by both depression and mania.

05.04 Altered Sexuality Processes

Neither manic nor depressed persons describe much satisfaction with sex; both may report decreased sexual desire. Some people engage in a great deal of sexual play, talk, or activity during manic or hypomanic episodes; however, this is usually outside the context of an intimate relationship.

05.05 Altered Social Interaction

Clients with mood disorders act out their internal discomfort in interpersonal relationships. For this reason, their ability to socialize is often impaired. These people engage in uninhibited people seeking and are outgoing and gregarious in social situations to the extent that they often make other people uncomfortable. When depressed, these people often withdraw and become socially isolated.

05.05.01 Social Intrusiveness   Individuals in this category tend not to recognize when they have crossed the lines of social convention. They intrude where they are not wanted and are generally seen as inappropriate. This is typical of the manic client.

05.05.02 Social Isolation/Withdrawal*   Persons in this category have given up in their attempts to develop or maintain relationships. Their level of discouragement or depression has caused them to turn inward upon themselves as an escape from reality. Withdrawal may assume autistic proportions in the depressed client.

---

*PND-I diagnosis also in NANDA list.

05.99 Potential for Altered Interpersonal Processes

05.99.01 Potential for Violence* Persons in this category give behavioral clues that give rise to concern that violence is possible. Therapeutic intervention at an early stage is helpful.

06. Human Response Patterns in Perception Processes

06.01 Altered Attention

Manic and depressed persons experience inattention and a decreased ability to concentrate: the manic individual, because of extensive attention to external stimuli, and the depressed person, because of excessive attention to internal stimuli. Both are distracted and unable to focus their attention on the task at hand. Similarly, clients with thought and organic disorders experience an inability to attend to environmental messages.

06.01.01 Distractability Manic clients with perceptual problems are easily distracted. They may seem to be engaged with another in an interaction and suddenly become involved elsewhere with little provocation.

06.01.02 Hyperalertness Clients in this category, generally manic, tend to be able to pick up on environmental stimuli not available to others.

06.01.03 Inattention Clients in this category either choose to ignore events around them or may be so flooded with anxiety as to be unable to attend. Manic or depressed clients may demonstrate this symptom but for different reasons. The manic client stays too busy while the depressed client remains disinterested.

06.01.04 Selective Attention Individuals in this category may attend only to those aspects that are of particular significance. Other stimuli are blocked out. Both manic and depressed clients may display this characteristic.

06.02 Altered Comfort Patterns*

06.02.01 Discomfort Manic clients may complain excessively of one discomfort or another, or they may ignore discomforts as they race from one thing to another. Depressed clients may ignore extreme discomfort, believing that they are unworthy of attention.

06.03 Altered Self-Concept

Persons with mood disorders experience severe alterations in self-concept. Exaggerated and diminished self-esteem

are opposite sides of the same coin, as exemplified by persons with bipolar disorders. When they are manic, these people tend to exaggerate their past accomplishments and experience a grandiose or inflated sense of themselves. When depressed, these same people can remember nothing they have ever done well and experience minimal self-esteem. Neither perspective is grounded in reality.

06.99 Potential for Altered Perception Processes

07. Human Response Patterns in Physiologic Processes

07.02 Altered Elimination Processes

Clients who are manic or depressed may have problems in this area due to inadequate or inappropriate food or water intake. Constipation may result in the depressed client who has a sharply limited amount of exercise along with limited food intake. The manic client may experience constipation as a result of limited food intake as well as diarrhea because of increased gastric motility due to increased vagal stimulation.

07.02.01 Altered Bowel Elimination*

  07.02.01.01 Constipation*
  07.02.01.02 Diarrhea*

07.06 Altered Nutrition Processes

Most clients with mood disorders experience some alteration in nutrition processes because they eat either more than or less than they normally need. Some depressed clients report a loss of appetite, while others overeat because they feel so bad about themselves. Hypomanic and manic clients pay little or no attention to nutrition. They may overeat during a period of agitation or forget to eat during a manic episode.

07.06.02 Altered Systemic Processes

  07.06.02.01 More than Body Requirements*
  07.06.02.02 Less than Body Requirements*

---

*PND-I diagnosis also in NANDA list.

08. Human Response Patterns in Valuation Processes

08.01 Altered Meaningfulness

Persons with mood disorders experience extended periods of hopelessness and helplessness. They feel overwhelmed and powerless to control their lives. They are lonely and distant from other people because they are either too depressed to reach out or because they are too manic to be in touch with themselves. In either case, they have nothing to share.

08.01.01 Hopelessness*

08.01.02 Helplessness

08.01.03 Loneliness

Planning and Implementing Nursing Interventions

General Relationship Principles

The psychiatric nurse treating persons with mood disorders must keep four general principles in mind.

1. Relating from a noncompetitive frame of reference
2. Emphasizing being rather than doing
3. Adopting a reality-oriented approach to thinking, feeling, and behaving
4. Developing realistic adult relationships and contracts for change

Regardless of the client's manic or depressive presentation and his or her specific human responses, psychiatric nurses must keep these underlying principles in mind while planning and delivering nursing care.

Relating from a Noncompetitive Frame of Reference

A noncompetitive frame of reference is essential for dealing with people who have been taught to experience themselves, their relationships, and their environments as competitive. These people tend to polarize issues and argue that such normal functions as thinking and feeling cannot be done simultaneously. They attempt to redefine treatment expectations in competitive terms with such statements as "But you told me not to work so hard" as justification for not completing a project at work and thereby jeopardizing a promotion. The nurse and client must confront this self-destructive process and explore the purpose for the redefinition of alternatives. Competition for who will win or who is in charge of the therapy must be avoided. These people are masters at winning or losing competitive battles, and neither outcome is beneficial.

Emphasis on Being Rather Than Doing

An emphasis on being rather than doing is an important strategy in working with people who present with so many behaviors that must be managed. As mentioned previously, the early competition with parents is eventually acted out by doing or not doing things successfully, and the person's worth and place in the world are externally defined by their accomplishments or lack thereof. Once this pattern is established, these people attempt to repeat the pattern and elicit a predictable response from significant others, including therapists. The nurse must get this message across: "I care about you, no matter who you are, or what you do or don't accomplish." Then the nurse must also deal with the behavioral manifestations of persons with affective disorders.

Reality-Oriented Approach

A reality-oriented approach to thinking, feeling, and behaving is the only way to ensure the safety and successful treatment of persons with affective disorders. Considerable time and energy must be spent confronting grandiosity, and clients must gradually learn to think about the consequences of their behavior. These clients need to internalize the message "You are capable of solving problems" as they confront their manic-depressive grandiosity. These people commonly have fears of never getting enough, always being depressed, driving people away, or not being able to "stand it." Such grandiosity is the justification for thinking, feeling, or doing certain things. Therefore, a great deal of time and attention are devoted to reality testing and obtaining information from other people about their experience of reality.

Developing Realistic Adult Relationships and Contracts for Change

The development of realistic adult relationships is initially modeled in the nurse-client relationship and gradually generalized to others in the client's environment. The goal revises the original construct of a fantasized nurturing par-

---

*PND-I diagnosis also in NANDA list.

Text continues on p. 454.

CASE STUDY: A Client with a Bipolar Disorder, Manic

Identifying Information	Name: Ronald B. Good

Age: 47

Address: 101 Pressure Drive
Columbia, SC 29206

Ethnic background: Caucasian

Religious preference: Baptist

Referring agency: Brought to ER by wife and police

Means of support: Self: Coach at Columbia High School
Wife: Teacher at Tangerine Elementary

Educational level: MS in education, Baylor University

Client's Definition of Present Problem

Ron angrily maintains that there is no problem. "If every one would just leave me alone so I can get ready for the big game, I'd be fine."

Emily, Ron's wife, reports that he has become increasingly agitated over the past two weeks while preparing for the local high school football championship game. "It's like he's possessed by a demon!" She reports that he has not eaten or slept for the past week and has become increasingly abusive to herself and the children. Yesterday he spent an entire day watching game films and shouting obscenities at people walking down their street.

History of Present Problem

Ron is the very competitive and successful head coach of the Columbia High Falcons. Since moving to Columbia in 1984, Ron has gained national visibility by turning the Falcons football team from losers into winners. Next Friday's regional championship game is the culmination of the Falcon's first undefeated season. His wife reports that Ron began having difficulty two weeks ago after he was interviewed by *Sports Illustrated.* He got into an argument with his two assistant coaches, who said they thought he was working the team too hard in practice. He became verbally abusive and threatened to have the principal fire them if they interfered with his championship training plan.

Although Ron never went to the principal, he began to work harder himself to prepare for the championship game. He designed new plays and watched game films in his spare time, refusing to talk with his assistants. At practice he began shouting at the players and would tell them to do two or three things at once. This new approach confused everyone, and then he would throw equipment around when they didn't follow his orders. "He acted like a stranger—a madman who frightened everyone." During the past week, Ron became more driven by his desire to win and his fear of losing. He isolated himself from his friends, wife, and children, returning home after midnight to watch game films. He refused to eat, called obscenities out the window at passersby, and became combative when friends and family expressed their concern. When he threatened his children with a baseball bat this afternoon, his wife called the police, who had to restrain him physically and brought him to the ER.

continued

Case Study (Continued)

Psychiatric History	Ron was hospitalized for one week for "physical exhaustion" four years ago. He saw a psychiatrist off and on during the following two years to help him deal with stress and pressures in his job. (He was coaching and selling real estate at the time.) He has not sought professional help since moving to Columbia. His wife reports two or three episodes of extreme energy and creativity during the past three years. For instance, last summer Ron and two friends worked night and day to build their new house in three months. "He was on top of the world and did a beautiful job. But then he was too exhausted to enjoy it."
Family History	
Parents	Ron's father, a 70-year-old retired postal worker currently living in Fayetteville, Arkansas, is described by Ron's wife as a hard-working, stern man whose major goal in life was to have his children do better than he did. He often worked two jobs while the children were young to earn enough to send his children to college. He continues to be very interested in Ron's success, and talks with him twice a week to give him advice. His mother is 69 years old and lives with her husband in Fayetteville, where she makes and sells quilts to supplement their retirement income. Both parents are in good health.
Siblings	Ron's younger brother (age 45) is a successful used car dealer in Columbus, Ohio, where he lives with his wife and two daughters. He reportedly shares Ron's drive to work hard. His younger sister (age 43) is a homemaker who lives with her husband and two children in Fayetteville, near her parents. She has assumed responsibility for attending to her parents, and Ron regularly sends her money to help out.
Extended Family	Ron sees his uncle, a bank manager in Columbia, regularly. His wife's parents and several aunts, uncles, and cousins live in Columbia, and Ron and Emily see a lot of her family. "They are all so proud of what Ron has accomplished."
Children	Ron and Emily have two sons, Ben (19 years old) and Alan (17 years old), and one daughter, Beth (14 years old). Emily reports that the children are happy and healthy, doing well in school and socially.
Social History	
Development	Ron's wife reports that he had a "normal childhood" and was loved by his parents, who are not demonstrative people. "They were tough, but they have always wanted the best for their children."
Education/Work	Ron was a goal-directed, excellent student. Has always wanted to teach and coach high school students. Ron is an excellent athlete who made the all-state teams in football, basketball, and baseball while getting all A's in high school. He played varsity football at Baylor and worked his way through graduate school as an assistant coach at Baylor. He is currently head coach at Columbia High and has begun receiving inquiries about coaching college football. His wife reports that Ron "likes what he is doing and is uncertain about coaching at the collegiate level." However, his father is encouraging him to continue climbing the ladder of success.

continued

Case Study (Continued)

Relationships/Support Systems	The family support system is extensive (see "Family History"). Ron and his family have numerous friends and colleagues in Columbia, many of whom have expressed concern about Ron's behavior in the past month.
Substance Use	None reported. Ron has begun drinking three or four beers per day over the past month.
Hobbies/Leisure Time	Ron works twelve to eighteen hours each day during the football season. He takes great interest in his sons and attends all of their sporting events. Ron enjoys fishing and hunting with his colleagues when he can get away.
Health History	In good health. Only known medical problem is high-normal blood pressure (140/90), which is being treated with a low-cholesterol diet.

Current Mental Status

General Appearance	Unshaven, disheveled, dressed in dirty flannel shirt and blue jeans with socks but no shoes. Combative and wild-eyed, frantic appearance. Struggling to get free of restraints. Very agitated and snarling at ER staff. Shouting obscenities at the door.
Sensorium	Incoherent responses to questions about time, place, and person. Knowledge, memory, and recall questionable. Judgment extremely impaired.
Emotions	Angry and extremely agitated. Alternately swearing and crying uncontrollably. Frantically scanning environment and appears frightened.
Moods	Rapid mood swings from excitement to anger to sadness to fear.
Voice and Speech	Loud swearing, growling, and snarling like an animal. Mostly incoherent, then sobbing, "I'm sorry, Daddy."
Motor Behavior	Kicking and thrashing about. Struggling against the restraints.
Thought Content	Incoherent.
Thought Process	Disorganized and easily distracted.

Other Significant Subjective or Objective Clinical Data

Medications	No prescription medications. Given 400 mg Thorazine IM in ER.
Suicide or Violence Potential	High potential for violence. Restraints will be continued and 300 mg Thorazine will be given IM every four hours until Ron is calm.
Summary	Ron is clearly experiencing a major manic episode that appears related to his increasing success as a coach, his recent interview with *Sports Illustrated,* and the pressure he feels to win the state football championship. His need to succeed and his fear of failure have resulted in a manic escalation over the past two to four weeks. Ron has history of a previous manic episode four years ago, and he has had several hypomanic episodes since.

continued

Case Study (Continued)

Diagnostic Impression

Nursing Diagnosis

01.01.05	Hyperactivity
01.03.01	Altered eating
01.03.02	Altered grooming
01.03.03	Altered health maintenance
01.03.04	Altered hygiene
01.04.03	Insomnia
02.01	Altered decision making
02.02	Altered judgment
02.06.01	Confusion
02.06.03	Disorientation
02.07.04	Obsessions
02.08.02	Altered concentration
02.08.03	Altered problem solving
02.99	Potential for altered cognition processes
04.02.01	Anger
04.02.02	Anxiety*
04.02.03	Elation
05.01.01	Altered nonverbal communication
05.01.02	Altered verbal communication
05.02.01.01	Aggressive/violent behaviors toward others
05.02.02.02	Bizarre behaviors
05.02.02.03	Compulsive behaviors
05.02.02.04	Disorganized behaviors
05.02.02.05	Unpredictable behaviors
05.03.01	Altered family role
05.03.02	Altered leisure role
05.03.03	Altered parenting role
05.03.06	Altered work role
05.04	Altered sexuality processes
05.05.01	Social intrusiveness
05.05.02	Social isolation/withdrawal
06.01.01	Distractability
06.01.02	Hyperalertness
06.01.03	Inattention
06.01.04	Selective attention
07.01.02	Altered cardiac circulation
07.06.02	Altered systemic processes
07.06.02.02	Less than body requirements*
07.99	Potential for altered physiologic processes

DSM-IIIR Diagnosis

Axis I: 296.44 Bipolar disorder, manic with psychotic features
Axis II: 301.00 Paranoid personality
Axis III: Borderline hypertension
Axis IV: 3—Moderate psychosocial stressors
Axis V: Current GAF: 10
            Highest GAF: 85

*PND-I diagnosis also in NANDA list.

CASE STUDY: A Client with Bipolar Disorder, Depressed

Identifying Information

Name: Marcia Maric
Age: 32
Address: 10 Up-Down Court
 Success, NY 12003
Ethnic background: WASP
Marital status: Single
Religious preference: Lutheran
Referring agency: Self
Means of support: Self, Executive with Cure-All Pharmaceuticals
Educational level: MBA, Harvard University, 1980

Client's Definition of Present Problem

Marcia states she is "afraid of losing control" of her behavior and emotions. She vacillates between "excitement and total lack of energy" since she was passed over for promotion six months ago, and has no energy for her friends or social activities. Unable to sleep through the night (only three to four hours sleep) for the month. Says she wants to "get back to normal," i.e., able to be happy and productive without worrying about unpredictable swings.

History of Present Problem

At age 32, Marcia was on the fast track within her corporation, having been promoted every two or three years to positions of increasing responsibility and authority. The next promotion Marcia expected was to associate vice-president for international sales, but she did not receive it. The reasons given to her for being passed over made no sense to Marcia. "We need new blood from outside the corporation." "You're too good at what you're doing; we couldn't afford to lose you from the new projects we're committed to." "You're young. There will be plenty of time for you to advance."

To Marcia, they all seemed like shallow excuses. On one level, she could agree with this logic. It certainly was not the end of the road for her. Yet, another part of her was convinced that she had not performed well enough to warrant the promotion. Yes, she had worked hard, giving eagerly of her time and energy to the corporation and enjoying the success that was personal and collective. But she could not shake the thought that they were not pleased with her work, that there was something wrong with her. And another part of her was furious, convinced that she had been sabotaged by her competitive male colleagues who could not tolerate one more reward for the woman who was more successful than those who played the game straight within the old boy network.

Marcia knew she had potential grounds for a sex discrimination case, yet she could not focus the energy that should have been available from her anger. She half-heartedly pursued opportunities with other companies, yet wound up turning down a lucrative advancement offer from the top corporation in the industry. Marcia was aware that her enthusiasm for work was dwindling. She was unable to convince herself that working evenings and weekends was worth it. But she could think of no better way to spend her free time. She also had no energy for friends, parties, concerts, plays, or cocktail parties. She thought to herself, "Others would kill for your position and success at this stage of your career. You have no

continued

Case Study (Continued)

	right to feel bad." Yet she did feel bad, and she finally decided to find someone to help her sort out her thoughts and feelings.
Psychiatric History	No prior hospitalizations. Reports obtaining tranquilizers from her general practitioner twice in past two years for what sound like hypomanic episodes of overwork and extreme agitation.
Family History	
Parents	Marcia's mother was a university professor of economics who died of cancer in 1982 at the age of 62. Her father was a neurosurgeon in private practice in Boston. He died of a heart attack in 1985, at the age of 67.
Siblings	None.
Extended Family	Marcia reports being close to one uncle (her mother's brother) who visits her two times each year while traveling on business.
Social History	
Development	Marcia reports normal growth and development as the only child of career-oriented parents. She was always the brightest child in the class and had to pretend she wasn't so smart so that the other kids would like her. She never lacked material things but describes a rather lonely childhood with respect to peer and social relationships.
Education/Work	Excellent student. BA, Radcliffe 1978; MBA, Harvard University, 1980. Graduated with honors and received numerous offers from top corporations. Accepted management position with Cure-All Pharmaceuticals because of the possibilities for rapid upward mobility.
Relationships/Support System	Although Marcia has no close friends or relationships, she reports numerous work and social contacts. She has decreased her social activities (concerts, plays, parties) in past four to six months.
Substance Use	Marcia engages in social drinking in moderation and has never smoked or used drugs. In the last month, she has been drinking more (2–3 oz) alone in the evenings.
Hobbies/Leisure Time	Marcia works twelve to eighteen hours/day. Although she used to socialize with her colleagues, she has been refusing invitations for the last two or three months. Prior to that, she attended about three work-related social events per week. In college, she enjoyed playing bridge and going to plays and concerts.
Health History	No known medical problems. Marcia has lost 10 pounds in past three months without dieting. Though thin, she reports excellent physical health. She jogs once or twice a week.
Current Mental Status	
General Appearance	Bright, poised, articulate, business executive. "Power dressed" in tailored suit and ruffled blouse. Carries herself like a confident woman who is used to being in charge.

continued

Case Study (Continued)

Sensorium	Oriented to time, place, and person. Knowledge, memory, recall, and judgment intact.
Emotions	Flat affect except when excited (e.g., when talking about work). Denies anger or depression.
Moods	Rapid mood swings between hypomanic and depressed affect.
Voice and Speech	Pressured to keep talking.
Motor Behavior	Very proper and controlled movements.
Thought Content	Normal. Denies thoughts of suicide or anger.
Thought Process	Presents herself and her ideas in a very controlled, organized manner, at times without affect. Appears pressured to keep talking. Reports increased difficulty concentrating on her work over the past month. Is working on three large marketing projects simultaneously. Demonstrates little insight into her current situation. Has difficulty reflecting on her own thoughts and feelings.

Other Significant Subjective or Objective Clinical Data

Medications	No prescription medications. Uses aspirin three or four times a week for tension headaches.
Suicide or Violence Potential	Not at this time. Will monitor as she gets in touch with her anger and sadness.
Summary	Bright, attractive career woman who is having difficulty dealing with perceived rejection and loss over recently not being promoted. Also, she has never dealt with grief over deaths of her mother (1982) and father (1985). She denies anger, guilt, or sadness.

Diagnostic Impression

Nursing Diagnosis

01.01.05 Hyperactivity
01.02.01 Inadequate diversional activity
01.03.01 Altered eating
01.97   Potential for altered activity processes
02.08.02 Altered concentration
02.08.03 Altered problem solving
02.99   Potential for altered cognition processes
04.02.01 Anger
04.02.02 Anxiety
04.02.05 Fear*
04.02.06 Grief*
04.03   Undifferentiated feeling pattern
04.97   Undeveloped emotional responses
04.97   Potential for altered emotional processes
05.01.01 Altered nonverbal communication
05.01.02 Altered verbal communication*
05.97   Potential for altered interpersonal processes

*PND-I diagnosis also in NANDA list.

continued

Case Study (Continued)

06.01.01 Distractability
06.03.03 Altered personal identity*
06.03.04 Altered self-esteem
06.03.05 Altered social identities
07.99   Potential for altered physiologic processes
08.01.02 Helplessness
08.01.03 Loneliness
08.01.04 Powerlessness*

DSM-IIIR Diagnosis

Axis I: 296.53 Bipolar disorder, depressed with melancholia
Axis II: 301.81 Narcissistic personality
Axis III: Recent weight loss without dieting
Axis IV: 3—Moderate stressors
Axis V: Current GAF: 65
              Highest GAF: 87

Nursing Care Plan

Nursing Diagnosis	Client Care Goals	Nursing Planning/ Intervention	Evaluation
05.01 Altered communication processes*	Eliminate pressure to keep talking.	Use conversation during treatment sessions to pace the client's rate and intensity of speech. Then lead her gradually to a more comfortable, conversational rate and intensity.	Engages in normal conversation. Reports feeling comfortable talking normally with others.
05.03 Altered role performance	Improve effectiveness/ productivity at work.	Set daily and weekly goals to help client with realistic time structuring (e.g., What can she realistically accomplish each day of the week?). Help client plan to negotiate revised expectations with immediate supervisor if necessary.	Client sets and accomplishes work goals three of five days a week.
05.05 Altered social interaction	Restore interest/pleasure in usual social activities.	Plan with client for two social activities per week. Help her select the people and activities that will make her most comfortable and during which she will receive positive strokes.	Plans and attends two social activities per week.
04.02 Altered feeling patterns	Experience and express full range of emotions.	Use therapeutic sessions (twice a week) to help client explore and express her	Experiences full range of emotions in personal, work, and social situations.

*PND-I diagnosis also in NANDA list.

continued

Case Study (Continued)

Nursing Diagnosis	Client Care Goals	Nursing Planning/ Intervention	Evaluation
		feelings about (1) loss of anticipated promotion, (2) loss of both parents within the past five years, and (3) her current work and social situation. Anticipate client will need permission and protection to help her confront her anger, guilt, and sadness. Obtain no-running (emotionally) and no-suicide contracts. Once denial of anger, sadness, and guilt has been eliminated, she should be able to experience joy/happiness more comfortably.	Reports feeling comfortable with herself and her feelings.
06.01 Altered attention	Improve ability to concentrate at work.	Talk with client about what is going on internally when she is having difficulty concentrating. (It is likely she is feeling agitated or pressuring herself to perform.) Help client set realistic expectations of herself. Encourage breaks and more contact with people to increase self-esteem and positive strokes.	Is able to concentrate on work for realistic periods of time. Takes morning and afternoon breaks and lunch with a friend or colleague.
01.01 Altered motor behavior	Decrease restlessness. Increase structured physical activity.	Help client plan to jog five mornings/week. Explore possibility of physical activity (tennis, racquetball, or health club) with friends.	Jogs five mornings per week. Reports being comfortable and in touch with her body.
01.03 Altered self-care	Improve appetite and reverse recent weight loss.	As client expresses feelings and deals with depression, her appetite will probably return. In the meantime, help her structure plans for three meals/day (2200 kcal) to regain weight. Help her select foods she enjoys and pleasant experiences (e.g., lunch with a friend) to support positive eating experiences. Give message that eating properly is one means of taking care of herself.	Eats three meals/day (2200 cal). Gains ten pounds. Reports improved appetite and enjoyment of food.

continued

Case Study (Continued)

Nursing Diagnosis	Client Care Goals	Nursing Planning/ Intervention	Evaluation
01.04 Altered sleep/ arousal patterns	Improve ability to sleep peacefully through the night.	Teach deep breathing and progressive relaxation techniques. Explore what client is thinking, feeling, and doing while unable to sleep. Help her express her denied feelings (should improve ability to sleep) and problem solve ways to be relaxed and quiet at night.	Gets six or seven hours of uninterrupted sleep each night. Reports sleeping comfortably.
05.03 Altered role performance	Increase structured physical activity and social activities with friends.	Explore possibility of physical activities (e.g., tennis, racquetball, or health club) with friends. Plan ways to meet people with common interests in music and theater.	Plans and attends two social activities per week. Reports enjoyment from social activities.

ent into a more realistic, adult approach to caring, nurturing, and relating to other people. Contracting within relationships is one way to accomplish this objective. A contract is a mutually agreed on set of expectations between two or more people about what each will contribute to the relationship. If conditions change, as they often do, the contract can be renegotiated. However, it always serves as a clear statement of what people can expect from each other at any given time.

Safe treatment of persons with mood disorders involves the use of several important contracts. The timing and significance of these nurse-client contracts vary depending on the issues presented by the client, but all should be considered potentially useful.

Social Control Contract   Social control contracts provide a good way to assess the client's ability to make and keep contracts. Since persons with mood disorders often present with problems of doing or not doing things, the nurse can begin by addressing practical problems related to time structuring. For example, a client may need help cutting back on an eighty-hour work week filled with overlapping committee meetings. The agreement may be to find ten free hours per week. Another client may require help obtaining employment, and the agreement may be to interview for three jobs in one week. The ability to make and keep contracts is essential for working with these people, and this expectation should be shared from the outset. Clients who are unwilling to make contracts do not usually

stay in treatment. Clients who are unable to keep contracts may require hospitalization for their own protection and safety.

No-Running Contract   The no-running contract is a direct way to address the personality structure of persons with mood disorders. This contract is essentially an agreement to deal with issues and not to run away or withdraw, either physically or psychologically. The importance of this contract is evidenced by the great anxiety most of these people experience while making the contract. Some are reluctant to make the commitment and say they feel trapped. The fact is that treatment work with these clients is not likely to succeed unless they agree to stay engaged with the nurse and confront uncomfortable issues previously ignored. The complementary messages delivered by the nurse are:

- Your problems can be solved
- Your feelings are not so overwhelming that you must run away
- You can stay and deal with issues

In this way, the nurse and client establish an alternative to grandiosity and discounting.

No-Secrets/No-Lies   Contract   The   no-secrets/no-lies contract is closely related to the no-running contract. Lies are active misrepresentations of reality, and secrets are the withholding of important information. Both are the primary mechanisms used by persons with mood disorders to maintain distance from other people. Because of their extensive use of denial, these people are often unaware of how greatly they distort reality. For example, they may deny being angry because they are out of touch with their own rage. One manic client denied ever having been depressed, even though she later reported having tried to kill herself on two occasions. The expectation that accompanies the no-lies/no-secrets contract is that it is possible to be aware of thoughts, feelings, and behaviors simultaneously, and that no aspect of oneself should be ignored or excluded.

No-Suicide/No-Homicide Contract A no-suicide/no-homicide contract is required to provide these people with the protection necessary to work on significant underlying issues. The nurse can ask a client to state, "I will not hurt or kill myself or anyone else, accidentally or on purpose, no matter what." It is important to watch and listen for any hesitation, changes in wording, or incongruence between what is said and how it is said. The nurse can ask the client to look directly at the nurse while making the contract. Once the client has made a clear and congruent commitment, the nurse says that she or he accepts the decision and is willing to help the client keep the contract.

Manic-depressive clients often deny the need for a no-suicide/no-homicide contract. They may not understand why it is so important, but they are usually willing to make the contract. They usually agree because their extensive use of denial has put them out of touch with the homicidal rage within the manic structure and the struggle for existence within the depressive structure. Even though these people are willing to make the initial contract, the contract may need to be repeated at a later time when they are more in touch with the feelings and thoughts of wanting to hurt themselves or someone else.

Clients with depressive disorders are usually aware of their own suicidal thoughts and depressed feelings and therefore appreciate the need for a no-suicide contract. They are, however, reluctant to give up the option of suicide as a solution to their pain and despair. It may take a number of discussions before they can believably commit to the contract. For these people the process of making the contract is a very important aspect of the treatment and is well worth the time and energy it takes to accomplish.

Specific Intervention Techniques

Specific intervention techniques vary significantly depending on the individual characteristics of the client and nurse, the setting in which the treatment is conducted, and the social supports available to the client and the therapeutic support available to the nurse (see Nursing Care Plan on

page 456). For example, in some settings all clients with bipolar disorders are routinely treated with lithium, and clients with depressive disorders are routinely treated with antidepressants. The role of the nurse—a very limited role indeed—is to administer medications, encourage compliance (see Research Note), and monitor their side effects.

In other settings, the nurse is one of several mental health professionals who work with clients and their families in community treatment centers. The nurse's role may be that of primary therapist conducting family groups and helping clients return to normal work, social, and family functioning. Nurses in in-patient settings may have little or no contact with the client's family but may instead be responsible for ensuring the client's safety during episodes of acute illness.

Because of this variation, the intervention techniques presented here are designed to provide a beginning list of considerations for nurses responsible for developing specific therapeutic interventions for clients with affective disorders. Table 18–2 contains a listing of the nursing diagnoses and related nursing interventions frequently used in working with clients with mood disorders.

Providing for Safety

Safety interventions are of primary importance for clients with affective disorders. As mentioned earlier, suicide is only one of many ways these people have of hurting themselves. Accidents, loss of jobs, and destructive relationships are often ways of acting out the same problem. When these clients demonstrate significant alterations in conduct/impulse control, motor behavior, or self-care activities, they may need to be hospitalized for their own safety and protection. Medication may also be used to alter behavior that is either too manic or too depressed. Clients who are actively suicidal must be protected in an environment that is free of all means of harming oneself. They may also require constant observation during certain periods. Hospitals should have policies and procedures for protecting clients who are actively suicidal. It is usually the responsibility of the nursing staff to provide this protection.

No-suicide contracts and other limit-setting, social control contracts are also useful in providing safety and protection. Once a client demonstrates a willingness to make contracts and an ability to keep them, social control contracts can be made specific to the needs of the individual.

One hypomanic woman said she was "picking up energy" from the car engine and radio while driving

Nursing Care Plan: The Client with Dysthymia

Nursing Diagnosis	Client Care Goals	Nursing Planning/ Intervention	Evaluation
05.01 Altered communication processes*	Increase frequency of conversations with other people.	Use conversation during treatment sessions to pace and lead client from monosyllabic responses to mutual sharing of information.	Initiates discussion and shares information comfortably with therapist.
05.05 Altered social interaction	Decrease social isolation and withdrawal from other people.	Contract with client to take her morning and afternoon breaks at work (doesn't usually take breaks) and say something to one co-worker each break. Once comfortable with conversations during breaks, contract to accept previously declined lunch invitation from the co-worker she likes who has plants in her window. Encourage client to buy a geranium for her own office.	Initiates two verbal exchanges with co-worker(s) each day for two weeks. Goes to lunch with co-worker. Buys a plant for her office.
04.02 Altered feeling patterns	Increase joy/happiness. Decrease guilt. Decrease sadness/depression.	Use therapeutic sessions (twice/week) to help client explore and express her feelings of guilt and self-hatred. A no-suicide contract is essential to provide protection/safety during this process. Reinforce permission to express these feelings verbally to therapist and not to act them out or take them out on herself. Gradually work toward expression of anger turned inward and obtain information about the cause(s) of her depression.	Expresses full range of emotions during therapeutic sessions. Reports feeling comfortable with herself and her feelings. Client is able to experience and report occasional joy/happiness.
05.03 Altered role performance	Involve client in pleasurable activities.	Since client currently reports no involvement in pleasurable activities, will need to begin slowly to help her gain experience. Once client is comfortable with treatment relationship, will plan to take her to local	Client can discriminate between pleasant and unpleasant activities. Engages in one pleasurable activity each week.

continued

Nursing Care Plan: The Client with Dysthymia *(Continued)*

Nursing Diagnosis	Client Care Goals	Nursing Planning/ Intervention	Evaluation
		shopping mall to observe a range of people and explore potentially pleasurable activities (e.g., shopping, eating ice cream, watching children). This wide range of stimuli should produce a positive experience on which to build.	
06.03 Altered self-concept	Increase self-esteem.	Begin with therapeutic relationship to communicate acceptance of client and her feelings. Encourage client to verbalize the negative messages she is likely using internally to put herself down so that they can be tested against reality. Teach her nonjudgmental approach to accepting herself the way she is. (This process will be gradual.)	Congruently expresses one positive statement about herself each session.
02.07 Altered thought content 08.01 Altered meaningfulness*	Eliminate suicidal ideation. Decrease hopelessness and loneliness.	Once no-suicide contract is obtained, encourage client to verbally express suicidal thoughts, feelings, and behaviors. Assess need for protection (e.g., crisis phone number, hospitalization) and discuss with client. Involve her in planning alternatives (e.g., calling a friend) to sitting home alone and thinking about killing herself. Gradually move toward decision to live and develop positive images about the future.	Makes congruent decision to live. Reports positive plans for future.
01.01 Altered motor behavior	Increase energy/decrease fatigue.	Plan with client for gradual increase in physical activity. Begin with walking— preferably one mile/day— then explore pleasurable physical activities with other people.	Walks one mile each day. Engages in social physical activity once a week.

*PND-I diagnosis also in NANDA list.

continued

and had received four speeding tickets during the previous six months. She agreed to drive no faster than 55 miles per hour and contracted to walk or take a cab if she was to "high" to drive safety. To keep her contract, she decided not to use the car radio or to pull off to the side of the road and breathe deeply until she was calm enough to drive. This contract saw her safely through a period of hypomanic agitation. The slower speed actually had a calming effect on her, and she now has a car with cruise control.

Once a client has demonstrated a willingness and ability to make and keep contracts, any alteration in conduct/impulse control, motor behavior, or self-care activities can be dealt with by means of a social control contract to ensure the client's physical safety. Then treatment can expand into other areas important to the client and nurse.

Providing for Understanding

Pace and lead is a general intervention that the nurse can use with any client who has an excess or deficit of an emotion or behavior. *To pace* simply means to match the rate at which the client is moving, talking, or feeling. Once that match or pace is established, the nurse can lead the client to a slower or faster pace, as required. For example, when establishing rapport with a depressed client who sits, stares, and shows no interest in talking, the nurse sits down near the client and "paces" the quietness. The nurse may begin leading by saying just a few words: "Quiet day, isn't it?" or "It's good to be with someone who appreciates peace and quiet." Before leaving, the nurse might say something like, "I assume that when you want something, you will tell me," thus creating the expectation that the client will be able to talk when the need arises. The nurse may need to repeat this approach several different times or for several days in a row before the client begins to respond, but the client will eventually respond. Once the client begins talking with the nurse, the nurse can gradually increase the rate of speech and the level of emotion expressed by carefully, slowly increasing the pace. The client is led through successive approximations to a new rate of speech and expression of affect.

Pacing and leading is also useful with manic clients who need to be slowed down. Their rapid, manic pace is obvious from their rate of communication, the pressure they feel to keep talking, their apparent need to keep moving and doing things, and their inability to sit still or rest. The pace and lead intervention is similar to that used with depressed clients. The nurse begins by matching the client's

Table 18–2
Nursing Diagnosis and Nursing Interventions

Nursing Diagnosis	Nursing Interventions
01. Activity process	
01.01 Altered motor behavior	Safety/protection
01.03 Altered self-care	Pace and lead
01.04 Altered sleep/ arousal patterns	Structured physical activity
	Contract for intake and weight program
	Relaxation/medication
02. Cognition processes	
02.01 Altered decision making	Contract for behavioral change
02.07 Altered thought processes	Reality confrontation
	Pace and lead
	Structured activities
04. Emotional processes	
04.02 Altered feeling patterns	Pace and lead
	Expand emotional experience
	Structured release/ confrontation
05. Interpersonal processes	
05.01 Altered communication processes*	Pace and lead
	Safety/protection
05.02 Altered conduct/impulse processes	Limit-setting/contracts
05.03 Altered role performance	Structured role activity work with significant others
05.04 Altered sexuality processes	Contract for behavioral change
05.05 Altered social interaction	Contract for social activities
06. Perception processes	
06.01 Altered attention	Structured activities (e.g., cards, games)
06.03 Altered self-concept	Reality confrontation
07. Physiologic processes	
07.06 Altered nutrition processes	Contract for intake and weight program
08. Valuation processes	
08.01 Altered meaningfulness*	Externalize/nonjudgmental approach

PND-I diagnosis also in NANDA list.

behavior. If the client is walking, the nurse walks fast and gradually slows the pace. If the client is talking, the nurse talks, laughs, and is very expressive before gradually diminishing the tone and affect so that a normal or serious discussion can take place.

One potential problem in pacing and leading people engaged in manic behavior is that others in their environment may wish to keep them animated. Manics who are not out of control can be entertaining and fun to be around socially, and others readily pick up the energy they transmit. The high level of energy and activity helps these clients and those around them to avoid their feelings and problems. Nurses may therefore have to make an extra effort to convince others to stop encouraging manic behavior. At times, manic clients are best treated in an isolated area or room where pacing and leading can be done more effectively.

Providing for Structure

Structured activities and contracts can be used to address a wide range of client problems. Alterations in motor behavior, role performance, self-care, sleep patterns, sexuality, emotional experience and expression, and even thought processes all respond readily to structured interventions. Clients who want to change and work with the nurse to make and alter behavioral contracts are good candidates for structured activities and goal-directed contracts. The nurse needs to remember that these clients tend to act out their difficulties by doing or not doing things, and the structured activities and behavioral contracts may become the stage on which they are able to act out and work through earlier unresolved issues.

Time structuring is often a good way to begin work with clients experiencing affective disorders because their difficulty with doing or not doing things is reflected in how they structure their days and spend their time. One can begin by asking these clients to keep an exact record of all their activities for one week and then thoroughly examine the written record together. This process usually makes clients much more aware of their use of time, the people with whom they spend time, and their feelings about the activities in which they are engaged. The record gives the nurse a wealth of quantitative and qualitative data about these clients and their lives. What are their regular physical activities? What are their usual work, social, and family role-related activities? What are their activity/rest patterns? Are they spending the necessary time for eating and

---

RESEARCH NOTE

Citation

Connelly CE: Compliance with outpatient lithium therapy. Perspect Psychiatr Care *1984;22(2):44–50.*

Study Problem/Purpose

"The purpose of this study was to identify the variables associated with patient compliance or noncompliance with a therapeutic regimen, which included lithium and regularly scheduled therapeutic appointments for the treatment of major affective disorders" (pp 44–45).

Methods

Subjects for this study were twenty-five clients from a large, federal psychiatric institution in a major Eastern city and fifty clients from a federally operated research facility in the suburbs of the same city. The mean age of the subjects was 47 (range = 21–74 years), 59 percent of the clients were female, and their mean number of years completed in school was 14.6 (range = 8–20 years). Fifty-one percent of the clients were treated individually and 49 percent were treated in group sessions.

A thirty-three item compliance questionnaire was administered to all subjects. Demographic data, therapeutic modality, lithium level, and number of scheduled and kept appointments were obtained from client records. "Patient compliance was operationally defined as serum lithium levels within recommended therapeutic range (0.5–1.5 mEq/L) and attendance at 75 percent or more of the scheduled therapeutic appointments for six months prior to completing the questionnaire" (p 47).

Findings

Fifty patients (67 percent) demonstrated compliance as evidenced by serum lithium levels and kept appointments, and only three patients (4 percent) were noncompliant according to both indices. "Lithium compliance was significantly greater among married patients and patients with higher levels of education. Appointment keeping compliance was positively associated with individual therapy and increased patients' perceptions of continuity, and negatively correlated with patients' perceptions of increased costs of treatment" (pp 49–50).

Implications

This study demonstrates the complex nature of client compliance with long-term treatment regimens. It is important to consider individual client characteristics, the treatment environment, client attitudes, and the type of treatment in nursing attempts to foster and enhance compliance.

sleeping? Do they have any regular sexual activity? Once both client and nurse have a common data base, they can discuss what they each feel and think about the information and begin to develop specific contracts for change.

Providing Emotional Confrontation and Cognitive Restructuring

Emotional confrontation and cognitive restructuring are intervention techniques for dealing with difficulties in feeling and thinking. Alterations in emotional response patterns and perceptual/cognitive response patterns are interrelated in clients with affective disorders. For this reason, both emotional confrontation and cognitive restructuring interventions are often done simultaneously. Emotional confrontation is a safe and structured way to let the client deal with emotions previously denied or considered overwhelming. At the same time, cognitive restructuring involves giving the client a new way to think about or understand the emotional experience. For example, a man who thinks that his anger is overwhelming may be asked to obtain feedback from other people about how they experience and deal with their own anger. The man can then compare that information with his own thoughts and feelings. At the same time, this client may also engage in a structured activity, e.g., racquetball, to express his anger safely and increase his range of emotional experiences.

Evaluation

Nursing diagnosis and treatment are intended to produce beneficial effects in the human responses to actual or potential health problems, which are the phenomena of concern for nurses. "It is the results of the evaluation of outcomes of nursing actions that suggest whether or not those actions have been effective in improving or resolving the conditions to which they were directed" (ANA 1980, p 12).

Nurses, clients, and significant others all participate in determining the treatment goals and outcomes for persons with mood disorders. Table 18–3 contains an example of the nursing diagnoses, treatment goals, and outcome criteria for the initial month of treatment with a client experiencing a manic episode. Outcomes are measured in terms of beneficial changes in human responses: biologic, emotional, cognitive, and motor behaviors.

Chapter Highlights

- People with mood disorders range from functional to dysfunctional depending on how comfortable they are

---

Table 18–3
Selected Nursing Diagnoses, Treatment Goals, and Outcome Criteria: Manic Episode

Nursing Diagnosis: 05.01 Altered communication processes

Goals	Outcome Criteria
To decrease quantity of speech	Engages in normal conversation
To decrease rate of speech	Engages in normal conversation
To decrease internal pressure to keep talking	Reports feeling comfortable talking normally with others

Nursing Diagnosis: 05.02 Altered conduct/impulse processes

Goals	Outcome Criteria
To decrease incidents of reckless driving to zero	Uses cruise control at 55 mph during freeway driving
	Has no citations for moving violations or accidents
	Passengers report client drives safely

Nursing Diagnosis: 05.03 Altered role performance

Goals	Outcome Criteria
To respond congruently within work and social situations	Jokes less and makes fewer puns
	Sits quietly in serious situations
	Listens to others when they are talking

Nursing Diagnosis: 06.01 Altered attention

Goals	Outcome Criteria
To increase attention span	Reads quietly for a half hour
	Completes sentences while conversing

Nursing Diagnosis: 06.03 Altered self-concept

Goals	Outcome Criteria
To decrease grandiosity	Makes reasonable appraisal of reality as confirmed by four other people
	Makes realistic statements about his or her own abilities

---

with themselves and how comfortable or accepting those in the environments are with the behavior.

- The DSM-IIIR psychiatric diagnosis is one helpful piece

of information in formulating a nursing diagnosis and treatment plan for clients with mood disorders.

- Nursing is the diagnosis and treatment of human responses to actual or potential health problems.

- Human responses are biologic, motor, emotional, and cognitive behaviors.

- A diagnosis is a predictable cluster or configuration of human responses.

- There is a great deal of similarity between the human responses of concern for psychiatric-mental health nursing practice and the diagnostic criteria used for determining a psychiatric diagnosis using DSM-IIIR. Human responses can be discussed using both systems simultaneously.

- Psychiatric nursing diagnoses for persons with mood disorders can be classified according to sociobehavioral response patterns, emotional response patterns, and perceptual/cognitive response patterns.

- Psychiatric nursing treatment of persons with mood disorders must be delivered from a noncompetitive frame of reference; with an emphasis on being rather than doing; with a reality-oriented approach to thinking, feeling, and behaving; and with the goal of developing adult relationships and contracts for change.

- A contract is a mutually agreed on set of expectations between two or more people about what each will contribute to the relationship.

- Specific intervention techniques for working with mood disordered clients vary significantly depending on the individual characteristics of the client and nurse, the setting in which the treatment is conducted, the social support available to the client, and the therapeutic support available to the nurse.

References

American Nurses' Association: *Nursing: A Social Policy Statement.* ANA, 1980.

American Psychiatric Association: *Diagnostic and Statistical Manual of Mental Disorders,* ed 3, revised. APA, 1987.

Arieti S: Manic-depressive psychosis and psychotic depression, in Arieti S (ed): *American Handbook of Psychiatry,* ed 2. Basic Books, 1974, pp 449–490.

Arieti S, Bemporad J: Psychological organization of depression. *Am J Psychiatry* 1980;137(11):1260–1365.

Beardslee WR, Bemporad J, Keller MB, Klerman GL: Children of parents with major affective disorder: A review. *Am J Psychiatry* 1983;140(7):825–832.

Beck AT: *Depression: Causes and Treatment.* University of Pennsylvania Press, 1967.

Beck A, et al: *Cognitive Therapy of Depression.* Guildford Press, 1979.

Belmaker RH, van Praag HM (eds): *Mania: An Evolving Concept.* Spectrum Publications, 1980.

Bowlby J: Grief and mourning in infancy and early childhood. *Psychoanalytic Study Child* 1960;15:9.

Chaisson M, Beutler L, Yost E, Allender J: Treating the depressed elderly. *J Psychosoc Nurs* 1984;22(5):25–30.

Davis JM, Maas JW (eds): *The Affective Disorders.* American Psychiatric Press, 1983.

Davison GC, Neal JM: *Abnormal Psychology.* Wiley, 1978.

Dixson DL: Manic depression: An overview. *J Psychiatr Nurs* 1981;19(6):28–31.

Freud S: *Mourning and Melancholia. Standard Edition of the Complete Psychological Works of Sigmund Freud,* vol 14. Hogarth Press, 1957.

Gordon VC, Ledray LE: Depression in women. *J Psychosoc Nurs* 1985;23(1):26–34.

Helm SB: Nursing care of the depressed patient: A cognitive approach. *Perspect Psychiatr Care* 1984;22(3):100–107.

Loomis ME, Landsman SG: Manic-depressive structure: Assessment and development. *Transactional Analysis J* 1980;10(4):284–290.

Loomis ME, Landsman SG: Manic-depressive structure: Treatment strategies. *Transactional Analysis J* 1981;11(4):346–351.

Meisenhelder JB: Self-esteem: A closer look at clinical intervention. *Int J Nurs Stud* 1985;22(2):127–135.

NIMH/NIH Consensus Development Plan: Mood disorders: Pharmacologic prevention of recurrences. *Am J Psychiatry* 1985;142(4):469–476.

Orsolits M, Morphy M: A depression algorithm for psychiatric emergencies. *J Psychiatr Diag Eval* 1982;4:137–145.

Schuckit MA: Genetic and clinical implications of alcoholism and affective disorder. *Am J Psychiatry* 1986;143:140–147.

Science News. May 24, 1986;129:324.

Seligman M: *Helplessness: On Depression, Development, and Death.* Freeman, 1975.

van Servellen GM, Dull LV: Group psychotherapy for depressed women: A model. *J Psychiatr Nurs* 1981;19(8):25–31.

Weitkamp L, Pardue L, Huntzinger R: Genetic marker studies in a family with unipolar depression. *Arch Gen Psychiatry* 1980;37:1187–1192.

Zung W: A self-rating depressive scale. *Arch Gen Psychiatry* 1965;12:63.

NINETEEN

Applying the Nursing Process for

Clients with Anxiety, Somatoform, and Dissociative Disorders

Marilynn Petit

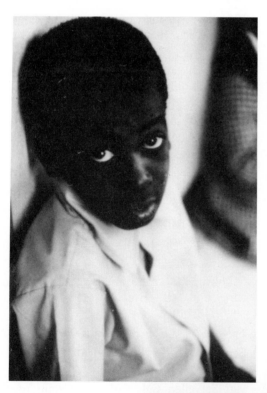
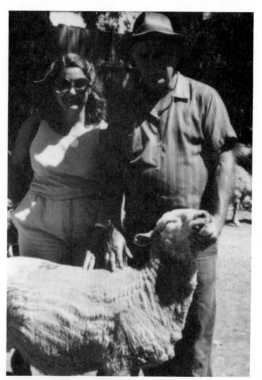
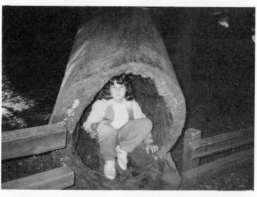

After reading this chapter, students should be able to

- Describe the historical and theoretical foundations pertinent to the understanding of anxiety disorders, somatoform disorders, and dissociative disorders.

- Compare and contrast clinical features characteristic to each of these disorders as delineated in DSM-IIIR.

- Apply the nursing process with clients with these disorders and their families.

- Assess clients who have symptoms of disabling anxiety, somatization, or dissociation.

- Formulate nursing diagnoses for clients experiencing an anxiety disorder, somatoform disorder, or dissociative disorder.

- Develop individualized nursing care plans for clients with these disorders, and their families.

- Implement appropriate nursing interventions for clients with these disorders and their families.

- Evaluate the effectiveness of nursing interventions for clients with these disorders and their families.

Other topics relevant to this content are: Basics related to anxiety, stress, and coping, Chapter 7; Crisis intervention for the acute stage of post-traumatic stress disorder, Chapter 29; Dissociative problems in victims of childhood sexual abuse, Chapter 25, Part II; Guidelines for teaching clients and families about antianxiety agents, Chapter 31; Psychopharmacologic treatment of anxiety (the antianxiety drugs), Chapter 31; Relaxation and stress management techniques, Chapter 32.

Imagine a different future.

abreaction
agoraphobia
anxiety
anxiety disorders
behavior modification
body dysmorphic disorder
compulsion
conversion disorder
depersonalization disorder
dissociative disorders
factitious disorders
generalized anxiety disorder
hypochondriasis
la belle indifférence
multiple personality
  disorder
narcoanalysis
obsession
obsessive-compulsive
  disorder
panic disorder with
  agoraphobia
panic disorder without
  agoraphobia
phobia
post-traumatic stress
  disorder
psychogenic amnesia
psychogenic fugue
simple phobia
social phobia
somatization disorder
somatoform disorders
somatoform pain disorder
systematic desensitization

The twentieth century has been called the "age of anxiety" (Auden 1947). Auden clearly saw the impact of **anxiety** in the modern era and its influence on day-to-day function. Though recognized as a separate psychologic entity only in relatively recent times, anxiety has influenced human behavior since the beginning of civilization. Only in the past fifty years, however, has anxiety been understood as central to the etiology of many types of emotional disorders. According to DSM-III, an estimated 2 to 4 percent of the population has at some time suffered from some type of anxiety disorder (DSM-III, p 225).

Anxiety exerts a powerful influence on the maturational process of individuals as they modify behaviors to be accepted in a given society. How people experience anxiety and what precipitates and relieves it are thought to be conditioned by the values and customs of a culture. In a sociologic context, then, the cultural milieu is central to the anxiety experience and must be considered in formulating a diagnosis and in developing treatment approaches and interventions.

A wide variety of problems face individuals today. These include adjustment to an increasingly technological environment in which the individual may be undervalued or overlooked. Standardization, centralization, and mechanization in business and personal life threaten individual identity and create anxiety. These phenomena need to be recognized as significant factors associated with the experience of anxiety.

Although anxiety is a universal experience, people vary in their ability to tolerate anxiety and anxiety-producing situations. This chapter explores the experience of individuals with anxiety disorders, somatoform disorders, or dissociative disorders. Although anxiety may be expressed in different ways, two factors are basic to the experience of all these persons:

1. The anxiety is sufficiently disabling and severe to cause major dysfunction in their lives.
2. A psychologic route of escape is used.

HISTORICAL AND THEORETICAL FOUNDATIONS

Anxiety Disorders

In the late nineteenth and early twentieth centuries, individuals with symptoms of anxiety were generally viewed as suffering from a primary physical illness. In America, for example, people in military hospitals during the American Civil War who suffered acute anxiety symptoms were diagnosed as having a functional disease of the heart, called "irritable heart," or DaCosta's syndrome, after the physician who described the condition (DaCosta and Mendes 1871).

Though psychiatrists and neurologists in Europe and America recognized anxiety as a symptom for several decades prior to the twentieth century, it was not viewed as a separate diagnostic entity. Instead, anxiety symptoms were grouped with other psychoneurotic symptoms such as depression and exhaustion under the label neurasthenia (Nemiah 1980). Sigmund Freud first conceptualized anxiety neurosis as a discrete clinical syndrome and came to regard anxiety as the fundamental problem in neurotic symptom formation, i.e., that physical symptoms are experienced as a result of anxiety (Freud 1936). In addition, Freud believed that understanding anxiety was essential to the development of a comprehensive theory of human behavior. Most anxiety, he reported, reflected unconscious signals of early childhood dangers. Neurotic behavior was the result of unconscious conflict—an attempt to find a compromise between the impulses of the id and the reality strivings of the ego. In other words, Freud saw anxiety as a sign of psychologic conflict resulting from the threatened emergence into consciousness of forbidden repressed ideas or emotions.

Anxiety disorders are characterized by a mixture of physical and psychologic symptoms, which are discussed later in this chapter. A rapid pulse, pounding heart, chest pain or tightness, and labored breathing are a few of the typical physical symptoms of anxiety. Psychologic symptoms include nervousness, apprehension, hyperalertness, and excessive vigilance. This diversity of symptoms leads to diversity of theoretical and treatment approaches.

Psychologic Approaches

In the past, attempts to understand anxiety disturbances were grounded in Freudian psychoanalytic theory and based nearly exclusively on the study of psychologic factors. The psychoanalytic approach to understanding mental disorders emphasizes the study of the mind, or psyche. Psychoanalytic frameworks suggest that mental disorder is the result of disturbed interpersonal dynamics, traumatic childhood experiences, and/or psychic conflict. Free association, dream analysis, and other interpretive techniques are used to study the disturbance. The treatment for these, usually milder, forms of mental disturbance is psychoanalysis or psychotherapy.

In psychoanalytic approaches, anxiety is seen as a sign of psychologic conflict resulting from the threatened emergence into consciousness of forbidden or repressed ideas or emotions. These repressed thoughts and feelings are considered unconscious aggressive and libidinal drives and their derivative emotions and fantasies. The individual fears expressing and discharging the forbidden impulses, which occur in four forms, according to the nature of their consequences:

1. Superego anxiety, in which the individual suffers from anxious expectation of guilt should he break his or her inner code of ethics and standards.
2. Castration anxiety, or fear of fantasized danger or injuries to the body or genitals.
3. Separation anxiety, or fear of losing the love, esteem, and caring of significant people.
4. Id or impulse anxiety, or fear of the complete annihilation of self.

Other analytic views, sometimes referred to as neo-Freudian, evolved from the work of Freud and differ about the nature of anxiety. Rank (1952) believed that anxiety can be traced back to birth trauma. Sullivan (1953) stressed the importance of the early relationship between the mother and the child and the transmission of the mother's anxiety to the child. Existential analysts viewed anxiety as the central feature of the human condition, and the fear of nonbeing as a primary human fear.

Proponents of psychologic frameworks for the understanding of anxiety note that although certain anxiety symptoms may often be related to neural and biochemical processes, the appearance and manifestations of anxiety syndromes cannot be traced to discrete neuropathologic lesions.

The psychoanalytic explanation of the development of phobia maintains that fear arises through a process of displacing an unconscious conflict to an external object that is symbolically related to the conflict. Thus, in becoming phobic, the individual fears an external object rather than an unknown internal source of distress. According to this model, the unconscious conflict must be brought into consciousness so that the real source of anxiety can be discovered and dealt with. Treatment takes the form of analysis or the less time-consuming psychodynamic psychotherapy.

Behavioral Approaches

Behaviorists (learning theorists) view anxiety as a learned response that can be unlearned. **Behavior modification** is the common name for the behavioral treatment that involves teaching clients new ways to modify their behavior. "Conditioning" techniques—using positive and negative reinforcements—are examples of modification techniques. Another usual method of treatment is **systematic desensitization** in which a client builds up tolerance to anxiety through exposure to a series of anxiety-provoking stimuli.

Behavioral approaches have perhaps been most effective in treating behavior disorders and disorders of impulse control such as overeating, excessive alcohol use, and nicotine dependence. However, behavioral approaches are also frequently effective in the treatment of anxiety and are widely used for modifying symptoms in phobic and obsessive-compulsive disorders.

Explanations of Phobia

Behaviorists believe that the cause of phobias is traumatic exposure to the avoided object, situation, or activity. The behavioral therapist believes that it is unnecessary to use analysis to induce the client to struggle with the anxiety. Instead, it is only necessary for the client to face the anxiety repeatedly until it becomes manageable. Many clinicians today consider behavioral psychotherapies the treatment of choice for most phobic disorders (Marks 1985). They are more efficient, less costly, and less time-consuming than other forms of insight-oriented psychotherapy treatment. Like some psychodynamically and psychoanalytically oriented therapists, behavioral therapists tend to avoid the use of medication because they believe that it may interfere with the client's ability to learn behaviors. In addition, recent research on phobic disorders suggests that phobic states not associated with panic episodes are best treated with nondrug modes of therapy (Swonger and Constantine 1983). These clients, they feel, do not respond well to anxiolytic (antianxiety) or antidepressant medication.

Explanations of Obsessions and Compulsions

According to learning theory on the development of obsessions, an original neutral obsessive thought is able to arouse anxiety because it becomes associated with an anxiety-provoking stimulus. In compulsions, a person discovers that a certain action relieves anxiety associated with the obsessive thought. The person repeats the action to achieve relief until eventually the act becomes fixed into a learned pattern of behavior.

Biologic/Physiologic Approaches

In the biologic approach to anxiety, treatment frequently revolves around drug therapy. (Drug therapy for anxiety is discussed later in this chapter.) Antianxiety drugs are among the most widely prescribed. These drugs may have serious long-term side-effects however, and it is important to carefully monitor their use.

Recent research in the function of the peripheral autonomic nervous system, the limbic system, and the hypothalamus has led researchers to speculate about a physiologic basis for anxiety. Much new knowledge is expected to be gained from this increased interest in possible physical-biologic explanations of anxiety disorders. At present, however, the relation of biologic processes to the experience of anxiety has not been completely explained.

Humanistic Interactionistic Foundations

The humanistic interactionistic framework that is adopted in this text implies that both the external situation and the inner state of mind need to be considered when assessing, diagnosing, and planning interventions. This nursing perspective identifies social and cultural as well as intrapersonal factors as important.

This perspective is particularly important in understanding the anxiety disorders, somatoform disorders, and dissociative disorders. Environmental stress—the "reality" concerns of the individual—and intrapsychic fears or conflicts cannot be adequately dealt with separately but only as they interact with one another. For example, clients suffering from a phobic disorder experience shame and helplessness as they attempt to cope with fears of annihilation in the presence of the dreaded object or situation. Interpersonal and functional withdrawal may occur, creating long-lasting disability.

This recognition has given rise to a multifaceted approach to the care of clients with these conditions.

Humanistic treatment approaches are integrative and may include the range of psychotherapeutic interventions, including psychotherapy (cognitive, behavioral, and/or dynamic), measures to develop or ensure effective social support systems, measures to reduce environmental stress, and psychopharmacologic treatment.

Somatoform Disorders

Somatoform disorders are those in which physical symptoms are present but evidence of physiologic disorder is not. The symptoms are thought to be linked to psychologic factors or emotional conflict. Conversion disorders, previously termed hysterical conversion reactions, were among the earliest disturbed coping patterns described by Sigmund Freud. They were often associated with the repressive sexual conventions and passive-dependent women's role of the Victorian period. One of Freud's most famous patients was Anna O., a woman whom he worked with in the 1880s in association with Josef Breuer. Anna O. was an intelligent, strong-minded woman of 21. After her father's illness and death, she had developed a set of symptoms including paralysis of the limbs, contractures, anesthesias, visual disturbances, disturbances of speech, anorexia, and a nervous cough. Anna had been very close to and fond of her father. She had nursed him on his deathbed. Using hypnosis as a primary tool, Breuer made the connection between inhibited sexuality and the production of symptoms such as Anna's that have no organic basis. Breuer and Freud described their clinical experiences in the treatment of hysteria in an 1895 volume entitled *Studies in Hysteria* (1966). This succinct book outlined a "theory of hysteria" that placed early repressed traumatic sexual experiences, such as seductions, at the root of hysterical symptoms. Later Freud was to modify this hypothesis by abandoning the notion of actual physical seduction and placing a new emphasis on the inner fantasy life of the child.

The Symbolism of Conversion Disorder Symptoms

The point of view advocated in this book leads us to search beyond repressed infantile sexuality for the meaning of conversion disorder. Some communication theorists believe that manifestations are really nonverbal body language intended to communicate a message to significant others. Sometimes the message is as general as "pay attention to me" or "take care of me." At other times the particular form that the *conversion of anxiety* takes actually symbol-

izes the nature of the specific underlying conflict. For example, a woman who wants to strike her children may develop a paralysis of her arm. A girl who feels guilty about reading erotic books may become blind. Both realize the primary gain of protection from their anxiety-provoking impulses, and both get secondary gains of attention and sympathy as well. These patterns are most likely to occur among clients who do not have more aggressive alternatives.

Other Behavioral Characteristics

Clients who deal with anxiety by converting it into physical symptoms usually show no other psychologic symptoms, e.g., disturbed thoughts or depressed moods. However, they are often said to exhibit subtler behavior patterns. Characteristics that have come to be associated with conversion disorder clients are self-dramatization, exhibitionism, narcissism, emotionalism, seductiveness, dependency, manipulativeness, childishness, and suggestibility. It is interesting to note, however, that these characteristics have usually been attributed to female clients by male psychiatrists.

Pain

Pain is associated with a great many disease processes, including many of the organ-specific somatoform disorders. Pain can be an adaptive or a maladaptive response. It often indicates real danger to the organism, but sometimes it interferes with functioning.

Consciousness, attention, perception, and cognition are all necessary for the experience of pain. According to modern theories of pain perception, humans have a control system over pain that operates as a "gate." Pain stimuli can be "allowed in" to or "shut out" from the cerebral cortex, depending essentially on the meaning the person attaches to the stimulus. This underscores the importance of meaning, symbol, and affect in the experience of pain sensation.

The basic schematic mechanism for so-called idiopathic pain is depicted in Figure 19–1. In psychoanalytic concepts, the unconscious conflicts are a result of traumatic or frustrating childhood experiences that are reawakened in adult life by an analogous stress or frustration. According to this theory, the person cannot express the affect that is aroused because of feelings of guilt, fear of loss of love, or fear of retribution. The affect is therefore repressed and transformed into physiologic correlates.

Dissociative Disorders

The dissociative disorders encompass a large group of interesting, uncommon, and sometimes bizarre conditions. In each of these disorders, there is a sudden, tem-

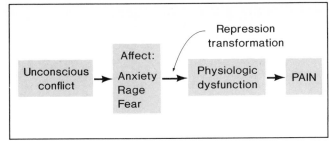

Figure 19–1
Schematic mechanism of idiopathic pain.

porary change in consciousness, identity, or motor behavior so that some part of one or more of these functions is lost.

Though awareness of the existence of dissociative phenomena extends far back in history, little was understood about their nature or cause. The phenomena were cloaked in superstition or mysticism during the Middle Ages or associated with "spells" or witchcraft. Because of the increasing scientific attention to the technique of hypnosis in the latter half of the nineteenth century, interest increased in the phenomena of dissociation. Hypnotic techniques were employed in exploring dissociative reactions.

Pierre Janet (1859–1947) was the first to develop the concept of the "splitting off" or dissociation of a part of consciousness. He believed that the individual needed to have a normal amount of "mental energy" for the maintenance of integrative mental processes. When the level of energy was high, integration was maintained. When it became low, however, the personality might cease to function as a unit and split or dissociate. Nearly any type of emotional illness could result, he thought.

Freud, in contrast, proposed the concept of repression to explain the loss of conscious awareness in dissociation. He then introduced the notion of the *dynamic unconscious,* a part of the mind in which affects or ideas that were unacceptable to a person were pushed from awareness or recall.

The basic concept of psychologic dissociation was accepted by Freud and other early analytic theorists. Conceptions and theories of the phenomenon of dissociation have continued to evolve during the twentieth century.

Current explanations of dissociation are based on Freud's dynamic concepts. The repression of ideas that leads to amnesia and other forms of dissociation is conceived as a way of protecting the individual from emotional pain arising either from disturbing external circumstances or internal psychologic conflicts. A dissociative reaction may be viewed as a flight from crisis or danger—a major psychologic route of escape from anxiety. Sometimes, as in states of fugue and multiple personality, the dissociated area takes over temporary direction and control of the entire personality. During such times, the individual may even appear to be functioning well to the observer.

Additional specific dynamic considerations relevant to dissociative disorders include the following ideas. In psy-

chogenic amnesia, the pattern is similar to conversion reactions except that the individual does not avoid some unpleasant situation by getting sick. Instead, the person does so by forgetting (repressing or suppressing) certain traumatic events or stresses. In multiple personality disorder there appears to be a deep-seated conflict between contradictory impulses and beliefs. A resolution is achieved by separating the conflicting parts and developing each into an autonomous personality.

PSYCHOPATHOLOGY

Anxiety Disorders

In this group of disorders, anxiety is either the predominant disturbance—as in generalized anxiety disorder—or anxiety is experienced as avoidance behavior when the individual attempts to master the symptoms—as in confronting the dreaded object or situation in a phobic disorder. When anxiety is not tied to a specific stimulus, it may be called *free-floating anxiety.* The anxiety disorders are categorized and described in Table 19–1.

People in anxiety states experience anxiety both as a subjective emotion and as a variety of physical symptoms resulting from muscular tension and autonomic nervous system activity. When acute, the anxiety rapidly drives the individual to seek help. When subacute or chronic, anxiety can lead to a number of somatic discomforts or disabilities. Heartburn, epigastric distress, diarrhea, and constipation may occur. Chronic muscular tension can lead to a variety of musculoskeletal aches and pains, e.g., backache, shoulder and neck pain, and headache.

Onset may be sudden or gradual. Some individuals experience an unexpected, incapacitating outbreak of acute anxiety, as in panic disorder. In others, anxiety may express itself through relatively mild somatic symptoms in which the existence of basic anxiety is missed unless specifically inquired about, as in generalized anxiety disorder.

Panic Disorder

An apparently common disorder, panic disorder is characterized by recurrent attacks of severe anxiety lasting a few moments to an hour. These attacks are not associated with a stimulus but instead seem to occur spontaneously or out of the blue. They may, however, become associated with certain situations, e.g., going into a shopping mall or driving a car. The person usually experiences somatic

Table 19–1 Classification of Anxiety Disorders	
Class/Disorders	**Features**
Panic disorder (with or without agoraphobia)	Recurrent panic attacks that may be unpredictable or may be associated with specific situations; symptoms such as dyspnea, sweating, palpitations, and chest pain or discomfort; often associated with agoraphobia
Generalized anxiety disorder	Generalized persistent anxiety without specific symptoms that characterize other anxiety disorders; symptoms generally involve motor tension, autonomic hyperactivity, and apprehensive expectation
Obsessive-compulsive disorder	Recurrent obsessions (persistent ideas, thoughts, images, or impulses that are ego-dystonic) or compulsions (repetitive and seemingly purposeful behaviors performed according to certain rules or in a stereotyped fashion and generally experienced as senseless and ego-alien)
Agoraphobia without history of panic disorder	Marked fear of being alone or in public places from which escape might be difficult or in which help might not be available; usually the person is afraid of having a limited symptom attack (a single or small number of symptoms)
Social phobia	Persistent irrational fear of situations in which an individual may be exposed to scrutiny by others and fear that the individual may behave in a humiliating or embarrassing manner
Simple phobia	Isolated fears focused on one situation or object
Post-traumatic stress disorder	The experience of a significant recognizable stressor or trauma followed by recurrent subjective reexperiencing of the trauma, a general numbing of responsiveness or reduced involvement with the external world, and two or more of several cognitive and somatic symptoms

symptoms such as palpitations, rapid pulse, nausea, diarrhea, dyspnea, and a feeling of choking or suffocation. The pupils are dilated, and the face is flushed. The person may feel dizzy or faint and often has a sense of impending doom or death. Restlessness is acute, and the person may make pleading, apprehensive appeals for help.

In its most advanced state, panic creates a symptom constellation totally mimicking severe cardiac disease. This symptom complex is seen most frequently in young adults and is called *cardiac neurosis.* Symptoms involved in cardiac neurosis are palpitations, tachycardia, chest pain, dyspnea, easy fatigability, dizziness, sweating, irritability, faintness, and a feeling of impending doom.

Panic attacks may occur on occasion in normal, healthy individuals with little or no remaining disability. The experience of having panic attacks is labeled panic disorder when the attacks occur frequently and when they interfere with the individual's social functioning at work, school, or in the family. Table 19–2 lists psychic and somatic features characteristic of a panic or anxiety attack.

Anticipatory fear of helplessness or of losing control during a panic attack is a common complication of the disorder. The individual frequently avoids situations evoking the fear, sometimes developing a phobic avoidance reaction. The DSM-IIIR states that a diagnosis of **panic disorder with agoraphobia** should be made when an individual experiences panic attacks and has phobic avoidance. In the absence of phobic avoidance, the condition is termed **panic disorder without agoraphobia.** This change reflects the fact that many investigators now believe that **agoraphobia** (the marked fear of being alone or in public places from which escape might be difficult or in which help might not be available) develops secondary to panic attacks (Klein 1980, Mavissakalian 1981) and that agoraphobia without panic attacks is uncommon (Spitzer and Williams 1984). These investigators suggest that the cause of agoraphobia is different from the cause of simple or social phobia. In addition, they note that agoraphobia with symptoms of panic attack is now treatable with some drugs. In contrast, simple or social phobias are not.

Panic disorder is often first noted in late adolescence or early adulthood. It may be limited to a single brief period lasting several weeks or months, recur several times, or become chronic. Though it is rarely incapacitating, the disorder can be severe. When complicated by agoraphobia, it can interfere greatly with individual functioning. Panic disorder is diagnosed much more frequently in women than in men, and some clinicians believe that sudden object loss and separation anxiety in childhood predispose to its development.

It has recently been noted that mitral valve prolapse may be an associated condition. According to DSM-IIIR, however, the occurrence of this condition does not rule out a diagnosis of panic disorder. Such physical disorders as hypoglycemia, hyperthyroidism, and amphetamine or caffeine intoxication must be ruled out before a diagnosis of panic disorder can be made.

Generalized Anxiety Disorder

Generalized anxiety disorder is considered less specific and less debilitating than panic disorder. It is characterized by pervasive, persistent anxiety of at least six months' duration but without phobias, panic attacks, or obsessions and compulsions. Chronic subjective feelings of nervousness and apprehension "for no reason" are experienced. Autonomic symptoms may be less frequent or less severe than in panic attacks.

There is little generally accepted information about age of onset, predisposing factors, cause of illness, prevalence, sex ratio, or familial pattern. Some authors note there appears to be a more equal sex ratio than in panic disorder. Also, generalized anxiety disorder is apparently more gradual than panic disorder (Anderson, Noyes, and Crowe 1984). Associated mild depressive symptoms are not uncommon in individuals with generalized anxiety disorder. Although impairment in social or occupational functioning is rarely more than mild, abuse of alcohol or other drugs may be a serious complication and may interfere with effective intervention.

Obsessive-Compulsive Disorder

Obsessive-compulsive disorder is classified with the anxiety disorders due to the anxiety symptoms that develop when an individual tries to resist an obsession or compulsion. Although compulsions are thought of as attempts to reduce tension, often the opposite eventually occurs as the individual becomes more and more agitated, unable to decide whether to stop or continue the compulsive act.

Obsessive-compulsive people usually fear that they will harm someone or something. They rely heavily on avoidance and are best understood in terms of their control needs. Individuals who develop obsessive-compulsive symptoms are characterized by high needs to control themselves, others, and their environment.

An **obsession** is a recurring thought that cannot be dismissed from consciousness. These thoughts are sometimes trivial or ridiculous, often morbid or fearful, and always distressing and anxiety provoking. An example of a strange but trivial obsession is that of a young adolescent man who could not get the rhyme "Snips and snails and puppydog tails" out of his mind. An example of a much more ominous obsession is that of a woman who could not stop thinking that she must kill her children to prevent a

| Table 19–2 |
| Common Features of Panic Attack |

Psychic	Somatic
Sudden onset of:	Sudden onset of:
Intense nervousness or apprehension	Tachycardia or palpitations
Feeling of impending doom or death	Chest discomfort
Mental confusion	Dyspnea
Feelings of unreality	Unsteadiness, dizziness, vertigo
Fear of going crazy or doing something uncontrolled during an attack	Sweating
	Choking or smothering sensations
	Faintness
	Hot and cold flashes
	Paresthesias
	Trembling or shaking

worldwide race war. Other common obsessive thoughts have to do with violence or contamination.

A **compulsion**, in contrast, is an uncontrollable, persistent urge to perform certain acts or behaviors to relieve an otherwise unbearable tension. There are two kinds of compulsive acts—those that give expression to the primary impulses, and those that are attempts to undo or control these impulses. The first kind is rare. Most compulsive acts are attempts to control or modify obsessions, either because compulsive persons fear the consequences or are afraid that they will not be able to control the primary impulse.

Typical compulsive acts are endless handwashing, checking and rechecking doors to see if they have been locked, and elaborate dressing and undressing rituals. Such defensive compulsive acts are used to contain, neutralize, or ward off the anxiety related to the primary impulse. In the case of the young man who could not dismiss the rhyme from his mind, compulsions that involved ritualistic washing of his genitals emerged to ward off the anxiety generated by his apparently silly obsession. The woman obsessed with thoughts about killing her children engaged in symbolic rituals of touching religious objects to repel evil influences through magical interventions by the saints. Such compulsive acts as counting and elaborately checking routine duties are frequently associated with the fear of failing or making a mistake, or with the need to be perfect.

Obsessions and compulsions have certain features in common.

- An idea or an impulse insistently, persistently, and impellingly intrudes itself into the person's awareness.

- A feeling of anxious dread accompanies the primary manifestation and often leads the person to take countermeasures against the forbidden thought or impulse.

- Both the obsession and the compulsion are ego-alien—i.e., foreign to one's self-perception.

- No matter how compelling the obsession or compulsion is, the person has enough insight to recognize it as irrational and experience it as a significant source of distress.

- Many of the personality traits associated with obsession and compulsion are highly valued in American culture. Success in many professions and occupations demands cautiousness, deliberateness, and rationality. These traits are usually associated with the tendency toward being obsessive or compulsive. When these personality traits are carried to an extreme, or when the balance between control and impulse expression leads to paralysis, they become a liability.

Obsessions and compulsions occur together in 75 percent of cases and usually follow a chronic course with waxing and waning of symptoms. In severe cases, extreme preoccupation or compulsive activity disrupts daily life. The disorder is believed to be quite rare, though obsessive-compulsive symptoms occur in approximately 14 percent of the general population (Marks 1981).

Obsessive-compulsive disorder is equally common in men and women. The usual age at onset is in the late teens to mid-twenties, though it has been diagnosed as early as childhood.

Phobic Disorders

Like the other anxiety disorders discussed in this chapter, a phobic disorder is a response to experienced anxiety. Unlike people with generalized anxiety disorder, however, whose anxiety is free-floating, people with phobias fear specific places or things. A **phobia** is a persistent and irrational fear of a specific object, activity, or situation that results in a compelling desire to avoid the dreaded object or situation. Nearly all phobic persons panic when in contact with the phobic situation. The fear is recognized by the person as excessive or unreasonable in proportion to the actual danger. Some common phobias are described in Box 19–1.

The major dynamic mechanisms of phobic disorders are thought to be displacement of the original anxiety from its real source and symbolization of the stressor in the focus of the phobia. The unconscious operations involved in phobias help the person control anxiety by providing a

---

Box 19–1
SOME COMMON PHOBIAS

Acrophobia: Fear of heights

Agoraphobia: Fear of leaving the familiar setting of the home; fear of open spaces

Ailurophobia: Fear of cats

Algophobia: Fear of pain

Avisophobia: Fear of birds

Byorthophobia: Fear of childbirth

Claustrophobia: Fear of closed spaces

Dementophobia: Fear of insanity

Ereuthophobia: Fear of blushing

Hemophobia: Fear of blood

Hydrophobia: Fear of water

Mysophobia: Fear of dirt, germs, contamination

Ophidiophobia: Fear of snakes

Pathophobia: Fear of disease

Pyrophobia: Fear of fire

Senilophobia: Fear of old age

Thanatophobia: Fear of death

Zoophobia: Fear of animals

---

specific object as a focus for anxiety. The phobic person can then control the intensity of the anxiety by avoiding the object with which the anxiety is associated.

A diagnosis of a phobic disorder is generally made when the avoidance behavior becomes so extreme or the problem so pervasive that it interferes with the person's normal functioning at home, work, or school.

DSM-IIIR divides the phobic disorders into three main types:

1. *Agoraphobia:* Fear of being alone or in public places

2. *Social phobia:* Fear of situations that may be humiliating or embarrassing

3. *Simple phobia:* Fear of specific things, e.g., animals, reptiles, heights, or darkness

Agoraphobia

Agoraphobia involves fear of being in public places from which escape might be difficult or in which help might not be available. The fears associated with agoraphobia are listed in Box 19–2. Often the individual fears leaving the safety of home, worrying that he or she might develop an incapacitating symptom, such as dizziness, loss of bowel or bladder control, or cardiac distress. Normal activities are increasingly curtailed as the fears dominate the individ-

Box 19–2
FEARS ASSOCIATED WITH AGORAPHOBIA

Being alone

Being in a crowded place

Being in a strange place

Driving, especially on major highways

Elevators

Enclosed places

Falling

High places or high buildings

Leaving home

Open spaces

Public speaking

Traveling by car, train, airplane

---

ual's life. Agoraphobic persons often limit travel and need a companion when away from home. If the phobic situation is endured, intense anxiety is experienced.

Agoraphobia without panic attacks (called agoraphobia without history of panic disorder in DSM-IIIR) is considered relatively rare. More usually, agoraphobics have spontaneous panic attacks (see panic disorder with agoraphobia discussed earlier in this chapter).

Most agoraphobics have a history of generalized anxiety or anxiety attacks at the onset of the phobic behavior. Some investigators believe others have had a significant depression preceding the onset of phobia (Cameron 1985, p 5). Onset is usually in the middle to late twenties. Agoraphobia is more frequently diagnosed in women than in men. Separation anxiety in childhood or sudden object loss appear to be predisposing factors. Depression, anxiety, rituals, minor "checking" compulsions, or rumination are frequently associated features.

The prognosis is variable. Some less severely disturbed individuals experience waxing and waning of symptoms and sometimes have periods of remission. The more severely impaired may suffer lifelong disability.

Social Phobia

The main characteristic of **social phobia** is a persistent fear and avoidance of situations in which the person may be exposed to scrutiny by others. The person especially fears he or she will act in an embarrassing or humiliating manner. Examples of social phobias are extreme fear of performing or speaking in public, making complaints, or writing or eating in front of others. Others include fear of interacting with the opposite sex, superiors, or aggressive individuals. Usually the individual has only one social phobia.

The prevalence of social phobia in the general population is apparently unknown (Cameron 1985, p 7), although it is reported as relatively rare in DSM-IIIR. In clinic populations, social phobia represents approximately 20 percent of phobias. Often appearing in late childhood or early adolescence, social phobia usually progresses to a chronic course. Some lessening of symptoms may occur in middle age. The course differs from agoraphobia, however, in that waxing and waning of symptoms are not common.

Sex ratio, familial pattern, and predisposing factors are yet unknown, although some investigators believe that the incidence is more evenly distributed between men and women than in simple phobia or agoraphobia (Tearnan and Telch 1984, p 168). Generalized anxiety, agoraphobia, or simple phobia may coexist with social phobia.

Simple Phobia

Sometimes referred to as "specific" phobias, **simple phobias** are more common than any other type of phobic disorder. Simple phobias are isolated fears focused on one situation or object, e.g., a fear of reptiles, darkness, or heights. This category of phobic disorders encompasses all phobias not included in the categories of agoraphobia or social phobia.

Simple phobias generally cause minimal impairment if the phobic object is rarely encountered and easily avoided, e.g., a fear of snakes does not seriously impair an individual living in a high-rise condominium. The phobia can, however, be incapacitating if the phobic situation is frequently encountered and not easily avoided, e.g., a fear of heights or elevators seriously incapacitates the individual living in a high-rise condominium.

Many simple phobias begin in childhood and subsequently disappear. Those that persist into adulthood rarely remit without treatment. Simple phobia is more often diagnosed in females than in males. Complications and predisposing factors are not well understood, and researchers disagree about the contribution of specific occurrences of conditioning of fear in these phobias (Ost and Hugdahl 1981).

Post-traumatic Stress Disorder

Although not included in the official psychiatric classification system until quite recently, **post-traumatic stress disorder** has been recognized as a psychologic disorder for many years. Older terms—*shell shock, battle fatigue,* and *war neurosis*—reflect an origin in combat situations. Post-traumatic stress disorder includes traumatic stress reactions to civilian and natural catastrophes as well, e.g., assault or rape, incest, skyjacking, and earthquakes.

Post-traumatic stress may be defined as the experience of a significant, recognizable stressor or trauma that is followed by recurrent subjective reexperiencing of the trauma. A general numbing of responsiveness followed by cognitive or somatic symptoms of irritability, anxiety, aggressiveness, and depression may follow (Cameron 1985, p 9). The stressor is generally outside the range of usual human experiences, although any environmental stimulus that is perceived as dangerous, whether it produces physical injury or not, can be sufficiently traumatic to precipitate a post-traumatic stress disorder (Scrignar 1984).

The course of post-traumatic stress disorder is variable. Most individuals who have suffered a significant stressor tend to have an acute reaction from which they recover spontaneously. In others, however, the reaction may be delayed or prolonged and eventually become chronic. Delayed onset is defined as symptoms occurring at least six months after the trauma. For example, many Vietnam veterans, upon return from combat, essentially relived their experience through recurrent nightmares. Other sleep disturbances, including insomnia, often occurred. "Psychic numbing"—emotional anesthesia in relation to other people and to previously enjoyed activities—was common. Some veterans reported difficulty in concentrating and remembering. Many veterans felt guilty about having survived when others did not or about actions they took to survive. When veterans were exposed to situations or events that resembled or symbolized the traumatic event, their symptoms often increased, and they felt even greater distress. Reactions such as these continue to disturb some Vietnam veterans even today. Box 19–3 lists common features of post-traumatic stress disorder.

Post-traumatic stress disorder can occur in people of any age, even children. Associated symptoms of depression and anxiety are common, as well as increased irritability, sometimes leading to unpredictable explosions of hostility with little or no provocation. A significant additional problem exists when alcohol or other substances are used in an attempt to maintain control and soothe emotions.

Somatoform Disorders

The essential features of somatoform disorders are physical symptoms suggesting physical disorders for which there is no positive evidence of organic or physiologic causes. Somatoform disorders are sometimes confused with physical disorders.

Somatoform disorders may also be confused with factitious disorders. Factitious means not genuine or natural. In the DSM-IIIR this category of disorders includes physical or psychologic symptoms that are consciously and vol-

---

Box 19–3
COMMON FEATURES OF POST-TRAUMATIC STRESS DISORDER

Aggressive behavior	Intrusive memories
Avoidance behavior	Memory impairment
Constricted affect	Nightmares
Depression	Panic attacks
Detachment	Phobic responses
Guilty rumination	Poor concentration
Hyperalertness	Repetitive dreams
Impulsiveness	Startle reactions
Insomnia	

---

untarily produced by the client. For example, a client may take anticoagulants to produce blood in the urine or dislocate a shoulder on purpose for no other reason than to assume a dependent role. The distinction between factitious and somatoform disorders is based on the determination that in factitious disorders the physical symptoms present are under voluntary control. In somatoform disorders, the physical symptoms are not under voluntary control. Both conditions must be thoughtfully assessed for the possible presence of a true, primary physical disorder.

Somatoform disorders include the following major clinical pictures described next and summarized in Table 19–3.

Somatization Disorder

Clients who have sought medical attention for recurrent and multiple somatic complaints of several years' duration but that are seemingly without physiologic causes are diagnosed as having somatization disorder. This problem usually begins before the age of 30 and has a chronic course often accompanied by anxiety and depressed mood. Clients believe they have been sickly for a good part of their lives and report lengthy lists of symptoms, including blindness, paralysis, convulsions, nausea and other gastrointestinal difficulties, and painful menstruation, among others.

Conversion Disorder

In conversion disorder, clients report loss or alteration of physical function that suggests a physical disorder but in fact is related to the expression of a psychologic conflict. Two mechanisms are thought to explain what a person "gets" from having a conversion disorder. The first, primary gain, helps the person to keep the psychologic need or conflict out of awareness. For example, a conflict about acknowledging a traumatic event one has seen may be expressed as "blindness." In this instance, the symptom can be a partial solution to the underlying conflict (not having to acknowledge witnessing the traumatic event because one has suddenly been struck blind). The second mechanism, **secondary gain**, helps the person to avoid a distressing, uncomfortable, or repugnant activity while, at the same time, receiving support from others. For example, a soldier with a paralyzed arm could hardly be expected to fire a gun and is also likely to receive sympathy for his paralyzed condition.

The problem usually begins in adolescence or early adulthood, although a conversion disorder may appear at any time during the life cycle. Regardless at what point it first appears, a conversion disorder can seriously impede one's normal life activities.

Somatoform Pain Disorder

In somatoform pain disorder, clients experience pain in the absence of physiologic findings and the presence of possible psychologic factors. Some of the clinical syndromes in which idiopathic pain may be the predominant complaint are conversion disorders, workers' compensation injuries, and masochistic personality styles. In conversion disorders, pain symbolizes the punishment for having an unacceptable wish, perhaps sexual or aggressive, aroused by a frustrating life situation. In workers' compensation cases, the client may unconsciously use pain, and the monetary compensation received for the suffering, to strike back against employers or others by whom the client feels unfairly treated. Some individuals seem to need to suffer to achieve any sort of gratification without guilt. They seem to assume they are otherwise unworthy of any pleasure. Often their entire lives are conducted according to a self-destructive pattern of expecting punishment and eliciting it from the environment.

Hypochondriasis

Clients with **hypochondriasis** are preoccupied with the fear or belief that they have a serious disease, which on physical evaluation is not present. The unrealistic fear or belief persists for a period of at least six months despite medical reassurance. This fear impairs the social or occupational functioning of the client.

Body Dysmorphic Disorder

Clients with **body dysmorphic disorder** are preoccupied with some imagined defect in physical appearance. The preoccupation is out of proportion to any actual abnormality. The belief is overvalued but not of delusional proportion.

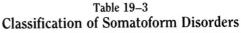

Table 19–3	
Classification of Somatoform Disorders	
Class/Disorders	**Features**
Somatization disorder	Many physical complaints or belief of having been sickly for several years before age 30; no organic or physiologic reason.
Conversion disorder	Loss or alteration in physical function due to psychologic factors; symptom is not consciously produced and is a culturally sanctioned response; not explainable by known physical disorder.
Somatoform pain disorder	Preoccupation of at least six months' duration with pain for which there is no organic or physiologic reason; if there is related reason, the complaint is grossly excessive.
Hypochondriasis	Preoccupation with having serious illness despite lack of pathology; duration of at least six months.
Body dysmorphic disorder	Preoccupation with an imagined defect in physical appearance out of proportion to actual physical abnormality.
Undifferentiated somatoform disorder	Multiple physical complaints with no physiologic basis; if physiologic basis exists, impairments or complaints are grossly excessive; duration in excess of six months.

Undifferentiated Somatoform Disorder

Clients have multiple physical complaints lasting at least six months for which no organic problem can be found after extensive evaluation. When there is related organic disease, the complaints or impairments are grossly excessive.

Dissociative Disorders

Dissociative disorders have, as their common base, the defense mechanism of dissociation, in which emotional significance and affect are separated from an idea, object, or situation. Dissociative responses are somewhat uncommon and often bizarre defensive reactions to stress. Dissociative disorders are complex and are usually difficult to distinguish from one another. They share one common characteristic. In any dissociative disorder, a cluster of recent, related mental events is beyond the client's power of recall but can return spontaneously to conscious awareness. Depersonalization disorder is included because the client loses the feeling of personal reality, an important component of identity. The most common forms of dissociative disorders are described here and summarized in Table 19–4. None is attributable to an organic mental disorder.

Multiple Personality Disorder

Clients with **multiple personality disorder** are dominated by two or more distinct personalities, each of which determines the nature of their behavior and attitudes while it is uppermost in consciousness. The transition from one personality to another is often sudden and dramatic. There are many popular stories about people with multiple personalities. Two of the best known are *Sybil* and *The Three Faces of Eve.* However, these portrayals are popularizations of a disorder that is not always so colorful. The belief that one has been taken over or possessed by another person or spirit may occur as the experience of the alternate personality's influence.

Psychogenic Fugue

A person with **psychogenic fugue** wanders, usually far from home and for days at a time. During this period, clients completely forget their past life and associations, but, unlike people with amnesia, are unaware of having forgotten anything. When they return to their former consciousness, they do not remember the period of fugue. Fugue clients are generally seclusive and quiet, and as a consequence their behavior rarely attracts attention. They may assume a completely new and apparently well-integrated identity during the fugue.

Psychogenic Amnesia

People with **psychogenic amnesia** suddenly become aware that they have a total loss of memory for events that occurred during a period of time that may range from a few hours to a whole lifetime. In *localized amnesia,* the most common form, a person forgets only specific and related past times, usually surrounding a disturbing event. *Selective amnesia* for some, but not all, of the events is less common. Least common are *generalized amnesia,* which encompasses the person's entire life, and *continuous amnesia,* in which the person cannot recall events up to a specific time including the present.

Table 19–4
Classification of Dissociative Disorders

Class/Disorders	Features
Multiple personality disorder	Adoption of two or more distinct personalities. Each personality at some time takes full control of the individual's behavior.
Psychogenic fugue	Sudden flight from the usual environment or place of conflict and the taking on of a new identity.
Psychogenic amnesia	A single episode of memory loss of important personal information due to psychologic reasons.
Depersonalization disorder	One or more episodes of feelings of unreality concerning the environment, the self, or both sufficient to produce significant impairment of social or occupational functioning.
Dissociative disorder, not otherwise specified	Experience of dissociative symptoms that do not meet the criteria for a specific disorder.

Depersonalization Disorder

The essential feature here is one or more episodes of alteration in the perception or experience of the self so that the usual sense of personal reality is temporarily lost or changed with subsequent social or occupational impairment. All the associated feelings are ego-dystonic.

Dissociative Disorder, Not Otherwise Specified (NOS)

This is a residual category to be used for disorders in which the predominant feature is a dissociative reaction that does not meet the criteria for any other specific dissociative disorder. An example is a child who enters a trancelike state following abuse or trauma or a person who enters a dissociated state following a period of brainwashing or thought reform.

THE NURSING PROCESS AND ANXIETY DISORDERS

Chapter 7 covers concepts of anxiety, stress, and coping that are relevant to the care of clients with anxiety disorders; it also covers the general anxiety continuum and the need to identify the level of anxiety. The subject of this section is the nurse's role with clients whose anxiety is severe enough to be classified as an anxiety disorder.

Assessment

Clients with anxiety disorders have impaired psychosocial and physiologic function. The feeling disturbances and physical and intellectual changes that take place as a result of extreme or chronic anxiety affect the client's work, school, and social functioning and frequently impair or threaten previously meaningful interpersonal relationships.

For the nurse with the humanistic interactionist philosophy espoused in this text, the goal is to restore the client's function within the family system and to restore intrapersonal health. Data gathered from both the client and family members are therefore essential to the assessment process.

The occurrence of acute anxiety and its related symptoms is common to a number of other physical conditions and acute medical emergencies. Therefore, a careful evaluation should always be conducted. A history and physical examination should rule out such conditions as hyperthyroidism and other endocrine problems, Ménière's syndrome, brain disorders, caffeine intoxication, and some medical emergencies (e.g., myocardial infarction).

Differentiation from other psychiatric diagnoses is difficult when anxiety and depression are mixed. The question "Which predominates?" can puzzle many practitioners and demands continued careful evaluation. Anxiety is part of many other clinical syndromes (e.g., schizophrenia and major affective disorders) and the medical diagnosis may be made on the basis of the dominant, most debilitating symptom.

Subjective Data

Clients with anxiety disorders may report a variety of physical and emotional symptoms. It is important to encourage clients to describe symptoms in their own words and to explain how the symptoms affect their daily activities. Clients with anxiety disorders may report emotional distress, cognitive and perceptual changes, somatic discomforts, or role impairments.

Emotional Distress

Clients with anxiety disorders may reveal a number of distressing emotional feelings, such as:

"I have a sense of impending doom—as if something terrible is going to happen."

"I feel helpless; vulnerable for no reason at all!"

"I just can't seem to enjoy life—everything bothers me."

Anger, guilt, feelings of worthlessness, and anguish are frequently associated with anxiety as well. When the anxiety is acute or extreme, as in panic disorder or in post-traumatic stress disorder, the client feels in immediate danger and may seek protection and reassurance from others. If the anxiety is too severe, however, they may become immobilized and unable to report their terrifying feelings at all, or they may refuse assistance and attempt to flee.

Sometimes clients with anxiety disorders may deny the existence of anxious feelings. They try to protect themselves by dissociating these feelings. The nurse needs to recognize clients' anxiety despite their denials. In such instances, careful observation of objective data is especially necessary to make a proper assessment.

Cognitive and Perceptual Changes

Clients frequently have difficulty concentrating and making decisions. Some clients report feeling as if they are "going in circles," unable to think through a problem to make a confident decision. They may worry about their effectiveness at work and fear losing their job as a result of these attention and judgment problems.

In the clinical situation, clients may ask the nurse to make decisions for them or to give directions. At the same time, however, they may express difficulty following through with suggestions, finding many loopholes or possible problems with the plan of action. Other clients become forgetful or misinterpret what they hear.

In extreme anxiety, as in a panic attack, the client is unable to assess a situation accurately and realistically. Such a client needs immediate attention from and orientation by the nurse. The client may later report having had a frightening feeling of personality disintegration.

Somatic Discomfort

Clients with anxiety disorders may complain of nausea, indigestion, headache, tightness in the neck or back, lack of appetite, a constant feeling of fatigue, or other psychophysiologic conditions. They may relate these somatic disturbances to having "bad nerves," or they may be unaware of any psychologic component of their discomfort.

The client with an obsessive-compulsive disorder who engages in repetitive activity, e.g., compulsive handwashing or hair-pulling, may report special health problems (tissue breakdown or hair loss) as a result of the actions.

Clients with post-traumatic stress disorder may report fitful sleep, terrifying nightmares, and a fear of returning to sleep.

Role Impairment

Clients may be aware of the impact that the emotional, cognitive/perceptual, and somatic changes have on their social, family, and work roles. They report worry about losing their job, being abandoned by loved ones, being unable to care for their families as they had once done.

A young mother despairs that she is unable to take her daughter out to the playground because her phobias prevent her leaving the house.

A middle-aged accountant, obsessed about tallying his firm's financial data, is unable to put it aside for the weekend and misses his son's football game. He experiences anger, guilt, and self-recrimination as a result.

Anxiety Disorders
Objective Data

In addition to noting general signs and symptoms of anxiety as discussed in Chapter 7, the nurse notes other specific physical, emotional, and intellectual changes.

Physical Findings

Clients with acute or extreme anxiety—e.g., clients with post-traumatic stress disorder, panic disorder, or phobic disorder when the phobic situation cannot be avoided—may experience a panic reaction and show extreme discomfort with the desire to flee. The nurse may observe acute physical changes, e.g., difficulty breathing, sweating, trembling, or vomiting, during these incidents. The nurse may note that the client is unable to verbalize or that verbalizations are confused and incoherent. During a panic episode, clients may be so frightened that they may refuse help at the moment and may require firm reassurance and protection until the episode wanes.

The nurse may note that the client with an anxiety disorder may develop long-term physiologic effects from the anxiety, e.g., susceptibility to viral infections, development of ulcer, hypertension, or asthma. Alcohol or other substance abuse may develop into a serious complicating problem when clients try to alleviate anxiety through chemical means.

Other physical findings may be the effects of ritualistic or compulsive activity, e.g., skin lesions in a client who obsessively picks at the skin.

Emotional Changes

Family and friends of a client with post-traumatic stress disorder may report personality changes in the client, e.g., increased irritability, suspiciousness, angry outbursts, and a tendency to blame others and to withdraw from them emotionally. The nurse may experience such reactions during the assessment interview. The nurse needs to persist in taking a careful history to trace the source of the emotional changes caused by the traumatic event.

Individuals with phobic and obsessive-compulsive disorders show a lack of emotional distress as long as the phobic object or situation is avoided or eclipsed by activity. The nurse may note little spontaneity or active involvement by the client during the assessment process.

Intellectual Deficits

Unrealistic or distorted perception of a real situation is common in anxiety states. During a panic attack, the client may distort or exaggerate details. The client may complain to the nurse about some seemingly insignificant detail. Clients may lose their ability to take in other pertinent data, and thus make errors in judgment.

In the interview, clients with an anxiety disorder are forgetful and unable to concentrate or pay attention to details. Errors in calculation and grammar are common.

Impact on Role Function

The symptoms of anxiety disorder affect social, work, and family relationships. It is important to understand the function that anxiety symptoms may have in the context of interpersonal relationships. Obsessive-compulsive acts, for instance, may become so pervasive that they take the place of relating to other people. In other cases, the obsessions and compulsions are used in negotiating interaction and social roles. It is not unusual for people to establish a reciprocal pattern of interaction based on obsessions.

Mr. O constantly complains that his wife does not keep the house clean enough. Actually he is using reciprocity to express his own wish to be untidy. He need never feel guilty, because he can blame the mess on his wife. In this rather convoluted way, Mr. O avoids some of the anxiety he would experience if he allowed himself to create some of the mess. His wife's messiness also enables him to spend time cleaning up the house, thus further undoing his own impulses. Finally, the housecleaning gives both Mr. and Mrs. O a focus for some level of interaction and communication—albeit a low one. As it turns out, this kind of wife is the perfect foil for a man with such a compulsive coping style. Mr. O would probably have difficulty establishing a safe relationship with someone as controlling and compulsive as himself. He can regard Mrs. O's sloppiness as somehow inferior because she obviously has difficulty managing. In this way he enhances his own shaky self-esteem. If Mr. O had nothing to complain about, he might well develop more severe problems, because he would be denied meaningful behavior patterns, and because his wife might demand a more mature relationship with him.

As this example suggests, nurses who plan intervention strategies for obsessive-compulsives and other individuals with an anxiety disorder should first assess the impact on the family system of intervening in one member's coping style.

Additional evidence of role impairment is noted when the client or family member reports that the client is having trouble at work. The client may be in jeopardy of losing his or her job due to poor performance. The individual with post-traumatic stress disorder, for example, may have been fired for absences, drug or alcohol abuse, or for outbursts of temper.

Many clients with a panic disorder report that fear of having a panic attack prevents them from seeking employment or from traveling to job interviews. For these individuals, as for many with severe phobic fears, normal activity may be greatly restricted.

Nursing Diagnosis

A comparison between PND-I and NANDA diagnoses for clients with anxiety disorders is given in Table 19–5. The following sections discuss their implications for the client and the nurse.

Impaired Emotional Experience

Apprehension, tension, and fright are emotional experiences common to clients with anxiety disorders. Anger and rage may occur when anxiety becomes excessive. A client with post-traumatic stress disorder, for example, may "fly off the handle" without apparent warning or provocation, reacting to an inner stimulus.

Feelings of distress, anguish, fear, hopelessness, and guilt may also accompany anxiety disorders. The focus of emotional expression may be impaired, i.e., clients may worry excessively, ruminating about what might go wrong in the future. They may express anxiety through worry about their physical well-being; somatic preoccupation or hypochondriasis may develop. The potential for substance abuse is high, and suicidal potential is increased. Sexual drive or behavior may be inhibited as well.

Alterations in Conduct and Impulse Control

Excessive anxiety can cause alterations in conduct and impulse control. Unpredictable behavior, such as seen in clients with post-traumatic stress disorder or panic disor-

der, occurs as the individual attempts to cope with the overwhelming fears. Individuals with an obsessive-compulsive disorder are unable to alter behavior, even though they may recognize it as harmful or unnecessary.

Clients with anxiety may turn to abusing drugs. In turn, drug abuse results in disordered conduct and impaired impulse control.

Impaired Role Performance

In clients with anxiety disorders performance in the family, at school, and at work is impaired. They may become less efficient and accurate in previously well-performed functions at work or school due to distractibility or other perceptual and cognitive difficulties. Clients may withdraw emotionally from formerly important and meaningful relationships, or they may become overly dependent on help from those around them. They may isolate themselves and avoid engaging in previously enjoyed activities and recreation. Excessive need for reassurance, decreased productivity, reduced creativity, impaired hygiene, and impaired home maintenance are all possible outcomes for the client with anxiety disorder.

A particularly debilitating consequence of phobic reaction is the incredible restriction it may impose. People who have several phobias concurrently, as is often the case, may become walled off and isolated from many normal activities. A housewife who is afraid of crowds and vehicles becomes gradually less able to carry out her responsibilities of grocery shopping, car pooling, and so forth. The multimillionaire Howard Hughes died a wasted recluse because he had grown so afraid of germs that he refused to leave his hotel room or wear clothing. Such people often consciously recognize the irrationality of their fears but cannot help experiencing them intensely.

Impaired Communication and Motor Behavior

Clients with anxiety disorders often have difficulty communicating. They may speak too quickly or too loudly and may overelaborate or talk about too many subjects at once, thereby confusing the listener. The client is easily distracted and may have trouble understanding explanations or retaining information. A client with severe anxiety may be incoherent, making verbal communication impossible.

Impairments in motor behavior are often related to hyperactivity and restlessness and place the client at risk of accidental injury. Writing skills are frequently impaired. Wringing of the hands, poor coordination, and the appearance of a startle reaction are motor behaviors asso-

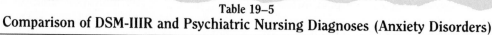

Table 19–5
Comparison of DSM-IIIR and Psychiatric Nursing Diagnoses (Anxiety Disorders)

DSM-IIIR Diagnoses	PND-I Diagnoses	NANDA Diagnoses
300.21 Panic disorder with agoraphobia	02.08.02 Alteration in concentration	Thought processes, altered; impaired concentration
300.21 Panic disorder without agoraphobia	04.02.02 Anxiety*	Anxiety
	04.02.05 Fear*	Fear
300.02 Generalized anxiety disorder	04.02.07 Guilt	Self-concept, disturbance in self-esteem
300.30 Obsessive-compulsive disorder	05.03 Altered role performance*	Role performance, altered
300.22 Agoraphobia without history of panic disorder	05.05 Altered social interaction*	Social interaction, impaired
		Sensory/perceptual alterations
300.23 Social phobia	06.01.01 Distractibility	Comfort, alteration
300.29 Simple phobia	06.02.02 Distress	
309.89 Post-tramatic stress disorder		

*PND-I diagnosis also in NANDA list.

ciated with anxiety disorders. The client with obsessive-compulsive disorder may perform bizarre repetitive acts, e.g., repeatedly washing the hands or counting, checking, and rechecking activity.

Alterations in Perception and Cognition

Alterations in perception and cognition may occur in clients with anxiety disorders. Anxiety reduces the client's ability to solve problems. Judgment, concentration, abstract thinking, and attention are impaired. The client is indecisive but at the same time may make decisions impulsively to relieve tension. In panic, the client may become disoriented, misinterpret reality, and distort the meaning of situations or events.

Loss of self-esteem and a lowered self-concept often result as the client loses previous skills and capacities.

Alteration in Circulation and Elimination

Alterations in circulation and elimination often occur as a result of stimulation of the autonomic nervous system. The client may experience increased blood pressure, rapid heart rate, dizziness, and palpitations as well as dry mouth, cold

or clammy hands, sweating, shortness of breath, and a bad taste in the mouth. Diarrhea or enuresis may occur, and digestion may be slowed.

In the client experiencing extreme anxiety or panic, these symptoms are intensified, and the client may faint or vomit. A medical emergency may arise if the client has an additional major health problem such as cardiac illness.

Impaired Sleep Pattern

Insomnia is a frequent response to anxiety. Nearly all clients with anxiety disorders complain of this phenomenon. Sleep may be further disturbed by nightmares or night terrors.

Planning and Implementing Interventions

Most mental health professionals believe that clients who cope with the stress of anxiety disorders can grow and change with therapeutic intervention. Nursing interventions for clients with anxiety disorders should be geared toward resolving the problems identified in the previous phases of the nursing process.

Promoting Emotional Comfort

Reducing Anxiety

The nurse should take direct measures to promote emotional comfort by reducing intense anxiety. During an acute panic attack, the client cannot engage in problem solving because perception is narrowed and disrupted to a great degree. The panic must be dealt with first. The interventions in Table 19–6 help the nurse control the client's panic. The goal is to reduce the client's immediate anxiety to more moderate and manageable levels, since learning cannot occur if the client is experiencing panic. The family of the distressed individual needs counseling about how to respond therapeutically in such events because they are often involved in or present during a panic episode.

A nurse can frequently detect subtle indications of mounting anxiety and intervene to prevent a severe attack. Some clients are adept at covering up their anxiety, but they usually transmit something to the sensitive observer. Often the nurse's own feelings of increased tension are a useful cue that the source of anxiety is in the client. Anxiety may make people excessively demanding. The nurse's response to the demands must take into account the consequences for the course of the client's anxiety. In some cases it may be reassuring to set limits and deny the request. In other cases such a response may place further stress on the client.

The nurse must know how to treat clients who suffer from prolonged anxiety. Here the intervention strategies are intended to help clients use their anxiety to learn about themselves and their coping strategies. This requires that the client endure the anxiety while searching out its causes. The client must then develop more effective and satisfying coping strategies to replace the old ones. To help clients learn to cope more effectively with anxiety, the nurse must first detect the anxiety, and second make thoughtful observations and responses that facilitate learning. Interventions for an anxious client are presented in Table 19–7.

The nurse who is working through this step-by-step intervention approach must avoid getting bogged down in the client's usual justification of his or her usual ways of coping. Often clients try to give plausible explanations for their ineffective anger, withdrawal, or somatization (automatic responses to anxiety; see Chapter 7). However, they do not explain the relief in terms of the factors that caused the anxiety. The temporary feelings of relief afforded by the usual coping patterns do not last long, because the needs or expectations that originally caused the symptoms still exist. They may even become more intense. Clients can begin to alter disturbed coping patterns only when they understand what their unmet needs are, what they did instead of fulfilling these needs, and what they felt then.

At this point, clients have two alternatives. They can reduce or change their hopes and expectations. Or they can try new tactics or resources to get their needs met. The nurse should discuss these options with the client and

RESEARCH NOTE

Citation

Hartfield MT, Cason CL, Cason GJ: Effects of information about a threatening procedure on patients' expectations and emotional distress. Nurs Res 1982;31(4):202–206.

Study Problem/Purpose

This study examined the effects of procedural and sensation information on subjects' expectations of a threatening procedure. The study was conducted to examine the effects of information about an impending threatening event (barium enema) on subjects' expectations and the intensity of their emotional response to the event.

Methods

In this quasiexperimental study, twenty subjects were assigned to receive either sensation or procedure information. Before receiving information, all the subjects completed a preinformation sensation inventory and the trait portion of the State-Trait Anxiety Inventory (STAI). A taped message of either sensation or procedural information was heard, followed by completion of the postinformation sensation inventory. After the barium enema, all the subjects completed a postprocedure sensation inventory and the state portion of the STAI.

Findings

There were no significant differences in either the expected sensations reported prior to hearing information or the responses provided after the procedure. There were significant differences, however, in reported expected sensations after hearing the information. Subjects receiving sensation information reported significantly less anxiety during the barium enema and their expectations were closer to their actual experiences than subjects receiving procedural information.

Implications

The results imply that sensation information enhances congruence between expected and experienced sensations, while procedural information does not. The results support the notion that emotional response is a function of congruency of expectation with actual experience. As congruency increased, emotional response, that is, anxiety, decreased. This finding indicates a need to further explore how sensation information modifies an individual's emotional response to a threatening situation.

It may be hypothesized that a cognitive reappraisal of a threatening event, by means of sensation information, may produce new coping skills.

negotiate a contract to work on one or both goals. Realizing either option often involves problem solving. Nurse and client must find ways to alter structural features of the client's environment to reduce or meet the need.

Mrs. K, a working wife and mother, played out a superwoman role by bearing 75 percent of the family respon-

---

Table 19–6
Interventions for Client in Panic

Step of Plan	Rationale
Assessment of Need	
Client is pacing and wringing her hands in a pointless, agitated manner. Tearfully she begs for help, says she is falling apart, can't concentrate, feels like she's going crazy.	
She is experiencing palpitations, chest pain, a feeling of choking, and trembling.	
Nursing Intervention Strategy	
1. Stay physically with client.	Often being left alone aggravates the client's panic.
2. Maintain calm, serene manner.	Anxiety is easily communicated from staff to client.
3. Use short, simple sentences and firm, authoritative voice.	Convey sense of ability to provide external controls.
4. Encourage client to move to a smaller physical environment, such as her room, to minimize the stimuli.	Client is already overwhelmed by stimuli.
5. Sometimes it is useful to focus client's diffuse energy on some physically tiring task such as moving furniture or scrubbing the floor.	Physical exercise can sometimes drain high levels of anxiety.
6. It may be wise to recommend that antianxiety medication be ordered for client.	Certain somatic interventions are highly specific and effective in relieving panic.

---

sibilities, only to find that her husband, from whom she expected appreciation and admiration, resented her and her accomplishments. Her unmet needs for his approval and love created automatic coping patterns of anger or depression, and he withdrew even further from her demands. Strategies for Mrs. K might include redistributing the work load more equitably, so that she no longer feels that she deserves any special appreciation, or helping her gain support and admiration from friends and relatives who find it easier to give than her husband does. Of course, Mrs. K could also seek and find another partner more responsive to her feelings and better able to meet her needs.

Nurses use a variety of psychotherapeutic techniques and skills in intervening with clients who experience states of anxiety. Progressive relaxation, meditation, "thought stopping" techniques, autogenic training, and imagery may be employed to help the individual learn new ways to reduce the disturbing affect. Other methods of helping clients reduce anxiety include helping them to reality test, because the person's sense of danger is often heightened out of proportion to actual danger. Development of goal-oriented contracts may help to reduce a client's sense of inner chaos by providing structure and direction.

Educating Clients in the Use of Medications

Education in the use of medications, when prescribed, is an essential role of the nurse. Recall that pharmacologic intervention is not considered the treatment of choice for most anxiety disorders. Clients should be aware of the major drugs used in management of acute anxiety and of their limitations and possible side-effects. The nurse needs to know that anxiety that is secondary to major medical illness or acute trauma (e.g., the death of a child) requires a different dosage than that prescribed for the primary treatment of anxiety.

Short-term use of higher dosage antidepressants has been found to help control panic attacks. For situational anxiety the benzodiazepine group of drugs have proven effective and relatively safe for periods of four to eight weeks. Antianxiety agents such as meprobamate (Equanil), diazepam (Valium), and chlordiazepoxide (Librium) or adrenergic blocking agents such as propranolol (Inderal) may be used.

Significant progress in pharmacologic treatments for agoraphobia with associated panic attacks has been made in the last decade. Pharmacologic agents, most notably the tricyclic antidepressants (TCAs), e.g., imipramine (Tofranil); the monoamine oxidase inhibitors (MAOIs), e.g., phenelzine (Nardil); and the second generation benzodiazepines (BZs), e.g., alprazolam (Xanax) have been found to be effective in reducing or eliminating panic episodes associated with agoraphobia (Sheehan 1985).

Although the antipanic drugs are primarily antidepressants, the existing evidence suggests that panic disorders and agoraphobia are responding to these drugs not because the disorders are types of depression. Instead, the therapeutic effect is thought to be the result of the side-effects on the vagal system.

Promoting Conduct and Impulse Control

Clients with Obsessive-Compulsive Disorders

Clients with obsessive-compulsive disorders avoid anxiety by engaging in compulsive acts and rigid thinking. Unless nurses are involved only in private practice, they will sooner or later encounter an obsessive-compulsive client whose problem is severe enough to require hospitalization.

Compulsive rituals are employed to undo and control anxiety. Therefore any interference with them must be carefully weighed and timed so as not to cause an escalation of the client's anxiety. For example, clients with washing compulsions may completely remove the skin from their hands, and nurses have successfully intervened by suggesting surgical gloves. However, it is not usually fruitful, and may be harmful, to prematurely interfere with a ritual unless it threatens the client's or another person's life or health. These clients often have a strong tendency toward negativism, which may cause them to become more firmly entrenched in their defenses if modifications are introduced prematurely. Nurses should attempt to develop an affirming, dependable relationship with clients before suggesting that they change their behavior patterns. The nurse must balance the value of intervening in behavior that protects clients from mental anguish against the need to prevent physical deterioration caused by the behavior.

Clients with Post-traumatic Stress Disorder

Clients with post-traumatic stress disorder frequently experience behavior or conduct disturbances as a result of the intense anxiety triggered by reexperiencing the trauma. When alcohol or other mood-altering drugs are used to relieve anxiety, they may contribute to destructive and impulsive acts. In the acute stage, crisis counseling is essential. Due to the chronic course of the illness and the many psychosocial problems associated with it, a comprehensive treatment approach is needed. Frequently clients experience disordered family relationships, physical disability, social and recreational disruptions, and impaired ability to work or attend school. They may experience symptoms and attitudes of demoralization that further hamper their functioning.

The goal of therapy in treating the client with post-traumatic stress disorder is to desensitize them to the memories of the traumatic events so that the ego, or coping functions, can gain mastery over the anxiety. The following interventions or techniques may be used; singly, or, more frequently, in combination.

- Education/explanation: Giving an explanation about the dynamics of the disability and a rationale of the

process of treatment. This helps engage the client's ego in treatment.

- Relaxation training: Typical training programs may include muscle relaxation and imagery. The emphasis is on providing new "tools" or skills that the person may use when faced with memories of the traumatic event.

Table 19–7
Interventions for Anxious Client

Step of Plan	Nursing Intervention
1. Observe client for increased psychomotor activity, anger or withdrawal, excessive demands, and tearfulness.	Verbalizations intended to help client recognize and name his experience as anxiety. "Are you feeling uncomfortable?" "Are you anxious or nervous now?" When client says "Yes," he is ready for step 2.
2. Connect feeling of anxiety with relief behavior. Client acknowledges, describes, and names feelings of nervousness or anxiety.	Ask client what he does to feel more comfortable when he feels anxious. When client understands that when he feels anxious he gets angry, withdraws, or somatizes, he is ready for step 3.
3. Investigate situation that immediately preceded feeling of anxiety.	Encourage client to recall and describe what he was experiencing immediately before he got anxious (including thoughts, actions, and other feelings).

4. Help client observe, describe, and analyze connections between what led to his anxiety and what happened after he felt anxious. Only through seeing all parts of this experience can client understand why he became anxious.

5. Formulate causes of anxiety. Help client state causes of the anxiety. Then help him observe and recall similar instances in his experiences of anxiety. Through such extensive discussions, client will eventually be able to recognize and perhaps alter his pattern of handling anxiety.

Source: Peplau H: Interpersonal techniques: The crux of nursing. Copyright © 1962, The American Journal of Nursing Company. Adapted with permission from the American Journal of Nursing, June, Vol. 62 No. 6.

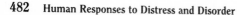

- Hypnosis or narcoanalyses (the injection of barbiturates or other drugs to induce partial anesthesia): These techniques have been used by some therapists to bring to consciousness repressed and suppressed material so that it can be integrated into the ego structure, where it will have a less powerful influence.

- Cognitive skill therapies: These include techniques such as "thought stopping," thought substitution, and providing the client with positive reinforcing statements. Cognitive restructuring of events giving new, less noxious interpretations may be used.

- Abreaction/systematic desensitization: A therapeutic effect may occur through emotional release or abreaction after recalling the painful repressed experience. Systematic desensitization in which the dreaded object, thought, or situation is introduced to the client in gradual amounts may be used as well. Systemic desensitization is discussed later in this chapter.

- Family conferences: Efforts are frequently needed to engage the family in working to resolve the many psychosocial effects caused by the trauma. If successful, the family may provide a crucial supportive function.

- Group treatment: The benefits of group membership have been clearly demonstrated in recent years. Vietnam veterans, Mothers against Drunk Drivers, and Women against Violence against Women are just a few of the growing number of self-help groups organizing to assist and support victims of trauma and violence.

- Exercise and nutrition: Maintaining a healthy physical state as an adjunct to other therapies is necessary to strengthen the body's adaptive efforts following trauma.

- Individual therapy: Individual psychotherapy can provide important ego supportive and/or cathartic benefits.

Recent advances in psychopharmacology have promoted the use of medication as adjuncts to psychologic forms of treatment for post-traumatic stress disorders. As is true for the other anxiety disorders, however, the nurse should be aware of the heightened potential for drug abuse among clients who suffer disorders of acute distress. The desire for immediate, total relief is powerful and may foster drug dependence and abuse.

BZs, TCAs, MAOIs, lithium, beta-blockers, alpha-adrenergic antagonists, and neuroleptics have all been reported to relieve symptoms of post-traumatic stress disorder, either partially or totally (Elledgrie and Bridges 1985). During the initial stage (four to eight weeks), the use of benzodiazepines may be helpful in the treatment of the anxiety, insomnia, and nightmares. Longer-term use, however, may lead to habituation and dependence and is a serious limitation to the use (Schuckit 1985). Most recently, prelimi-

nary investigations are being conducted using the beta-adrenergic blocker propranolol (Inderal) and the anticonvulsant clonazepam (Clonopin) in an effort to avoid the side-effects of the benzodiazepines (Burris 1983).

In those instances where depression is a major factor, one of the cyclic antidepressants or an MAOI may be used. Sleeplessness, another common feature, is best treated with a behavioral approach first (e.g., relaxation techniques, imagery, muscle relaxation, and exclusion of daytime naps). Sedatives are discouraged except for very brief use. The nurse's goal is to help the client reestablish the ability to sleep naturally and cope with stress without the use of drugs.

Promoting Effective Role Performance in Clients with Phobia

Clients with phobic disorders attempt to avoid anxiety by binding it to a specific object or situation. Many people manage to lead successful productive lives by binding their anxiety up in this way. Others, though, may experience severe restriction in their activities, and their performance at work, home, or school may be greatly compromised. It is essential to recognize that forcing clients to come into contact with the feared object or the basic source of their anxiety can create in them an intense, disorganizing flood of panic.

Most clinicians agree that phobic coping patterns are highly resistant to most insight-oriented therapies. These therapies require that clients confront and at least temporarily experience some of their originating anxiety. It is not surprising that they are ineffective with phobic clients, since the phobic's style is basically one of *avoidance*. In recent years, however, some relatively dramatic symptomatic improvements have been made using techniques derived from behaviorist learning theory. The most commonly used interventions are desensitization and reciprocal inhibition.

In *systematic desensitization*, the client is exposed serially to a predetermined list of anxiety-provoking situations graded in a hierarchy from the least to the most frightening. See Box 19–4. Through techniques of progressive relaxation, the person becomes desensitized to each stimulus in the scale and then moves up to the next most frightening stimulus. Eventually the stimulus that originally provoked the most anxiety no longer elicits the same painful response. For example, a man who is irrationally afraid of ordinary earthworms might first talk about earthworms until the topic no longer evokes the same anxiety. Then he might be shown pictures of earthworms until he masters that level of closeness—and so on, increasing contact until he can actually hold a live earthworm in his hand.

In *reciprocal inhibition*, the anxiety-provoking stimulus is paired with another stimulus that is associated with an opposite feeling strong enough to suppress the anxiety. Through the use of antianxiety medications, hypnosis,

Box 19–4
DESENSITIZATION HIERARCHY FOR PHOBIC FEAR OF HEIGHTS

1. Develop ten to twelve scenes of increasing approximation to the fear. Example:

   Tell the client to imagine:

   a. "You are going up the kitchen stepladder; walk to the third rung and look around."
   b. "Now you are going up to the top rung. You are up to the top. Look around at the cupboards. Look at the floor."
   c. "Now you are on the second floor of an office building. You walk toward the window and look out."

2. Continue in this manner, advancing the scene to nearer approximations of the fear each time the client is able to visualize without undue anxiety.

   "Now you go to the top of the World Trade Center. You go over to the guard rail and look straight down."

3. The final steps of the desensitization process include encouraging the client to try some of these behaviors in real life, after the simulations have been successful.

meditation, yoga, or biofeedback training, clients are taught how to induce in themselves both psychologic and physical calm. Once they have mastered these techniques, they are taught to use them when faced with the anxiety-provoking hierarchy of stimuli.

Two other behavior-based interventions may also be used. In *cognitive restructuring* or *"relabeling,"* the client is encouraged to relabel a frightening situation, object, or activity. Closely linked to learning theory, this intervention is based on the belief that anxiety stems from erroneous interpretations of situations. In *exposure* or *"flooding,"* the client is repeatedly brought in prolonged contact with those situations that usually evoke distress or rituals until discomfort in their presence subsides.

Using behavioral conditioning techniques to rid the client of a phobia merely eliminates the symptom without removing the original stressor or conflict. If clients give up a phobic reaction without learning a more effective coping strategy, they can usually expect some alternative and equally troublesome disturbed pattern to emerge.

Promoting Effective Communication and Improved Motor Behavior

Nursing interventions that reduce anxiety, e.g., those identified in Tables 19–6 and 19–7, are important general measures that promote more effective communication and motor behavior.

Clients with an obsessive-compulsive disorder require patience and an unhurried attitude from the nurse in response to their particular problems with details and ruminations. It is frustrating to try to communicate with people who cope by developing an obsessive-compulsive reaction. If we use the customary techniques of paraphrasing and reflecting, these clients will say that we have failed to get the details right. They will then go on to correct, qualify, and clarify what we've said. Curiously, this pedantic striving for accuracy produces greater vagueness and confusion. It is as if parallel conversations are going on. Clients hear only themselves repeating and correcting insignificant details and completely lose the overall meaning of the message.

Promoting Safety Needs of Anxious Clients

Due to lack of coordination or tremors, anxious clients may be prone to accidents. The nurse needs to counsel clients not to perform potentially dangerous activities, e.g., driving a car, when anxiety is high. The nurse may advise them to move more slowly or to go over instructions carefully when undertaking a new task or when using tools.

Promoting Optimum Circulation and Elimination

Like communication and motor behavior, circulation and elimination processes improve when anxiety is reduced. Interventions previously discussed are important steps for the nurse to take. Additionally, attention to proper nutrition and adequate activity are necessary, because clients with anxiety frequently overlook their self-care and health needs. Walking, participating in sports, or developing new hobbies and interests promote physiologic functions and need to be part of a comprehensive nursing treatment plan.

Promoting Sleep

Nonpharmacologic nursing measures to promote sleep should be used before medications. These may include any of a variety of relaxation methods. A currently popular method is the use of audio tapes. Like imagery, they provide a relaxing atmosphere—listening to the sounds of a beach or of birds in a wooded forest is soothing and sleep-promoting to some individuals.

The nurse may suggest the client try reading in bed, drinking warm liquids, or taking a warm tub bath prior to retiring. (See Box 28-3, Visualization for the Bath.) The

Text continues on p. 488.

CASE STUDY: Client with Panic Disorder with Agoraphobia

Identifying Information

Mrs. R is 43 years old, married, Irish Catholic, and mother of four daughters in their late teens or early twenties. Until very recently she had been employed as a secretary at a local pediatrician's office. She has a high school education and recently attempted attending community college, hoping to fulfill a lifelong dream of getting a college degree. She was referred to the psychiatric out-patient clinic for follow-up counseling by the emergency department of the local general hospital where she had been rushed in acute distress the prior evening with symptoms of a panic attack.

Client's Definition of Present Problem, Precipitatory Stresses, Coping Strategies, Goals for Care

At the time of the panic attack, Mrs. R believed she was having a heart attack and feared she was dying. She reported racing heartbeat, sweating, and feeling faint. She could not identify any events, thoughts, or feelings that were precipitants to the incident; it seemed to her to occur "out of the blue." She wanted relief from her fears of a medical emergency and felt unable to cope with the severity of the symptoms of the attack: "I tried to talk myself out of it; to tell myself it would go away, but it only got worse."

History of Present Problem

Mrs. R reported she had had similar attacks over the years and that she had always been reassured of her medical and cardiac health, but when these attacks occurred, she "feared the worst" and "lost all perspective." The attacks could last from two minutes to two hours. Her daily routine had become quite restricted as she now sought to have one of her daughters or her husband with her when she went out of the home due to fear of an attack. She sometimes could make it to school on her own but only with great effort, forcing herself to go. She did not feel comfortable when alone in her home and could not go to sleep if the other family members were not home. As an aside, she wondered what she would do when all the girls were off in college and she had no "sidekick." She felt ashamed and angry about her growing disability and often tried to cover up her fears to friends and family.

On interviewing the family, the nurse was able to gather information about a number of significant recent life events preceding the panic episode:

1. Recent major surgery. A hysterectomy occurred four weeks earlier.
2. Loss of her employment due to her hospitalization. She was abruptly terminated from her position at a new job due to too many absences.
3. Recent discovery that her oldest daughter was taking birth control pills.
4. The upcoming anniversary date of her father's sudden death from a heart attack.

Psychiatric History

Mrs. R had never been hospitalized before for a psychiatric condition, although she had been to the emergency room on three prior occasions with symptoms of panic attack. She had seen a therapist years ago when the attacks first occurred, "about the time I left home to marry." She did not follow up with the therapist, however, saying she felt ashamed ("I've always been a strong and effective person!"), that the episodes were not so severe then, and that she found relief from panic attacks after she had the children.

continued

Case Study (Continued)

Family History	Both Mrs. R's parents died within the past six years. She was especially close to her father and the second anniversary of his death was approaching. Mrs. R's mother was considered a "homebody"; she rarely left the house and took part in social activities only if they occurred at the family home. Mrs. R suddenly wondered if her mother had "these fears" too. She did not feel close to her mother in her adolescence, and there were many conflicts over her growing independence. She remembered feeling hurt that her father would not stand up to her mother and "protect me" when she felt her mother was in the wrong or especially harsh. Mrs. R had four older sisters and one older brother. They were "always around," and she realized only after she married "how important that was" to her feelings of security.
Social History	Mrs. R had always been considered a "doer" and an achiever, "someone people came to for help with problems, not the other way around!" She liked her new position as secretary for a pediatrician's office but felt angry at being terminated from the position due to her many absences. In addition to her absences due to her gynecologic problems she acknowledged that her fears she would have a panic attack at work were interfering with her attendance as well.
	She reported she had begun to curtail social and recreational activities, preferring to stay at home where she was most comfortable. She noticed she was "living through the kids" rather than participating actively in golf and church activities as she had previously done with her husband.
	Her relationship to her husband she described as emotionally warm and supportive. Although she sometimes resented his being away from her, she recognized this as part of her "problem" with being alone.
	Her primary relationships had been with her husband and children. She talked of facing the "empty nest" as her daughters, one by one, left for work or college. She "was shocked" to discover that her oldest daughter was using birth control pills but had "gotten over it," concluding that she was being old-fashioned and judgmental "like my mother."
Significant Health History	With the exception of chronic gynecologic problems leading to the recent hysterectomy, Mrs. R reported a history of good health. She had no allergies or other chronic illnesses. Her only other hospitalizations were to have her children. The recent hospitalization had been more physically taxing than she expected, and the fact that she was not allowed to return to work after her recovery came as a blow: "Going back to work would have been good for me. I felt discarded."
Current Mental Status	Mrs. R presented as an attractive, carefully groomed woman looking her stated age. She sat erect in the office chair, appearing somewhat tense. She answered questions cooperatively, but at times with some hesitation and as if expectant of criticism or judgment from the interviewer. She would say, for example, "Well how would *you* feel?" in response to an inquiry abut her emotional reaction to a significant event.
Sensorium	She was oriented to time, place, and person. She exhibited a good fund of knowledge, appropriate for her education and experience. Her memory was intact and recall good. She had no difficulty with calculations. Her judgment was unimpaired. During times of panic, however, sensory and perceptive awareness was greatly impaired.

continued

Case Study (Continued)

Feelings	Affect appeared normal, with occasional evidence of anger in the form of irritability and light sarcasm. Mood was within normal limits.
Voice and Speech	Speech was normal in flow and volume. It appeared pressured at times when she attempted to correct an impression she believed the interviewer held.
Motor Behavior	Posture was at times rigid, but she relaxed somewhat as she became more comfortable with the interview.
Thought Content	There were no delusions, ideas of reference, or hallucinations. Obsessive worry about the occurrence of panic episodes and of her safety were present. Embarrassment and shame over her symptoms were apparent. Suicidal or homicidal thoughts were denied.
Thought Processes	Associations and abstractions were appropriate and there was no evidence of thought process disorder or difficulty in concentration, except during acute panic, at which times concentration was impaired and thought processes were disorganized.
Defenses	Some guardedness toward the interviewer was noted. Rationalization, overintellectualization, and avoidance were other coping and defense mechanisms used.
Insight	Insight into the meaning of the current situation was minimal.
Other Significant Subjective or Objective Clinical Data	Mrs. R was considering the use of a trial of antipanic medication, despite "hating the idea" of medication.

Diagnostic Impression

Nursing Diagnosis
(PND-I/NANDA)

06.02.02 Distress
/Comfort, altered

02.08.02 Alteration in concentration
/Thought processes altered, impaired concentration associated with panic attack

05.97 Undeveloped interpersonal processes
/Coping, ineffective individual

05.03 Altered role performance
/Role performance, altered

05.05.02 Social isolation
/Withdrawal

04.02.02 Anxiety
/Anxiety

04.02.05 Fear
/Fear

04.02.07 Guilt
/Self-concept, disturbance in self-esteem

06.01.01 Distractibility
/Sensory/perceptual alterations associated with panic attack

DSM-IIIR Multiaxial Diagnosis

Axis I: 300.21 Panic disorder with agoraphobia
Axis II: None
Axis III: Gynecologic disorder, under treatment
Axis IV: Psychosocial stressors: recent hysterectomy, acute event; loss of employment, acute event; recent knowledge of daughter's use of birth control, acute event; upcoming anniversary of father's sudden death, acute event
Severity: 3-moderate
Axis V: Current GAF: 42
Highest GAF past year: 76

continued

Case Study (Continued)

Nursing Care Plan

Nursing Diagnosis (PND-I/NANDA)	Client Care Goals	Nursing Planning/ Intervention	Evaluation
06.02.02 Distress /Comfort, altered	The client will experience less discomfort, including dyspnea, tachycardia, sweating, fear, and anxiety.	1. During a panic attack: a. Maintain calm manner. b. Stay physically with the client. c. Acknowledge that he or she will not die. d. Use short, simple sentences and firm, authoritative voice. e. Consider calling the client's attention to some physically tiring or repetitive task in order to focus energy away from fears. f. Consider use of antianxiety medication as an adjunct to psychologic measures. 2. Consider use of specific psychologic treatment approaches: desensitization, hypnosis, "flooding," and imagery therapy to help client master the phobic fears.	The client will be without symptoms of dyspnea, tachycardia, sweating, fear, or anxiety.
05.03 Altered role performance /Role performance, altered	The client will expand activities of daily living.		Client no longer has altered life-style. Client is able to conduct normal activities at home, work, or school.
05.05.02 Social isolation/ withdrawal /Social isolation	The client will be able to travel away from home.	See No. 2 above.	Client will travel away from home whenever he or she desires.
04.02.02 Anxiety 04.02.05 Fear 04.02.07 Guilt /Self-concept, disturbance in self-esteem	The client's feelings of fear, anxiety, or guilt will lessen.	3. Recommend dynamic, insight-oriented psychotherapy if unconscious conflicts appear to be motivating force behind mood and affect changes. 4. Educate client on the proper use of medication, if prescribed.	Client no longer complains of feeling fearful, anxious, or guilty. Client verbalizes an understanding of medications and uses them correctly.

continued

Case Study (Continued)

Nursing Diagnosis (PND-I/NANDA)	Client Care Goals	Nursing Planning/ Intervention	Evaluation
02.08.02 Alteration in concentration /Thought processes, altered, impaired concentration	The client will be able to concentrate better.	5. Teach client self-relaxation therapy to reduce early signs of anxiety and symptoms. See also No. 2 above.	Client reports that she can concentrate better.
05.97 Undeveloped interpersonal processes /Coping, ineffective individual	The client will develop effective coping strategies.	6. Assist client in identifying and using own resources and social supports to broaden activities. See also Nos. 2 and 5 above.	Client reports and demonstrates use of effective coping strategies, e.g., use of relaxation techniques. Client no longer uses excessive avoidance. Client is able to use social supports and has broadened her activities.
06.98 Altered perception process, not otherwise specified /Coping, ineffective individual	The client will gain mastery over incidents of panic.	See Nos. 1, 2, and 5 above.	Client reports feeling able to manage incidents of anxiety. Client demonstrates use of relaxation techniques.
06.03.01 Altered body image* /Self-concept, disturbance in body image	The client will not fear that she is dying.	7. Encourage verbalization of fears. Validate that fear of dying is a subjective experience.	Client reports no fear of dying.
01.99 Potential for altered activity processes (associated with potential to abuse medication) /Health maintenance, altered	The client will not abuse substances.	See No. 4 above.	The client uses medication in correct and safe manner.

PND-I diagnosis also in NANDA list.

client with post-traumatic stress disorder may fear going to sleep because of nightmares. Having another member of the family nearby and aware of the client's fear may be reassuring.

Promoting Effective Perception and Cognition

To function more effectively and independently, the client needs to know about normal anxiety and about anxiety disorders. Providing accurate information at the right time and in an appropriate manner is an essential nursing function. Other strategies the nurse uses when seeking to promote effective perception and cognition include the following:

- The nurse may use adjuncts to verbal communication to stimulate memory and retention of information, e.g., use of visual aids or role playing.
- Problem-solving vignettes may be practiced as a way of improving judgment and insight.
- The nurse may need to identify misperceptions that the client holds as a result of a narrowed perceptual field. The nurse can help the client by offering such comments as, "I wonder if you've considered this possibility?" or "Perhaps if we tried this tack?"
- The nurse helps the client reality test, i.e., helps the client to explore his or her opinions based on validated experience rather than on emotional needs that block accurate perception of reality.

Emotional Comfort

Clients should be without evidence of acute or intense anxiety and be able to perform activities of daily living independently when appropriate. Clients will verbalize feeling less anxious, and there will be a decrease in somatic complaints. They will state they feel more comfortable.

Fewer symptoms of physiologic distress, e.g., racing pulse, diaphoresis, or hyperventilation, will be present. Clients will be without signs of increased psychomotor activity. They will no longer complain of tearfulness, feelings of rage, or impatience. When appropriate, they will more readily engage in interactions with others. Phobic clients will be better able to tolerate the presence of the feared object, activity, or situation without experiencing panic or the need to flee.

Conduct and Impulse Control

The obsessive-compulsive client will be able to limit or cease performing compulsive rituals; for example, a client with a handwashing compulsion will wash his hands no more than four times a day.

Clients will demonstrate the ability to continue with necessary activities even though some anxiety is present. They will be less likely to panic or flee. Family members will report that the client is "more like himself/herself," and that he or she is less agitated, driven, or explosive in conduct.

Role Function

The client will be able to attend work or school on a regular basis. Family members report that relationships at home have improved and that the client is once again taking responsibility for activities within the family.

Clients will report engaging in recreational or social activity and independently performing self-care. They will express feeling more comfortable about their performance at home, work, or school. The phobic client will be able to function in daily activities with less restriction or interference from any feared object, activity, or situation.

Communication and Motor Behavior

Clients will state satisfaction with their communication; they feel heard and understood. They will report being able to perform usual small motor tasks, such as writing, in a competent manner. There will be open lines of communication between client and nurse and client and family. Clients will report no tremors and will not have accidents due to poor motor coordination.

Circulation and Elimination

Clients will report feeling energetic. Somatic complaints will decrease, and clients will report engaging in daily physical activity. Vital signs will be normal and weight will be stable.

Sleep

Clients will sleep through the night without medication or with appropriately prescribed medication. They will have fewer nightmares or wake less frequently throughout the night.

Cognition and Perception

Clients will be able to correctly recall information that was taught by the nurse. They will begin to make decisions about their health care and ask questions about the anxiety process.

Clients will be able to describe what led to anxiety and what happened after they felt anxious. They will be able to state the cause of anxiety and will be able to recall similar instances. They will verbalize techniques to reduce anxiety.

The client will correctly verbalize the use, side-effects, and limitations of medications used. Clients will verbalize increased awareness of their environment.

THE NURSING PROCESS AND SOMATOFORM DISORDERS

Assessment

Assessment of the client with a somatoform disorder is complex because of the wide-ranging biopsychosocial factors involved.

Subjective Data

The client with a somatoform disorder reports physical symptoms for which there is no positive evidence of organic or physiologic cause. Clients with hypochrondriacal illness, for example, may return many times to the outpatient clinic or emergency room, demanding to be reexamined or retested. They feel sure that they are suffering from some major illness that has been undetected. They are not reassured by the lack of physical findings and may go from doctor to doctor hoping to find someone who will validate their fears.

In conversion disorder, the individual has loss of function or an alteration in function. They may be unable to walk, for instance, complaining, "I woke up this morning with no feeling in my legs; for some reason they won't move." Examination reveals normal sensitivity however, and again, no reason for the apparent loss of function. Interestingly, however, this client with conversion disorder seems unconcerned about the presenting problem despite its apparent severity. The attitude of la belle indifférence, literally "beautiful indifference," is characteristic of these clients who show an inappropriate lack of concern about their disabilities.

Clients with somatization disorder or hypochondriacal disorder, in contrast, are overly dramatic and emotional in telling about their symptoms and pain. They report the history in vivid detail and colorful language but often pay more attention to how the symptoms have affected relationships in their lives than in giving careful description of the nature, character, location, onset, and duration of the symptoms.

In body dysmorphic disorder, the client may request unnecessary operations, for example, demanding cosmetic surgery for an imagined or greatly magnified defect in appearance.

Careful interviewing by the nurse frequently uncovers a stressful life situation with which the client is not coping, suggesting that the preoccupation with somatic disorder is a way of avoiding underlying conflict. Helping the client to identify and talk about this is a crucial beginning to psychotherapeutic intervention.

Objective Data

Physical examination reveals no evidence for the physical symptoms of the client. Laboratory findings likewise do not substantiate organic or physiologic disorder. Despite this, the client may have undergone many exploratory procedures without relief or diagnosis.

Family members often report the client is moody, self-centered, or demanding. They feel alienated from the client and are frustrated with the client's chronic preoccupation with physical symptoms. In a hospital setting, these clients often create scenes that bring them the attention they need without regard for the needs of either fellow clients or staff. Nurses frequently find it difficult to be kind, understanding, and nonjudgmental with these clients. Nurses who cannot cope with their own reactions to these clients cannot work with them effectively. It may help to remember that these clients do not intentionally produce their symp-

toms, neither do they appreciate the effects of their behavior on other people. Nurses who appreciate the whole story can sometimes feel more empathy for a client's coping style.

Nursing Diagnosis

A comparison between PND-I and NANDA diagnoses for clients with somatoform disorders is given in Table 19–8. The following sections discuss their implications for the client and the nurse.

Impaired Communication

Clients with somatoform disorders have an impaired ability to communicate their needs. Though they may be highly verbal, careful listening reveals many gaps, oversimplifications, overdramatizations, and overgeneralizations in their communications. The symptoms are considered nonverbal substitutes for the expression of underlying conflict that they feel unable to master.

The nurse considers the nonverbal communication function of the symptom itself. Symptoms of blindness, deafness, pain, numbness, itching, swelling, vomiting, paralysis, and so forth may be communicating something as general as "take care of me," "pay attention to me," or "I want out of these responsibilities." Specific symptoms may have more exact or symbolic meanings. The "blind" person may be saying, "I don't want to see something, because not having to see it allows me to escape my feelings about it." The client with an upcoming marriage may suddenly develop acute pain in the genital area as a way of saying "I'm afraid of becoming sexually involved."

Alterations in Role Performance

The manipulative and dependent traits of the client with a somatoform disorder lead to impairment in social, work, and family relationships and to diminished performance in these roles. Friends and relatives eventually tire of their demands and become less available for support. Clients become emotionally isolated because their self-absorption makes them unable to respond appropriately to the needs of others.

Work performance suffers from frequent absences due to imagined illness. Preoccupation with their health uses up creative energy that could otherwise be directed toward their work.

Impaired Emotional Experience

Clients with a somatoform disorder experience anxiety, anger, and feelings of helplessness. They may feel these

| | Table 19–8 | |
| Comparison of DSM-IIIR and Psychiatric Nursing Diagnoses (Somatoform Disorders) | | |
DSM-IIIR Diagnoses	**PND-I Diagnoses**	**NANDA Diagnoses**
300.70 Body dysmorphic disorder	01.01 Altered motor behavior	Anxiety
300.11 Conversion disorder	01.03 Altered self-care*	Coping, ineffective individual
300.70 Hypochondriasis	01.04.04 Nightmares	Fear
300.81 Somatization disorder	02.03.03 Knowledge deficit*	Knowledge deficit
307.80 Somatoform pain disorder	04.02.02 Anxiety*	Comfort, alteration in: pain
300.70 Undifferentiated somatoform disorder	05.01 Altered communication processes*	Impaired physical mobility
	05.01 Altered communication process*	Powerlessness
300.70 Somatoform disorder NOS	05.02.02 Dysfunctional behaviors	Self-care deficit
	05.03 Altered role performance	Self-concept, disturbance in body image
	06.02.03 Pain*	Self-concept, disturbance in role performance
	06.03.01 Altered body image*	Sensory/perceptual alterations
	07.02 Altered elimination processes*	Sleep pattern disturbance
	07.04 Altered gastrointestinal processes	
	07.05 Altered neurosensory processes	
	08.01.04 Powerlessness*	

PND-I diagnoses also in NANDA list.

emotions acutely and demonstrate these feelings excessively, as in somatization disorder and hypochrondriacal disorder. Paradoxically, they may show an uncanny lack of feeling where more would be expected, as in the blithe reaction to loss of physical function in conversion disorder.

The emotional life of the client becomes increasingly constricted. The focus of emotional experience becomes somatic concerns, and they no longer experience meaningful emotional connections with other persons, activities, and events. Range of expression of emotion may be limited to making demands, manipulation, and symbolic manifestation of anxiety.

Alterations in Perception and Cognition

These clients show selective inattention, i.e., they filter out stimuli as a response to anxiety. Their judgment is often impaired as a result of keeping ideas and events out of awareness. In a further effort to prove their ideas, they distort reality and tend to ramble. It is evident to the nurse

that their conclusions are not logical. They may distort memory or show selective memory as well.

Clients with somatoform disorder have an impaired body image; they sense that they are weak or vulnerable physically. They incorrectly perceive sensory data. For example, if they have abdominal discomfort, they believe they have cancer rather than common indigestion.

Planning and Implementing Interventions

Once organic problems have been ruled out and a client's behavior is confirmed as representing an example of a somatoform disorder, effective intervention involves:

- Recognizing and understanding the life problem or adjustment the client is facing
- Recognizing and understanding the client's self-perception as helpless to cope
- Helping the client learn more effective ways of adapting

These steps may be accomplished by insight-oriented or supportive psychotherapy, behavior modification, hypnosis, or any of several other psychologic, as well as some physical, therapies. None can claim superior effectiveness, and new approaches and techniques are indicated when traditional ones prove inadequate.

It is important to recognize that many clients with somatoform disorders are highly resistant to change. Progress may be slow and recovery partial.

Promoting Effective Communication

After assessing the meaning behind the client's communication patterns, the nurse can plan intervention strategies that enhance the client's functional verbal communication and self-esteem to the point where the client feels ready to face problems.

It is usually necessary to help these clients tone down their characteristic extravagances and to express respectful skepticism regarding their oversimplifications and overdramatizations. A communication and feelings group will give the client the opportunity to receive feedback about the effect his or her behavior has on others.

Promoting Improved Role Performance

Working with the family as well as with the client is especially important for clients with somatoform disorders. The nurse educates the family and the client about the disorder, stressing the importance of avoiding unnecessary surgery or medical procedures. Supporting self-sufficiency, encouraging independent functioning, and reducing the possibility of secondary gain by not focusing on physical symptoms are attitudes the family, as well as the nurse, need to adopt. The nurse assumes a matter-of-fact, supportive attitude, with optimistic expectation that the client will return to functioning in work, family, and social roles.

Promoting Effective Emotional Expression

The goal of counseling clients with somatoform disorders is to assist them in verbally expressing their conflicts, rather than acting them out in symptomatic behaviors. The aim of long-term, or insight therapy, is to promote effective emotional expression by exploring the sources of anxiety. Supportive therapy seeks to improve self-esteem, perhaps through such measures as expanding clients' interest in their environment.

In general, the nurse tries to avoid reinforcing the client's symptoms. A well-known psychiatric axiom that applies to clients in this general category is "ignore the symptoms but never the client." To concentrate on the physical symptom by trying to get a "paralyzed" client to walk or a "blind" client to see again is to give the symptom more importance than it merits, thus increasing the secondary gain associated with it. Ultimately this merely makes it harder for the client to relinquish the symptom.

Promoting Improved Perception and Cognition

The nurse helps clients improve their capacities of perception and cognition by supporting general measures to reduce anxiety and improve communication of needs. In addition, the nurse maintains a calm, unhurried attitude toward the client and helps by listening and maintaining an objective and undistorted view of reality while avoiding a premature challenge to the client's symptoms and complaints.

As the client's defenses reduce, the nurse proposes other ways that the client may understand his or her condition, e.g., suggesting a psychologic explanation for a physical complaint.

Evaluation

Communication

Clients will more regularly express feelings and conflicts verbally. They will have fewer physical complaints and fewer somatic symptoms.

Role Performance

Clients will attend work regularly without frequent absences due to illness or interference due to worry about physical health. They will be more interested in outside activities and may begin to engage in socialization and recreation. Family and friends will report being more satisfied with their relationship with the client and will be more willing to interact with the client socially.

Emotional Expression

Clients will be less demanding, manipulative, and attention-seeking in interaction with others. They will appear less anxious and will talk of subjects other than their current physical status. They will appear less helpless and more able to participate in and make responsible decisions about their health care. For example, they may carry out a plan of treatment without voicing innumerable objections or worries.

They will appear more interested and involved in the activities and attitudes of others and more aware of the impact of their own behavior.

Perception and Cognition

The nurse will note that the client distorts and misinterprets reality less frequently. Conversation with the client will "flow," with fewer monologues by the client and more natural dialogue between client and nurse. Judgment, insight, and memory will improve as a result of reduced defensiveness in perception and cognition. Clients may report feeling more positive about their bodies. They will be more assertive in physical activities because they no longer tend to feel so vulnerable.

THE NURSING PROCESS AND DISSOCIATIVE DISORDERS

Assessment

The major areas to focus on in assessment are identity, memory, and consciousness.

Subjective Data

Clients with dissociative disorders often report sudden loss of memory of events. Clients may report, for example, that they cannot recall certain important personal events or information. They may not recall aspects of their own identity, e.g., how old they are and where they reside.

Sometimes amnesia is only partial, and clients remain conscious of what happened although they report that they feel no control over it. In instances where amnesia is more or less complete, the "lost" memories can be recovered under certain therapeutic circumstances or they may return spontaneously.

If a client has sustained loss of his or her own reality, the nurse may discover that the client has adopted an entirely new identity.

If motor behavior is affected in dissociative disorder, clients or their families may report wandering episodes in which they physically traveled away from home. Clients with depersonalization disorder may report fears that they are going crazy and have great secondary anxiety. In instances of multiple personality disorder, the original personality typically is not aware of the existence of the different personalities, although the secondary personalities may be aware of the original personality as well as of each other and may report this awareness to the nurse.

Objective Data

The nurse conducts a careful assessment of the client's physical condition because of the possibility of organic causes for the dissociative disorder, e.g., brain tumor. Many of the

---

Table 19–9
Differentiation of Postconcussional Amnesia and Psychogenic Amnesia

Properties of Postconcussional Amnesia	Properties of Psychogenic Amnesia
1. History of a head injury	1. No history of head injury
2. Retrograde amnesia does not extend beyond a week into the past.	2. Retrograde amnesia extends indefinitely into the past
3. Amnesia disappears slowly and memory is not completely restored for events that occurred during the amnesic period	3. Client can recover suddenly with total restoration of memory

---

behaviors exhibited by a client with a dissociative disorder resemble organic conditions, including postconcussional amnesia and temporal lobe epilepsy. Tables 19–9 and 19–10 summarize the major differentiating points.

The nurse's observations of the character, duration, frequency, and context of the dissociative disorder contain crucial firsthand data. Physical examinations are not continued as part of the long-term intervention program, however, because they reinforce the symptoms and provide secondary gain. Therefore the completeness and accuracy of the initial physical assessment is of the utmost importance.

A psychosocial assessment is conducted to help discover the fundamental source of the anxiety as early as possible. Although many episodes of dissociation appear to

---

Table 19–10
Differentiation of Temporal Lobe Epilepsy and Dissociative Trances

Properties of Temporal Lobe Epilepsy	Properties of Dissociative Trances
1. Presence of positive electroencephalographic evidence of temporal lobe dysfunction	1. No such evidence
2. Usually does not occur in conjunction with other patterns	2. Often occurs with other behavior (stigmata, sleepwalking)

occur spontaneously, there may be a definite history of a specific, shocking emotional trauma or a situation charged with painful emotions and psychologic conflict. Family or friends may provide clues to the client's conflict and should be included in the psychosocial data gathering.

Nursing Diagnosis

A comparison between PND-1 and NANDA diagnoses for clients with dissociative disorder is given in Table 19–11. The following sections discuss their implications for the client and the nurse.

Clients with dissociative disorder may experience sudden memory loss, disorientation, loss of personal identity, and alteration in state of consciousness. Clients with psychogenic amnesia have partial or total inability to recall or identify past experiences. In a client with depersonalization disorder, feelings of unreality and estrangement can be severe and painful. These can affect the client's perception of the physical and psychologic self and of the world around him or her. Parts of the body or the entire body may seem foreign. Dizziness, anxiety, and distortion of time and space are common.

Role Impairment

Unexplained disappearances, absences from work, unreliability, and unpredictability are common manifestations of

Table 19–11
Comparison of DSM-IIIR and Psychiatric Nursing Diagnoses (Dissociative Disorders)

DSM-IIIR Diagnosis		PND-I Diagnoses		NANDA Diagnoses
300.14	Multiple personality disorder	01.01	Altered motor behavior	Anxiety
300.13	Psychogenic fugue	01.04	Altered sleep/arousal patterns*	Communication, impaired: verbal
300.12	Psychogenic amnesia	02.03.03	Knowledge deficit*	Coping, ineffective individual
300.60	Depersonalization disorder	02.05.01	Amnesia	Family process, alteration in
300.15	Dissociative disorder NOS	02.05.03	Long-term memory loss	Fear
		02.05.04	Short-term memory loss	Hopelessness
		02.06.01	Confusion	Knowledge deficit
		04.02	Altered feeling patterns	Parenting, alteration in
		05.01	Altered communication processes*	Post-trauma response
				Powerlessness
		05.03	Altered role performance*	Self-concept, disturbance in role performance
		05.05	Altered social interaction*	
		06.03.03	Altered personal identity*	Self-concept, disturbance in personal identity
		06.03.05	Altered social identity	
		06.04	Altered sensory perception*	Sensory/perceptual alterations
		07.05.01	Altered levels of consciousness	Sleep pattern disturbance
		08.01.01	Hopelessness*	Social interaction, impaired
		08.01.02	Helplessness	Social isolation
		08.01.03	Loneliness	Spiritual distress
		08.01.04	Powerlessness*	
		08.02.01	Spiritual distress*	

*PND-I diagnosis also in NANDA list.

dissociative disorders. Of course, the social or occupational functioning of the client is adversely affected.

Symptoms of depersonalization lead to limited or superficial involvement with others and to withdrawal or disengagement in past work or social pursuits. As expected, relationships become highly complicated and disorganized when a client has multiple personalities.

Alteration in Conduct and Impulse Control

In addition to amnesia, a fugue state may occur in clients with dissociative disorders. In this state, clients defend against perceived danger by active flight. They may wander away from home. Days, weeks, or sometimes even years later they may suddenly find themselves in a strange place, not knowing how they got there and with complete amnesia for the period of the fugue. Along with this unpredictable behavior they may adopt a new identity and life pattern.

Planning and Implementing Interventions

In choosing intervention strategies for clients with dissociative disorders, the treatment team must decide whether to alleviate the troublesome symptom or reintegrate the anxiety-producing conflict. Some teams emphasize the disruptions in day-to-day functioning occasioned by dissociative disorders. These include unexplained disappearances, absences from work, unreliability, and unpredictability. The dread associated with them justifies intervention strategies designed to change the disruptive behavior pattern. Others believe that new problems are created by removing the so-called symptoms without considering how they help the client control internal anxiety and maintain some balance in external social life.

Nurses should keep in mind that although clients may complain about the difficulties associated with their symptoms, the symptoms often form the basis of relationships with other significant people in their lives. These clients' roles in social groups are likewise built around their coping styles. If we remove these coping styles, we must offer clients more effective and satisfying ways to handle anxiety and to be supported in their social network. Such a learning task usually requires long-term psychotherapy. However, we can alleviate symptoms using strategies of behavior modification.

Promoting Improved Perception and Cognition

Strategies for identifying the source of anxiety that underlies the perceptive and cognitive impairments in clients with dissociative disorders include those for recovering unconscious content, such as free association or dream

description. At times more active strategies are used. These may include projective psychometric tests (Rorschach, Thematic Apperception Test), and hypnosis, with or without intravenous administration of sodium thiopental (Pentothal). These techniques are more likely to be employed by psychoanalysts or clinical psychologists.

Supportive insight therapy may be used with the goal of surfacing and integrating traumatic experiences and learning new ways of coping with future anxiety. This is especially relevant for those clients in whom the dissociative phenomena arise primarily against a background of intrapsychic or subjective conflict.

Promoting Effective Role Performance

Inclusion of family members in a therapeutic family counseling relationship may be indicated to help them learn new ways of dealing with the client. As stated earlier, considerable secondary gain is often associated with dissociative behavior: The client can use the illness to escape responsibility and get special treatment. Families may need support in learning to avoid reinforcing dissociative behavior by acting as the source of secondary gain.

Environmental manipulation may be an indicated intervention. For example, it may be necessary to assist the client in problem solving with the goal of minimizing other stressful aspects of the environment. In learning to confront and become desensitized to the underlying conflict, the client will experience some anxiety and discomfort. This anxiety must be kept within manageable limits. Therefore, more obvious and alterable sources of stress and anxiety should be minimized.

Promoting Improved Conduct and Impulse Control

The nurse may use such measures as psychotherapy (if prepared as a clinical specialist), environmental manipulation, and behavior modification to help the client with a dissociative disorder cope more effectively with impairments of conduct and impulse, e.g., unpredictable and bizarre behavior. Treatment may prove to be long term and progress may be slow. The establishment of a supportive therapeutic alliance between the client and the nurse and the family and the nurse is crucial. The nurse helps the family and client to understand the periodic occurrence of symptoms and guides them in supporting improved behaviors.

Evaluation

Perception and Cognition

Clients will no longer experience sudden memory loss, disorientation, loss of identity, or alteration in state of consciousness, or they will experience it less frequently. They will be able to correctly recall and identify past experiences.

Role Performance

Clients will experience increased satisfaction with family and work relationships. Involvement with others will occur more often and will be more fulfilling. They will experience increased success at work or school. They will be able to attend work or school regularly, without unexplained absences due to dissociative episodes.

Conduct and Impulse Control

Clients will no longer exhibit bizarre or unpredictable behaviors, or they will experience them less frequently. For example, incidents of being missing from home without explanation will occur less frequently or not at all.

Chapter Highlights

- The theoretical frameworks of major importance in the study of anxiety disorders, somatoform disorders, and dissociative disorders include the psychologic, behavioral, and biologic.

- Anxiety disorders, somatoform disorders, and dissociative disorders may be considered disturbed coping patterns and are characterized by loss of freedom to make choices, presence of conflict, repetition despite ineffectiveness, feelings of distress or pain, and the potential for secondary gain.

- In anxiety disorders, anxiety is either the predominant disturbance or is experienced when the individual attempts to master the symptoms.

- Clients with anxiety disorder experience anxiety both as a subjective emotion and as a variety of physical symptoms resulting from muscular tension and autonomic nervous system activity.

- Somatoform disorders are characterized by physical symptoms for which there is no positive evidence of an organic or physiologic basis.

- Dissociative disorders encompass a large group of uncommon and sometimes bizarre conditions in which there is sudden, temporary change in consciousness, identity, or motor behavior so that some part of these functions is lost.

- Nursing assessment to determine the extent of disability in anxiety disorders, somatoform disorders, or dissociative disorders includes, but is not limited to, assessment of subjective emotional experience, presence of physiologic symptoms, alteration in conduct and impulse control, impairment in role performance, and alteration in perception and cognition.

- Nursing diagnoses for clients with these disorders concern: impairment in emotional experience, e.g., feelings of distress, fear, anger, or anxiety; alteration in sleep, elimination, circulation, and motor behavior; inappropriate use of or abuse of medication; impaired communication; lack of knowledge about the disorder and its treatment; and distorted perception of the environment.

- Nursing interventions for clients with anxiety disorders, somatoform disorders, and dissociative disorders and their families are integrative and may include the range of psychotherapeutic interventions including providing psychotherapy, increasing social supports, reducing environmental stress, advocating the use of stress reduction strategies, and administering psychopharmacologic treatment.

- Nursing evaluation for clients with anxiety disorders, somatoform disorders, or dissociative disorders should include assessment of physical and psychologic symptoms, the client's subjective report of emotional feelings, the clients ability to understand and practice anxiety-reducing skills, demonstration of increase in cognitive capacities, and freedom from restriction in life-style.

References

American Psychiatric Association: *Diagnostic and Statistical Manual of Mental Disorders,* ed 3. APA, 1980.

American Psychiatric Association: *Diagnostic and Statistical Manual of Mental Disorders,* ed. 3, revised. APA, 1987.

Anderson DJ, Noyes R, Crowe, RR: A comparison of panic disorder and generalized anxiety disorder. *Am J Psychiatry* 1984;141:572.

Andreasen NC: Posttraumatic stress disorder, in Kaplan HI, Sadock BJ: *Comprehensive Textbook of Psychiatry/IV.* ed 4. Williams & Wilkins, 1985, pp 918–924.

Auden, WH: *The Age of Anxiety.* Random House, 1947.

Beck A, Emery G: *Anxiety Disorders and Phobias: A Cognitive Perspective.* Basic Books, 1985.

Braun BG: *The Treatment of Multiple Personality Disorder.* American Psychiatric Press, 1986.

Breier A, et al: Agoraphobia with panic attacks. *Arch Gen Psychiatry* 1986;43(11):1029–1036.

Breuer J, Freud S: *Studies in Hysteria.* Avon Books, 1966.

Burris BT: *Symposium on PTSD.* New York: American Psychiatric Association Convention, 1983.

Cameron O, Hudson C: Influence of exercise on anxiety levels in patients with anxiety disorders. *Psychosom* 1986;27(10):720–722.

Cameron OG: The differential diagnosis of anxiety. *Psychiatr Clin North Am* 1985;8(1):3–23.

DaCosta JM: On irritable heart: A clinical study of a form of functional cardiac disorder and its consequences. *Am J Med Sci* 1871;61:17.

Davis J: Treatment of a medical phobia including desensitization administered by a significant other. *J Psychosoc Nurs* 1982;20(8):6–11.

Ettedgrie E, Bridges M: Posttraumatic stress disorder. Symposium on Anxiety Disorders. *Psychiatr Clin North Am* 1985;8(1):89–103.

Farrington A: Obsessive-compulsive disorder. *Nurs Mirror* August 17, 1983; pp vii–viii.

Freud S: *The Problem of Anxiety*. Norton, 1936.

Goodwin DW, Guze SB: *Psychiatric Diagnosis*. Oxford University Press, 1984.

Hallowell AI: The social function of anxiety in a primitive society. *Am Sociol Rev* 1941;7:869–881.

Insel T, Akiskal H: Obsessive-compulsive disorder with psychotic features: A phenomenological analysis. *Am J Psychiatry* 1986;143(12):1527–1533.

Klein DF: Anxiety reconceptualized. *Compr Psychiatry* 1980;21:411.

Konikow N: Hysterical seizures or pseudoseizures? *J. Neurosurg Nurs* 1983;15(1):22–26.

Lim D: Behind closed doors. *Nurs Mirror* April 21, 1982;50–51.

Marks IM: *Cure and Care of Neurosis*. John Wiley and Sons, 1981.

Marks IM: Behavioral psychotherapy for anxiety disorders. *Psychiatr Clin North Am* 1985;8(1):25–35.

Mavissakalian M, Barlow DH: Phobia: An overview, in Mavissakalian M, Barlow DH (eds): *Phobia: Psychological and Pharmacological Treatment*. Guilford Press, 1981.

Nemiah JC: Anxiety states (anxiety neurosis), in Kaplan HI, Sadock BJ: *Comprehensive Textbook of Psychiatry/IV*. ed 4. Williams & Wilkins, 1985, pp 883–894.

Nemiah JC: Dissociative disorders (hysterical neurosis, dissociative type). In Kaplan HI, Sadock BJ: *Comprehensive Textbook of Psychiatry/IV*. ed 4. Williams & Wilkins, 1985, pp 942–957.

Nemiah JC: Obsessive-compulsive disorder (obsessive-compulsive neurosis), in Kaplan HI, Sadock BJ: *Comprehensive Textbook of Psychiatry/IV*. ed 4. Williams & Wilkins, 1985, pp 904–917.

Nemiah JC: Phobic disorders (phobic neuroses), in Kaplan HI, Sadock BJ: *Comprehensive Textbook of Psychiatry/IV*. ed 4. Williams & Wilkins, 1985, pp 894–904.

Nemiah JC: Somatoform disorders, in Kaplan HI, Sadock BJ: *Comprehensive Textbook of Psychiatry/IV*. ed 4. Williams & Wilkins, 1985, pp 924–942.

Olson M: The out-of-body experience and other states of consciousness. *Arch Psychiatr Nurs* 1987;1(3):201–207.

Ost L, Hugdahl K: Acquisition of phobias and anxiety response patterns in clinical patients. *Behav Res Ther* 1981;19:439.

Pasnau RO: *Diagnosis and Treatment of Anxiety Disorders*. American Psychiatric Press, 1984.

Peplau, H: Interpersonal techniques: The crux of nursing. *Am J Nurs* 1962;62.

Rank O: *The Trauma of Birth*. Robert Brunner, 1952.

Rogers B, Nickolaus J: Vietnam nurses. *J Psychosoc Nurs* 1987;25(4):11–15.

Schaffer D: Recognizing multiple personality patients. *Am J Psychotherapy* 1986;40(4):500–510.

Schuckit M: Anxiety treatment progress. *The Psychiatric Times* (June) 1985;3.

Schwartz G, et al: Anxiety disorders and psychiatric referral in the general medical emergency room. *Gen Hosp Psychiatry* 1987;9(2)87–93.

Scrignar CB: *Post-Traumatic Stress Disorder: Diagnosis, Treatment, and Legal Issues*. Praeger Publisher, 1984.

Sheehan DV: Monoamine oxidase inhibitors and alprazolam in the treatment of panic disorder and agoraphobia. Symposium on Anxiety Disorders. *Psychiatr Clin North Am* 1985;8(1).

Sonneberg SM, Blank AS Jr, Talbott JA: *The Trauma of War: Stress and Recovery in Viet Nam Veterans*. American Psychiatric Press, 1985.

Spitzer RL, Williams JBW: Diagnostic issues in the DSM-III classification of the anxiety disorders, in Grinspoon L (ed): *Psychiatric Update*. American Psychiatric Press, 1984, pp 23–26.

Stein M: Panic disorder and medical illness. *Psychosom* 1986;27(12):833–838.

Stinnett J: The functional somatic symptom. *Psychiatr Clin North Am* 1987;10(1):19–33.

Stoudemire A, Sandhu J: Psychogenic/idiopathic pain syndromes. *Gen Hosp Psychiatry* 1987;9(2):79–85.

Sullivan HS: *The Interpersonal Theory of Psychiatry*. W.W. Norton, 1953.

Swonger A, Constantine L: *Drugs and Therapy: A Handbook of Psychotropic Drugs*, ed 2. Little, Brown, 1983.

Tearnan B, Telch M: Phobic disorders, in Adams H, Sutker P (eds): *Comprehensive Handbook of Psychopathology*. Plenum Press, 1984, Chapter 7.

TWENTY

Applying the Nursing Process for
Clients with Gender and Sexual Disorders

Deborah Frank

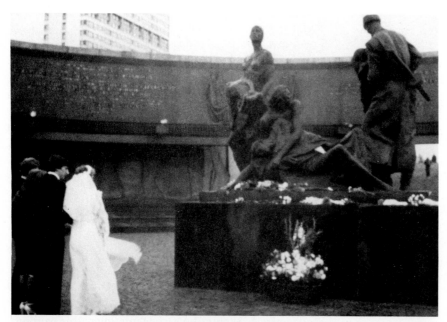

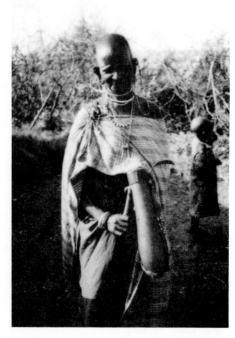

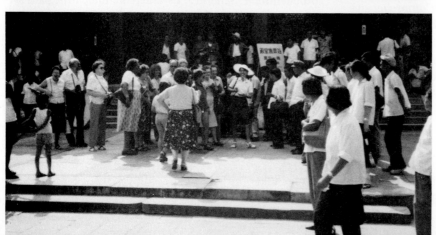

Learning Objectives

After reading this chapter, students should be able to

- Identify their own values and beliefs related to variations of sexual expression

- Apply theories of sexuality when providing nursing care with clients to promote, maintain, or regain sexual health

- Describe etiologies of various gender and sexual disorders

- Identify potential side-effects of selected prescription and nonprescription drugs that may affect sexual function

- Assess clients' sexual health status

- Elicit a detailed sexual history in which clients express specific sexual concerns

- Formulate nursing diagnoses for clients expressing sexual concerns or having potential for sexual health problems

- Identify principles common to most treatment plans for gender and sexual disorders

- Apply a nursing model for intervening with clients to promote sexual health

- Describe the nurse's role in providing interventions for clients who are experiencing gender or sexual concerns

- Evaluate nursing interventions to promote sexual health with the purpose of making referrals, when needed, to a qualified sex counselor or therapist

Cross References

Other topics related to this content are: AIDS and high-risk sexual behaviors, Chapter 26; Developmental aspects of sexuality throughout the life cycle, Chapter 6; Incest, and rape and rape counseling, Chapter 25, Part II.

Consider your own personal vision.

Key Terms

bestiality
bisexuality
dyspareunia
ego-dystonic homosexuality
excitement phase
exhibitionism
female sexual arousal
    disorder
fetishism
frotteurism
gender identity
gender role
heterosexuality
homosexuality
hypoactive sexual desire
    disorder
inhibited female orgasm
inhibited male orgasm

lesbianism
libido
male erectile disorder
orgasm phase
paraphilia
pedophilia
plateau phase
premature ejaculation
resolution phase
sexual aversion disorder
sexual desire
sexual masochism
sexual sadism
transsexualism
transvestic fetishism
vaginismus
voyeurism
zoophilia

All humans are sexual beings. Regardless of gender, age, race, socioeconomic status, religious beliefs, physical and mental health, or other demographic factors, human beings express their sexuality in a variety of ways throughout their lives.

Human sexuality is difficult to define. "Maleness, femaleness, sensuality, sense of self, ego, perception of self in relationship to the world and others, the quality or state of being sexual, the condition of having sexual activity or intercourse, the expression or receiving and expressing sexual interest are all connotative of human sexuality" (Monat 1982, p 1). Sexuality is an individually expressed and highly personal phenomenon whose meaning evolves from objective and subjective experiences. Physiologic, psychosocial, and cultural factors influence a person's sexuality and lead to the wide range of attitudes and behaviors seen in humans. There are no normal, universal sexual behaviors. Satisfying or "normal" sexual expression can best be described as whatever behaviors give pleasure and satisfaction to those involved without threat of coercion or threat of injury to others.

Sexual health is an individual and constantly changing phenomenon falling within the wide range of normal healthy expressions of human sexual thoughts, feelings, needs, and desires. The World Health Organization (WHO) defines sexual health as the "integration of the somatic, emotional, intellectual, and social aspects of sexual being, in ways that are positively enriching and that enhance personality, communication and love" (WHO 1975). An individual's degree

Kevin Huchshorn is acknowledged for her contributions in the preparation of this chapter.

of sexual health is best determined by that individual, sometimes with the assistance of a qualified professional. It is helpful for some to view sexual health on the wellness-illness continuum, which allows for changing biopsycho-sociocultural factors and varied sexual attitudes, values, and needs.

NURSING AND SEXUAL HEALTH CARE

Sexual health care is a relatively new area of involvement for psychiatric nurses. Until recently, sexuality has not been viewed as falling within the scope of treatment. Currently, sexuality is increasingly recognized as an important component of a holistic approach to humans and their overall health status. Nursing is a legitimate and appropriate discipline to provide sexual health care. The close and often extended relationships that psychiatric nurses have with clients and families foster the rapport necessary to discuss this private area of clients' health status.

Nursing roles in the area of human sexuality are evolving gradually. The prerequisites for psychiatric nurses involved in nursing activities related to human sexual functioning include:

1. Having concrete and comprehensive knowledge about sexual function and dysfunction

2. Having skill in communication techniques

3. Being comfortable with their own sexual values and expressions

4. Being willing and able to explore and separate personal values and attitudes from those of clients

5. Becoming proficient in using the nursing process to assess, diagnose, intervene, and evaluate care to promote optimal sexual health.

Unfortunately, human sexuality is a subject historically characterized by myth and controversy. This history has hindered both the delivering and receiving of services that promote sexual health and well-being. Although scientific knowledge has expanded immensely in the past decade, modern Americans continue to view sex and sexuality with discomfort. Our confusion is complicated by our traditional religious and social values. Nurses may hold some of these negative attitudes and biases. Psychiatric nurses must confront these negative, inappropriate, or stereotypic ideas and opinions before they can meet professional standards of care in helping clients attain optimal sexual health.

Basic to nursing is the notion that the nurse's personal beliefs should not influence the quality of care given a client. It is easier for nurses to live up to this standard if they engage in values clarification before providing sexual health care. One way for nurses to clarify their values is to respond to a sentence completion exercise about sexuality such as the following. Nurses complete the statements with their own beliefs and then may choose to discuss their responses with peers.

> The practice of masturbation is . . .
>
> When I think about homsexuality I feel . . .
>
> I feel premarital sexual relations are . . .
>
> I think abortions are . . .
>
> When I think of oral sex I feel . . .
>
> If I see nude pictures or explicit sex acts I feel . . .
>
> My attitude about love and sex is . . .
>
> I feel extramarital affairs are . . .
>
> The sex acts I believe are wrong or abnormal are . . .
>
> If a client of the same sex talks about sex with me I feel . . .
>
> If a client of the opposite sex talks about sex with me I feel . . .

Giving nonjudgmental nursing care does not mean that the nurse has to agree with others' beliefs and values about sexuality. However, self-awareness can help psychiatric nurses respect their clients' sexual rights and needs.

HISTORICAL AND THEORETICAL FOUNDATIONS

Human sexual behavior has been studied from various theoretical perspectives. The most significant of these include the (a) historical, (b) psychoanalytic, (c) behavioral, (d) actuarial, (e) sociologic, (f) cultural, and (g) biologic approaches.

Historical Foundation

One takes a historical approach by examining past sexual behaviors and identifying patterns and influences that have led to present behaviors. In Western society sexual practices have been strongly influenced by Christianity, which traditionally associated sexual activity closely with reproduction. Certain Christian doctrines also equated sex with evil and chastity or celibacy with good. During the Middle Ages and long after, women were thought to be virginal, pure, and "untainted" by physical desires. Prostitution flourished and was generally condoned by society to protect "honest" women from man's "baser" nature. This view of sexual behavior has remained a significant factor over centuries.

The discovery of effective safe contraception and the women's rights movement, which challenged the traditional view of women as passive, nonsexual creatures, are relatively recent events. The sexual revolution that was spurred by the work of Masters and Johnson allowed men and women greater freedom to talk about their sexual experiences and feelings. Women, especially, began to redefine their sexuality. Thus, in less than a generation, society has been forced to adapt to new sexual values and beliefs. This adjustment has resulted in understandable controversy between church and state, men and women, and parents and children. Today, many clients are concerned about their sexuality because of conflicting cultural, religious, and personal values.

Psychoanalytic Foundation

Sigmund Freud is the originator of the theoretical perspective that identifies sexuality as the most important factor in the development of the human personality. Freud believed that most psychologic problems and dysfunctions evolve from conscious and unconscious sexual issues, mainly sexual frustrations. This theory made significant contributions to the understanding of human sexuality. Among Freudian concepts are (a) children are sexual beings; (b) attraction to the parent of the opposite sex is a normal part of growth and development; (c) all individuals experience sexual desire on conscious and unconscious levels; (d) sexual desires influence behavior, and (e) human sexuality encompasses more than physical arousal and responses (Geer et al. 1984).

Behavioral Approach

Behaviorists focus on the influence of past experiences on present behaviors. The emphasis is on actual behaviors that can be observed and recorded—what people say and do in the context of actual sexual situations. In this view, individuals learn how to behave sexually from life experiences, e.g., parent and peer interactions, education, media influences, and other methods of learning. This approach is especially helpful in understanding sociocultural, ethnic, and gender similarities in sexual behavior while allowing for individual differences. No one is assumed to have had precisely the same life experiences.

Actuarial Approach

In the actuarial approach, human sexuality is classified according to demographic data. Statistics are generated from surveys and interviews designed to identify the correlation between type and frequency of sexual behavior and

such demographic variables as age, gender, marital or other types of relationships, religious activities, social class, and educational level. In this approach, little attention is paid to extremes of behaviors, and individual differences are not stressed. It is used for descriptive reports that do not attempt to interpret or predict behavior.

Sociologic Foundation

These theories describe human sexuality in terms of the social conditioning that directly influences a person's behavior. For example, contemporary sexual practices can be linked to affluence, which permits greater flexibility in gender roles. "Social movements . . . have sexual effects, . . . the women's movement, the youth movement . . . and gay liberation [have affected] sexual expression. [Other influences on sexual behaviors are] the trend toward deemphasis on gender differences demonstrated in dress, education, and occupational roles and the increasing sexual explicitness of the American media as evidenced in magazines, television, and movies . . ." (Geer et al. 1984).

Cultural Approach

In this view, widely divergent patterns in sexual behaviors and meanings appear to be culture specific. For example, the Western practice of lip kissing varies tremendously in frequency and meaning across cultural boundaries. Findings of cultural differences strongly challenge stereotypic beliefs about the basic nature of men and women. Recognition of cultural variety promotes tolerance and understanding of individual differences in sexual behavior. This perspective can be especially useful for nurses working with clients of various cultures.

Biologic Foundation

Those who take a biologic approach are concerned with physiologic aspects of human sexual response: biochemical, genetic, hormonal, vascular, neuromuscular, and anatomic factors. The sexual response cycle, from arousal to resolution, is of major importance here. Psychosocial and cultural variables are considered in relation to their effect on physical sexual response. The following section details this approach.

Sexual response is a culmination of physical and emotional stimulation that is interpreted as pleasurable and sexually arousing. Healthy individuals of all ages are capable of sexual response. For instance, infant boys may respond to physical stimulation with erections, and couples in their eighties have sexual intercourse. Further, when asleep, males and females experience erections or lubricate every eighty to ninety minutes and may also experience nocturnal orgasm.

The nurse needs knowledge about anatomy and physiology of the body during sexual arousal and the factors that may influence one's response. This knowledge helps the nurse clarify any misconceptions, myths, or questions clients may have about their sexual function. Figure 20–1 depicts female and male sexual anatomy. Table 20–1 summarizes sexual anatomy.

Masters and Johnson (1966) and Helen Singer Kaplan (1979) have suggested models describing phases of sexual response. The contribution of Masters and Johnson to the understanding of human sexual response is considered a milestone in the field of sexual research. They were the first to describe, under direct laboratory observation, physiologic sexual response patterns. They recorded the responses

of 382 women and 312 men in more than 10,000 sexual experiences and identified a four-phase response of excitement, plateau, orgasm, and resolution. See Figure 20–2. Kaplan brought an integrated psychodynamic/physiologic viewpoint to her conceptualization of a three-stage model of sexual response. Her model includes a desire phase (prior to excitement), excitement, and orgasm. This is depicted in Figure 20–3.

The two major physiologic changes occurring in sexual response are increased *neuromuscular tension* (myotonia) and *increased vasocongestion*. These changes occur in response to sensory stimulation of the autonomic nervous system (ANS). Both parasympathetic and sympathetic branches of the ANS influence sexual organ responses. For instance, erection and lubrication are thought to be under parasympathetic control, whereas ejaculation is under sympathetic control. The brain is often considered the most important sexual organ as it interprets physiologic as well as psychologic stimuli as arousing. It has been suggested that sexual centers within the limbic system in the brain allow the stimulation received through the ANS to be identified as pleasurable. These centers can also enhance or diminish the spinal reflex centers in the lower spinal cord that produce reflex erection or lubrication. Thus, a male might lose a reflex erection produced by a tactile stimu-

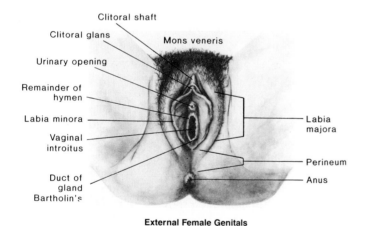

External Female Genitals

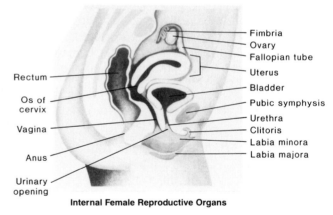

Internal Female Reproductive Organs

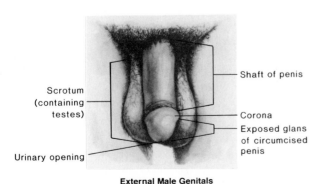

External Male Genitals

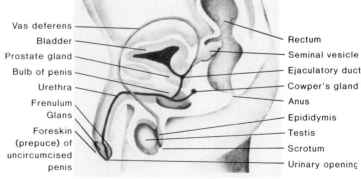

Internal Male Reproductive Organs

Figure 20–1
Female and male sexual and reproductive anatomy.

Table 20–1 Summary of Sexual Anatomy	
Structures	**Comments**
Female mons and labia	These are fatty tissues. The mons lies over the pubic bone and is sensitive to pressure. The labia surround the vaginal opening.
Clitoris	Sole function is to receive and transmit sexual stimuli. It is .25 to 1 inch long. It has a high density of nerve endings and is highly sensitive to touch.
Vagina	The vaginal opening is sensitive to stretch. The vaginal barrel contains fewer nerve endings, most of which are in the outer one-third.
Uterus	A pear-shaped hollow muscle organ that contracts during orgasm.
Penis	Has three cylinders of spongy tissue, two corpora cavernosa, and one corpus spongiosum. The head or glans of the penis is highly sensitive to touch. Circumcision does not appear to affect sensitivity of the glans. The average penis is 3–4 inches long and increases to 6.25 inches when erect. There is little difference in the size of the erect penis among males.
Scrotum	Sac of skin under the penis that contains the testes.
Sperm	Made in the testes and are mixed with seminal fluid to yield ejaculate.
Breasts	Female breasts are considered erotic in our society. Nipple sensitivity is present in both men and women.
Other body parts— mouth, anus, buttocks, skin	Other body parts are sources of arousal and considered erotic during sexual activity.

lation if his emotional interpretation from the higher centers in the brain is negative (e.g., fear or anxiety).

Among the physical influences underlying sexual response is the role of sex hormones. Androgen (testosterone) is necessary for male sexual desire and for ejaculation. Also, ovarian hormones (estrogen and progesterone) in the female influence sexual activity and response levels. However, the nature of this influence is less clear than the influence of testosterone on males. Thus, the specific facilitating or inhibiting roles of sex hormones remain open to controversy, because it is difficult to separate the role of hormones from the influence of learned sexual behavior.

Phases of Sexual Response

The phases of sexual response presented here are an adaptation of both the Masters and Johnson and Kaplan models. These stages include desire, excitement, plateau, orgasm, and resolution. Tables 20–2 and 20–3 summarize the physiology of female and male sexual response. It should be noted that the sexual response cycle is similar regardless of how one is stimulated. For example, both physical and psychologic stimulation exhibit the same phases of sexual response, although the intensity, length, and subjective

pleasure associated with each phase may differ. Likewise, sexual response is similar in both men and women and heterosexuals and homosexuals.

Desire Phase

Sexual desire, or **libido**, is the drive to seek out or be receptive to sexual activity or interaction (Kaplan 1979). This arousal is triggered by physical, psychologic, and environmental factors. For instance, the person who is being physically touched may feel increased desire and encourage further caressing. Thinking about sexually arousing fantasies can be a source of psychologic arousal. Being in a setting that is perceived as arousing, e.g., having a romantic dinner, might also arouse sexual desire. Thus, the desire phase is initiated under a variety of circumstances from a variety of cues that are erotic to that individual. If the person experiences the desire as a positive feeling and the opportunity is available, he or she will likely be motivated to seek out continued sexual arousal.

Excitement Phase

The **excitement phase** is the body's initial response to sexual stimulation. The first sign of physiologic arousal in the

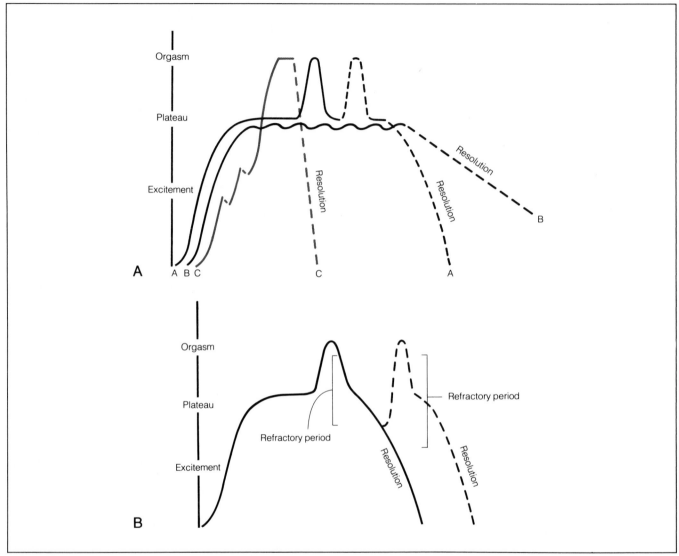

Figure 20–2

A, Female sexual response cycle. Masters and Johnson identified three basic patterns in female sexual response. Pattern A most closely resembles the male pattern, with the exception of the possibility of one or more orgasms without dropping below plateau level of sexual arousal. Variations may include an extended plateau with no orgasm (line B), or a rapid rise or orgasm (line C) with no definitive plateau and a very quick resolution. B, Male sexual response cycle. Only one male response pattern was identified by Masters and Johnson. However, men do report considerable variation in their response patterns. Note the refractory period: Males do not have a second orgasm immediately after the first.

Source: Masters WH, Johnson VE: Human Sexual Response. Little, Brown, 1966. Reprinted by permission of the Masters & Johnson Institute, St. Louis, MO.

female is lubrication, which begins almost immediately. Lubrication results from a process called transudation. As a result of vasocongestion, moisture seeps across the vaginal lining into the vaginal barrel. The woman may not realize she is lubricating until sexual arousal continues and the moisture increases. Lubrication does not necessarily mean a woman is emotionally or physically ready for sexual intercourse. Other changes that need to occur are the expansion of the inner two-thirds of the vagina with the pulling upward of the cervix and uterus so that the penis will not hit the cervix upon penetration and thrusting. The labia increase in size from vasocongestion, and the nipples become erect from increased muscle tension.

For males, erection is the first major sign of excitement. The penis is not muscle or bone but vascular, spongy tissue. Rapid vasocongestion of the erectile tissue causes

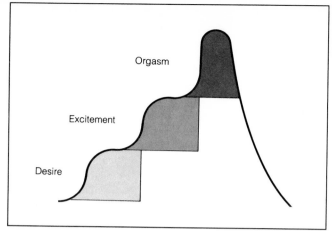

Figure 20-3
Kaplan's three-stage model of the sexual response cycle. This model is distinguished by its identification of desire as a prelude to sexual response.

Source: Figure based on HS Kaplan's Three-Stage Model of the Sexual Response Cycle. Disorders of Sexual Desire. Brunner/Mazel, 1979. Reprinted with permission.

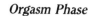
the penis to become erect. At the same time, the blood flow out of the penis is partially blocked so that the erection is maintained. Thus, the firmness of the erection varies as blood flows in and out of the penis. This variation in the erection is more noticeable among older men and is a normal physiologic response. Men, too, experience increased muscle tension during excitement including nipple erection and sensitivity.

Plateau

With continued physical and emotional arousal, sexual tension builds in the **plateau phase.** Increasing vaginal vasocongestion forms an orgasmic platform. This tissue swelling narrows the vaginal opening so that it will grip the penis. The width or length of the penis is not critical for pleasure to be experienced during coitus because the vaginal opening accommodates any size. The clitoris also becomes engorged and very sensitive. It retracts under the clitoral hood but can be stimulated indirectly by movement of the clitoral hood or by touch of the mons area. Increase in breast size and the development of a "sex flush" (a measleslike rash) are also characteristic of this phase.

When males reach plateau, the head of the penis (the glans) grows larger. The testicles also enlarge from vasocongestion. The male may emit a small amount of a clear fluid thought to be from the Cowper's glands, which may contain sperm. If a man is using a condom for birth control, he needs to put it on during the early plateau phase before vaginal penetration to ensure effective contraception.

Both men and women experience increased muscle tension in this phase resulting in elevated blood pressure, pulse, and respirations as well as tension in the thighs, buttocks, and abdomen.

Orgasm Phase

The **orgasm phase** is marked by a reflex response of rhythmic contractions of the internal and external organs and pelvic muscles. These occur at intervals of eight tenths of a second. This reflex response is controlled by spinal nerve centers. Women may describe orgasm as a feeling of spreading pleasurable warmth, tingling, or throbbing. In the past, a distinction was made between clitoral and vaginal orgasms. Most sex researchers strongly believe that all orgasms produce the same physiologic response regardless of the method of stimulation. Subjective pleasure may be different, depending on which kind of stimulation—vaginal or clitoral—the woman prefers. However, the entire pelvic musculature, including the uterus and vagina, is involved in orgasm regardless of the stimulation that preceded it.

Men have a two-stage phase of orgasm—emission and ejaculation. During emission, reflex contractions of internal smooth muscles force semen into the urethra and close the sphincter to the bladder (to prevent retrograde ejaculation or a backward flow into the bladder). During the ejaculatory phase, muscular contractions propel the semen out of the urethra. These contractions are similar to those of female orgasm.

There have been reports that women ejaculate. This ejaculation was linked to stimulation of a particular area, the Graffenberg spot (or G-spot), which is thought to be analogous to the prostate gland. Although women report specific areas of vaginal sensitivity, there remains much controversy about female ejaculation and the G-spot because subsequent research has failed to replicate these findings (Geer et al. 1984).

For both men and women, increased muscle tension throughout the body during orgasm elevates blood pressure, pulse, and respiration rates. However, this increase in vital signs is present only for a few seconds. Thus, this elevation does not pose a problem for most clients with cardiac disease. Both men and women may also experience increased involuntary muscle contractions in other parts of the body, lessened voluntary muscle control, anal sphincter contraction, carpopedal spasm, and involuntary pelvic thrusting.

Resolution Phase

The **resolution phase** is the time when internal and external organs return to their preexcitation state. The time of onset appears to differ for men and women. Immediately after one orgasm, women have the physical capability to have further orgasms if continued interest and stimulation are present. Men do not have this ability. Rather, men experience a refractory period or recovery time during which

	Table 20–2 Physiology of Female Sexual Response	
Phase	**Body Part**	**Response**
Excitement	Vagina	Lubrication within ten to thirty seconds of effective stimulation. Barrel lengthens, inner two-thirds distends. Irregular expansive movements of walls late in phase; wall color changes to darker, purplish hue.
	Labia majora	Thin and flatten against perineum in nulliparous women; become markedly distended with blood in multiparous women.
	Labia minora	Expand markedly in diameter.
	Clitoris	Shaft increases in diameter through vasocongestion, elongates in some women (less rapidly than vaginal lubrication occurs; vaginal lubrication, not clitoral erection, is the "neurophysiologic parallel" to penile erection). Vasocongestion of glans varies from barely discernible to two-fold expansion of glans, depending on whether stimulation is direct or indirect and on individual variations in anatomy.
	Uterus	Pulled slowly up and back if initially in normal anterior position.
	Breasts	Nipple erection due to involuntary contracting of nipple muscle fibers. Vein patterns in breast extend and stand out. Actual breast size increases and areolae markedly engorge toward end of phase.
	Sex flush	In some women, a rash appears between the breastbone and navel late in this phase or early in the plateau phase.
	Myotonia	Initial total-body responses include increasing restlessness, irritability, and rapidity of voluntary and involuntary movement. *Myotonia* (muscular rigidity) increases in long muscles of arms and legs; abdominal muscles involuntarily tense; involuntary contractile rate of muscles between ribs increases, increasing respiratory rate.
	Other	Heart rate and blood pressure increase.
Plateau	Vagina	Marked vasocongestion further reduces central opening of the outer third by at least one-third. Base of vasocongestion encompassing outer third of vagina and engorged labia minora is called the *orgasmic platform,* which "provides the anatomic foundation for the vagina's physiological expression of the orgasmic experience" (Masters and Johnson 1966), and is regarded as a sign that plateau stage has been reached. Further increase in inner width and depth of vagina during this phase is negligible. Production of lubrication slows, especially if phase is prolonged.
	Labia majora	No further changes.
	Labia minora	Vivid color changes; nulliparous from pink to bright red; multiparous from bright red to deep wine. Orgasm invariably follows if stimulation continues once this "sex-skin" color change occurs.
	Clitoris	Retracts from normal position late in phase; withdraws; at least 50 percent overall reduction in length of total clitoral body by immediate preorgasmic period.
	Uterus	Full elevation is reached.
	Breasts	Markedly increased areolar engorgement. Unsuckled breast increases one-fifth to one-fourth over unstimulated size by end of phase; little or no increase in breast that has been suckled.
	Sex flush	Spreads over breasts in some women; may have widespread body distribution by late plateau stage on those affected.
	Myotonia	Overall increase. Involuntary facial contractions, grimaces, clutching movements; involuntary pelvic thrusts late in phase near orgasm.
	Other	Hyperventilation develops late in phase. Further increase in heart rate and blood pressure.

continued

Phase	Body Part	Response
Orgasm	Vagina	Strong, rhythmic contractions of orgasmic platform (three to fifteen), beginning at intervals of eight-tenths of a second and gradually diminishing in strength and duration; may be preceded by spastic contraction lasting two to four seconds. Inner vaginal area remains essentially expanded.
	Labia	No changes.
	Clitoris	Retracted and not observed.
	Uterus	Contracts irregularly.
	Breasts	No specific reaction.
	Sex flush	Peaks.
	Myotonia	Muscle spasms and involuntary contraction throughout the body. Loss of voluntary control.
	Other	Hyperventilation, heart rate, and blood pressure peak. Urinary meatus will occasionally slightly dilate, returning to usual state before orgasmic platform contractions have ceased. Rectal sphincter sometimes rhythmically contracts involuntarily.
Resolution	Vagina	Central opening of orgasmic platform rapidly increases in diameter by one-third. Cervix and upper walls of vagina descend toward vaginal floor in minimum of three to four minutes. Vaginal color returns to pre-excitement state, usually in about ten to fifteen minutes. Occasionally production of lubrication continues into resolution phase; suggests remaining or renewed sexual tension.
	Labia majora	Rapidly back to pre-excitement levels if orgasm; slowly if only plateau levels were reached.
	Labia minora	Sex-skin color returns to light pink within five to fifteen seconds after orgasm. Further color loss is rapid.
	Clitoris	Returned to pre-excitement position within five to fifteen seconds after cessation of orgasmic-platform contractions. Vasocongestion of glans and shaft usually disappears five to ten minutes after orgasm, ten to thirty minutes in some women; may take several hours if plateau phase but no orgasm.
	Uterus	Cervical os dilates early in phase; observable in nulliparous women.
	Breasts	Rapid detumescence of areolae. Nonsuckled breasts lose size increase in about five to ten minutes. Superficial vein patterns may last longer.
	Sex flush	Rapidly disappears from body sites in almost opposite sequence of apperance.
	Myotonia	Obvious muscle tension usually disappears within five minutes of orgasm. Overall myotonia resolves less rapidly than superficial or deep vasocongestion.
	Other	Heart rate and blood pressure return to normal. Hyperventilation ends early in stage. A sheen of perspiration appears over the bodies of some women.

Table 20–2 *(Continued)*
Physiology of Female Sexual Response

Source: De Lora JS, Warren CAB: Understanding Sexual Interaction. *Houghton Mifflin, 1977, pp 43–46; developed from Masters W, Johnson V:* Human Sexual Response. *Little, Brown, 1966. Reprinted by permission of the Masters & Johnson Institute, St. Louis, MO.*

they cannot have orgasm. The male may maintain some penile engorgement. He may then continue to stimulate his partner to orgasm. The length of the refractory period is influenced by a variety of factors, including age (increasing length as men get older) and personal or cultural expectations about frequency of sexual performance.

The entire resolution phase may last thirty minutes. If orgasm has occurred, the process takes less time. When orgasm is not experienced and there has been prolonged arousal, the person may feel a pelvic heaviness or fullness due to vasocongestion. Sometimes this person experiences nocturnal orgasm and thus completes the resolution phase.

Table 20–3 Physiology of Male Sexual Response		
Phase	**Body Part**	**Response**
Excitement	Penis	First physiologic response to effective stimulation is erection, within three to eight seconds; erection may wax and wane throughout excitement phase.
	Scrotal sac	Decreases in internal diameter; outer skin tenses and thickens; dartos-layer muscle fibers contract. Localized vasocongestion.
	Testes	Elevate toward perineum; if phase is prolonged, may redescend and reelevate several times. Spermatic cord shortens.
	Breasts	Nipple erection and tumescence develop in some men late in phase; remain throughout rest of sex cycle.
	Sex flush	Sometimes appears late in phase. Occurs or fails to occur with wide variation in same individual and between individuals.
	Myotonia	Observed late in phase. Similar to female pattern. Both voluntary muscle tension and some involuntary.
	Other	Heart rate, blood pressure, and respiration increase as sexual tension increases. Rectal sphincter contracts irregularly after direct stimulation.
Plateau	Penis	Increase in coronal area of glans due to increased vasocongestion. Glans deepens in color in some men.
	Scrotum	No further reactions.
	Testes	Continue to increase in size until about 50 percent larger than in unstimulated state. Further elevate until in pre-ejaculatory position against perineum.
	Sex flush	First appears late in plateau more frequently than in excitement phase. Indicates high levels of sexual tension.
	Myotonia	Voluntary and involuntary tensions increase. Pelvic thrusting becomes involuntary late in phase. Total body reactions of male and female quite similar.
	Other	Further increases in heart rate and blood pressure. Hyperventilation appears late in phase.
Orgasmic (Ejaculatory)	Penis	Ejaculatory contractions along entire length of penile urethra. Expulsive contractions start at intervals of eight-tenths of a second and after three or four reduce in frequency and expulsive force. Final contractions are several seconds apart.
	Scrotum	No specific reactions.
	Testes	No reactions observed.
	Myotonia	Loss of voluntary control. Involuntary contractions and spasms.
	Other	Heart rate, blood pressure, and hyperventilation peak. Degree of sexual tension is frequently indicated by intensity and duration of hyperventilation. Involuntary contractions of rectal sphincter.
Resolution	Penis	Two stages: Rapid reduction in size to about 50 percent larger than in unstimulated state; less rapid if excitement or plateau stages have been intentionally prolonged. Slower disappearance of remaining tumescence, especially if sexual stimulation continues to take place.
	Scrotum	One of two patterns: Rapid decongestion, or decongestion occurring over one or two hours. Typically, but not true of everyone, individuals consistently follow one pattern or the other. In general, within the individual pattern, the more prior stimulation has occurred, the longer the resolution process.
	Testes	Rapid or slow resolution relative to scrotal pattern.
	Breasts	Loss of nipple erection if present; may occur slowly.

continued

Table 20–3 (Continued) Physiology of Male Sexual Response		
Phase	Body Part	Response
	Sex flush	Disappears rapidly in reverse order of appearance.
	Myotonia	As in female, rarely lasts more than five minutes, but not lost as rapidly as many of the signs of vasocongestion.
	Other	Heart rate and blood pressure return to normal. Perspiration sometimes appears on soles of feet and palms of hands. Hyperventilation resolves during refractory period. Ejaculation cannot again occur until this refractory period has passed.

Source: De Lora JS, Warren CAB: Understanding Sexual Interaction. *Houghton Mifflin, 1977, pp 46–48; developed from Masters W, Johnson V:* Human Sexual Response. *Little, Brown, 1966. Reprinted by permission of the Masters & Johnson Institute, St. Louis, MO.*

Other Considerations

The length, intensity, and duration of the phases of sexual response vary among persons and from one sexual episode to the next. One may not always experience each phase from desire to resolution. Not all men or women experience orgasm or ejaculation each time they engage in sexual activity. For instance, variations in levels of women's sexual needs and responses are now acknowledged as valid individual patterns. Women need not respond the same way each time they have sex to feel fully satisfied. (Bernhard and Dan 1986). Further, men may experience erection and gain pleasure from caressing without ejaculation. Helping clients identify their own sexual desires and needs frees them from imposed notions of how often they should have sex and how many orgasms constitute satisfaction.

Sexual Response and Aging

Nurses often do not see the aging individual as needing sexual expression or activity. The vast majority of persons have the capacity to respond sexually throughout life. In older people, the body responds more slowly and sometimes less intensely during each phase, but satisfaction is still experienced. For example, a 70-year-old woman may have less lubrication than she did when she was 20, and an elderly male may not get an erection as quickly as he did when he was 20. However, both can still experience the total sexual response. The major predictors of satisfying sexual activity in later years are good health, an interest in experiencing sexual pleasure, and a history of regular sexual activity. The lack of a partner or chronic illness can be reasons for a change in the sexual activity of the elderly. The nurse should be aware that elderly clients may have questions about sexuality and should not assume sexual concerns are irrelevant to this group.

Sexual Response and Reproduction/ Contraception

Pregnancy/Fertility/Infertility

For couples desiring a child, the major purpose of sexual activity may be to conceive. Timing sexual intercourse to coincide with ovulation and achieving ejaculation may become more important than experiencing enjoyment during the phases of sexual response. The pair may take a mechanical, objective approach to their sexual activity during this time. This approach can inhibit the emotional component of sexual response and in turn the physiologic response. Of course, desire for a child does not prevent enjoyment of the sexual interaction.

Some partners may not conceive even after numerous attempts over a long time. This lack of success can influence sexual response negatively, especially for clients undergoing infertility treatment. In a comprehensive review of the literature on this topic, Frank (1984) notes that people being treated for infertility may experience a lack of desire, difficulty in becoming excited (lubricating or getting an erection), and difficulty ejaculating or having orgasm. These problems seem to stem from low self-esteem, frustration, pressure to perform sexually at a particular time, and fear of not being able to achieve ejaculation and conception. Such feelings interfere with the couple's ability to interpret sexual stimuli as arousing, making it difficult for the naturally occurring physical response to build sufficiently for them to complete the sexual response cycle. Nurses providing health care to clients who are trying to conceive need to assess the effects on sexual activity.

The pregnant female experiences much variation in sexual response. Physical and emotional changes resulting from pregnancy can inhibit or intensify desire and sexual activity. Generally, couples may experience lessened interest or activity during the first and third trimesters of pregnancy. For instance, the woman in her first trimester may feel nauseated and fatigued, thus lessening her interest in and physical energy for sexual interaction. In the third trimester, the father may fear hurting the fetus if he initiates sexual intercourse, and this fear may inhibit his desire. The second trimester is generally associated with increased sexual responsiveness. These changes may be due in part to positive emotional states, such as looking forward to taking on new roles of father and mother. In addition, the pregnant woman may have intensified pelvic and genital sensations as the blood supply increases in the pelvic area. These physical changes can increase her desire for sexual expression.

Sexual activity during pregnancy is usually safe and satisfying. However, because each woman's experience of pregnancy is different, nurses should encourage pregnant women to seek guidelines about sexual activity from a physician. Desire for sexual activity after the child is born varies among women and may differ between men and women. New mothers feeling pelvic soreness, fatigue, and concern about mothering may lack interest in sexual expression. In contrast, fathers who feel closer to the mother because of the birth of the child often desire sexual intimacy. Discussion about sexual needs and alternative modes of expression is critical for these couples (Lenz et al. 1985).

Contraception

When sexually active partners do not wish to risk pregnancy, a reliable and satisfactory method of contraception is critical. The decision to use a particular method is based on many factors. Four major considerations are the clients' views of the morality or immorality of contraceptive use, medical safety with minimal side-effects, reliability, and ease of use. Use of a contraceptive can permit enjoyment of sexual response without fear of pregnancy. Because the various contraceptives have advantages and disadvantages, nurses need to assess clients' contraceptive use and its effects on their sexual response.

PSYCHOPATHOLOGY OF GENDER AND SEXUAL DISORDERS

Gender Identity Disorders

Gender identity is a term used to describe an individual's personal or private sense of identity as masculine, feminine, or ambivalent. Gender identity is a sex role assign-

ment usually based in identification of external genitals. This identity is established between the ages of 18 months and 3 years.

Gender role describes the public behaviors that demonstrate the individual's perceptions of his maleness or her femaleness. These behaviors are specific to sociocultural environment and are also influenced by age, race, and other demographic factors.

Theories of Gender Development

Biologic Imperative

How do gender identity and gender roles develop? One contemporary theory rests on the notion that for the most part anatomy is destiny: Because men and women are biologically different, they have innately different characteristics and styles of interacting. In this view, the fetus has a biologic mechanism that directs it to become male or female.

Cognitive Switch

Another theory is that children are born more or less neutral, but that one of the central developmental tasks of childhood is to label oneself male or female. According to this theory, a *cognitive switch* occurs at age 3 or 4. After this point, the process of acquiring gender identity is irreversible.

Social Learning and Labeling

A third theory is advocated in this text. This theory focuses on social learning. It holds that gender identity and roles are continuously constructed and maintained through the life span. The stability of one's gender identity depends on biologic differences, but it also depends on everyday situations that continuously provide expectations, demands, and feedback for one or another conception of oneself.

Sexual expression refers to those sex role behaviors that a person exhibits as a result of his or her gender identity and role. Many modes of sexual expression are learned and developed throughout life as the person attempts to define and meet sexual needs. Table 20–4 identifies typical kinds of sexual expression. Obvious sexual activities, including fantasy, self-stimulation, and coitus, are only a part of sexual expression. Behaviors that meet one's emotional needs for self-esteem, a sense of belonging, intimacy, and appreciation and respect from others are also forms of sexual expression. The concepts of love and sex are not synonymous, but it is generally believed that sexual activity motivated by feelings of affection increases the resulting emotional satisfaction. This combination of shared affection and sexual activity can lead to a desire for marriage or parenting. In this way, the family unit is promoted, and

Table 20–4	
Typical Sexual Activities	
Activity	**Comments**
Kissing	Of another's lips, breasts, ear lobes, or other body parts that are considered erotic
Breast stimulation	Enjoyed by both men and women
Hand stimulation by partner	Usually involves caressing another's genitals with one's fingers or palm of the hand
Cunnilingus	Oral stimulation of the female genitals
Fellatio	Oral stimulation of the male genitals
Coitus	Sexual intercourse or penetration of penis into the vagina; may be done in a variety of positions that the couple find arousing
Anal intercourse	Penile penetration of the partner's anus
Masturbation	Self-stimulation using one's hand, a vibrator, an object, or other arousing method; may be done alone or in the presence of partner
Sexual fantasy	Use of thoughts about specific sexual experience, romance, other partners, or various erotic themes that enhance the person's sexual arousal

survival of the human species is ensured. From birth, children are exposed to love and affection and develop their own patterns of sexual expression as part of their growth and development.

An individual's moral or spiritual identity also has a strong impact on sexual expression. The "rightness" or "wrongness" of certain behaviors are shaped by societal values, which in turn are strongly influenced by moral and spiritual beliefs. Conflict is often apparent between actual sexual behaviors and stated moral values in our modern society. This conflict exists partly because religious beliefs from the eighteenth and nineteenth centuries have survived while technology and values have changed dramatically. Many individuals experience moral or spiritual conflicts about their sexual expression, which may cause guilt, confusion, and diminished sexual health. Figure 20–4 is a developmental conceptualization of the complex set of factors that influence the development of gender identities, gender roles, and sexual conduct.

Transsexualism

DSM-IIIR identifies **transsexualism** as a disorder of gender identity in which persons have consistently strong feelings that their biologic and psychologic genders are at odds. For these individuals, sexual anatomy is not consistent with internal feelings of masculinity or femininity. Instead, they feel trapped in the wrong body. Most transsexuals report that they have always felt this way. Typically, transsexuals do not view themselves as homosexuals in sexual preference. Rather, they seek partners of the sex opposite that of their psychologic gender identity. Transsexuals crossdress to make their outward appearance consistent with their gender identity.

Transsexualism is caused, in part, by psychologic conditions and experiences that confuse learning about gender roles. It also appears to be related to the influence of sex hormones during fetal development. Transsexualism may also be more likely to develop in cultures where rigid stereotyping of sex roles allows little flexibility in expression of masculinity or femininity. Many adult transsexuals seek hormonal therapy or sex-change surgery to become comfortable with their sexual identity.

Two- to five-year follow-up adjustment studies of those having undergone sex-change surgery show that about two-thirds of these clients improve in life functioning after their surgery. Those changing from female to male seem to fare better after surgery than those changing from male to female, possibly because male-to-female socialization is more difficult than female-to-male socialization (Abramowitz 1986).

Surgery appears to be decreasing in frequency as a treatment method. This trend may be associated with the cost and practical difficulties of the complex procedures involved. However, society may be developing more tolerance for nonstereotypic sex role behavior, thus allowing transsexuals to express their sexuality without the need for surgical interventions.

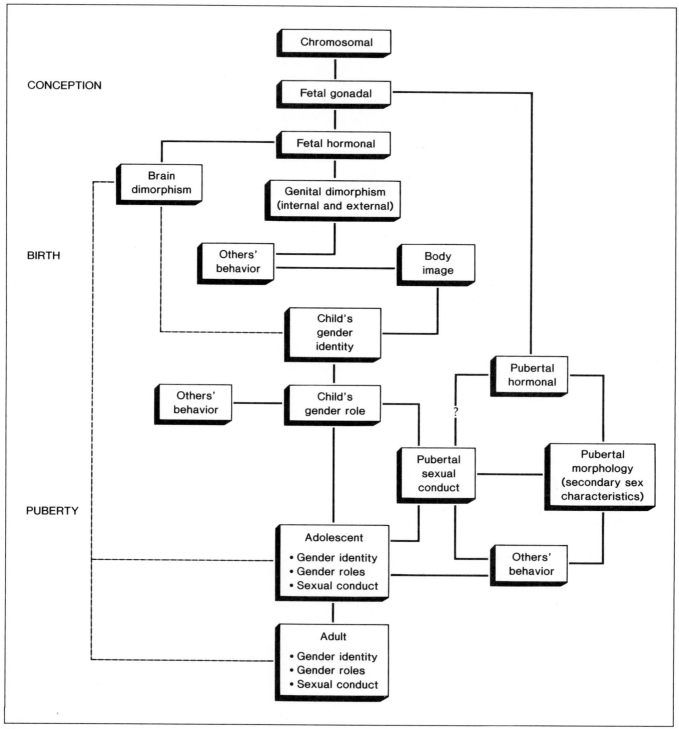

Figure 20–4

Development of gender identities, gender roles, and sexual contact. The question mark signifies an effect not demonstrated (that hormonal changes produce sexual conduct or eroticism in any direct way) and the dashed line suggests weak connection.

Source: Based on Money J, Erhardt A: Man Woman/Boy Girl. *Johns Hopkins University Press, 1973. © 1973 The Johns Hopkins University Press.*

These disorders occur in children who feel persistent and intense distress about their biologic gender. They state an intense desire to be of the other sex. Girls insist that they are boys, that they have a penis, and that they will not grow breasts or menstruate. These girls demand to wear boys' underwear and clothing and wish to urinate in a standing position. Similarly, boys demand to wear girls' underwear and clothing. Boys express intense dislike of their penis and voice the desire to grow breasts. This classification by the DSM-III refers only to children who have not reached puberty and who express these symptoms persistently (DMS-IIIR 1987).

Gender identity disorder may also occur for the first time in adolescence or adulthood. In addition to persistent discomfort and a sense of inappropriateness about one's assigned sex, the person engages in persistent cross-dressing. Cross-dressing may range from the occasional wearing of a single item of clothing of the other sex, to dressing entirely as a member of the opposite sex.

Some persons with this disorder may once have had transvestic fetishism but no longer experience sexual arousal with cross-dressing. Others may be homosexuals who cross-dress. The disorder is also thought to be common among female impersonators (DSM-IIIR, p 76).

Alternative Patterns of Sexual Expression

In the United States, the norm for sexual expression is heterosexuality, sexual activity with others of the opposite sex. Homosexuals, bisexuals, and transsexuals violate this norm since they engage in sexual relations with people of the same sex. **Homosexuality** is sexual activity with others of the same sex. **Bisexuality** behavior is sexual activity with people of both sexes.

Until fairly recently, most people in the United States assumed that there were only three categories of sexual behavior—homosexuality, heterosexuality, and bisexuality—and that everyone fell into one or another of the three. Typically, only heterosexuals were assumed to be normal. Homosexuals and bisexuals were perverted objects of pity or scorn, in need of psychiatric attention and perhaps of institutionalization. Modern sex research has disproved this assumption. Kinsey and other sex researchers use a seven-point scale to rate people along a continuum. One extreme on this continuum represents exclusive heterosexuality; the other, exclusive homosexuality. According to the continuum idea, however, homosexuals are defined as people who engage only in physical homosexual acts. It is probably more accurate to recognize that there is not just one kind of homosexuality. There are many different ways to organize a homosexual preference into a commitment and an ongoing life-style.

Male Homosexuality

Some men who have experienced homosexual fantasies label themselves as "gay." Others who have experienced these fantasies do not. Sexual behaviors of homosexual males include fellatio, anal intercourse, oral-anal contact, hand stimulation, friction or rubbing the penis against the partner's body, the use of vibrators and dildos for anal stimulation, and insertion of the fingers into the anus. Many homosexual men have modified their sexual activities because of the AIDS epidemic in the direction of lower risk behaviors (see Chapter 26).

In order for a homosexual to join the gay community, he must "come out." The gay subculture can be extremely important to a homosexual, because it provides places, such as gay bars, to meet lovers, and because it can also supply a cadre of supportive persons. However, the public gay culture is often limited in its emotional diversity. Homosexuals who have not "come out" are referred to as "closet queens."

Many people believe that a male homosexual may be easily recognized because he is effeminate. Some homosexuals do indulge in extravagant mannerisms or appear in "drag" (women's clothes). However, many homosexuals are indistinguishable from other men. In sum, homosexuality is as varied as heterosexuality in its cultural, social, and sexual aspects.

Lesbianism

Like male homosexuality, **lesbianism** can be defined as a form of sexual behavior between females, an emotional preference, a part of one's identity, or a social role. As a form of sexual behavior, lesbianism can include masturbation, cunnilingus, rubbing the genitals against the partner's body, and use of vibrators and dildos on the internal or external sexual structures. Very little is known about the psychologic and social characteristics of lesbians. Many lesbians are married women with children who are secretive about their lesbian affairs.

Lesbians may play lovemaking and social roles with each other. A "butch" plays the masculine role, and a "femme" plays the feminine role. In some instances—in prison, for example—partners play either a butch or a femme role exclusively. In other lesbian relationships, neither partner plays a specifically masculine or feminine role. The sexual and social roles can vary with the setting.

Many lesbians do not belong to any lesbian community or group. However, several types of lesbian communities are emerging. These include the lesbian bar community, the overt lesbian feminist activist community, lesbian affiliations with the gay male community, and lesbian familial organizations in single households and communes.

Bisexuality

In contemporary society many people are declaring a bisexual identity. It is possible that this trend is influenced by the mass media and by popular bisexual role models coming forward and talking about their sexual preference. The most notable aspect of bisexuality is its increasing institutionalization as an alternative life-style and identity.

Ego-Dystonic Homosexuality

In recent decades the religious conception of homosexuality as "evil" was partially replaced by the medical conception of it as "sick." Until the 1970s homosexuality was on the American Psychiatric Association's diagnostic list of categories of mental illness. After a great deal of conflict among psychiatric professionals, the list was revised to include only ego-dystonic homosexuality. This diagnosis applies to the person who has weak heterosexual desire but consistently states the wish for a heterosexual relationship and explicitly states distress with homosexual arousal (DSM-IIIR 1987).

Although ego-syntonic (acceptable to the self) homosexuality is no longer officially an illness, psychiatrists still tend to search for a cause and cure. The medical view of homosexuality is based on the assumption that people are born with a tendency to be heterosexual. It is probably accurate to say that human sexual behavior varies widely and that it depends on learning and social experiences as well as on inborn tendencies. Homosexual men and women can feel very comfortable about their sexual preference, but the intolerant and rejecting attitude of others may cause them stress. Further, homosexuals experience psychosocial coping difficulties as do heterosexuals. These clients would not be appropriately described as having ego-dystonic homosexuality. It is imperative that psychiatric nurses be aware of their own feelings about homosexuality so that they can accurately assess the causes of any concerns homosexual clients express.

Paraphilias

Paraphilias are a group of psychosexual disorders classified by the DSM-IIIR that include sexual behaviors most persons would define as unusual, deviant, or perverse. These behaviors must have been ongoing for at least six months. To achieve full sexual arousal and satisfaction, the paraphiliac requires the presence of a specific object or must engage in a specific activity; e.g., receiving or inflicting pain or having sexual activity with a nonconsenting partner (DMS-IIIR 1987). The person, usually a male, depends on the object or activity for sexual arousal. Various paraphilias are defined in Table 20–5. Often the person feels guilt, shame, low self-esteem, or anxiety after the sexual experience. Sometimes the paraphiliac experiences erectile failure in ordinary adult sexual interactions.

The causes of paraphilia are not clearly known. Prenatal effects of the androgens might diminish the adult's

Table 20–5
Paraphilias

Term	Definition/Description
Exhibitionism	Intentional exposure of one's genitals to a stranger or unsuspecting person is accompanied by sexual arousal and masturbation either during or after the exposure.
Fetishism	The presence of an object, e.g., shoes, hair, or panties, is required for sexual response.
Frotteurism	Intense sexual arousal is associated with acts or fantasies of rubbing up against a nonconsenting person.
Pedophilia	The sex object is a child. Manipulation or fondling of the child's genitals is usually involved.
Sexual masochism	Experiencing emotional or physical pain, real or fantasized, is necessary for sexual arousal.
Sexual sadism	Inflicting emotional or physical pain/humiliation, real or fantasized, is necessary for sexual arousal.
Transvestic fetishism	Cross-dressing (most often a heterosexual male dressing in female clothes) is required for sexual arousal prior to masturbation or coitus.
Voyeurism	An unsuspecting person (usually a woman) is watched while that person is undressing, grooming, or having sexual interaction. The voyeur often masturbates during or after the episode.
Zoophilia (bestiality)	Animals are the actual or fantasized participants in sexual activity.

capacity for normal arousal and thus make that person more vulnerable to becoming a paraphiliac (Money 1980). Psychodynamic theorists suggest that the sexual development of the person is confused and that the paraphiliac behavior defends against castration and separation anxiety (Kaplan and Sadock 1985). Also, the behavior may compensate for feelings of immaturity and fears of rejection in establishing and maintaining adult sexual relationships. Behavioral theorists postulate that early sexual experiences in which the person associated a particular object or act with sexual arousal can condition the person to respond to that stimulus by becoming aroused. Once the initial association is made, repeated fantasy or actual use of the object in sexual activity (usually masturbation) reinforces its arousing nature. For instance, a boy may try on his mother's panties and get an erection. The erection is felt as pleasurable. The next time the boy is masturbating, he remembers the panties and uses them or fantasizes about them when masturbating. With repeated experiences, seeing the panties or putting them on becomes a sexual stimulus. Finally, some people demonstrate paraphiliac behavior only when they are in the acute phase of another psychiatric illness or are under extreme stress.

A **pedophiliac** is an adult who persistently associates sexual arousal and activity with stimuli involving one or more children age 13 or younger (DSM-IIIR 1987). Pedophilia warrants specific discussion since it involves a victim and is a crime. All sexual relationships between adults and children are viewed as criminal in the United States. The courts consider these acts nonconsensual because minors are presumed to have insufficient knowledge of the consequences of their acts to give meaningful consent. In many states, the penalty for the offending adult is life imprisonment; in a few states, the penalty is death. Pedophiliac activity can include genital touching, nudity, kissing, digital penetration of the vagina or anus, or oral sex. Attempts at actual sexual intercourse are rare. Most acts are committed by a person known to the child, e.g., a family member, neighbor, or friend.

The causes of pedophilia are similar to the causes of other paraphilias, previously described. Pedophiles are usually unable or unwilling to seek sexual gratification with adults. They are often sexually and socially immature and have problems in their marriages and jobs. Children are less threatening sexual partners than adults are. Like other paraphiliacs, the pedophile often feels shame and guilt after the sexual encounter. Some pedophiles have antisocial motivations. They inflict aggression and sexual abuse for the excitement of acting against social norms. Such pedophiles feel no guilt about their actions.

The nurse often has the opportunity to identify victims of the pedophile. Disturbed sleeping, eating, and play patterns as well as regressive behavior, angry outbursts, and withdrawal can be the child's reactions to sexual abuse (Federation 1986). The nurse has a legal and professional responsibility to report sexual abuse of a child to the appropriate legal and social welfare agencies.

Sexual Dysfunctions

The diagnosis of *sexual dysfunction* describes people who experience changes in sexual function that are unsatisfying or causes for concern (Carpenito 1983). Effective sexual functioning is psychophysiologic. For this reason, organic and emotional (individual and relationship) factors influence effective response. Lo Piccolo and Stock (1986) suggest that the majority of sexual dysfunctions are both physical and psychologic in origin. Major categories of organic causes include physical illness, neuromuscular disorders, endocrine disorders, and drug-induced effects. Emotional influences include anxiety, guilt, or fear about sexual interactions or response. Also, relationship conflicts and communication problems that result in anger, disappointment, or fear of rejection related to the partner can cause sexual dysfunction.

The DSM-IIIR (1987) classifies sexual dysfunctions according to the phase of the sexual response cycle that is affected. The dysfunction may be a lifelong problem or an acquired one. Dysfunctions are either generalized to all sexual interactions and settings, or are situational—i.e., occurring in a specific setting with specific types of sexual activity (DSM-IIIR 1987).

Disorders of Sexual Desire

Hypoactive Sexual Desire Disorder

Kaplan (1979) contributed to the identification of **hypoactive sexual desire disorder** (HSD) as a clinical problem. This disorder can occur in both males and females. Typically, clients verbalize a lack of interest in sexual activity and report little sexual interaction with their partner and sometimes little self-stimulation. Usually the partner expresses dissatisfaction with the sexual relationship and is often the one who initiates the seeking of help. The client feels asexual, lacks motivation to seek sexual expression, feels "turned off," and often complains about sexually unattractive aspects of the partner. These symptoms are a way to suppress or control sexual feelings and arousal.

A physiologic factor associated with lack of desire is abnormally low sex hormone levels. For instance, a man with a low testosterone level may lack interest in and motivation for sexual expression. Relationship and intrapersonal concerns can also contribute to hypoactive desire. Disappointment or anger with one's mate, fears of closeness and intimacy with one's partner, or guilt and anxiety related to sexual activity are major psychologic factors contributing to HSD. Typically, clients have little insight into the association between their lack of sexual desire and their negative feelings about the relationship.

Sexual Aversion Disorder

Sexual aversion disorder is a severe distaste for sexual activity or the thought of sexual activity, which then leads to avoidance of sex. It occurs in both men and women. Intense emotional dread of an impending sexual interaction also can cause physiologic symptoms of anxiety, e.g., sweating, increased heart rate, or extreme muscle tension. The client then stops the sexual interaction or prevents it from even beginning. Primary causes of sexual aversion are: a history of sexual trauma, a pattern of constant sexual pressuring by the partner, gender identity confusion or intense negative feelings about sexual activity (Masters et al. 1982).

Female and Male Sexual Arousal Disorder

Lack of lubrication and failure to attain and then maintain an erection are the major disorders of the excitement phase. In **female sexual arousal disorder**, the woman may complain of dryness or discomfort when having sexual intercourse. She and her partner may express a need for additional lubrication. The man with **male erectile disorder** may have difficulty becoming firm or may lose his firm erection during sexual activity. Some men lose their erection just prior to attempting sexual intercourse. In instances where lubrication and erection are adequate, a persistent or recurring lack of sexual excitement or pleasure is another diagnostic criterion for sexual arousal disorder.

Both male and female excitement phases can be inhibited by physiologic factors that interfere with the vasocongestion necessary for lubrication or erection to occur. Some researchers estimate that organic causes account for at least one-third of male erectile problems (Lo Piccolo and Stock 1986). For instance, neurologic changes associated with diabetes may inhibit sexual excitement.

Psychologic factors may also be the primary cause of dysfunction in arousal disorders. Having intense anxiety and fear about one's ability to perform sexually is the most prominent cause of erectile failure or inadequate lubrication. Masters and Johnson (1970) describe the *spectator role* in association with these fears. *Spectatoring* occurs when the person engaged in a sexual interaction monitors and evaluates sexual performance and progress in a distant, noninvolved manner. Thinking in an objective intellectual manner can reduce the person's spontaneity and involvement in the sexual interaction so that pleasurable stimuli are not perceived as arousing. In turn, the person is not physically or emotionally aroused. Consequently, there is inadequate lubrication or loss of erection. When a person constantly evaluates his or her performance and arousal is not proceeding as the person thinks it should, anxiety and fear can inhibit excitement further. The fears of inadequate sexual performance are then realized in a self-fulfilling prophecy.

Sometimes, sexual arousal disorders are caused by factors in the relationship, e.g., inadequate communication with the partner. The person's partner does not provide the necessary physical stimulation for lubrication or erection to occur, but the person does not express what kind of caressing is desired. A woman may not communicate her sexual needs because she fears rejection or feels embarrassed. A man sometimes hesitates to ask for genital caressing because he feels he should be able to get an erection spontaneously or feels his partner does not want to caress his penis.

Orgasm Disorders

Inhibited Female Orgasm

Inhibited female orgasm is persistent or recurrent delay in or absence of orgasm in the female during sexual activity that appears to be adequate in focus, intensity, and duration (DSM-IIIR 1987). Women who attain orgasm during sexual play but not during sexual intercourse are *not* considered as having an orgasm disorder. Women who have the ability to attain orgasm but simply have not learned to experience one have been described as preorgasmic (Barbach 1980).

Orgasm disorder is a commonly recognized problem, perhaps because the recent cultural openness about female response has prompted women (and their partners) to discuss sexual response and seek orgasm if they have not been orgasmic.

Some physiologic causal factors related to anorgasmia are noted in Table 20–6. Physical illnesses, hormonal influences, or drugs that interfere with desire and arousal may also inhibit orgasm. In the healthy female, a lack of information or negative attitudes about female sexual response often contribute to orgasm disorder. Barbach (1980) notes that some women believe there is only one "normal" way to have sexual activity and orgasm (e.g., through sexual intercourse with the male on top). This attitude restricts the physical stimulation the woman may request or receive. Further, the woman's perception of her sexual response may be clouded by guilt, shame, and anxiety. Women who believe their sexual role is passive may receive inadequate physical stimulation and may also be emotionally uninvolved in the sexual interaction. They do not become sufficiently aroused to have orgasm. Finally, some women may fear loss of control or excessive vulnerability, which prompts them to stop sexual activity before experiencing orgasm.

Male Orgasm Disorders

Men may experience two different orgasm disorders: **premature ejaculation** and **inhibited male orgasm**. Premature ejaculation is somewhat subjective in definition. Different

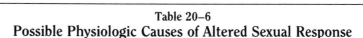

Problem/Associated Medication	Phase of Response		
	Desire	Excitement	Orgasm
Alcoholism	—	Inhibit	Delay
Antabuse	—	—	Delay
Antihistamine	—	Inhibit lubrication	—
Antihypertensive medications	—	Inhibit	Inhibit
Bilateral oophorectomy	Inhibit	—	—
Diabetes	—	Impair	Retrograde ejaculation; delay
Estrogen therapy	—	Inhibit males; increase lubrication	Delay in males
Fatigue	Decrease	—	—
Hysterectomy	—	—	—
Multiple sclerosis	—	—	Inhibit
Ostomies	—	Inhibit	—
Parkinson's disease (L-dopa)	Increase	—	—
Perineal or radical prostatectomy	—	Inhibit	—
Physical illness (acute)	Decrease	—	—
Prostatectomy	—	—	Retrograde ejaculation
Renal disease	Decrease	Inhibit	Delay
Spinal cord injuries	Inhibit	Inhibit	Retrograde ejaculation; delay or inhibit
Steroid therapy	Increase	—	—
Testosterone therapy	Increase	—	—
Tubal ligation	—	—	—
Ulcers	Decrease	—	—
Vascular disease	—	Inhibit	—
Vasectomy	—	—	—

Table 20–6
Possible Physiologic Causes of Altered Sexual Response

clients have different notions of how long arousal and stimulation should last before ejaculation. However, when a man does ejaculate too quickly, he and his partner often feel frustrated. The partner may feel the man is ejaculating intentionally, and the man often feels guilty and inadequate for having the premature response.

There is very little empirical information about the mechanisms that cause premature ejaculation. Possible influences include the man's inability to perceive his arousal level accurately, a lowered sensory threshold due to infrequent sexual activity, early conditioning of rapid ejaculation from self-stimulation or hurried instances of sexual intercourse, or extreme anxiety during the sexual interaction, resulting in the sympathetic nervous system activity that triggers ejaculation.

The opposite problem is inhibited orgasm. The man with this disorder can maintain an erection for long periods (e.g., an hour) but has extreme difficulty ejaculating within the vagina during sexual intercourse. Some men are able to ejaculate with self-stimulation or with hand stimulation by the partner, whereas others have great difficulty ejaculating with any type of stimulation. This disorder occurs much less frequently than premature ejaculation does.

Organic causes that inhibit sexual desire or excitement

can prevent the male from reaching an adequate arousal level for ejaculation. Some neuromuscular diseases (e.g., multiple sclerosis) inhibit male orgasm.

Emotional causes of inhibited orgasm include fear of pregnancy, performance pressure, and anxiety and guilt about engaging in sexual activity. Also, the man may become physically aroused quickly but not allow enough time for emotional arousal. Finally, anxiety about not ejaculating can adversely affect the sexual relationship and both partners' ability to enjoy the sexual interaction.

Sexual Pain Disorders

Vaginismus

Vaginismus is an involuntary spasm of the outer one-third of the vaginal muscles that makes penetration of the vagina painful and sometimes impossible. The woman often experiences desire, excitement, and orgasm with stimulation of the external sexual organs. Attempts at intercourse, however, elicit the involuntary spasms. She may also have similar difficulty undergoing pelvic exams and inserting tampons or a diaphragm.

The partner of the vaginismic woman often becomes fearful and anxious about hurting her or may become resentful and believe she is having the spasms on purpose. The mate may develop sexual desire, arousal, or orgasm disorders as a result of these negative feelings and interpretations.

Causes of vaginismus are thought to be psychophysiologic. The vaginismic response may develop initially as a protection against anticipated pain. It has been associated with experiencing sexual trauma such as rape or incest, extreme fears of pregnancy, intense guilt about engaging in sexual intercourse, and a high level of religiosity. The DSM-IIIR diagnosis of vaginismus is not appropriate when a physical disorder is the exclusive cause of response.

Dyspareunia

Both men and women can experience dyspareunia, or painful intercourse. It is associated with many physiologic causes, and in women, especially those that inhibit lubrication. Thus, skin irritations, vaginal infections, and use of medications that dry vaginal secretions can cause women to experience discomfort with intercourse. Pelvic disorders, such as infections or tumors, can result in painful intercourse. Similarly, in males, infection or inflammation of the glans penis or other genitourinary organs can cause pain with coitus. Also, some contraceptive foams and creams irritate the penis.

Although there are multiple physiologic causes of dyspareunia, the emotional response to the painful experience can bring on, worsen, or perpetuate sexual dysfunction. Fear and anxiety in anticipation of pain can undermine the person's ability to feel pleasurable sexual responses. Dyspareunia is a DSM-IIIR (1987) diagnosis when the condition is not caused exclusively by lack of lubrication or by vaginismus.

THE NURSING PROCESS AND CLIENTS WITH GENDER AND SEXUAL DISORDERS

Assessment

The psychiatric nurse finds numerous opportunities to apply the nursing process to promote sexual health. Assessment of sexual status is part of a thorough and comprehensive assessment of a client's general health.

Subjective Data

The sexual history provides subjective assessment data needed for formulating nursing diagnoses. The nurse elicits sexual information much as she or he elicits a general nursing history. However, special attention should be given to planning a setting where privacy and uninterrupted time are available. Such a setting helps clients feel comfortable discussing these private aspects of their lives. It is helpful to begin the interview by explaining why the nurse is asking about sexuality. For example, the nurse might say, "Sexuality is a part of people's lives. People often have questions about sexual activity when they have changes in their health. I'd like to take this time to talk with you about your sex life."

The nurse should move from general to specific questions. This gradual focus on specific sexual behavior allows clients to develop trust and rapport with the nurse. Initially, questions can relate sexuality to health status. Open-ended questions encourage clients to expand on their sexual experiences and concerns. The nurse should reassure clients that it is normal to have sexual concerns and questions. For instance, the nurse might say, "It is common for many people to feel concerned about. . . . Do you have any questions?" By restating the client's response, the nurse encourages him or her to expand on feelings. Box 20–1 lists an inventory of questions that the psychiatric nurse can ask as a part of a general nursing history. Questions to ask if the client does identify a sexual problem or disorder are also included. Remember that psychiatric clients often take medications that can affect sexual desire or sexual behavior (see Table 20–8).

Box 20–1
SEXUAL HISTORY

1. When you were growing up, how did you learn about sex?

2. In general, how satisfied are you with your current sexual activity?

3. How would you describe your current sexual activity?

4. What, if anything, would you change about your sexual activity?

5. How, if at all, do you think your current state of health/illness has affected your sex life?

6. Are you taking any medications? Do you think these affect your sexual activity?

7. Do you have any concerns about birth control?

8. Do you feel any physical or emotional discomfort during sexual activity?

9. Do you have any questions or concerns about masturbation . . . homosexuality. . . ?

10. Do you have questions or concerns about any sexual experiences?

11. Do you want to talk about any other questions or concerns?

Additional questions to ask if the client identifies a sexual problem.

1. How would you specifically describe your sexual problem?

2. When did this problem start?

3. How often does this problem occur?

4. Under what circumstances does it happen?

5. What are your ideas as to its cause?

6. How has the problem affected your partner (if appropriate)?

7. How have you tried to solve it?

Sources: Mims F, Swensen M: Sexuality: A Nursing Perspective. McGraw-Hill, 1980; Webb C: Sexuality, Nursing, and Health. John Wiley, 1985.

Objective Data

Objective data include the nonverbal behaviors observed by the nurse, laboratory data, test results, medical diagnoses, physical examination results, and other documented sources such as the chart.

Objective data may also include results of physiologic assessment of sexual function. The nocturnal penile tumescence (NPT) procedure provides a direct measure of

---

RESEARCH NOTE

Citation

Frank D, Downard E, Lang A: Androgyny, sexual satisfaction and women. J Psychosoc Nurs and Ment Health Serv 1986;24:10–15.

Study Problem/Purpose

The purpose of this study was to explore the relationship between women's sex role personality traits and sexual satisfaction.

Methods

The subjects were 155 women who responded to an anonymous survey distributed by nursing students and returned by mail. Almost 90 percent of the subjects were between the ages of 21–45 and had a minimum of some college education. About half were married. Subjects were asked to recall their most recent satisfying and unsatisfying sexual experiences. They were then asked to rate the importance of seven factors in determining each outcome. These factors included: the woman's own sexual skill or ability, her effort or involvement, the partner's sexual skill or ability, the partner's efforts or involvement, situational factors or luck, the extent to which it is easy (or difficult) to feel sexual satisfaction, and the quality of the overall relationship. Women also completed the BEM Sex Role Inventory as a measure of their sex role traits: androgynous, feminine, and masculine.

Findings

Results indicated that these women viewed their personal efforts, their partner's efforts, and the quality of their relationship as major influences of sexual experience outcomes. Also, women's beliefs that they had the capacity to experience orgasm when they tried were positively associated with a history of orgasm. Sex role personality traits of masculine, feminine, or androgynous did not exert a direct influence on perceptions about sexual experiences.

Implications

The researchers suggested that a couple's agreement with *how* sex roles are expressed may be more critical to satisfaction levels than individual personality traits. Nursing assessment should include eliciting perceptions about the extent of involvement in the sexual relationship and the quality of the relationship. Assessment and interventions should also be directed toward fostering a positive sexual self-concept in women to build confidence about their ability to attain sexual satisfaction.

erectile capacity. The device measures penile engorgement that occurs during sleep. NPT measurement is considered the best available method to determine if a man's erectile difficulties are physiologic. If so, there is minimal penile engorgement during sleep. Men whose erection difficulties appear to be psychologic in origin have normal engorgement during sleep. Although the NPT procedure is an important source of objective data, its results are not always reliable. Research findings report 28 to 42 percent error in accuracy (Conte 1986).

Physiologic assessment of female sexual function is accomplished by use of vaginal plethysmographs or probes. These devices are inserted into the vagina and measure vasocongestion of the vaginal wall tissue.

Several sophisticated and expensive laboratory tests are designed to assess sexual function. For instance, testosterone and estrogen blood levels may be measured. However, laboratory data must be interpreted with caution since test results are not always reliable indicators of clients' actual sexual behavior. Thus clients' self-reports of sexual performance, feelings, and values (the subjective data) are of prime importance in assessment. The nurse evaluates and interprets the data to formulate actual and potential nursing diagnoses.

Nursing Diagnoses

There are various models for classifying nursing diagnoses related to gender and sexual disorders. Table 20–7 lists those diagnoses proposed by the ANA work group formed to identify phenomena of concern to psychiatric nurses.

Table 20–7
Comparison of DSM-IIIR and Psychiatric Nursing Diagnoses

DSM-IIIR	PND-I Diagnoses	NANDA Diagnoses
302.60 Gender identity disorder of childhood	02.03.03 Knowledge deficit*	Activity intolerance
302.50 Transsexualism	04.99 Potential for altered emotional processes	Sexuality, altered patterns
302.85 Gender identity disorder of adolescence or adulthood, nontranssexual type	05.01 Altered communication processes*	Family processes, altered
302.85 Gender identity disorder NOS	05.04 Altered sexuality processes	Self-concept, disturbance in: body image, self-esteem, personal identity
302.40 Exhibitionism	05.05.02 Social isolation/withdrawal*	
302.81 Fetishism	06.02 Altered comfort patterns	
302.89 Frotteurism	06.03.02 Altered gender identity	Role performance, altered
302.20 Pedophilia	06.03.04 Altered self-esteem*	
302.83 Sexual masochism	07.03.02 Altered hormone regulation	Coping, ineffective family
302.84 Sexual sadism	08.02.01 Spiritual distress	
302.30 Transvestic fetishism	08.03.01 Conflict with social order	Coping, ineffective individual
302.82 Voyeurism		
302.90 Paraphilia NOS		Knowledge deficit
302.71 Hypoactive sexual desire		Sexual dysfunction
302.72 Female sexual arousal disorder		Social isolation
302.72 Male erectile disorder		Spiritual distress
302.73 Inhibited female orgasm		
302.74 Inhibited male orgasm		
302.75 Premature ejaculation		
302.76 Dyspareunia		
302.79 Sexual aversion disorder		
306.51 Vaginismus		
302.70 Sexual dysfunction NOS		
302.90 Sexual disorder NOS		

*PND-I diagnoses also in NANDA list.

Because sexual disorders have many causes, nursing diagnoses that describe other aspects of clients' health status also identify etiologies of sexual problems. These related NANDA nursing diagnoses are also listed in Table 20–7.

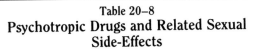

Sexual Dysfunction

The nursing diagnosis of sexual dysfunction is used to describe those who experience actual or potential changes in sexual function that are unsatisfying or causes for concern (Carpenito 1984). These changes in sexual activity may be related to physical alterations in clients' health states. The emotional response to an illness or physical problem can also prevent optimum sexual functioning.

Feelings of low self-esteem, negative changes in body image, or undesired role changes can inhibit desire for sexual activity. Physical limitations may necessitate changes in sexual practices or kinds of stimulation that the individual or couple may not accept. Instead, the person or couple compare present sexual responses negatively to past experiences. Other clients or partners may fear sexual activity will cause further physical harm and avoid sexual expression for this reason. Finally, clients may use physical problems as an excuse to stop unwanted sexual expression.

Psychologic Problems and Sexual Dysfunction

Many clients with psychiatric diagnoses or coping problems experience sexual dysfunction or have the potential to experience it. The cause of the sexual dysfunction can be related to psychotropic medications prescribed as a part of the treatment regimen (see Table 20–8). For instance, a wide variety of antipsychotic and antidepressant drugs inhibit or delay orgasm or ejaculation. In addition, the signs and symptoms of the client's psychosocial difficulties may secondarily result in sexual dysfunction.

Clients who feel worthless or view themselves with a sense of failure may have inhibited sexual desire. Some clients may perceive themselves as sexually undesirable partners. This perception can generate anxiety in sexual interactions that prevents arousal during the excitement phase of sexual response. People with low self-esteem may also avoid sexual relationships. Extreme feelings of guilt may lead to sexual problems. Guilt about engaging in sexual activity or experiencing sexual pleasure may inhibit any phase of sexual response.

Sexual Acting Out

Sexual acting out is a term used for clients with sexual behavior disturbances. It can also describe clients with disturbed conduct or impulse control. Sexual acting out can include such behaviors as making sexually provocative remarks, flirting inappropriately, attempting to touch others sexually, masturbating in public, exhibiting one's genitals,

Table 20–8 Psychotropic Drugs and Related Sexual Side-Effects	
Category	**Reported Side-Effects**
Antianxiety	Changes in desire
Anti-Parkinsonism	Increased desire Levodopa may inhibit ejaculation
Antipsychotic	Breast engorgement in men and women Menstrual irregularities Changes in desire Erectile or lubrication difficulty Delayed or inhibited orgasm (Haldol has no specific adverse effects noted)
Tricyclic antidepressants	Breast engorgement in men and women Testicular swelling Changes in desire Erectile/lubrication difficulties Inhibited orgasm
MAO inhibitors	Changes in desire Erectile/lubrication difficulties Delayed or inhibited orgasm

Sources: Biomedical Information Corporation: The Psychiatrist's Compendium of Drug Therapy. *Biomedical Information Corporation, 800 Second Avenue, New York, 10017, 1984; Seagraves R: Female orgasm and psychiatric drugs.* J Sex Educ Ther *1985;11:69–71.*

engaging in extramarital affairs, or being promiscuous (McFarland and Wasli 1986).

When assessing sexual acting out, nurses must consider many factors. Clients may have a need to test their sexual attractiveness. This testing could occur in clients having changes in body image or low self-esteem. Clients who have inadequate coping skills to deal with social situations or to develop interpersonal relationships may make offensive sexual overtures in an attempt to establish relationships. Some clients may alleviate feelings of intense anxiety by inappropriate sexual behaviors, e.g., public masturbation, exhibitionism, or voyeurism. Increased sexual drives may underlie such client behaviors as multiple sexual relationships, inappropriate sexual remarks, or sexual touching of others.

For some clients, such acting out may cause feelings of shame, guilt, and embarrassment. Others lack desire to control their sexual impulses and feel no guilt about any of their sexual behavior.

Clients who act out sexually can have problems in interpersonal relationships. Partners may feel coerced, used, or not considered in the sexual interaction. Partners may also feel betrayed or angry when the clients have sexual interactions with others. Thus, sexual acting out often threatens the satisfaction and stability of interpersonal relationships.

Planning and Implementing Interventions

Nurses play several roles in promoting sexual health. The Mims-Swensen Sexual Health Model (1980) identifies four levels at which nurses can intervene, consistent with their comfort and knowledge.

The *life experience level* of intervention describes a minimal level of effective practice. Interventions are based solely on nurses' own personal experiences. Interventions may be appropriate for clients who share similar life experiences. However, clients holding different values or demonstrating different behaviors may perceive interventions based on the nurses' life experiences as irrelevant.

The *basic level* of intervention to promote sexual health is grounded in nurses' self-awareness combined with a nonjudgmental respect for others' sexual beliefs, practices, and concerns. Nurses at this level have some knowledge about human sexual function. The knowledgeable and nonjudgmental nurse can intervene as a facilitator for clients needing to talk about their sexuality.

The nurse practicing an *intermediate level* of intervention synthesizes knowledge, self-awareness, communication skills, and the use of the nursing process. Nurses are validators of normal sexual behavior and accept the range of sexual expression in our society. Teaching about sexual response is another intervention to resolve client concerns. Teaching is often directed at helping clients understand their stage of sexual development. For instance, teenagers and young adults frequently require accurate information regarding anatomy and physiology, sexual desire, and contraception. Counseling interventions are also implemented in the intermediate level. Counseling is not merely giving advice. The nurse counselor helps clients clarify their sexual problems and decide on alternatives to resolve the problems. Some specific sexual counseling strategies are listed in Table 20–9.

The Mims-Swensen Sexual Health Model identifies the *advanced level* as requiring that nurses have specialized preparation and knowledge of sexual and gender disorders.

Nurses at this level practice sex therapy, develop and present formal education programs, and do sex research. Most nurses refer clients who require sex therapy. Nurses who do function in the sex therapist role should meet the qualifications for practice identified by the American Association of Sex Educators, Counselors, and Therapists (AASECT), which differentiate sex counseling from sex therapy. *Sex counseling* helps clients incorporate their sexual knowledge into satisfying life-styles and socially responsible behavior. *Sex therapy* is a highly specialized, in-depth treatment to help clients resolve serious sexual problems, especially some sexual disorders (AASECT 1979). The resource list in this text gives the address of AASECT, which will provide details about qualifications for specialized practice. In addition, AASECT publishes a national directory of professionals certified to provide sex education, counseling, or therapy. This directory is a resource for nurses referring clients who need sex therapy.

Sex Therapy

There are a variety of approaches to the treatment of sexual disorders. Masters and Johnson (1970) originated the use of a two-person team (a male and female cotherapy model) to treat couples on a short-term basis. Their two-week, daily intensive treatment format revolutionized treatment for sexual problems. Before that, treatment often took years, was done only by psychiatrists, and had varied effectiveness.

The therapy of Masters and Johnson is based on several principles. The focus of treatment is the couple's relationship, with emphasis on their communication. Fears of performance and anxiety about sexual response are discussed with the couple. Behavioral exercises are assigned to overcome these concerns. Education about the physiology of sexual response and the natural processes of sexual function is also emphasized.

Since the introduction of the dual sex team format, many other modes of sex therapy have developed, including individual, couple, and group treatment with one or two sex therapists. The duration of treatment programs also varies. Treatment programs may be for heterosexual or homosexual individuals with sexual dysfunction and sometimes sexual deviations. The effectiveness of these programs depends on the client's needs and the therapists' skill. Helen Singer Kaplan's model of therapy (1979) is one such treatment alternative. In this lengthened form of sex therapy, therapists and clients seek to understand the multiple hidden causes of the sexual disorder. Deep-seated psychologic difficulties are resolved through a psychodynamic approach to sex therapy. One or two therapists can be involved.

Sex therapy programs have these components in common:

1. *Giving permission and reassurance* about the normality of sexual thoughts, fantasies, and behaviors. Per-

Table 20–9
Interventions for Sexual Difficulties

Sexual Difficulty	Guidelines for Therapeutic Intervention	Sexual Difficulty	Guidelines for Therapeutic Intervention
Male erectile disorder	Reestablish a climate of comfort and acceptance for sexual interaction. Encourage client to masturbate and enjoy touch and body stimulation in general.		The emphasis is not on achieving orgasm but on learning erotic preferences. The couple is instructed to use the side-by-side position, which enables both partners to move freely with emphasis on slow, exploratory thrusting. The goal is to develop an ability to enjoy pelvic play with the penis inside the vagina.
Premature ejaculation	The man or woman is instructed to stimulate the erect penis until the premonitory sensations of impending orgasm are felt. Then penile stimulation is abruptly stopped. This process is repeated to lower the threshold of excitability and make the client more tolerant of the stimuli. Sometimes the woman uses the squeeze technique: At the point of orgasm, she squeezes the head of the penis with thumb and first two fingers for 3 to 4 seconds. This stops the urge to ejaculate. The couple is also instructed in ways to reduce friction in the vagina by limiting the frequency of thrusts or the movement within the vagina.	Vaginismus An involuntary tightening or spasm occurs in the outer third of the vagina that can be so severe as to make intercourse impossible.	The initial step is physical demonstration of her involuntary vaginal spasm to the woman by inserting an examining finger into her vagina. Then Hegar dilators in graduated sizes are inserted by the man into the woman's vagina. At first she manually controls his insertion of the smallest dilator. Later he can insert larger dilators following her verbal instructions. After larger dilators are successfully inserted, she is instructed to retain the dilator for several hours each night. Most involuntary spasms can be relieved in three to five days with the daily use of dilators. In addition to physical relief from spastic constriction, therapy is directed toward alleviating the fear that led to the onset of symptoms.
Inhibited female orgasm	Intercourse is avoided. Nongenital caressing exercises begin, with man and woman alternating as the initiator of a session of caressing, thus sharing responsibility for sexual interaction. Next, genital stimulation is added to provide positive sexual experiences without intercourse. When intercourse is attempted, the woman is instructed to assume the superior position and insert the man's penis into her vagina. When setbacks occur, the couple is advised to rely on sexual techniques that do not involve intercourse. The couple is advised to assume a nondemand position for female stimulation. The woman is to place her hand lightly on her partner's to indicate her preference for contact.	Sexual acting out	Identify increased levels of anxiety. Openly discuss meanings of behaviors. Give feedback about inappropriate behavior. Discuss appropriate ways to meet sexual needs. Reassure clients you are not rejecting them but the behavior.

Source: Compiled from Masters W, Johnson V: Human Sexual Inadequacy. Little, Brown, 1970, pp 30–56. Reprinted by permission of the Masters & Johnson Institute, St. Louis, MO.

CASE STUDY: A Client with Premature Ejaculation

Identifying Information

Mr. Blackborn is a 32-year-old married male admitted to the acute care mental health unit two weeks ago. This is his first hospitalization, which was prompted by vague suicidal thoughts related to financial stress. He has increasingly felt the pressure of managing his plumbing business. The loss of a prized plumbing contract precipitated feelings of inadequacy, low self-esteem, and hopelessness. During his hospitalization on the mental health unit, Mr. Blackborn identified strategies to cope with this stress. He initiated contact with a financial advisor and was exploring arrangements for refinancing his business. He explored the relationship of job success to his feelings of self-esteem. Mr. Blackborn now verbalized a renewed sense of self-worth and confidence that he could cope with the business pressure more effectively. He had made an appointment for follow-up counseling at the outpatient clinic. On this day of discharge, before his wife came, the client approached Nurse Kelly to talk

Mr. Blackborn told Nurse Kelly that he was looking forward to discharge, but that he was wondering how he would react to his wife. He had fears about his sexual performance. He stated that he was feeling better about himself regarding his work situation but that he was unsure if he could handle arguments with his wife if he failed in bed again.

Client's Definition of Present Problem, Precipatory Stresses, Coping Strategies, Goals for Care

Mr. Blackborn states that when he and his wife have sex, he "comes too quickly." He expressed concern that his wife might expect this hospitalization to have helped their sexual relationship, but he did not have that expectation. The major concern Mr. Blackborn voiced was coping with his wife's reactions if he again failed in lovemaking. He asked the nurse about her perception of a need for sex counseling. He had always resisted the idea of a counselor when his wife had suggested it, but now thought he might be willing to try to work on this problem. His stay in the mental health unit had allowed him to see he could be helped by others, not just solving problems only by himself.

History of Present Problem

He said that he and his wife both enjoyed sex but that she was frustrated because it was over so quickly and left her unsatisfied. He also was frustrated about this and knew he "let her down" when he "came" too fast. He had always been quick to ejaculate. However, it seemed that over the years, his wife had become less tolerant of the situation. She felt she was missing something. Mr. Blackborn said he ejaculated quickly almost every time he had sexual intercourse. Sometimes he could manage to have insertion of his penis into her vagina for one or two seconds before ejaculating but usually, immediately upon trying to have intercourse, he would ejaculate. He thought it was caused by his "nature." His wife had read that the situation can get better after being married awhile, but it had not seemed to. He had tried to distract himself during lovemaking or have his wife not stimulate him in an effort to last longer. This worked sometimes but not always. He had never sought help professionally for his sexual concerns.

Psychiatric History

No prior psychiatric history.

continued

Case Study (Continued)

Family History	Mr. Blackborn has been married to the same woman eight years. They have two children, a boy of two and a girl of six. He is self-employed as a plumber, a business that he has been in for about a year.
Sexual history	Mr. Blackborn related that he had learned most of his sexual information from kids in school and from health classes. His parents had said little about sexuality except that he should treat girls with respect. He had known that sex before marriage was wrong and that his parents would be upset if he had sex before marriage and they found out. He felt his sexual development was normal in growing up, much like the other boys he knew.
	He and his wife have sexual intercourse two times a week except during the time when he was under stress before this hospitalization. Then, he had little interest. His frequency of sexual interaction was less than once a month. He would like to be more interested in sex and be confident that he could last long enough to satisfy his wife. He had no concerns about birth control since his wife had a tubal ligation. He did not experience physical pain with sexual arousal.
	His masturbation history was of self-stimulation beginning at about age 9. He masturbated once or twice a week, usually when he felt tense. Masturbation served as a physical relaxant for him. Also, he masturbated quickly, ejaculating within one or two minutes. This pattern had been consistent from adolescence through adulthood. He admitted feeling little guilt about masturbation since he felt he needed to do this for relaxation.
Significant Health History	No current or past medical problems. The client was not taking any medications upon discharge. He had taken antianxiety medications while in the hospital but had agreed with his psychiatrist that these were not needed at home.
Current Mental Status	During the interview, Mr. Blackborn maintained eye contact and talked openly. He smoked while describing his sexual concerns but did not appear overanxious. He was alert and oriented, giving an accurate historical account of his sexual problem. His speech was sometimes halted, as he appeared to be thinking of how to express his thoughts about this private topic. He told the nurse it was hard to talk to someone about sex; he had not done this before. Mr. Blackborn did not appear to be delusional or hallucinating. He appeared organized and relevant in his discussion of his concerns. However, the client lacked insight into the causes of his sexual difficulties and had little knowledge of how to proceed to change his sexual interaction. His attitude was cooperative and suggested motivation for changing his situation.

Diagnostic Impression

Nursing Diagnosis— *(PND-1/NANDA)*	05.04	Altered sexuality processes /Sexual dysfunction
	02.03.03	Knowledge deficit* /Knowledge deficit
DSM-IIIR Mutiaxial Diagnosis	Axis I	302.75 Premature ejaculation
		296.22 Major depression, single episode, moderate

PND-I diagnosis also in NANDA list.

continued

Case Study (Continued)

Axis II   None
Axis III   None
Axis IV   Psychosocial stressors: financial and work concerns; marital discord
              Severity: 3
Axis V   Current GAF: 61

Nursing Care Plan

Nursing Diagnosis (PND-I/NANDA)	Client Care Goals	Nursing Planning/ Intervention	Evaluation
05.04 Altered Sexuality Processes/ Sexual dysfunction	Client will verbalize feelings. Client will initiate discussion with wife. Couple will agree to a meeting with the nurse. Couple will accept referral to sex counselor.	Encourage expression of feelings. Offer feedback about appropriateness of feelings. Explore client's view of sexual expression in his marital relationship. Validate importance of concerns with client. Elicit detailed sexual history. Explain need for mutual problem solving with wife. Encourage client to talk with wife about concerns when she comes. Initiate discussion with wife alone, if they agree, to assess her perceptions of the problem. Offer to hold discussion with he and wife for mutual problem solving.	Document client's verbalization of feelings in chart. Document that client initiated discussion with wife. Couple will meet with the nurse. Record in chart that couple accepted referral to sex counselor. Sex counselor will report to nurse that couple kept the appointment.
02.03.03 Knowledge Deficit* /Knowledge deficit	Client will verbalize understanding of sexual function. Client will ask questions to clarify understanding of treatment. Client and wife will verbalize feelings about seeking therapy.	Assess client's knowledge of sexual function. Explore client's definition of premature ejaculation. Explain anatomy and physiology of sexual response as needed. Provide information about the definitions and causes of premature ejaculation.	Document client's understanding of sexual function. Document in chart the feelings the client expressed about seeking sex therapy. Record summary of the couple's meeting with the nurse.

*PND-I diagnosis also in NANDA list.

continued

Case Study (Continued)

Nursing Diagnosis (PND-I/NANDA)	Client Care Goals	Nursing Planning/ Intervention	Evaluation
	Couple will select a referral source. Couple will select one new way to express sensuality and affection.	Provide information about treatment approaches and treatment effectiveness. Provide information about the process of sex therapy. Identify community resources for referral. Offer to meet with the couple to provide information to the wife and answer additional questions they may have. Encourage the couple to explore alternative ways of expressing sensuality in addition to sexual intercourse (caressing, oral or hand stimulation, kissing). Refer couple to sex counselor; make the appointment before they leave.	Record the referral source selected by the couple. Couple will report to sex counselor they have tried one new way of expressing affection.

mission strategies assume the behavior is neither against the law nor involves the nonconsent of another.

2. *Providing information and education* about sexual functions. Specific information is given about the client's particular needs. Some programs also offer a pre-planned package of information that clients may choose or be required to review.

3. *Facilitating attitude change* related to sexual behavior or one's recognition that, as a partner, one participates in the sexual dysfunction and should share the therapy.

4. *Reducing performance concerns.* Strategies to reduce concern include sensate focus exercises during which partners caress each other to experience emerging feelings instead of focusing on attaining orgasm. Other strategies are prohibiting coitus for a period of time and teaching assertive skills or social skills to improve social and sexual confidence.

5. *Increasing communication and effective sexual technique* by identifying methods of communication the couple can use to enhance intimacy and sexual pleasure.

6. *Examining life-style problems.* Sexual expression may not be given any priority. Children and work can often become excuses for infrequent or unsatisfying sexual experiences. Having sex at unsuitable times or under unsatisfactory circumstances can also perpetuate sexual problems.

7. *Structuring sexual experiences* to diminish anxiety, to increase the repertoire of arousing stimuli and sexual techniques, and to treat specific dysfunctions. Structured sexual experiences are more effective when assigned after discussion of feelings and attitudes.

Research has not yet shown which components are critical for an effective outcome; perhaps all are necessary to some.

Evaluation

Methods of evaluating nursing interventions to promote sexual health depend on the criteria specifying desired outcomes. Evaluation criteria should be realistic and measurable. Criteria can be expressed from the point of view of what the client says (Webb 1985). For example

Client will verbalize an understanding of . . .

Client will ask relevant questions about . . .

Client will explain . . . in his own words.

Another method to assess outcome is to evaluate client actions. Clients may agree to talk with their partners about a subject of concern, carry out a specific suggestion, or read a suggested book. To evaluate changes in clients' feelings and attitudes, the nurse can rely on direct observation or on client reports. For instance, a client may state she feels less anxious or more comfortable in the sexual interaction. Or a client may appear calm and relaxed when discussing sexuality with the nurse.

Evaluation of interventions should be a process shared with clients. When nurses or clients feel there has been only partial improvement, alternative interventions need to be identified. Referral to a specialized sex counselor or sex therapist is often an appropriate intervention at this time.

Chapter Highlights

- All humans are sexual beings throughout their life spans; sexual expression is an integral facet of clients' overall health and well-being.

- People have the right to express their sexual needs and desires in ways that reflect their personal value system and life-style.

- Clients have the potential for optimal sexual health through acquiring knowledge about sexuality and having the opportunity to communicate concerns and problems.

- Nurses must be able to accept and respect the client's sexual beliefs, attitudes, and behaviors as equal in value though possibly different from their own personal beliefs, attitudes, and behaviors.

- Gender disorders have multiple causes. Environmental, cultural, and learning influences determine the severity and intensity of the disorders.

- Sexual disorders have psychophysiologic causes. Disorders are classified according to the phase of sexual response that is primarily affected.

- Nurses are appropriate providers of sexual health care by virtue of life experience, self-awareness, communication skills, theoretical knowledge, use of the nursing process, and the unique characteristics of the nurse-client relationship.

- Nurses are responsible and accountable for the delivery of effective sexual health care that includes accurate assessment, diagnosis, education, counseling, and referral.

- Nurses should take a sexual history to assess general sexual health and, if indicated, gather detailed information about specific sexual problems.

- Nursing diagnoses of sexual health status include the major classifications of sexual dysfunction and sexual acting out. Nursing diagnoses of changes in physical or emotional health often are directly associated with diagnoses of changes in sexual health.

- To gauge the effectiveness of nursing interventions for sexual problems, the nurse can evaluate how well the client has absorbed education and what changes the client reports or the nurse observes.

- Nurses may function in the specialized and expanded roles of sex therapist, researcher, and formal educator after advanced preparation that includes in-depth education and supervised experiences.

References

Abramowitz S: Psychosocial outcomes of sex reassignment surgery. *J Consult Clin Psychol* 1986;54:183–189.

American Association of Sex Educators, Counselors, and Therapists: *AASECT Code of Ethics.* AASECT, 1979.

Barbach L: *Women Discover Orgasm.* The Free Press, 1980.

Bernhard L, Dan A: Redefining sexuality from women's own experiences. *Nurs Clin North Am* 1986;21:125–136.

Carpenito L: *Nursing Diagnosis: Application to Clinical Practice.* Lippincott, 1983.

Conte H: Assessment of Sexual Dysfunction. *J Consult Clin Psychol* 1986;54:149–157.

Crooks R, Baur K: *Our Sexuality,* ed 3. Benjamin/Cummings, 1987.

Federation S: Sexual abuse: Treatment modalities for the younger child. *J Psychosoc Nurs Ment Health Serv* 1986;24:21–24.

Frank D: Counseling the infertile couple. *J Psychosoc Nurs Ment Health Serv* 1984;22:17–24.

Frank D, Downard E, Lang A: Androgyny, sexual satisfaction, and women. *J Psychosoc Nurs Ment Health Serv* 1986;24:10–15.

Geer J, Heiman J, Leitenberg H: *Human Sexuality.* Prentice-Hall, 1984.

Glazebrook C, Munjas B: Sex roles and depression. *J Psychosoc Nurs* 1986;24(12):9–12.

Kaplan H: *Disorders of Sexual Desire.* Brunner Mazel, 1979.

Kaplan H, Saddock BJ: *Comprehensive Textbook of Psychiatry, IV.* ed 2. Williams and Wilkins, 1985.

Lenz E, Soeken K, Rankin E, Fischman S: Sex role attributes, gender, and postpartal preceptors of the marital relationship. *Adv Nurs Sci* 1985;7:49–62.

Lo Piccolo J, Stock W: Treatment of sexual dysfunction. *J Consult Clin Psychol* 1986;54:158–167.

Masters W, Johnson V: *Human Sexual Response.* Little, Brown, 1966.

Masters W, Johnson V: *Human Sexual Inadequacy.* Little, Brown, 1970.

Masters W, Johnson V, Kolodny R: *Human Sexual Inadequacy.* Little, Brown, 1970.

McFarland G, Wasli E: *Nursing Diagnoses and Process in Psychiatric Mental Health Nursing.* Lippincott, 1986.

Meyer JK, Schmidt CW Jr, Wise TN: *Clinical Management of Sexual Disorders.* American Psychiatric Press, 1986.

Mims FH, Swensen M: *Sexuality: A Nursing Perspective.* McGraw-Hill, 1980.

Monat KK: *Sexuality and the Mentally Retarded.* College Hill Press, 1982.

Money J: *Love and Love Sickness.* Johns Hopkins, 1980.

Seagraves R: Female orgasm and psychiatric drugs. *J Sex Educ Ther* 1985;11:69–71.

Stoller RJ: *Perversion: The Erotic Form of Hatred.* American Psychiatric Press, 1986.

Valois R, Kammerman S: *Your sexuality: A personal inventory.* Random House, 1984.

Webb C: *Sexuality, Nursing and Health.* John Wiley, 1985.

World Health Organization: Education and treatment in human sexuality. *The Training of Health Professionals,* World Health Organization Technical Report Series, no. 572. WHO, 1975.

TWENTY-ONE

Applying the Nursing Process for

Clients with Personality Disorders

Judy Banks Campbell
Noreen King Poole

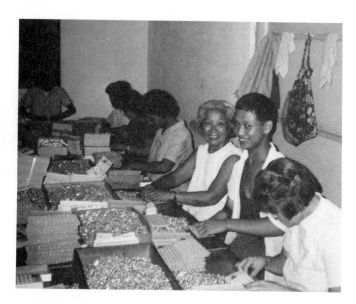

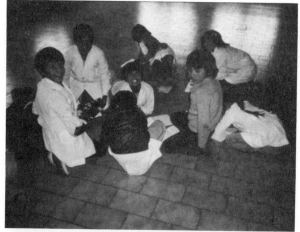

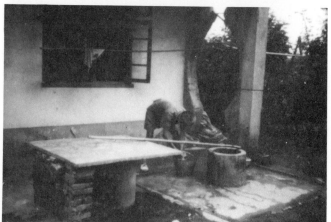

After reading this chapter, students should be able to

- Differentiate personality traits and styles from personality disorders

- Compare and contrast characteristics of various personality disorders

- Correlate DSM-IIIR with the nursing process in providing care for clients with personality disorders

- Apply the nursing process in a variety of clinical settings with clients identified as having personality disorders

- Distinguish developmental characteristics of the major personality disorders

- Relate theoretical concepts, which are supported by research, to the nursing assessment, diagnoses, planning, implementation, and evaluation of clients who have personality disorders

- Apply the nursing process in caring for clients who manifest angry and/or manipulative behavior

- Discuss positive and negative effects of the nurse's emotional responses to clients who have personality disorders

Cross References

Other topics relevant to this content are: Chronicity, Chapter 22; Communication techniques, Chapter 11; Defense mechanisms, Chapter 7; Growth and development, Chapter 6; Nursing process, Chapter 4; Psychiatric theories, Chapter 5.

Decide what your personal responsibilities are.

Key Terms

antisocial personality disorder
anxious-fearful group of personality disorders
avoidant personality disorder
Axis II
borderline personality disorder
compulsive personality disorder
denial
dependent personality disorder
dramatic-erratic group of personality disorders
dysphoria
eccentric group of personality disorders
ego dystonic
ego syntonic
histrionic personality disorder
hypervigilance
narcissistic personality disorder
omnipotence
paranoid personality disorder
passive-aggressive personality disorder
personality disorders
psychodynamics
schizoid personality disorders
schizotypal personality disorder
splitting
trait

Frank consistently compliments his female coworkers. They, in turn, prepare his lunches, lend him money, and make excuses for his sloppy work performance.

Alice interrupts a supervisory meeting to borrow a stapler. She is surprised when her behavior is criticized.

Whenever Keith is asked a personal question, he responds, "Why do you want to know?"

Jill contributes to daily team conferences only when her input is solicited. She prefaces her comments with, "You probably won't think this is important, but. . . ."

Lance offers detailed descriptions of his personal life to anyone who will listen. Quickly bored with his monologues, his listeners do not return for "seconds."

All these people demonstrate persistent behavioral patterns that do not significantly interfere with their lives but may charm, annoy, or frustrate others. Such behavioral patterns may be called personality traits or styles, and they often define the uniqueness of the individual. These life-long patterns are exhibited in a variety of social and personal experiences, and generally anxiety is absent (Eaton et al. 1976). These relatively stable patterns, however, may become rigid and maladaptive, cause significant personal distress, and impair social functioning. When this happens, these personality traits or styles are called **personality disorders**. Since people with personality disorders experience problems in living rather than clinical symptoms, they may not seek professional help unless there is extreme external stress (DSM-IIIR 1987).

The psychiatric nurse encounters people with personality disorders in a variety of settings, including the workplace, counseling centers, general hospitals, and forensic facilities. As Widiger and Frances (1985) point out, the essential features of personality disorders are (a) chronicity, (b) pervasiveness, and (c) maladaptation. All three features must be present to make a psychiatric diagnosis. However, the psychiatric nurse must be aware that personality disorders are extreme exaggerations of personality traits or styles. (A *trait* is a peculiar or unusual mannerism, whereas a *style* is a characteristic way of coping with the environment.) Although the DSM-IIIR delineates diagnostic criteria for personality disorders in the Axis II category, human beings rarely manifest clusters of behaviors that have distinct boundaries. Furthermore, persons with personality disorders may or may not view their life-styles as abnormal or intrusive.

If we assume a common developmental course for the emergence of a person's personality, different levels of adjustment may occur. Consequently, one individual may view peculiarities as "natural" or "eccentric" (**ego syntonic**) and seek no change, while a second person may feel tension and conflict as the behaviors become increasingly rigid and lead to difficulties in a variety of social activities (**ego dystonic**). The person may begin to view a characteristic once valued as unique as a weakness. This changed perspective leads to dissatisfaction and disequilibrium, which motivate the person to seek therapy. Our society contributes to such lack of insight by discouraging direct confrontation and feedback about self-defeating behaviors, thus delaying intervention.

Personality disorders may coexist with extreme psychopathology, considered under DSM-IIIR Axis I groupings. In addition, under stress, the individual with a personality disorder may progressively deteriorate even to the point of psychosis.

COMMON FEATURES OF PERSONALITY DISORDERS

Three major clusters of personality disorders guide psychiatric nurses in diagnostic, treatment, and research issues (see Table 21–1). These clusters are (a) eccentric, (b) dramatic-erratic, and (c) anxious-fearful. The eccentric category includes paranoid, schizoid, and schizotypal personality disorders. The histrionic, narcissistic, antisocial, and borderline personality disorders are included in the dramatic-erratic group. The final cluster groups avoidant,

dependent, compulsive, and passive-aggressive personality disorders in the category **anxious-fearful**. These clusters establish criteria for distinct disorders based upon the presence or absence of symptoms that do not characterize major thought, perceptual, or mood disorders. Because individuals often have personality characteristics that overlap DSM-IIIR Axis II categories, mental health professionals are encouraged to use multiple Axis II diagnoses when necessary. As the psychiatric nurse becomes familiar with the **psychodynamics** and behaviors of people with personality disorders, the following common features emerge:

- Restricted or exaggerated development of a particular pattern or trait
- Restricted or exaggerated moral development
- Restricted or exaggerated problem-solving skills
- Seriously impaired ability to develop meaningful interpersonal relationships and communications
- Difficulty in adjusting to social or occupational relationships
- Defensive coping strategies against real or perceived threats to the sense of self
- Lifelong pattern of responding that is consistent in most situations and that becomes accentuated under stress
- Self-stabilizing and self-perpetuating level of functioning despite distorted coping strategies
- Exaggerated or restricted affective responses to the environment, e.g., overly sensitive, unemotional, "cold"
- Conflict with others, either in the immediate family or in society
- Lack of awareness that others view the life-style as different or unusual

HISTORICAL AND THEORETICAL FOUNDATIONS

Our styles of perceiving, thinking, and responding shape our ability to adapt and defend our sense of self (Shapiro 1965). Biologic, developmental, and experiential factors determine a person's general life-style, which affects his or her style of defense. If we accept that each human being is unique in biologic endowment, mental capacity, and environmental stimuli, then it follows that early object relations (e.g., material things, actions, people, and symbols) give rise to behavioral responses that defend the person from threats to the self (Schaefer and Lamm 1986, p 18). As the individual experiences life, his or her adaptive-defensive operations solidify, ultimately crystallizing into an automatic response style. When the response style is based on misperceived or distorted object relations, a personality disorder may emerge. Given these premises, the psychiatric nurse using a humanistic interactionist model

Table 21–1
Clusters of Personality Disorders

Eccentric	Dramatic-Erratic	Anxious-Fearful
Paranoid	Borderline	Avoidant
Schizoid	Histrionic	Dependent
Schizotypal	Narcissistic	Obsessive compulsive
	Antisocial	Passive-Aggressive

Source: Adapted from American Psychiatric Association: Diagnostic and Statistical Manual of Mental Disorders, *ed 3. APA, 1987, p 337.*

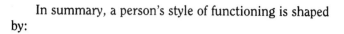

views clients with personality disorders as people whose communication and behavior are greatly influenced by past experiences, a need to maintain self-direction and control, and a unique style of interpreting their world. The following example demonstrates how an office worker defends her rigid response pattern:

Martha, a 49-year-old secretary, is a perfectionist and shows exaggerated loyalty to her company. Most of her energies are directed toward work and being indispensable to her employer. She consistently takes work home at night and weekends, even postponing her vacation to complete elaborate, detailed reports. Martha's relationships with co-workers focus on work only; she is unable to socialize with co-workers without experiencing extreme anxiety. Consequently, others view her as rigid, isolated, cold, and tense. They try to avoid relating to her. When during a performance evaluation her employer pointed out her defensive peer relationships, Martha became irritable and pressured, stating, "I was not hired to socialize. Those people who complain should be doing their work and earning the paychecks they receive."

Martha's definition of any situation is based on her narrow view of the world and her purpose in it. When confronted with her behavior, she does not attend to personal issues but rather focuses on the technical details of the situation. Martha justifies her position by falling back on the rules and regulations that reinforce her own moral convictions. Even with her distorted strategies, Martha is able to achieve stable functioning. As a result, people interacting with Martha generally choose not to confront the frustrating behaviors. Instead, they accept her "peculiarities" as a trade-off for her work performance. The likelihood that Martha will change her response style is minimal unless she experiences deep dissatisfaction and begins to examine her own personality traits.

In summary, a person's style of functioning is shaped by:

- Original biopsychosocial characteristics
- Object relations
- Reinforcement of behavioral responses

Table 21–2 illustrates the developmental concepts identified above and their interaction. It is only when we acknowledge the individual's response style and definition of a situation that we can identify the subjective meaning of a thought, feeling, or behavior for that person.

Little systematic research has been conducted on the causes or treatment of personality disorders (Widiger 1985). Furthermore, debate continues about the developmental course of personality disorders. Some theorists argue that their course of development is different from that of anxiety-related and psychotic forms of maladaptation. Other theorists see personality disorders as belonging in a developmental continuum that includes personality disorders, anxiety-related disorders, and psychoses. Table 21–3 illustrates the response patterns associated with the personality disorders discussed in DSM-IIIR.

CLUSTERS OF PERSONALITY DISORDERS

In 1980, DSM-III grouped the personality disorders into three clusters (see Table 21–1). In presenting the nursing care plans for clients with personality disorders, we shall follow this organization. In addition, DSM-IIIR designates a residual category of personality disorders to include people who meet some of the criteria for more than one personality disorder but who do not manifest sufficient responses in any one category to be assigned an Axis II diagnosis.

Eccentric Personality Disorders

The paranoid, schizotypal, and schizoid personalities are identified as "odd or eccentric" in the DSM-IIIR (1987, p 337). The major features of these disorders are social detachment and consequent impairment in social and occupational functioning. These disorders are frequently observed in family members of schizophrenic persons (Kendler et al 1984). People with these disorders have been identified as having more cognitive style impairments than people with the disorders in the other DSM-III clusters (Torgersen 1984, Widiger 1985). The eccentric disorders

---

Table 21–2
Factors Influencing Style of Functioning

Factor	Definition	Example
Original biopsychosocial characteristics	Unique endowment of qualities, e.g., physical form, mental ability, and social group	An 8-year-old Korean child is adopted by white American parents. The child experiences rejection from his classmates because of his physical characteristics. Consequently, he begins to avoid situations, and he scrutinizes others' behavior for hidden motives.
Object relations	Interaction between the individual and objects in the environment, e.g., people, material things, symbols	An upwardly mobile professional couple demand perfection and conformity from their 7-year-old daughter. They discourage fantasy and creativity. The daughter procrastinates and follows directions half-heartedly in coping with her parents' demands.
Reinforcement of behavioral responses	A reward or punishment that strengthens or weakens a person's responses	A highly anxious mother gives in to her child's demands when the child has a temper tantrum; she fails to respond positively to the child's "good" behaviors. The child rarely makes polite requests, but interrupts, screams, and shouts for attention.

Interaction of Factors

The medicine man of the Hopi Indians sometimes uses meditation to diagnose illnesses. He may even use a crystal ball as his focal point during meditation. At other times the Hopi medicine man chews roots of jimsonweed (datura) to go into a trance as he meditates. The ensuing hallucinations are believed by the Hopis to be visions of the evil that caused the sickness. After the meditation, he prescribes an appropriate herbal treatment, e.g., fever is "cured" by a plant that smells like lightning. Indeed, the Hopi phrase for fever is "lightning sickness" (Spector 1985).

Table 21–3
Response Patterns Associated with Personality Disorders (DSM-IIIR)

Type	Characteristics	Type	Characteristics
Eccentric Styles			preoccupations. Is suspicious and hypersensitive to real or imagined criticism. Isolates self from society.
Paranoid	Is pervasively and unjustifiably suspicious and mistrustful, as evidenced by jealousy, envy, and guardedness. Is hypersensitive and usually feels mistreated and misjudged. Restricts feelings, as evidenced by lack of humor, absence of sentimental or tender feelings, and pride in being cold and unemotional.	**Dramatic-Erratic Styles**	
		Histrionic	Is overly dramatic and reactive, and responds intensely. Engages in attention seeking, self-dramatization, and irrational outbursts of emotion. Is perceived by others as shallow, self-indulgent, vain, demanding, dependent, and inconsiderate. Is prone to manipulative threats and gestures.
Schizoid	Is emotionally cold and aloof. Shows indifference to the praise or criticism of others. Has no desire for social involvement and a tendency to be reserved and reclusive.		
Schizotypal	Manifests various oddities of thought, perceptions, speech, and behavior, such as ideas of reference, bizarre fantasies, and	Narcissistic	Has grandiose sense of self-importance. Is preoccupied with fantasies of unlimited success, power, beauty, brilliance, etc. Needs attention and admiration.

continued

Table 21–3 *(Continued)*
Response Patterns Associated with Personality Disorders (DSM-IIIR)

Type	Characteristics	Type	Characteristics
	Is indifferent or reacts to criticism with rage, feelings of inferiority, or humiliation. In relations with others, expects special favors. Takes advantage of others; shifts between overidealizing others to disregarding them. Lacks ability for empathy.	**Anxious-Fearful**	
		Avoidant	Is hypersensitive to rejection and interprets innocuous events as ridicule. Is unwilling to become involved with others unless given a guarantee of acceptance. Withdraws socially in interpersonal and work roles. Desires affection and acceptance. Has low self-esteem and is overly dismayed by personal shortcomings.
Borderline	Is impulsive and unpredictable in areas of life that are self-damaging. Has unstable but intense interpersonal relationships involving manipulation of others. Displays temper inappropriately. Has unstable moods (including rage); is uncertain about identity, and intolerant of being alone. May inflict physical damage on self. Has chronic feelings of boredom and emptiness.	Dependent	Passively allows others to assume responsibility for major areas of life. Subordinates own needs to those on whom client depends to avoid possibility of having to rely on self. Lacks self-confidence.
		Obsessive compulsive	Is overconscientious, overmeticulous, and perfectionistic. Is excessively concerned with conformity. Adheres rigidly to strict standards. Is prone to self-doubt, unhappiness, and worry. Has limited ability to express warm and tender emotions; is preoccupied with trivial details, rules, schedules, and lists.
Antisocial	Engages in behavior that causes conflict with society, e.g., theft, vandalism, fighting, delinquency, truancy. Is unable to sustain consistent work or to function as a responsible parent or spouse. Cannot maintain enduring attachment to sexual partner. Lacks respect or loyalty; is irritable and aggressive. Manipulates others for personal gain, does not plan ahead, lacks guilt, does not learn from past experiences, blames others.	Passive-aggressive	Resists demands for adequate functioning through indirect methods, e.g., procrastination, dawdling, stubbornness, intentional inefficiency, and forgetfulness.

are the most peculiar and reflect the most maladaptive defensive styles.

The Nursing Process and Paranoid Personality Disorders

Nursing Assessment: Defining Characteristics of the Paranoid Personality

Suspiciousness and Mistrust Suspiciousness and mistrust reflect an attitude of doubt toward the trustworthiness of objects or people. The suspicious person is usually preoccupied with being maneuvered, tricked, or framed. Suspiciousness is also a way of thinking and includes such manifestations as expectations of trickery or harm, guardedness, secretiveness, jealousy, doubt of others' loyalty, and overconcern with hidden motives and special meanings. For example, the suspicious person may perceive a birthday gift as a trick to create an obligation.

Rigidity Paranoid people are inflexible in their perception of the world. They are preoccupied with their expectations of others and relentlessly try to confirm these expectations, often through argumentation. Rational arguments and contrary information are closely examined, but with prejudice. The paranoid person justifies a position by excessive rationalization. Any evidence refuting the original notion is rejected. It is not unusual for a paranoid person to suspect people with opposing ideas. The paranoid person goes to great lengths to prove a point, making mountains out of molehills. A need to be in control and have power is another characteristic, as is a preoccupation with the rank and status of themselves and others.

Hypervigilance   The hypervigilant individual is a keen, penetrating observer, far more attentive and acute than the ordinary person (Shapiro 1965, p 58). Constant sensitivity to nuances in social relations, interpretation of both open and hidden attitudes of others, and scrutiny are modes of operation.

Following a bomb threat, a unit clerk carefully observes and documents all packages brought into the ICU by staff and visitors, anticipating that someone will bring weapons into the unit.

Distortions of Reality   Although paranoid people may perceive facts accurately, they invest them with a special significance. In this way, they create a private reality. They have a special interest in hidden motives, underlying purposes, special meanings, and the like. They do not necessarily disagree with the average observer about the existence of any given fact, only about its meaning and significance. Therefore, even severely paranoid people can recognize various essential facts well enough to achieve a limited adjustment to the normal social world. At the same time, however, they continue to interpret substantial portions of this world autistically. They often have difficulty distinguishing real from imagined offenses. The individual's distorted attitudes antagonize others and may lead to real discrimination.

A paranoid woman is quick to detect signs of anger, jealousy, and rejection in the actions of her co-workers. She magnifies these negative aspects and overlooks such positive behaviors as humor, support, and empathy. Eventually, her co-workers begin to snicker when she makes public statements, and they gossip about her.

Projection   Paranoid people attribute to external figures their own intolerable motivations, drives, or feelings. Some psychiatric theorists believe that paranoid people use projection to attribute to others the evil intentions that they themselves feel. In this way, the idea that one may be harmed really reflects the individual's own wish to harm others.

Nancy's idea that her boyfriend is seeing another woman may reflect her wish to terminate their relationship.

Restricted Affect   Lack of emotional expressiveness and spontaneity are observed in paranoid people. These individuals often appear cold, humorless, and devoid of tender, sensitive feelings. They pride themselves on remaining objective and rational. They frequently use intellectualization and rationalization to avoid affective experiences. Some paranoid people may appear friendly, but in fact, this friendliness is a "script" that helps them adapt to social situations or achieve their goals.

The Process of Exclusion   As a consequence of the paranoid person's antagonism, suspiciousness, and restricted object relations, tension develops between the person and significant others. The persistent strain on relationships cause others to define the paranoid person as more than simply "different." Instead, the individual is described as unreliable or untrustworthy, and others begin to interact according to their perceptions. These behaviors reinforce the suspicions and beliefs of the paranoid person. The effects of this process include:

- Blocked communication, which increases the process of exclusion
- Emergence of a crisis, which formally excludes the paranoid person
- Reinforcement of the paranoid person's beliefs, interpretations, or ideas of reference

See Box 21–1 for an example of a paranoid person's behavior and recommended nursing interventions.

Because paranoid persons are generally intelligent, persuasive, and creative in justifying their beliefs, these clients may adapt in one of two ways. The person may join quasipolitical groups, esoteric religions, or quasiscientific organizations that reinforce his or her interpretations of reality. Or the paranoid person may join organizations that challenge societal norms and trends in an effort to direct and thus control hostile feelings.

Nursing Diagnosis

After gathering objective and subjective data about the paranoid client's behavior, the nurse categorizes the information into problem areas designated as nursing diagnostic categories. It is critical to involve the client in all steps of the treatment planning process in order to enhance participation and promote planned changes. DSM-IIIR psychiatric diagnoses, and current NANDA and PND nursing diagnoses for the paranoid client are shown in the nursing care plan on the following pages. The general nursing diagnostic groupings that follow for this client focus on psychosocial needs only. They reflect a synthesis of themes in specific PND-I and NANDA categories. The psychiatric nurse develops individualized care plans to address the unique needs of each client assessed.

Coping, Ineffective Individual The client demonstrates impairment of adaptive behaviors in meeting life's demands. The paranoid personality may exhibit these forms of ineffective coping, among others:

- Suspiciousness
- Limited affect
- Reluctance to confide in others
- Carrying grudges
- Pessimistic regard for others

Thought Processes, Altered The paranoid client experiences impaired cognitive functioning without loss of reality contact. Behaviors often observed include:

- Preoccupation with theories of conspiracies
- Hypervigilance and hypersensitivity
- Misinterpretation of benign remarks as threats
- Egocentricity
- Perseveration
- Impaired problem solving

Communication, Impaired The predominant communication dysfunctions of the paranoid personality are distortions and overuse of defense mechanisms related to high levels of fear and anxiety. Communication impairments include:

- Failure to interpret messages accurately
- Stereotyping others
- Judgmental attitudes toward others
- Failure to listen actively
- Arrogance
- Aggressiveness
- Overuse of defense mechanisms of denial, rationalization, projection, and intellectualization

Planning and Implementing Interventions

Nursing interventions with the paranoid client center around mutual decision making. The goal of all interventions is to diminish the client's pervasive suspiciousness, distortions of thought, communication problems, and resulting

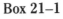

Box 21–1
NURSING INTERVENTIONS USEFUL WITH THE PARANOID CLIENT

Jim, a 39-year-old engineer, suspects that his employer is withholding significant data from him pertaining to an important job assignment. Jim began to question others about the reliability and integrity of his boss. Jim went to the plant one Sunday morning without authorization. A security guard found him going through the filing cabinets of his employer, who confronted him the following day and sent him to the employee assistance program nurse. During the interview, Jim states, "I knew he [the employer] was dishonest from the start. He never could give me a straight answer. As soon as I was almost on him, he sets me up to lose face and maybe my job."

Nursing Responses

- Remain calm, nonthreatening, and nonjudgmental in all interactions.
- Give clear information regarding confidentiality and job-related consequences of counseling sessions.
- Assist client to identify and verbalize feelings.
- Respond to suspicious ideas by focusing on feelings, e.g., "It must be distressing . . ."; "You see him as vindictive . . ."
- Do not interpret client's beliefs or argue with him about them.
- Include client in formulating the treatment contract.
- Focus on ideas that are reality based.
- Inform client of the emotional cues he gives to others, e.g., suspiciousness, intimidation, contempt. Encourage him to validate your perceptions.

---

impairment of role performance. See the following pages for a detailed nursing care plan for the paranoid client.

Evaluation

Coping, Ineffective Individual It is unlikely that the paranoid client will give up coping responses developed over a lifetime. Consistently used interventions, however, should reduce anxiety and allow the client to identify at least one significant person as trustworthy. At the least, the client should be able to relax sufficiently in the presence of the nurse to explore how his or her coping modes have created

Text continues on p. 540

Nursing Care Plan: The Client with a Paranoid Personality Disorder

Nursing Diagnosis (PND-I/NANDA)	Client Care Goals	Nursing Planning/ Interventions	Evaluation
06.01.02 Hyperalertness 06.01.24 Selective attention 04.02 Altered feeling patterns 05.03 Altered role performance /Coping, ineffective individual (associated with responses such as exclusion; restricted, controlled affect, guardedness, seclusiveness, and secretiveness) 05.05 Altered social interaction /Social isolation	The client will diminish suspicious behavior and establish effective and satisfying relationships with staff and significant others.	(Ineffective Coping) 1. Respect the client's privacy and preferences as much as is reasonable. 2. Give feedback to client based on observed nonverbal cues of responsiveness, e.g., eye movement, posturing, voice tones. 3. Point out inconsistent behaviors such as affect/ verbalization. 4. Provide a daily schedule of activities and inform client of changes as needed. 5. Help client identify adaptive diversionary activities, e.g., leisure, recreation, in one-to-one sessions and groups. 6. Encourage client to evaluate how his or her behaviors led to the current crisis. 7. Gradually introduce client to group situations. 8. Use role playing techniques to help client identify feelings, thoughts, and responses that are experienced in stressful situations.	1. Attends and spontaneously participates in short one-to-one sessions and activity groups (less than 1 hour). 2. Initiates one-to-one sessions with assigned staff member. 3. Approaches other clients and staff without encouragement. 4. Identifies personal behaviors that precipitated hospitalization. 5. Demonstrates a variety of moods appropriate to situation encountered. 6. Attends to individual and group tasks without attaching unusual meanings to them. 7. Identifies support systems outside the therapeutic relationship.
02.02 Altered judgment 02.08.03 Altered problem solving 02.07.02 Ideas of reference /Thought processes, altered (associated with suspiciousness, rigidity, distortions of reality, projection, and hypersensitivity)	The client will develop a sense of reality that is validated by others.	1. Tell the client firmly and kindly that you do not share his or her interpretations of an event, while acknowledging his or her feelings. 2. Follow through on commitments made to client (e.g., contracts).	1. Focuses on ideas that are reality based. 2. Accepts positive feedback without questioning motives or hidden meanings. 3. Accepts responsibility for own feelings and thoughts without attributing them to

continued

Nursing Care Plan: The Client with a Paranoid Personality Disorder *(continued)*

Nursing Diagnosis (PND-I/NANDA)	Client Care Goals	Nursing Planning/ Intervention	Evaluation
		3. Assign the same staff member to work with the client to establish consistency and trust.	others, e.g., makes "I" statements.
		4. Give positive reinforcement for successes in a matter-of-fact manner.	4. Remains in a group activity for the duration of the activity.
		5. Respond honestly to the client at all times.	5. Realistically applies the problem-solving process, including making plans for after discharge.
		6. Refocus conversation to reality-based topics and set limits on the duration and frequency of suspicious concerns during one-to-one sessions and groups.	
		7. Do not argue with illogical assertions but simply point out that you do not share the same beliefs.	
05.01 Altered communication processes 04.98 Altered emotional processes not otherwise specified /Communication, impaired: verbal (associated with argumentativeness, critical comments about others, arrogance, aggressiveness, and defensiveness)	The client will express thoughts and feelings verbally in a nonaggressive manner.	1. Use an objective, matter-of-fact approach with client. 2. Use concrete, specific words rather than global abstractions. 3. Give feedback concerning behavior. 4. Identify feelings presented by client during interactions. For example, "I notice some reluctance on your part to tell me about that"; or "From the way you are looking at me, I wonder if you think I'll break my promise?" 5. Direct client to clarify the person or object when pronouns are used. 6. Keep verbal and nonverbal messages clear and consistent.	1. Expresses feelings without intellectualizing. 2. Consensually validates perceptions of events with a staff member or significant others. 3. Makes assertive nonjudgmental statements to staff and other clients. 4. Responds to feedback without rationalizing, projecting, or intellectualizing.

continued

Nursing Care Plan: The Client with a Paranoid Personality Disorder *(continued)*

Nursing Diagnosis (PND-I/NANDA)	Client Care Goals	Nursing Planning/ Interventions	Evaluation
		7. Conduct brief one-to-one sessions daily (avoid prolonged sessions).	
		8. Encourage client to express feelings through creative modes (e.g., drawing, writing) and to discuss the same.	
		9. Involve in communication skills groups, e.g., assertiveness training, current events.	

problems in living and to identify ways to avoid future conflicts with others.

Thought Processes, Altered   Consistency and structure help direct the client's thoughts to here-and-now reality. The nurse can use role modeling to reach this goal, i.e., the nurse tests reality appropriately to encourage the client to do the same. When the client begins to voice doubts about his or her own interpretations or begins to identify alternative interpretations, the nurse is in a position to reinforce the client's achievements. Many paranoid clients simply learn not to discuss their illogical or irrational beliefs with others.

Communication, Impaired   The client should learn to make global statements concrete and to clarify verbal expressions. The client may learn to defuse anxiety-producing situations by making "I" statements rather than responding aggressively and judgmentally. Creative modes of expressing feelings are perceived as an acceptable, nonthreatening outlet. Behavior in groups should reflect the client's increasing ability to accept varying opinions without attaching personal significance to them.

The Nursing Process and Schizoid-Schizotypal Personality Disorders

Nursing Assessment: Defining Characteristics of Schizoid and Schizotypal Personalities

Persons with schizoid and schizotypal personality disorders generally have a detached and aloof social style. The schiz-

otypal personality, however, has more cognitive impairments than the schizoid personality does. There is a range of adjustment in clients with these personality disorders. Some are fairly well-adjusted individuals who are loners; others live out their lives in protective environments, e.g., group homes, mental hospitals, and prisons. When conducting nursing assessments, the nurse needs to rule out the possibility of a crisis response or chemical dependency.

Lifelong Patterns of Social Isolation   These individuals show a preference for solitary interests and occupations. They have a history of being loners and are indifferent to feedback and insensitive to others.

Blunted Affective Response   The person may appear cool, aloof, humorless, "in a fog," bored, and perhaps even mentally retarded although the IQ would negate this assumption (Cameron and Rychlak 1985).

Detachment from the Environment   The individual appears absent-minded, daydreams, is vague about goals and indecisive, and lacks social skills.

The schizotypal personality demonstrates eccentricities in communication and behavior not seen in the schizoid personality. Examples include (a) such oddities of thought as magical thinking and ideas of reference; (b) altered perceptions, e.g., illusions, depersonalization, and derealization; and (c) speech alterations, e.g., circumstantiality (giving detailed, factual but nonessential information), digression, and metaphorical speech patterns.

Some researchers have found that schizoid and schizotypal personality disorders are significantly more common among relatives of schizophrenic clients. At this time, however, there is no substantial evidence that these personality disorders are early indicators of a future schizophrenic process (Kendler et al. 1984, Torgensen 1984).

Rhoda is a 50-year-old homeless female seen in the emergency room of a large metropolitan hospital. She was brought in after experiencing a hypoglycemic episode in the lobby of a museum. Rhoda's appearance is unkempt and eccentric. She is wearing three layers of clothing and mismatched shoes. She has many sores, bruises, and insect bites on her arms and legs. Her hair is matted and infested with lice. Rhoda reports living under the stairwell of a "friend's" house and finding food in trash bins at grocery stores and restaurants. During the nursing admission interview, Rhoda makes frequent inappropriate grimaces and mutters to herself about getting "back home." She avoids answering the nurse's questions and states, "I don't need any help. I have my own remedies that work just fine. Leave me alone." Following stabilization of her condition, Rhoda is released to the streets against medical advice.

Nursing Diagnosis

Persons in the schizoid-schizotypal personality categories are not a danger to themselves or others, a criterion used to authorize long-term hospitalization. They are frequently found among "street people" or marginal individuals called "bag ladies," although some have the financial reserves to lead more adaptive life-styles. They are often brought to the attention of health professionals as a result of cluttered, negligent life-styles that are considered asocial, unaesthetic, and unhygienic. Assessment of these clients may be hampered by their preference for independence, in spite of the negative consequences such "freedom" may have. If the psychiatric nurse is able to sustain a relationship with these clients, the following NANDA nursing diagnoses are often the basis for guiding nursing care (NANDA and PND-I diagnoses are compared in this chapter's care plans).

Coping, Ineffective Individual   These clients have a narrow range of coping skills and tend to resist acquiring new skills if they must give up their independence as a result. Ineffective coping may be identified from the following problems:

- Social isolation
- Inadequate social skills
- Lack of ongoing support systems

Communication, Impaired   Schizoid-schizotypal clients have minimal verbal and nonverbal interactions with others. Typical behaviors may include but are not restricted to:

- Aloofness
- Restricted affect
- Indifference or excessive social anxiety

Self-Care Deficits   These deficits are characteristically seen, particularly in those clients who live on the streets. All aspects of activities of daily living may be involved, including:

- Inadequate hygiene
- Bizarre grooming
- Presence of vermin
- Failure to seek health care or adhere to prescribed regimens

Nutrition, Altered   Nutritional alterations may be the result of lack of knowledge, inadequate living arrangements, or lack of interest and motivation. Nutritional alterations often lead to physical problems that precipitate visits to emergency rooms and neighborhood clinics. The nurse may be identifying the following problems in this category:

- Obesity
- Anorexia
- Malnutrition
- Dehydration

Home Maintenance Management, Altered   Impaired home maintenance includes all aspects of one's ability to make the environment healthful and safe. Problem areas are:

- Inadequate housing or lack of housing
- Inadequate sanitation facilities
- Rodent- or vermin-infested living quarters
- Inability to manage finances
- Insufficient income or lack of income

Planning and Implementing Interventions

The nursing care plan for the client with a schizoid or schizotypal personality disorder is on the following pages. The goal of nursing interventions is to provide an uncomplicated, supportive environment that is safe and nonthreatening to the client. It is hoped that this approach will prevent deterioration and will enhance the client's level of adaptation and functioning. Because the schizoid and schizotypal personalities have extreme difficulty with emotional commitments, the nurse must be watchful of stressful conditions that could precipitate a psychotic episode.

Nursing Care Plan: The Client with a Schizoid-Schizotypal Disorder

Nursing Diagnosis (PND-I/NANDA)	Client Care Goals	Nursing Planning/ Interventions	Evaluation
05.03.02 Altered leisure role 05.05.02 Social isolation/ withdrawal /Coping, ineffective individual (associated with social isolation, inadequate social skills, lack of support system)	The client will increase level of attachment to available social support systems.	1. Provide client with schedule of daily activities (in-patient and day treatment programs). 2. Approach client for one-to-one sessions on a daily basis. 3. Assign same staff members to client to develop rapport and trust. 4. Encourage client to attend and participate in group activities, beginning with those that involve limited interaction and progressing to those of a more verbal nature. 5. Enlist client's cooperation in identifying needs and participating in treatment plan, including goal setting and planning.	1. Participates in ongoing support systems offered by community mental health clinic. 2. Initiates at least one interaction with a staff member daily.
05.01.02 Altered verbal communication /Communication, impaired: verbal (associated with detachment, aloofness, and lack of spontaneity) 04.97 Undeveloped emotional responses	The client will increase effective interactions with others.	1. Link with case management system at community mental health clinic. 2. Involve in nonthreatening verbal group activities, e.g., current events, social skills groups, leisure skills. 3. Focus on low-stress topics to encourage normal speech.	1. Selects one activity for the group three times weekly. 2. Remains out of room at least six hours daily. 3. Speaks for ten minutes without introducing circumstantial material.
01.03.02 Altered grooming* 01.03.04 Altered hygiene* /Self-care deficit: dressing/ grooming /Self-care deficit: bathing/ hygiene	The client will maintain adequate hygiene and grooming.	Set up bathing/grooming schedule for client and assist client with tasks, daily.	1. Bathes and changes clothing at least three times weekly. 2. Prepares dirty laundry

*PND-I diagnosis also on NANDA list.

continued

Nursing Care Plan: The Client with a Schizoid-Schizotypal Disorder *(continued)*

Nursing Diagnosis (PND-I/NANDA)	Client Care Goals	Nursing Planning/ Interventions	Evaluation
07.06 Altered nutrition processes* /Nutrition, altered: less than body requirements (associated with malnutrition, deficit in normal weight, and vitamin deficiencies)	The client will maintain adequate nutrition, hydration, and elimination.	1. Monitor and record client's intake daily. 2. Refer for dietary consult and implement recommendations. 3. Schedule and assist with PE. 4. Administer dietary supplements, as ordered. 5. Discuss with client the minimum requirements for an adequate diet and ways to obtain these necessary foods. 6. Monitor bowel patterns daily.	1. Eats three balanced meals daily. 2. Participates in a complete physical exam within 48 hours of hospitalization. 3. Gains 2–3 lbs weekly while hospitalized. 4. Takes vitamin supplements as ordered. 5. Reports any problems of elimination to nursing staff.
03.03 Altered home maintenance* /Home maintenance management, impaired (associated with inadequate housing, inability to manage finances, lack of sanitation)	The client will be physically safe postdischarge.	1. Refer to social services for assessment and HRS link-up. 2. Provide client with list of emergency services, e.g., crisis hotline, Salvation Army, shelters for homeless.	1. Accepts social service plan to locate adequate housing, food, and medical care. 2. Accepts referral to human services for evaluation and support.

PND-I diagnosis also on NANDA list.

Evaluation

Although health care providers often address the needs of schizoid-schizotypal persons, it is difficult to persuade them to cooperate with and adhere to structured treatment plans after they are discharged from in-patient settings or halfway houses. In structured settings, these clients perform on the fringe of the group, needing encouragement and reinforcement to become involved in self-care, meal planning, and leisure activities.

Coping, Ineffective Individual These clients may not achieve dramatic behavioral and personality changes. If, however, the client is able to maintain a therapeutic alliance with the psychiatric nurse as an outpatient in individual or group settings, the goal of increasing the client's level of attachment may be met.

Communication, Impaired If the client remains linked with the support system, increasing levels of interaction

should occur. Any appropriate verbal or nonverbal response by the client may indicate motivation and progress toward meeting the goal of effective communication. By focusing on low-stress topics during interactions, (e.g., weather, travel, current events, games, cards) and using clear, concise speech, the nurse encourages the client to use more direct and meaningful speech patterns.

Self-Care Deficit Some of these clients carry all their belongings with them and frequently bathe in bus terminal restrooms. For this reason, it may be difficult to teach and monitor adequate self-care activities. The nurse can help those clients who are not homeless to maintain adequate hygiene by assisting the client in developing weekly schedules for self-care activities.

Nutrition, Altered Linking these clients with meals-on-wheels or congregate dining facilities following discharge from in-patient settings not only facilitates adequate nutrition but also encourages increased social interactions.

Because many of their physical problems are the result of poor nutrition, the nurse should use a variety of resources to teach nutritional concepts, e.g., pictures, activity groups, cooking classes, and outings to grocery stores.

Home Maintenance Management, Impaired Because the schizoid or schizotypal client values independence highly, any interventions must take into account the client's preferences and former life-style. If the client has a history of transience, giving him or her a list of community resources may prevent life-management crises. Guardianship by government agencies may be necessary and desirable if the client is incompetent to care for himself or herself.

Dramatic-Erratic Personality Disorders

The borderline, histrionic, narcissistic, and antisocial personality disorders are identified in DSM-IIIR as "dramatic, emotional, erratic" dysfunctions. Individuals with these disorders are often in conflict with society due to their impulsive behavior. Impulsive people view the world as a discontinuous, fragmented conglomerate of opportunities, frustrations, and affective experiences. They live in the present. They lack the ability to examine hunches and to formulate long-range plans. They act decisively without critical evaluation of consequences. Intellectual and emotional goals are focused on achieving immediate gain and satisfaction. This lack of impulse control and inability to delay gratification often result in both verbal and nonverbal outbursts of anger, which may be self- or other-directed. Indeed, clients with dramatic-erratic personality disorders may experience rapid escalation of anxiety when their own angry impulses are not controlled by others. Table 21–4 illustrates some common angry behaviors and offers guidelines for nursing interventions.

Most researchers agree that psychologic fixations in the genital stage of development account for many of the behaviors noted in this cluster of disorders (Cameron and Rychlak 1985). Specifically, parental deprivation; inadequate, excessive, or inconsistent discipline; and failure of the child to develop integrated cognitive, affective, and behavioral modes in early life may lead to these disorders. Clients have generalized feelings of low self-esteem, need to control people and situations, and are unable to delay gratification. In response, dramatic-erratic clients tend to interact by negatively manipulating others. While manipulation is a standard response in the repertoire of people with these personality disorders, its occurrence escalates with increased stress. Table 21–5 illustrates some manipulative behaviors and offers guidelines for nursing interventions.

Common features of the dramatic-erratic cluster of

Box 21–2
COMMON FEATURES OF DRAMATIC-ERRATIC PERSONALITIES

- Labile affective responses
- Intense episodes of anger/rage
- Self-centeredness/egocentricity
- Unstable personal relationships
- Superficiality, exploitiveness, and manipulativeness
- Lack of empathy for others
- Inability to postpone gratification
- Boredom or need for constant attention
- Poor judgment
- Failure to learn by experience
- Failure to assume responsibility for behavior
- Poorly integrated sexual identity
- Ability to test reality and absence of major thought or affective disorders

---

personality disorders are summarized in Box 21–2. Due to its instability and the potential for transient psychotic symptoms, the borderline personality disorder is discussed first.

The Nursing Process and Borderline Personality Disorders

Nursing Assessment: Defining Characteristics of the Borderline Personality

Although the person with a borderline personality disorder is unstable in a variety of areas, e.g., relationships, mood, and self-image, no single feature is invariably present. Of the eight criteria in DSM-IIIR, at least five must be observed to diagnose this disorder. Although some theorists characterize borderline personality disorders as occupying a place on a continuum between neurotic and psychotic disorders, a great deal of research data are being compiled to identify causative factors (Cameron and Rychlak 1985). To date, the data lend support to Mahler's concepts of separation-individuation (Mahler et al. 1975) as the psychodynamic basis of this disorder. Benner and Joscelyne (1984) also suggest that the borderline personality is the foundation for the multiple personality disorder.

Among those researchers seeking a biologic basis for the borderline personality, Loranger and Tulis (1985) report that compared to nonborderline clients, a significantly higher number of borderline clients have a family history of alcoholism. These authors speculate that a biologic or genetic

Table 21-4
Nursing Guidelines for Working with Angry Clients

Defining Characteristics	Nursing Interventions
Nonverbal	
Glaring, piercing stares	Use a calm, unhurried approach
Tight facial muscles	Do not touch indiscriminately
Facial flushing	Respect personal space
Distended neck veins	Use active listening skills
Hyperalertness	Remain aware of personal feelings
Knitted brows	Use statements to provide feedback and to identify sources of anger, e.g., "I notice your fists are clenched . . . what's happening?"
Tense body posture	
Arms crossed over chest or placed on hips	Set verbal limits on behavior
	Use adult-adult rather than parent-child communications
Finger pointing	Offer time-out periods/one-to-one sessions in a quiet area
Fist clenching, waving, or pounding	Assure client that the staff will not allow the client to hurt self or others
Slamming, throwing, or punching inanimate objects	Observe for escalation of anger (increased activity, verbal and nonverbal acting out)
Irritability	Institute precautions against suicide, homicide, assault, or escape, as indicated
Overreaction; temper outbursts	Document patterns of acting out, including trigger situations
Intimidation	Discuss alternate means of releasing tension and physical energy
Physical assault/injury to animals or persons	Provide physical outlets to reduce tension, e.g., exercise, punching bags, gardening, clay, music, art (avoid competitive or contact sports)
Homicide/suicide ideation, plan, or gesture	Offer medication if appropriate
	Be prepared to use seclusion and restraints
	Recognize client's potential to act on threats
Verbal	Initially ignore derogatory statements
Derogatory statements and sarcasm	Protect other clients from verbal/physical abuse
Malicious gossiping	Clearly communicate and enforce unit regulations concerning acting-out behavior
Angry voice tone	Postpone discussion of anger and consequences of acting out until client is in control
Pressured speech	
Shouting, screaming, cursing	Role model appropriate assertions of angry feelings, e.g., "I dislike it when . . ."
Overly critical, impatient	State desire to assist client to maintain/regain control
Threatening	Hold client responsible for behavior; remind client that he or she can make choices
Scapegoating	Do not argue or criticize
Negativity	Give feedback regarding client's ability to maintain control in similar situations
Statements such as, "You make me mad. I could kill you."	Do not threaten punitive action
	Involve in treatment planning
Overuse of defense mechanisms of denial, rationalization, projection, and displacement	Use contracts for behavioral control, including seeking out staff people when feelings emerge
	Teach assertive skills, relaxation, imagery, thought stopping, thought control, etc.

Table 21–5
Nursing Guidelines for Working with Manipulative Clients

Defining Characteristics	Nursing Interventions
Nonverbal	
Smiling to excess	Assign one staff member as primary resource person
Touching inappropriately	Provide for staff conferences on a regular basis
Crying, whining in public	Allow sufficient time to develop a relationship
Appearing confused and helpless	Use group and peer supervision for staff
Drawing attention to self (e.g., falling, dramatic displays of somatic problems, etc.)	Provide for consistency in limit setting
	Make limits realistic with enforceable consequences
Gift giving	Give reasons for limits and consequences
Tardiness	Identify personal feelings, e.g., anger, frustration, discomfort, rescuer needs, in response to client's behavior
Selective forgetting	Model respect, honesty, openness, and assertiveness
Refusal to participate in activities	Avoid power struggles and focus on need for self-control
Seductive dressing, eye movements, body language	Seek times to interact with client when he or she is not acting out
Decreased frustration tolerance	Confront client each time manipulation occurs
Self/other destructive acting out	Describe impact of client's manipulation in an unemotional way, e.g., "I feel angry when you scream at me in front of all the staff members."
Verbal	Explore the meaning and effects of the client's manipulations
Compliments, flattery	Discuss with the client alternative ways of dealing with people or situations
Sarcasm	Do not express nonverbal amusement (e.g., eye rolling, smiling) when the client manipulates others
Threats	
Demanding behavior	Avoid accepting gifts
Induction of guilt, e.g., "I thought we had a relationship of trust."	Explore meaning of gift giving with client
	Enlist client's participation in treatment plan
Excessive criticism of others	Encourage control over routine ADL decisions
Wheeling and dealing	Encourage participation in group activities in both member and leader roles
Bargaining for special privileges	Assist client to write a self-assessment identifying both assets and liabilities
Being overly solicitous of others	Remove limits from treatment plan when client adheres to objectives consistently
Requesting exemption from rules, e.g., "Couldn't I have my medication just one hour earlier?"	Evaluate effectiveness of limit setting
	Jointly develop contracts for behavioral change
Mimicking therapeutic responses used by staff, e.g., "I have a feeling you're angry with me."	If client refuses to comply with contracts or treatment recommendations, avoid negotiating; enlist staff team to resolve issues
Confronting staff in the presence of other clients	Offer support to other clients who may be targets of manipulations
Lying	Involve both client and significant others in identifying and managing manipulative behavior
Reporting great "insights" early in the relationship	Teach stress-reduction techniques (e.g., guided imagery, relaxation, thought-stopping)
	Involve in assertiveness training and problem-solving
Telling the nurse what he or she "wants" to hear	Practice role rehearsal skills

continued

Table 21–5 *(Continued)* Nursing Guidelines for Working with Manipulative Clients	
Defining Characteristics	**Nursing Interventions**
Using information about others to exploit them	See previous page
Excessive involvement in the problems of others	
Aggressive questioning about personal matters	
Rationalizing, projecting, and minimizing blame for behavior	
Self-pity	
Role reversal	

component may account for their findings. Also lending support to the biologic theorists, Andrulonis et al. (1980), in an intensive study of clients with borderline syndromes, report organic involvement, including histories of minimal brain dysfunction and episodic dyscontrol syndromes among their subjects.

Surprisingly, little research has been conducted in the area of family interactional patterns that may predispose to the borderline personality disorder. Feldman and Guttman (1984) recommend further research in this area based upon findings that indicate that biparental failure, rather than failures during the separation-individuation process with the primary caregiver, may lead to the development of symptoms. Biparental failure is evident in those homes where the male parent fails to offset the child's troubled relationship with the mother by providing positive experiences for the child. For example, the male parent fails to become involved in day-to-day parenting, generally lacks interest in the child, gives little approval, is passive, or affectively neglects the child.

The following subjective and objective nursing assessment criteria for clients with borderline personality disorders have been adapted from the DSM-IIIR diagnostic criteria.

Instability or Unpredictability The individual with a borderline personality disorder has fluctuating responses in a variety of situations that are subjectively interpreted and often distorted. This individual often makes such comments as, "I did it. I don't know why I did. I just did." Impulsiveness may be observed in such habits as spending money, sexuality, substance use, eating habits, shoplifting, and frequent job changes.

Unstable Interpersonal Relationships The client's failure to resolve the separation-individuation process described by Mahler et al (1975) is reflected in this individual's attitudes toward self and others. Normal autism and symbiosis are necessary before the separation-individuation process, referred to as "psychological birth," can begin. The inability to unify the "good and bad" objects into one whole is demonstrated by the inability to integrate the self as both "good and bad" or to separate or individuate from the maternal object (see Table 21–6).

The sense of self originates with the earliest mother-child interactions. If the mother is not sensitive and attuned to the child's needs, she fails to confirm the child's emerging sense of reality. Consequently, the child distorts reality and develops an unreal "as-if" personality that shifts to meet the demands of cues in the outer world (Brainerd 1978, Mahler et al 1975). The implications for the child's later relationships include such behaviors as:

- Manipulation of others
- Pitting individuals against one another
- Intense attachment
- Explosive separations
- Sudden shifts in attitude toward others perceived as good or bad
- Clinging, demanding
- Controlling, exploitive behavior
- Sadism or masochism in close relationships
- Relationships motivated by a need to avoid being alone rather than the need to be with others
- Lack of empathy

<table>
<tr><td colspan="5" align="center">Table 21–6
Separation-Individuation Subphases</td></tr>
</table>

Age	Subphase	Task Versus Failure	Expected Behaviors
5 months	Differentiation	Separation ("hatching") versus increased autistic behavior such as: rocking, bland affect, autoerotic stimulation, and intense stranger anxiety	Is increasingly alert Makes tactile exploration of mother Uses transitional objects to replace mother Compares mother visually with other humans Shows stranger anxiety Begins to separate from maternal object
9 months 10–18 months	Practicing (early) Practicing (late)	Separation ("expansion") versus withdrawal, apathy, and desperate crying	Crawls away while holding on Is capable of upright locomotion Keeps mother "in sight" Is exuberant Continues to use transitional object for comfort Retains memory when person or object is out of sight (object permanence)
15–18 months	Rapprochement 1. Beginning 2. Crisis	Establishing optimal distance to maintain psychologic equilibrium versus inability to integrate positive and negative aspects about self and others: "splitting"	Clamors for mother's attention Shadows mother/darts away Shares objects with mother Plays imitation games Has reactions to strangers Has temper tantrums Is shy with strangers Shows ambivalence (clings/pushes) Is indecisive Perceives caretakers as "good" and "bad" Is able to make requests
21 months	3. Resolution		Has wider emotional range Develops verbal language Learns simple rules Expresses wishes and fantasies through symbolic play Begins to establish gender identity Fears loss of love object and/or approval
36 months	Consolidation 1. Individuality 2. Object constancy	Achieving self-boundaries, unifying good/bad aspects of self and others, developing a permanent sense of significant others (object constancy)	Tolerates separation from mother for longer periods Engages in fantasy play; role playing

continued

		Table 21–6 *(Continued)*	
		Separation-Individuation Subphases	
Age	**Subphase**	**Task Versus Failure**	**Expected Behaviors**
		versus ongoing ambivalence, impulsiveness, intense affective extremes, manipulation	Shows increased interest in adults other than mother
			Develops a sense of time
			Attains gender identity
			Plays purposefully
			Communicates verbally
			Tests reality
			Can delay gratification

Source: From The Psychological Birth of the Human Infant: Symbiosis and Individuation, *MS Mahler, F Pine, A Bergman. Copyright © 1975 by Margaret S. Mahler. Reprinted by permission of Basic Books, Inc., Publishers.*

- Diminished capacity to evaluate others realistically
- Transient, brief, close relationships.

Intense Anger Borderline individuals, unable to tolerate their own "bad" self-image, project it onto others and rage against those negative attributes. As a consequence of childhood disappointments and frustrations related to insensitive and inadequate parenting, the borderline client seethes with intense, unexpressed rage. This rage may be directed at anyone who demonstrates the negative attributes that the borderline client sees in himself or herself. However, anger is greatest toward those people who remind the client of nurturing/frustrating parents. Schwarz and Halaris (1984) suggest that this may explain why it is so difficult to maintain these clients in therapy. Borderline clients tend to instigate problems as they become involved in therapeutic relationships. The anger may be observed in accusations, frequent displays of temper, inability to control anger (acting out), irritability, sarcasm, argumentativeness, devaluing others, and overreaction to minor irritants. (See Table 21–4 to review manifestations of anger and nursing guidelines.)

Identity Diffusion Erikson (1964) coined the term *identity diffusion* to describe the failure to integrate various childhood identifications into a harmonious adult psychosocial identity. The borderline person displays behaviors that show confusion about values and goals in life. Deutsch (1965) describes these individuals as "as-if" people, who assume roles and characteristics of others in a chameleon-like fashion. They persuasively imitate or "play act" others' behaviors. Indeed, they may become "copies" of the people

with whom they associate. These clients cannot genuinely experience feelings and emotions; the core personality of the borderline client is hollow. They do not assume responsibility for their actions but project blame and credit onto others.

Problems of identity diffusion are also apparent in the areas of sexual intimacy and gender identity. Sexual intimacy is disturbed as a result of the person's fears of being engulfed and destroyed or abandoned by another. An approach-avoidance conflict emerges as a consequence of the mother having thwarted independence and rewarded dependent behavior during the rapprochement subphase. As a result, the borderline client develops two major fears: the fear of abandonment, which leads to clinging behavior, and fear of engulfment, which leads to distancing from others. The client desperately wants intimate relationships but is terrified of losing the self. These fears are reminiscent of the early choice between mother's love and autonomy, which is the core of the borderline conflict. This conflict is managed by using the primitive dissociation defense, also called *splitting,* which is discussed later in this chapter. Gender identity disturbance may be manifested by the selection of rejecting or abusive partners, the preference for homosexual relationships while maintaining a heterosexual life-style, bizarre fantasies, and transsexualism (Akhtar 1984).

Another area of identity diffusion is temporal discontinuity, which is manifested by a searching for one's origins or keeping detailed chronologic journals. Borderline individuals seem unable to integrate past, present, and future into a continuum. They may frantically plan for the future while reminiscing about past events. These behaviors often lead to difficulty in choosing long-term goals, making career choices, and reassessing personal values.

Affective Instability   The failure to resolve object permanence issues is also related to the inability of the borderline person to maintain a consistent, satisfying, affective state. Characteristic of this individual are intense fluctuations of mood, normally of short duration (a few hours to a few days); intense, discrete episodes of depression with accompanying suicidal ideation and gestures; and hypomanic or elated episodes.

Feelings of Emptiness and Aloneness   Individuals with borderline personalities report hollow, empty feelings, lack of peaceful solitude, a sense of being disconnected, and anhedonia (absence of pleasure in performing ordinarily pleasurable acts). The person may attempt to combat these feelings by compulsive eating, drinking, drug abuse, sexual encounters, and self-mutilation. It is believed that excessive anxiety associated with unresolved separation-individuation issues underlies these behaviors (Perlmutter 1982).

Self-Damaging Acts   Impulsiveness, together with identity disturbances, often leads to self-destructive behaviors. Borderline persons are often depressed, but they may make self-destructive gestures to affirm their reality and relieve tension rather than to express a wish to die. Additional self-damaging behaviors include self-mutilation (cigarette burns, cutting, taking drug overdoses), recurrent accidents, and physical fights.

Overuse of Primitive Defenses   According to Lego (1984, p 419), borderline persons consistently use the following defenses:

- Primitive dissociation (also called **splitting**): The opposing affective states of love and hate are kept separate to avoid contamination. The borderline client fears that the bad aspects (hate) will poison the good aspects (love).

  A borderline nursing student loves her instructor during clinical instruction when she receives individual attention but detests the same instructor in the role of distant lecturer.

- Projective identification: The client projects his or her feelings onto another, thereby justifying expressions of anger and self-protection.

  A borderline client accuses a second client, whom she dislikes, of disliking her. The borderline client refuses to attend any activities at which the other client is present.

- Primitive idealization: The client assigns unrealistic powers to an individual on whom he or she is dependent.

  A client tells the nurse, "You are the perfect nurse; I always know nothing bad can happen when you're around."

- Omnipotence: **Omnipotence** is made evident by fantasies of greatness or exaggerated importance.

  In response to a question about a suicidal gesture, a client states, "Don't worry. I knew I wouldn't die."

- Devaluation: The client criticizes another to defend against a sense of inadequacy.

  A client repeatedly criticizes those nursing staff members who do not have master's degrees as being "nontherapeutic."

- Denial: **Denial** occurs when disturbing thoughts and feelings are kept out of conscious awareness.

  A nursing student was expelled from school for academic and clinical incompetence. When the new term began, she attempted to register for the next nursing class. She acted dumbfounded when told she could not register.

Distortions of Reality   When identity diffusion reaches panic proportions, the borderline individual may experience the following:

- *Depersonalization:* A feeling of strangeness or unreality about one's self.
- *Derealization:* A feeling of disconnectedness from the environment.

A client with multiple cigarette burns reports no pain or discomfort and smiles when the lesions are being cleaned and dressed.

Due to the nature of the borderline personality, the aim of therapy is generally to resolve the immediate crisis and then develop a long-term therapeutic alliance. The long-standing history of affective instability, impulsiveness, and intense, immature relationships leads to persistent maladaptive behavior. The following NANDA nursing diagnoses are integral parts of any nursing care plan for these clients. (More precise PND-I diagnoses are compared with the general NANDA categories in this chapter's care plans.)

Self-Concept, Disturbances in: Personal Identity   Persons diagnosed with borderline personality disorders experience feelings of self-devaluation because of failure to negotiate the rapprochement subphase of separation-individuation. Self-concept disturbances may be identified from the following problems:

- Chameleonlike behavior
- Superficial interactions
- Intense but disruptive relationships
- Play-acting roles
- Mood swings

Coping, Ineffective Individual   These clients tend to overuse primitive defenses to the extent that learning adaptive coping skills is highly impaired. Behavior frequently observed includes:

- Splitting, projection, and regression
- Devaluation or idealization of others
- Potential for chemical dependency
- Persistent sense of boredom and loneliness
- Inadequate responses to life stresses and expectations

Violence, Potential For   Because of the borderline client's mood swings, limited problem-solving strategies, and self-concept disturbances, the following problems may be observed:

- Intense and often contagious rage
- Impulsiveness
- Self-mutilation or suicidal gestures
- Hostile, threatening verbalizations
- Property destruction

Planning and Implementing Interventions

The nursing care plan for the client with a borderline personality disorder is on the following pages. When providing care, the nurse must be alert to the often intense feelings that the borderline client may precipitate in the nurse. These feelings (e.g., anger, guilt, overgiving, rescuing, rig-

idity) may cloud the nurse's judgment and lead to decisions that the client may interpret as abandonment, distancing, engulfment, or lack of empathy.

RESEARCH NOTE

Citation

Schulz PM et al: The impact of borderline and schizotypal personality disorders on patients and their families. Hosp Community Psychiatry 1985;36:879–881.

Study Problem/Purpose

To measure the impact of borderline pathology on clients and families and to ascertain their views about the etiology of the disorder, the degree of burden compared to chronic medical illnesses, and specific troublesome traits in order to design services for needs identified.

Methods

Using the Schedule for Interviewing Borderlines, the authors selected 31 clients identified as having borderline personality disorder, schizotypal personality disorder, or both. They and 35 family members completed the Family Attitudes Toward Personality Disorder Questionnaire (FAPDQ), which addresses the presumed etiology of borderline and schizotypal personality disorders and ranks five factors as possible causes.

Findings

There were significant differences in the responses of patients and family members on the etiology of the disorders. However, both groups agreed that the disorder led to a considerable burden on the family unit—similar to and slightly more than a serious physical illness, yet less than ratings by relatives of schizophrenic clients in a previous study. Families indicated that the burden was correlated with antisocial acts such as drunkenness and substance abuse, absenteeism, and promiscuity. Chronic economic problems associated with having a borderline or schizotypal individual in the family concerned both the clients and family.

Implications

Borderline and schizotypal clients and their families often know little about the disorder but are keenly aware of the psychologic and social stress suffered by the family unit. Results suggest that both clients and families would benefit from further education about the disorders and behaviors, which cause embarrassment and burden.

Text continues on p. 556

Nursing Care Plan: The Client with a Borderline Personality

Nursing Diagnosis (PND-I/NANDA)	Client Care Goals	Nursing Planning/ Intervention	Evaluation
05.04 Altered sexuality processes 04.02.01 Anger 04.02.02 Anxiety* /Anxiety 02.98 Altered cognition processes not otherwise specified 02.07.03 Magical thinking 06.03.02 Altered gender identity 06.03.03 Altered personal identity* /Self-concept, disturbance in: personal identity (associated with history of physical and sexual abuse) 06.03.04 Altered self-esteem* /Self-concept, disturbance in: self-esteem 06.03.05 Altered social identity 02.08.01 Altered abstract thinking 02.08.03 Altered problem solving 02.05.02 Distorted memory 02.02 Altered judgment	The client will identify and resolve the immediate crisis and initiate the development of a secure sense of self.	1. Develop a consistent treatment plan involving all staff. 2. Encourage staff to discuss feelings directed toward client in staff meetings. 3. Encourage client to discuss his or her body image. 4. Assist client to deal with loss of body image associated with history of abuse. 5. Help client to examine belief systems and identify how perceptions and beliefs influence responses. 6. Encourage client to write an autobiography and give feedback. 7. Encourage client to set daily objectives and assist in meeting goals. 8. Give positive reinforcement of achievement of goals. 9. Have client evaluate personal progress weekly. 10. Point out to client when affective responses are inappropriate and/or incongruent to situations. 11. Assist client to identify rewards of both appropriate and inappropriate responses. 12. Encourage participation in a variety of group situations.	1. Behaves and dresses appropriately in social situations. 2. Develops a realistic view of self by identifying strengths and weaknesses. 3. Explores how beliefs and perceptions of situations influence responses and roles played. 4. Establishes goals that can be reached in a specified time period. 5. Identifies consequences of behaviors. 6. Evaluates personal progress. 7. Sustains a situation-appropriate mood, i.e., absence of mood swings. 8. Discusses modes of sexual expression and ways of achieving satisfaction.

*PND-I diagnosis also on NANDA list.

continued

Nursing Care Plan: The Client with a Borderline Personality *(continued)*

Nursing Diagnosis (PND-I/NANDA)	Client Care Goals	Nursing Planning/ Intervention	Evaluation
		13. Assist to accept disappointments by altering thoughts with such statements as, "It would be nice if . . ." rather than magnifying losses.	
		14. Confront client with various ways in which he or she denies pleasure.	
		15. Discuss with client ways to change feelings and behavior.	
05.03 Altered role performance 04.98 Altered emotional processes not otherwise specified /Coping, ineffective individual (association with destructive behavior toward self and others; use of defenses such as splitting, projecting, and regression; verbal manipulation)	The client will demonstrate moderate and stable means of expressing feelings and relating to others.	1. Assign nonjudgmental staff to work with client; maintain consistency. 2. Schedule frequent staff meetings; establish behavioral expectations. 3. Schedule family meetings if possible. 4. Inform client of acceptable behavior and unit rules. 5. Enforce limits when client attempts to manipulate. 6. Delegate to one staff member the final authority and responsibility for the treatment plan. 7. Use problem-solving techniques to help the client make changes. 8. Point out to client when he or she is experiencing both positive and negative responses toward the same person. 9. Challenge client's idealizations of staff.	1. Develops a therapeutic relationship with at least one staff member. 2. Verbally acknowledges both positive and negative characteristics about self and others. 3. Explores responses to other's behavior and relates these responses to feelings about oneself. 4. Describes feelings rather than somatizing them. 5. Identifies situations in which manipulation is employed and verbalizes the consequences. 6. Identifies and uses modes of responding that are assertive and responsible. 7. Engages in constructive and satisfying activities during free time. 8. Sustains a meaningful relationship without using primitive defenses such as

continued

Nursing Care Plan: The Client with a Borderline Personality *(continued)*

Nursing Diagnosis (PND-I/NANDA)	Client Care Goals	Nursing Planning/ Intervention	Evaluation
		10. Point out discrepancies in client's behavior.	projection and splitting.
		11. Tell client you do not feel the way he or she imagines that you do.	9. Explores past use of chemicals as a means of coping.
		12. Draw a parallel between how you respond to the client's behavior and how others are likely to respond.	10. Takes time to process a problem, using problem-solving skills rather than acting impulsively.
		13. Remain neutral to client's comments, being neither flattered nor offended.	11. Sustains a long-term therapeutic relationship.
		14. Do not seek client's approval.	
		15. Explore feelings and experiences rather than making interpretations.	
		16. Use group techniques to teach responsibility for self.	
		17. Use role play to demonstrate adaptive communications.	
		18. Teach client to recognize needs requiring immediate attention and those that may be delayed.	
		19. Avoid rescuing or rejecting client, rather deal with the behavior that is manipulative.	
		20. Have client maintain a journal for discussing daily experiences, feelings, and responses; use the journal to proceed with the relationship.	
		21. Use a "transitional object" (e.g., appointment card, postcard) when out of	

continued

Nursing Care Plan: The Client with a Borderline Personality *(continued)*

Nursing Diagnosis (PND-I/NANDA)	Client Care Goals	Nursing Planning/ Intervention	Evaluation
		town or out of touch with the client.	
05.02.01.02 Aggressive/ violent behaviors toward others* 05.02.01.03 Aggressive/ violent behaviors toward self* /Violence, potential for: self-directed or directed at others (associated with inability to verbalize frustration and anger, history of impulsive self-mutilating acts, hostile and threatening verbalizations)	The client will eliminate destructive acting-out behavior, e.g., suicidal/ homicidal threats and gestures.	1. Assess history of previous self-mutilation. 2. Observe behavior and document every shift. 3. Utilize suicide precautions as necessary. 4. Tell client that staff will not permit him/her to injure self or others. 5. Contract with client to notify staff members when suicidal/self-mutilating thoughts occur. 6. Assist client to identify alternatives to self-destructive behavior. 7. Explore self-destructive fantasies. 8. Assist to identify situations in which self-destructive ideas occur. 9. Explore relationships in the past that have been hostile. 10. During one-to-one sessions when client verbalizes anger, point out that client's anger is not caused by the current situation, but by perceptions of things in the past. 11. Modulate amounts of warmth shown to the client. 12. Explore means of expressing anger in a constructive manner.	1. Verbalizes feelings of anger and frustration when they occur. 2. Requests time-out periods, physical activities, and p.r.n. medications when anger cannot be defused by verbalizing. 3. Identifies precipitants to feelings, e.g., rejection, separation, loss, disappointment. 4. Seeks out staff member with whom to discuss anger or releases anger in constructive activity. 5. Identifies alternatives to self-mutilating behavior. 6. Uses "I" statements when dealing with anger and frustration.

PND-I diagnosis also on NANDA list.

continued

Nursing Care Plan: The Client with a Borderline Personality *(continued)*

Nursing Diagnosis (PND-I/NANDA)	Client Care Goals	Nursing Planning/ Intervention	Evaluation
		13. Encourage verbal expression of anger and give positive reinforcement for same.	
		14. Explore with client how energy from angry feelings may be positively directed, i.e., motivation for change, problem solving, etc.	
		15. Deal with client's transference phenomena, which are expressions of anger and hatred.	
		16. Utilize treatment contracts between client and team with mutually agreed upon goals.	
		17. Give consistent feedback for goal achievement or lack thereof.	

A client presents herself as a pathetic victim of involuntary hospitalization. As a result, the staff becomes guilt-ridden and prematurely grants an out-of-hospital pass. The client, in turn, acts out her sense of abandonment by making a serious suicide attempt.

Responding to seductive, angry, or solicitous behavior in either a negative or rescuing manner may reinforce the inappropriate responses of the client. An ideal therapeutic relationship is one in which the nurse: (a) maintains a matter-of-fact but caring approach, (b) establishes and maintains consistent, firm limits, (c) makes regular appointments, and (d) mobilizes the healthy aspects of the client's personality.

As with all clients with personality disorders, the nurse should use clinical supervision, staff counseling sessions, and team meetings to identify the client's underlying dynamic issues and to work toward decreasing distortions in communications between the client and others.

Wendy is a 27-year-old dental hygienist who comes from a blue-collar family and gives a history of physical and sexual abuse as a child. Her biologic parents were divorced when she was a young child; two younger brothers are addicted to opiates and have had many legal problems related to drug use. Wendy's chemical use was sporadic and primarily recreational until completion of college. At age 18, she married a laborer to escape her home situation. She became pregnant twice but aborted both times. Wendy was divorced at age 20. Prior to her divorce, she lived with her second husband, a chef of Hispanic origin who sought a traditional male-dominated home life. This relationship was marked by verbal and physical abuse, withholding of financial support, sexual indiscretions, and alcohol and cocaine use. Wendy became pregnant three times during this six-year marriage, aborting each fetus prior to five months' gestation.

Wendy presents as a slim, well-groomed, and well-developed young woman with generously applied makeup. She is consistently cheerful on initial contact; she minimizes problems with her husband and is involved in many outside activities. Although she has maintained residence in the community and has worked for eight years in the same dental office, she has no close friends, claiming that her husband forbids socializing. Her primary outlet is physical activity. She jogs, bicycles, plays tennis and racquetball, and does daily aerobic exercises. She seeks out sports that involve contact with the opposite sex and always wears designer sports attire when not working.

Throughout the two-year dental hygiene program, Wendy was identified as being very intelligent but manipulative. Instructors documented patterns of tardiness, absenteeism, illness, and accidents in every course. When instructors confronted her behaviors, Wendy gave elaborate rationalizations, which often appeared implausible. However, Wendy was able to meet all course requirements and completed the program as scheduled.

Three weeks prior to taking state board examinations, Wendy cut both wrists, lacerating the tendons and requiring immobilization. She had left her husband, and her new boyfriend had evicted her from his home. She denied any intent to kill herself but stated, "I couldn't help it. I was so confused and desperate." She was able to write the examinations but demonstrated indifference to her injuries by such expressions as, "Oh, I hurt myself." Classmates reported feeling surprised and shocked by both the behavior and her response to it.

After receiving her license, Wendy was employed by a large health maintenance organization. During this time, her supervisor confronted her several times for wearing seductive clothing and makeup. She became very friendly with male clients and saw some of them socially outside the office.

Wendy established residence with a female friend on a house-sharing basis but consistently had difficulty meeting her financial obligations for home maintenance. This placed increased strain on their relationship. Wendy's chemical addiction became apparent to her employer within six months. Her rapid mood swings, irritability, and absenteeism led to a confrontation and subsequent admission to a substance-treatment facility. Wendy denied chemical dependency during the first week, displaying intense mood swings and angry outbursts at the staff. When she threatened suicide if not released from the program, she was committed to a psychiatric program.

Within twenty-four hours of admission, Wendy became very calm and identified herself as a "hygienist" to other clients. She participated in all program activities but assumed a therapist role. She lacked insight into her behavior, intellectually accepted "alcohol" as her problem, and requested to be reassigned to the substance-treatment facility. As it was determined that she was no longer actively suicidal, the transfer was made.

When she returned to the unit of her choice, she talked incessantly about the poor standard of care on the psychiatric unit. She focused on staff deficiencies and praised the performance of the substance-treatment staff. She was confronted almost daily about her seductive attire and decision to socialize only with male clients. She attempted to pit one staff member against another and, indeed, had some success. A social worker cried because she felt helpless when Wendy was transferred to the psychiatric unit, while an alcohol counselor raged about Wendy's manipulation of him.

Wendy's treatment program consisted of daily groups and one-to-one sessions, including occupational, recreational, and music therapies, and psychotherapies. Because of the anxiety and depressive components of her disorder, her physician ordered 5 mg of thiothixine (Navane) three times daily. She continued to receive thiothixene until her discharge.

Wendy remained in the treatment facility for five weeks. At the time of discharge, she demonstrated increased consistency of mood, the ability to verbally identify consequences of her behavior, and some capacity for discussing the anger she felt in daily situations. She would not consider long-range goals, especially those pertaining to employment or living arrangements. During her last week on the unit, she called her Alcoholics Anonymous sponsor, who invited Wendy to live with her until Wendy could reestablish herself. A one-year follow-up showed Wendy working as an office manager and public relations coordinator for a busy dental clinic in a large metropolitan area. She was still actively working in her recovery program.

Evaluation

Although borderline clients often appear relatively healthy, the nurse may find it difficult to maintain a therapeutic alliance with them because of their intense and contagious affects, impulsiveness, and the intense feelings they trigger in others. The quality of object relationships, especially that between the therapist and the client, is crucial to the outcome of therapy.

Self-Concept, Disturbance In   Successful integration of fragmented aspects of the borderline client's personality ("healing the split") depends upon the client's ability to remain in a sustained therapeutic relationship (Platt-Koch 1983). Among clients who do remain in therapy, those who demonstrate likeability, warmth, reliability, interest in people, talents, and social as well as occupational skills have the most favorable treatment prognosis (Woollcott 1985).

Coping, Ineffective Individual   The use of primitive defenses may be replaced by more adequate problem-solving skills over time. The client who has innate cognitive and psychomotor talents should be encouraged to sublimate feelings of intense rage into productive outlets (e.g., art, music, dance). Receiving positive reinforcements for these achievements may enhance the development of effective coping strategies.

Violence, Potential For   According to Woollcott (1985), those clients who are most infantile and regressed (as opposed to those who have more narcissistic features) tend to achieve greater affective stability. The nurse can confront the client's anger during one-to-one sessions by comparing the client's responses to those of others. This strategy may cause the client to think before acting.

The borderline person has established patterns of responding to others in any situation. This pattern may sabotage the client's objectives. Furthermore, these clients usually terminate therapy when the acute crisis has ended. Among the factors that influence the likelihood of successful change are:

- The severity of the client's emotional deprivation
- The rigidity of the client's personality structure
- The client's ego strengths
- The client's motivation to change
- The nurse's skill and commitment
- Social support systems in the client's family or milieu that favor the desired change

The Nursing Process and Histrionic Personality Disorders

Nursing Assessment: Defining Characteristics of the Histrionic Personality

Persons with histrionic personalities show a lifelong tendency for dramatic, egocentric, attention-seeking response patterns. Their seeming lack of sincerity and of emotional commitment contributes to disturbances in interpersonal relationships. These people appear to be continually "on stage" and acting a role. Their extensive use of coping patterns based on repression, denial, and dissociation leads them to deal with problems as though they do not exist.

Dramatic, Exhibitionistic, and Egocentric Responses   Responses are characterized by exaggerated emotional expression; craving for attention, activity, and excitement; overreaction to minor stressors; irrational emotional outbursts; and temper tantrums.

Difficulty Sustaining Interpersonal Relationships   Histrionic clients constantly need love, reassurance, and validation of existence because of their feelings of dependency and helplessness. For this reason, histrionic persons have problems with significant relationships. These individuals are likely to manipulate others to hold on to a love object while being highly inconsiderate and lacking empathy.

Sexual Expression   The histrionic person is generally provocative and seductive and uses sexual expression to manipulate and control others in relationships. The client is often unaware of this flamboyance and how others perceive it. Individuals are often competitive with those of the same sex and seductive with the opposite sex. This personality disorder is more frequent in women than men. In males, it may be associated with a homosexual arousal pattern.

Dysphoric Moods   Dysphoria is a sense of disquiet or restlessness. Histrionic persons may experience depression when their demands for attention and affection are not met. They may act out in a suicidal fashion. Often, these individuals behave frivolously, acting silly and making nuisances of themselves.

Cognitive Dimensions   Histrionic personalities are much more interested in creative or imaginative pursuits than in analytical or academic achievements. They tend to be impressionable and highly suggestible and tend to look to authority figures for magical solutions to problems.

Health Patterns   Regression and the development of somatic and/or dissociative disorders are frequent among histrionic people. These disabling symptoms may serve the purpose of calling attention to the person. They generally occur when an audience is present or when an unpleasant situation is anticipated. Substance use, depression, seizurelike activity, blackouts, falling, dizziness, or reactive psychoses may lead to hospitalization.

Linda, a 33-year-old woman who is twice divorced, was observed at the out-patient clinic responding flirtatiously to male staff members. She was neatly groomed but dressed in a low-cut peasant blouse, a tight mini-skirt, and bright red knee-high boots. When called by the female therapist for her appointment, Linda screamed that she had waited too long, complaining loudly about patients' rights to rapid treatment. She quickly captured the attention of others in the waiting room. Then Linda feigned dizziness and "fell" as she arose from her chair. During the ensuing session, Linda complained that several men had made passes at her on the bus. When the therapist pointed out that her manner of dress was a probable factor, Linda accused her of being jealous. Linda terminated the interview at that point and left the office, slamming the door behind her and stating, "My problems are physical, and no one cares whether I live or die. You'll be sorry for treating me this way!"

Nursing Diagnosis

Although histrionic clients may look and act as though they have few problems, major dysfunctions are present. Nursing diagnoses may include the following:

Injury, Potential For   The dramatic, impulsive responses of histrionic clients may lead to injuries or suicidal gestures. Problems often include:

- Increased potential for accidents, e.g., falls and automobile accidents
- Self-inflicted injuries/suicide attempts
- Misdiagnosis of physical illness

Coping, Ineffective Individual   Ineffective coping is manifested by behavior resulting from high anxiety levels, limited judgment, and need for attention and reassurance. Behaviors often observed include:

- Seductiveness (e.g., in dress, makeup, mannerisms, conversational tone and content)
- Substance use
- Manipulation of others, lack of consideration
- Emotional lability
- Low frustration tolerance
- Irresponsibility, vanity, silliness, frivolity
- Lack of insight
- Overuse of denial

Planning and Implementing Interventions

Nursing care for the histrionic client closely resembles that for borderline persons. Since many health professionals view these clients as feigning illness, it is imperative to carry out a thorough physical assessment. In addition, the potential for self-injury is a risk. Suicidal assessment should be a component of daily interviews when the client is in crisis. Treatment plans need to emphasize that staff should

avoid paying attention to the sexual provocations of these clients. Positive reinforcement for appropriate behavior should be stressed.

Evaluation

Even when intervention strategies are implemented consistently, histrionic clients tend to manifest more denial than clients with other disorders in the dramatic-erratic clusters. The treatment plan should emphasize the nurse's need to remain objective.

Injury, Potential For   When acting-out behavior is eliminated, the potential for self-destructive acts should be decreased. The client, however, may develop a conversion or dissociative reaction that impedes optimal functioning and forces others to pay attention to his or her needs.

Coping, Ineffective Individual   It is not unusual for histrionic clients to exaggerate all aspects of living and loving. If the client can learn to be less conspicuous and to express emotions appropriately, then many seductive, attention-seeking behaviors will diminish. There is always the possibility that when the client's needs for affection and attention are thwarted, vulnerability to depression may increase.

The Nursing Process and Narcissistic Personality Disorders

Nursing Assessment: Defining Characteristics of the Narcissistic Personality

Persons with narcissistic personalities have difficulty regulating self-esteem and self-expression (Masterson 1981). Jacobson (1979, p 431) advises that the term *narcissism* should apply to clients whose self-esteem is too low, as well as inappropriately high. Characteristics most frequently observed include a sense of entitlement, interpersonal manipulations, lack of empathy, and indifference toward others.

Grandiosity   Grandiosity is evidenced by expressions of exaggerated self-importance, self-absorption, and egocentricity. This inflated self-concept may be a compensation for feelings of diminished self-worth. Isolating a child from the feedback of others and the parents' failing to mirror the child's behavior may contribute to this disorder. *Mirroring* or "mirror images" reflect what the parents think of and how they treat the child. When coming in contact with people outside the home, the child may discover a discrepancy between the way others treat him or her and the mirror image developed at home. Excessive boasting may result from this inconsistency in self-concept.

Preoccupations The narcissistic person is generally preoccupied and fantasizes about power, success, idealized love, morals, and intelligence. These behaviors may be the result of overidealization of the child by the parents.

Exhibitionism Exhibitionistic behavior is evidenced by the constant seeking of support and admiration from others. Because of their limited interests, these clients perseverate about themselves to the point of boring others.

Vacillation of Affective Response In spite of the narcissistic individual's extensive use of rationalization for failures, there is an underlying sense of rage, shame, and diminished self-esteem. The perceptive nurse may observe cool indifference, emptiness, humiliation, uncontrolled anger, or desire for revenge.

Dysfunctional Interpersonal Relationships Persons who have narcissistic personalities feel entitled to special favors and attention. Further, they refuse to assume mutual responsibilities in relationships. They tend to exploit others and disregard their rights. Kernberg (1975) emphasizes that chronic, intense envy and defenses against envy lead to idealization or devaluation of others. Responses to others may include lack of empathy, mistrust, lack of intimacy, accusations of incompetence, or demands for unattainable perfection.

Socialization In addition to having problems forming and sustaining interpersonal relationships, the narcissistic person may experience occupational divergences. Kohut (1971) describes work inhibitions as peculiar to this group. In contrast, Cameron and Rychlak (1985, p 460) note that these individuals often assume active leadership roles, putting their power needs to work and attacking the established working order. One may also consider the effect of the culture on the development of socialization skills. The post–World War II philosophy of "looking out for number one" may well have contributed to the rise of identification of narcissistic disorders and their recent inclusion as a diagnostic category in DSM-III (Widiger 1985).

Sexual Expression Perverse sexual fantasies, promiscuity, or homosexuality may be associated with this disorder. There may be confusion regarding sex-role behavior as a result of learned defenses against libidinal and ego needs conflicts (Wilson and Prabucki 1983, p 1237).

Roy is a 40-year-old male nurse who seeks professional counseling after dropping out of a graduate nursing program. He presents as a slender, well-groomed individual with marked effeminate behaviors (e.g., voice tones, inflections, posturing). Roy makes it clear upon initial contact that he is "gay," although he has a wide circle of both heterosexual and homosexual friends. Indeed, he devotes the first thirty minutes of the session to recounting sexual exploits and venting anger that concern about AIDS is limiting the availability of sexual partners in his community. He states that he had a live-in relationship with one partner for 15 years but that recently his partner became discontented with Roy's need to "party." Consequently the two are not "communicating." Roy defends his desire to seek out a variety of sexual partners by focusing on his personal needs and the "lack of consideration" of his friend.

When questioned about dropping out, Roy rationalizes his failure by blaming it on a "hostile major professor" and further proclaiming, "I know more than she does." He describes himself as the "leader" in his group of six graduate students and interprets this to mean that they have great respect for him.

He tells the therapist that he attempted to call two nurse friends following his withdrawal from school. He dramatically and self-righteously expresses anger and disappointment that they were not available to him. (One was vacationing out of state and the other was hospitalized for major surgery.) When the therapist inquires how his friend was doing following surgery, Roy responded, "How should I know? That's not my problem. She never bothered to call me back."

Roy requests that the therapist set up Saturday morning appointments (no office hours were normally scheduled on this day), because he became very tired in the afternoons and always took a nap. When the therapist refuses to meet this request, he becomes angry and shouts, "You're just like all the rest of them. No one considers my needs! I'll see to it that your supervisor hears about this and I'll let all my friends know how incompetent you are as a therapist."

Nursing Diagnosis

Like people with histrionic and borderline personality disorders, narcissistic people have problems associated with disturbed self-concept and coping abilities. The following dysfunctional behavior may be observed:

Self-Concept, Disturbance In

- Self-centeredness
- Exaggerated sense of importance and intelligence

- Setting unrealistic goals
- Indifference to the feelings of others
- Interpersonal exploitiveness

Coping, Ineffective Individual

- Excessive use of denial of shortcomings, rationalization of errors, and projection of blame
- Inconsistent and intense emotional responses to interpersonal relationships
- Occupational dysfunctions
- Preoccupation with or fantasies of power
- Exhibitionism

Planning and Implementing Interventions

The objectives for care of the narcissistic client are to help the client accept feedback without defensiveness and rationalization, to increase his or her capacity to tolerate frustration and disappointment, and to help the client appreciate the rights and needs of others. Interventions are geared toward using the therapeutic alliance to work through feelings of abandonment, rejection, shame, and self-doubt, thereby heightening self-esteem. Heterogeneous group therapies have been successful with some narcissistic clients (Wong 1980). However, the client often terminates both individual and group work prematurely.

Evaluation

The goal is for the narcissistic individual to learn how to empathize with others by recognizing that it is not necessary to be right all the time—i.e., that imperfections in self and others exist. Although some clients develop positive roles through the use of creativity and humor, most substitute hypochondriacal behavior and a sense of emptiness and lowered self-esteem for previous behaviors and feelings.

The Nursing Process and Antisocial Personality Disorders

Nursing Assessment: Defining Characteristics of the Antisocial Personality

The antisocial personality was one of the earliest to be identified. It has been labeled *psychopathy, sociopathy,* and *moral insanity.* Without question, it is the most researched and validated of these disorders (Widiger 1985, p 623). Yet, understanding of the syndrome and successful treatment of these individuals have not progressed to a marked degree (Reid 1985). One reason is that most antisocial persons do not seek medical help but often come to the attention of authorities because of criminal activity. Such criminal behavior creates anger toward the person committing it, which precludes medical research support. It is difficult to

identify the antisocial personality disorder as an illness when the behaviors are seemingly intentional, antagonistic, and self-serving.

Some clinicians are concerned about the term *antisocial* because it connotes criminality. In fact, the behaviors may be adaptive in people with certain life-styles, e.g., in the transient pieceworker, in people holding high-risk jobs, and even in the chronically mentally ill (Cameron and Rychlak 1985, Reid 1985, Travin and Protter 1982). The nurse must remember that manipulation, which is a hallmark of the antisocial client's behavior, may be a normal, nondestructive mode of meeting one's needs. However, when used to control others, manipulation interferes with interpersonal relationships. In antisocial clients, the drive to manipulate others is paramount, as these clients feel a need to be "number one" at all times.

The essential features of the antisocial personality, according to the DSM-IIIR, include:

- A history of continuous and chronic antisocial behavior in which the rights of others are violated
- A pattern of antisocial behavior that begins before the age of 15 and persists into adult life
- A failure to sustain adequate role performance over a period of several years

The antisocial behavior is not due to severe mental retardation, schizophrenia, or manic episodes.

It is estimated that 3 percent of American men and 1 percent of American women have antisocial personalities, although many researchers predict that the latter figure will increase as female life-styles become more like those of the male population (Reid 1985, Rowe 1984). There may also be a relationship between conduct and attention deficit disorders during the prepubertal years and the later development of antisocial personality syndrome. Although Schlesinger (1980) differentiates the psychopath, antisocial personality, and sociopath according to types and motives of criminal activities, all syndromes are classified as antisocial personality disorders in this chapter.

The study of developmental considerations has been hampered by the fact that the majority of investigators have used prisoners as research subjects. Although many criminals are sociopaths, not all sociopaths are found in prisons.

Physiologic Factors   Researchers, in an effort to identify biologic markers, have found that antisocial persons have a history of hyperactivity in childhood, a high rate of nonspecific electroencephalographic (EEG) abnormalities, and autonomic nervous system dysfunction manifested by high arousal states. The dysfunctional arousal of the autonomic nervous system may help to explain the early risk-taking behaviors (Cloninger 1978). In 1978, Rowe reported that brain trauma was a possible precursor to this disorder. More recently, depletion of serotonin and 5-HIAA (the metabolite of serotonin) has been associated with some forms of primitive aggression in mammals. Likewise, impulsive physical violence in humans (including violent suicide) has been negatively correlated with levels of 5-HIAA in cerebrospinal fluid. These data are consistent with the finding that antisocial behavior frequently peaks in late adolescence and young adulthood, when 5-HIAA levels are usually lowest (Reid 1985, p 832).

Cognitive Factors   Cognitive development is impaired to the extent that the individual is dominated by interests that are immediate and personally relevant (Shapiro 1965). This would account for the cunning abilities of the antisocial person to capitalize on others' vulnerabilities and quickly achieve personal goals. Gorenstein (1982, p 377) reports that although antisocial persons are able to acquire new ideas, they tend to act in ways that have been previously reinforced. This researcher believes that impaired *cognitive flexibility* characterizes the thinking processes of these persons. Perhaps the long-term planning deficiencies seen in this group are partially explained by this data.

Cognitive theorists, using measures of skill acquisition, hypothesize that developmental arrest of the antisocial personality occurs between the ages of 7–11. During this time, the normal child lacks the ability to reverse roles and seeks retribution for transgressions, showing little empathy or guilt. Around the age of 13, the normal child develops reciprocity with others and is able to abstract and be an empathic partner in a relationship. The antisocial person, however, remains narcissistic and intolerant of the rights of others.

Psychodynamic Factors   Psychodynamic theorists propose that antisocial individuals use primitive, global defenses such as projection and splitting to distance themselves from others. The antisocial person stabilizes his or her identity by using these defenses and filling life with action and stimulation to blot out affect and anxiety. Hence, the nurse may observe a "caricature of love" (Cleckley 1964) as the antisocial person playacts relationships (Reid 1985).

Social Factors   Social considerations in the development of antisocial personality disorder include:

- Failure of early identification experiences
- Excessive, harsh, inconsistent, or overpermissive discipline
- Lower socioeconomic level
- Lack of nurturing
- History of broken homes
- Alcoholic or antisocial parents
- Numerous parent surrogates
- Parental and or community rejection (self-fulfilling prophecy)
- Positive reinforcement of acting out or antisocial behavior during early childhood

Subtle encouragement of a child's antisocial behavior to bolster pathologic family stability has also been identified by Reid (1985) and is consistent with family systems theory.

It is most likely that the antisocial personality disorder has multiple causes. The nurse is cautioned not to make hasty judgments regarding the issue of criminality versus illness. If one views psychopathy as an internal defect, the antisocial person does not feel satisfaction with this disruptive life-style. Nonetheless, it is wise to consider the adaptive nature of this disorder, as well as its encouragement in an increasingly pleasure-seeking Western culture. The public anger aroused by antisocial persons and their behavior is likely due to fear and a sense of powerlessness to stop or prevent their actions (Figure 21–1). The following example illustrates the typical behavior of an antisocial person who has become disruptive without overt criminality.

Jack is a handsome, charming man of 38 who was the vice-president of a prominent general construction company. Jack is the second of three boys. Both his parents were alcoholics, and his father had spent many years putting together unsuccessful business deals. Jack was encouraged and applauded by his father, even as a child, whenever he outsmarted someone else, particularly those in authority, such as teachers and police. Jack's first legal involvement occurred at the age of 14, when he stole a neighbor's car and went joyriding. His charm and persuasiveness, as well as his neighbor's perception that Jack was a neglected child, kept the neighbor from pressing charges. Jack continued to be involved in antisocial activities, financing his college education by stealing and selling exams and dealing drugs on campus.

Jack initially sought consultation due to marital problems arising from his repeated acts of infidelity and lying. His third wife was contemplating divorce after finding a two-carat diamond engagement ring in his briefcase. He heatedly denied the ring was for someone else. He did not give it to his wife, however, stating, "You spoiled the surprise." The few people who know him well in social and work relationships view Jack as unreliable, unethical, unpredictable, and insincere. They call him a "pathological liar." Three months prior to this visit, Jack had been caught embezzling over $300,000 from the construction company. His response to the discovery was, "Somehow there's been a big misunderstanding on the part of the accountants." He was

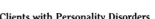

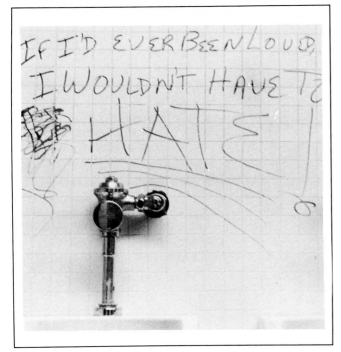

Figure 21–1
People with antisocial personality disorders are storm centers in their social relations and sometimes thrive on the trouble they create. Underlying their behavior and attitudes may be feelings they seldom express.

able to charm the company owner out of pressing charges against him. Jack paid back only a part of the embezzled funds, citing high entertainment and travel expenses on company business for his need for the money.

When news of the embezzlement reached the community, Jack denied the story and stated, "He [the owner] is jealous of my intelligence and was looking for a way to get rid of me." After leaving this company, Jack formed his own business. He again engaged in illegal and unethical business practices. He spent large sums skydiving, flying to Switzerland to ski, and having cosmetic surgery. He became preoccupied with both his own and his wife's appearance. He demanded that she have cosmetic surgery, dye her hair, and wear tinted contact lenses to alter the color of her eyes. Jack had several hair transplants and exercised excessively. As the marriage began to deteriorate, Jack began to use cocaine and drink alcohol daily. On one occasion, while intoxicated, he beat his wife severely because "she was losing her sex appeal." He told the therapist during the first interview, "Any problems we have are due to my wife's behavior; I'm here only to please her."

Jack canceled appointments for both his second and third sessions, stating, "My tax accountants have to spend some time with me. The IRS thinks I've cheated them out of some money."

Lifelong patterns of antisocial behavior often emerge during childhood and adolescence. However, this diagnosis is not applied to people younger than 18. DSM-IIIR criteria for the antisocial personality disorder are shown in Box 21–3. The following subjective and objective data have been adapted from this source:

- Has impaired superego (conscience) development associated with faulty identification process
- Is relatively free of anxiety; shows free-floating anxiety only when under external stress
- Is unable to defer pleasure; wants immediate gratification
- Cannot feel guilt, although easily verbalizes or play-acts a remorseful role
- Lacks interest in morals or values
- Is impulsive without considering the alternatives or consequences
- Is insincere and lies
- Uses people as objects for gratification of needs and discards them when they are no longer useful
- Commits frequent sexual indiscretions
- Lacks responsibility for commitments, including marriage, family, and occupation
- Manipulates situations and people for personal gain without concern for the rights or feelings of others
- Is extroverted; makes good first impressions due to charm and persuasiveness
- Is financially and emotionally dependent on others but fears intimacy
- Has few close friends but many casual relationships
- Changes jobs frequently, has long periods of unemployment, and is belligerent
- Has poor school and work history
- Abuses or is dependent on drugs
- Is intellectually competent; however, does not profit from experience or mistakes
- Is often involved in socially unacceptable or criminal activities, including crimes of violence such as rape
- Has no major disorders of thought, affect, or brain function

Nursing Diagnosis

Despite the quantity of assessment data, the primary nursing diagnoses for the antisocial client are ineffective individual coping and self-concept disturbance. These problems are often observed:

Box 21–3
DIAGNOSTIC CRITERIA FOR 301.70 ANTISOCIAL PERSONALITY DISORDER*

A. Current age at least 18.

B. Evidence of Conduct Disorder with onset before age 15, as indicated by a history of *three* or more of the following:

1. Was often truant

2. Ran away from home overnight at least twice while living in parental or parental surrogate home (or once without returning)

3. Often initiated physical fights

4. Used a weapon in more than one fight

5. Forced someone into sexual activity with him or her

6. Was physically cruel to animals

7. Was physically cruel to other people

8. Deliberately destroyed others' property (other than by fire-setting)

9. Deliberately engaged in fire-setting

10. Often lied (other than to avoid physical or sexual abuse)

11. Has stolen without confrontation of a victim on more than one occasion (including forgery)

12. Has stolen with confrontation of a victim (e.g., mugging, purse-snatching, extortion, armed robbery)

C. A pattern of irresponsible and antisocial behavior since the age of 15, as indicated by at least *four* of the following:

1. Is unable to sustain consistent work behavior, as indicated by any of the following (including similar behavior in academic settings if the person is a student):

   a. Significant unemployment for six months or more within five years when expected to work and work was available

   b. Repeated absences from work unexplained by illness in self or family

   c. Abandonment of several jobs without realistic plans for others

2. Fails to conform to social norms with respect to lawful behavior, as indicated by repeatedly performing antisocial acts that are grounds for arrest (whether arrested or not), e.g., destroying prop-

erty, harassing others, stealing, pursuing an illegal occupation

3. Is irritable and aggressive, as indicated by repeated physical fights or assaults (not required by one's job or to defend someone or oneself), including spouse- or child-beating

4. Repeatedly fails to honor financial obligations, as indicated by defaulting on debts or failing to provide child support or support for other dependents on a regular basis

5. Fails to plan ahead, or is impulsive, as indicated by one or both of the following:

   a. Traveling from place to place without a prearranged job or clear goal for the period of travel or clear idea about when the travel will terminate

   b. Lack of a fixed address for a month or more

6. Has no regard for the truth, as indicated by repeated lying, use of aliases, or "conning" others for personal profit or pleasure

7. Is reckless regarding his or her own or others' personal safety, as indicated by driving while intoxicated, or recurrent speeding

8. If a parent or guardian, lacks ability to function as a responsible parent, as indicated by one or more of the following:

   a. Malnutrition of child

   b. Child's illness resulting from lack of minimal hygiene

   c. Failure to obtain medical care for a seriously ill child

   d. Child's dependence on neighbors or nonresident relatives for food or shelter

   e. Failure to arrange for a caretaker for young child when parent is away from home

   f. Repeated squandering, on personal items, of money required for household necessities

9. Has never sustained a totally monogamous relationship for more than one year

10. Lacks remorse (feels justified in having hurt, mistreated, or stolen from another)

D. Occurrence of antisocial behavior not exclusively during the course of Schizophrenia or Manic Episodes.

Source: Reprinted with permission of the American Psychiatric Association: Diagnostic and Statistical Manual of Mental Disorders, ed 3, revised. APA, 1987, pp 344–346.

Coping, Ineffective Individual

- Altered participation in society
- Verbal and nonverbal manipulation
- Destructive behavior toward self and others
- Overuse of defense mechanisms of denial, splitting, projection, rationalization, and intellectualization
- Impaired problem-solving abilities

Self-Concept, Disturbance In

- Altered self-esteem evidenced by affective disturbances (grandiosity, depression)
- Lack of responsibility, accountability, or commitment
- Lying
- Distancing relationships
- Nonparticipation in therapy
- Impulsiveness

Planning and Implementing Interventions

Because antisocial people manipulate others so successfully, it is unlikely that these individuals will seek change unless faced with severe external stress. In clinical situations, the nurse's responses to these clients are critical to developing and maintaining a therapeutic alliance as well as preserving the hospital or prison milieu. Box 21–4 illustrates some guidelines for developing a relationship. It is important to recognize, however, that these clients identify unit power structures and pit staff members against one another. Since these clients tend to be intelligent and charming, staff may fail to identify manipulations or excuse these behaviors. In addition, these clients may often actively resist directives while appearing to be compliant. Short-term therapy is usually ineffective, and long-term hospitalization or incarceration may be indicated.

In general, the nurse must present the "brick wall" against which the client can butt (Dighton 1986) as the antisocial person attempts to manipulate others to achieve his or her ends. Because of the charm, facade of superiority, and persuasiveness of these people, nurses sometimes assume the roles of nurturers and rescuers. Nurses should never give out telephone numbers, assign special privileges, or make themselves available to these clients outside the therapeutic relationship. The clients have life-long patterns of victimizing others.

Evaluation

Extensive studies indicate that antisocial clients: (a) do not respond to drug therapy, (b) remain in psychodynamic therapies only long enough to decrease their anxiety and ingratiate therapists, and (c) respond to cognitive-behavioral therapies only as long as someone is available to reinforce the desired behaviors. Court-ordered hospitalization

---

Box 21–4
NURSING GUIDELINES: ANTISOCIAL CLIENTS

- Use a concerned but matter-of-fact approach.
- Set, communicate, and maintain consistent rules and regulations for all clients.
- Do not argue, bargain, or rationalize.
- Confront inappropriate behaviors without anger, punitiveness, or personalization.
- Do not seek approval.
- Set limits on all interactions.
- Be alert for flattery or verbal attacks.
- Do not permit client to dictate therapeutic regimen.
- Using contracts and relaxation techniques, teach client how to delay immediate gratification and impulsiveness.
- Teach client to redirect thrill-seeking impulses into socially acceptable outlets, e.g., race car driving versus speeding.
- Use peer pressure (e.g., groups, buddy systems) to modify manipulative behaviors.
- Use reinforcing techniques to achieve desired behaviors.
- Role model self-discipline.
- Participate in staff meetings and clinical supervision to work through transference and countertransference phenomena.

---

tends to be more successful than voluntary treatment because the antisocial individual is generally highly manipulative and may easily disrupt the milieu or leave the facility. Some therapeutic success has been observed with back-to-nature, survival programs in which survival depends on developing skills and relationships with others (Reid 1985).

Some antisocial people "burn out" in later life (over age 35), giving up extreme forms of antisocial responses. Narcissism continues, but family stability and occupational adaptation are evident in about 25 percent of the population (Cloninger 1978). These people do not become model citizens, but they tend to avoid the criminal and welfare systems.

When evaluating short-term in-patient objectives, the nurse looks for the following client behaviors as evidence that coping abilities and self-concept are within normal boundaries.

Coping, Ineffective Individual

- Increased impulse control and ability to delay gratification
- Decreased verbal and nonverbal manipulations
- Adherence to unit rules and regulations
- Acceptance of personal responsibility and accountability for actions

Self-Concept, Disturbance In

- Realistic identification of assets and liabilities
- Identification of personal problem areas
- Absence of aggression directed to self or others
- Assertive communications with others

A nursing care plan for a client with an antisocial personality disorder is on pages 568 and 569.

Individuals with personality disorders who present primarily as anxious or fearful may be diagnosed as **avoidant, dependent, obsessive compulsive,** or **passive-aggressive** under the criteria established in the DSM-IIIR. Anxious-fearful persons generally experience both social and occupational impairments as a result of their restricted affect, nonassertiveness, problems expressing feelings, unrealistic expectations of others, and impaired decision making and problem solving. These individuals tend to have arrested development during the oral or anal stages of psychosexual development (Cameron and Rychlak 1985). Developmental precursors to these disorders include early anxiety associated with parental attitudes and fears of abandonment and rejection. Overly critical, demanding, and punitive parenting practices coupled with diminished opportunities to express feelings may be contributing factors. The lifestyle of the anxious-fearful person is characterized by intense emotional repression and behaviors that are socially isolating and self-defeating. Because the behaviors of the disorders in the anxious-fearful cluster tend to overlap, common features of these conditions are shown in Box 21–5.

Box 21–5
COMMON FEATURES OF ANXIOUS-FEARFUL PERSONALITIES

Aloof, Ambivalent Social Style

The anxious-fearful person restricts social contact to those individuals typified as safe and nonrejecting. Because they anticipate rejection and criticism from others, their relationships may be either clinging or detached.

Restricted Affect

The affective responses of anxious-fearful persons range from insensitivity to the feelings of others to overconcern and oversensitivity to the evaluation by others. The inability to express underlying feelings is generally based on a fear that others will reject them unless they are perfect. The avoidant and dependent personalities tend to see themselves as inferior to others and subordinate their needs accordingly. In contrast, the compulsive and passive-aggressive personalities view authority as overly restrictive; consequently, they are insensitive to others' needs.

Fear of Success or Failure

Active or passive avoidance of responsibility characterizes all the anxious-fearful personalities. Resistant behavior may be deliberately avoidant as seen in dependent and avoidant persons. The behavior may be covert, as evidenced by the compulsive person's obsessive attention to details, leading to ineffective overall performance. Passive-aggressive persons set themselves up to fail by dawdling, intentional forgetting, and procrastination.

Fear of Loss of Control

When a person's quest for autonomy is thwarted at an early age, response patterns manifested by rigidity are often noted. The needs to control, to have guarantees of others' love, to avoid relaxation and fun, and to maintain structure and orderliness are seen in anxious-fearful people. These responses seem to provide some reassurance of predictability and control in their lives.

Fear of Embarrassment

Persons with all the personality disorders in the anxious-fearful cluster manifest response patterns indicating low self-esteem and lack of self-confidence. An insignificant act by a waitress or salesperson may be construed as rejecting or overly solicitous.

Difficulty with Decision Making

Related to low self-esteem and fear of criticism is a fear of making an incorrect choice or recommendation. Consequently, anxious-fearful people either tend to focus on details and procrastinate, or they may give responsibility for decision making to others.

Negativity

Anxious-fearful people view the world as potentially disappointing. They exude an air of pessimism, irritability, sulkiness, discontent, and submissiveness that colors all their interactions. They tend to dampen everyone's spirits, thus confirming their perceptions and expectations.

The Nursing Process and Avoidant Personality Disorders

Nursing Assessment: Defining Characteristics of the Avoidant Personality

The essential features of the avoidant personality are fear and hypersensitivity to potential rejection and shame. These people withdraw socially although they avidly desire affection and acceptance. They want guarantees that people will uncritically accept them. Their avoidant behavior results in their often visiting public places, e.g., movies, museums, and ballparks, simply to experience the presence of other people because they do not enjoy being alone. When in public places, however, they maintain a safe distance from others. For example, in a movie theater one can be physically close to people without any intrusion on personal space. Avoidant people devalue their own achievements. They appear overly serious, humorless, and painfully shy. Speech is often slow, and they do not express feelings. Thought content is generally serious.

Mary Jane is a 27-year-old single female who sought counseling due to feelings of loneliness and lack of friends. She describes herself as having grown up on a Midwest farm where she was "pretty much a homebody." In high school she made good grades but did not participate in any extracurricular activities. She studied library science in college and admits to receiving secondhand pleasure from reading about the experiences of others. Historical novels are her favorites. She is currently employed as a reference librarian in a large aerospace company where she has minimal contact with other people. She says she wants to establish both male and female friendships but feels afraid that "people will laugh" at her. Mary Jane joined the company bowling team at the suggestion of a coworker but quit after the first evening because she felt she would "hold them back." Mary Jane rationalized her decision by stating, "I think I would be more comfortable pursuing an intellectual hobby."

Although the schizoid and avoidant personalities have many similar characteristics, the avoidant person's motivation to form a therapeutic relationship differentiates the two. The avoidant person also tends to lead a fairly productive life, particularly regarding occupation and self-care maintenance.

Nursing Diagnosis

Social isolation and self-concept disturbances are the major nursing diagnoses for the avoidant client. The social isolation is self-induced, and the feelings that promote distancing are very painful.

Social Isolation

- Feelings of being "different"
- Lack of significant purpose
- Insecurity in public
- Verbalized fears of rejection

Self-Concept, Disturbance In

- Inability to accept positive reinforcement
- Inability to evaluate one's own worth realistically
- Belittling oneself in daily activities
- Condemning oneself for failing to develop adequate social skills

Planning and Implementing Interventions

Intervention strategies are focused on developing a therapeutic alliance with the client. In this relationship, the nurse confronts clients' illogical beliefs about themselves and their perceptions of others. Systematic desensitization techniques are useful in helping the clients bridge the gap in forming social relationships. Behavioral techniques, e.g., contracting with the client to network with others in support groups and employment activities, may also be useful. Underlying any intervention strategies should be the knowledge that avoidant personalities, because of their intense fear, are prone to episodes of depression, phobias, and periods of intense inner-directed rage. Consequently, the nurse should be prepared to prevent and deal with intermittent crises as psychodynamic issues are uncovered.

Evaluation

Unless the cycle of timidity and fear in social situations is interrupted, avoidant clients continue to reinforce their apprehension by their own interpersonal restraint. Cognitive-behavioral therapies are often useful in helping these clients look at their own behaviors and the erroneous meanings that they may assign to the comments of others.

The Nursing Process and Dependent Personality Disorders

Nursing Assessment: Defining Characteristics of the Dependent Personality

The essential features of the dependent personality include lack of self-confidence, inability to make decisions, and inability to function independently. In sharp contrast to the avoidant person, dependent people cling to others and

Nursing Care Plan: The Client with an Antisocial Personality

Nursing Diagnosis (PND-I/NANDA)	Client Care Goals	Nursing Planning/ Interventions	Evaluation
05.02 Altered conduct/ impulse processes 04.98 Altered emotional processes not otherwise specified 06.98 Altered perception processes not otherwise specified 06.01.04 Selective attention 02.02 Altered judgment 02.08.01 Altered abstract thinking 02.08.03 Altered problem solving 02.04 Altered learning processes 02.05 Altered memory /Coping, ineffective individual (associated with inability to delay gratification, manipulation of others, failure to learn behaviors, overuse of defensive mechanisms including denial, projection, rationalization, intellectualization, splitting)	The client will assume personal responsibility for behavior and its consequences.	1. Develop a plan for dealing with manipulative behavior and instruct all staff to use the same approaches. 2. Help client to identify patterns and consequences of manipulative behavior by pointing them out when they occur. 3. Set firm, consistent limits and expectations of behavior and review these with the client. 4. Discuss with client what he or she hopes to achieve by manipulations. 5. Listen matter-of-factly when client verbalizes frustration, annoyance, etc., at the limits established. 6. Observe for escalating behavior of a violent nature (assault, suicide) and take precautions as necessary. 7. Encourage client to identify consequences of behavior. 8. Contract with client to express feelings verbally without acting out. 9. Teach client differences between immediate needs and those which can be delayed. 10. Establish privilege system based on compliance with treatment program activities. 11. Point out to client defensive behaviors and	1. Verbally identifies manipulative responses. 2. Identifies unfulfilled needs that lead to manipulation of others. 3. Delays immediate gratification when appropriate. 4. Develops appropriate outlets for aggressive impulses. 5. Verbalizes the consequences of actions. 6. Develops alternative strategies for dealing with frustration. 7. Minimizes use of defense mechanisms of denial, projection, splitting, rationalization, and intellectualization.

continued

Nursing Care Plan: The Client with an Antisocial Personality *(continued)*

Nursing Diagnosis (PND-I/NANDA)	Client Care Goals	Nursing Planning/ Interventions	Evaluation
		encourage expression of underlying feelings.	
		12. Assist client to write behavioral options for dealing with situations of anger, frustration, or desire.	
		13. Give consistent feedback and positively reinforce appropriate behaviors.	
		14. Identify personal feelings about client and the behaviors they manifest; use clinical supervision to deal with issues.	
		15. Use peer pressure to modify manipulative behaviors.	
05.01.02 Altered nonverbal communication*	The client will exercise honesty and increased impulse control within societal guidelines.	1. Help client assess strengths and weaknesses via feedback, peer reviews, verbal dialogue in one-to-one sessions and journals, and "homework" tasks of a self-evaluative nature.	1. Realistically identifies assets and liabilities.
05.01.01 Altered verbal communication* /Communication, impaired: verbal			2. Uses self-control and appropriate judgment in meeting short-term objectives.
05.98 Altered interpersonal processes not otherwise specified		2. Give positive reinforcement when client is able to delay gratification.	3. Refrains from deceitful communications, e.g., lying, breaking promises, "stretching" the truth, intentional forgetting.
05.02.01.02 Aggressive/ violent behaviors toward others		3. Help client to problem solve, identifying alternative actions and probable consequences.	
05.02.01.03 Aggressive/ violent behaviors toward self		4. Confront client with lies and insist upon truthfulness in all interactions.	4. Develops and maintains a support system that encourages adherence to group norms and mutual respect.
05.03.01 Altered family role		5. Be firm and courteous when client becomes angry and/or hostile.	
05.03.06 Altered work role		6. Role play situations, demonstrating direct and adaptive responses.	
05.04 Altered sexuality processes /Self-concept, disturbance in (associated with impulsivity, lying, failure to meet role expectations, sexual indiscretions, lack of support system)			

*PND-I diagnosis also in NANDA list.

passively accept their dictates and leadership. Dependent people view themselves as "helpless" or "stupid" and seek out dominant others or objects to lean on for guidance, control, and support as well as for "permission" to behave. The dominant other/object relationship stems from the normal life-sustaining bond between mother and infant. In dependent people, this normal symbiotic relationship has been excessively prolonged, impairing their capacity for thinking, feeling, and responding on their own. They believe they must be taken care of and consequently rely on others to mirror their feelings to them. Dependent people subordinate their desires and needs to the wishes of others in order to maintain relationships. They often appear friendly, helpful, and indispensable. When the dominant other or object is unavailable, or perceived as unavailable, dependent persons experience intense anxiety. This may lead to feelings of unhappiness, anger, resentment, or depression. It is also noteworthy that significant others may eventually respond to dependent people with anger and resentment because of their continuous clinging and ingratiating behaviors.

The early childhood environment, which is characterized by premature separation from parents, neglect, overprotection, or lack of parental responsiveness, may predispose to dependent personality disorders (Moyer and Snider 1984). Like people with other personality disorders discussed in DSM-IIIR, the dependent person may have multiple Axis II diagnoses. The following example illustrates how a dependent client might behave.

Marie is a 40-year-old single parent of two teenage daughters. She has gained seventy pounds since her divorce two years ago. Currently, Marie is sporadically attending a group for displaced homemakers, where she has shared a great deal of information about herself. She states that she is essentially a "homebody" and feels most satisfied when baking, cooking, and sewing for her daughters. Marie describes her secondhand pleasure in their activities, including ballet, gymnastics, and modeling. In fact, Marie becomes visibly saddened when she discusses her daughters' eventual departure for college. When her daughters expressed concern about Marie's weight gain and general health, Marie giggled and said, "Better to be fat and jolly than skinny and mean." Marie has made no attempt to develop new friendships or social outlets since her divorce. She is poorly groomed and haphazardly dressed, in contrast to her impeccably groomed daughters. When confronted by group members about her priority setting and the need to direct some energy toward herself, Marie responded, "My life is devoted to

my daughters; their needs are more important than mine, and that's why I agreed to make the thirty costumes for their dance recital next week."

Nursing Diagnosis

Nurses frequently avoid or voice dislike for dependent clients because of their cloying, clinging, and demanding behaviors. This avoidance response tends to reinforce these clients' perceptions that other people are unwilling to help and that they are unable to help themselves. As a result, clients increase their clinging responses because they know no other way to behave. This increased clinging only leads to further avoidance by others. The primary nursing diagnoses and problem areas are as follows:

Self-Concept, Disturbance In

- Is verbally and nonverbally compliant
- Lacks initiative
- Avoids decision making or changes mind frequently
- Is unable to meet own needs independently
- Is unwilling to make assertive requests of others for fear of rejection
- Belittles personal assets and abilities

Self-Care Deficit

- Altered activities of daily living, e.g., grooming, hygiene, and nutrition
- Self-indulgence in food, alcohol, and drugs
- Inattention to medical and dental needs

Planning and Implementing Interventions

The goal of nursing interventions is to help the client achieve independent functioning. Guidelines for nursing interventions are shown in Box 21–6.

Evaluation

Dependent personalities commonly experience crises when the dominant support system is altered. During crisis episodes, these clients may be open to cognitive-behavioral strategies, but the outlook for major personality restructuring is dim. Instead, dependent people tend to transfer dependency needs to others.

The Nursing Process and Obsessive Compulsive Personality Disorders

Nursing Assessment: Defining Characteristics of the Obsessive Compulsive Personality

The obsessive compulsive individual demonstrates anxiety and fearfulness by behavior that shows fear of losing control over situations, objects, or people. The obsessive compulsive personality strives at all times to keep the world predictable and organized. The major features of this disorder are an excessive dedication to work, productivity, and perfectionism to the exclusion of feelings and pleasure. The obsessive compulsive individual may be likened to a drill sergeant in the military who is rigid, serious, detail oriented, and stingy with emotions.

A focus on trivial details often leads this person not only to "miss the forest for the trees, but [also] fail to see the tree while counting its leaves" (Eaton et al. 1976, p 106). Although these people may be highly praised for their organizational skills and work ethic, eventually their rigidity causes them to fear making mistakes. Consequently, they postpone making decisions. They tend to resent authority but rarely express this resentment openly. Instead, they may engage in passive-aggressive behavior, e.g., procrastination and stubbornness. To manage their procrastination, obsessive compulsive people often initiate work on a project far in advance of the due date, as shown in the following example:

Peter set himself a deadline in early fall for ordering his family's Christmas gifts. His family found this deadline something of an annoyance. Yet Peter persisted in his attempts to get commitments from everyone about what they wanted. Often, he would mislay his early purchases by the time Christmas arrived, and he would rush out to do last-minute shopping anyway.

Peter appears to be concerned with his family and interpersonal relationships, but he is really more concerned with meeting the Christmas deadline and checking off his list than in his relatives' enjoyment of their gifts.

Box 21–6

NURSING INTERVENTION GUIDELINES FOR DEPENDENT PERSONALITIES

- Evaluate the client's ability to perform self-care activities; encourage grooming and personal hygiene.

- Anticipate the client's needs *before* he or she demands attention through inappropriate responses by scheduling regular sessions with the client.

- Help the client identify assets and liabilities, including plans for change; emphasize strengths and potential.

- Encourage the client to take responsibility for own opinions; point out when the client negates own feelings or opinions.

- Encourage the client to verbalize feelings of anxiety related to independent functioning.

- Encourage the client to talk about how needs for affection, control, and responsibility are currently being met.

- Share your observations of the client's manipulative behavior with him or her. For example, a client may offer to accompany a physically impaired client to a group activity in order to minimize the amount of time spent in productive therapy.

- Set realistic limits about what can and cannot be done for the client.

- Using group therapy to provide support, emphasize that the client is not alone in experiencing fear of failure or of success.

- Work through feelings of disappointment with the client when new behaviors are not immediately successful.

- Explore with the client the consequences of behaviors; for example, clinging tends to result in avoidance by others.

- Discuss personal responsibilities and make the client aware that he or she has choices.

- Teach the client problem-solving techniques, including goal setting, making alternative responses, and evaluating consequences.

- Provide opportunities for client to have successful experiences and encourage participation in such activities.

- Help the client develop a realistic time frame in which independent living activities (e.g., getting a job or apartment) will be achieved.

- Do not do for the client what he or she is capable of doing without help.

- Give positive reinforcement for successful achievements.

- Teach and role model assertive behavior; teach client to develop strategies for confrontations by others.

- Prevent secondary gains from negative statements about self by refocusing interactions.

- State goals for nursing care in terms the client and staff can understand.

- Involve staff members in conferences and clinical supervision to deal with transference and countertransference issues.

Although Peter suffers under the pressure of his deadlines, he sets them for himself. He functions as his own overseer, issuing commands, directives, reminders, warnings, and admonitions about what should be done. People like Peter are also keenly aware of society's and other people's expectations, of the threat of possible criticism, of the weight and direction of authority, of rules, regulations, and conventions, and of a great collection of moral or quasimoral principles. These people feel required to fulfill unending duties, responsibilities, and tasks that are, in their view, not chosen, but simply there.

Compulsive people do not view taking work home and working long hours as an imposition, since work organizes their lives and binds their anxiety. Indeed, the compulsive person will make work out of pleasurable activities, as the following example shows:

Jennifer planned her European vacation in meticulous detail. She scheduled exhausting daily tours and activities from 6:30 A.M. until 12:00 PM. Jennifer planned to visit every attraction available as quickly as possible. So as not to waste time, she wrote her postcards to her family while she rode tour buses. The cards were crammed with information about weather, prices of goods and services, menus, and daily time tables. She wrote nothing about how she felt or what she was experiencing. Upon returning home, she spent two weeks cataloging all her photographs and typing short paragraphs to accompany each photo. She passed her album around at work during lunch hour expecting that her co-workers would read all the captions. She became insulted and irate when several co-workers flipped through the album quickly. Jennifer found it difficult to forgive them for "slighting" her in this way.

When a co-worker was planning a trip, Jennifer suggested that he record details of the trip in a diary so that he could compile an album similar to her own. Jennifer was not aware of the resentment, hurt, and irritation her behavior generated in others.

Specific defining characteristics of the obsessive compulsive personality are listed in Box 21–7. However, the nurse should always consider how clients will react to the realization that years of denying themselves satisfaction, working hard, saving, and restricting the quality of life have not produced the expected rewards (e.g., career advancement, status, promotions). This realization often leads to the potential for depression, especially during middle life. As the following example shows, the obsessive compulsive

---

Box 21–7

DEFINING CHARACTERISTICS OF THE OBSESSIVE COMPULSIVE PERSONALITY

- Shows excessive dedication to work
- Is sensitive to criticism and rejection
- Is preoccupied with organization, details, procedures, and rules
- Is a perfectionist
- Is indecisive and ambivalent
- Demands conformity to his or her standards
- Resists authority of others
- Excludes pleasure; makes work out of play
- Is moralistic and judgmental about self and others
- Concentrates on minute details and trivia
- Restricts emotional expression
- Is stingy with both emotions and material objects
- Harbors anger and resentment against others
- Shows little empathy
- Expresses anger indirectly
- Is status conscious
- Fears making mistakes
- Has potential for depression

---

person may even postpone acting on major decisions to avoid the reality of life without work.

Millie, a 61-year-old college professor, seeks counseling one year prior to her planned retirement. She complains of insomnia, weight loss, and pervasive anxiety about "what life will be like without anything to do." Millie is retiring early because she feels that in spite of twenty-five years of loyal service to the university and diligent work, she has been passed over repeatedly for promotion to the position of department chairperson. Millie is an unmarried, slender woman who is meticulously dressed in very conservative clothing.

During the interview, she says that she made most of her own clothing and purchased only items that were on sale. In describing her daily activities, Millie states that she is a "hard worker who always took things home to finish." She voices resentment that neither the department chairperson nor other faculty did likewise. Millie says that she spent more than ten years caring for an elderly mother because "my sister didn't have time for her." Millie devoted a great deal of time to church and university activities. The therapist's impression is that Millie performed these functions out of duty rather than for spontaneous enjoyment or satisfaction. Millie states that she volunteered to be secretary of the local humane society because she knew she could keep the detailed records better than any of the other members.

When questioned about her relationships with other faculty, Millie says that she communicated with them by memos to avoid being misquoted. She further states that she kept copies of all these memos because "They can't keep things straight most of the time." Millie becomes visibly angry when relating a recent experience: She overheard two colleagues ridiculing a memo requesting, six months in advance, that guest lecturers be permitted to use the colleagues' parking spaces. When challenged about the lack of immediacy of her request, Millie states that she has "stopped speaking to them [the faculty] entirely." When the therapist questions Millie about her interests for retirement, Millie says, "I don't really know; I've never had time for frivolous activities." By the end of the session, Millie has become indecisive about whether she should retire, after all.

The obsessive compulsive personality evolves from the need to exert control and autonomy over one's bodily functions and the world during the second stage of psychosexual development. The struggle with parental figures over bowel control and the resultant anxiety and frustration may lead to characteristics of stinginess, pompous bookishness, and touchiness. Consequently, there is a lifelong struggle for independence, which is hampered by equally strong feelings of inadequacy, self-doubt, and ambivalence toward authority figures (Cameron and Rychlak 1985).

Interestingly, excessively conscientious, rigid people often exhibit a contradictory pattern of slovenliness, which is also compulsive. Thus, a compulsive housewife may scrub her kitchen floor daily but allow bags of garbage to accumulate and become infested with maggots.

If one looks to learning and behavioral theories for explanations for the obsessive compulsive personality, it is clear that society positively reinforces the ritualistic patterns that the person uses to adapt to the world. It is also likely that the parents of the obsessive compulsive individual disciplined the child excessively during the early years of development. Whether a compulsive response is adaptive or symptomatic depends on: (a) its effectiveness and (b) the person's ability to modify the response when it is inappropriate.

Nursing Diagnosis

"Coping, ineffective individual" is the primary nursing diagnosis with obsessive compulsive clients. This is evidenced by responses that show restricted cognitive, affective, and motor behavior. "Social isolation" related to resentment, self-doubt, and exclusion of pleasure is the other major nursing diagnosis.

Planning and Implementing Interventions

The goal is to help clients examine and evaluate their lifestyles and goals so that they can modify troublesome compulsive traits. The nurse intervenes to help these clients express dissatisfaction with their lives and to encourage realistic planning for future changes. Guidelines for nursing interventions are shown in Box 21–8.

Evaluation

As always, when evaluating any client with a personality disorder, the nurse must consider the potential for major psychiatric conditions such as depression and anxiety-related disturbances. Even though people with obsessive compulsive personalities often seek treatment for subjective distress, the course of treatment may be drawn out and ineffective due to the rigidity of their defensive operations. If the nurse confronts the obsessive compulsive behavior directly, the client might develop acute psychiatric conditions because of intense anxiety.

The Nursing Process and Passive-Aggressive Personality Disorders

Nursing Assessment: Defining Characteristics of the Passive-Aggressive Personality

The DSM-IIIR (1987) definition of and criteria for identifying the passive-aggressive personality disorder are substantially different from those in the 1980 edition. Box 21–9 shows the new DSM-IIIR criteria for diagnostic purposes. Resistant behaviors often observed are listed in Box 21–10. Simply stated, passive-aggressive behavior is the indirect expression of anger.

All passive-aggressive behaviors are eventually self-defeating. Consider the dynamics presented in the following example:

A nurse is asked to work overtime to cover a very short-staffed unit. If she chooses to accept the assignment willingly and does her best, she receives the approval of her employer. If she flatly refuses the assignment, she avoids the work but possibly risks her job. Her third option is to compromise in a mutually satisfactory way with her employer. However, if she chooses to respond in a passive-aggressive manner, she will stay, do the work hurriedly and carelessly, and complain frequently about how unfair the employer is. By choosing the passive-aggressive option, she forfeits the advantage of winning approval but still has to do the task.

> ## Box 21–8
> ## NURSING INTERVENTION GUIDELINES FOR OBSESSIVE COMPULSIVE PERSONALITIES
>
> - Confront nonconstructive, compulsive responses gently and be alert for anxiety when the client is confronted.
> - Discuss the importance of these responses with clients.
> - Show approval of recreation and enjoyment.
> - Do not demand that clients engage in leisure or recreational activities (clients will "work" at them instead of enjoying them).
> - Make a contract with the client stating how much time during one-to-one sessions will be used to discuss obsessive thoughts or rituals; gradually decrease the time allotted to these activities.
> - Help clients identify feelings of anxiety generated in stressful situations and their usual responses to this anxiety.
> - Help the client identify alternative coping methods to deal with stressful situations.
> - Help the client identify and differentiate between "shoulds" (behaviors expected by others) and "wants" (desirable activities).
> - Explore activities that were or are pleasurable or satisfying.
> - Plan activities and interventions around pleasurable memories.
> - Encourage physical activity.
> - Encourage verbalization of feelings, especially those of anger and resentment.
> - Provide examples of appropriate ways to handle emotion through role modeling, skills training, and group activities.
> - Discuss with clients how to recognize changes in themselves.
> - Monitor levels of compulsive behavior after initial baseline assessment.
> - Give gentle feedback, identifying weaknesses as well as strengths.
> - Provide progressive opportunities to make decisions.
> - Encourage clients to evaluate progress in meeting goals.

The example demonstrates the underlying dynamics of the passive-aggressive person. It is believed that early during the person's childhood, the parents were assertive or aggressive toward the child but blocked the child's need to express anger. In addition, the child's dependency needs were not met through nurturing and protective parental behavior. Consequently, the child learned to deal with anger by passively responding to those in authority with seemingly polite and undemanding behavior. This behavior, however, is marked by inefficiency and subtle resistance. Because these passive-aggressive maneuvers (which were unconsciously selected to protect the person from fear of abandonment) are so irritating to others, a self-defeating situation is perpetuated. Significant people continue to withdraw from the passive-aggressive person, who then increases the use of these maladaptive responses (Mahler et al 1975).

> ## Box 21–9
> ## CRITERIA FOR PASSIVE-AGGRESSIVE PERSONALITY DISORDER
>
> Clients who are passive-aggressive tend to passively resist demands requiring adequate social and occupational performance. A diagnosis of passive-aggressive personality disorder may be made if the client consistently demonstrates five or more of the following behaviors:
>
> - Puts off jobs that need to be done and thus misses deadlines (procrastination)
> - Deliberately works slowly or does a bad job on those tasks that he or she really doesn't want to do
> - Protests, unjustifiably, that others make unreasonable demands on him or her
> - Claims "forgetfulness" to avoid meeting obligations
> - Becomes pouty, sulky, irritable, or argumentative when asked to do something that he or she does not want to do
> - Overestimates the value of his or her work, i.e., thinks that he or she is doing a much better job than others think is being done
> - Becomes resentful when others offer useful suggestions to enhance his or her productivity
> - Obstructs task accomplishment by failing to do his or her share of the work
> - Is unreasonably critical or scornful of those persons in positions of authority
>
> *Source: Adapted from American Psychiatric Association:* Diagnostic and Statistical Manual of Mental Disorders, *ed 3, revised. APA, 1987, pp 358–359.*

The major nursing diagnosis for passive-aggressive clients is "coping, ineffective individual." Problem behaviors have been identified in Box 21–10.

Planning and Implementing Interventions

The nursing care plan for clients with a passive-aggressive personality is on the following pages. In addition to implementing the interventions in the care plan, the psychiatric nurse may find it helpful to teach the families of passive-aggressive clients how to interact with and relate to their significant others in order to disrupt ineffective patterns

---

Box 21–10
RESISTANT RESPONSES OF PASSIVE-AGGRESSIVE PERSONALITIES

- Is stubborn and complies half-heartedly
- Is inefficient
- Is forgetful
- Procrastinates
- Is negative
- Is pessimistic
- Is sarcastic, makes snide remarks
- Is envious, resents others
- Dawdles
- Is sullen and moody
- Sees self as a victim of circumstances
- Assumes no responsibility for control of situations
- Is subtly antagonistic
- Complains chronically
- Sulks and pouts
- Is critical of advice or direction from others
- Avoids open hostility or expressions of anger
- Sabotages the work of others
- Is chronically late
- Is verbally abusive toward others
- Has repeated educational, vocational, and social failures
- Is crude and rude in social situations, e.g., cracks gum, does needlework, belches, is flatulent or falls asleep during working meetings
- Deliberately dresses inappropriately for social or occupational activities
- Has frequent somatic complaints or disability claims

---

of behaving. In general, the dawdling, resistant behaviors of the passive-aggressive personality are best viewed as ineffective coping strategies. In specific situations, passive-aggressive responses may be adaptive. For example, a prison inmate who openly complies with authority may be at high risk of violence by other inmates. In this situation, slowdowns and careless workmanship would satisfy the authorities without antagonizing the other inmates. Consequently, the nurse must assess the client's responses within the context of the situations in which they occur. The following example shows how one therapist learned to cope with a passive-aggressive client.

Greg, a 22-year-old medical student, visits the university counseling service requesting assistance with time management. During the initial interview, he was soft-spoken, submissive, and polite, but his affect was sullen and pouting. He was evasive when asked for information concerning his daily activity schedule, making such comments as, "Well, sometimes I spend a lot of time thinking about how easy my classmates have it and how hard I have to work." Greg initially contracted to work on a list of problems, and he cooperated with the therapist. However, by the third session he had not only established a pattern of arriving late but also was interrupting role playing and counselor modeling, stating, "The real problem is something else." When the therapist tried to focus him on one problem at a time, Greg would become angry, sulk, and make whining complaints about not being "understood." He repeatedly "forgot" to do his homework assignments, stating, "I would have done it, but . . . ." By the fourth session, the therapist was feeling helpless and demoralized by Greg's habitual partial compliance. It was only after the therapist sought clinical supervision and cut back on the demands she made on Greg that a successful therapeutic alliance was established.

Evaluation

Two factors influence the outcome of therapeutic strategies. The first is the degree of insight the client and family have concerning the passive-aggressive behavior. The second is the attitude of the family system toward assertiveness or open aggression. If insight is lacking and the attitude toward change is negative, then the passive-aggressive person will go through life feeling frustrated and victimized. These individuals will never comprehend the part they play in their own misery.

Nursing Care Plan: The Client with a Passive-Aggressive Personality

Nursing Diagnosis (PND-I/NANDA)	Client Care Goals	Nursing Planning/ Interventions	Evaluation
06.01.03 Inattention 06.01.04 Selective attention 02.05.02 Distorted memory 02.02 Altered judgment /Coping, ineffective individual (associated with cognitive responses such as procrastination, half-hearted agreement, and forgetfulness) 04.98 Altered emotional processes not otherwise specified 05.02.02 Altered conduct /impulse processes /Coping, ineffective individual (associated with affective responses such as sulking, pouting, irritability, and moodiness) 05.03 Altered role performance /Coping, ineffective individual (associated with behavioral responses such as belching in public, leaving room early, cracking gum during meetings, habitual lateness)	The client will develop assertive strategies for coping with stress.	1. Establish a relationship based upon mutual responsibilities, minimizing authoritarian approaches. 2. Assess client's perceptions of his or her situation, including underlying assumptions. 3. Evaluate if client's perceptions of situations are realistic. 4. Deal initially with minor problems to generate successful experiences. 5. Give feedback to client on his or her ability to create and control successful experiences. 6. Involve client in setting short- and long-term objectives and stick to the plan of action. 7. Avoid focusing on negative responses, e.g., whining, tantrums, angry outbursts. 8. Point out to client when hostility is being shown in a passive rather than in an open, assertive manner. 9. Use active, directive approaches in helping the client identify and express feelings. 10. Discuss ultimate positive and negative consequences of choice. 11. Model assertive responses for the client.	1. Verbalizes the belief that he or she can control the outcomes of a situation. 2. Identifies feelings of anxiety in stressful situations. 3. Uses appropriate assertive responses in a variety of situations without experiencing undue anxiety. 4. Verbalizes anticipated outcomes of assertive behavior. 5. Identifies and uses coping responses that are not passive-aggressive to reduce anxiety.

continued

Nursing Care Plan: The Client with a Passive-Aggressive Personality *(continued)*

Nursing Diagnosis (PND-I/NANDA)	Client Care Goals	Nursing Planning/ Interventions	Evaluation
		12. Encourage client to try different approaches to problem solving.	
		13. Use cognitive approaches, e.g., homework assignments, journals, explanation of illogical beliefs.	
		14. Involve in assertiveness training groups.	
		15. Avoid arguing with client when he or she offers excuses for passive-aggressive behavior; focus on the meaning that "giving in" has for client.	
		16. Teach anxiety-reducing and relaxation techniques.	
		17. Use humor to defuse argumentativeness and resistant behavior.	
		18. Use clinical supervision or staff meetings to work through transference and countertransference phenomena.	

Chapter Highlights

- When personality traits (consistent, enduring response patterns) become inflexible, maladaptive, and cause social or occupational impairments, they may be diagnosed as personality disorders.

- Personality disorders are modes of functioning that include ways of thinking and perceiving, ways of experiencing emotion, and modes of subjective experience that are generally consistent patterns over broad areas of living.

- Personality disorders are characterized by life-style responses that may create problems both for clients and, to some extent, for society.

- Personality disorders are best understood as defensive modes of living rather than as psychiatric illnesses.

- Examples of personality disorders include three major DSM-IIIR clusters, as follows: (a) eccentric, (b) dramatic-erratic, and (c) anxious-fearful.

- The eccentric life-style is generally associated with people who are emotionally cold, aloof, guarded, and seclusive and who exhibit various degrees of odd behavior.

- The dramatic-erratic life-style is generally associated with people who are impulsive, demonstrative, emotionally labile, needy, lacking in empathy, and unmindful of the consequences of behavior.

- The anxious-fearful life-style is generally associated with people who are hypersensitive, fearful of losing control, and lacking in spontaneity.

- The interactionist view of personality disorders focuses on those complex processes of perception and interpretation of people and the situations in which we encounter each other.

- Nursing interventions for clients with personality disorders are based on the understanding that defensive operations such as anger and manipulation allow the client to avoid anxiety and maintain an ego syntonic state.

References

Agras WS: *Behavior Modification Principles and Clinical Applications.* Little Brown, 1978.

Akhtar S: The syndrome of identity diffusion. *Am J Psychiatry* 1984;141:1381–1385.

American Psychiatric Association: *Diagnostic and Statistical Manual of Mental Disorders,* ed 3. APA, 1980.

American Psychiatric Association: *Diagnostic and Statistical Manual of Mental Disorders,* ed 3, revised. APA, 1987.

Andrulonis PA, et al: Organic brain dysfunction and the borderline syndrome. *Psychiatr Clin North Am* 1980;4:47–66.

Benner DG, Joscelyne B: Multiple personality as a borderline disorder. *J Nerv Ment Dis* 1984;172:98–104.

Brainerd CJ: *Piaget's Theory of Intelligence.* Prentice-Hall, 1978

Braverman B, Shook J: Spotting the borderline personality. *Am J Nurs* 1987;2:200–203.

Cameron N, Rychlak JF: *Personality Development and Psychopathology: A Dynamic Approach.* Houghton Mifflin, 1985.

Chitty KK, Maynard CK: Managing manipulation. *J Psychosoc Nurs Ment Health Serv* 1986;24:8–13.

Cleckley H: *The Mask of Sanity.* Mosby, 1964.

Cloninger CR: The antisocial personality. *Hosp Prac* (Aug) 1978;97–106.

Cull A, Chick J, Wolff S: A consensual validation of schizoid personality in childhood and adult life. *Br J Psychiatry* 1984;144:646–648.

Deutsch H: *Neuroses and Character Types.* International Universities Press, 1965.

Dighton S: Tough-minded nursing. *Am J Nurs* 1986; 86:48–51.

Eaton Jr MT, Peterson MH, Davis JA: *Psychiatry,* ed 3. Medical Examination Publishing, 1976.

Ellis A: *Humanistic Psychology.* McGraw-Hill, 1973.

Erikson EH: *Childhood and Society.* Norton, 1964.

Feldman RB, Guttman HA: Families of borderline patients: Literal-minded parents, borderline parents, and parental protectiveness. *Am J Psychiatry* 1984;141:1392–1396.

Frank H, Paris J: Recollections of family experience in borderline patients. *Arch Gen Psychiatry* 1981;38:1031–1034.

Frosch J: The Psychosocial Treatment of Personality Disorders, in Frosch J (ed): *Current Perspectives on Personality Disorders.* American Psychiatric Press, 1983.

Gallop R: The patient is splitting: Everyone knows and nothing changes. *J Psychosoc Nurs Ment Health Serv* 1985;23:6–10.

Garfinkel T: A reconsideration of psychotherapy of narcissistic personality disorder. *Am J Psychoanal* 1982; 42:207–220.

Genetic traits predispose some to criminality. *U.S. News* (Sept) 1985;54.

Gorenstein E: Frontal lobe functions in psychopaths. *J Abnormal Psychology* 1982;91:368–379.

Haaken J: Sex differences and narcissistic disorders. *Am J Psychoanal* 1983;43:315–324.

Hickey BA: The borderline experience: Subjective impressions. *J Psychosoc Nurs Ment Health Serv* 1985;23:24–29.

Jacobson G: Personality disorders, in Lazare A (ed): *Outpatient Psychiatry.* Williams and Wilkins, 1979, pp 431–437.

Johnson AG: *Human Arrangements: An Introduction to Sociology.* Harcourt-Brace Jovanovich, 1986.

Kendler KS, Gruenberg AM: Genetic relationship between paranoid personality disorder and the schizophrenic spectrum disorders. *Am J Psychiatry* 1982;139:1185–1186.

Kendler KS, et al: A family history study of schizophrenia-related personality disorders. *Am J Psychiatry* 1984; 141:424–427.

Kernberg O: *Borderline Conditions and Pathological Narcissism.* Aronson, 1975.

Kohut H: *Analysis of the Self.* International Universities Press, 1971.

Lego S (ed): *The American Handbook of Psychiatric Nursing.* Lippincott, 1984.

Loomis ME, Horsley JA: *Interpersonal Change: A Behavioral Approach to Nursing Practice.* McGraw-Hill, 1974.

Loranger AW, Oldham JM, Tulis EH: Familial transmission of DSM-III borderline personality disorder. *Arch Gen Psychiatry* 1982;39:795–799.

Loranger AW, Tulis EH: Family history of alcoholism in borderline personality disorder. *Arch Gen Psychiatry* 1985;42:153–157.

Mahler MS, Pine F, Bergman A: *The Psychological Birth of the Human Infant: Symbiosis and Individuation.* Basic Books, 1975.

Masterson JF: *The Narcissistic and Borderline Disorder.* Bruner/Mazel, 1981.

McEnany GW, Tescher BE: Contracting for care: One nursing approach to the hospitalized borderline patient. *J Psychosoc Nurs Ment Health Serv* 1985;23:11–18.

Moyer RL, Snider MJ: Interpersonal problems of adults, in Howe J, et al (eds): *The Handbook of Nursing.* Wiley, 1984, chap 37.

O'Brien P, Caldwell C, Transeau G: Destroyers: Written treatment contracts can help cure self-destructive behaviors of the borderline patient. *J Psychosoc Nurs Ment Health Serv* 1985;23:19–23.

Perlmutter R: The borderline patient in the emergency department: An approach for evaluation and management. *Psych Quart* 1982;54:190–197.

Perry JC, Flannery RB: Passive-aggressive personality disorder: Treatment implications of a clinical typology. *J Nerv Ment Dis* 1982;170:164–173.

Platt-Koch LM: Borderline personality disorder: A therapeutic approach. *Am J Nurs* 1983;83:1666–1671.

Reid WH: The antisocial personality: A review. *Hosp Community Psychiatry* 1985;36:831–837.

Rowe CJ: *An Outline of Psychiatry.* Brown, 1984.

Schaefer RT, Lamm RP: *Sociology.* McGraw-Hill, 1986.

Schlesinger LB: Distinctions between psychopathic, sociopathic, and anti-social personality disorders. *Psychol Rep* 1980;47:15–21.

Schwarz G, Halaris A: Identifying and managing borderline personality patients. *Am Family Physicians* 1984;29:203–208.

Shapiro D: *Neurotic Styles.* Basic Books, 1965.

Slavney PR, Teitelbaum ML, Chase GA: Referral for medically unexplained somatic complaints: The role of histrionic traits. *Psychosomatics* 1985;26:103–109.

Smoyak SA: Borderline personality disorder (editorial). *J Psychosoc Nurs Ment Health Serv* 1985;23:5.

Spector RE: *Cultural Diversity in Health and Illness.* Appleton-Century-Crofts, 1985.

Standage K, et al: An investigation of role-taking in histrionic personalities. *Can J Psychiatry* 1984;29:407–411.

Togersen S: Genetic and nosological aspects of schizotypal and borderline personality disorders. *Arch Gen Psychiatry* 1984;41:546–554.

Travin S, Protter B: Mad or bad? Some clinical considerations in the misdiagnosis of schizophrenia as antisocial personality disorder. *Am J Psychiatry* 1982;139:1335–1338.

Waldinger R: Intensive psychodynamic therapy with borderline patients: An overview. *Am J Psychiatry* 1987; 144(3):267–274.

Widiger TA, Frances A: Axis II personality disorders: Diagnostic and treatment issues. *Hosp Community Psychiatry* 1985;36:619–627.

Wilson JP, Prabucki K: Psychosocial antecedents of narcissistic personality syndrome. *Psychol Rep* 1983; 53:1231–1239.

Wong N: Combined group and individual treatment of borderline and narcissistic patients: Heterogeneous versus homogeneous groups. *Int J Group Psychother* 1980; 30:389–404.

Woollcott Jr P: Prognostic indicators in the psychotherapy of borderline patients. *Am J Psychotherapy* 1985;39:17–29.

PART FOUR

Contemporary Clinical Concerns

TWENTY-TWO

The Chronically Mentally Ill

Linda Chafetz

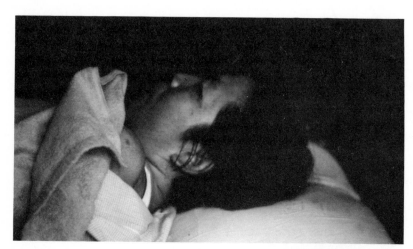

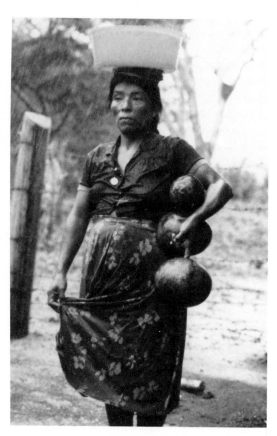

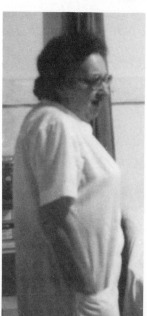

Learning Objectives

After reading this chapter, students should be able to

- Define psychiatric chronicity

- Identify psychiatric disorders that often involve chronicity

- Discuss ways in which ideas about chronic disorders have changed historically

- List three or more problems of the chronically mentally ill in the community

- Identify factors that burden families of the chronically mentally ill

- Discuss the treatment issues in care of homeless clients

- Describe the characteristics of effective support programs in the community

Key Terms

chronically mentally ill
chronic disorders
dual diagnosis
ghettoization
homelessness
new chronic patient
pervasive impairment
psychiatric chronicity
psychoeducational
    approaches
residential instability
resource management
social causation
social reaction
social selection
stress-vulnerability models
transinstitutionalization

Mr. Lloyd comes to the crisis clinic with the chief complaint of: "I need a place to sleep." He states that he has been in this area for several weeks, after leaving his former residence (a boarding home in another city) "because people's voices were getting too loud." Since his arrival in this city, he says he has managed by sleeping "in the park." He is dressed in wet, soiled clothing and appears cold and frightened. He claims he would like to return to a residential placement, but he cannot elaborate on this since he is very anxious and tired.

The term **psychiatric chronicity** refers to persistent functional impairment due to a mental disorder. **Chronic disorders** include illnesses that carry a high potential for impairment. It may appear repetitive to discuss chronicity here, since contributions throughout this text discuss the nursing process in long-term psychiatric illnesses. Why would it be important to add another chapter focused on psychiatric chronicity?

Despite all we know about diagnosis and treatment of specific disorders, psychiatric chronicity remains one of the most puzzling phenomena in psychiatric nursing. We cannot always predict which client will experience a disabling course of illness or consistently explain variations in individual treatment response. We have difficulty sorting out biologically determined aspects of illness from problems reflecting environmental factors or social learning. We know that, given adequate community resources, the chronically mentally ill benefit from a combination of pharmacologic, therapeutic, and environmental interventions. In the absence of these resources, we also know that chronicity tends to go hand in hand with social and economic disadvantage. The isolation and poverty of many of the community-based mentally ill have become urgent issues for our society in general, and for mental health nurses in particular.

Take action.

To understand this situation and respond better to the complex needs of the chronically mentally ill, we need to consider the phenomenon of chronicity as a nursing issue in its own right. This chapter begins with a discussion of the psychiatric problems that follow a chronic course, their common features, and the number of people affected by them. It reviews historical meanings of psychiatric chronicity and the problems of the chronically mentally ill today. Next it presents the theories used to explain some of these problems and the current service models that respond to the needs of the severely mentally ill. The chapter concludes by discussing the meaning of psychiatric chronicity to individuals and the humanistic-interactive perspective that can guide the nursing process.

CHRONIC DISORDERS

Schizophrenic Illnesses

Schizophrenic illnesses account for the largest subgroup of the chronically mentally ill and dominate much of the literature on psychiatric chronicity and disability. As Chapter 17 explains, schizophrenia is considered a spectrum disorder, or a broad clinical category including subgroups of related problems. It follows that while most schizophrenic illnesses follow a chronic course, they involve different types of functional impairment.

Some persons experience acute symptoms, such as hallucinations and delusions. Others may have deficits in social and self-care skills, sometimes called *negative symptoms.* Clients differ in response to and tolerance of psychoactive medications. A proportion of these clients experience only *intermittent* illness, but many experience *progressive* loss of functional ability and have more extensive treatment needs.

This client's history of psychiatric treatment dates to his adolescence. He left high school because of what his family called learning and emotional problems. Since age 22, he has been hospitalized as an adult a total of four times. His first admission occurred in his home state in 1981, after he developed acute psychotic symptoms while living in a residential placement. He was diagnosed as schizophrenic and spent six weeks on a locked unit before discharge to a half-way house. Since 1981, he has required readmission on almost a yearly basis: two weeks in 1982 in the state of Washington, one month in 1983 in Oregon, six weeks in 1984 in Oregon, eight days in 1985 in California. He has

been treated with antipsychotic medications and responds favorably. He has always been discharged the moment his acute symptoms subsided and before a rehabilitative program could begin.

Recurrent Mood Disorders

Major mood disorders account for a smaller proportion of the chronically mentally ill than schizophrenic disorders do, since mood disorders do not always recur and do not necessarily imply serious functional impairment (see Chapter 18). Nevertheless, protracted and recurring depressions, mood swings, and hypomanic episodes can seriously erode functional level. Bipolar mood disorders are recurrent by definition, and carry a risk of impairment between acute episodes (APA 1987).

Progressive Organic Illness

Progressive organic mental disorders (such as Alzheimer's disease) affect a growing part of our society. A large proportion of persons with these diagnoses reside in nursing homes or other institutional settings (Chafetz et al. 1983). Persons with milder impairment or intact social resources often remain in community settings, where psychosocial and environmental interventions can help them maintain optimal levels of function as long as possible.

Other Potentially Disabling Disorders

Other psychiatric problems that do not usually involve serious functional impairment account for a small proportion of the chronically mentally ill. Personality disorders, described in Chapter 21, are long-term problems by nature. Severe personality disorders, such as borderline and paranoid subtypes, may follow a chronic disabling course. While substance abuse occurs among our general population and does not always lead to chronic psychiatric problems, long-term alcohol and drug abuse may produce a range of chronic psychiatric problems, both "functional" and organic. **Dual diagnosis** clients, e.g., depressed persons with drug or alcohol dependence, may experience chronic disability related to multiple and interrelated problems.

Common Features of Chronic Psychiatric Illness

Chronic disorders have common features, including the tendency to affect the personality in a pervasive sense. **Pervasive impairment** means impairment in multiple areas of function that produces global difficulties rather than a single symptom or problem. For example, we sometimes refer to schizophrenic disorder as a thought disorder, to call attention to what some consider a central disturbance in cognition. Yet the client with a schizophrenic diagnosis shows more than disordered thoughts. The clinical picture also includes problems in other areas. A delusion of persecution generally involves more than a false idea. It produces anxious, fearful affect and bizarre or inappropriate behaviors. A severe depressive episode involves a primary disturbance of mood and feelings. However, the depressed mood also distorts a person's ideas about self and the world and can alter behavior with others.

Pervasive impairment does not necessarily recede when acute symptoms subside. The problems that persist during nonacute phases of illness—often called residual symptoms—also have a pervasive quality. It is not generally one long-term residual symptom that affects the individual but a set of problems in such areas as social interaction and family relationships, occupational functioning, community living, and personal care skills.

Joe Lloyd is currently without any stable place to live. He states he is afraid to go to a shelter and that he feels safer going to a park to sleep, and "panhandling for food." He seems to follow an exhausting schedule of walking between dawn and dusk.

When asked if he has any friends, Mr. Lloyd refers to "people who help me out with food." He appears to have no viable social support system.

Bizarre or eccentric behavior can be all too apparent, even to a layperson. However, withdrawal, apathy, and impaired social skills also indicate chronicity. It is not clear to what extent these behaviors should be attributed to the illness process itself, to medication, or to environmental factors. Whatever their basis, they can interfere with function as pervasively as more "active" signs of illness.

Unpredictability and Vulnerability

Chronic illnesses tend to follow a changeable or oscillating course. Even disorders with a fairly clear prognosis (such as serious organic impairment) involve highs and lows of function that are difficult to predict. Persons with recurrent mood disorders or schizophrenic diagnoses are vulnerable to acute exacerbations and unanticipated rehospitalization. Fear of such relapses sometimes compels clients to avoid environmental stressors, scale down or restrict their activities, and reduce the amount or quality of their interpersonal contacts (see Figure 22–1). A protective withdrawal from overstimulation reduces the risk of relapse, but it may also restrict and diminish the quality of life.

Epidemiologic Considerations

When most of the chronically mentally ill resided in state mental hospitals, census data made it relatively easy to estimate their numbers. Since the transition to community-based care, this task has become more complex. Many people remain in institutions (psychiatric hospitals and nursing homes) for long-term care, but they account for only a segment of the chronically mentally ill, most of whom are now dispersed in a variety of community living situations and treatment settings.

To resolve the problem of counting the chronically mentally ill, Goldman, Gatozzi, and Taube (1981) employed three overlapping criteria. The first, chronic diagnosis, uses information about the prevalence of major mental disorders to estimate the size of the population. The second, duration of hospital treatment, counts census data from institutional settings for the mentally ill. The third, disability, looks at the numbers of people receiving disability benefits for psychiatric disorders through federal pro-

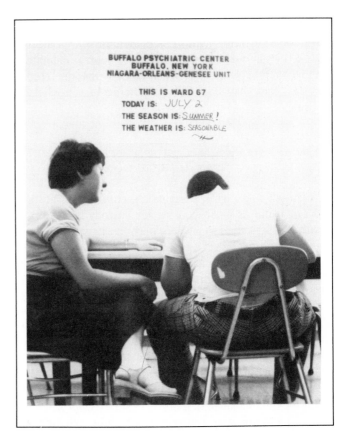

Figure 22–1
Withdrawal from the threat that a one-to-one relationship may bring is an often temporary, but important, coping method for clients with lowered self-esteem.

grams. Using these criteria, the chronically mentally ill include between 1.7 and 2.5 million people, of whom 800,000 to 1,500,000 reside in the community (Goldman et al. 1981). This makes psychiatric chronicity a major public health problem affecting a large and varied part of our society.

HISTORICAL PERSPECTIVES: CHANGING MEANINGS OF CHRONICITY

The term *chronic mental illness* once evoked images of incurability and hopelessness. It implied placement in a distant and forbidding psychiatric institution, a setting for people who could not be helped by active treatment. If family and friends hoped for the person's eventual release, they also realized that such institutions often became the person's permanent home.

To nurses and other mental health professionals, the term *chronic* meant custodial care. Nursing care of the chronically ill meant work in settings with little emphasis on active treatment, except for practices employed to reduce agitation and excitement of the acutely ill. Treatments such as physical restraint, hydrotherapy, and insulin or electric shock therapy were efforts to control poorly understood and frightening symptoms. When acute symptoms receded, nursing care, like daily living, adhered to a predictable routine.

Preinstitutional Care

As Chapter 40 explains, the public mental health hospital did not begin as an institution for custody and confinement. It represented an advance in the treatment of serious psychiatric disorder. Prior to the nineteenth century, the United States had no organized system for care of the mentally ill. The indigent insane were consigned to poorhouses or prisons rather than to settings for the sick or disabled.

The *moral treatment movement* described in Chapter 2, considered a psychiatric disorder an illness and proposed its treatment in a therapeutic environment. Hospitals grounded in this philosophy were located in calm, restorative surroundings, frequently far from cities. Enthusiasm about psychiatric hospitals contributed to a movement for their expansion. Reformers such as Dorothea Dix noted the number of indigent insane who remained in poorhouses and prisons because of an absence of state-funded hospitals. By the end of the nineteenth century, a public hospital system was charged with the protection and treatment of the chronically mentally ill.

State Hospitals

As Chapter 40 explains, the state mental hospital system did not live up to expectations. The early emphasis on active treatment gave way to a model of custodial care. The quality of custodial care declined as well, making institutional environments depersonalizing and regimented. One cause of this decline was disenchantment with moral treatment, which did not yield consistently positive results. Another was overcrowding, due at least in part to immigration and industrialization. As the character of the population changed, the social distance between attendants and clients increased. Rural locations of state hospitals, once intended to restore the mentally ill to health, increasingly isolated them and removed the problem of psychiatric chronicity from public view.

Hospital Reform

As discussed in Chapter 40, reform of public hospitals became an issue after World War II. State governments bore the costs of operating these facilities and looked favorably on alternatives to expensive institutional care (Chafetz et al. 1983). Accounts of conditions within institutions generated indignation and contributed to public support for hospital reform. Some reports depicted extreme abuse and neglect of long-term clients (Deutsch 1948). Mental health professionals wondered whether these institutional environments actually caused the withdrawn and dependent behavior seen among long-term residents (Chafetz et al. 1983).

New Treatments for Community-Based Care

Crisis intervention and milieu therapies developed after World War II offered alternatives to custodial care and held out hope for active treatment of the seriously mentally ill. At the same time neuroleptic medications came into use, providing an effective treatment for acute psychotic symptoms. Existing medications could sedate the acutely ill, but they did not act as selectively on disturbances in the perceptual and cognitive systems (see Chapter 32). Mental health professionals hoped that medication regimens would make the chronically mentally ill amenable to therapy and rehabilitation in community settings.

Legislation to Support Deinstitutionalization

During the mid-1950s state mental hospitals began to report a drop in resident census, which was to persist during the next two decades. As Chapter 40 explains, legislation at the federal and state levels accelerated this deinstitutionalization process. The Community Mental Health Centers Act, passed by Congress in 1963, established a network of federally assisted mental health centers offering emergency, hospital, and outpatient care, as well as rehabilitation and community education and consultation. Various state statutes also shaped local treatment systems. Patients' rights statutes limited the amount of time a person could be treated in restrictive surroundings (see Chapter 39). Federal programs that provided income to the disabled were extended to include the chronically mentally ill (Aid to the Totally Disabled, later renamed Supplemental Security Income). The psychiatrically disabled would also be eligible for public insurance coverage (Medicare, Medicaid) to reimburse providers for their care.

Hopes for Community-Based Care

The 1960s were a time of optimism about the benefits of community living for the mentally ill. Many behaviors associated with chronicity were considered at least partial reactions to the institutional environment. Community treatment seemed to offer a way to prevent or avoid these types of problems. Perhaps because of these high expectations for treatment, community mental health services placed more emphasis on therapeutic services than on assistance with fundamental supports, such as housing, income, and general medical care.

Today few of the mentally ill face long-term institutionalization. Certain severe and disabling illnesses continue to require twenty-four-hour care on a more-or-less permanent basis. For example, in 1981 more than 700,000 nursing home residents in the United States had primary or secondary diagnoses of organic mental disorders (Goldman et al. 1981). Certain state hospital clients, perhaps those with particularly disabling disorders, remained in long-term state mental hospitals for one year or more. Nevertheless, most current psychiatric services were provided in community settings (ambulatory settings and psychiatric units of community mental health centers or general hospitals) or in short-term (three months or less) psychiatric facilities. By the early 1980s, state and county hospitals reported a permanent census of 140,000 compared to 560,000 in 1955 (Chafetz et al. 1983).

THE CHRONICALLY MENTALLY ILL TODAY: NEW ISSUES

Limits of Medication Management

Medication regimens have become the mainstay of treatment programs for the chronically mentally ill. Research on the efficacy of medication, particularly neuroleptic regimens in schizophrenia, demonstrates that these agents reduce rates of relapse and hospital readmission. However,

they have not been problem free. As Chapter 32 explains, drug regimens demand compliance, tolerance of temporary side-effects, and acceptance of the risk of long-term problems such as tardive dyskinesia. Secondary effects of medications can be uncomfortable. They can also be embarrassing, since their effects on motor behavior (for example, muscular stiffness, a shuffling gait) are visible to others (Estroff 1981).

In addition, psychoactive medications do not cure severe mental illness. Medications do not work with equal success for every individual or solve all the problems of chronic disorder. Many individuals who use psychoactive medications competently continue to experience some symptoms. For example, it is possible to suppress acute symptoms of schizophrenic illness without changing deficits in the area of social skills.

Persistence of Disability

Independence and autonomy are such cherished values in this culture that they permeate our treatment policies. Community mental health systems in many regions of the United States emphasized the importance of self-support and gainful employment whenever possible. Clients, families, and communities sometimes held such high expectations about independence that they considered even mild disability to be a form of failure.

However, surveys of the chronically ill suggest a low rate of competitive employment and indicate that expectations for autonomy may be unrealistic for some clients. A 1982 survey of the chronically mentally ill found only one quarter to be employed, while less than half held full- or part-time competitive jobs (Tessler et al. 1981). These figures reflect conditions in the job market, as well as individual disability. General unemployment tends to increase competition for jobs that might fit the skills of the mildly disabled.

Programs such as Supplemental Security Income (for the disabled) address the financial needs of some of the chronically mentally ill. Such programs simply provide a small, fixed income, however, and do not address the need for vocational programs and other meaningful activities for clients in the community.

Limits of Outpatient Therapies

As community-based systems developed, outpatient services formed their core, and rates of ambulatory service use climbed dramatically. Clinics offered some services for the severely ill (such as medications and day treatment), but they also provided individual, family, and group treatments to the larger population. Individuals with less severe or persistent problems accounted for part of the 120 percent rise in outpatient visits reported in national statistical data (Chafetz et al. 1983). In fact, some of the chronically mentally ill failed to connect with ambulatory services or to follow through consistently with outpatient treatment.

During the early deinstitutionalization period, poor coordination between state hospital and community mental health systems seemed to contribute to problems of outpatient follow-up. Hospital discharges sometimes occurred rapidly without adequate attention to aftercare. In certain areas reports described "dumping" of former clients in communities, providing them with little more than a referral to continuing care.

Today we recognize that traditional outpatient programs (therapeutic services, generally on an appointment basis) may not meet the needs of all the varied population of chronically mentally ill. While some clients use traditional outpatient care modalities, others require broader support services and do not benefit from psychotherapy. Some of the more successful outpatient services for this group emphasize coordination of comprehensive and continuous services, rather than traditional therapies alone (Test and Stein 1978).

The Enduring Need for Acute Care

The chronically mentally ill continue to require access to acute care. Twenty-four-hour emergency and crisis units, in-patient services, and outreach programs were mandated in community mental health statutes to provide for people with problems exceeding the resources of the outpatient sector, such as dangerous behavior, suicidality, or grave disability. Many community health planners hoped to use hospitals as a last resort, treating only the most urgent problems in expensive acute care components of the service system.

In-Patient Services

Despite the goal of diverting clients from twenty-four-hour settings, a segment of the chronically mentally ill require periodic hospitalization. While long-term hospital *residency* (twelve months or more) has dropped dramatically during the past three decades, a large number of clients enter psychiatric in-patient facilities annually. However, the amount of time the average client spends in the hospital has fallen to less than ninety days (Chafetz et al. 1983).

Crisis and Emergency Care

Community-based psychiatric emergency services have also expanded. Crisis and emergency units are the point of entry into the mental health system for clients requiring hospitalization. These walk-in services also provide primary care to individuals who cannot or will not use traditional ambulatory services. Reviews of emergency service client populations indicate a high proportion of chronic diagnoses, combined with other problems such as poverty, social isolation, and histories of poor compliance with outpatient care (Bassuk and Gerson 1979).

Difficult-to-Treat Patients

A subgroup of the chronically mentally ill appears to be particularly dependent on acute treatment services. Known as "revolving door," "recidivist," "chronic crisis," and "difficult-to-treat" patients, these clients reappear with disturbing frequency in acute care settings.

Some new chronic patients may have characteristics of severe personality disorders, rather than classic symptoms of the major mental illnesses (Schwartz and Goldfinger 1981). Others, particularly younger adults, seem to reject ongoing care because they find it inappropriate or unappealing. For example, they may feel alienated from services developed for older long-term clients (Pepper et al. 1981). Many isolated younger adults seem to "slip through the cracks" of the mental health system, until their problems have become too advanced to ignore. At this point some may be detained for psychiatric observation on an involuntary basis. This can reinforce a sense of alienation from mental health services (Segal and Baumohl 1980).

Community Residence

Deinstitutionalization is sometimes described as a change in "locus of care," but it would be just as accurate to call it a change in "locus of residence." Psychiatric hospitals once functioned as homes for the majority of chronically mentally ill. Although they were not adequate homes, they acknowledged clients' needs for food, clothing, and shelter. The community mental health movement created new treatment settings without a parallel emphasis on new places to live and new sources of social support. This transitional oversight had profound repercussions for the chronically mentally ill, their families, and their communities.

Family Residence and Family Burden

A series of reports reviewed by Goldman (1984) suggest that one third of the chronically mentally ill live with relatives. Family residence offers many obvious benefits, but it also makes special demands on the household. Even partial or episodic disability in an adult member can strain family resources and feelings.

Stress of Caregiving

Where families assume a caregiving or supervisory function, they take on roles that involve additional stress. Medication supervision often raises concerns about policing the client. Liaison activities with health and social services take time and effort since they often demand negotiation of services within complex and poorly coordinated systems. These activities can also involve frustration, since mental health and social welfare systems are designed to communicate with clients as individuals, not their relatives. Families may feel rebuffed if they act on behalf of the clients and negligent if they leave them to fend for themselves. If acute illness recurs, it may raise intense feelings in the family, including fears of betraying the client by calling for outside help, doubts about what might have been done to prevent recurrence, and bitter disappointment about the relapse.

Emotional Burden

In fact emotional problems seem to burden families of the chronically ill as heavily as practical or economic concerns. Families report distress about behaviors they consider "embarrassing" or inappropriate. They also describe problems with the stigma of psychiatric illness (Goldman 1984). One of the saddest problems for families is guilt about the psychiatric illness. Many psychodynamic theories of mental disorders stressed the etiologic importance of family factors (communication patterns, child-rearing practices). This sometimes contributed to a sense of guilt among members of clients' families. In fact current psychiatric research counters the notion that family interaction *causes* chronic disorders, although family factors often influence course of illness (Falloon et al. 1984). Guilt not only adds to the emotional burden but also distances families from sources of support and assistance.

Demographic Factors and Residence

Marriage rates for the chronically mentally ill fall far below norms for the general population. For example, in a national sample of the chronically mentally ill receiving community support services, only 12 percent were currently married (Tessler et al. 1982). For single adult clients, family dependence means dependence on families of origin, generally parents. As the chronically mentally ill near middle age, their parents may be elderly and ill equipped to manage a home for them. Older clients may have no living relatives.

Aging or illness of other members of a household may influence a family's ability to maintain the client at home. Practical concerns also play a role. Nuclear families often live in homes that are too small to accommodate an additional adult. It may be difficult for even concerned relatives

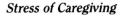

to make room for an extra person. Geographically mobile families may become scattered. There may be no relatives in the client's community who are able to share a stable home.

Whatever the precise factors operating in each case, a large proportion of the chronically mentally ill cannot reside with members of a natural social network, and require other kinds of living arrangements.

Residential Placements

One community response to the presence of the chronically mentally ill has been proliferation of proprietary boarding homes and residential placements. Benefits from the federal Supplementary Security Income program (or other disability or general assistance programs) often pay only residential costs, leaving very little in the way of extra funds for personal use.

These placements vary in size and quality, making it difficult to generalize about them. Some boarding arrangements provide a warm, stable environment for residents and encourage autonomy. Others, however, fall far below standards that should be applied to living environments for the disabled. Even satisfactory boarding facilities may provide limited opportunities for active treatment and community participation. For this reason the movement of the chronically mentally ill to proprietary boarding homes is sometimes called **transinstitutionalization**, referring to movement from one custodial setting to another.

Community Exclusion and "Ghettoization"

Boarding homes and other group residences for the mentally ill sometimes cluster in neighborhoods where few opportunities for community participation or integration exist. Movement to marginal urban districts has been called **ghettoization** (Chafetz et al. 1983), since it reflects containment of a disadvantaged group within special areas. It applies to more than boarding homes. For example, many of the chronically mentally ill reside in central city areas where single room rentals can be found.

Single room rentals have become a dwindling resource in many cities. Conversion of resident hotels to other uses reduces the overall housing supply, and obliges the chronically mentally ill to compete with less stigmatized or disabled groups for limited resources. Loss of low-cost rentals has been linked to increasing **residential instability** (moving from place to place) among the chronically mentally ill, and to their merging with the urban homeless (Chafetz and Goldfinger 1984, Baxter and Hopper 1982).

Homelessness and Chronicity

Over the past decade homelessness has become a national problem that touches the lives of a broad and diverse population. The U.S. Department of Housing and Urban Development estimates the homeless to number from 250,000 to 300,000 people; advocacy groups estimate their number at between two and three million people (DHHS 1983). "Street people" or "bag ladies" who have no form of acceptable shelter form the most visible segment of the undomiciled. Another group, perhaps a larger one, moves among temporary forms of lodging such as public or charitable shelters, short-term hotels, transient private housing, and institutions (Chafetz and Goldfinger 1984).

The proportion of the chronically mentally ill among the homeless is a matter of some controversy. Although a high percentage of the homeless appear to have psychiatric problems, their intolerable living conditions might explain their distress or disturbance. For example, it is difficult to imagine the experience of street dwelling without feeling suspicion, resentment, and depression. Physical hardships endured by the homeless also have significant effects on mental status. However, reports from many parts of the United States suggest that the chronically mentally ill are at risk for homelessness. As a result they are all the more vulnerable to severe environmental stressors (Chafetz and Goldfinger 1984).

Clinical Problems and Barriers to Care

Data obtained on the homeless mentally ill to date indicate that they are clinically heterogeneous, with a range of psychiatric disorders. They share social isolation, poverty, and the medical illnesses their living conditions impose. These multiple and interrelated problems require concerted services, yet the homeless often fail to receive any ongoing care because homelessness itself reduces the individual's ability to comply with or fit easily into standard mental health programs.

The homeless experience medical problems related to malnutrition, poor hygiene, and exposure. Psychiatric services are often ill-equipped to deal with their general health problems, and tend to refer the client elsewhere for medical treatment and follow-up. Very few psychiatric or medical clinics provide bathing facilities or meals. Instead, the client may be confronted with multiple referrals for multiple problems and feel unable to cope with any of them.

This failure to cope can reflect individual confusion or disorganization, but even well-organized people may be deterred by obstacles in the treatment system. For example, the homeless must often walk to scheduled appoint-ments with multiple agencies in different, possibly distant areas. Referring undomiciled clients to medical facilities, psychiatric clinics, and social services denies the interactive nature of their immediate problems and their need for rapid and comprehensive care.

The homeless require subsistence services above all, yet they may be unable to negotiate complex social welfare systems without help. Regulations may appear overwhelming in systems that never anticipated or planned for their needs. For example, in some areas people without a local address cannot obtain public assistance. This "catch 22" regulation blocks the homeless from programs that would help them obtain housing. Application procedures and interviews consume large amounts of time. Yet waiting long hours in the social service office may mean missing a place in line for a bed or a meal. If the homeless attend to their survival needs, they may be unable to act like "good patients" and conform to rules and regulations.

Attitudes Toward Homeless Clients

A regrettable consequence of this situation is the image the homeless acquire with social service and mental health providers. They appear to be "noncompliers," "manipulators," or simply "poor risks" for investment of time and energy (Goldfinger and Chafetz 1984, Segal and Baumohl 1980). These ideas make working with this population even more difficult, and reduce the possibility of engaging the homeless in services that might address their very serious problems. Effective programs for the undomiciled must begin with acceptance of their alienation and suspicion and with interventions to build trust, beginning with efforts to meet subsistence needs (Goldfinger and Chafetz 1984).

THEORETICAL PERSPECTIVES

Explaining the Problems of the Community-Based Mentally Ill

Looking at psychiatric chronicity today, it is clear that not every individual faces the hazards and dangers of the homeless. Some of the chronically mentally ill manage well in existing treatment programs, participate in social and occupational activities, and demonstrate that serious disorder need not be synonymous with social withdrawal or poverty.

It seems equally clear, however, that the chronically mentally ill comprise a population at risk for extreme social disadvantage. Their vulnerability raises many questions for mental health professionals. These questions have particular relevance for nursing, because of its foundation in community health and its history of service to the disadvantaged.

We must ask what factors, if any, increase the risk of isolation and alienation. We must question the ways in which clinical problems seem to beget social difficulties. Above all we need to develop a theoretical perspective on these problems that can guide the nursing process and enable us to prevent or reverse a loss of social and economic resources. Such a perspective would consider factors within the individual, the social environment, and the treatment system that make some people extremely vulnerable to poor clinical outcomes, exclusion from community living, isolation, and poverty.

Social Resources and Psychiatric Disorder

The relationship between social resources and chronic psychiatric disorder has preoccupied clinicians and social scientists since the beginnings of psychiatric epidemiology.

Although many studies in this area focus on persons diagnosed as schizophrenic, we can, with some caution, apply it to the chronically mentally ill in general.

Studies spanning several decades note that social resources (as indicated by factors such as marriage, educational level, occupation, and income) tend to correlate with less chronic outcomes, seen in reduced incidence or duration of hospitalization (Turner and Gartrell 1978). This means that one kind of advantage (better clinical status, personal well-being, and competence) seems to go hand in hand with other kinds of advantages (e.g., having a marriage, a job, educational attainment). More recent research on social network and social support systems also suggests a relationship between social assets and clinical outcomes.

RESEARCH NOTE

Citation

Chafetz L, Goldfinger SM: Residential instability in a psychiatric emergency setting. Psychiatr Q 1984;56(1): 20–34.

Study Problem/Purpose

This study examined the phenomenon of residential instability, or the absence of consistent and acceptable housing, among a psychiatric emergency service clientele. The majority of clients in the sample suffered from chronic and severe illness. The research was exploratory, with three major objectives: to develop a demographic and clinical profile of a representative sample of emergency clients; to identify the proportion who could be considered residentially unstable; and to identify the degree to which residential status influenced clinical factors at the time of psychiatric emergency care.

Methods

This was a descriptive study based on data obtained from clinical records. A representative sample of 124 cases was obtained on the basis of admission during observation periods distributed over all times of the day and week. The clinical record for each case was reviewed immediately following the emergency assessment. Brief questions to admitting clinicians clarified information from written records.

Findings

Cases were divided into three groups according to level of residential instability. The urban homeless who lacked any form of shelter were in the High category and accounted for 17 percent. The Moderate group (29 percent) included persons with some form of shelter, which fell short of a stable residence. The residentially stable accounted for 54 percent.

The High and Moderate groups were demographically and diagnostically similar to clients with stable housing. They were compared in terms of symptom ratings. Although they differed significantly from others in several symptom areas, they were far more like other cases than different. The symptoms that distinguished them, such as social isolation, are problems that might reflect homeless or transient living conditions. They appeared clinically and demographically diverse, indicating that residential instability affects a broad segment of the mentally disordered. Treatment histories suggested that loss of housing could be an episodic event for many of the cases in the study, and that the risk may involve a larger group than those who lose housing at a given point in time.

Implications

This exploratory study provided a descriptive, cross-sectional view of the mentally disordered in psychiatric emergency care. It could not provide answers to questions about the causes of homelessness. Rather it indicates the dimensions of the problem and the type of clients affected. The data suggest that at a given time almost half the clients in this setting are inadequately housed. Since they are similar to other cases in demographic and clinical terms, the research also suggests that a large and varied group may be at risk for residential loss. The first and most evident implication is the need for emergency shelter. However shelter units are not enough for individuals in psychiatric crisis. Clinicians must develop assessment, treatment, and referral procedures that meet the multiple and interrelated needs of the residentially unstable. The study also implies the need for community support programs that offer both shelter and treatment.

Social Selection, Social Reaction, and Social Causation

The reason for these relationships remains a matter of some debate. One point of view considers poor treatment outcomes a function of *individual factors.* From this perspective, severity of illness reduces individual ability to maintain interpersonal and economic assets. This social selection hypothesis places the locus of causation within the individual and sees social disadvantages as results of illness (Turner and Gartrell 1978).

Could the direction of this relationship be reversed? Could social characteristics cause poor clinical outcomes? The poor, the powerless, and the socially isolated are more likely than others to bear the negative consequences of *psychiatric labeling.* They are hospitalized more frequently and for longer and are more likely to receive custodial care than advantaged clients. This is the social reaction hypothesis. In contrast to the social selection hypothesis, it places the site of causation in the social environment (Turner and Gartrell 1978).

Community studies have also attempted to examine the persistent relationships between mental illness (particularly schizophrenia) and socioeconomically deprived environments. Epidemiologic studies dating back to the 1930s demonstrate that rates of mental illness rise in socially disorganized parts of the central city and drop in more affluent or socially integrated areas (Faris and Dunham 1939). More recent reports continue to document the movement of the mentally ill to marginal areas (Baxter and Hopper 1981). A social causation explanation considers urban poverty and alienation as stressors that help produce psychiatric disorder. However, the same phenomenon has been explained in terms of social selection, by explaining that sicker and more isolated people "drift down" to pockets of urban poverty.

The Service System and Social Resources

Social disadvantage and isolation have been tied to the mental health system itself and its lack of flexibility. The most successful programs for the chronically mentally ill have sometimes selected clients with superior treatment histories and intact social resources (Braun et al. 1981). The system as a whole may respond best to clients who "fit" into programs, people who resemble the ideal client that treatment settings anticipated. Others, less attractive or less able to fit into existing programs, receive less attention.

Segal and Baumohl (1980) use the concept of "social margin" to describe patients who seem to slip through the cracks of the mental health system. *Social margin* refers to attributes and assets a person can trade on to obtain services, material, and interpersonal resources, which indicate that the individual will be able to use services and remain in treatment. People who appear to be "bad risks," including the transient mentally ill and volatile younger chronic clients, receive little follow-up. This means that those with multiple needs sometimes receive the least support. In this sense, the system actually contributes to clients' clinical and social difficulties.

Chronicity as a Biopsychosocial Phenomenon: A Holistic View

The concepts of social reaction, social causation, and social selection play a role in the ongoing debate about "nature versus nurture" in psychiatry. This debate concerns the comparative importance of innate factors (the illness, personal competence) and environmental factors (child-rearing practices, social resources) in incidence and course of chronic psychiatric illness. We have witnessed many swings of the pendulum, in this discussion, with biologic or social theories gaining prominence at different points in history.

During the early deinstitutionalization period, professionals and laypeople widely believed that some of the more unfortunate effects of long-term illness, e.g., withdrawal and loss of initiative and social skills, were caused by the institutional environment. The persistence of some of these problems in community settings has rekindled debate on how they come about and on how much responsibility for chronicity should be borne by the individual and how much by the social and physical surroundings.

Recent advances in biologic psychiatry (see Chapter 9) make it impossible to consider psychiatric chronicity a purely social construction. Since biologic processes appear to play a role in both incidence and course of illness, it is difficult to dismiss them in discussions of social adjustment. At the same time, knowledge is increasing about the effects of environmental variables on functional adaptation, even where clear biologic factors may be operating. Psychiatric chronicity appears to be a complex *biopsychosocial* phenomenon, determined by multiple factors and amenable to different types of interventions.

Stress, Vulnerability, and Chronic Illness

Recent research on schizophrenia suggests that constitutional vulnerability (schizophrenic *diathesis*) interacts with environmental factors to influence rates of relapse. Persons with a low vulnerability (low genetic risk, less neurophysiologic predisposition) require a higher level of environmental stress to exhibit symptoms than highly vulnerable individuals do. Stress-vulnerability models consider schizophrenic episodes to result from an interaction between internal and environmental factors (Falloon et al. 1984).

Although stress-vulnerability models have been elaborated for the study of the course of schizophrenic illness, this holistic perspective also contributes to our understanding of psychiatric chronicity in a more general sense. Persons with major affective illnesses are also vulnerable, with demonstrable physiologic changes during major depressive or manic episodes. At the same time, the course of affective illness suggests great sensitivity to social and environmental factors. Stressful life events, for example, often interact with individual vulnerability to precipitate recurrence of acute illness.

Patients with dementias like Alzheimer's disease have clear-cut organic pathology. Yet the functional level of clients with milder symptoms of organic illness reflects an interplay between cognitive deficits and environmental supports or stressors. For example, clients with cognitive impairment can be destabilized by abrupt changes in their environments and often respond positively to environmental supports.

The stress-vulnerability perspective can guide us in the planning of nursing care. It helps us identify individual vulnerability without "blaming the victim." When we focus exclusively on environmental determinants of well-being, we ignore very real intrapersonal problems; when we consider individual factors in isolation, we run the risk of overlooking or underestimating determinants of behavior in the interpersonal and physical milieu. For example, an exclusive focus on individual psychopathology can mask the fact that we sometimes oblige the most vulnerable people (the chronically ill) to tolerate extreme levels of environmental stress and deprivation (such as homelessness). Rather than promoting an exclusive emphasis on pathology, this perspective directs our thinking toward matching people with environmental resources.

THE NURSING PROCESS AND THE CHRONICALLY MENTALLY ILL: SOME SPECIAL CONSIDERATIONS

The nursing process with the chronically mentally ill addresses individual problems and environmental supports.

Comprehensive Data Collection

Information about the individual should include functional level, specific areas of impairment (such as self-care and hygiene, community living, social or family relationships, and control of inappropriate behavior), and current psychiatric treatment. The data collection process should also focus on the types of events or experiences that the individual client finds stressful or difficult.

Comprehensive data collection focuses simultaneously on the environment, looking not only at problems but at supports that protect the client. Attention to the environment should occur in any settings where nursing care is

delivered: family home, boarding facility, apartment, or hospital.

Diagnosis and Planning

The psychiatric nurse analyzes information about client and environment to identify areas where nursing intervention may buffer environmental stress, increase support, or decrease individual vulnerability. Nursing care plans will vary according to the setting where care is delivered. Psychiatric nurses in hospitals, for example, care for clients experiencing acute exacerbations of illness who need environmental protection and symptomatic treatment. Nurses who are clinical specialists in a community setting may have a case load of outpatients with different needs. In both situations, nursing diagnoses and nursing care plans can reflect a comprehensive view of the person in his or her environment.

Interventions with Individuals

Many specific interventions to reduce individual vulnerability are discussed at length in the chapters on diagnostic groups. Medication regimens, psychotherapeutic services, social skills training, and psychosocial rehabilitation (day treatment, vocational training, and other types of before and after psychosocial rehabilitation) emphasize control of an illness process, or development of skills to correct individual deficits in behavior.

It should be emphasized that many clients seem to benefit from interventions that address functional problems, such as referrals to socialization groups or vocational rehabilitation programs. These approaches promote development of specific community living skills. This differs from a traditional psychotherapeutic orientation, which assumes that personal growth or evolution will lead to better coping or function. In fact, at least among persons diagnosed as schizophrenic, intense psychosocial interventions may actually increase vulnerability to relapse (Falloon et al. 1984). It appears that for at least a subgroup of the chronically mentally ill, treatment should focus on areas of functional impairment, working toward realistic goals within these areas.

Providing Environmental Support

Social networks tend to be smaller among people with psychiatric disabilities, yet clients rely heavily on these networks for practical or instrumental assistance (Falloon et al. 1984). Social networks serve a vital function in helping vulnerable individuals live in the community. To prevent the erosion of support that often accompanies chronicity, nurses and other mental health professionals have turned their attention to interventions that "support the supporters."

Family Support

Family therapies once placed the responsibility for the client's illness on the family itself (for example, communication patterns in clients diagnosed as schizophrenic). Our increasing awareness of the biologic bases of major mental disorders and growing recognition of the family burden these disorders impose have shifted attention to support of natural support networks.

While the idea that families engender chronic illness may have been discredited, family factors remain important determinants of illness outcomes. A family's ability to cope with psychiatric chronicity appears to influence the course of schizophrenic illness and possibly other disorders (Falloon et al. 1984). The management of "expressed emotion" in families is currently the subject of rigorous research (see Chapter 17). It appears that when families modify their type and amount of contact with a chronically ill member, the risk of acute exacerbation may diminish. This **psychoeducational** approach to care minimizes blame for the illness by educating family members about its biologic bases. It offers constructive ways to help manage schizophrenic disorders and perhaps other cases of psychiatric chronicity.

Relatives who maintain a disabled member in the household and assume caregiving responsibilities (such as medication supervision and maintenance of a safe environment) may require very practical assistance. Information about homemaking or legal services can be as welcome as information about treatment. Family caregivers often face seemingly insurmountable obstacles when they plan vacations and trips. Respite services (or short-term placements to relieve the family of the burden of care) allow families the help they require to continue in a caregiving role. Such services have been widely recommended as a way to reduce family burden and enhance the quality of life for both patient and relatives on a long-term basis.

Nurses working with families of the chronically mentally ill need to become attuned to their concerns about the future and their inability to control or predict changes in the client's status that affect the household. Families may express ambivalence about caregiving. For example, they may want to promote the client's autonomy yet feel discomfort or guilt about the type of living situation the

client is able to maintain independently. Clear information and nonjudgmental attitudes from nurses and other providers can do much to alleviate a family's distress and assure them that there may not be a perfect way to deal with their problems. In addition, self-help groups and advocacy organizations formed by families of the mentally ill promote sharing and support for common problems.

Supporting Nonkin Networks

Family resources may not be the best solution for every individual with chronic psychiatric illness. Family relationships may be full of conflict; the family's responsibilities may preclude psychiatric caregiving; or the client may simply prefer an independent living situation. Under these circumstances, the client's network of interpersonal resources goes beyond the family.

People residing in proprietary boarding homes and residential hotels benefit from contacts with managers and fellow residents. Despite the problems described in some residential placements, there are conscientious and competent managers who occupy a pivotal position in the individual's support system. Like families, these "support persons" need access to assistance from providers. For example, residential care managers or hotel staff are more willing to retain a difficult or volatile patient in their facility if they feel that outreach and emergency services are available. In a similar sense, clients with strong links to health care and social service systems place fewer demands or inappropriate burdens on support systems in residential placements.

The chronically mentally ill sometimes establish support systems that seem idiosyncratic. Clients living in hotels or other urban rentals, for example, may benefit from casual contacts with local merchants, workers in local restaurants or meal services, or other neighborhood residents. Clients may feel closer to other recipients of psychiatric services than to the larger community. In a study of the community-based mentally ill, Estroff (1981) notes that "insiders," or other clients, feel a special rapport or sense of mutual understanding.

It is important for psychiatric nurses to recognize that clients have their own life experiences and preferences, which should be respected. Although the literature indicates that chronic mental illness alters social networks, there is no basis for active intervention to alter the individual's social support system. Overintrusive or interventionist approaches of this kind may in fact contribute to rather than alleviate environmental stress.

This does not mean that nurses and other mental health professionals should follow a hands-off policy about environmental conditions that appear inadequate or even intolerable (as in the case of isolated, dirty, or even dangerous places to live). It does mean that interpersonal environments should be assessed from the client's perspective, with understanding of his or her unique needs and preferences.

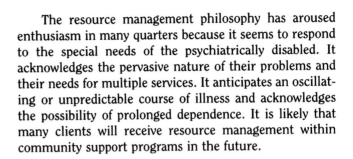
The chronically mentally ill contend with what is sometimes an unpredictable and oscillating course of illness. Unlike acute health problems with a clear resolution, chronic psychiatric disorders may change over time. These changes can occur in reaction to shifting individual factors (for example aging and changes in general health status) and external factors (living conditions and events). Where mental health nurses have the opportunity to work with clients over time (as in community clinics), they can monitor changes over time. In this sense, nursing evaluation identifies shifting needs and matches them with resources.

TRENDS IN COMMUNITY TREATMENT

Comprehensive Models

Comprehensive service models being developed for the chronically mentally ill go beyond psychiatric treatment in a narrow sense. They offer a range of support services to correct some of the problems of deinstitutionalization and promote quality of life in the community. The "basic and specialized needs of the chronically mentally ill," identified in *Toward a National Plan for the Chronically Mentally Ill* (DHHS 1980), include shelter in a range of structured to independent settings; food, clothing, and household management; income management and financial support; meaningful activities; transportation, general medical, and mental health services; habilitation and rehabilitation; vocational and social services; and integrative services that bring together and coordinate other areas of care.

Community Support and Case Management

One of the integrative services mentioned in this list is **resource management** or "case management." The concept of resource management is fundamental to a community support program model of care. This model was developed through the Federal Community Support Program (a demonstration project with federal-state collaboration that began in 1978) and employs a case manager to coordinate therapeutic and support services.

The role of the resource or case manager is to assess the total needs of the chronically ill individual, establish goals, and obtain the set of services required to meet them. Since service needs can change over time, the goals and referrals for a given client will be subject to change. In contrast to conventional treatment, however, clients remain in contact with the same provider throughout alterations in their clinical status.

The resource management philosophy has aroused enthusiasm in many quarters because it seems to respond to the special needs of the psychiatrically disabled. It acknowledges the pervasive nature of their problems and their needs for multiple services. It anticipates an oscillating or unpredictable course of illness and acknowledges the possibility of prolonged dependence. It is likely that many clients will receive resource management within community support programs in the future.

A HUMANIST INTERACTIVE PERSPECTIVE

Integrated and comprehensive programs hold considerable promise for the chronically ill, but they also involve risks. In an effort to provide comprehensive care, mental health care providers may turn to *brokerage of services* rather than treatment of the seriously ill. A humanist interactive perspective can help the care provider avoid this undesirable outcome.

Recognizing Personal Characteristics

No matter what range or constellation of services the client requires, they must be delivered in a manner that is meaningful to the individual. Meaning is a function of factors such as culture and ethnicity, age, sex, values, and beliefs about health and illness. For example, if the chronically mentally ill require supportive environments, no fixed set of characteristics make an environment supportive in a general sense. Diagnostic differences alone suggest a variety of environmental needs. In addition, the chronically mentally ill have diverse social and cultural backgrounds and individual tastes and preferences about life-styles. Interpersonal factors, such as dependence or closeness, and more material environmental properties, such as crowding or noise, have different meanings for different people. In fact environmental needs rarely remain static for any person, and the mentally disordered, like anyone else, experience dynamic changes related to their own growth and development. We cannot say that a person lives within supportive surroundings if personal characteristics and individual potential for change are not acknowledged.

In the same sense, although we may assume that psychosocial stressors influence the course of illness, events will be more or less stressful to individuals according to their personal meanings. The client or the client's family, for example, can often identify the events that "trigger" acute illness episodes. These events may not appear universally stressful, but they have personal significance.

To go beyond the brokerage or provision of resources and services and respond to each person's needs, psychiatric nurses must develop rapport with the individual, working to develop trust and understanding. Through this interactive approach the nurse can assess each person's individual and unique needs. The nursing process, for the chronically mentally ill as for other client groups, occurs through a human exchange and shared understanding. As a humanistic, interactive process, it involves both acceptance of the client's problems and consideration of his or her potential for change and growth.

Overcoming Obstacles to Humanistic Care

It is sometimes difficult for nurses to maintain a humanistic perspective on care for the severely ill. Like some clients' families, perhaps like some of the chronically mentally ill themselves, nurses may interpret long-term impairment or relapse as treatment failure and invest the idea of chronicity with negative meanings. We may consider the persistence of disorder as a sign of the client's unwillingness to cooperate or of our own inability to deliver effective services. In either case, the message is one of disappointment, adding to the client's loss of self-esteem, alienation, and loneliness.

Nurses occupy a very important position in mental health systems with regard to the chronically mentally ill. Because of nursing's traditional concern with such issues as self-care, environmental support, and family-oriented health services, psychiatric nurses can apply their skills to the planning of care more easily than mental health professionals prepared for narrower psychotherapeutic activities. To promote humanistic and effective nursing care of the chronically ill, hospitals and other health care agencies may need to consider ways to support nursing staff, counter feelings of failure or hopelessness, and promote individualized and respectful treatment of individuals who experience psychiatric chronicity.

Chapter Highlights

- Chronicity has to do with function, not simply diagnosis. Disorders described as chronic psychiatric illnesses carry a high potential for long-term impairment in function.

- Chronicity was once associated with hopelessness. Its meaning has changed with advances in treatment, but it continues to burden the client and the support system.

- The chronically mentally ill often require comprehensive services that meet a range of treatment and support needs.

- The chronically mentally ill constitute a very vulnerable population. They may suffer from social isolation, poverty, and inadequate housing.

- All people with mental disorders are not homeless, and all the homeless are not mentally disordered. However, psychiatric chronicity increases vulnerability to loss of social resources such as housing.

- The relationship between social disadvantage and chronicity has been explained in many ways. A holistic view considers both individual vulnerability and environmental stressors.

- A humanistic interactive perspective in psychiatric nursing focuses on the meaning of chronicity to the individual and its effects within the context of the person's life.

References

American Psychiatric Association: *Diagnostic and Statistical Manual of Mental Disorders,* ed 3, revised. APA, 1987.

Bachrach LL: A conceptual approach to deinstitutionalization. *Hosp Community Psychiatry* 1978;29(9):126–131.

Bassuk EL, Gerson S: Into the breach: Emergency psychiatry in the general hospital. *Gen Hosp Psychiatry* 1979;1:31–43.

Baxter E, Hopper K: *Private Lives/Public Spaces: Homeless Adults in the Streets of New York City.* Community Service Society, 1981.

Baxter E, Hopper K: The new mendicancy: Homeless in New York City, *Am J Orthopsychiatry* 1982;52:393–408.

Braun P, Kochansky G, Shapiro R, Greenberg L, Gudeman JE, Johnson S, Shore MF: Overview: Deinstitutionalization of psychiatric patients, a critical review of outcome studies. *Am J Psychiatry* 1981;138:736.

Chafetz L, Goldfinger SM: Residential instability in a psychiatric emergency setting. *Psychiatr Q* 1984;56(1):20–34.

Chafetz L, Goldman HH, Taube CA: Deinstitutionalization in the United States. *Int J Mental Health* 1983;11(4):48–63.

Deutsch A: *The Shame of the States.* Harcourt Brace, 1948.

Department of Health and Human Services Steering Committee on the Chronically Mentally Ill. *Toward a National Plan for the Chronically Mentally Ill.* DHHS, December 1980.

Estroff SE: *Making It Crazy: An Ethnography of Psychiatric Clients in an American Community.* University of California Press, 1981.

Falloon IRH, Boyd JL, McGill CW: *Family Care of Schizophrenia.* Guilford Press, 1984.

Faris REL, Dunham HW: *Mental Disorders in Urban Areas.* University of Chicago Press, 1939.

Goldfinger SM, Chafetz L: Developing a better service delivery system for the homeless mentally ill, in Lamb HR (ed): *The Homeless Mentally Ill: A Task Force Report of the American Psychiatric Association.* APA, 1984.

Goldman HH: Mental illness and family burden: A public health perspective. *Hosp Community Psychiatry* 1984; 33:557–560.

Goldman HH, Gatozzi AA, Taube CA: Defining and counting the mentally ill. *Hosp Community Psychiatry* 1981; 32(1):21–27.

McCausland M: Deinstitutionalization of the mentally ill: Oversimplification of complex issues. *ANS* 1987;9(3):24–33.

Mechanic D: The challenge of chronic mental illness: A retrospective and prospective review. *Hosp Community Psychiatry* 1986;37(9):891–896.

Pepper B, Kirshner MC, Ryglewicz H: The young adult chronic patient: Overview of a population. *Hosp Community Psychiatry* 1981;32:463.

Schwartz SR, Goldfinger SM: The new chronic patient: Clinical characteristics of an emerging subgroup. *Hosp Community Psychiatry* 1981;32:470.

Segal SP, Baumohl J: Engaging the disengaged: Proposals on madness and vagrancy. *Social Work* 1980;25:358–365.

Surlos R, McGurrin M: Increased use of psychiatric emergency services by young chronically mentally ill patients. *Hosp Community Psychiatry* 1987;38(4):401–405.

Tessler RC, et al: The chronically mentally ill in community support systems. *Hosp Community Psychiatry* 1982; 33(3):208–211.

Test LI, Stein MA: Community treatment of the chronic patient: Research overview. *Schizophrenia Bull* 1978; 4(3):350–364.

Turner RJ, Gartrell JW: Social factors in psychiatric outcome: Toward the resolution of interpretive controversies. *Am Social Rev* 1978;43:368–382.

TWENTY-THREE

Psychophysiologic Conditions

Mary-Eve Zangari

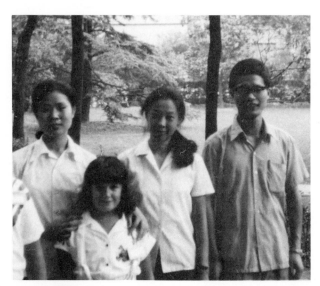

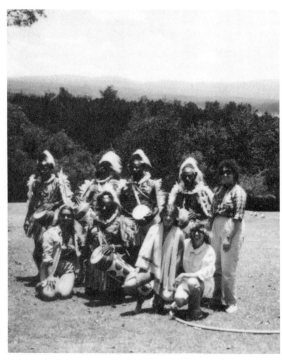

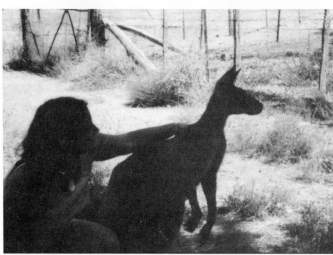

After reading this chapter, students should be able to

- Explain the multicausational concept of illness
- Define the term *psychophysiologic disorders*
- Relate psychologic and physiologic factors to the syndromes presented in this chapter
- Choose specific nursing interventions to augment the client's medical regimen

Cross References

Other topics related to the content in this chapter are: Caring for clients in a general hospital setting, Chapter 24; Influence of anxiety and stress on coping, Chapter 7; Psychobiology, Chapter 9; Stress-management techniques, Chapter 28.

Key Terms

Axis III
cardiac neurosis

pychophysiologic disorders
type A personality

This chapter and the chapter that follows present material about the intriguing ways in which our bodies and our minds interact to produce a variety of behaviors and symptoms. **Psychophysiologic disorders** (containing both physiologic and psychologic components) are those that have an important emotional component in their onset and course. Examples are peptic ulcer, ulcerative colitis, and asthma.

Because all illnesses may ultimately be termed psychophysiologic, a holistic theory of illness serves as a basis for understanding all human disorders. By appreciating the complex, interwoven pattern of emotional and physical elements that clients present, the nurse can more fully comprehend the essential unity of the body and the mind.

Clients who come to the attention of health care professionals because of physical complaints frequently have their psychologic needs neglected. Often, those unmet needs may be contributing to the complaint, may be the primary cause of symptom development, or may be the reason for the client's decision to seek help. Even though the most technologically advanced diagnostic and treatment approaches are applied, ignoring the psychologic components of illness can be disastrous. Such psychologic components can undermine medically appropriate treatment.

Therefore, in all illness, and certainly in those discussed in this chapter, a holistic approach is necessary if each facet of the client's overall problem is to be addressed. For each of the disorders, we suggest nonmedical interventions that reduce stress while increasing the client's understanding and control over troublesome symptoms. Promoting healthy life-styles and advocating life-style modification are important nursing responsibilities regardless of the clinical area in which nurses practice.

HISTORICAL AND THEORETICAL FOUNDATIONS

The relationship between the mind and the body has always been a subject for speculation. Early humans had a holistic approach to disease, making no distinction between physical and mental illness. From Socrates we have, "As it is not proper to cure the eyes without the head, nor the head

Peace activism ranges from changing nations and international relations to changing individuals and interpersonal relationships.

Portions of the material in this chapter were contributed to the second edition by Andrew Skodol.

unconscious feelings produce gastric hypersecretion, and eventually a peptic ulcer.

without the body, so neither is it proper to cure the body without the soul." And from Hippocrates, "In order to cure the body it is necessary to have a knowledge of the whole of things." Then, during the Middle Ages, medicine became dominated by mysticism and religion. Sin was thought to be the cause of disease. In reaction to this view, and in conjunction with the scientific discoveries of the Renaissance (autopsy and microscopy), the study of the psyche was completely divorced from the study of medicine. In the nineteenth century, the rift was deepened by further scientific advances. It was thought that all disease must be associated with structural cell changes. Hence, the disease and not the client was the focus. Now, in the twentieth century, we have come full circle, and the mind and body are again united. How they are united is still unknown, although many theorists have attempted to explain the nature of the relationship.

The Specificity Model

One theory is the specificity model of Franz Alexander (1950). According to Alexander, specific types of emotional conflict cause anxiety in the individual. In defending against this anxiety, the individual regresses to an earlier psychologic and physiologic stage of development. For instance, a person may regress into the oral receptive stage, in which there is an unconscious wish to be fed by the mother. This results in gastric hypersecretion. If the person has a vulnerable duodenal mucosa, peptic ulcer may result. The following case example illustrates how the specificity model is applied.

Linda, a 20-year-old nursing student, has been diagnosed with a small peptic ulcer, treatable with diet and medication. Because she mentioned that she was having difficulties at school, she is also referred to the psychiatry service, where she meets with a psychoanalytically inclined therapist. He asks Linda about her childhood and discovers that she was cared for by her grandmother while both her parents were away at work during the day. Later, Linda had to take care of a younger sister and brother after school and on weekends. The student says she never had a "real childhood" and doesn't ever remember her mother being there when she needed her. According to Alexander's model, the therapist would deduce that Linda has a dependency conflict deriving from her early childhood. Current academic stress causes her to wish for a time when she was protected and nurtured by her mother. These

Other investigators made further attempts to relate specific personality characteristics to certain diseases. People with ulcerative colitis were found to be passive, conforming, and dependent. Those with hypertension had counterdependency strivings. Diabetic people were passive, needed affection, and wished to be cared for. Women with dysmenorrhea were infantile and expressed hopelessness and self-denial. Cancer clients were found to be selfless and undemanding (Sachar 1975).

On closer scrutiny, the specificity theory is not very specific after all. Certain emotional states, such as dependency, appear to be common to all disorders. Furthermore, research does not indicate whether dependence is a cause or an effect of the disease process. Another criticism is that some of the relationships described above have been based on faulty physiologic premises. For instance, ulcerative colitis was thought to be caused by an inability to express anger openly. Instead, the client's rage "explodes" in uncontrollable bouts of diarrhea. It was believed that the frequent evacuations caused inflammation of the bowel lining. However, recent research has shown that *before* the persistent diarrhea appears, small ulcerations are already forming in the bowel (Sachar 1975).

The Nonspecific Stress Model

A second theory is the nonspecific stress model of Gustav Mahl (1953). Unlike Alexander, who focused on specific types of emotional conflict, Mahl theorized that the psychosomatic process can be activated by any stressful event, such as an earthquake, or a more subtle intrapsychic event, such as a fear of elevators. Whatever the source of the stress, the physiologic responses are identical for everyone. These physiologic responses have also been studied by Selye (1950, 1976). They include gastric and cardiovascular hyperfunctioning and hormonal changes, such as increased adrenal steroid secretion. A person who experiences chronic stress may develop a biologic symptom, the nature of which will be determined by organ susceptibility and early learning experiences involving pathologic responses.

This nonspecific model can be applied to the same case study that was used to illustrate Alexander's specificity model. Linda, the nursing student, still has a small peptic ulcer, but with this model it is explained differently.

Linda experienced the usual school stresses along with the rest of her classmates. But Linda develops an ulcer because her stomach is particularly vulnerable to stress. She may naturally produce an excess of hydrochloric acid, or her stomach lining may have some congenital defect. Along with organ susceptibility, Linda may have a parent who also had a peptic ulcer. She may have seen a parent react to stress with abdominal disturbances and learned to react in a similar manner.

This viewpoint is consistent with the clinical research data that have been gathered from studying people under stress. However, this theory fails to account for the influence that meaning and symbol have in an individual's interpretation of stressful events.

The Individual Response Specificity Model

A third theory is the individual response specificity model formulated by Lacey, Bateman, and Van Lehn (1953). According to this model, individuals tend to show highly characteristic and consistent physiologic responses to a wide range of stimuli. This model contradicts the nonspecific model in which everyone is seen as responding in much the same way to stress. Instead, according to the individual response model, there are "cardiac reactors," "gastric reactors," and "hypertensive reactors."

To illustrate this model, we return to Linda and her peptic ulcer.

Linda always has indigestion when she becomes upset. However, Monica, her roommate, never has indigestion. Instead, she frequently has migraine headaches.

This theory is compatible with the previously mentioned theories of organ susceptibility and early learning experiences. Because it encompasses much of the current research data, this theory has become increasingly popu-

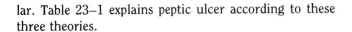

lar. Table 23–1 explains peptic ulcer according to these three theories.

The Multicausational Concept of Illness

It is readily apparent that the preceding models do not fully illuminate the relationships between emotions and physical functioning. By taking some other factors into account, researchers developed a more useful model. Some of these factors are presented in the research by Holmes and Rahe (1967), Mutter and Schleifer (1966), and Rahe and Arthur (1978). These studies show that physical illness is commonly preceded by stressful life changes. Their findings thus indicate that emotions have a role in all disease processes. The studies further suggest that physical disorders, like mental disorders, are related to social class. Furthermore, individuals in similar social situations defined those situations differently and consequently had different reactions to the similar situations.

Several basic considerations emerge from these findings.

- The concept of separation of mind and body is not useful in understanding the total disease process.
- Stress comes in many forms—psychologic, physiologic, and sociologic—and is a causative factor in all illness.
- Stress is perceived differently, depending on the individual and the specific context.

There seems to be no doubt that meaning and symbol function in humans as the mediating mechanism between emotion and physiology, although the nature of the process

---

Table 23–1
Peptic Ulcer Explained by Three Different Theories

Model	Stimulus	Biologic Responses
Specificity model	A specific unconscious conflict, e.g., dependency needs	Regression to oral receptive stage and increase in hydrochloric acid secretion results in peptic ulcer.
Nonspecific stress model	Any internal or external stress	General stress response (e.g., increased blood pressure and adrenaline secretion) results in peptic ulcer because stomach is most susceptible organ.
Individual response specificity model	Any internal or external stress	Individual predisposition as a "gastric reactor" results in peptic ulcer.

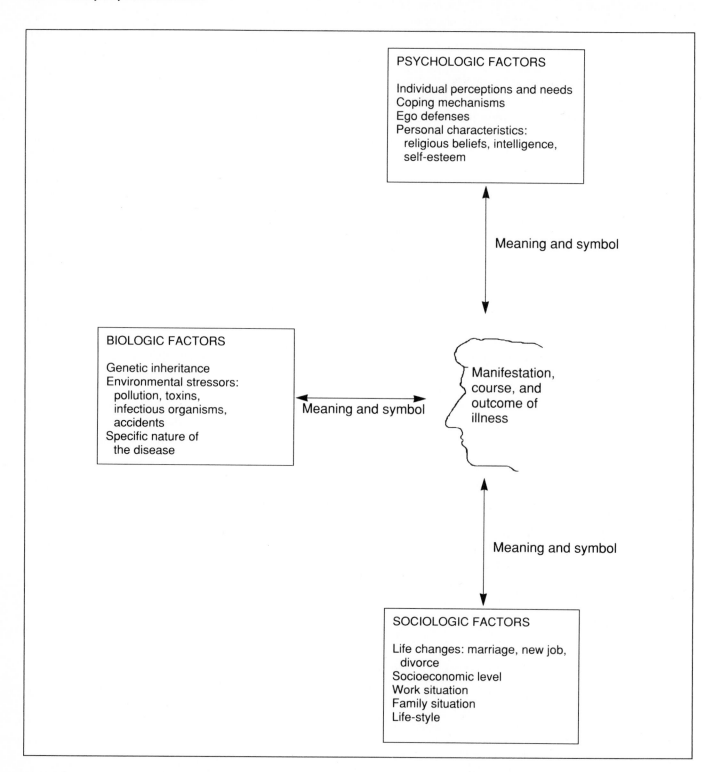

Figure 23–1
Multicausational concept of the illness process. The phrase *meaning and symbol* in the figure refers to the fact that the client interprets all experiences in a highly individualized manner according to their specific meaning for that client and their broader meaning in the client's culture.

remains undefined. Figure 23–1 and the following clinical example illustrate these ideas.

Peter G, 5 years old, was admitted for the fourth time in six months for an acute asthma attack. While Peter was being treated medically, his parents waited in the family room. Mrs. G sat crying and wringing her hands while Mr. G paced the floor with a strained expression on his face. A staff nurse was able to talk to them and trace the sequence of events leading up to Peter's admission to the hospital.

It was a Saturday afternoon, and Mr. and Mrs. G had been arguing about whether to send Peter to kindergarten in the fall. Two points of view had emerged. Mr. G was all for it. He wanted Peter to grow up quickly and leave his "babyish ways" behind. Mrs. G was against it. Peter was the baby of the family, and Mrs. G felt that her husband was always pushing him to do things too advanced for a 5-year-old. Peter had awakened from his nap to hear his parents shouting at each other. The quarrel ended abruptly when Peter started to wheeze, and both parents rushed to his bedside, united in their concern for him.

What factors brought on Peter's asthma attack at that particular time? The biologic factors include Peter's physiologic makeup. His mother had been a child asthmatic. She and Peter are both allergic to chocolate, eggs, feathers, and dust. Peter inherited certain genetic features that make him susceptible to certain environmental stressors, in this case, the specific allergens. Sociologic components of Peter's illness revolve around his family's functioning. Mr. and Mrs. G have different viewpoints on what Peter's role in the family should be. Their conflicts create a second source of stress for Peter. A third component is Peter's psychologic state. A 5-year-old boy views the integrity of his family as extremely important, and parental conflicts may threaten his sense of security. Peter had discovered that his parents rallied together when he was ill.

In view of these contributing factors, the treatment plan for Peter should not end when Peter stops wheezing. To reduce the number of such emergencies, caregivers need to devise a long-range treatment plan. This plan should encompass the physiologic, psychologic, and sociologic components of Peter's asthma attacks.

DSM-IIIR Classification

The preceding sections might seem to indicate that all diseases are psychophysiologic in nature. Many health professionals do believe so; others adhere to more simplistic theories or do not apply holistic concepts to their practice.

The psychophysiologic disorders appear in DSM-IIIR as "Psychological Factors Affecting Physical Condition." Any physical condition can be cited. Those commonly included because of the striking clinical evidence are peptic ulcer, asthma, bowel disorders, cardiovascular disorders, arthritis, allergy, headache, and certain endocrine disorders. The physical condition or syndrome is noted on **Axis III** of the multiaxial evaluation system. Until 1968, and today in some circles, the term *psychosomatic disorder* was used as the official nomenclature. The new terminology is more consistent with the "systems" approach to clients who have illness with marked organic and emotional components.

The revised DSM-IIIR classification of these problems allows for the consideration of the role of psychologic factors that lead up to, worsen, or perpetuate *any* physical illness. Therefore, even disorders not traditionally viewed as psychosomatic or psychophysiologic can be evaluated according to the new model. The revised classification is expected to encourage greater collaboration between mental health professionals, and strictly medical professionals in the treatment of ill persons.

PSYCHOPHYSIOLOGIC DISORDERS

The following sections review the characteristics of syndromes traditionally considered psychophysiologic disorders. For most of the syndromes, an exact etiology is unknown. Current research focuses on the complicated interrelationships among such factors as stress, personality, environment, and hormones. Psychoanalytic theories are presented when applicable.

Peptic Ulcer

Peptic ulcer has been one of the most thoroughly studied psychophysiologic illnesses. Still, many questions remain unanswered. Peptic ulcer incidence rises in response to stress (e.g., in times of war) and is prevalent among those persons with stressful life-styles (e.g., city dwellers, air traffic controllers, and police officers). Peptic ulcers seem to run in families. Other related causational factors are nutritional deficiencies, allergies, remote infections, alcohol and caffeine ingestion, and situations prompting prolonged responses of anxiety and resentment.

Peptic ulcers of the duodenal type occur three to six times more often in men than in women. Most persons with duodenal ulcer secrete excess acid. Among people with the gastric type of ulcer, 50 percent secrete normal or less than normal amounts of acid. This evidence illustrates the mixture of emotional and psychologic factors involved in ulcer formation and in the progression of the illness. The following clinical example illustrates this point.

A 42-year-old trial lawyer, married and the mother of two children, is referred for consultation by her gastroenterologist following her third hospitalization for duodenal ulcer disease. Her ulcer disease was first diagnosed four years ago, but an upper gastrointestinal (GI) series at that time showed evidence both of an active ulcer and of scarring secondary to previously healed ulcers. The gastroenterologist has requested the consultation for help in considering the possibility of surgery, prompted by the seriousness of the bleeding episode that precipitated the client's last admission and by the fact that she seems to "ignore pain." His referral note indicates that he sees no clear connection between the bleeding episodes and her highly stressful occupation.

The client appears exactly on time for her appointment; she is neatly and conservatively dressed. She presents an organized, coherent account of her medical problem and denies any past or immediate family history of significant mental disorder. She appears genuinely worried by her recent hospitalization, frightened by the prospect of surgery, and doubtful that speaking to a psychiatrist will produce any meaningful help. As she points out, "Ulcers are supposed to be related to stress, and that just isn't true with me." She then produces a detailed, written outline of her professional life over the past five years side by side with a chronology of her ulcer attacks. Indeed, there seems to be no temporal relationship between her attacks and several dramatic and highly taxing court cases in which she has appeared.

During the second evaluation session, the client discusses her background. She is the oldest of four children and the clear favorite of her father, also an attorney. He communicated a strong expectation that she would become a lawyer and that she would succeed in his field. The client sees herself as having fulfilled this expectation admirably and displays a rare smile while describing several of her more dramatic courtroom triumphs. There is no evidence that she experiences these difficult cases as stressful; in fact, she seems to enjoy them.

She married a law-school classmate, who is also quite successful and who works noncompetitively in an unrelated legal field. Their marriage seems sound. As she begins to talk about her two sons, aged 8 and 4, the client becomes noticeably more tense and appears much more concerned and upset than usual while describing minor crises they have experienced with friends or in school. With great surprise, she discovers that the chronology of these crises corresponds clearly to five of her seven ulcer attacks, including all of those that resulted in hospitalization. She admits that despite being upset by her sons' problems, she finds it difficult to share her concerns about parenting with her husband or friends. At the end of the session she comments: "You'd have made a good lawyer. I'm glad I'm not arguing against you." She herself suggests that some further sessions may be in order.*

The classic ulcer personality type is said to be competitive and aggressive, and appears lean and hungry. Psychoanalysts explain these characteristics as defenses against dependency needs. These traits have not been consistently demonstrated by research. Other psychologic constructs have more obvious validity.

Gastric functioning becomes intimately tied to dependency needs in humans through the feeding process from earliest infancy. The baby's mouth and digestive system are its early means of relating to the external world and its principal sources of gratification and frustration. Through complex learning processes, humans associate feeding and being taken care of and nurtured in a general sense. The mouth, through biting and chewing, also becomes the first mechanism through which the human infant can express anger and disappointment at being frustrated. It is well known that gastric secretion increases when infants and children are emotionally involved in either a positive or a negative sense.

Along with medical and surgical treatments, the care of these clients may include stress management techniques designed to decrease stress or the response to it. Psychotherapy may be appropriate if a dependency conflict exists and the client wishes to resolve it.

Bowel Disorders

Ulcerative colitis and Crohn's disease are chronic inflammatory disorders whose etiology remains unknown. They are characterized by diarrhea, abdominal pain, anorexia, fever, weight loss, vomiting, urgency to defecate, and incontinence. In severe cases, an ileostomy or colostomy may be necessary.

Clients with ulcerative colitis are said to display a compulsive personality style with the following features:

---

*Adapted from Spitzer, R L et al: *DSM-III Casebook.* American Psychiatric Association, 1981, pp 23–24.

- Neatness
- Orderliness
- Punctuality
- Indecisiveness
- Emotional guardedness
- Humorlessness
- Conscientiousness
- Obstinacy
- Conformity
- Moral rigidity
- Worry

According to psychoanalytic theory, ulcerative colitis develops in early childhood, usually as a result of a relationship with a controlling, domineering mother who makes the child feel overwhelmed, helpless, and rejected. Such a pattern of rearing often leads the individual, once adult, to feel that relationships to important others are always threatened, highly dependent on his or her performance in meeting the demands or expectations of others, and constantly colored by impending disapproval, especially by authority figures. The client feels helpless to cope and unable or forbidden to express the emotions associated with this frustration.

Contemporary researchers say that the psychologic traits these clients display are similar to those of clients with other chronic illnesses, with dependency being the most common trait. In many cases, onset and flare-ups seem linked to stressful life events, e.g., separations, failures, and disappointments.

Regardless of the source of the client's illness, treatment should focus on present troublesome areas. Hence, the plan may include individual psychotherapy, family therapy, and environmental manipulation along with the medical regimen. These persons do best when they are involved in solid and long-term supportive relationships with their nurses and physicians.

Cardiovascular Disorders

The cardiovascular system is a sensitive indicator of emotional arousal, whether fear, anger, or pleasurable excitement. High levels of stress are suspected to have harmful effects on the heart and vascular system, especially if stress is chronic or repeated. Experience, learning, and symbolic meaning, along with their emotional content, can influence the heart rate, heart rhythm, and blood pressure. These cardiovascular changes can in turn create emotions, mostly unpleasant, that affect perception and ideation by means of a feedback loop.

A number of factors have been identified as associated with high risk of heart disease. They include genetic, physiologic, social, and psychologic factors:

- Family history of heart disease
- Diet high in saturated fats, cholesterol
- High level of blood cholesterol, triglycerides, sugar, uric acid
- Hypertension, diabetes, hypothyroidism, renal disease, gout
- Low level of physical activity
- Heavy smoking and eating
- High-pressured life-style (type A personality)

The highly competitive, driving **type A personality** displays the classic constellation of personality characteristics associated with coronary disease, angina pectoris, and myocardial infarction. Adverse conditions in the client's environment, either social or economic, can also create the stress that leads to cardiac dysfunction.

Essential hypertension, cardiac dysrhythmias, and so-called cardiac neurosis are three syndromes of cardiovascular functioning with major psychologic inputs. The classical hypothesis in hypertension has been that people have conflict between their dependent and aggressive inclinations. This causes chronic repression of all displays of anger or resentment. The repressed emotions are eventually transformed into disorders of blood pressure regulation. Although this specific hypothesis has been difficult to prove, experiments have shown that fear, anger, frustration, and guilt all cause rises in diastolic blood pressure in vulnerable individuals. Likewise, anxiety, hostility, depression, interpersonal conflict, and disruptive life events have all been shown capable of precipitating dysrhythmias, e.g., sinus tachycardia, paroxysmal atrial tachycardia, and both atrial and ventricular ectopic beats.

Cardiac neurosis is a syndrome consisting of cardiac distress, exercise intolerance, easy fatigability, respiratory discomfort, and dizziness. These features are very similar to those found in panic disorder and mitral valve prolapse.

The treatment of cardiac disease must be multifaceted. In addition to medical or surgical treatment, other approaches involve stress management, relaxation training, biofeedback, and behavioral interventions to help people give up smoking. More efforts are being geared toward prevention, including programs by industry and corporations to promote healthy life-styles among employees.

Asthma

Asthma is among the most widely studied psychophysiologic illnesses of the respiratory system. Because breathing is essential to life, there has been much speculation about the emotional and symbolic significance that can become attached to the processes of air exchange. Asthma is characterized by labored breathing and wheezing resulting from spasm, secretions, and swelling in the bronchial tree.

There are allergic, immunologic, and emotional inputs to asthmatic attacks. The emotional components may lead directly to alterations in bronchus size. They may also affect the allergic and immunologic systems through hypothalamic nuclei in the central nervous system.

According to psychoanalytic theory, the typical asthmatic client is very dependent because of an exaggerated fear of loss of the mother induced early in infancy. These clients are therefore sensitive to separations or threats of separation, real or imagined, from people to whom they are attached. The asthmatic attack is interpreted as a repressed cry for a lost mother. It is unclear, due to the absence of controlled studies, whether the asthmatic's dependency and need for love are the cause or the result of the disease. Asthmatic persons may be extremely frightened by the attacks, particularly in childhood. This may make them feel more helpless and vulnerable. In response, they adopt a clinging style of relating. The emotional and the physical aspects of the illness seem to interrelate in a complex system of feedback loops. See the case history of Peter G on page 603 for an example of these concepts.

Each person with asthma must be assessed individually to determine what group of factors are contributing to the disease process. A treatment plan may include, along with medication, family therapy, relaxation training, behavior modification, and hypnosis.

Arthritis

Rheumatoid arthritis (RA) has long been identified as an illness that is strongly influenced by emotional life. Written records over 1500 years old attest to this. Basically, RA is a progressive inflammatory disease primarily of the joints, with unknown causes. Family prevalence studies indicate a genetic predisposition to the disease.

Psychologic stresses are thought to precipitate attacks and flare-ups. The mechanism of transformation from idea or affect into tissue alteration appears to be by hormonal and autonomic nervous system pathways. Specifically, growth hormone, sex hormones, thyroid hormone, and adrenal corticosteroids all change in states of emotional arousal, and all are involved in the production of connective tissue, especially collagen. The hypothalamus and the limbic system also mediate. Heredity and stress may operate in inverse proportion, according to a study by Rimon (1960). Rimon found that arthritic clients without genetic predisposition developed the illness under severe stress,

and others with a heavy genetic loading developed it despite little evidence of life conflict. In a follow-up study, Rimon and Laakso (1985) found that in those persons who developed RA amidst serious emotional trauma, later flare-ups were also linked to such circumstances.

In another study, Baker (1982) studied the relationship between stressful life events and the onset of RA. Baker suggests that severe emotional stress can bring on RA by decreasing the body's resistance to a virus, which then activates an autoimmune response.

People with RA appear to have difficulties with control, especially of hostility. Most clients appear to be overcontrolled, highly responsible, sensitive to criticism, and self-sacrificing. The diagnosis cannot be based on personality type, however, because there are many exceptions to the rule. Physical findings, deformities, subcutaneous nodules, and blood studies remain the criteria for identification.

A treatment plan for the arthritis client may include pain control, surgery, drugs, vocational counseling, occupational therapy, and interventions to alleviate or prevent depression and to deal with hostility more directly.

Headache

The experience of headache resulting from emotional tension is common. Headaches may be divided into the following types:

1. Vascular headache of migraine type
2. Muscle contraction headache
3. Combined vascular–muscle contraction headache
4. Delusional, depressive, conversion, or hypochondriacal headaches
5. Structural or disease-related headaches

Structural or disease-related headaches arise from:

- Systemic infections
- Primary or metastatic tumors
- Hematomas
- Abscesses
- Cranial infections
- Cranial nerve inflammations
- Eye, ear, nose, sinus, or tooth diseases

The mechanism of vascular headache seems to involve the release of various vasoactive substances in the brain, such as serotonin, catecholamines, histamine, bradykinin, and prostaglandins. This release frequently occurs with stress. In genetically susceptible individuals, the substances cause vasodilation and inflammation of the arterial walls. There are generally early warning symptoms of migraine attacks. These range from mood changes and gastrointestinal upset to gross neurologic findings in the visual and contralateral sensorimotor systems. A number of upsets in physiologic functioning can actually be migraine equivalents. These include nausea and vomiting, diarrhea, tachycardia, cyclical edema, vertigo, periodic fever, pain, depression, confusion, and insomnia. Another mechanism of tension-induced headache is muscular contraction in the neck, shoulders, face, or scalp. These are steady, persistent headaches with no warning signs and commonly feel like a "band wrapped around the head." Some theorists support the notion that headache sufferers are likely to maintain rigid control over emotions, feel hostility toward others, use introjection as a defense, and be perfectionists.

Interventions are based on the diagnosis and the contributing factors that have been identified. Possible treatments include measures that increase circulation, e.g., massage or heat application; use of medications; alterations in diet, rest, and exercise patterns; psychotherapy; biofeedback; transcendental meditation, hypnosis; relaxation; and other stress management approaches (Kneisl and Ames 1986).

Endocrine Disorders

A large number of disorders of endocrine functioning are associated with psychologic factors. Studying the endocrine system has particular significance for psychiatry, because there is a close relationship between the emotions and a variety of active chemical substances released in tissues by nerve impulses. In physical medicine, the feedback loop has long been accepted as the model for the functioning of the endocrine organs.

Extensive research on the endocrine feedback system has led to a sophisticated model that includes three kinds of feedback loops. The levels of circulating hormones released by endocrine glands, such as the thyroid or sex glands, are controlled by long feedback loops that send information to the cerebral cortex and limbic system. Short feedback loops of pituitary hormones affect the hypothalamus. Very short loops of releasing hormones from the hypothalamus determine their own production and control. Studies on the relationship of emotions to endocrine function have shown that:

- Various neurotransmitters affect hormone-releasing factors.
- Psychoactive drugs whose action is mediated by neurotransmitters also affect the release of releasing factors.
- Stress stimulates the autonomic nervous system, which can stimulate the adrenal medulla to produce epinephrine or the pancreas to secrete insulin.
- Corticosteroid production of the adrenal cortex increases greatly during acute psychotic episodes of schizophrenic clients.

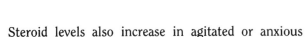
- Steroid levels also increase in agitated or anxious depressive people.

RESEARCH NOTE

Citation

Woods, NF, Most, A, Longnecker, GD: Major life events, daily stressors, and perimenstrual symptoms. Nurs Res 1985; 34:263–267

Study Problem/Purpose

This study sought to determine the relationship of major life events and daily stressors to perimenstrual symptoms.

Methods

The subjects were 100 nonpregnant, randomly selected women, ages 18–35, from varied racial and socioeconomic backgrounds. Three tools were used to collect data: The Menstrual Distress Questionnaire was used to assess the presence and severity of symptoms associated with the menstrual cycle. Subjects used the health diary to record daily experiences and health problems. Stressful life events were measured by Holmes and Rahe's Schedule of Recent Events.

Findings

The results of this study provide modest support for the relationship between stressors and perimenstrual symptoms. The symptoms of negative affect, performance impairment, and pain were made worse by stressful life experiences.

Water retention was not associated with major stressful life events. Overall, women who lead a steadily stressful life experience more troublesome symptoms than those with relatively low-stress lives and only incidental intervals of stress during their menstrual phase. These findings are consistent with those of other studies on this subject.

Implications

Premenstrual syndrome has become an area of intense inquiry. Special treatment centers are addressing the wide variety of symptoms that women may experience during their menstrual cycle. This study adds to the data suggesting that psychologic factors alone do not account for the mood changes, pain, and fatigue of the syndrome. However, since women who lead highly stressful lives may be at risk for more frequent and severe perimenstrual symptoms, stress-reduction interventions are recommended as part of the nursing care plan for these clients.

Table 23–2
Normal Developmental Alterations in Endocrine Function

Development	Physical Evidence	Psychologic Aspects
Puberty	Age, growth spurt, changes in fat and muscle proportions and distribution, changes in genitals, changes in secondary sex characteristics, menarche	Changes in popularity, prestige, self-confidence; increase in moodiness, hostility, depression, interpersonal difficulties
Menstruation	Menstrual bleeding cycles, cramps, backaches, headaches, alterations in estrogen-progesterone ratio	Irritability, mood swings, tension, depression
Postpartum	Pregnancy and delivery, vast prior increases in progesterone and estrogen levels during pregnancy fall to normal within ten days, changes in fluid and electrolyte balance, increased prolactin secretion	Emotional lability, body image changes, self-esteem issues, anxiety about adequacy as mother, sensitivity to father's responses to mother and baby
Menopause	Cessation or irregularity of menses, hot flashes, low levels of estrogen secretion	Anxiety, depression, irritability, decreased sexual interest, end of reproductive era, increased physical illness, loss of youth, issues of children being grown, parents dead or infirm, husband changing

It seems fair to conclude that the emotional centers of the brain—the cortex and limbic systems—are intimately tied to the endocrine organs, through the axis of the hypothalamus and the anterior pituitary. Their secretions act as communication messengers. It is not surprising, then, to find expressions of emotional arousal through endocrine changes and major effects on emotional states from endocrine diseases. These are both, in fact, common.

The major normal, developmental changes in the endocrine system are shown in Table 23–2, and disease-induced changes are summarized in Table 23–3. Adequately preparing a person for developmental changes by offering accurate information about likely physical and emotional alterations can help prevent severe psychiatric disturbances during these periods. Reliable support and open channels of communication are necessary. New coping strategies can be successful, if their ingenuity, timing, and presentation are appropriate.

Adrenal dysfunction characteristically produces prominent mental as well as distinctive physical symptoms. Thyroid disorders commonly are accompanied by cognitive or emotional changes. Stress has been implicated, though inconclusively, in the precipitation of thyrotoxic crises. Stress may influence the course of diabetes, either directly by promoting a flare-up or indirectly by causing the client to neglect a usually rigid medical regimen. So many mental symptoms are associated with hypoglycemia that many clients are classified and treated as "classic neurotics."

It is evident that numerous problems can be caused by endocrine dysfunction. The treatment approach must be individualized to meet the client's physical and psychologic needs.

Skin Disorders

Allergic illnesses, particularly those involving the skin, have been shown to have psychologic elements in etiology or course. The skin, with its critical sensory functions, becomes symbolically identified with the ego, or the part of an individual's psychologic makeup that mediates between the outside world and internal states. Itching (pruritus), excessive sweating (hidrosis), urticaria, and atopic dermatitis are all commonly classified as psychophysiologic conditions.

A variety of stressful or emotional states are associated with flare-ups of allergic skin disorders. Attempts have been made to correlate the following specific ones with individual disorders:

- Generalized pruritus: aggression
- Genital and anal pruritus: sexuality (heterosexual and homosexual)
- Hyperhidrosis: anxiety
- Urticaria: anger
- Atopic dermatitis: longing for love

	Table 23–3	
	Disease-Induced Alterations in Endocrine Function	
Disease	**Physical Symptoms**	**Mental Symptoms**
Cushing's syndrome (adrenal cortex hyperfunction)	Truncal obesity, moon facies, abdominal striae, hirsutism, amenorrhea, hypertension, osteoporosis, weakness	Impotence, decreased libido, anxiety, increased emotional lability, apathy, insomnia, memory deficits, confusion, disorientation
Addison's disease (adrenal insufficiency)	Weakness, fatigue, anorexia, weight loss, nausea and vomiting, pigmentation of skin, hypotension	Depression, irritability, psychomotor retardation, apathy, memory defect, hallucinations
Hyperthyroidism	Staring, exophthalmos, goiter, moist warm skin, weight loss, increased appetite, weakness, tremor, tachycardia, heat intolerance	Anxiety, tension, irritability, hyperexcitability, emotional lability, depression, psychosis, or delirium
Hypothyroidism	Dull expression, puffy eyelids, swollen tongue, hoarse voice, rough dry skin, cold intolerance	Psychomotor retardation, decreased initiative, slow comprehension, drowsiness, decreased recent memory, delirium, stupor, depression or psychosis
Diabetes mellitus	Polydipsia, polyuria, polyphagia, weight loss, blurred vision, fatigue, impotence, fainting, paresthesia	Stupor, coma, fatigue, impotence
Hypoglycemia	Tremor, light-headedness, sweating, hunger, nausea, pallor, tachycardia, hypertension	Anxiety, fugue, unusual behavior, confusion, apathy, psychomotor agitation or retardation, depression, delusions, hallucinations, convulsions, coma
Premenstrual syndrome	Headache, breast engorgement, lower abdominal bloating, GI complaints, increased sweating, craving for sweets, other appetite changes	Irritability, depression, anxiety, emotional lability, fatigue, crying spells

In truth, these affective states and conflicts are seen in normal, neurotic, and other psychophysiologic states. Nurses should therefore be cautious about accepting pathogenic mechanisms and explanations.

The location of the lesions has, historically, had symbolic significance. Thus, conflict over an extramarital affair has been associated with dermatitis in the wedding ring area. Head and face locations have been classically associated with conflict over affective display. Affliction of the hands is associated with practical or professional conflicts. A genital distribution is associated with sexual concerns.

RESISTANCE TO INTERVENTION

Behavior therapy, biofeedback, hypnotherapy, and psychotherapy have all been used with success with appropriate clients. However, despite the wealth of psychosocial interventions available to persons with psychophysiologic disorders, many clients are resistant to approaches that are not strictly medical. Some reasons for this are:

- These clients are believed to lack insight, since they express conflict through somatic complaints rather than verbalization.

- In psychoanalytic terminology, clients are said to suffer from a large number of pregenital conflicts—conflicts over unresolved dependency and aggressive wishes. This makes them difficult to relate to interpersonally.

- These clients focus steadfastly on their somatic complaints, apparently indicating that alternative defense mechanisms are unavailable or inadequate.

- They are rarely highly motivated to heighten their self-awareness, which is the goal of many forms of psychotherapy.

- Even when they are somewhat motivated, they may be unable or unwilling to delay gratification and thus are impatient with the slow process of growth usually required in psychotherapeutic work.

For these reasons, traditional psychotherapy is not the most useful intervention. Approaches that enhance medical and surgical intervention and allow the client's primary bond to remain with nonpsychiatric health care providers are more successful. Programs geared toward stress management are very useful because they present stress as part of the human condition and the participants do not feel labeled as having psychiatric problems.

Chapter Highlights

- The multicausational concept of illness acknowledges the biologic, psychologic, and sociologic components of the illness/disease process.

- Psychologic factors should always be considered among those factors that lead up to, worsen, or perpetuate any physical illness.

- Ignoring the psychologic components of illness can undermine appropriate treatment.

- Psychophysiologic disorders are those that have an important emotional component in their onset and future course.

- The psychophysiologic disorders in particular illustrate the complicated interactions of mind, body, and environment because they present physical symptoms with a strong psychologic component.

- Syndromes in which physical and psychologic factors interact by means of feedback loops include peptic ulcer; asthma; arthritis; headache; and certain bowel, cardiovascular, endocrine, and skin disorders.

- Promoting healthy life-styles and advocating life-style modification are important nursing responsibilities.

- Regardless of the clinical area in which they practice, nurses must have a knowledge of stress management approaches to offer clients a useful plan of care.

- Many clients resist the idea that emotions may play a part in their disorders. Therefore, the plan of care should be thoughtfully managed by a health care professional that the client trusts.

References

Alexander F: *Psychosomatic Medicine: Its Principles and Application.* W. W. Norton, 1950.

American Psychiatric Association: *Diagnostic and Statistical Manual of Mental Disorders,* ed. 3. APA, 1980.

American Psychiatric Association: *Diagnostic and Statistical Manual of Mental Disorders,* ed 3, revised. APA, 1987.

Arthritis and Related Rheumatoid Disease: *Nurs Clin North Am* 1984;19:entire volume.

Baker GHB: Life events before the onset of rheumatoid arthritis. *Psychother Psychosom* 1982;38:173–177.

Bohachick P: Progressive relaxation training in cardiac rehabilitation: Effect on psychologic variables. *Nurs Res* 1984;33:283–287.

Burckhardt CS: The impact of arthritis on quality of life. *Nurs Res* 1985;34:11–16.

Caplan G: Mastery of stress: Psychological aspects. *Am J Psychiatry* 1981;138:413–420.

Conte HR, Karasu TB: Psychotherapy for medically ill patients: Review and critique of controlled studies. *Psychosomatics* 1981;22:285–315.

Engel GE: Clinical application of the biopsychosocial model. *Am J Psychiatry* 1980;137:535–544.

Fuller E (ed): When endocrinopathies affect behavior. *Patient Care* 1984;18:55–68.

Gallon RL (ed): *The Psychosomatic Approach to Illness.* Elsevier Biomedical, 1982.

Green SA: *Mind and Body: The Psychology of Physical Illness.* American Psychiatric Press, 1985.

Holmes TH, Rahe RH: The social readjustment scale. *J Psychosom Res* 1967;11:213–218.

Kaplan HI, Sadock BJ: *Comprehensive Textbook of Psychiatry.* Williams and Wilkins, 1985.

Knapp PH, Mathe AA: Psychophysiologic aspects of bronchial asthma, in Weiss et al: *Bronchial Asthma: Mechanisms and Therapeutics.* Little, Brown, 1985.

Kneisl CR, Ames SA: *Adult Health Nursing: A Biopsychosocial Approach.* Addison-Wesley, 1986.

Lacey, JI, Bateman, DE, Van Lehn, R: Autonomic response specificity. *Psychosom Med* 1953;15:8.

Mahl GF: Physiological changes during chronic fear. *Ann NY Acad Sci* 1953;56:240.

Mennies JH, et al: Overview of adult allergy. *Nurs Pract* 1985;16:19–23.

Minuchin S: *Family Kaleidoscope.* Harvard University Press, 1984.

Mutter AZ, Schleifer M: The role of psychological and social factors in the onset of somatic illness in children. *Psychom Med* 1966;28:333–343.

Osofsky HJ, Blumenthal SJ (eds): *Premenstrual Syndrome: Current Findings and Future Directions.* American Psychiatric Press, 1985.

Pollock SE: Human responses to chronic illness: Physiologic and psychosocial adaption. *Nurs Res* 1986;35:90–95.

Rahe R, Arthur R: Life change and illness studies: Past history and future directions. *J Human Stress* 1978;4:3–15.

Rahe R, et al: Simplified scaling for life change events. *J Human Stress* 1980;5:22–27.

Rimon R: A psychosomatic approach to rheumatoid arthritis. *Acta Rhumatol Scand* [Suppl] 1969;13:1–154.

Rimon R, Laakso RL: Life stress and rheumatoid arthritis. *Psychother Psychosom* 1985;43:38–43.

Sachar EJ: Current status of psychosomatic medicine, in Strain J, Grossman S (eds): *Psychologic Care of the Medically Ill.* Appleton-Century-Crofts, 1975, pp 54–56.

Schwab JJ: Psychosomatic medicine: Its past and present. *Psychosomatics* 1985;26:583–593.

Selye H: *The Physiology and Pathology of Exposure to Stress.* Acta, 1950.

Selye H: *The Stress of Life.* McGraw-Hill, 1976.

Shaver JA: Biopsychosocial view of health. *Nurs Outlook* 1985;33:186–191.

Sparacino J: Blood pressure, stress, and mental health. *Nurs Res* 1982;31:89–94.

Sparacino LL: Psychosocial considerations for the adolescent and young adult with inflammatory bowel disease. *Nurs Clin North Am* 1984;19:41–49.

Spitzer RL, et al: *DSM-III Casebook.* American Psychiatric Association, 1981.

Stein MA: Biopsychosocial approach to immune function and medical disorders. *Psychiatr Clin North Am* 1981;4(2):203–220.

Wolpe J: Behavior therapy for psychosomatic disorders. *Psychosomatics* 1980;21:379–385.

TWENTY-FOUR

Psychosocial Nursing in the Nonpsychiatric Setting

Mary-Eve Zangari

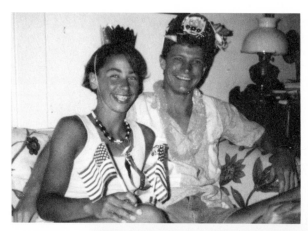

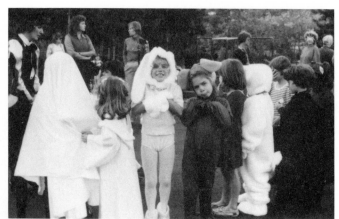

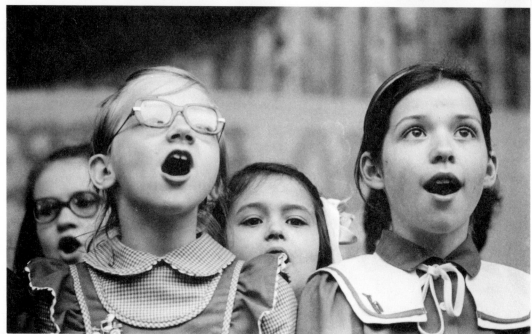

Learning Objectives

After reading this chapter, students should be able to

- Discuss the coping tasks of the hospitalized client
- Evaluate the usefulness of the client's coping skills
- Explain the process of helping clients to develop effective coping skills
- Describe the role and functions of the psychiatric nursing consultant

Cross References

Other topics relevant to this content are: Coping strategies, Chapter 7; Crisis management, Chapter 29; Death and dying, Chapter 37; Family dynamics, Chapter 33; Hostility and aggression, Chapter 27.

Key Terms

anticipatory guidance
body image
consultant
consultant-liaison psychiatry
intensive care syndrome
  (ICU psychosis)

liaison nurse
phantom experience
phantom pain

Nurses working in general hospitals face the challenge of combining what futurist Naisbett has called "high tech and high touch." They must not only keep abreast of the latest technology, but also must apply it with an understanding of the emotional and psychologic ramifications for each client.

Nurses have always practiced holistically, paying attention to their clients' families, life-styles, values, and beliefs. In health care in general, the trend is toward the delivery of more humanistic care. Some of the change is in response to the demand of the public for more personalized and effective health care. Another influence is the steady accumulation of research that points to a biopsychosocial model of illness. Among hospitalized persons in general, studies indicate that 30 to 60 percent have significant psychologic problems secondary to their medical illness (Strain 1982).

Chapter 23 presented the theoretical base for a holistic approach to all physically ill persons. Here we apply the nursing process to the psychosocial needs presented by clients in nonpsychiatric settings. This chapter also describes the process of coping with the stresses of hospitalization.

To aid nurses in delivering care to clients with diverse psychosocial needs, many general hospitals have added psychiatric nurse clinical specialists to their staffs. This role has helped nurses to apply psychiatric nursing principles to their work with the general hospital client. Clinical examples in this chapter demonstrate the application of theory to practice.

THE HOSPITAL EXPERIENCE

Hospitalization As a Crisis

Illness and hospitalization can be viewed as crisis situations for clients and their families. This section discusses what the nature of this crisis is, how clients and their families

People at peace offer a means to a peaceful world.

---

*Portions of this chapter were contributed to the second edition by Carol Ren Kneisl.

- Having strangers sleep in the same room
- Having strange machines around
- Having nurses or doctors talk too fast or use words they can't understand
- Not getting pain medication when they need it
- Thinking they might lose a kidney or some other organ
- Thinking they might have cancer

The scale consists of forty-nine events, a sober reminder of the number of stressors a hospitalized person confronts.

In addition to this lack of customary support systems and the fear of bodily injury, they suffer a psychologic reaction to hospitalization. Clients are expected to assume the *sick role* described by Parsons (1951). While occupying this role, they are exempt from responsibility and from their normal social role obligations. They are expected to depend on others, not to be self-directed. Essentially, clients can be left almost totally without their usual supports, including the coping mechanisms on which they usually rely.

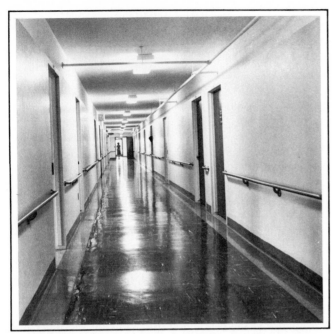

Figure 24–1
Hospitals can be cold and lonely places in which physical needs only are attended to. Psychosocial concepts must be incorporated into nursing practice in general hospital settings.

Coping with Illness and Hospitalization

How does someone manage to survive so many obstacles? Several authors have made excellent studies of the coping processes of the physically ill (Lambert and Lambert 1985, Miller 1983, Moos 1977, Weisman 1978). Moos (1977, p 12 to 14) identifies seven coping skills common to clients with a variety of physical problems.

1. Denying or minimizing the seriousness of a crisis
2. Seeking relevant information
3. Requesting reassurance and emotional support
4. Learning specific illness-related procedures
5. Setting concrete limited goals
6. Rehearsing alternative outcomes
7. Finding a general purpose or pattern of meaning in the course of events

These coping skills are behaviors that can be practiced and learned. They can be used at various times and in no special order or sequence. Sometimes they are labeled "positive," as in the case of the diabetic who learns to inject her own insulin. When a person constantly bombards the staff with questions about his or her treatment, the skill may be labeled "negative." Coping with illness is a *process* that takes place over time. It necessitates the guidance of the hospital staff to help the client develop a workable coping style. The nurse must identify the client's present coping skills, evaluate their effectiveness, and intervene if necessary to help the client develop new methods of coping. This process is called **anticipatory guidance**.

can learn to cope, and how nurses can facilitate the coping process.

Hospitals are ideal places in which to see crisis brewing. The emergency room and the cardiac and intensive care units are designed specifically for clients who are experiencing an unexpected illness or accident. However, general medical and surgical floors, where clients are admitted by schedule, also include clients in states of crisis.

Any hospitalization is extremely stressful. Clients are in a strange environment away from their customary supports of family and friends (Figure 24–1). They literally fear for their lives. Never knowing from minute to minute what to expect, they are subjected to all sorts of indignities. Usually no one informs them of procedures more than a few minutes ahead of time, and what is worse, they are the last to know the results of their many tests. In a large teaching hospital, the client has a specialist for everything and consequently may not develop a supportive relationship with any one physician or nurse. These clients are constrained to lie passively in bed, while the parade of hospital personnel work on their various parts. In 1975, Volicer and Bohannon developed the Hospital Stress Rating Scale, which ranks stressful events that are commonly experienced by hospitalized persons such as:

The following questions help the nurse explore clients' coping styles:

- What has bothered you most about this illness?
- How has it been a problem for you?
- What have you done (or are you doing) about the problem?
- Is this helping?
- What has been the most difficult thing you've had to face until now?
- What did you do then?
- Whom do you rely on most, or expect will be most helpful to you?
- In general, how do things usually turn out for you?

The nurse can also evaluate the client's coping style by assessing key areas: Is the client emotionally distressed by anxiety, depression, and hostility? How does the client deal with significant others? Does the client's coping style interfere with *necessary* medical or surgical treatment or with other components of the treatment plan?

There are many approaches available to nurses who want to guide their clients toward optimal coping. Among them are:

- Being knowledgeable about the usual responses to a given illness so that the client's behavior can be properly evaluated
- Accepting the client's feelings and behavior as the best response the client can make at the present time
- Educating the client and the client's significant others about the reactions the client and others may have to the illness
- Knowing what the client is likely to be struggling with (i.e., the developmental tasks at the client's age and stage of life)
- Allowing the client the opportunity to try out new ways of being (e.g., talking about feelings with the nurse)
- Listening to clients solve problems out loud and providing feedback without giving direct advice
- Teaching such skills as relaxation and assertiveness
- Giving information (e.g., the relationship between anxiety and pain)
- Providing referrals to other resources (e.g., self-help groups, specialists, or other clients)
- Helping the client to manage the hospital environment, thereby increasing the client's sense of control and competence
- Developing written contracts with clients
- Separating the nurse's own personal responses from those of the client

Clients who develop effective coping styles will be strengthened in many ways. They will feel more capable of dealing

with future problems, and, should the current illness prove to be chronic, will have developed the beginning skills to cope with a lifelong source of stress.

APPLYING THE NURSING PROCESS WITH CLIENTS IN THE GENERAL HOSPITAL SETTING

In the following sections, the nursing process is described as applied to selected clinical examples. Many of these examples include the input of a consulting psychiatric nurse.

The Demanding Client

Ruth was a resident of a home for the permanently disabled. She had been admitted to the hospital for a possible bowel obstruction. She was 65 and had lived most of her life in a wheelchair. Her body was misshapen from cerebral palsy, and she had no use of her legs or left hand. Recently she had developed arthritis in her right hand and could use it only for short periods each day. She had also been born with megacolon and was obsessed with the use of various laxatives. Ruth's appearance belied the fact that she was very intelligent, although humorless, as the staff soon found out.

According to the staff, Ruth was the "worst client they'd ever had." Ruth wanted to direct her own care in meticulous detail. She had to be bathed at a certain time and in a certain sequence, out of bed in time for breakfast and dressed by her own idiosyncratic method. It took two nurses one half hour to make her bed—they declared they needed a ruler to make sure the bedclothes hung precisely even. Medications were a real problem. Ruth had many p.r.n. medicines and constantly experimented with various combinations of laxatives, antispasmodics, and tranquilizers. No matter how one tried to please Ruth, she always found some fault with her nurse for the day, until finally she had been through the entire staff, and they all dreaded seeing her name on their assignment list.

Since Ruth aroused such strong feelings from the staff, the psychiatric nurse clinical specialist was consulted to ensure an objective plan of care.

Assessment

Discussions aimed toward connecting Ruth's behavior with theory to understand the *meaning* of her actions and attitude.

Ruth's demanding attitude was a life-style that had been exaggerated by the current hospitalization. The consultant helped the staff understand Ruth's behavior by looking at the underlying dynamics. Ruth had a distorted body image that reached back to her childhood, when she was confined to her bedroom and had to deal with body casts and braces. She had had to rely on others all her life and apparently had never resolved this dependency issue. To counteract her rage at being so helpless, she devised ways to control her environment by making incessant demands on others. In this way she vented her anger toward those with normal bodies. At the same time, she felt as if she had some degree of control over her surroundings. Ruth had behind her a lifetime of maladaption to her handicap, and it was not to be expected that she would change overnight. In fact, the current loss of functioning of her right hand constituted a crisis situation for Ruth. Behind Ruth's demands lay a myriad of feelings: anger, helplessness, frustration, jealousy, fear, and ambivalence.

Diagnosis

Here is a list of some of the nursing and psychiatric diagnoses that apply to Ruth:

- Obsessive compulsive personality disorder (DSM-IIIR)
- Impaired social interaction (NANDA)
- Disturbance in self-concept: body image (NANDA)
- Ineffective individual coping related to loss of right hand function (NANDA)
- 02.07.04 Obsessions (PND-I)
- 06.03.01 Altered body image (PND-I)
- 08.01.02 Helplessness (PND-I)

Planning and Implementing Interventions

In this situation, the consultant found herself performing a *parallel process*. This means that she was fulfilling parallel needs for both the staff and the client. She would meet with Ruth and allow her to *vent her feelings* of anger and frustration—some of which were justified and some of which were distortions of reality—toward the staff and the world in general. She encouraged Ruth to use her coping mechanism of intellectualization to recognize how she distorted reality because of fear and frustration.

At the same time the clinician *worked with the staff,* allowing them to express their feelings about Ruth. These feelings were also justified. Here, the clinician worked toward helping the staff recognize their anger at the client—a very difficult task for most nurses. Once the anger has been identified, steps can be taken to control it. Otherwise nurse and client engage in a no-win battle over control. The clinician demonstrated that anger was acceptable between nurse and client. She taught the staff how to *set limits* without being punitive or feeling guilty. This is also a difficult task for nurses who often feel they must fulfill everyone's wishes without paying any attention to their own needs.

A demanding person *needs* to have limits set and to be treated in a consistent and nonconflicted manner. Thus Ruth's nurse conveyed to her that she wanted to make her as comfortable as possible, but that she couldn't spend a half hour making and remaking the bed until she got it just right. It was OK for the nurse to tell Ruth when she was angry, to be clear about what had provoked the anger, and to demonstrate that this did not mean that she would abandon or punish her. The staff and clinician hoped that Ruth would begin to learn how to handle her own anger.

A client as difficult as Ruth always arouses feelings that nurses usually find unacceptable for themselves. But before we can accept anger from a client, we must learn to accept it in ourselves and learn that it will not overwhelm us. Working with demanding clients involves looking behind the external behavior for the reasons that are always there, although not always obvious.

In summary, the key interventions were:

1. Daily meetings between Ruth and consultant
2. Weekly meetings between staff and consultant
3. One staff nurse assigned to Ruth to coordinate *all* care
4. Limit-setting approach discussed with Ruth and consistently used by all staff

Evaluation

By the end of one week, tension on the unit had visibly decreased. There were fewer outbursts of anger from Ruth; staff was no longer hostile toward her. Ruth was discharged without further incident.

The Client in Pain

Many nurses remember receiving an order to give an injection of sterile water for pain. Feeling guilty about carrying out such an order, we wondered why the client would "pretend" to be in pain. Who'd *want* to get injections, anyway?

The whole issue of pain and the use of medication to alleviate it is laden with myths and value judgments. References are made to psychogenic pain versus "real" pain. In fact, pain is both an objective and a subjective experience. A nurse can observe pain behaviors like wincing, limping, or splinting. And a nurse can listen to a client's reports of feeling pain. How a client manifests pain depends on many factors. These include the client's background, previous experiences with pain, family's attitude toward the expression of pain, immediate environment, illness, and emotional state. The nurse's perception of a client's pain depends on the same factors. A nurse who thinks that people should suffer in silence will be intolerant of a client with a low pain threshold. It is important to realize that whether it is labeled psychogenic or physiologic, the client *experiences* the same pain.

An accompanying factor is the emotional component of pain. Anxiety, depression, guilt, anger, and hostility can all be associated with the experience of pain and can, in fact, become indistinguishable from one another.

A familiar cartoon shows a client sitting on a stretcher, his sleeve rolled up, his eyes shut tightly, waiting for the nurse to give the injection. As she rubs the client's arm with alcohol, the client lets out a scream of pain and relief, only to discover that the worst is yet to come. The cartoon's point is that the expectation can be much more painful than the actual experience, and that one can actually *feel* the emotion of anxiety.

In the general hospital, the nurse encounters pain in all its variations, from the post-cardiac-surgery client, to the cancer client with pathologic fractures, to the adolescent who has just had a tonsilectomy. Each client has an individual response to particular stimuli. Therefore, the nurse should evaluate each client's needs individually. Here is a case in point.

Mr. S had been a client on the oncology service for eight months. He had come to America from his home in Brazil when he discovered that he had a mandibular tumor. He had heard that the United States had the most advanced methods of chemotherapeutic and surgical treatment of cancer. During his eight months of hospitalization, Mr. S had undergone numerous courses of chemotherapy and four operations. Now he was ambulatory and self-sufficient. He had facial scars and a left-sided facial paralysis, but he could communicate clearly. His treatment had come to a standstill, and the doctors were planning discharge. However, Mr. S complained of constant severe pain that he reported kept him awake all night and prevented him from thinking about anything else. At this point the psychiatric nurse clinical specialist was asked to see Mr. S and help with the discharge planning.

Assessment

The consultant suggested a comprehensive assessment of Mr. S's situation. This involved learning about his family background, his present relationship to his family, his plans for the immediate and distant future, and his perception of his illness. It also involved obtaining a detailed account of his pain experience.

Mr. S had left all his friends and relatives in Brazil. He was divorced and had a 12-year-old daughter. In Brazil, he had held a university position, but he was not interested in returning either to his job or to his family. His reasons were not very clear, but he kept saying that he wanted to get a doctoral degree and a teaching position in the United States. He had written to several universities to inquire about their programs but had not made any definite plans. Apparently, money was no problem, but Mr. S repeatedly returned to the issue of his pain. This pain kept him from making progress—he couldn't rest until he knew whether the pain was from another tumor growing in his jaw. For this reason he felt he had to stay in the hospital for further tests.

Diagnosis

Two key nursing diagnoses in this situation are:

- Ineffective individual coping (NANDA)
- 06.02.03 Altered comfort pattern: pain (PND-I and NANDA)

Mr. S's pain behavior was related to his fear of dying, his fear of rejection due to disfigurement, his fear that he had lost his status and role in his own country, and his fear of leaving the hospital. All these issues were considered in his treatment plan.

Planning and Implementing Interventions

A coordinated approach was planned with the primary nurse as the client's primary contact. First, she obtained information about Mr. S's medical status and asked the physicians to communicate clearly to Mr. S his present condition and his prognosis. He was told that there was no evidence of another tumor, that no further treatment was indicated at this time, and that they were willing to help him make plans for discharge. Next, the nurse carefully evaluated the client's pain behavior. Exactly where was the pain? When was it most severe? What medications helped most? What activities made it worse or better? Together with Mr. S, the staff nurses, and the physicians, the consultant implemented a plan whereby Mr. S could gradually be weaned from his present analgesics. The client was also taught how to meditate and use distraction and relaxation techniques. Underlying the entire plan was the relationship formed between Mr. S and the primary nurse. It was understood that Mr. S had developed a strong dependency on the hospital and indeed believed that he could not survive outside its walls. The nurse aimed to reduce this dependency gradually, guiding Mr. S through the process of regaining his autonomy.

In summary, the key interventions were:

1. Evaluate pain
2. Learn status of tumor
3. Wean client from analgesics
4. Teach client meditation and relaxation techniques
5. Increase client's independence gradually

Evaluation

Within one month, Mr. S returned to Brazil to his former position, needing only a nonnarcotic analgesic.

The Dependent Client

Some degree of dependency is a normal, necessary, and expected part of the person's new role as client. In order to be cured, clients allow us to take control of most of their bodily functions. They obediently open their mouths for the thermometer at six in the morning. They cooperate while we record everything they eat, drink, and eliminate. They answer questions in minute detail about their most intimate parts. Dependency and regression are aspects of their new role that allow clients to tolerate hospital life.

American culture values self-reliance and independence. But when we become ill, it becomes socially acceptable to ask for help. In fact, this is exactly what is expected. But sometimes the system backfires, and instead of giving up the sick role after the appropriate convalescent period, the client continues to act helpless. Whether or not clients return to their prior level of functioning depends on many factors. These include the length and severity of the illness, the client's personality, the client's family situation, and the attitude of the nursing staff, as illustrated in the following case.

Mrs. C was admitted to a neurology unit amid rumors that she probably had Guillain-Barré syndrome, a rare disease that sometimes ends in total paralysis. The nurses were afraid to leave her bedside, expecting that at any moment she would stop breathing. After the official diagnosis had been made, Mrs. C was intubated and transferred to the intensive care unit, where she remained for four weeks. When she returned to the neurology unit, the nurses met a severely regressed young woman who needed complete and total nursing care. Mrs. C was off the respirator, and she was able to blink her eyelids. Otherwise she could move her limbs only with excruciating pain. Imagine the sensation one feels when one's leg has fallen asleep and one is trying to move it—that was only a fraction of what Mrs. C felt.

At first the nurses were awed and sympathetic. Mrs. C had survived. Now the staff's goal was to return her to her former role as a wife and mother. After several weeks, however, staff members became disillusioned. It seemed that Mrs. C did not always share the staff's grand design for her rehabilitation. She cried that getting out of bed was too painful. She couldn't possibly brush her own teeth. At times Mrs. C was too exhausted even to talk and seemed scarcely better than she had been on admission.

Assessment

The psychiatric nursing consultant began to meet with the staff to discuss Mrs. C's lack of progress. It was established that the nurses were anxious for her to improve because they wanted to deny the extreme severity of Mrs. C's illness. The woman had suffered a catastrophic event, and it reminded the nurses that sickness is often meaningless and uncontrollable. Staff members discussed their need to control her progress. In their heads, they had formulated a time chart on which to record Mrs. C's expected progress. It was very difficult to accept that the client didn't meet their expectations, because to them this meant that they were failures as nurses. It is interesting to observe that the nurses' need for control was actually aggravating the client's dependency. Mrs. C was to give up her dependency according to the nurses' schedule! This is like demanding that someone "be spontaneous!"

Another factor in the case was the prolonged period of immobility and complete helplessness that Mrs. C had experienced. Her regression had been severe, and she needed time to relearn how to function on her own. This was a fearful and bewildering period for Mrs. C and her family. For the first time, she contemplated how close she had come to death. Because Mrs. C had been mercifully unconscious for much of the time in the ICU, this period was analogous to a rebirth for her. Psychologically and physically she had to learn to live again.

Diagnosis

The following nursing diagnoses apply to the psychologic problems Mrs. C experienced:

- Anxiety, related to fear of death (PND-I and NANDA)
- Powerlessness related to illness and health care environment (PND-I and NANDA)
- Ineffective individual coping (NANDA)

Planning and Implementing Interventions

Out of weekly nursing care conferences with the consultant, the staff developed a plan that allowed the client to gradually increase her independence. The staff allowed Mrs. C to "pace" herself and gave her increased attention for her progress.

In summary, the key interventions were:

- Weekly care conferences with consultant
- Schedule and priorities developed in collaboration with Mrs. C
- Use of behavior modification principles

Evaluation

Because the nurses were insightful and perceptive enough to recognize their part in the situation, and because Mrs. C had the desire to regain her former role, this case had a satisfactory ending. When the nurses were able to let go of their own objectives, Mrs. C gained the ability to progress at her own rate.

The Client's Family

Hospital personnel speak of "the client with breast cancer," as if that phrase defined the target of their treatment. It may be more appropriate and accurate to talk about "the family of the client with breast cancer." This is because family members constitute a system, each part of which affects the functioning of all the other parts. Each family member fills a certain role, and if one member is hospitalized, that role is left vacant. The remaining members must make adjustments to compensate for the missing role.

The illness of a family member constitutes a family crisis. A crisis represents a turning point, the outcome of which can be adaptive or maladaptive depending on the

contributing factors. The consultant is often called on when the nursing staff believe that the client's family is not making a positive contribution to their efforts to treat the client. That is what happened in the following case.

Mrs. W was recovering from a stroke that had left her aphasic and with right-sided weakness. Her treatment included physical therapy, speech therapy, and a weight-reduction, low-salt diet. The client, a widow, had been living alone at the time of the stroke. Luckily, her daughter had found her collapsed on the kitchen floor and had brought her to the hospital.

Mrs. W's daughter and son visited her every night, bringing her presents of candy, fried chicken, and potato chips. They literally spoon-fed her and were horrified when the nurse suggested that Mrs. W show her family how she could feed herself. The nurses were angry, believing that the family was encouraging Mrs. W to remain dependent and spoiling her weight-reduction diet.

Assessment

The consultant was asked for suggestions on how to deal with Mrs. W's family.

One evening during dinner, the consultant dropped in on Mrs. W and her family. She commented to the children that they showed great concern for their mother, and that it must sometimes be a strain to visit the hospital every night when they had families of their own. The son nodded agreement, but the daughter's eyes filled with tears and she asked to talk to the clinician alone. She began to tell her how guilty she felt about her mother's stroke. She had not visited Mrs. W for several weeks prior to the accident, saying she was too busy. When she finally had visited, it was to find Mrs. W unconscious. If only she'd been a better daughter! Now the barrage of food and attention became understandable. Mrs. W's children needed to assuage their guilt over what they believed to be neglect of their mother. The consultant made it clear that the staff did not view them as neglectful and indeed needed their help in rehabilitating Mrs. W.

Diagnosis

The major nursing diagnosis in this instance was ineffective family coping, a NANDA diagnosis.

Planning and Implementing Interventions

Mrs. W's family was included in a care planning session in which family members were designated certain tasks. The primary nurse determined which members were interested in and capable of giving her bed baths and back care and feeding her.

Evaluation

The family became very helpful to both Mrs. W and the nursing staff, allowing the client to progress more rapidly. They felt they had been an important part of her recovery and had been allowed to stay close to her during the long hospitalization.

Another situation frequently encountered is that of the angry, demanding family. They complain about the nursing care, ask to talk to the supervisor, and may even ask to see the hospital administrator. This behavior is one way a family can cope with the rage and impotence they feel. It is not acceptable to express anger toward the ill family member, although many spouses *do* experience anger. A wife is angered and frightened by her heavy new responsibilities and by the possibility of her husband's death. She cannot express this anger to her husband. Nor can she direct it toward the doctors, who seem to have the power of life and death. Often she takes her feelings out on the nurse, who is less threatening and more accessible. A husband whose wife is ill is also angry and frightened and feeling particularly left out in caring for his wife. He may overcompensate by keeping a close watch on the care the nurses are giving.

Nurses can provide this kind of family with a safe place to express their anger, fear, and frustration. They can let these families know that their feelings are not unusual and that the nurse doesn't find them selfish or insensitive. The staff can also be helped to understand the meaning of the family's behavior. This often leads to a decrease in hostility and allows everyone to spend more energy on adaptive methods of coping.

The nursing staff are often instrumental in helping the family cope successfully.

Ella came in four times a week to visit her mother, Mrs. R. This client was 87 and had suffered a severe stroke three months ago. She had been hospitalized all that time, awaiting placement in a nursing home. Ella was upset that she couldn't take her mother home, but she had a full-time job and realized that she couldn't give her mother the proper care. Mrs. R was fully bathed every morning by the nursing staff. Nevertheless, Ella always gave her mother a complete bath on each visit, checking her carefully for any sign of pressure ulcers and finishing off with a cloud of dusting powder. Often one of the nurses would assist Ella with the second bath. The staff did not consider this a comment on their ability to give adequate care. Instead, they recognized the pleasure Ella received in caring for her mother. Mrs. R was eventually discharged to a nursing home.

Several months later the staff learned that Ella was a client on the psychiatric unit. Mrs. R had died, and Ella had reacted with a psychotic episode. One of the nurses went to visit Ella on the psychiatric ward. Ella immediately recognized her and embraced her warmly. Excitedly, she began to ask the nurse, "Didn't I take good care of my mother? She never had a sore on her body when she was here!" Then she told how the nursing home staff had refused to let her bathe her mother, and how one day she had discovered an ugly pressure ulcer on Mrs. R's hip. Shortly thereafter, Mrs. R had died.

This example illustrates the powerful bonds that exist between family members. These bonds are strained when one member becomes seriously ill. Nurses can help maintain the integrity of the family unit, thus providing the client with this very crucial element of support.

The Client in the Intensive Care Unit

Throughout this chapter we have emphasized the importance of recognizing that the hospitalized client is under stress, and that this stress is both physiologic and psychologic. Because the stress is multidetermined, we have stated that meeting the client's physical needs alone will not restore the client's equilibrium. In an intensive care unit—that is, in any specialized acute care area such as cardiac care or respiratory care—the stress is magnified many times because the client's life is acutely threatened. All efforts are directed toward keeping the client's body functioning, a task that involves using sophisticated machinery and highly trained personnel. It is understandable that amid these valiant efforts, the client's psychologic state may well be overlooked. However, now that the intensive care unit is no longer a novelty, more attention is being paid to making it a more humane place for clients, their families, and the staff.

Clients in these units commonly develop an ICU psychosis, or intensive care syndrome. These terms are not exact and may refer to any combination of the following: depression, withdrawal, anxiety, hallucinations, delusions, paranoia, and delirium. A typical case is described below.

Mr. W, a 55-year-old man, was admitted with a possible myocardial infarction. After forty-eight hours in the unit, he began to call for the nurses constantly. He would clutch their hands and plead with them to stay at his bedside. He would cry when the technicians came to draw blood, or when he received injections. Mrs. W reported that her husband could not keep track of her visits and was very much afraid that he would be left in the hospital all alone. This behavior lasted twenty-four hours. At that point Mr. W was transferred out of the unit onto a general medical floor. His progress thereafter was uneventful, and there was no recurrence of any confused behavior.

Assessment

The stresses on such a client can be divided into three categories: environmental, psychologic, and physiologic. The following list includes some stressors that belong in each category.

1. Environmental stressors
   a. Sensory overload from constant noise, lights, unfamiliar treatments
   b. Sensory deprivation from immobility, restraints, bandages
   c. Lack of familiar orienting cues such as clocks, calendars, windows, meals, radio, television
   d. Close proximity to other clients who are also very ill
   e. Constant attendance by physicians, nurses, and technicians
   f. Lack of personal belongings
2. Psychologic stressors
   a. Fear of mutilation or death
   b. Little or no understanding of medical jargon or procedures
   c. Separation from family and friends
   d. Separation from familiar environment
   e. Depersonalization and physical exposure
   f. Powerlessness
   g. Pain
   h. Inability to release tension in accustomed fashion
3. Physiologic stressors
   a. Metabolic changes
   b. Decreased cardiac output
   c. Neurologic status
   d. Fever

   e. Electrolyte imbalance
   f. Drugs
   g. Pain
   h. Length of time spent on pump or under anesthesia
   i. Sleep deprivation

Diagnosis

Among the relevant nursing diagnoses for clients in the intensive care unit are:

- Delirium (DSM-IIIR)
- 01.01.04 Altered motor behavior: hyperactivity (PND-I)
- 04.02 Altered feeling patterns, e.g., anger, anxiety (PND-I)
- 06.04 Altered sensory perceptions (PND-I)
- 02.02 Altered judgment (PND-I)
- 02.06.01 Confusion (PND-I)

Planning and Implementing Interventions

All clients in acute care areas experience some of these stressors. What can be done to reduce the occurrence of an ICU psychosis? Obviously, the stressors themselves should be eliminated, if possible. Many intensive care units are now being remodeled to create a less frightening environment for the client. When structural alterations are not feasible, other innovations can be made, such as adding color and pictures, arranging beds for maximum privacy, and turning lights down at night. In essence, any manipulation of the environment that will reduce stress and increase positive meaningful sensory input is helpful.

Clients and their families should be adequately prepared if circumstances permit. Clients who know what they can expect are much less frightened by the strangeness of the unit. Ideally, clients should meet some of the staff who will be caring for them. A familiar face is a welcome sight to someone who is recovering from anesthesia or waking from a fitful sleep.

Clients should be provided with consistent nursing personnel. This will diminish the process of depersonalization and isolation that always occurs to some degree in an intensive care unit. Family members can be encouraged to visit as the situation permits. An often overlooked feature is a room where family members can spend their many hours of waiting.

There is one way to reduce client stress in the acute care areas. This is to attend to the frustrations and needs of the staff. Work in a high-pressure unit affects staff dramatically, causing a high turnover rate and sometimes intrastaff conflict. The nursing staff should identify ways in which they can support one another. This may range from weekly meetings with the psychiatric nursing consultant to regular intrastaff volleyball games. It is crucial that the staff have some means of dealing with the enormous pressures they face. Perhaps this is where the consultant can be most helpful—as a vital link in the chain of support.

In summary, the key nursing interventions are:

1. Educational preparation of clients (see the Research Note)
2. Use of orientation devices, e.g., clocks, windows
3. Reducing environmental stressors
4. Support provided for family
5. Staff support sessions

Evaluation

Mr. W's problems ended upon transfer out of the unit. With appropriate interventions, his "syndrome" could have been prevented or minimized.

The Client with Overt Sexual Behavior

Sexual acting out is psychiatric jargon for sexual behavior sometimes seen in the general hospital. For example, male or female clients may make flirtatious comments, attempt to touch or hold a male or female nurse, boast about sexual experiences, or deliberately expose their genitals while bathing or changing. One sees a wide range of reactions toward this kind of behavior from the staff. Some nurses react by chastising clients verbally and then shunning them or reporting them to a supervisor or doctor. Other nurses simply ignore it, or do not notice it, or do not consider this kind of behavior important enough to comment on. Part of the reason for these varied responses to sexual behavior lies in the differences among clients and the perceptions and values of staff members. A young, attractive man who flirts with the female nurses may be acceptable, while a paunchy middle-aged man who exhibits the same behavior may be labeled a sex maniac. A young woman client who wears makeup and sexy nightgowns may be criticized, whereas an elderly woman who habitually exposes herself may be virtually ignored.

Another reason for staff members' varied responses is that regressive behavior in the hospital is expected and even encouraged. *Regression* means that the client role includes, among other things, loss of identity, especially one's sexual identity. Clients are dressed in flimsy hospital gowns, they are left lying naked under the sheets on a stretcher, and they are examined without much attention to discretion or modesty. Because the system encourages sexual regression, a client's acting out may not be seen as anything unusual.

A third factor to consider is the attitude of the individual nurse about his or her own sexuality. These personal values will determine how nurses view the client's behavior and how they will choose to interact with the client who acts out sexually. The following case history illustrates many of these points.

Mr. H was a 19-year-old male who had been admitted for a crush injury of the right hand. He was a frequent drug abuser, lived in a slum area, and was unemployed. From the beginning, he was not a popular client. He complained constantly of pain and demanded narcotics by name and dosage. No amount of medication seemed to hold him for very long, and he began threatening to call his friends and have them bring in the drugs he needed. Indeed, some shady-looking visitors were often seen in Mr. H's room. This unpleasant situation reached crisis proportions when Mr. H hung a pornographic poster in his room. At this point the staff called the psychiatric nursing consultant, and a staff conference was arranged.

Everyone was noticeably unnerved by the situation and needed to verbalize individual reactions to seeing the poster. One nurse had demanded that he take it down immediately. This confrontation had ended in a heated argument between the nurse and the client, and the poster was back on the wall the next day. Another nurse had quickly averted her eyes and pretended not to have noticed it. Thereafter, she avoided entering his room. A third nurse, alone on the night shift, became very frightened when Mr. H asked to have his back rubbed. She spent a very uncomfortable eight-hour shift, feeling both afraid and guilty. The consultant accepted and understood all these reactions. However, none of them had proved a useful intervention.

Assessment

The consultant now explored with the group some of the possible dynamics behind Mr. H's behavior. Mr. H was only 19, an age when one's sexuality is extremely important. But both his injury and the hospitalization were threats to his image of himself as an active sexual male. The clinician discussed several issues. She explained the depersonalization and desexualization of a hospitalized client. Added to this, she pointed out, is the powerlessness and dependence of the client role. Many clients, especially unpopular ones, also experience emotional and touch deprivation. Another important concept in understanding Mr. H was the insult to his body image. What was his perception of himself without the use of his right hand? Also, what sexual significance did his right hand have for him?

Diagnosis

Appropriate nursing diagnoses are:

- Potential for disturbance in self-concept secondary to change in body image and self-esteem (NANDA and PND-I)
- 06.02.03 Altered comfort pattern: pain (PND-I and NANDA)

Planning and Implementing Interventions

The staff responded readily to these ideas. They began to see Mr. H as someone who was trying to maintain some control and self-esteem in a situation that was very threatening to him. It was decided that the staff would talk to him on a one-to-one basis and state their true reactions to his poster: "Mr. H, I feel very uncomfortable being in your room since you hung that poster. I would appreciate it if you'd keep it in a more private place." Mr. H soon complied, and overall relationships improved rapidly as other suggestions were made. These included allowing Mr. H time to be alone with his girl friend; being more aware of his need for privacy; and giving him more control over his daily activities.

These new policies resulted in more open communication with the client in other areas as well. The nurses explained to Mr. H that they wanted to keep him pain-free, but that it was impossible to assess the effects of analgesics when he was suspected of taking drugs on his own.

In summary, the key interventions used with Mr. H were:

1. Use of assertive communication by staff nurses
2. Meetings with the nurse consultant to plan nonjudgmental approach
3. Increased client control over activities

Evaluation

The medication issue remained a problem, but the nurses felt much less judgmental and were better able to tolerate Mr. H's behavior. This interaction with the consultant allowed the staff to explore some of their own values about

sexuality. It also showed them how these values affected their ability to give optimal client care.

The case example on the next page illustrates some further issues in dealing with the sexual concerns of clients.

RESEARCH NOTE

Citation

Owens JF, Hutelmyer CM: *The effect of preoperative intervention on delirium in cardiac surgical patients.* Nurs Res 1982;31:60–62.

Study Problem/Purpose

This study tested the hypothesis that clients who are educated preoperatively about the possibility of unusual sensory or cognitive experiences will postoperatively not have such experiences or will feel comfortable or in control of the experiences if they occur.

Methods

The subjects were sixty-four adults with no psychiatric or organic brain disease who were undergoing elective cardiac surgery. The experimental group was given information about delirium and instructions to inform the staff should they have any of these experiences. The control group received no information about delirium. After surgery all clients were interviewed to elicit evidence of cognitive or sensory disturbances. Charts were also searched for relevant data.

Findings

Sixty-eight percent of all clients were found to have had at least one unusual sensory or cognitive experience. Twenty-five of thirty-two clients in the control group and nineteen of thirty-two in the experimental group reported these experiences. When studied for degree of comfort with the unusual experiences, the experimental group was significantly more comfortable, with twenty-two of the clients reporting that they had an understanding of the event.

Implications

Preoperative teaching about the possibility of delirium and instructions should it occur should be a part of the surgical routine. Such preparation will lessen the psychologic stress of having a sensory or cognitive disturbance. Nurses can apply such anticipatory guidance to other situations where the client may be frightened by unusual or unexpected occurrences.

Mr. M, a 68-year-old man, had been on the unit for four weeks. During this time he had received cancer chemotherapy, and he was now in a state of remission. The psychiatric nursing clinical specialist had not been consulted for this particular client, but while she was spending time on the unit, she noted some unusual behavior. Mr. M would pinch the nurses whenever they got near enough. They would respond by making a disapproving face that Mr. M couldn't see, or by completely ignoring him. He also made suggestive remarks, which the staff also ignored. On one occasion, Mr. M approached the consultant, saying he wanted to kiss her for "good luck." The consultant thought it important to understand the meaning of his behavior. Reading his chart, she learned that he had been impotent for the last six months.

Because the consultant already had a good working relationship with the staff, she approached them with the data she had gathered, instead of waiting for them to consult her. A staff conference was held. At this conference the nurses discussed why they had not taken direct measures to deal with Mr. M's behavior. An important point was that the staff consisted mostly of newly graduated female nurses. Several nurses said they thought they were the only ones that Mr. M was bothering and felt that they personally had done something to provoke him. Others said they were afraid that the doctors or nursing supervisors would laugh if they voiced their concerns. Another issue was documentation—they were uncertain whether such behavior should be noted in the client's chart. Was this information important? Would it be harmful to the client to document his behavior?

It became clear that the nurses were missing the meaning of Mr. M's behavior because they became uncertain and embarrassed when the behavior was overtly sexual. Looking further, they could see the behavior as a defense against the actual impotence Mr. M was experiencing. The consultant developed a therapeutic relationship with Mr. M, who subsequently ceased his sexual acting out but became depressed instead. He and the consultant began working their way through the natural grieving process he had to undergo in relation to having cancer.

As this example illustrates, it is important for nurses to understand that all client behavior has meaning. It also points again to the all-important task of exploring your own sexuality in order to understand the sexual behavior of clients during hospitalization.

The Noncompliant Client

The noncompliant client is both poorly understood and poorly tolerated. Many people fall under this label: the man with a recent myocardial infarction who refuses to stay in bed; the new diabetic who won't test his urine; the hypertensive who forgets to take her medicine. These clients may verbally state their understanding of the prescribed regimen, but their behavior indicates an underlying problem. Research indicates that at least one-third of clients studied did not follow their prescribed regimen (Young 1986). Noncompliance also causes frustration for the nurse whose task it is to promote the highest possible level of client learning and functioning.

Mrs. Schwartz is a 54-year-old woman who has been diabetic since age 30. She is divorced, has no children, and lives alone in a small apartment. She works as a cashier in a parking lot. Over the years, she has controlled her diabetes with diet and later with insulin. Recently she injured her left foot but did not seek treatment for several weeks until her foot became black and swollen. Now she is hospitalized for a below-the-knee amputation of her left leg. Mrs. Schwartz is very aggressive and controlling. Because she has been diabetic for so long, she views herself as an expert and taunts the younger nurses about their ignorance on the subject of diabetic teaching. Mrs. Schwartz does not comply with the hospital routine; instead she follows her own regimen of self-care, which is not sound in principle.

Assessment

There is always a reason for noncompliance, although neither the nurse nor the client may initially understand the dynamics involved. Many nurses respond to such clients with anger and impatience, which serves only to increase the distance between client and nurse. It is admittedly very difficult to watch self-destructive behavior that thwarts what we believe to be the correct therapeutic route. The nurse can reach an understanding of the client's behavior only through careful thought and observation.

In general, the factors that contribute to noncompliance can be summarized as follows:

- *Psychologic*—lack of knowledge; clients' attitudes, beliefs, and values; denial of illness and other defense mechanisms; personality type (rigid, defensive, etc.); very low or very high anxiety levels

- *Environmental and social*—lack of support system; other problems that distract from health care; finances, transportation, and housing

- *Characteristics of the regimen*—demands too much change from client; not enough benefit realized; too difficult, complicated; distressing side-effects; leads to social isolation and stigma

- *Properties of the provider-client relationship*—faulty communication; client perceives provider as cold, uncaring, authoritative; client feels discounted and treated like an "object"; both parties engage in struggle for control.

The example of Mrs. Schwartz illustrates many of the above factors. Her psychologic profile includes long-standing rigidity. She is extremely independent and strong-willed. Presently, she has the added need for control to compensate for the loss of her leg. This client should not be expected to accept a new regimen from an unfamiliar hospital staff. The fact that Mrs. Schwartz lives alone and has no family will contribute to her difficulty in learning new behaviors because she will have no one to *reinforce* her new behaviors. Also important is the nature of the regimen itself. If Mrs. Schwartz follows the regimen set out for her, will she see results quickly, and will those results be worth the effort of following the plan?

In addition, the nurse must examine the nature of the relationship with the client. Research points out that clients respond negatively to nurses and doctors who are cold, disapproving, rigid, and controlling. Mrs. Schwartz could easily engage with such a nurse in a battle for control. An added detriment would be a frequent turnover of nurses, none of whom feel responsible for the client, and hence do not form a stable relationship with her.

Diagnosis

Relevant medical and nursing diagnoses are:

- Noncompliance with medical treatment (DSM-IIIR)
- Noncompliance related to diabetic regimen (NANDA)
- Powerlessness (NANDA and PND-I)
- Disturbance in self-concept secondary to change in body image (NANDA and PND-I)

Planning and Implementing Interventions

Mrs. Schwartz's noncompliance can be dealt with through contracting. One nurse could be assigned to her for the duration of her hospitalization. This would foster mutual communication, commitment, and understanding. Nurse and client would explore the *client's* goals, which would undoubtedly include prevention of further complications. They could establish what steps to take to meet the goals.

As the steps are discussed, the nurse should acknowledge Mrs. Schwartz's self-care activities and ask her to

review the basics of a diabetic regimen. Since the client's goal is to reduce complications, she should agree to review this material with the nurse. Mrs. Schwartz will probably respond to being treated like an individual, not like another client who "needs diabetic teaching." Ideally, in this atmosphere of mutual respect, the client can relearn some important principles without having to admit that she has been amiss in her own routine.

Evaluation

Even when nurses understand the dynamics leading to noncompliance and take measures to prevent it, clients may not always respond to their efforts. In these circumstances, nurses must deal with their own feelings of frustration. Resolution of this frustration will come only when the nurse accepts that clients are ultimately responsible for their own actions.

The Client with Body Image Alteration

Because every illness results in some change in body image, this is an important concept for all nurses in health care settings to consider. The body image is the individual's concept of the shape, size, and mass of his or her body and its parts. This image allows a person to evaluate the space the body occupies and to move about freely in the environment. It is the internalized picture a person has of the physical appearance of the body. Sensations arising inside the body and the attitudes and responses of others influence the individual's concept of his or her own body. In this way, body image is closely allied with self-concept or self-image. Changes in the body image are threatening. Of necessity, people attempt to maintain the integrity of their own bodies.

The body image extends beyond the physical body. Objects of daily use that are intimately connected with the body surface, such as a cane, dentures, clothes, a tattoo, makeup, and jewelry, are incorporated into the body image. Without these, a person may feel incomplete and anxious. Objects connected with and symbolizing a profession, such as the policeman's gun or the nurse's cap, may be even more intensely incorporated into the body image, not only by the wearer but by the public as well.

All these factors form an inner mental diagram called the body image. This diagram is fluid and dynamic—it changes in response to the current sensory and psychic stimuli it receives.

Assessment

Certain consistent elements are important in evaluating the significance of the body image and its alteration.

First, body characteristics that people have from birth or acquire early in life seem to have less emotional significance for them than those that arise in adolescence or later. The boy born lacking a limb formulates an image of himself that accounts for the limb's absence. His healthy self-concept naturally excludes that limb from the "me." Children with crossed eyes, buck teeth, or disfiguring facial birthmarks often similarly incorporate these features into their body images. The school nurse or teacher who recommends correction of such a "defect" is often astounded by the resentment that greets this well-meant suggestion. Attempts to change a characteristic are unwelcome and resisted because they require changing the loved "me."

A second factor to consider in evaluating the significance of alterations in body image is that a defect, handicap, or change in body function that occurs abruptly is far more traumatic than one that develops gradually. For example, crippling arthritis that eventually impairs the use of an extremity is less disturbing than traumatic amputation of an extremity during an auto accident. A person has time to adjust to the effects of arthritis on body function and body image, whereas the person whose extremity has been suddenly amputated is not allowed the healing effects of time. This person suddenly discovers the absence or loss of function of a loved part of self.

Third, the location of a disease or injury greatly affects the emotional response to it. Internal diseases are generally less distressing than external diseases that can be seen by the person and by others. For example, radical head and neck surgery, with its consequent disfigurement, is devastating to the body image and to the psyche, since the face is one of the primary means by which people communicate. Most people focus on the face in interacting with others. When that face becomes less pleasing to the eye, radical changes in body image are also necessary.

People generally experience a great threat when the genitals or breasts are involved in change. Breast surgery is of particular significance to many women, for breasts symbolize femininity and sexual attractiveness in Western culture. In men, such surgical procedures as circumcision and inguinal hernia repair pose a far more disturbing threat to the body image than major operations such as gastrectomy or cholecystectomy. Fears about sexuality and virility are reawakened and reinforced when illness or injury threatens genital areas. Those parts of the body are important to people's mental view of themselves as men or women.

Diagnosis

Diagnoses that may be given to persons with body image problems are:

- Depersonalization disorder (DSM-IIIR)
- 06.03.01 Altered body image (PND-I and NANDA)
- 06.03.04 Altered self-esteem (PND-I and NANDA)

Planning and Implementing Interventions

Individuals develop new body images when they *interact* with the new body part. Nurses can begin this process with the client.

Mrs. M has returned from the operating room after undergoing an above-the-knee amputation. When she is alert enough, the nurse orients Mrs. M and tells her that her stump is now bandaged and will be changed tomorrow. The nurse encourages Mrs. M to look at her leg and touch the dressing. The nurse herself uses touch frequently in changing the stump dressing. She is gentle and caring toward this "new" body part. Mrs. M and her family will soon be involved in looking at Mrs. M's stump and learning to dress and care for it.

Nurses need to be aware of their own reactions toward clients' altered bodies. A nurse who can accept his or her own body's imperfections accepts those of a client more readily.

It is important for nurses who may work with "repulsive" body alterations to learn to *look past* the unpleasantness to the person inside the body. Nurses who can accomplish this find that over time the initially unbearable becomes secondary to the nurse-client relationship that develops.

Mourning a Body Image Alteration or the Loss of a Body Part

Loss is the general theme in all body image alterations. To cope with the loss of a loved person, loved object, or loved body part, a person must mourn. Clients may need to be helped to acknowledge the loss in order to move from a stage of shock and disbelief into developing awareness. Health professionals sometimes believe that ignoring or minimizing the loss is helpful to clients and their families. This is not true. Those who fail to acknowledge the loss or minimize it hinder grief work.

Clients need a supportive person to help them move toward the resolution phase of mourning. It may be necessary to create opportunities for discussing the disability, its meaning to the client, the problem of compensating for the loss, and the reaction of persons with whom the client will come in contact. Attitudes of disapproval, repulsion, or rejection toward a person with a physical disfigurement or defect hinder the person's social adaptation. Nurses can help family and friends to overcome such attitudes, if they experience them, by creating similar opportunities for them to discuss their fears and concerns.

Providing Anticipatory Guidance

Anticipatory guidance aims to help people cope with a crisis by discussing the details of an impending stressful occurrence and solving problems before the event occurs. Anticipatory guidance is needed not only for clients but also for the significant persons in their lives, both family and friends. It is believed that anticipatory guidance lays the foundation for effective grief work. It consists of brief psychotherapeutic intervention to discuss the meaning of the body part to the client and significant others, their beliefs and feelings concerning previous losses they have experienced, and the beliefs they hold about the body image. A discussion of the phantom phenomenon should be included for all clients who experience the loss of a body part. The **phantom experience** can be defined as the sensation of feeling a part of the body that is no longer there. The phantom limb phenomenon is the most well known. It is far more common than is generally believed. Phantom limb experiences increase markedly if amputation occurs after the client is 4 years of age and they are almost universal when the client is age 8 or older.

Phantom experiences occur in an attempt to redefine the lost part and to maintain the stability and integrity of the body image. In fact, some theorists view the phantom as an indication of a stable body schema. Too stable a body schema can prove troublesome, however, when the individual recognizes that the phantom is unreal and that others do not share the perception of it. Problems also arise when the phantom is experienced as painful.

Although phantoms are considered universal, phantom pain is relatively rare and is considered psychopathologic. People experiencing them have described the pain as acute, burning, grinding, tearing, and crushing. The severity of the pain may account for the high incidence of addiction to narcotics and suicidal tendencies among persons with painful phantoms. Therapeutic preparation of a person who is to undergo amputation can help prevent the painful phantom.

The nonpainful phantom eventually disappears, although there are recorded instances in which phantoms have persisted for as long as twenty years. Phantoms of the upper limb are generally stronger and last longer than phantoms of the lower limb. They often begin to disappear through a process known as *telescoping*—i.e., the hand or the foot appears to be shrinking toward the stump. The final parts to disappear are usually the thumb, the index finger, and big toe.

Remember also to explore the client's fears and to determine how the client wishes to dispose of the body part to be amputated. Fantasies and superstitious beliefs about amputated parts of the body can increase a client's anxiety and discomfort.

Evaluation

Nursing interventions for a client with altered body image are successful if the client is able to express thoughts and feelings about body changes, to look at and touch a body deformity, to participate in self-care related to the body part, and to discuss the alterations in life-style (if any) resulting from the body change.

ROLE OF THE PSYCHIATRIC NURSING CONSULTANT

Almost every general hospital has some kind of mental health professional available to work with clients directly or to support and educate the staff toward handling clients' emotional problems. Here, we discuss the role of the psychiatric nurse in the consulting role.

History of Consultation in the Hospital Setting

Physicians were the first to practice **consultation-liaison psychiatry**—providing psychiatric consultation to clients in the general hospital—based on the previously discussed concepts of psychophysiologic medicine and preventive psychiatry. Liaison psychiatry originated in the late 1950s. Paralleling this trend, psychiatric nurses also began to act as consultants to their colleagues in medical and surgical settings. At first, the liaison nurses remained based on their psychiatric units, providing indirect assistance when it was requested. Later, they began to work directly with clients and their families. Currently, psychiatric nurse clinicians perform both direct and indirect consultative functions. (See the work of Caplan [1970] and Lewis and Levy [1982] for in-depth information on the consulting process.)

Qualifications of the Consultant

The psychiatric nurse **consultant** should be prepared at the graduate level. Some graduate programs are specifically geared to liaison nursing and provide clinical experiences in a general hospital setting. Other programs are oriented toward the community mental health center or the psychiatric in-patient unit. In any case, the consultant's education includes classroom and supervised clinical experiences in individual, group, and family therapy, since all these modes are used in practice. Most graduate programs include courses in organizational theory in which the principles of power and influence and planned change are emphasized. A hospital is an incredibly complex organization, and the greater the preparation of consultants, the better they can withstand the bureaucratic onslaught. A successful consultant needs a solid theoretical and experiential base, along with confidence, competence, and concern.

Consultants who have actual staff nursing experience in a nonpsychiatric general hospital setting have an invaluable advantage over the inexperienced clinician. They have first-hand knowledge of the day-to-day problems facing the staff nurse: what is it like to rotate shifts; having to work weekends; being the only registered nurse in charge of forty clients; dealing with complaints from x-ray, dietary, and operating room departments—and on top of it all, having clients say they would get better service for less money in a hotel down the street. It is definitely true that nursing educators and administrators gain respect by having "paid their dues." Consultants with staff experience start out with two advantages. They are *nurses,* and they share a common background of experience with their consultees.

Guidelines for the Consultation Process

The consulting psychiatric nurse usually works according to the classic consultation process developed by Caplan. The staff nurse who seeks a nurse consultant's help can expect the relationship to be guided by the following precepts:

- Mental health consultation is a process of interaction between two professionals with respect to a client or a program for clients.

- Ideally, the consultant has no administrative responsibility for the consultee's work. He or she is under no compulsion to alter the consultee's handling of the case.

- The consultee has no obligation to accept the consultant's ideas or suggestions.

- The basic relationship between the two is egalitarian. This allows the consultee to accept or reject what the consultant says and to incorporate any ideas the consultee feels are appropriate to the situation.

- Consultation can take various forms. These include individual and group consultation and work with staff as well as with clients, depending on the particular situation.

- The exact form of the consultation is made explicit in the contract—a verbal or written agreement between consultant and consultees.

- The goals of consultation are to help the consultees improve their handling or understanding of the current work problem and to generalize this learning to future similar situations.

- The consultative process is not therapy, but it can be therapeutic. Increasing a consultee's competence in the work situation gives the consultee an overall sense of accomplishment and self-worth (Caplan 1970, pp 28–30).

Chapter Highlights

- Nurses working in general hospitals face the challenge of combining "high tech" and "high touch."

- Illness and hospitalization can be viewed as crisis situations for clients and their families.

- Hospitalized clients can be left almost totally without their usual supports, including the coping mechanisms upon which they usually rely.

- The nurse must identify the client's present coping skills, evaluate their effectiveness, and intervene if necessary to help the client develop new methods of coping.

- Clients who develop effective coping styles will feel more capable of handling future problems and, should the current illness prove to be chronic, will have developed the beginning skills to cope with a lifelong source of stress.

- Working with demanding clients involves looking behind the external behavior for the reasons that are always there, although not always obvious.

- A comprehensive assessment and a coordinated approach is needed for the client in pain.

- Although some degree of dependency is a normal, necessary, and expected part of a person's new role as client, it is essential to help clients regain their former independence and autonomy.

- The illness of a family member constitutes a crisis for a family. The nursing staff are often instrumental in helping the family cope successfully.

- The stress of hospitalization is magnified many times for the client in the intensive care unit because the client's life is actually threatened.

- Nurses must explore their own sexuality to understand the sexual behavior of clients during hospitalization.

- There is always a reason for a client's noncompliance with the treatment regimen; this reason can be understood only through careful thought and observation.

- Clients who undergo a body image change should be provided with anticipatory guidance and the opportunity to prepare for the body image alteration or mourn the loss of a body part.

- In complex client situations, nurses may need input from case conferences and nurse consultants to remain objective and to attend to all aspects of the client's problems.

References

Baer CL (ed): Patient compliance: Issues and outcomes. *Top Clin Nurs* 1986;7:entire issue.

Bohannon-Reed R, et al: Staying human under stress: Stress reduction and emotional support in the critical care setting. *Crit Care Nurse* 1983;3:26–30.

Brown L: The experience of care: Patient perspectives. *Top Clin Nurs* 1986;8:56–62.

Caplan G: *Theory and Practice of Mental Health Consultation.* Basic Books, 1970.

Caplan G: Mastery of stress: Psychosocial aspects. *Am J Psychiatry* 1981;138:413–420.

Cohen-Cole S, Stoudemire A: Major depression and physical illness. *Psychiatr Clin North Am* 1987;10:(1):1–17.

Diagnostic and Statistical Manual of Mental Disorders, ed 3, revised, APA, 1987.

Fife BL: Establishing the mental health clinical specialist role in the medical setting. *Issues Ment Health Nurs* 1986;8:15–23.

Fitzpatrick R, et al: *The Experience of Illness.* Tavistock, 1984.

Green C: How to recognize hostility and what to do about it. *Am J Nurs* 1986;86(11):1230–1234.

Groves JE: Taking care of the hateful patient. *N Engl J Med* 1978;298:883–887.

Hart CA: Psychiatric mental health nursing consultation: A two-model system in the general hospital. *Issues Ment Health Nurs* 1982;4:127–147.

Lambert VA, Lambert CE: *The Impact of Physical Illness.* Prentice-Hall, 1979.

Lambert VA, Lambert CE: *Psychosocial Care of the Physically Ill.* Prentice-Hall, 1985.

Lewis A, Levy JS: *Psychiatric Liaison Nursing.* Prentice-Hall, 1982.

Liptzin B: The geriatric patient and general hospital psychiatry. *Gen Hosp Psychiatr* 1987;9(3):198–203.

Miller JF: *Chronic Illness.* F. A. Davis, 1983.

Montgomery C: How to set limits when a patient demands too much. *Am J Nurs* 1987;87(3):365–366.

Moos R (ed): *Coping with Physical Illness.* Plenum, 1977.

Moos R: *Coping with Physical Illness: New Perspectives.* Plenum, 1984, vol 2.

Norris CM: Body image, in Carlson CE, Blackwell B (eds): *Behavioral Concepts and Nursing Intervention.* Lippincott, 1978.

Parsons T: *The Social System.* The Free Press, 1951.

Perry SW, Heidrich G: Placebo response: Myth and matter. *Am J Nurs* 1981;81:720–725.

Pollock SE: Human responses to chronic illness: Physiologic and psychosocial adaption. *Nurs Res* 1986;35:90–95.

Relling-Garskof K: Transferring the past to the present. *Am J Nurs* 1987;87(4):477–478.

Strain JJ: Needs for psychiatry in the general hospital. *Hosp Community Psychiatry* 1982;33:996–1001.

Strauss A: *Chronic Illness and the Quality of Life.* Mosby, 1975.

Turk DC, Kerns RD: *Health, Illness, and Families.* John Wiley & Sons, 1985.

Volicer BJ, Isenberg MA, Burns MW: Medical-surgical differences in hospital stress factors. *J Human Stress* 1977;June:3–13.

Volicer B, Bohannon M: A hospital stress rating scale. *Nurs Res* 1975;24:352–359.

Wallen J, et al.: Psychiatric consultations in short-term general hospitals. *Arch Gen Psychiatr* 1987;44(2):163–168.

Weisman AD: Coping with illness, in Hacket TB, Cassem NH (eds): *Handbook of General Hospital Psychiatry.* Mosby, 1978.

Whitley MP: Seduction and the hospitalized person. *J Nurs Educ* 1978;17(6):34–39.

Wright LK: Life-threatening illness. *J Psychosocial Nurs* 1985;23:6–11.

Young SM: Strategies for improving compliance. *Top Clin Nurs* 1986;7:31–39.

Zangari M, Duffy P: Contracting with patients in day-to-day practice. *Am J Nurs* 1980;80:451–455.

TWENTY-FIVE

Violence and Victimatology

Part I   Violence and Victimatology in the Psychiatric Setting

Anastasia Fisher

Part II   Violence and Victimatology: Rape and Intrafamily Abuse

Karen Lee Fontaine

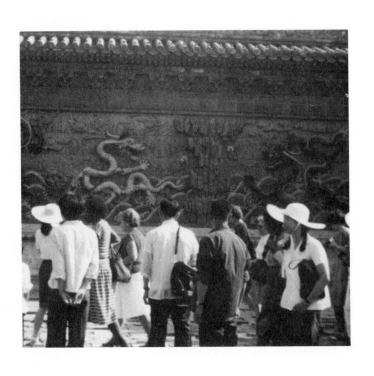

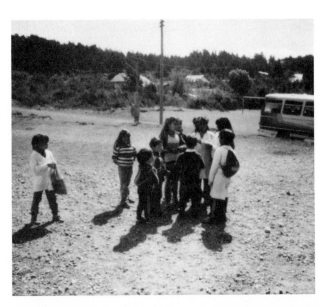

PART I   VIOLENCE AND VICTIMATOLOGY IN THE PSYCHIATRIC SETTING

Anastasia Fisher

Learning Objectives

After reading this part, students should be able to

- Define three theoretical frameworks useful in understanding violence

- Identify and describe strategies for managing violent behavior

- Define in-patient psychiatric violence

- Assess a client's potential for violent behavior

- Plan nursing interventions for clients assessed as violent

- Explain staff responses to violent assault

- Recognize the factors that increase staff vulnerability to violent assault

Cross References

Other topics relevant to this content are: Ethics, Chapter 10; Legal issues, Chapter 39; Milieu therapy, Chapter 31; Rape, abuse, and suicide, Chapter 25, Part II.

Key Terms

assault
deflection and neutralization of blows
evasive techniques
restraints
seclusion
show of force
standard therapeutic holds
victimatology
violence

There are relatively little data on institutional violence or systematic description of the frequency, types, or consequences of assaults on nursing personnel (Lanza 1983). The three reasons generally offered for this deficiency are (1) a lack of nursing research in the area, (2) the tendency to deny the frequency and severity of resulting injuries, and (3) the tendency to hold nurses accountable for the assaults (Levy and Hartocollis 1976).

The information that does exist tells us not only that institutional violence occurs frequently, but also that psychiatric nurses are the most frequent victims of psychiatric client assault (Fottrell 1981, Lanza 1983). A study of formal incident reports determined that almost five times as many assaults occurred as were reported (Lion et al. 1981). The reasons postulated by the authors for the underreporting of assaults were: staff expectations of assault, the effort required to complete the report, and the admission of a performance failure. The authors also speculated that staff feared legal investigation of the event.

A survey of university-affiliated psychiatrists working within various settings reported that 42% have been assaulted by their clients during their careers (Madden et al. 1976). Another study noted that 24 percent of therapists—including psychiatrists, psychologists, and social workers—were assaulted during a year by one or more clients (Whitman et al. 1976). Conservative estimates suggest that clinicians can expect 7 percent to 10 percent of in-patients to be assaultive just prior to or shortly after admission to a psychiatric unit (Craig 1982), and that one in four therapists may be assaulted at some time during their careers (Whitman et al. 1976). Whatever the precise dimensions of psychiatric violence, mental health professionals have the responsibility for its prediction, prevention, and management.

The author of this part prefers the use of "patient" to "client" in institutional work. Client is retained for the text's overall consistency.

For the purpose of this chapter, psychiatric client violence is defined as behavior by a psychiatric in-patient that threatens or actually harms or injures persons or destroys property (APA 1974). Although there are no simple approaches to the topic of violence, several frameworks can be used to stimulate our thinking about in-patient psychiatric violence.

THEORETICAL FOUNDATIONS

Descriptive frameworks are ways to organize our thoughts, observations, and intuitive notions into coherent patterns. They do not explain the causes of violence on a case-by-case basis or tell us what to do about it. Because of the complexity of individuals, situations, and interactional components to violence no one framework is sufficient. It is necessary to approach psychiatric violence from a variety of perspectives. The frameworks useful in understanding psychiatric violence are the importation theory, situationism, and an interaction model.

Importation

The "importation" theory reflects the position that the client brings or imports certain values, attitudes, and behavior patterns conducive to violence into the treatment setting (Armstrong 1978). Most of the literature on violence represents this position, identifying such client characteristics as social and cultural factors, psychiatric diagnosis and personality traits, and demographic characteristics. The social and cultural conditions often associated with violent behavior include:

- Low socioeconomic status
- A history of childhood abuse
- Life experiences from a subculture condoning or expecting the use of violence to resolve conflicts
- A history of violent behavior

Research findings on the role of psychiatric diagnosis in the production of violent behavior are conflicting and unclear. Violent behavior has been observed across the entire spectrum of diagnoses, but violent clients are more likely to have a diagnosis of schizophrenia, personality disorders, psychotic organic brain syndrome, or mental retardation (Lion et al. 1981, Tardiff and Sweillam 1980, 1982). Most current thinking suggests that the degree of psychopathology, or severity of the illness, is the more significant

contributor to violent behavior, not the specific diagnostic classification. A central psychodynamic theme repeatedly described in the literature is that violent clients perceive themselves to be hopeless and powerless (APA 1974; Lion et al. 1981). Violent clients are also three to four times more likely than nonviolent clients to have attempted suicide at least once (Tardiff 1983).

Age and sex are the demographic characteristics typically included in research on psychiatric client violence. Young males tend to be overrepresented in the samples. Whether this reflects a subculture that condones violence or the frustration of a deprived status is not clear.

Of all the characteristics noted, the only one found to be predictive of future violence is a history of violent behavior. This generalization requires some modification since a past episode of violent behavior in the community appears to be the best predictor of future violence in the community and a past event of violent behavior in the hospital setting is a good indicator of a future event in the same setting (Steadman 1981).

If one were to use the importation theory to construct a profile of a client most likely to exhibit violent behavior, it might look like the following. He would be a young male (under 44 years of age) from a subculture or minority group that condones the use of violence to resolve conflicts (APA 1974, Tardiff and Sweillam 1982). He would be poor, have little formal education, and possess few employment skills and poor verbal communication skills (APA 1974, Tardiff and Sweillam 1980). He would come from a home in which there was violence or parental deprivation. His parents would have had problems with alcoholism, and he would have experienced abuse as a child. He would have engaged in some expression of violent behavior in the recent past. His psychiatric diagnosis would be anything from psychiatric conditions such as schizophrenia or organic brain syndrome to a severe personality disorder. He would exhibit severe psychopathology and impairment in function. He would see himself as helpless and powerless. He would have a history of at least one previous suicide attempt.

In-Patient Management Strategies

The in-patient management strategies suggested by the importation theory include verbal techniques, medications, behavioral techniques, seclusion, and restraint. Typically these strategies are targeted to individuals who are currently violent or are perceived to be imminently dangerous. However, such strategies are also common in the long-term management of violent behavior.

The overall goal of these strategies, whether considered individually or used in combination, is to strengthen the client's ability to control himself or herself. Implementation of these management strategies must be considered within the context of the principle of least restrictiveness. This principle requires that staff demonstrate attempts to use less restrictive measures of control before resorting to more restrictive interventions. For example, staff must document their efforts to intervene with a client using verbal strategies before they intervene physically.

Verbal Technique

Forming a verbal alliance with the potentially violent client is often the first step to containing the violent behavior. Two common errors occur during the initial efforts to intervene with the potentially violent or violent client (Nigrosh 1983):

1. Confusion between control and confrontation
2. Overemphasis on supportive concern characterized by statements such as, "I know how you feel and I'm here to help"

It is important to convey control in the situation by using clear, calm statements, and a confident physical stance rather than through remarks or cues that can be interpreted as challenging the client. A confrontive, aggressive, or threatening manner or a tendency to overidentify with the client's experience can make the staff member a target of violence.

Several strategies are suggested as guidelines to assist in establishing quick rapport and alliance with the potentially violent client. Clinical judgment and the situation must dictate the appropriateness of their use. Some violent behavior occurs impulsively and without warning. Most episodes, however, involve an escalation of behavior, and are therefore more amenable to verbal intervention. An example of verbal intervention useful in working with some potentially violent clients is summarized in Table 25–1. The overall goals of these verbal techniques and positional strategies are to establish a relationship that minimizes the client's projection on the helper, and to protect the

---

RESEARCH NOTE

Citation

Jones MK: Patient violence: Report of 200 incidents. J Psychosoc Nurs *1985;23(6):12–17.*

Study Problem/Purpose

This study examined the demographic characteristics and environmental influences that contribute to violent behavior by clients in institutional settings.

Methods

The descriptive study was conducted in an in-patient and out-patient unit of an acute medical/surgical 290-bed hospital, which included 75 psychiatric beds and a 206-bed nursing home. All employees, including trainees and students in these settings submitted a "Report of Aggressive Behavior" if they witnessed aggressive physical contact with an intent to do harm. Staff had no direct contact with clients but were sometimes interviewed to supplement missing data. Client charts were reviewed to validate age, race, and diagnosis.

Data were collected using "The Aggressive Incident Report." This report included the following information: age, race, and diagnosis of the assaultive individual; time, date, place, and target of the violence; physical harm; use of alcohol, drugs, or weapons; environmental mood; number and gender of staff; number of clients in the area; number of persons needed to control the client; and care required after the incident.

Two hundred incidents of violent behavior involving 119 clients were reported over a 5½-year period. Violent incidents were tabulated at six-month intervals to examine trends.

Findings

Of the 119 clients, 76 were involved in a single incident of violence, with 34 individuals involved in more than one incident. These 34 clients were responsible for 120 incidents of violence, or 60 percent of the total 200 reported violent episodes. The most violent individuals were found in the sample from the nursing home and the psychiatric unit.

The majority of incidents occurred during the day in the psychiatric and medical/surgical areas, while the largest number in the nursing home occurred at night. It appears from the data that short staffing conditions tend to increase the potential for violent behavior. The use of alcohol or street drugs was reported in 14 percent of the violent episodes.

Psychiatric clients in this study were between 20 and 40 years old and diagnosed psychotic with substance abuse. Increased activity was found to be the single most significant environmental factor contributing to violent behavior, with a cluster of violent episodes occurring at mealtime and bedtime. Staff was the most frequent victim.

Implications

Studies describing the actual incidents of violence in institutional settings increase our knowledge and ability to predict, prevent, and manage violent behavior. The present study is significant because it presents a model for the systematic analysis of violent behavior useful to clinicians and administrators within institutional settings.

Although daily use of neuroleptic medication is the most widely used treatment for the control of violent behavior in institutional settings, it is important to recognize that pharmacologic agents alone are not the answer to violence (Lion 1983). Whether these medications are being prescribed in response to the degree of psychotic symptomatology or in response to the violent behavior remains an issue for future research.

Choice of neuroleptic medication is often a function of the clinician's preference and the client's medication history. Among those medications routinely used are haldoperidol (Haldol), chlorpromazine (Thorazine), thioridazine (Mellaril), and thiothixene (Navane). Long-acting injectable fluphenazine (Prolixin) and haloperidol are used with clients discharged to the community to be followed as out-patients, as well as with clients who have histories of noncompliance. Dosages vary for each medication. Younger clients with previously documented histories of violent behavior tend to receive higher doses of neuroleptic medications. Refer to Chapter 32 for a thorough analysis of antipsychotic medications, frequent side-effects, and treatment of their symptoms.

Behavioral Techniques

Various behavioral strategies established around the principle of progressive isolation are often attempted before initiation of seclusion and restraint. The therapeutic intent of this technique is to reduce disruptive stimulation and provide the client with a contained, well-defined space for reassurance, protection, and defense. Depending on unit construction the client can be encouraged to seek quiet refuge at the back of the unit or in his or her individual room. Isolation can progress from the back of the unit, to the client's room, to open seclusion or a quiet room as indicated. These strategies are typically used in conjunction with the medications previously mentioned and to avoid the more aggressive and restrictive procedures of seclusion and restraint.

When efforts to contain the client's behavior using verbal techniques separately or in combination with administration of medications and behavioral techniques do not prevent the violent behavior, or if an assault occurs without warning, staff must intervene to restrain the client physically and protect the milieu.

Seclusion and Restraint

Seclusion and restraint are techniques used to contain violent clients who do not respond to less restrictive verbal, chemical, or behavioral interventions. Using seclusion or restraint as punishment, divorced from the treatment interests of the client, cannot be justified and represents a serious mismatch between the needs of the client and those of the treatment setting (Soloff 1983).

Table 25–1

Verbal Techniques and Positional Strategies to Use With Potentially Violent Clients

Techniques of Staff	Goal of Intervention
1. Approach the client from the side, symbolically facing what the client faces. Do not stand face to face with the potentially violent person.	1. Focusing the interaction away from the client-staff dyad can decrease the tendency of the violent person to project and externalize the attack.
2. Avoid direct eye contact.	2. Avoid becoming a target of the client's violent expression.
3. Center the verbal content on the figures or issues of concern to the client. For example, if the client states, "The nurse said I'm too sick to leave the hospital," a response such as, "That's a real drag," will likely be more effective than "I can see how you must be upset by that." The latter statement draws attention back to the client and staff member (Nigrosh 1983).	3. Deflect attention away from the staff member as a potential target for the violent behavior.
4. Express affect similar to the client's. For example, when responding to the client's anger at not being allowed to leave, state, "That really is crummy."	4. Avoid sounding too clinical. Identify and verbalize some part of the client's feelings toward the object(s) or person(s) of concern to the client (Nigrosh 1983).

---

client's already damaged self-esteem as much as possible, thereby decreasing the potential for violent behavior.

Sometimes verbal techniques are insufficient to contain the situation, particularly when the violent behavior occurs impulsively. In these instances, additional interventions—including medications, behavioral techniques, and seclusion and restraint—can be used with or instead of the verbal strategies just presented.

Facilities using seclusion and restraint as a means of controlling violent behavior generally require staff attendance at assault training programs. These programs teach hospital policies and procedures for dealing with assaultive clients, including legal and clinical documentation requirements, as well as appropriate physical contact skills for use with violent psychiatric in-patients. While all courses in contact skills must emphasize the concept of team building, variations do exist. Some courses emphasize situation-specific skills, such as **standard therapeutic holds** and "release from hair pull," while others provide practice for more general strategies such as **evasive techniques** and **deflection and neutralization of blows** (Nigrosh 1983). The most comprehensive programs provide analysis and opportunities to role play interview situations, as well as other non-contact techniques, in addition to specific contact skills training. Evidence in the literature indicates an association between participation in staff training programs and not being assaulted. In other words, nursing personnel who participate in staff training workshops are less likely to be assaulted than staff who do not participate (Infantino and Musingo 1985).

Whichever type of program is offered, it is important to provide monthly on-unit reviews for each shift. These reviews, emphasizing the team orientation, provide opportunities for practice, role modeling, and evaluation of performance. In addition, it is important that these physical contact skills be integrated into a larger training program that places the physical interventions into proper clinical perspective.

The decision to use medication, seclusion, or restraint to control violent behavior depends on an understanding of the individual client. For example, the use of repetitive neuroleptic medication to control violent behavior in an organically impaired client would not be as desirable as using restraint or seclusion as the first intervention option. On the other hand, involuntary medication may be preferred to the use of seclusion and restraint in the case of a schizophrenic client whose violent behavior is a response to paranoid delusions.

Techniques of Seclusion and Restraint Psychiatric nurses have a major responsibility in the decision to seclude and restrain as well as in caring for the client while in seclusion and restraints. Once the decision has been made to seclude and restrain a potentially violent client, a "leader" is chosen from among the available staff. The leader is responsible for designating roles to be played by the remaining staff and for directing the steps in the seclusion-restraint procedure. Choice of the leader is important and can be based on numerous factors, including familiarity with the client. It is important to remember that the goal in the procedure is to gain maximum cooperation from the client and minimize violence. For example, one would not choose a large male staff member to confront a psychotic client in homosexual panic (Tardiff 1984a).

After a leader is chosen a sufficient number of person-

nel must be gathered. This support staff should convey confidence and calm reflecting a detached, professional approach to a familiar procedure. The staff should avoid intimidating language and physical stances as these behaviors may provoke the client's potential for violence. It is often sufficient to have the support staff gather around the leader the first time the client is approached. This **show of force** may be intervention enough and the client may comply without further escalation. It is important for the client to perceive that sufficient strength is available to control his or her behavior. From the staff's perspective, the show of force provides confidence with minimal physical risk to staff, client, and the remaining milieu (Tardiff 1984a).

One staff member is assigned responsibility for managing the unit environment and other clients. This person is responsible for supporting and calming the other clients, who may become anxious during the procedure. In addition, the area near the seclusion room must be cleared of clients or physical obstructions to minimize the potential of injury.

Once the unit environment is safe, the team approaches the potentially violent client. The leader offers a clear, brief statement of the purpose and rationale for seclusion or restraint. For example, the client is told that his or her behavior is out of control and that time in seclusion is required to help him or her regain control. The other team members position themselves around the client for easy access to the client's limbs. The leader then asks the client to walk into the seclusion room accompanied by staff. At this point, further discussion or negotiation should be avoided as it frequently aggravates the situation. The behavioral options given to the client must be kept simple, clear, and minimal. Time allowed for client cooperation must be brief, measured in seconds rather than minutes, to avoid an escalation of the behavior into an uncontrolled episode of violence (Tardiff 1984a).

If the client does not begin to walk toward the seclusion room, on cue from the leader, the team members positioned around the client move in to restrain the client physically. Using practiced techniques the team brings the client to the ground and restrains each limb at the joint.

Once the client is safely controlled on the ground, additional staff may be needed to transport the client to the seclusion room where mechanical restraints can be applied. These clients can be carried in the recumbent position with arms pinned to sides, legs held at the knees, and head controlled. Other clients may be walked into the seclusion room with staff maintaining adequate control over both arms.

In the seclusion room the client is routinely positioned on the bed on his or her back. Street clothes are removed and the client is placed in a hospital gown. Belts, shoes, jewelry, and glasses are removed to avoid self-injury. If the client is to be restrained, one limb at a time is secured in the restraint with staff announcing as each limb is secured and pressure released. The client's head should be secured until all staff members have withdrawn their holds to reduce the chance of staff being bitten by the client. Medications are frequently injected at this time. Once the client is safely restrained and medicated, the leader reassures the client that he or she will be carefully monitored and the staff will assess his or her capacity for control. Then the team can exit one at a time, with the final member moving backward out of the seclusion room door, which is then quickly locked.

The final step in the seclusion or restraint process is a rehash of the procedures and techniques used. During the rehash staff must be allowed to express their emotional reactions to the episode. The client community should also be given an opportunity in community meetings or other forums to ventilate their feelings and verbalize their concerns about the restraint and seclusion procedure. Clear therapeutic rationales for the use of seclusion or restraint should be openly discussed with the client community (Tardiff 1984a).

Care of the Client in Seclusion and Restraint Once a client requires seclusion or restraint, observations of the client's behavior are to be made every 15 minutes by nursing staff. These checks include a description of the client's behavior (e.g., yelling or sleeping), as well as routine care activities, including meals, circulation checks, and toileting needs. When the client is quiet, these checks should be conducted by nursing staff entering the seclusion room and participating in a verbal exchange with the client. The content of these dialogues should be documented, paying particular attention to a reduction in the client's symptoms, responsiveness to limits, capacity to discuss options, and increased capacity to tolerate frustration. Documentation of these behavioral checks and routine physical care activities are required and can be accomplished in a checklist format. A sample of a nursing care checklist is presented in Figure 25–1.

Release from Seclusion and Restraint Clients may be released from seclusion and restraint when the goals of the intervention have been accomplished, that is, when the client's behavior is under control and no longer poses a danger to self, others, or the milieu. The decision to release from seclusion or wean from restraint and seclusion is based on an assessment of data gathered while the client is in seclusion. The ability of the client to control his or her behavior has been observed many times during the course of seclusion or restraint and is the basis for the decision to release. Each time nursing staff enter the seclu-

sion room for the purpose of feeding, bathing, or toileting the client, responsiveness to verbal direction can be assessed. If a client has been secluded and not restrained, the first entries into the seclusion room should always be preceded by specific behavior requests. For example, the client should be asked to sit on the bed before staff will enter. The capacity of the client to follow simple directive statements is a first step in gathering assessment data for making a decision to release (Tardiff 1984a).

The release process follows a behavioral course that can be outlined in the nursing care plan. The initial step may be opening the seclusion room door for brief periods of time and monitoring the client's tolerance. With the door open, the client is expected to remain in the room and converse with staff across the open door. Deviation from the stated expectations of staff leads to a relocking of the door and a requirement to begin the process again. Once the client has demonstrated cooperation with medications, meals, hygiene care, and interaction with staff from an open seclusion setting, staff can consider a return to the client's room and the milieu. A sample nursing care plan for clients in seclusion is presented on page 638.

The client in restraints should be released from restraints gradually. There are many different types of restraints, from cloth camisoles and posey belts to locked leather restraints. Locked leather restraints are frequently used in acute psychiatric facilities. These restraints are secured to the frame of a bed that is often bolted to the floor of the seclusion room. A restraint is applied to each limb of the client and locked. With this type of restraint it is possible to vary the placement based on an assessment of the client's need for external control. It is common when assessing the client's capacity for control to move gradually from a condition of four-point restraints (two ankle, two wrist), to three-point restraints (two ankle, one wrist), to two-point restraints (opposite ankle and wrist). This strategy allows the staff a margin of safety while providing the client gradual release. Once released from restraints, clients require the same assessment as indicated above for individuals in seclusion (McCoy and Garritson 1983, Soloff 1983, Tardiff 1984b).

Limitations of Importation Theory

Although the in-patient management strategies of verbal techniques, medication, behavioral techniques, seclusion, and restraint are among the most frequently used, the importation theory on which they are based has limited value. Knowing the numerous individual characteristics that are the basis of the importation theory has not helped in predicting psychiatric client violence. In spite of its popularity the importation theory is limited because the characteristics identified are not descriptive of all clients who are violent, and not all clients fitting this profile exhibit violent behavior. The two frameworks discussed next address dimensions excluded by the importation theory and define the problem of violence in terms of the environment or

Date _____ Time in _____

Renew R/S order at _____

Seclusion only _____

Type of restraint _____

Client I.D.

Level of search:
I. Clothing and belongings _____
II. In hospital gown _____
III. Body search _____

Time every 15 minutes	Check circulation q 15 min.	Fluids offered every hour	Exercise/limb massage q hour	Hygiene needs assessed q 2⁰	Need for elimination assessed q 2⁰	Observations (include client behavior, sleep, etc.):	Staff Initials

CRITERIA FOR RELEASE MET

Time	Accepts limits	Tolerates frustration	Contracts	Other	Staff initials

Initials	Staff signatures/title	Initials	Staff signatures/title

Figure 25–1
Nursing care checklist for clients in seclusion or restraint.

Nursing Care Plan: Clients in Seclusion

Nursing Diagnosis (PND-I/NANDA)	Client Care Goals	Nursing Planning/ Intervention	Evaluation

*05.02.01.02 Aggressive/ violent behaviors toward others /Potential for violence directed at others	Client will gradually gain control of impulses during episode of seclusion.	1. Provide clear and firm limits to supplement the client's lack of internal controls.
		2. Assess client's ability to respond to limits:
		  a. Instruct client to sit on bed before staff enters seclusion room.
		  b. Evaluate client's cooperation taking oral meds.
		  c. Graduate from locked to open seclusion room during the next 2 hours if client can tolerate.
		3. Teach client alternative ways to deal with assaultiveness.
		4. Use medications as ordered for increasing control.
		5. Restrain if client demonstrates violent behavior toward others.
			Client will be able to verbalize one option to hitting others before he/she is released from seclusion room, i.e., talking, requesting meds, requesting a "quiet place."

06.01.02 Hyperalertness	Client will be able to tolerate environmental stimuli.	1. Provide a low stimulus environment of seclusion room. 2. Graduate from locked to open seclusion during next 2 hours if client can tolerate.	Behavioral observation of client over the next 2 hours will indicate tolerance of open seclusion door, staff contact, following instructions.
01.03.01 Altered eating* /Self-care deficit: feeding	Client will maintain an adequate intake of food and fluid.	1. Offer client food and fluids at meal time. 2. Offer supplemental fluids every 2 hours while client is in seclusion. 3. Physically assist client with eating and drinking if necessary. 4. Document client's actual intake of food and fluids.	Documentation will show that client was offered food and fluids at least every 2 hours and will provide a record of client's actual intake.

continued

Nursing Care Plan: Clients in Seclusion (*Continued*)

Nursing Diagnosis (PND-I/NANDA)	Client Care Goals	Nursing Planning/ Interventions	Evaluation
01.03.06 Altered toileting* /Self-care deficit: toileting	Client's need for toilet facilities will be met.	1. Offer client opportunity to use bathroom facilities every 2 hours or as requested. 2. Physically assist client in meeting toileting needs if necessary. 3. Document client's use of facilities.	Documentation will indicate that client was offered facilities at least every 2 hours.
01.03.04 Altered hygiene /Self-care deficit: bathing/ hygiene	Client will have hygiene needs met during seclusion.	1. Offer client opportunity to wash face and hands. 2. Offer client dental hygiene after meals, at bedtime, or on request. 3. Provide client with clean gown and linens if needed or requested.	Interview with client at time of release from seclusion will indicate client had opportunity to brush teeth, change gown, etc.

*PND diagnoses also in NANDA list.

the interactional process as integrated components contributing to violence.

Situationism

Situationism proposes that violence is a response to the unique, coercive, and regimented hospital environment in which the client feels devalued and dehumanized (Armstrong 1978). Research conducted in this area suggests the environmental elements that contribute to the violence process on in-patient psychiatric units are space and location, time of day, unit construction, staffing patterns, activity levels, and population composition.

Space and Location

Space and location factors include territoriality, privacy, overcrowding, and place of the incident (Depp 1983, Dietz and Rada 1983, Kinzel 1970). The concept of territoriality involves defense of physical objects or the space a client

has identified or "staked out" as his or her own. For example, often a client will "claim" a special chair on the unit only for a new client to come along and sit in it. The resulting conflicts over special territory also raise the issue of privacy.

Overcrowding

Overcrowding is also related to the issue of privacy. Evidence suggests that assaultive clients have unusual and consistent difficulty tolerating people near them or touching them (Depp 1983, Kinzel 1970).

Place on the Unit

Observation of the location or place on the unit where assaults take place can be instructive. For instance, one recent study of assaults on a forensic service revealed that most assaults occurred in the dining room during mealtime (Dietz and Rada 1983). In another study the highest number of incidents occurred in the corridors or in clients' rooms with fewer assaults occurring in the dining room (Quinsey and Varney 1977). The difference in results appeared to be related to institutional policy. In the first example, all clients except those in seclusion were required to go to the dining room for meals, while in the second instance access to the dining room was obtained only after the client had demonstrated the ability to handle that social environment.

Specific management strategies suggested by these data include options such as structural enlargement of communal ward areas, or diversion of some clients to alternative areas at times of highest use (Dietz and Rada 1983). The frequency of dining room incidents might be reduced by staggering mealtimes, seating fewer clients at a table, or increasing selectivity over which clients go to the dining room. On units where assaults are highest in client rooms, consideration might be given to issues of negotiating ward census, structural changes providing a higher proportion of single rooms, and flexibility in moving clients to decrease density or establish a better match of roommates.

Time of Day

The example of mealtimes and incidents in the dining room indicate that the time of day may be closely linked to the location of violent incidents. Although the times of highest assaults have varied across research studies, assaults appear to occur with greatest frequency at the times and places with the highest level of interaction among clients (Dietz and Rada 1983).

Architectural Design

Another reported precondition for violence is architectural designs that create blind spots and opportunities for non-observation. Research suggests, however, that rather than a lack of staff monitoring contributing to violence, fights between clients occur around scarce items that require sharing, often creating an atmosphere of competition (Depp 1983). Placement of the radio, telephone, piano, or washer and dryer in out-of-the-way places (to decrease noise on the unit) often contributes to incidents. Mirrors have been used effectively to cope with particular architectural design problems in psychiatric units. But how a unit and staff choose to handle scarce items is far more complex and is related not only to institutional policy and unit philosophy but also to individual clinical judgment. Many units monitor these items, either through using signup procedures or by locking them up and distributing them at the discretion of the staff or a member of the client government. The significant issue is developing an awareness that loca-

tion of these items often creates areas where violence occurs. Sometimes the simple installation of one additional client telephone or a minor structural alteration on a unit can significantly reduce the number of incidents.

Staffing Patterns

The relationship between staffing patterns and violence is not well understood. The notion of optimal staffing, often cited as a prerequisite for attainment of treatment objectives, is ambiguous and appears more complex than "more staff equals less violence." Whether a given hospital milieu has sufficient staff to manage potentially violent clients depends on the amount of care required by the total client population at that period of time. Most units are prepared to deal with a certain amount of acting-out, disorganized, agitated, or violent behaviors, but beyond that they may become overwhelmed.

Although a number of studies have attempted to clarify the relationship between staffing patterns and violence, they have generated conflicting results. Some have found increased numbers of assaults on days with higher staffing levels (Depp 1983, Kalogerakis 1971). The researchers attributed this finding to the idea of activity level (see the next section) or the potential for physical coercion that occurs with an increased presence of staff authority. Other researchers exploring the problem of understaffing and its relationship to psychiatric violence have found that the presence of one or two staff members is associated with a significant decrease in violent episodes (Rogers et al. 1980). In this case it is not clear whether staff passively provide an audience that inhibits violent behavior or whether staff actively model more acceptable role behaviors (Cobb 1984). In addition to confusion over optimum numbers of staff, there is controversy over the relationship between client violence and nursing staff gender. It has been suggested that female staff are less likely to provoke violence than male staff (Levy and Hartocollis 1976).

Because of the difficulty comparing across studies due to differences in unit and staffing compositions, the relationship between staffing and violence remains unclear. It is likely that the staffing question will not be answered through study of such survey characteristics as number or gender of staff, but by pursuing an understanding of the quality, content, and variations in staff to client interactions.

Activity Level

Activity level refers to the requirement that clients participate in therapeutic activities. As mentioned previously, peak times for violent incidents tend to be mealtimes and periods of concentrated treatment programming. In both situations there is a high concentration of clients, and performance and participation are demanded. Ways of handling the problems suggested by activity level include scheduling, coordinating, and withdrawing. Scheduling staff breaks and mealtimes during client meals can create a situation of temporary understaffing on the unit. Whether this contributes to staff anxiety that is communicated to clients is not clear, but staggering mealtimes for clients and staff is a simple alternative and may prevent violent behavior. Coordinating client activities with the nursing staff schedule, although a tedious process, is an important consideration.

Staff who are expected to cajole or coerce clients into participation often create a situation where the client feels trapped and striking out becomes the only defense. Sometimes the most valuable intervention with any client—but particularly with one who is agitated, angry, and frightened—is temporary withdrawal. This allows the client quiet time free from the anxiety of interpersonal demands. Making frequent, short, individualized contact with the client is more reassuring and will go further in de-escalating a situation than forcing the client to attend a community meeting or other activity where his or her behavior is likely to be the focal point of the community's discussion. Individualizing the milieu activities of clients may be as important to advancing their treatment and preventing violence as the proper medication regimen.

Client Population Composition

The last element evolving from the situationism framework is client population composition, which involves the risks and benefits of establishing segregation or special units for violent clients. This raises clinical as well as ethical issues. Designation within a facility of one unit for "assaultive clients," while creating a homogeneous treatment unit, may actually establish an assaultive unit. On the other hand, admitting violent clients to all units contributes to an increased risk from assault for more vulnerable clients. Although the latter is by far the most popular and pragmatic approach, danger of serious injury to other clients by ward violence is a factor of growing concern in many hospitals (Depp 1983).

It has been suggested that much of the violent and disruptive behavior within settings reflects the success with which the institutional environment conveys the message that clients are expected to act violently (Dietz and Rada 1983). This is particularly true in forensic services, but every treatment unit contributes to these messages either implicitly or explicitly. Physical characteristics of a unit such as the posted notice "High Assault Risk" on the front door of the unit or the storage of leather restraints in plain view, alert clients as well as staff to potential problems.

While it is important to attend to issues such as space and location, time of day, unit construction, etc., their contribution to psychiatric violence is not well understood. However, the situationism framework provides an additional perspective from which to understand violence and generate assessment data. These data can then be used to plan interventions for individuals that take into account the environmental component in violent behavior. The major

limitation of the situationism framework is that it fails to account for the vast majority of clients in these settings who do not engage in violent behavior. Like the importation framework, this perspective fails to address the complexity of psychiatric violence. The framework discussed next emphasizes client-staff interaction as a contributing element in psychiatric violence.

Interaction

Emphasizing the interactional process as the trigger or cue for violent assault, this framework concentrates on client and staff interaction. The specific interactional processes identified as cues to violence between staff and clients tend to cluster around three elements: (1) provocations, (2) expectations, and (3) conflicts. While the emphasis here is on client-staff violence, and these elements have been noted typically in relation to this specific interactional pattern, they may also be important in understanding client-client violence.

Provocation

Several studies suggest that provocative styles of interaction contribute to violence (Hatti et al. 1982, Madden et al. 1976, Ruben et al. 1980, Straker et al. 1977). In each of these studies the therapist interviewed thought he or she had done something to trigger the violence. These provocations to violence were described as frustrating clients by not granting requests regarding hospitalization or medications and making the client do something he or she was unwilling to do, such as attend group activities.

Individual therapist's behaviors that increase the likelihood of assault are irritability, a tendency to speak up when angry, and a tendency to fight when confronted with physically threatening situations (Ruben et al. 1980). Although nurses may not know what part they play in the violent encounter, repetitive incidents of assault or threats of assault on the same nursing staff member may provide clues. A tendency in staff toward a controlling, rigid authoritarian, and intolerant stance toward clients increases vulnerability to assault (Soloff 1983). These attitudes are often communicated unwittingly through tone of voice, physical demeanor, or choice of language. Abusive language or actual assault on clients may provoke a violent defense from clients. These provocations and abusive interactions increase nurses' vulnerability to violent assault. Strategies for providing supervision and staff support will be discussed in the next section. At this point it is important to suggest that some nurses may not be able to work successfully with certain types of clients at certain times.

Nurses working with the violent need to monitor themselves and each other with regard to the following:

- Their ability to use anger constructively and not to take the anger of clients personally
- Their capacity for clear verbal communication
- Their capacity for self-analysis
- Their capacity to listen
- Their capacity both to establish and maintain empathic linkages with clients and to disengage
- Their capacity to understand their fears and anxieties about violence
- Their belief that violent psychiatric clients are treatable

Nurses with long-standing difficulties in these areas and the previously mentioned controlling interpersonal style may be more successful in other clinical settings.

In addition to the behavior styles and provocations that increase vulnerability to violence, two major staff expectations have been associated with psychiatric violence:

1. Expectations that clients will act violently
2. Expectations that clients are hopeless and cannot be treated

Expectations

Within the hospital setting, persistent expectations and fears of assault may set up a self-fulfilling prophecy (Levy and Hartocollis 1976, Straker et al. 1977, Whitman et al. 1976). Seeing the danger of being assaulted as part of the work hazard in psychiatric nursing (Duvall 1984) and expecting to be assaulted at work are related but separate experiences. A greater need for staff vigilance in recognizing that they work with assaultive individuals is necessary, but this does not require that assaultive behavior be expected or acceptable. The client may interpret such attitudes to mean that violence is not serious (Madden 1983).

Staff hopelessness about clients has also been associated with psychiatric violence. As noted previously, the major presenting psychodynamic theme describing violence-prone individuals is their self-perception as hopeless and powerless. It is believed that communications by staff supporting these perceptions provides another interpersonal cue to violence (Depp 1983).

Conflicts

It has long been suggested that conflicts between staff can become the basis for acting-out behavior in clients (Stanton and Schwartz 1954). As a result of staff conflicts over philosophic splits or competitive rivalries, clients can be scapegoated into behaving violently as a mechanism for releasing ward tension (Straker 1977).

In conjunction with provocations, expectations, and staff conflicts, it is important to consider the concept of timing; knowing when to engage in interaction is as crucial as knowing how to engage. Single episodes of provocation, assault expectations, or staff conflicts may have no adverse effects, but repeated interactions involving these dynamics may culminate in violence.

In-Patient Management Strategies

Management strategies specific to the interaction framework focus on the client-staff dyad, rather than the individual client or the environment. Among the strategies are provision for clinical supervision, staff development opportunities, and staff meetings. These techniques will be discussed in the next section.

This final management approach is based on integration of the frameworks of importation, situationism, and interaction. This integrated approach to managing in-patient psychiatric violence recognizes violence as a response to the complex social processes between actors. Using this integrated approach to understand psychiatric in-patient violence has implications for assessment, planning, intervening, and evaluating the nursing care delivered to these clients.

Figure 25–2 is a comprehensive violence assessment tool addressing clinical, situational, and interactional factors that will assist the nurse in collecting and organizing data. This tool seeks information relevant to each of the frameworks presented. Information from the assessment tool can be used to plan meaningful, individualized integrated interventions designed to decrease the incidence of violent behavior.

These interventions can be coordinated around the factors that most significantly contribute to increasing the individual's potential to violent behavior. The client and his or her family are important sources of information. Interview questions about the violent client's history should be open and direct much as though one were questioning a suicidal individual. The client should be asked how much he or she has thought about violence, what he or she has done about it, what weapons are available to him or her, what preparations have been made, how close he or she has come to being violent, and what is the most violent thing he or she has done (Monahan 1981).

The assessment tool can be used to gather data throughout the hospitalization or during multiple hospitalizations adding data with each admission. Nurses should not become discouraged if the data prove difficult to obtain. At this time, few practitioners use such a comprehensive framework when thinking about violence.

Integrated Management Approach

Clustering around three considerations—the client, the unit, and the staff—the integrated strategies capitalize on contributions from the importation, situationism, and interaction frameworks. These strategies emphasize negotiation, collaboration, and sensitivity to the multiple meanings each actor brings to the situation. Although the strengths and limitations of this approach to management have yet to be discovered, the strategies emphasized are compatible with the theoretical frameworks presented.

Client-Focused Strategies

The five client-focused strategies discussed below represent an extension to the strategies mentioned in the previous discussion of the importation framework.

History Taking

It is important to begin by taking comprehensive violence histories on admission. In taking the history nurses should think of each acute violent episode as an event in a life history and establish a longitudinal picture of violence in and out of the hospital. The goal of the history is to find patterns or trends in the violent behaviors to understand the conditions in which an individual is likely to act violently. (See Figure 25–2.)

Planning

With a comprehensive history functioning as assessment data, active treatment planning and goal setting with the client is the next step. Nurses can begin to address and minimize the coercive regimentation of the hospital environment by developing a sensitivity to the individual's habits, strengths, and perceived needs. A treatment plan reflecting awareness of the client's capacity and tolerance for participation in therapeutic activities, as well as specific "cues" to violent behavior, is the goal.

Role of Catharsis in Treatment

When planning the client's treatment, be cautious in using catharsis as a way of handling the violent feelings of an individual. Encouraging clients to hit punching bags and pillows may actually increase emotions and lead to violent acts. Consultation with the therapist involved in the client's treatment is required before recommending or initiating this technique. Teaching the client how to talk about vio-lence and develop options to the violent behavior is a more useful intervention.

Rehash Violent Episodes

If a violent act occurs on the unit, use a rehash format for client witnesses to the violence, as well as with the individual client(s) involved if possible. A rehash is a small, spontaneous group led by staff that discusses what happened, the outcome, and the feelings of the community members about the incident (see the section "Seclusion and Restraint"). The goal is to decrease anxiety, increase understanding about violence and its management, and reduce the potential for others in the client group to behave violently.

Reintegration

If a client assaults another client or a member of the staff, it is important to reintegrate that client with the individual he or she has assaulted. If the client has been secluded after the incident, this reintegration can begin after the client has regained control but before release from the seclusion room. Too often no effort is made to establish a therapeutic understanding of the events of the assault. Failure to reintegrate the individuals involved in the violent act can result in lingering anxieties for them and the larger milieu.

Unit-Focused Strategies

The six strategies presented here provide nurses with additional management strategies and are consistent with the situationism framework.

Unit Philosophy

Nurses can help develop a unit philosophy of prevention of violent behavior. No one professional discipline can assume responsibility for the prevention of violent behavior. It is important to articulate a unit philosophy that identifies shared responsibility among all disciplines for the maintenance of acceptable client behaviors.

Unit Policies

Nurses can also help establish and regularly evaluate unit policies regarding the management of violent incidents. The policies should include client consequences for violent behavior and a careful delineation of areas of responsibility

I.   Clinical history

   A.   Diagnosis at discharge
       Axis I: _____

               _____

       Axis II: _____

               _____

   B.   Age: _____
   C.   Sex: ___ M ___ F
   D.   Admitting status
       ___ 72-HR hold   ___ Vol.
       ___ 14-DAY cert.   ___ Other
       ___ Temp conservatorship
   E.   Previous experience in seclusion/restraint
       ___ Yes   ___ No
       Reaction to seclusion/restraint

       _____

       _____

       _____

F.   Age at onset: _____
G.   Psychotropic medications:
   ___ Taking prior to admission
   ___ Not taking prior to admission

   Medications:

   _____

   _____

   _____

   _____

   Previous criminal history
   ___ Yes   ___ No

   _____

   _____

I.   Use of ETOH/street drugs
   ___ Yes   ___ No

   _____

   _____

   _____

II.   Violence history

   A.   Previous institutional violence   ___ Yes   ___ No

       Type of institution: _____   Date(s): _____ _____
       Number of incidents: _____   _____ _____
       Type of violence:

Against person	___ Yes	___ No	Date	_____
Family	___ Yes	___ No	Date	_____
Stranger	___ Yes	___ No	Date	_____
Inmate/client	___ Yes	___ No	Date	_____
RN/LPT/MD	___ Yes	___ No	Date	_____
Other	___ Yes	___ No	Date	_____
			Who	_____
Weapon used	___ Yes	___ No	Date	_____
Against property	___ Yes	___ No	Date	_____
Type	_____			
Verbal threat (only)	___ Yes	___ No	Date	_____

       Situational factors: Time of day   _____
                       Location   _____
       Engaged in therapeutic activity   ___ Yes   ___ No
               Type of activity   _____
       Other factors   _____

                        _____

                        _____

       Interactional factors: Engaged in interaction with victim ___ Yes ___ No
                       Type of interaction _____

                       _____

                       With whom: _____
                       Content of conversation, request:

                       _____

                       _____

Figure 25–2
Violence assessment tool.

Response to violence: Medications   ___ Yes   ___ No
                        Type and dose: _____
                                         _____
                                         _____

                        Seclusion only   ___ Yes   ___ No
                    Seclusion/restraint   ___ Yes   ___ No
                    Milieu management   ___ Yes   ___ No
                        Combination   ___ Yes   ___ No
                            (list)   _____
                                          _____
                                          _____

Client's response to intervention(s):   _____
_____
_____

B.   Community violence
     Previous violence: ___ Yes ___ No
     Number of incidents: _____   Date(s):   _____ _____
                                               _____ _____
                                               _____ _____

     Type of violence: Against person   ___ Yes   ___ No   Date _____
                             Family   ___ Yes   ___ No   Date _____
                             Stranger   ___ Yes   ___ No   Date _____
                         Inmate/patient   ___ Yes   ___ No   Date _____
                           RN/LPT/MD   ___ Yes   ___ No   Date _____
                             Other   ___ Yes   ___ No   Date _____
                                                                  Who _____
                          Weapon used   ___ Yes   ___ No   Date _____
                        Against property ___ Yes   ___ No   Date _____
                             Type   _____
                        Verbal threat (only) ___ Yes ___ No   Date _____
     Situational factors: ETOH   ___ Yes   ___ No   Amount _____
                          Street drugs   ___ Yes   ___ No
                             Type   _____
                                          _____

                          Time of day   _____   Activity _____
                                                                  _____
                            Location   _____ _____
                          Other factors   _____
                                                     _____

     Interactional factors: Engaged in interaction with victim ___ Yes ___ No
                        Type of interaction: _____
                                               _____
                                               _____

                          Others present: _____

     Content of conversation, request, argument, or dispute: _____
                                               _____

among the disciplines in the management of violence in the milieu.

Team Approach

Staff members should develop a unit attitude of collaboration and negotiation and a team approach to prevention and violence management. Developing a consensus about the unit's position on violent behavior and its consequences that is consistent with unit policy will decrease arguments and anxieties among staff and clients.

Record Keeping

Comprehensive unit record keeping regarding violent incidents is important. In addition to the formal unusual occurrence reports with their administrative orientation, it is useful to collect clinical documentation on incidents, which will provide a basis for structured clinical audits. Contents of the clinical documentation include identification of the who, what, where, when, and how of a violent act. These notations are behavioral rather than interpretive and serve multiple purposes, including:

- Increasing understanding of violence by looking for patterns among episodes
- Teaching and clinical supervision
- Establishing and revising policy
- Conducting research

Clear Authority

While no one person or discipline can prevent and manage violent behavior alone, there must be a clearly identifiable authority in decision making around the violent incidents. Nurses who have responsibility for milieu management must have authority for decisions regarding violence management. This authority requires clear articulation and support from unit leadership and departmental administration.

Review Committee

A unit-based committee should be established for periodic review of incidents, policies, and mechanisms for handling client and staff issues around violent incidents. All the disciplines on the unit should be represented, with nursing as chair.

Staff-Focused Strategies

The following staff strategies are suggested as the last element in the integrated management model. These staff strategies are compatible with and complementary to the client and unit strategies outlined.

Supervision

The department should provide ongoing clinical supervision with an expert in management of in-patient violence.

In-Service Education

Continuous in-service training on violence will help staff:

- Understand ways in which they increase their vulnerability to assault
- Develop provocation profiles of staff members to increase sensitivity and awareness among the staff
- Role play conversations with the violent
- Practice teamwork for physical restraint procedures
- Promote a safe, nonblaming environment for them to discuss their experiences of working with violent clients
- Develop sensitivity to the effects their own experiences of violence have in their daily work

These discussions are not a license to act in abusive or punishing ways toward clients or other staff members.

Research

Nursing staff should encourage and participate in nursing research in the area of psychiatric violence and establish contact with doctoral programs in nursing, inviting interested researchers to discuss their studies and providing them access to the unit.

Rehash

Nurses can encourage and ritualize the use of rehash after each incident to understand, not blame, those involved in the episode. These sessions can focus on identifying precipitants to the violence, reinforcing the client's own control, and working together as a team. The overall goal of the rehash sessions is improved competence and confidence for staff.

Support for Victims

Staff victims of violence need a safe, supportive environment. When nursing staff are assaulted on the unit, establishing a "buddy system" with another nursing staff person may decrease the isolation and denial of the incident (Lanza 1983, 1984). In addition, providing emotional support for the staff may decrease the potential for retaliation.

Evaluating Effectiveness of Strategies

There are many elements to consider in evaluating the effectiveness of strategies for violence management. As suggested by the three theoretical frameworks, individual characteristics of the actors, conditions in the social environment, and the interactional styles of both clients and staff contribute to violent behavior. In spite of these theoretical understandings of violent behavior and efforts to implement management strategies that decrease the likelihood of its occurrence, we are not yet able to predict with certainty when someone will act in a violent manner. The fact is that violence occurs in our health care settings and that psychiatric nurses are victims of assault from psychiatric in-patients.

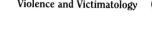

ick 1982). Whether these responses are typical of members from other disciplines or across different work settings is a subject for further research. It is apparent, even from the scarce information available, that for many nursing personnel, being assaulted on the job has serious personal and professional ramifications.

VICTIMATOLOGY

The study of victims of violent assault, whether from psychiatric in-patients or other sources, is called victimatology. This section focuses on the psychiatric nurse as the target of violence from psychiatric in-patients. Literature on client-nurse violence is almost nonexistent (Lanza 1983). Although much more research must be conducted on client-nurse violence, the limited information available reveals three general issues:

1. Staff reactions to the assault
2. Impact on the institutional setting
3. Services required by the victims

Staff Reactions

Two interesting and contradictory findings reported by Lanza (1983) are:

1. Reactions of staff members who have been assaulted can last much longer than the time they are away from work.
2. Staff members often report having no reaction to the assault.

These findings suggest that client-nurse assaults can result in acute or immediate response as well as long-term sequelae for the staff member. In addition, denial of any reaction may be the most frequent immediate response to the assault, possibly due to fear of being overwhelmed by the event if it were acknowledged.

Among the emotional reactions reported by staff who were assaulted are anger, anxiety, irritability, depression, shock, disbelief, apathy, self-blame, fear of returning to work and of other clients, disturbed sleep patterns, and other somatic symptoms, as well as a change in relationship with their co-workers and feelings of professional incompetence (Engel and Marsh 1986, Lanza 1983). In one study of psychiatric nurses physical violence in the work place was most frequently cited by the respondents as the reason for leaving the psychiatric nursing profession (Mel-

Institutional Implications

When violence occurs in the context of the work environment, it has an impact on the setting. Although it is difficult to draw clear distinctions between the consequences for the individuals and the impact on the institution, there are several identifiable implications for the work setting. When either physical or emotional injuries occur, staff often lose time from the work place. Efforts to replace a worker temporarily increase the budget. Morale is often lower among the remaining staff, who frequently share guilt and a sense of responsibility for the incident. Other staff members can also experience increased fear and vulnerability after an incident, which decreases their own effectiveness.

Often an incident of violence provokes an overemphasis on control among staff due to their increased fears. This attitude of control takes precedence over treatment and sound clinical judgment. These measures and efforts to overcontrol can actually increase the staff's vulnerability to future assaults.

The staff may also limit their interactions with certain clients who they perceive as likely to be violent. This withdrawal and avoidance coupled with staff anxiety can also increase their vulnerability to assaults.

Institutional Services

Staff victims of psychiatric assault require in addition to the emotional support of their unit leadership and co-workers a variety of services. These services can be provided through the employee health service and/or an employee assistance program. Among the services that can be made available are opportunities for medical attention, trauma-crisis counseling, legal advice, and information regarding insurance, workers' compensation, and rights to health and safety in the workplace (Engel and Marsh 1986). Due to the number of incidents occurring in health care settings, many institutions have developed a policy and procedure for filing assault charges against a client. While this remains controversial, and nursing personnel report ambivalent feelings about using this option, it is being used more frequently and is considered a major institutional support for staff (Hoge and Gutheil 1987, Sales et al. 1983).

Much of our understanding of staff victims of psychiatric violence is speculative. Recognizing that staff assaults occur and assuming a multidimensional response approach are important first steps. As research studies increase our knowledge about the phenomena of staff victims, their needs, and the impact on the institutional setting, more specific interventions will evolve.

Part I Highlights

- Violence is a complex human behavior with individual, environmental, and interactional components.

- In-patient psychiatric violence represents a specific type of violent behavior.

- A theoretical understanding of violence will help staff design management strategies.

- Nurses are frequent targets of in-patient psychiatric violence.

- Comprehensive assessment and treatment planning can decrease the likelihood of violent behavior among psychiatric in-patients.

- Nurses frequently deny the impact and significance of a violent assault by psychiatric clients.

- Psychiatric nurses are in a key position to contribute a unique perspective on psychiatric violence.

- Not all violence is committed by psychiatric clients and not all psychiatric clients are violent.

References

American Psychiatric Association: *Clinical Aspects of the Violent Individual*. Task Force Report No. 8. U.S. Government Printing Office, 1974.

Armstrong B: Conference report: Handling the violent patient in the hospital. *Hosp Community Psychiatry* 1978;140:301–304.

Cobb BA: *A Descriptive Correlational Study Exploring the Relationship Between Adult Psychiatric Patient Role Strain and Violence in an Inpatient Setting*, thesis. University of California, San Francisco, California, 1984.

Craig TJ: An epidemiologic study of problems associated with violence among psychiatric inpatients. *Am J Psychiatry* 1982;139:1262–1266.

Depp FC: Assaults in a public mental hospital, in Lion JR, Reid WH (eds): *Assaults Within Psychiatric Facilities*. Grune and Stratton, 1983, chap 2.

Dietz PE, Rada RT: Interpersonal violence in forensic facilities, in Lion JR, Reid WH (eds): *Assaults Within Psychiatric Facilities*. Grune and Stratton, 1983, chap 3.

Duvall J: Violence is hazard for psych nurses. *American Nurse*, June 1984, p 4.

Engel F, Marsh S: Helping the employee victim of violence in hospitals. *Hosp Community Psychiatry* 1986;37:159–162.

Fottrell E: Violent behavior by psychiatric patients. *Br J Hosp Med*, January 1981, pp 28–34.

Hatti S, Dubin WR, Weiss KJ: A study of circumstances surrounding patient assault on psychiatrists. *Hosp Community Psychiatry* 1982;33:660–661.

Hoge SK, Gutheil TG: The prosecution of psychiatric patients for assaults on staff: A preliminary empirical study. *Hosp Community Psychiatry* 1987;38:44–49.

Infantino JA, Musingo S-Y: Assaults and injuries among staff with and without training in aggressive control techniques. *Hosp Community Psychiatry* 1985;36:1312–1314.

Kalogerakis MG: The assaultive psychiatric patient. *Psychiatr Q* 1971;45:372–381.

Kinzel AF: Body-buffer zones in violent prisoners. *Am J Psychiatry* 1970;127:99–104.

Lanza ML: The reactions of nursing staff to physical assault by a patient. *Hosp Community Psychiatry* 1983;34:44–47.

Lanza ML: A follow-up study of nurses' reactions to physical assault. *Hosp Community Psychiatry* 1984;35:492–494.

Levy P, Hartocollis P: Nursing aids and patient violence. *Am J Psychiatry* 1976;133:429–431.

Lion JR: Special aspects of psychopharmacology, in Lion JR, Reid WH (eds): *Assaults Within Psychiatric Facilities*. Grune and Stratton, 1983, chap 19.

Lion JR, Snyder W, Merrill GL: Underreporting of assaults on staff in a state hospital. *Hosp Community Psychiatry* 1981;32:497–498.

Madden DJ: Recognition and prevention of violence in psychiatric facilities, in Lion JR, Reid WH (eds): *Assaults Within Psychiatric Facilities*. Grune and Stratton, 1983.

Madden DJ, Lion JR, Penna MW: Assaults on psychiatrists by patients. *Am J Psychiatry* 1976;133:422–425.

Maier G et al.: A model for understanding and managing cycles of aggression among psychiatric inpatients. *Hospital Community Psychiatry* 1987;38:5:520–524.

McCoy SM, Garritson SH: Seclusion: The process of intervening. *J Psychosocial Nurs Mental Health Serv* 1983; 21:8–15.

Melick ME: *Factors Associated With Psychiatric Nurse Turnover: A Report on an Exit Survey and Some Recommendations*. Funded by Grant No. 5T23MH15378-04. Manpower programs for a changing mental health system, National Institute of Mental Health, January 1982.

Monahan J: *Predicting Violent Behavior: An Assessment of Clinical Techniques*. Sage Publications, 1981.

Nigrosh BJ: Physical contact skills in specialized training for the prevention and management of violence, in Lion JR, Reid WH (eds): *Assaults Within Psychiatric Facilities.* Grune and Stratton, 1983.

Quinsey VC, Varney GW: Characteristics of assaults and assaulters in a maximum security hospital unit. *Crimes and Justice* 1977;5:212–220.

Rabkin JG: Criminal behavior of discharged mental patients: A critical appraisal of the research. *Psychol Bull* 1979; 85:1–27.

Rogers R, Ciula B, Cavanaugh JL: Aggressive and socially disruptive behavior among maximum security psychiatric patients. *Psychol Rep* 1980;46:291–294.

Ruben I, Wolkon G, Yamamoto J: Physical attacks on psychiatric residents by patients. *J Nerv Ment Dis* 1980; 168:243–245.

Sales BD, Overcast TD, Merrikin KJ: Worker's compensation protection for assaults and batteries on mental health professionals, in Lion JR, Reid WH (eds): *Assaults Within Psychiatric Facilities.* Grune and Stratton, 1983.

Soloff PH: Seclusion and restraint, in Lion JR, Reid WH (eds): *Assaults Within Psychiatric Facilities.* Grune and Stratton, 1983.

Stanton AH, Schwartz MS: *The Mental Hospital.* Basic Books, 1954.

Steadman HJ: Special problems: The prediction of violence among the mentally ill, in Hays JR, Roberts TK, Soloway KF (eds): *Violence and the Violent Individual.* Spectrum, 1981.

Straker M, et al.: Assaultive behaviors in an institutional setting. *Psychiatr J Univ Ottawa* 1977;II:185–190.

Tardiff K: The use of medication for assaultive patients. *Hosp Community Psychiatry* 1981;33:307–308.

Tardiff K: A survey of assault by chronic patients in a state hospital system, in Lion JR, Reid WH (eds): *Assaults Within Psychiatric Facilities.* Grune and Stratton, 1983.

Tardiff K: *The Psychiatric Use of Seclusion and Restraint.* American Psychiatry Press, 1984a.

Tardiff K: Violence: The psychiatric patient, in Turner JT (ed): *Violence in the Medical Care Setting.* Aspen, 1984b.

Tardiff K, Sweillam A: Assault, suicide and mental illness. *Arch Gen Psychiatry* 1980;37:164–169.

Tardiff K, Sweillam A: Assaultive behavior among chronic psychiatric inpatients. *Am J Psychiatry* 1982;139:212–215.

Whitman RN, Armao BB, Dent OB: Assault on the therapist. *Am J Psychiatry* 1976;133:426–429.

PART II   RAPE AND INTRAFAMILY ABUSE

Karen Lee Fontaine

Learning Objectives

After reading this part, the student will be able to

- Discuss the incidence of rape and intrafamily physical and sexual abuse

- Discuss theories related to the dynamics of rape, intrafamily physical abuse, and intrafamily sexual abuse

- Identify the behavioral, affective, cognitive, physiologic, and sociocultural characteristics related to rape trauma syndrome, intrafamily physical abuse, and intrafamily sexual abuse

- Repudiate myths about rape and intrafamily violence with facts about rape and intrafamily violence

- Assess a client and family behaviorally, affectively, cognitively, physiologically, and socioculturally

- Formulate appropriate nursing diagnoses for rape victims, victims of intrafamily physical or sexual abuse, and their families

- Plan and implement interventions for victims of rape or intrafamily physical or sexual abuse and their families

- Evaluate the effectiveness of nursing interventions for these clients and their families

Cross References

Other topics relevant to this content are: Anxiety disorders, Chapter 19; Elder abuse, Chapter 36; Family dynamics and family therapy, Chapter 33; Growth and development, Chapter 6; Human sexuality and sexual disorders, Chapter 20; Multiple personality, Chapter 19; Posttraumatic stress disorder, Chapter 19; Substance abuse, Chapter 16.

Key Terms

acquaintance (or date) rape
anger rape
incest
intrafamily physical abuse
intrafamily sexual abuse
power rape
rape
rape trauma syndrome
sadistic rape

Violence that is demonstrated as rape or occurs as physical or sexual abuse within the family is a national health problem that confronts psychiatric nurses as well as nurses in many different clinical settings. Victims are seen in the community, in pediatric units, in intensive care units, in medical-surgical units, in maternal care settings, in ambulatory care facilities, in geriatric units, and in psychiatric settings.

Nurses need to be able to assess and provide appropriate intervention for the emotional consequences, as well as the physical trauma, of the rape victim. Nurses may be called on to give legal evidence in the prosecution of a rapist. Within the community, nurses can establish, or refer victims to, support groups. They can also become active in increasing public awareness of rape through formal and informal teaching activities. This unique position of nurses allows them to be active in the prevention of rape and treatment of its victims.

Nurses also need to be involved in the prevention, detection, and treatment of intrafamily violence. Development of the knowledge base and the ability to identify factors that contribute to intrafamily violence will enable the nurse to assist in prevention by providing public education and becoming active in changes in public policy. This knowledge, along with increased awareness of the extent of the problem, will help nurses arrive at earlier, more accurate detection of intrafamily violence. Nurses also need to comply with state laws on the reporting of violence and referral for treatment. Some nurses with advanced education in family therapy are part of the therapy teams that intervene with violent families.

Portions of this chapter appeared in another form in Cook JS, Fontaine KL: *Essentials of Mental Health Nursing*. Addison-Wesley, 1987.

RAPE

Rape is a crime of violence second only to homicide in its violation of a person. The issue is not one of sexuality but one of force, domination, and humiliation. In this text, rape refers to any forced sex act with the key factor being lack of adult consent. Legally, the definition varies from state to state. In many states, rape is defined as forced sexual intercourse against a female who is not married to the perpetrator. Other states have broadened the definition to include other sex acts. The legal climate in regard to marital rape is beginning to change. In many states a husband cannot be charged with rape if he sexually assaults his wife. But other states have recognized that rape can be committed within a marriage and that the husband can be prosecuted.

From the perspective of the victim, rape occurs very suddenly. There is often no warning of the attack, which most frequently occurs between 6 PM and midnight. However, the majority of rapes are not sudden and impulsive; indeed, 60 to 75 percent of all rapes are well planned.

The perpetrators often use guns or knives and may tie the victim or use verbal intimidation, such as a threat of death. Some victims attempt and are able physically to resist. Others may reason or plead with the perpetrator. However, fear of death combined with the suddenness of the event makes many victims unable either to flee or to fight.

Victims of Rape

There is no typical rape victim although, of reported rapes, 93 percent of the victims are female, and 90 percent of the perpetrators are male. One can be a victim of rape at any age, from childhood through old age. The average age of female children who are raped is 7.9 years, and in 80 percent of the cases, the perpetrator is someone the child knows. The rapist may attack strangers, acquaintances, friends, or family members. With increased awareness of the possibility of rape, women are becoming more sensitive to preventive measures. Since this means being suspicious of men in potential rape environments, all women and men are, in one sense, victims of rape. Women have become fearful for their safety, and men, in general, are the recipients of this fear and suspicion. Thus, everyone is affected, at least indirectly, by the crime of rape.

Male victims of rape are just beginning to come to the attention of the general public. As with females, rape of males can occur at any age. The myth of male rape has been that it occurs only where heterosexual contact is not possible, such as in prisons or in isolated living conditions. As more male rape victims report the crime, however, this myth has been exploded. Male rape is not a homosexual attack. Again the issue is one of violence and domination

rather than one of sexuality. Some rapists, who define themselves as heterosexual, will rape both males and females; at times, they rape whoever is available.

In the past, men have been afraid to report rape for fear of being ridiculed or not believed. As was true for females in the past, society has a tendency to blame the male victim by saying such things as, "He must have thought you were trying to pick him up," "You must have made him angry," or "You could have resisted if you had really wanted to." Male rape victims undergo the same emotional trauma that female victims do, and they need the same protection, interventions, and understanding that is provided for female victims (Seeley 1985).

Incidence of Rape

It is difficult to determine the incidence of rape since it is the most underreported crime. Because of shame and fear of being blamed, victims have been hesitant to report and testify (Resick 1983). It is projected that one woman out of every six will experience an attempted rape sometime in her lifetime, and one woman out of every eight will be forced to submit. Between the ages of 16 and 19, females are at the highest risk for being raped. Nonwhite victims are more likely to be raped at an earlier age, with the highest risk being between 12 and 19 years of age. The highest risk for white victims is between the ages of 20 and 34. Most often, the rapist is of the same race as the victim (Warner 1980).

Rape Trauma Syndrome

Rape trauma syndrome was first described by Burgess and Holmstrom (1979) as a two-phase syndrome of *disorganization* (the acute phase) and *reorganization*. An intermediate phase, *outward adjustment,* was proposed by others (Golan 1978). These phases and the rape victim's accompanying responses are described in Table 25–2. The characteristics of rape victims in each of these phases are discussed next.

Behavioral Characteristics

Many victims of rape do not report the crime. Sometimes this is due to guilt or embarrassment about what has occurred. Other victims are fearful of how their families

Table 25–2 Phases of the Rape Trauma Syndrome	
Phase	**Response**
Acute phase	Fear, shock, disbelief, desire for revenge, anger, denial, anxiety, guilt, embarrassment, humiliation, helplessness, dependency; victim may seek help or may remain silent.
Outward adjustment phase	Victim appears outwardly composed, denying and repressing feelings; for example, she returns to work, buys a weapon, adds security measures to her residence, and denies need for counseling.
Reorganizational phase	Victim experiences sexual dysfunction, phobias, sleep disorders, anxiety, and a strong urge to talk about or resolve feelings; victim may seek counseling or may remain silent.

Source: Niehaus MA: Rape, in Griffith-Kenney J: Contemporary Women's Health. Addison-Wesley, 1986, p 226.

real," "I must be dreaming. This couldn't have happened," or, "I just can't believe this has happened to me."

Doreen, a graduate student at the local university, was brought to the hospital by the police who found her running down the street half clothed. In the hospital she was able to tell the staff that she had been raped by her date, Mike, another graduate student. She exhibited outward calmness but kept repeating "This cannot have happened to me. My friends introduced us and he seemed so nice." She was unable to decide who to call to take her back to the dorm or what to tell her friends about what had happened.

Nurses need to recognize that underneath the appearance of being in control and calmness is a person in acute distress. The victims' need to control should be supported until they are able to manage the reality of their situation. Nurses who assume that the calmness indicates no distress will miss the victims' needs for emotional support and intervention.

There may be long-term behavioral characteristics of rape victims. Some are prone to crying spells that they may or may not be able to explain. Some may have difficulty maintaining or forming interpersonal relationships, especially with people who remind them of the perpetrator. Many victims develop problems at work or school. Some report nightmares and have difficulty sleeping. Others develop secondary phobic reactions to people, objects, or situations that remind them of the rape (Resick 1983). A woman who is a victim of marital rape suffers additional problems. Often she must continue to interact with her rapist because she is dependent on him. She may be forced to pretend, to herself and to other family members and friends, that the rape never occurred. Until it becomes more socially acceptable and legally feasible to report marital rape, many of these victims will suffer in silence.

or the police will react to the information. Some perpetrators threaten victims by saying they will return to rape them again if the police are notified. Since many of the crimes are committed by acquaintances or friends, victims fear they will not be believed. This has been termed the *silent reaction*. It dooms the victim to experiencing the rape trauma syndrome without the help of support systems.

Some rape victims respond immediately with agitated and nonpurposeful behavior. They are brought to the emergency room emotionally distraught and unable to respond to questions about what has occurred. So great is their level of anxiety and fear that they may be unable to follow simple directions.

Other rape victims may return home and shower or bathe before notifying the police or going to the emergency room. In the past, this behavior has been viewed with suspicion of a false charge of rape. It is now recognized that people who have been violated by rape experience extreme feelings of helplessness. Often, this cleaning up behavior is an attempt to regain control of the self and return to the normality that was so suddenly disrupted.

The majority of victims appear in good control of their feelings and behavior immediately after the rape. This appearance of outward calmness usually indicates a state of numbness, disbelief, and emotional shock. Statements may be made such as, "This whole thing doesn't seem

Affective Characteristics

Victims of rape suffer immediate and long-lasting emotional trauma. After a period of shock and disbelief, many of them experience episodes of anxiety and depression. Anxiety arises when people's integrity has been threatened or assaulted, and depression may be a response to losses that people incur. Rape victims have been threatened, both physically and emotionally. They have experienced losses in the areas of autonomy, control, safety, and self-esteem. Thus, anxiety and depressive reactions in response to rape are not unusual (Warner 1980).

Many victims feel ashamed and embarrassed about the rape since sexual behavior is normally an intimate, private act. They often feel unclean or contaminated. These feelings are unique to victims of rape as opposed to victims of other crimes. To have to share specific details of the rape with police officers and in a courtroom may be humiliating, particularly since women have been socialized not to talk about sexual behavior in public. Victims who do not report rape generally say it was too private or personal for them to be able to talk about it with strangers.

Rape victims feel physically and emotionally violated. The loss of control over their bodies and their autonomy leads to feelings of helplessness and vulnerability. They may feel alienated from friends and family, particularly if there is not a strong supportive network. Feeling anger is a healthy response to the violation that has occurred, but the energy of anger needs to be appropriately discharged so that the victim does not later become consumed with fantasies of revenge.

Cognitive Characteristics

During the actual rape, some victims use the defense mechanisms of depersonalization or dissociation to cope with the attack. By perceiving the attack as "not really happening to me" the victims protect their sense of integrity. Other victims rely on denial to block out the traumatic experience. The use of these defense mechanisms may continue through the initial treatment of the victim and should be supported until the person is able to face the reality of the attack (Resick 1983).

Victims often enter the emergency room in a state of confusion. They may have great difficulty concentrating and appear unsure of exactly what has occurred. This confusion and uncertainty must be interpreted not as evidence that a rape did not occur, but as an indication of emotional shock. Moreover, the victim's problem-solving and decision-making abilities are greatly reduced during the immediate aftermath of the rape as the result of a high level of anxiety and fear.

Some victims are unable to discuss the attack at all. Some may not even be able to report the rape until the next day when they feel better prepared to cope with the event and the subsequent procedures. Other victims will be very much concerned about whom among their family and friends they should tell. They may be uncertain about how significant others will react to the information that a rape has occurred. They also may not know how to tell others about the experience and may depend on the nurse for guidance and support.

There may be a period during which victims blame themselves for the rape. This self-blame may be heard in statements such as, "If only I had taken a different way home," "I should have been able to escape because he didn't have a gun," or "I should have fought harder than I did." This personal responsibility may also be felt by a marital rape victim. Statements may be made such as, "If I were a better wife, he wouldn't have raped me," or "If I tried harder to please him sexually, he wouldn't have to force me."

Some victims develop obsessional thoughts about the rape, which may be severe enough to interfere with daily functioning. Some, though not obsessed, experience periodic flashbacks of the event. Others are preoccupied with thoughts of future danger, and dreams of a violent nature are common.

Rape may profoundly affect one's beliefs about the environment. If the assault occurred in the victim's home, the normal feeling of safety within the home will most likely be disrupted. Some victims fear retaliation by the perpetrator for reporting the crime, especially when the rapist is known to the victim. Fears may be generalized to all men or all strange men, particularly in young female victims. Women who have been raped by their husbands often state that their ability to trust the husband or any other man has been destroyed (Warner 1980).

Physiologic Characteristics

Rape usually results in a number of physical injuries. Most likely the vagina or rectum will be sore and swollen. There may be tearing of the vaginal or rectal wall from forceful insertion of the penis or a foreign object. The throat may be traumatized from forced oral sex. The victim may also be beaten, stabbed, or shot. Profuse bleeding as well as injuries to vital organs may be a critical problem.

Female victims of child-bearing years may become pregnant as a result of the rape. Victims of all ages and both genders may contract a sexually transmitted disease from the perpetrator. This could be transmitted to mucous membranes in the vagina, rectum, mouth, or throat.

In addition to the immediate physical trauma, there may be serious, long-term physiologic effects. Insomnia or anorexia may be experienced for a long time after the event. Some victims may complain of fatigue or generalized aches and pains, and some may experience gynecologic problems. There may also be long-term effects of a beating, stabbing, or shooting. Victims are also at risk for developing a psychophysiologic disorder in response to a chronic high level of anxiety and fear.

Future sexual functioning may also be adversely affected by a rape. The possibility of developing a sexual dysfunction depends on the quality of sexual experience and relationships before the attack, the behavior used to cope with the attack and the quality of future relationships. Women victims of marital rape often have more difficulty adjusting sexually in a subsequent relationship. Nearly all adult rape victims need to withdraw from sexual activity for a time. For some, the period of celibacy is necessary to reestablish control and autonomy. Others may choose abstinence because they feel unclean or contaminated. Both the victim and the sexual partner need to understand that the need for closeness and nondemanding physical contact continues. Giving comfort through touch will decrease the partner's feelings of rejection and the victim's feelings of self-blame or uncleanness (Warner 1980).

Sociocultural Characteristics

Families experience many of the same thoughts and feelings as the rape victim. They may talk about guilt, doubts, fears, hatred toward the perpetrator, and feelings of helplessness. They need to be educated about the nature and trauma of the rape and the immediate and long-term potential reactions of the victim. They need support and direction in how to help the victim.

Many cultural myths have surrounded the crime of rape for a long time. Examples of these myths and the facts that nurses can use to dispel them are presented in Box 25–1. In the past fifteen years, great strides have been made to abolish these myths from the legal system and to treat rape as the crime of violence it is.

Changing the personal belief system of the general public has been a slower process. Many people continue to believe the rape myths that blame the victim rather than the perpetrator. In one study, 50 percent of both women and men accepted the myths without question. The greatest predictors of acceptance of the myths were rigid gender role stereotyping and the acceptance of interpersonal violence by the participants in the study (Burt 1980). Thus people who are more flexible in gender roles and abhor violence are more likely to support the victim and blame the perpetrator.

Box 25–1
RAPE MYTHS VS. RAPE FACTS

Myth: Sexual assault is caused by uncontrollable sex drives.

Fact

Sexual assault is an act of physical and emotional violence, not of sexual gratification. Men assault to dominate, humiliate, control, degrade, terrify, and violate. Studies show that power and anger are the primary motivating factors.

Myth: Women provoke sexual assault, and sex appeal is of prime importance in selecting targets.

Fact

Women who have been sexually assaulted range in age from infants to the elderly. Appearance and attractiveness are not relevant. A man assaults someone who is accessible and vulnerable.

Myth: Women are usually sexually assaulted by strangers.

Fact

Studies show that the majority of those sexually assaulted are acquainted with their assailants.

Myth: Most sexual assaults are interracial.

Fact

As a national average, more than 90 percent of all sexual assaults occur between people of the same race, although attacks by men of color against white women are given more publicity. There is evidence of racial bias in our legal system: Although men of color are estimated to constitute a small proportion of sexual assailants, they are 48 percent of those convicted and 80 percent of those jailed for assault.

Myth: Sexual assault is unplanned and spontaneous.

Fact

Studies show that a majority of sexual assaults are planned in advance.

Myth: Women make false reports of sexual assault.

Fact

Statistics show that 2 percent of reports of alleged rape are unfounded; this is the same proportion as for all other crimes.

Myth: Men do not have to be concerned about sexual assault because it affects only women.

Fact

Men, both straight and gay, suffered 10 percent of the sexual assaults treated last year at the San Francisco Sexual Trauma Services. In addition, men have wives, friends, mothers, and daughters who may someday need help coping with the aftereffects of sexual assault. Lastly, rape will not cease until men stop raping.

Source: Adapted from Resources Against Sexual Assault. *Rape Prevention Education Program, University of California, San Francisco, 1987, pp 5–6.*

Intrapersonal Theories

Rape is a crime of violence generated by issues of power and anger rather than by sexual drive. The intrapersonal perspective views rapists as emotionally immature persons who feel powerless and unsure of themselves. They are incapable of managing the normal stresses of everyday life. The causes of rape are multidetermined, but the dynamics of the act are that perpetrators abuse their own and others' sexuality as a method of discharging anger and frustration. From this perspective, there are three types of rape: the anger rape, the power rape, and the sadistic rape.

The **anger rape** is distinguished by physical violence and cruelty to the victim. The rapist believes he is the victim of an unjust society and takes revenge on others by raping. He uses extreme force and viciousness to debase the victim. The ability to injure, traumatize, and shame the victim provides an outlet for his rage and temporary relief from his turmoil. Rapes occur episodically as the rage builds up and he strikes out at others to relieve his pain.

In the **power rape**, the intent of the rapist is not to injure the victim but to command and master another person sexually. The rapist has an insecure self-image with feelings of incompetency and inadequacy. The rape becomes the vehicle for expressing power, potency, and might. Seeing the victim as a conquest, the rapist temporarily feels omnipotent.

The **sadistic rape** also involves brutality. The use of bondage and torture is not an expression of anger but a necessary ingredient for the rapist to become sexually excited. The assault is eroticized and is sexually stimulating. For this person to achieve sexual gratification, an unwilling sexual partner who will resist his advances is necessary. Rape becomes a source of excitement in his life (Groth and Birnbaum 1980).

Interpersonal Theories

Some rapists are unable to develop intimate and strong relationships with other men and women. The relationships they do have are unequal and characterized by a lack of mutuality and an inability to share. With this model for relationships, the rapist sees no need for consent to sexual activity, particularly within a marital relationship. The husband may view the rape as merely a disagreement over sexual activity. Unless he is extremely brutal, the wife may not regard the forced sex as an assault and rape either. Both of them may view sexual relationships as exploitive rather than a process of mutual sharing. If the wife has said she does not want to engage in sex and the husband uses force, her control and autonomy have been violated. When sex occurs without consent, it is, in fact, rape. What appears to be a conflict over sex in the marriage is actually a conflict over power and the right to consent to or refuse a given activity (Finkelhor and Vllo 1985, Burt 1980).

Sociocultural Theories

The acceptance of interpersonal violence in a culture contributes to a higher incidence of rape within that culture. Society's approval of the use of intimidation, coercion, and force to achieve one's goals promotes an excessive level of violence. It becomes an issue of power and strength rather than a consideration of individuals' rights.

Rigid gender role expectations and stereotypes may be correlated with the incidence of rape. When women are considered inferior to men, there is tacit approval given for coercion and force. These stereotypes support the false beliefs that at times women deserve to be raped, that they may want or need to be raped, and that it does not cause them much physical or emotional damage.

More than half of sexually abused women are the victims of **acquaintance rape**, or **date rape**. Rape by an acquaintance, friend, lover, boyfriend, or husband fits this category. Some of the reasons that are thought to account for acquaintance rape are sociocultural and are based on societal attitudes toward females. These stereotypes are perpetuated when, in instances of acquaintance rape, the woman's actions, rather than the man's, are questioned. It is believed that elimination of stereotypes and sexism will decrease men's use of rape as a way to demonstrate power and control (Resick 1983, Groth and Birnbaum 1980). Russell (1975, p 16) describes it this way:

> Rape is the ultimate sexist act. It is an act of physical and psychic oppression. Eradicating rape requires getting rid of the power discrepancy between men and women, because abuse of power flows from unequal power.

Steps that men can take to reduce rape are presented in Box 25–2.

Agism, which defines the older person as weak and incompetent, is a correlate to the crime of rape. Older people, especially those who are socially isolated or live alone, are seen as easy victims. Some older people, believing the myth that only young women are raped, do not protect themselves as well as they could. Older people are more vulnerable if they have established patterns of daily activities that can be readily observed. If they depend on walking or public transportation, they can be more easily accosted, particularly if their vision and hearing are impaired. Moreover, they may have neither the physical strength to resist a rape nor the ability to outrun the rapist.

Prevention and Resistance

Awareness, trusting intuitive feelings, and assertive behavior are the key to preventing rape. While awareness can be

---

Box 25–2
STEPS MEN CAN TAKE
TO PREVENT RAPE

- Tell other men that you do not think rape jokes are funny.

- Set time aside to talk with the women in your life about working toward equal relationships.

- Confront men who are harassing women on the street or at a party.

- Point out sexist comments and behavior to your friends and co-workers.

- Be aware of situations that increase a woman's vulnerability. How would you respond if you witnessed an intoxicated woman at a party being escorted by two or three men to a bedroom?

- If a woman says no to your sexual advances, respect that no at face value. Do not accept the myth that no means yes.

- In a dating or intimate relationship communicate clearly how you feel and what you want. Do not assume that your date or partner feels the same way. Respect the other person's feelings and needs.

- Learn new skills to help you express your anger in constructive, rather than destructive, ways.

Source: Adapted from Resources Against Sexual Assault. *Rape Prevention Education Program, University of California, San Francisco, 1987, p 4.*

---

taught, it may be more difficult for women to rely on their intuition or to apply assertive behavior because they do not want to appear suspicious or unfriendly. However, being polite and friendly may signal to the rapist that one is an "easy mark" and unlikely to resist. Rape prevention strategies in various environmental settings are presented in Box 25–3.

There is no one easy answer to the question of how one should behave if attacked. According to the Rape Prevention Education Program at the University of California, research indicates that while an immediate aggressive response increases one's possibility of escape when rape is threatened, it can sometimes slightly aggravate the situation (*Resources Against Sexual Assault,* 1987). Suggestions for resisting attack are discussed in Box 25–4.

Before rape victims are assessed or treated, they need to be informed of their rights, which include the right to have:

- A rape crisis advocate accompany them to the hospital

- Their personal physician notified

- Privacy during the assessment and treatment process

- Family, friends, or an advocate present during the questioning and examination

- Confidentiality maintained by all staff

- Gentle and sensitive treatment

- Detailed explanations and consent for all tests and procedures

- Referrals for follow-up treatment and counseling

The nurse functions as an advocate for rape victims in supporting these rights.

Assessment

Rape victims need first to be assessed physically from head to toe for any serious or critical injuries that may have resulted from the assault. With the victim's permission, a vaginal examination is performed for treatment and legal proceedings. Again with permission, photographs of the injuries may be taken for legal documentation (Foley 1984). The physical assessment process must be carefully documented in writing to assist with possible prosecution of the perpetrator. Guidelines to assist with physical assessment are given in Box 25–5.

The victim's mental status then needs to be assessed. Behavioral, affective, and intellectual responses to the traumatic event need to be gathered. A sociocultural assessment provides additional data for planning appropriate interventions. Guidelines for assessing the rape victim's mental status are given in Box 25–6.

Victims who present a controlled style may be able to respond to assessment questions, but those in a state of emotional shock and disbelief may find it difficult to engage actively in the assessment process. The method by which the nurse completes the assessment obviously depends on the person's response to the trauma.

Nursing Diagnosis

The central NANDA diagnosis for clients who have been raped is rape trauma syndrome. This is a general category for clients experiencing the syndromes described in Table 25–2. Several other nursing diagnoses may also be appro-

Box 25–3
RAPE PREVENTION STRATEGIES

At Home

In an apartment or house:

- Good locks on doors and windows make it difficult for assailants and burglars to get in. If you have a deadbolt, use it. For information on window locks and other home security measures consult the crime prevention unit of your local police department.

- When you're home alone, pull the shades or curtains after dark. If you let someone in and have second thoughts, be assertive: (1) tell him to leave; (2) leave if you can; (3) call a friend or neighbor and ask her or him to come over; (4) pretend you're not alone; mention a family member or a friend who is sleeping or about to return.

- Make sure hallways, entrances, garages, and grounds are well lighted. (Timers or photosensitive devices may be installed to conserve electricity.) Leave porch light on all night. When away from home at night or if you expect to return after dark, leave an interior light on in a room or two with shades drawn, and leave a radio on.

- Install a peephole in your door.

- When someone is at your door, never open it without first asking who's there. Repair and sales people, police and survey takers carry identification; ask to see it and then call the company to verify before letting the person in. If someone wants to use your phone, make the call for him, while he waits outside.

- Leave spare house keys with a friend, not under the doormat, in planter boxes, etc.

- Get to know your neighbors so you can get help if necessary and are familiar with who's coming and going in the neighborhood.

- List last name and two initials only on mailbox and door and in phone book. Consider not listing your address in the phone book.

- Avoid giving out information about yourself or making appointments with strangers over the phone.

- Have a preconceived escape plan.

In residence halls and student housing:

- Living groups are only as safe as the residents make them. *Take your share of responsibility.* Always keep outside doors locked. Ask strangers to wait outside while you get their friends. Lock your room when you

leave—even if only for a few minutes. Look out for one another.

In Public Places

On the street:

- *Be alert.* Look around you; be aware of who else is on the street; make it difficult for anyone to take you by surprise.

- Wait a few minutes in order to walk or bike with others. If you have a choice, don't walk alone.

- Stay on populated, well-lighted streets when you can.

- If possible, avoid dark or concealed areas—consider open areas—walk in the street if it appears to be safer.

- If you think someone is following you:
    — Turn around and check so you're not caught off guard.
    — Cross the street, change direction.
    — Walk or run toward people, traffic.
    — Consider confronting the man with a loud, firm voice, "Don't follow me!"
    — Do anything necessary to enter an occupied building; throw something through a window if necessary.

- If a car follows you or stops, do not approach the car. Change directions, walk or run toward other people, stores, or a house.

In the car:

- Park in well-lighted areas at night; pay for parking. Check the street before leaving the car.

- Walk to your car with key ready.

- Check the backseat before you get in to make sure no one is hiding there.

- While driving, keep doors locked so no one can jump in at a red light.

- Keep enough gas in your tank for emergencies.

- If you're followed by another car, drive to a police or fire station, or hospital emergency entrance or any open business or gas station. DON'T go home or to a friend's home. If necessary, call attention to yourself by honking the horn or speeding.

- If your car breaks down, lift hood, put on flashers,

continued

Box 25–3 (continued)

and wait inside with the doors locked. Ask people who stop to call the California Highway Patrol (or AAA if you are a member).

- Don't stop for a stranded motorist; call the California Highway Patrol, local police, or sheriff's department, who can help him.

Elevators:

- Trust your intuition; if you feel uncomfortable you don't have to get on or off.
- Stand near the controls. If necessary, you can press all the buttons or use the telephone.

Jogging:

- Be aware.
- Try to avoid jogging alone, even in daylight.
- Stay on well-lighted paths in open areas.
- Vary your route.
- Be suspicious of people you pass many times.

Hitchhiking:

Hitchhiking increases your vulnerability to sexual assault. However, if you do risk it:

- Consider taking rides only from women.
- Ask first where a driver is going before you volunteer

your destination; never go with someone who offers to take you wherever you want to go.

- If there is more than one man in a car, do not accept a ride.
- Always jot down the license number of the car.
- While entering the car, check to be sure there is an inside handle to the door on the passenger side.
- Mention that someone is waiting for you and will be anxious if you are late.

Using public transportation:

- If possible, wait for buses at well-lighted stops.
- *Be alert* so you can't be grabbed from behind.
- If possible, join other people at a nearby stop.
- If anyone bothers you on the bus:
  — In a loud, firm voice say "Leave me alone!"
  — Let other riders and the bus driver know what's happening.
  — If the bus is radio dispatched, ask the driver to call the police.
  — Don't get off in an isolated area.
- Notice who else gets off at your stop. If someone is following you, practice the tips for street safety.

Source: Adapted from Resources Against Sexual Assault. *Rape Prevention Education Program, University of California, San Francisco, 1987, pp 13–17.*

---

priate, depending on the client's needs and the results of both physical and mental status assessment.

There is no corresponding DSM-IIIR diagnosis. Rape is, however, mentioned specifically as the type of trauma that may result in post-traumatic stress disorder. Rape victims may also experience one of the anxiety disorders or sexual dysfunctions discussed in DSM-IIIR.

Planning and Implementing Interventions

Nursing actions appropriate to the three phases of rape trauma syndrome are summarized in Table 25–3.

Acute Phase

Physical and mental status priorities must be quickly established by the health care team. Attention must then be

given to long-range physical, emotional, social, and legal concerns of the victim.

It is advantageous to the client to have a primary nurse assigned in the emergency room. The client needs a warm, accepting, understanding, and respectful relationship with the nurse. If police officers are involved, the nurse needs to act as an advocate in helping the client decide when to talk with the police about the rape. The nurse needs also to provide breaks in the questioning if the client appears overwhelmed and distressed by the interview. A nursing care plan for the acute phase is given on page 663.

Outward Adjustment Phase

Nurses may have contact with a rape victim or her or his family in the outward adjustment phase in their roles as school or industry nurses or mental health counselors or in their roles as citizens and community members.

Box 25–4
SUGGESTIONS FOR RESISTING ATTACK

- Evaluate the situation for possible ways of escape. If one method doesn't work, try another, and another; often women have had to try several before one worked.

- Resist only as long as you feel it is safe to do so. If resistance proves to be too dangerous, stop. It may be less dangerous, however, to risk minor injury in order to escape than to remain in an assault situation.

Women have deterred assailants in a variety of ways. Talking and thinking about what you might do if attacked increase your chances for successfully defending yourself. We provide the following brief list to stimulate your thinking.

Verbal

- Deep, guttural yell that is simply a startling sound, not any word.

- Yell directions, e.g., "Call the police, this man is after me!"

- Yell "fire" rather than "help" or "rape." Though our intent is not to hide sexual assault from the community, yelling "fire" is more apt to bring a response, because people are concerned with protecting their own property. If *you* ever hear a yell of "help" or "rape," take it seriously and respond.

- Do something unpredictable.

- Assertive verbal confrontation, e.g., "Leave me alone!" "Stop bothering me!"

- Make noise, e.g., throw a heavy object through your window if someone attempts to enter your home.

Physical

- Escape, or put something between you and him.

- Run.

- Fight (see information on self-defense).

- Use available objects as weapons.

- Use tear gas. In the State of California you must take a class to obtain a license to carry tear gas legally. We recommend taking a class that informs you of the drawbacks of tear gas as well as the situations in which it is effective. Using tear gas is one of several options and cannot be relied on to work in every situation. It works best when used in conjunction with physical self-defense techniques.

Only the person being attacked can decide whether resistance or submission is the safer thing to do. If you do submit, it doesn't mean you asked for it, enjoyed it, or wanted it. Rather, you chose the best survival technique available to you at the time.

Self-Defense Classes

As previously mentioned, an immediate aggressive response is more likely to result in rape avoidance than in further violence. We urge women to take classes in street-fighting techniques that can be learned in a relatively short period of time. The benefits of learning self-defense include increased options for self-protection, self-confidence, and verbal and nonverbal assertiveness skills. If you decide to resist physically, know how to do it effectively. The Rape Prevention Education Program recommends classes that combine street-fighting techniques with sexual assault prevention information.

Source: Adapted from Resources Against Sexual Assault. *Rape Prevention Education Program, University of California, San Francisco, 1987, pp 19–21.*

Encouraging, but not forcing, mental health counseling on rape victims and their families may help them cope with their feelings during this time.

Reorganization Phase

Many victims have a strong urge to discuss their feelings and experiences during the reorganization phase. Rape counseling may be especially helpful during this phase.

Three phases of rape counseling have been identified by Foley and Davies (1983):

1. *Self-exploration* revolves around establishing a rela-

tionship with the client and helping the client verbalize thoughts and feelings.

2. *Self-understanding* focuses on working to identify the source of the feelings and exploring the behaviors the client can undertake to resolve feelings.

3. *Action* involves making specific, often step-by-step, plans for action and testing out alternatives. A major emphasis in this phase is the client's resumption of control over her or his own life.

Some clients may find family therapy or social networking activities such as women's groups or self-defense

---

Box 25–5
PHYSICAL ASSESSMENT OF THE RAPE VICTIM

Complete a head-to-toe physical assessment with particular attention to the following:

Head

Evidence of trauma
Facial bruises
Facial fractures
Eyes: swollen, bruised, hemorrhages

Skin

Bruises
Genital trauma
Rectal trauma

Musculoskeletal

Fractures of the ribs
Fractures of arms/legs
Dislocated joints
Impaired mobility

Abdomen

Bruises or wounds
Evidence of internal injuries

Other

Have physical injuries such as scratches, bruises, and cuts been recorded and photographed?
Have fingernail scrapings been taken and preserved?
Has blood typing been done?
Have smears for sexually transmitted diseases been taken of the mouth, throat, vagina, and rectum?
Have combings of the pubic hair been made and preserved?
Has genital trauma been recorded and photographed?
Has rectal trauma been recorded and photographed?
Have semen specimens been preserved?
When was the client's last menstrual period?
Has the clothing been inspected for rips, blood, and stains?
Has the clothing been preserved?

Box 25–6
NURSING HISTORY TOOL FOR ASSESSMENT OF THE RAPE VICTIM

Behavioral Assessment

Is the client able to respond verbally to questions?
Is the client able to follow simple directions?
Has the client bathed, douched, changed clothes, or done any self-treatment before coming to the hospital?

Affective Assessment

Which of the following emotions is the client experiencing? Describe with objective and subjective data.
Disbelief
Shame
Embarrassment
Humiliation
Hopelessness
Vulnerability
Anxiety
Fear
Guilt
Anger
Depression
Alienation from others

Cognitive Assessment

Evidence of defense mechanisms.
Is the client confused?
Has the client been informed of her rights?
Describe the client's attention span.
Is the client able to describe what occurred?
Is the client able to make decisions?
Who has the client informed about the rape? Family? Friends? Police?
Does the client need assistance in telling others?
Is the client blaming self for the attack?
Is the client experiencing flashbacks to the attack?
What does this event represent to the client?

Sociocultural Assessment

Who and where are the available support systems for the client? Family? Friends? Advocate? Clergyperson?
Is the client in need of temporary shelter?
Does the client know about available counseling?

---

classes helpful in addition to, or as a substitute for, rape counseling.

Evaluation

The long-term goal of intervention with rape victims is that they return to their prerape level, or a higher level, of functioning. Three general outcomes must occur if the crisis is to be resolved in an adaptive fashion (Warner 1980):

1. Verbalization of accurate cognitive perceptions of the rape

2. Emotional equilibrium

3. Adaptive coping behaviors

Crisis intervention is terminated when the evaluation process determines that the client has met the outcome criteria. Some clients will need or desire long-term counseling to adjust to the trauma of rape.

INTRAFAMILY VIOLENCE— PHYSICAL ABUSE

Family violence, although a centuries-old practice, gained public attention in the 1970s as a social problem of magnitude. Before that time, the beating of children, wives, and the elderly was often justified as a means of necessary

discipline. Those who would intervene had no legal basis on which to do so. The problem is illustrated in the case below.

In 1874 a church worker in New York City was contacted by the neighbors of a local family. This family had a 9-year-old named Mary Ellen as an indentured servant in their household. Neighbors reported that the

---

RESEARCH NOTE

Citation

Burgess AW, Hartman CR, Wolbert WA, Grant CA: Child molestation: Assessing impact in multiple victims. Arch Psychiatr Nurs *1987;1(1):33–39.*

Study Problem/Purpose

The purpose of this study was to ascertain the impact of child molestation among twelve young girls who had been sexually abused on a school bus by the driver.

Methods

The study sample comprised twelve girls, ranging in age from 6 to 9 years, who had been abused over a four-month period while riding a school bus. The children and their parents were interviewed to collect data on the present functioning of the child at home and at school and to review with the parents any symptoms and concerns. Data were also collected to assess how the child retrospectively structured the experience of sexual abuse through (1) attributions and (2) drawings.

Attributions were explored by asking specific questions such as: "Why do you think this happened to you?" "Why do you think the man did this to you?" and "Why do you think he kept doing it to you?" These and other attribution questions were designed to reveal how the children presently explain their personal responsibility to themselves, to what extent they believe themselves to be vulnerable, to what extent they perceived the events as controllable, and what they did to survive the assault.

Each child was also asked to make a sequence of seven drawings—favorite weather, herself at a younger age, herself at her current age, her family doing something, the sexual abuse event, a house and a tree, and a "free" drawing. The drawings were designed to elicit the child's mood state, body image and self-esteem, perception of her social support network, memory and recall of the event, and the degree of anxiety she felt about the abuse.

Data analysis was by a drawing assessment tool with a standardized list of characteristics for interpreting the

drawings, and analysis of the attribution questions according to specific criteria for each question. Six clinicians rated the drawings and the children's responses to the attribution questions.

Findings

The data suggest that in order to survive molestation, children dissociate complex units of social behavior. When the children were asked to recall what happened, the unresolved molestation event disrupted and impaired their performance and social interaction as demonstrated through the series of drawings. Blocking on questions, anxiety, and confusion were reported. The children manifested varying degrees of symptoms of post-traumatic stress disorder. The findings suggest possible deviations in later life such as: (1) excessive passivity, (2) self-appraisals that could be linked to guilt and depression, (3) the fragmentation and isolation of body parts in drawings suggests that internalization of the trauma may be a precursor to psychotic reactions or multiple personality, and (4) the acting-out behaviors, both sexual and aggressive, direct attention to possible links to later socially deviant behavior patterns.

Implications

The data suggest that both children who are victims of sexual molestation and their parents need intervention to avoid developmental lags. Parents generally handled the sexual abuse event by limiting discussion of it in the home, leaving both the daughters and their parents to cope as best they could. The researchers suggest that the following interventions be employed: (1) individual counseling with art for the child victim, and (2) group and art-work follow-up intervention for both the children and their parents. Intervention is crucial at those times of social disclosure when court actions are in process to correct distortions and begin to "move the child from a victim position to that of an active survivor." The child in whom an unresolved suppressed traumatic event surfaces is at risk for delayed post-traumatic stress disorder.

Table 25–3
**Nursing Actions Appropriate to Phases of the
Rape Trauma Syndrome**

Phase	Nursing Action
Acute phase	Creating a safe milieu
	Explaining the sequence of events in the health care facility
	Allowing the victim to grieve and express feelings
	Providing care for significant others
Outward adjustment phase	Providing advocacy and support at the level requested by the victim
	Providing assistance to significant others
Reorganizational phase	Establishing a trusting relationship
	Assisting the victim to understand her or his role in the assault
	Clarifying and enhancing the victim's feelings
	Assisting the victim in planning for the future

*Source: Adapted from Niehaus MA: Rape, in Griffith-Kenney J:
Contemporary Women's Health. Addison-Wesley, 1986, p 229.*

child was beaten daily, stabbed with scissors, and tied to a bed. When the church worker tried to intervene, she found that there was no legal way to rescue Mary Ellen from the people who were mistreating her. United States laws did not provide for the rescue of battered children. However, the church worker was persistent in her efforts, finally going to the Society for the Prevention of Cruelty to Animals (SPCA) for help. Using the rationale that Mary Ellen was a member of the animal kingdom, the SPCA authorities were able to remove the child from the couple's home and bring them to trial, where the wife was sentenced to one year in prison. This led to the founding in 1875 of the New York Society for the Prevention of Cruelty to Children, the first such organization of its kind in the United States.

More recent public attention to family violence has been due mainly to the efforts of feminist organizations.

Intrafamily physical abuse, violence within the family, occurs within all strata of society. The myth is that physical abuse occurs only among the poor and undereducated, but in reality physical abuse also occurs among white-collar workers and professionals. In the past these problems among wealthy or prominent people were kept hidden from the general public. With an increase in national concern, however, more publicity is being given to cases of intrafamily physical abuse at all levels of society (Jackson 1985).

Although the image of the nuclear family in American culture is one of agreement, happiness, cohesiveness, and harmony, this ideal public image is often in conflict with the underlying reality of abuse and violence within the family. In fact, the family home may be the most dangerous place to live since violence is more likely to occur within the family than between strangers. Children are beaten by their parents, brothers and sisters beat one another, spouses beat each other, and even elderly parents are beaten by family members. Beatings often escalate into more severe violence with 25 percent of all murders occurring within the family unit (Thorman 1980, Straus and Hotaling 1980).

Incidence of Physical Abuse

Child Abuse

Each year approximately 3.8 percent of children between the ages of 3 and 17 are beaten, which places the number at two million physically abused children (Humphreys and Campbell 1984). As the general public has become more aware of the problem, more cases are being reported, but these are probably only a small percentage of the total. To know if the actual rate of incidence is increasing is impossible because of lack of historical data. Laws mandating the reporting of child abuse were not passed in all 50 states until 1968 (Straus et al. 1980).

The sex of the child does not appear to be significant in the incidence of abuse. Of those children under the age of three who are abused, as many as 25 percent die from the abuse. Some studies say the most dangerous age for abuse is 3 months to 3 years. Other studies say the incidence of abuse increases during adolescence. By the time the abuse is discovered and reported, most acts of violence have been going on for one to three years (Thorman 1980, Straus et al. 1980).

Mothers are more physically abusive to their children than fathers. Several explanations are given for this higher incidence of violence. Mothers typically spend a greater amount of time with their children and thus experience greater parental stress in raising them. Because the culture judges the mother's competency as a parent on the behavior of her children, she is more likely to use physical force to obtain the obedience of her children so that others will see her as an adequate, responsible parent. The third factor is that having children does not generally interfere with the father's career plans, but it often does interfere with

Nursing Care Plan: The Victim of Rape During the Acute Phase

Nursing Diagnosis: 04.01.01 Rape trauma syndrome/Rape trauma syndrome*
Goal: Client will return to prerape level of functioning within six weeks.

Intervention	Rationale	Expected Outcome
Give client time to respond to simple questions.	Anxiety decreases the ability to perceive input and slows the responsive time.	
If client is unable to express feelings, acknowledge the difficulty (e.g., "I understand that it is difficult for you to describe your feelings right now. That's okay. You may be able to talk about them later.").	Support defense mechanisms until client is able to cope with the reality of the situation.	
Communicate your knowledge and understanding of usual emotional responses to rape (e.g., "People usually experience a number of feelings such as anxiety, fear, embarrassment, guilt, or anger.").	Client needs to be reassured that these feelings are a normal reaction to rape.	Client identifies and expresses feelings about the rape.
Encourage client to talk about the rape.	Talking with others will assist client through the stage of disbelief.	Client talks about the rape.
Identify distortions related to self-blame or guilt.	Beliefs of personal responsibility and fault interfere with resolution of the syndrome.	Client identifies self as a victim.
Identify specific coping behavior client used during the rape (e.g., screaming, fighting, talking, blacking out).	Identifying behavior as an adaptive mechanism to survive will increase self-esteem and decrease feelings of guilt.	Client identifies adaptive behavior.
Encourage client to discuss the personal meaning of the rape.	Clarification of specific fears or concerns will assist nurse in formulating additional interventions.	Client verbalizes anticipated problems.
Help client identify and arrange immediate concerns in order of importance.	Focusing on immediate problems decreases sense of confusion and the feeling of being overwhelmed.	Client identifies most important concerns.
Assist client to use the problem-solving process in developing solutions to concerns.	The problem-solving process will increase feelings of control.	Client develops short-term plan for concerns.
Support client's making own decisions and acting in own behalf.	Decision making will help client regain feelings of control and autonomy.	Client makes necessary decisions.
Assist client to identify who to tell and how to tell about the rape.	Anticipatory guidance will assist client in using available support systems.	Client uses significant others for support.
Discuss beliefs about postcoital contraception and abortion if appropriate.	Pregnancy may be a realistic outcome of the rape. Clients need to be provided with information about available choices.	Client verbalizes understanding of available choices.

continued

Nursing Care Plan: The Victim of Rape During the Acute Phase (*Continued*)

Intervention	Rationale	Expected Outcome
Discuss need for follow-up medical evaluation and treatment for sexually transmitted diseases.	Providing client with information about potential physical problems will help ensure prevention of disease.	Client verbalizes importance of medical care.
Provide anticipatory guidance about common physical, emotional, and social reactions to rape.	Client needs to know what to expect and needs guidelines for need for additional counseling.	Client acknowledges understanding of potential reactions.
Provide written list of referrals to community resources.	Crisis intervention counseling may decrease long-term impact of rape.	Client verbalizes need for short-term counseling.
Make follow-up phone contact within two to four days.	Client may need additional support to follow through on formulated plans.	Client implements immediate plans.

*PND-I/NANDA diagnoses.

the mother's career plans. Thus, having children in the home may interrupt a mother's career and threaten her self-image.

Sibling Abuse

The most common and unrecognized form of family violence occurs between siblings. Many people assume it is natural and even appropriate that children use physical force with one another. Statements are made such as, "It's a good chance for him to learn how to defend himself," "She had a right to hit him. He was teasing her," or "Kids will be kids." These attitudes teach children that physical force is an appropriate method of resolving conflict among themselves. Sibling violence is highest in the early years and decreases with age. In all age groups girls are less violent toward their siblings than are boys.

Spouse Abuse

National attention to spouse abuse is more recent than the concern for child abuse. The woman's movement in the 1970s brought the issue into the public domain. In 1976 efforts were begun to establish resources for battered wives. There has been a continuing focus on providing counseling and shelters and passing new laws to protect the abused spouse.

How many adults are abused by their spouses or live-in partners is unknown. The statistics range from 11 to 34 percent of the population. It is believed that as many as 80 percent of the cases are unreported because the victims are ashamed, feel responsible, or fear reprisal in the form of increased violence (Resick 1983). One out of every six couples in the United States will commit at least one act of violence against each other in any given year. That incidence rises to one out of every three couples when the entire length of the relationship is considered (Straus et al. 1980).

In couples filing for divorce, it is generally found that most abuse cases involve violence by husbands. In the cases where both partners are violent, it is unknown what proportion are women acting in self-defense. Women are more vulnerable to violence because of their disadvantage in size and strength and their social and economic dependence on men.

Elder Abuse

National attention to the abuse of the elderly by family members is just beginning. Elder abuse may take the form of having basic physical needs neglected. Some elderly people are psychologically abused by verbal assaults, threats, or isolation. Some are financially exploited by their relatives through theft or misuse of property or funds. Others are beaten and even raped by family members.

The rate of elder abuse is unknown because many older people are ashamed to admit that their children have abused them and often fear retaliation if help is sought. At present, between 4 and 11 percent of older persons are being abused. The majority of the victims are between the ages of 59 and 90. Older women are more likely to be abused and account for 75 percent of the reported cases. Two-thirds of the abusers are over the age of 40, and half of them are either sons or daughters of the victims. Spouse abuse accounts for 12 percent of the cases among the elderly, with the remaining abusers being other relatives such as grandchildren, siblings, nieces, and nephews. As the proportion of elderly increases in this country, it is likely that abuse of the elderly will become a greater problem (Sengstock and Barrett 1984).

Characteristics of Intrafamily Violence

Behavioral Characteristics

Acts of violence within the family range from a light slap, to a severe beating, to a homicide. Hitting or spanking children, with 84 to 94 percent of all parents using this form of discipline at some time in the life of a child, is condoned and even approved of as being necessary and good for the child. Many parents, however, do not realize that these underlying messages are given to the child (Straus et al. 1980):

- If you are small and weak, you deserve to be hit.
- People who love you hit you.
- It is appropriate to hit people you love.
- Violence is appropriate if the end result is good.
- Violence is an appropriate method of resolving conflict.

Parental violence can become extreme and often becomes chronic in that it occurs periodically or regularly. Many times, it ends in the death of the infant or child.

A young father was convicted in the death of his six-month-old daughter. He had beaten her to death because she would not stop crying (Father convicted, 1985).

The boyfriend of the mother of a two-year-old boy was charged with the boy's murder. While caring for the child, the boyfriend bit him on the face, abdomen, and buttocks. The child bled to death from deep bite wounds into the abdominal cavity (O'Connor 1985).

The father of a 17-year-old young man was convicted of solicitation to commit murder. There was evidence of previous physical abuse with the son testifying that

he had been beaten with a broomstick and a hose, and at one point his father had held a cocked, loaded gun to his head. Previously, the father told the son: "I can't wait until you die. When you die, I'll put your name on my trucks to show my appreciation" (Rossi 1985).

Acts of violence between adult family members fall along the same continuum with women committing fewer violent acts than men. Women do more hitting, kicking, and throwing of objects when involved in violent conflict with men. The acts that men commit against women are more dangerous and result in more severe injuries. Men are likely to push, shove, slap, beat up, and even use knives or guns against their wives or girlfriends (Straus et al. 1980). In one study (Giles-Sims 1983) of abused women, it was found that 50 percent of the abusing men had threatened their partners with a knife or gun, and 25 percent had actually assaulted their partners with a knife or gun.

There is real danger that women may be killed by a violent male family member. A study of 538 women murdered in 1981 found that 29 percent of these women were killed by their current husbands or boyfriends. If the data had included former husbands or boyfriends, the percentage would have been higher. In one study of domestic killings, there was a history of wife abuse in 71.9 percent of the murders. Women are more likely to kill their husbands or boyfriends as an act of self-defense when battering has been a continual problem in the home (Campbell 1984a).

A pattern of behavior usually develops in violent families. The first incident may be precipitated by frustration or stress. If a pattern of violence is to be avoided, the victim must immediately refuse to accept the violence. Outside help may be necessary to put a stop to the behavior. If the victim submits to the violence, physical force, without the stimulus of frustration or stress, becomes a way of relating to one another, and the pattern becomes resistant to change. Intrafamily violence is typically cyclic. Conflict escalates into a violent episode. After the episode, the perpetrator, feeling regret and shame, begs for the victim's forgiveness. The victim stays in the system because the perpetrator promises to reform and perhaps because of material rewards for remaining. During the next episode of conflict, the cycle begins again, and violence becomes a stable pattern of family behavior (Giles-Sims 1983).

Michael, age 45, is a very successful physician. During recent divorce proceedings, he has confessed to beating his wife Maria, periodically. At times, he would yank her around by the hair or hold her out of a second-story window and threaten to let her fall. During each of Maria's three pregnancies, Michael would beat her, particularly in her abdomen, saying he wished he could kill both her and the unborn child. This periodic abuse has continued throughout the 20-year marriage but was kept a family secret until the divorce proceedings.

Many victims of abuse attempt to cope by becoming compliant. They try to placate the abuser hoping that conflict will not escalate into physical abuse. However, the more submissive the victim becomes, the more severe and frequent the abuse becomes. If victims are dependent on the security of the home, they often accept the abuse rather than risk disruption of the family. Some victims, immobilized by fear, are unable to leave the abuser. Others attempt to leave but are tracked down and forced back into the home by the abuser. Both fear and inability to escape contribute to further compliant behavior in the victim.

Affective Characteristics

Physically abusive people are often described as extremely jealous and possessive. They view other family members in terms of property and ownership. Within a culture that historically condones violence as a method of protecting property rights, these people believe violence is an acceptable method of maintaining the family unit. Extreme jealousy can escalate to hostility toward the victim and even the entire world as the abuser feels forced to defend his or her rights of ownership.

Some abusers have strong dependency needs and fear the loss of intimate relationships. They may beat a child because of the competition for the love and attention of their spouse. Some men are so dependent and fearful of loss that when their wives attempt to become more independent, they respond with violence.

Closely related to the dependency needs of abusers is the feeling of inadequacy. Abusers use violence in an attempt to prove to themselves and others that they are superior and in control. The use of physical force temporarily decreases their fears of inadequacy and compensates for the lack of other internal resources. People who feel inadequate in relationships may use violence to create emotional distance and thereby avoid the fears of closeness and intimacy (Thorman 1980, Giles-Sims 1983).

Victims may be immobilized by a variety of affective responses to the abuse. In one study, it was found that 25 percent of the victims felt guilty, 50 percent felt helpless, and 75 percent experienced feelings of depression (Resick 1983). The feelings of guilt and self-blame may be expressed in statements such as, "If I were a better wife, he wouldn't beat me," or "If I hadn't talked back to my mother, she wouldn't have hit me." Victims who feel responsible for the abuser's behavior may also experience guilt if they are unable to change the pattern of violence within the family. Many victims feel helpless to prevent the violence and fear greater injury or death if they attempt to defend themselves. Guilt can contribute to distorted thinking and depression, which further immobilize the victim from leaving or seeking help for the family system.

Cognitive Characteristics

Many abusive people have perfectionistic standards for themselves and members of their families. There is a sense of rigidity and an obsession with discipline and control. This inflexibility decreases their ability to find alternative solutions to conflict. Some abusers are self-righteous, believing it is their right to use physical force to get others to comply with their wishes. Many abusers lack understanding of the effect of their behavior on the victims and may even blame their abusive behavior on the victims. Inadequate self-esteem contributes to feelings of impotency and the use of power to counteract this negative self-evaluation.

Many parents who abuse their children suffered emotional deprivation when they themselves were children. As a result, they may have unrealistic expectations of their own children. Anger may turn to violence when the children are unable to fulfill the unrealistic emotional needs of the parent.

Other parents may have minimal information about children's growth and development and unrealistic expectations of what the child is capable of performing. In this situation, child abuse may begin—for example, when the child is not toilet trained by the age of 9 months, an unrealistic expectation on their part.

Victims of abuse often begin with or develop an inadequate self-esteem. Victims who are beaten begin to believe that the violence itself is evidence of personal worthlessness. This distorted thinking process contributes to guilt and a toleration of the violence.

Some victims believe they are helpless to change the pattern of domination or to leave the relationship. Some victims rationalize that the perpetrator was not responsible for the abusive actions, but that the behavior was the result of a high level of stress or too much alcohol. The belief in reform is a common characteristic among victims. When the abuser promises never to strike again, the victim is seduced by the hope of reform and the belief that perhaps this was the last incident of violence. Wives who believe the responsibility for maintaining the family unit belongs to women may stay in a battering relationship in an attempt to keep the family together. This responsibility may also be a factor for women who submit to abuse out of the fear that the children will become victims if they do not submit (Resick 1983, Campbell 1984a).

Physiologic Characteristics

A variety of injuries may be inflicted on victims of physical abuse. In general, small children may be retarded in the areas of growth and development. For victims of all ages, any combination of the following characteristics may be observed (Humphreys 1984, Campbell 1984b):

- There may be bald patches where hair has been pulled out, or there may be subdural hematomas from blows to the head.

- The eyes may be bruised or swollen, or the victim may have hemorrhages into the eyes.

- The skin, genitals, and rectal areas may be bruised or burned and may show scars of past injuries.

- Fractures, or evidence of previous fractures, may be present, particularly of the face, arms, and ribs.

- Joints are often dislocated, especially in the shoulder, when the victim is grabbed or pulled around by the arm.

- Intra-abdominal injuries are common, especially in pregnant women.

- Neurologically, the victim may have areas of parasthesias or numbness from old injuries, and their reflexes may be hyperactive from neurologic damage.

Sociocultural Characteristics

The abuser's family of origin is an important factor in understanding intrafamily violence. Violence is often perpetuated by each generation in the family unless circumstances occur that alter the family dynamics.

Much of adult behavior is determined by childhood experiences within the family system. Parents model marital interactions and parent-child interactions for their children. When the children grow up and form their own nuclear families, there is an unconscious attempt to recreate the same form of interactions within the new family system. Negative patterns are often repeated because they represent security despite the pain involved (Barash 1979). Thus, the experience of violence in the family of origin teaches the individual participants that the use of physical force is appropriate. Violence becomes integrated into the dynamics in such a way that violence and love are fused, or violence is perceived as morally right when used to achieve good results (Straus and Hotaling 1980). There is evidence that some adult abusers were emotionally neglected or abandoned as children. Since early security and dependency needs were not met, these adults are unable to meet their own children's needs for affection and trust (Thorman 1980).

Traditional gender roles affect the use of violence within the family. Violent families are more likely to enact sex-role stereotyping and to have a hierarchical family structure. Some men get caught up in compulsive masculinity whereby they feel a need to be tough, strong, aggressive, and nonemotional. These husbands see an egalitarian marital relationship as evidence of a lack of masculinity. They tend to marry women who are younger, less educated, and less economically productive in an attempt to support their superior position. In addition, they may view women as childlike and needing to be overprotected.

When the position of dominance or leadership is threatened by the wife or the children, violence is more likely to occur. Men whose sense of masculinity does not depend on positions of superiority or who are able to adapt to egalitarian relationships are less likely to use violence against their wives and children (Resick 1983, Giles-Sims 1983, Campbell 1984a).

The violent family is often socially isolated. In some families, the isolation precedes the violence. With few network support systems, the isolated family is less able to manage life stresses and may resort to violence in an attempt to cope with frustration. For other families, the social isolation is a response to the violence. Family members, ashamed of what is occurring, withdraw from interactions with others. This withdrawal prevents the humiliation that might occur if the violence became known to others.

Many violent families have experienced a high number of significant life events (see Chapter 7) before the onset of physical abuse. This bombardment of stress places a great deal of strain on the family's ability to adapt to change. When emotional, physical, or financial resources are drained, violence may erupt within the family system.

It is difficult for many women to leave an abusive relationship. Many women are financially dependent on their abusive husbands. If they have outside employment, they are unlikely to earn as much as their male counterparts. If there are children involved, they may desperately need financial child support, and many fathers do not honor this obligation and default on the payments. The burdens of child care have traditionally been assigned to the mother. Lack of affordable and adequate child care facilities is a major problem for the single mother seeking employment. Single parents may experience some social disapproval because of the separation or divorce. The cultural norm continues to be that two parents are always better for the children than one parent.

The criminal justice system has been unable to decrease significantly the amount of intrafamily violence in America. Police officers and lawyers have minimal or no training in crisis or family violence intervention. There may be long delays in obtaining court orders or peace bonds to protect the victims. Court cases are often rescheduled, causing long delays in legal relief. The victims need advocates in the court so that they are not revictimized by the trauma of the judicial system (Straus and Hotaling 1980, Giles-Sims 1983). Male and female defendants are often treated differently by the courts. Walker (1984, p 205) points out this difference in cases involving family violence: "Women who kill their husbands are more likely to be charged with first degree murder, while men who kill their wives are more likely to receive a manslaughter charge." Changes must be made within the criminal justice system to allow all victims legal relief from family violence.

Theoretical Perspectives

There is no single cause of family violence. Violent behavior takes many forms and has many origins. Aggressive behavior involves the internal and external systems of both the abuser and the victim. This multidimensional approach to understanding family violence includes biologic, intrapersonal, social learning, sociologic, and system theories.

Biologic Theories

The *instinctivist theory* suggests that people possess a natural fighting instinct that preserves the species. The animal kingdom is cited as proof that it is natural to protect territory and prey on smaller or weaker victims. Many authorities refute this theory stating that it confuses hunting for food with indiscriminate violence. Animal fighting for territory or mating privileges does not contain the cruelty that characterizes human violence. In addition, most animal groups work to keep fighting incidents at a minimum.

The *neurophysiologic theory* proposes that the limbic system and the neurotransmitters are implicated in violent behavior. It is thought that an increase in norepinephrine, dopamine, and serotonin increases irritability and may result in various types of aggression. Stimulation of the lateral and medial hypothalamus in animals produces attack behavior, whereas stimulation of the dorsal hypothalamus results in escape behavior. It is also thought that the septal area of the limbic system normally has an inhibiting influence, since lesions that destroy the septal region cause ferocious and vicious behavior in animals. Research is also continuing into the increased tendency toward violence in women experiencing premenstrual syndrome (PMS). The decrease in progesterone before menstruation is implicated in the symptoms of increased irritability and hostility that some women experience premenstrually.

Substance abuse, especially of alcohol, is often implicated in violent behavior. In some people, alcohol may decrease the normal inhibitions against violence and thereby increase the probability that violent behavior may occur. With high alcohol levels, people have a decreased verbal ability, an increased fear of attack from others, and a decreased recognition of their own inappropriate behavior. These factors may contribute to a violent outburst (Campbell 1984d, Montague 1979).

Intrapersonal Theories

The intrapersonal theories suggest that the cause of violence lies in the individual personalities of the abusers. It is thought that aggression is a basic drive within the personality and that people who are violent are unable to control the impulsive expression of anger and hostility. People who feel helpless or inadequate may use physical force in an attempt to defend themselves and increase their low self-esteem. Other explanations involve personality traits or disorders. Abusers are often obsessive-compulsive, jealous, suspicious, paranoid, or sadistic. Violent behavior may be used to enforce absolute discipline, protect one's "property," or protect one's self from being attacked (Giles-Sims 1983, Campbell 1984d).

Social Learning Theory

The social learning theory proposes that violence is a learned behavior rather than an instinctive behavior. It is believed that stimulation of the neurophysiologic mechanisms for violence are under cognitive control. Both the abuser and the victim learn their roles during childhood. Children learn about violence by observation, being a victim, or behaving violently themselves. If the use of violence is rewarded by a gain in power, the behavior is reinforced. If there is immediate negative reinforcement within the family, a decrease in violent behavior will occur (Walker 1984, Campbell 1984d). In addition to family models, the media have many models of violence to which children are exposed. Westerns, cartoons, police shows, and adventure movies all demonstrate that "good" people use force to achieve "good" ends. Much of the violence in the media does not even attempt to rationalize the use of force for "good" ends but rather is just endless, senseless cruelty of one human being to another. With these types of family and media examples, children develop values that tolerate and accept violence between people.

Sociologic Theory

The social environment can place additional stress on the family unit. Violent families tend to be multiproblem families that have experienced a prolonged series of significant life events such as illnesses, accidents, economic crises, and the entrance of new persons such as babies or aged parents. Factors such as underemployment, unemployment, and poverty contribute to feelings of anger and deprivation. When financial, physical, or emotional resources are limited and strained there is a greater probability that conflict will end in violence.

Identifiable factors contribute to the abuse of elders within the family. With the trend to smaller family size, there are fewer family members to share in the care of older parents, and with the longer life expectancy, the number of years of caring for a dependent parent have increased. As people live longer, they often develop many medical problems, and the cost of medical care can be a financial burden.

Middle-aged adults often look forward to freedom from the demands and responsibilities of child care. Before this freedom can be experienced, an aged parent may move into the family system, and the adult children may find themselves limited socially and economically. The feeling of being caught between their children's needs and their parent's needs, with no time for themselves, may contribute to the abuse of elderly parents. Some daughters and sons have difficulty redefining the relationship with their parents. For them to see the parent as dependent, rather than all powerful and resourceful, is difficult. A great deal of anger may be generated when aged parents can no longer be a source of support for the adult child.

When older parents move into the homes of their adult daughters and sons, the level of intrafamily stress may rise. The physical environment may become crowded with few places or opportunities for privacy. Power struggles often ensue with strong differing opinions on how the household should be managed. The subsequent increase in stress and frustration may be a contributing factor in the abuse of the elderly (Sengstock and Barrett 1984).

Family Systems Theory

System theorists believe violence does not occur in isolation but results from the interrelationships between people, events, and behavior. This theory describes the process of intrafamily violence in the following way (Giles-Sims 1983):

- The taboo against violence is broken.

- A rise in expectations of further violence occurs.

- The family system denies that violent behavior is deviant.

- The abused person does not label himself or herself as a victim.

- Violent behavior is reinforced when it produces the desired results.

The abused child may be the scapegoat in a dysfunctional family system. One particular child may be labeled as the deviant member of the family. In this situation, marital conflict is displaced onto the scapegoated child, who becomes the target of hostility and violent attacks.

In the enmeshed family system, boundaries may be diffused with a resulting increase in stress and conflict. Family member roles may be constantly shifting. If the parents are unable to meet each other's needs for support and affection, they may turn to the child for this type of

adult love. Each parent then begins to view the child as his or her special support system, and the parents begin to compete for the child's attention. When the child is unable to meet all the emotional needs of the parents, frustration builds and often ends in violent behavior. This type of family system may become disorganized and chaotic when the parents are unable to provide consistent leadership functions.

A closed family system is characterized by rigidity, inflexibility, and highly repetitive patterns of behavior. Input from larger social systems such as friends or community resources is discouraged and avoided. Solutions to problems must be found within the family system, whose resources are eventually depleted. The closed family system is rigid in its authoritarianism; it needs children who conform and comply with the family rules. When children begin to question the rules or challenge the power structure of the family, violence may be used to reinforce the authoritarian structure (Thorman 1980).

The Nursing Process and Intrafamily Physical Abuse

Assessment

Nurses in all clinical settings must routinely assess clients for evidence of violent attacks. Considering the extent of the problem of intrafamily violence, one or two introductory questions should be asked of every client. In assessing a child, the nurse may ask, "Moms and dads try to help their children learn how to behave well. What happens to you when you do something wrong?" In assessing an adult, the nurse may ask, "One source of stress in all our lives is family disagreements. Could you describe how disagreements affect you?" If the responses to these questions are indicative of violence, a detailed assessment, based on the nursing history tool in Box 25–7 and the guidelines for physical assessment in Box 25–8, needs to be conducted. Obviously, the assessment must be adapted to the client's age, gender, and family situation.

Because there is an increased incidence of violence toward pregnant women, nurses in these clinical settings must routinely look for evidence of violence through history taking and physical assessment. There are more incidents of beating during pregnancy than of either diabetes or placenta previa; indeed, one out of every fifty pregnant women women is physically abused (Humphreys and Campbell 1984).

Privacy must be ensured when conducting the assessment interview. It may be difficult for the client to admit to the reality of family violence until a level of trust has

---

Box 25–7

NURSING HISTORY TOOL FOR ASSESSING VICTIMS OF FAMILY VIOLENCE

Behavioral Assessment

Tell me about how people communicate within your family.
What types of things cause conflict within your family?
How is conflict managed or resolved?
Who in your family loses control of themselves when angry?
Have you received verbal threats of harm?
Have you ever been threatened with a knife or gun?
In which ways have you been at the receiving end of a family member's violent outbursts? Slapped? Hit? Punched? Thrown? Shoved? Kicked? Burned? Beaten up?
Is there a history of need for emergency medical treatment?
In what ways have you attempted to stop the violence?
Have you attempted to leave the situation in the past?
What occurred when you attempted to leave?
Describe the use of alcohol in the family.
Describe the use of drugs in the family.

Affective Assessment

Who do you think is responsible for the use of physical force within the family?
In what way is this person(s) responsible?
How much guilt are you experiencing at this time?
Tell me about your fears. Lack of security? Financial problems? Child care problems? Living apart from spouse? Further physical injury?
What kinds of factors contribute to your feeling of helplessness to leave or stop the abuse?
How hopeless do you feel about your situation?
How would you describe your level of depression?

Cognitive Assessment

Describe your strengths and abilities as a person.
If you were describing yourself to a stranger what would you say?

What are your beliefs about keeping your family together?
Tell me about your reasons for remaining in this situation. Promises of reform? Material rewards?
Do you believe/hope the violence will not recur?
What are your expectations of how children should behave?
What rights do parents have with their children?
What rights do spouses have with each other?
What are the rules about physical force within your family?

Sociocultural Assessment

How did your parents relate to each other?
Who enforced discipline when you were a child?
What type of discipline was used when you were a child?
What was/is your relationship like with your mother?
What was/is your relationship like with your father?
How did you get along with your siblings?
In your present family, who is the head of the household?
How are decisions made in your family?
How are household jobs assigned in the family?
Describe the recent and current stresses on the family. Unemployment? Financial problems? Illness? New family members? Deaths or separations? Child rearing problems? Change in job status? Increase in conflict? Change in residence?
Who can you turn to for support in times of stress?
Describe your social life.
What types of contact have you had with the legal system? Phoned police? Peace bonds? Obtained a lawyer? Court cases? Protective services?

---

been established with the nurse. Many clients are fearful the nurse will respond in a judgmental manner against the victim for being abused or remaining in the situation and against the abuser. The client needs to be assured of the nurse's genuine desire to assist the entire family system (Sengstock and Barrett 1984).

Nursing Diagnosis

Nursing diagnoses appropriate for the family in which physical abuse occurs are:

NANDA

- Coping, ineffective family: disabled

- Coping, ineffective individual

- Family processes, altered

- Alteration in parenting

- Powerlessness

- Self-concept, disturbance in: self-esteem

- Violence, potential for: directed at others

- 05.02.01.02 Aggressive/violent behaviors toward others
- 05.03.03 Altered parenting role
- 05.05.02 Social isolation/withdrawal
- 06.03.04 Altered self esteem
- 08.01.04 Powerlessness

Obviously, other nursing diagnoses would be appropriate depending on the individual family's needs.

Planning and Implementing Interventions

The majority of people involved in intrafamily violence are disturbed by this behavior and would like it to end. Even though they want help in stopping the abuse, they may not know how to seek the assistance they need. It is extremely important that the nurse be nonjudgmental in interactions with all family members. The abusers feel condemned by society at large and may therefore be distrustful of the motives of the nursing staff. Initially, the victims may be unwilling to trust the nursing staff because of family shame and fears of being accused for remaining in the violent situation. It is vital that nurses not impose their own values on the family by offering quick and easy solutions to intrafamily violence.

Treatment of violent families requires a multidisciplinary approach with a broad range of interventions. Nurses, social workers, physicians, family therapists, vocational trainers, police, protective services personnel, and lawyers need to coordinate their skills to intervene effectively. The family is the most open and accepting of professional intervention during periods of crisis. When the violent family is identified during a crisis period, they should be immediately referred for multidisciplinary treatment. They will be most open to developing new patterns of behavior in the four to six weeks following the crisis. If no interventions are made during that time, they are likely to return to the familiar patterns of interaction, including the use of physical force (Campbell 1984c).

Nurses need to be knowledgeable about the laws regarding the reporting of physical abuse. In all fifty states, nurses are required by law to report suspected incidents of child abuse, and in every state there is a penalty—civil, criminal, or both—for failure to report child abuse. The state laws vary for reporting abuse of adults and the elderly (Munro 1984). If trust is to be maintained, the family needs to be told that a report is being made to protective services. Nurses need to know the procedures that follow a report of abuse so that the family can be adequately informed of the process. Many families are fearful that the only function of protective services is to remove family members from the home; in fact, protective services can be very supportive to the family by offering counseling and other social services.

Nurses in all clinical settings are able to intervene with violent families at the basic level shown in the nursing care

---

> **Box 25–8**
> ## PHYSICAL ASSESSMENT OF THE VICTIM OF FAMILY VIOLENCE
>
> Complete a head-to-toe physical assessment with particular attention to the following:
>
> ### Head
>
> Evidence of trauma
> Evidence of hematoma
> Bald patches on scalp
> Facial bruises
> Facial fractures
> Eyes: swollen, bruised, hemorrhages
>
> ### Skin
>
> Swelling or tenderness
> Bruises
> Burns
> Presence of scars from burns or injuries
> Genital trauma
> Rectal trauma
>
> ### Musculoskeletal
>
> Fractures of the ribs
> Fractures of arms/legs
> Dislocated joints
> Impaired mobility
>
> ### Abdomen
>
> Bruises or wounds
> Evidence of internal injuries
>
> ### Neurologic
>
> Reflexes
> Parasthesias
> Numbness
> Pain

plan on page 672. The referral process is a vital component of nursing care since the family will need multidisciplinary interventions to halt the use of physical force within the family. (See Resources in Appendix C.)

Evaluation

Nurses in acute care settings may not have the opportunity for long-term evaluation of the family system. Sengstock

Nursing Care Plan: The Victim of Family Violence

Nursing Diagnosis: Ineffective family coping: disabling, related to inability to manage conflict without violence
Goal: Family will resolve conflict without the use of violence

Intervention	Rationale	Expected Outcome
Teach communication skills to family: • Blocks that occur • Active listening with feedback • Clear and direct communication • Communication that does not attack personhood of family members	Improved communication skills will enable family to resolve issues before they escalate to the point of violence.	Communication is more direct and clear. Family members actively listen to one another.
Discuss how violence is learned and transmitted from generation to generation.	Identifying violence as a learned behavior supports interventions aimed at learning new alternatives.	Family members verbalize need for violence to be stopped now if it is not to be perpetuated.
Discuss how disagreement in a family is inevitable.	Counteract myth that happiness will occur only when there is no conflict.	Family identifies the normality of conflict.
Explore with family the democratic process.	The more democratic the family structure in decision making and conflict resolution, the less likely that violence will occur.	Family verbalizes understanding of democratic process.
Using a minor, nonemotional family problem, have family solve the problem in a democratic manner.	Once the process is learned, family can transfer this knowledge and ability to solve other problems.	Family uses democratic process.
Discuss nonviolent ways of expressing anger.	Learning alternative modes of expression of anger will decrease incidence of violence.	Family identifies alternative modes of expressing anger.
Have family identify times and places that each member can have privacy and time alone.	Quiet time alone will decrease the stress and tension of family members.	Family establishes private times for family members.

Nursing Diagnosis: Ineffective individual coping related to being a victim of violence
Goal: Client will manage feelings and physical disorders related to violence

Intervention	Rationale	Expected Outcome
Listen carefully to client's difficulties, and treat client with respect.	Respect and attentive listening will increase client's feelings of worth.	
Give verbal recognition of client's hesitancy to trust staff.	Victims of abuse have difficulty trusting because they have often been judged as failures by society.	Client identifies fears of trusting staff.
Assist client in identifying feelings related to being the recipient of violent behavior.	Clients may initially use denial or disassociation of feelings to cope with the situation. They need to understand the normality of strong negative feelings.	Client decreases use of denial, identifies feelings.
Assist client in identifying ambivalent feelings (e.g., love/hate, hopelessness/hopefulness, or terror/security).	Clients need to understand the normality of ambivalence to decrease the confusion that may be caused by these feelings.	Client verbalizes understanding of ambivalent feelings.

continued

Nursing Care Plan: The Victim of Family Violence (*Continued*)

Intervention	Rationale	Expected Outcome
Discuss how stress is related to psychophysiologic disorders.	Client needs to make the connection between physical symptoms and family problems.	Client verbalizes understanding of physical illness and stress.
Refer to physician for diagnosis and medical intervention of psychophysiologic disorders.	Adequate medical care must be provided for clients with these disorders.	Client follows up on medical care.
Prepare client for any referrals that are made.	Preparation will increase likelihood of client accepting help.	Client follows through on referrals.

Nursing Diagnosis: Alteration in family process related to use of violence to maintain family relationships
Goal: Family will maintain the family unit without the use of violence

Intervention	Rationale	Expected Outcome
Assist family in seeing that the use of violence is a family problem, that is, that all members are involved in maintaining the violent behavior.	Family members may want to focus only on the abuser as the problem individual. Understanding interactional patterns that maintain the violence is necessary to prevent further violence.	Family identifies each member's role in maintaining the dysfunction.
Assist family in problem solving alternative behaviors for each family member.	Changes in behavior in part of the family system will result in changes throughout the entire system.	Family identifies possible changes in behavior.
Help family redefine intrafamily relationships as ones in which physical force is unacceptable.	Most violent families are not violent with friends or strangers. They need support to enforce those same limits within family.	Family defines family as a nonviolent place of refuge.
Assist family to see relationship between developmental crises and coping with physical force.	Anticipatory guidance will decrease use of violence as a method to cope with expected changes in family.	Family verbalizes understanding of future crises.
Encourage family to formulate alternatives for coping with elderly parent in the home. • Investigate day care centers. • Investigate extended care centers. • Enlist help from other family members. • Investigate short-term care so family can take vacation.	Decreasing the stress of total care for elderly parent will decrease use of violence within the home.	Family develops plans to provide relief.
Refer for family therapy.	Long-term therapy may be necessary to restructure family as a nonviolent family.	Family follows through on referral.

continued

Nursing Care Plan: The Victim of Family Violence (*Continued*)

Nursing Diagnosis: 05.03.03 Altered parenting role/Parenting, altered and related to physical abuse of children*
Goal: Parents will not abuse their children in the future

Intervention	Rationale	Expected Outcome
Express concern for all family members including parents.	When parents understand the nurse is also concerned about them, they will be more willing to become actively involved in treatment.	Parents verbally recognize nurse is nonjudgmental.
Give recognition for positive parenting skills.	Recognition of positive aspects will increase parents' feelings of worth.	Parents identify areas of strengths in parenting.
Give recognition that use of violence is a desperate attempt to cope with children.	Recognition of parents' care and concern for their children will increase the likelihood of active participation in treatment.	Parents identify need to cope more effectively.
Discuss with parents how they were punished as children.	Recall of effects of violence in their own childhood will increase motivation for treatment.	Parents discuss childhood experiences.
Teach parents about normal growth and development of their children.	Unrealistic demands on children often result in violence in an attempt to have children comply beyond their developmental ability.	Parents verbalize knowledge of growth and development.
Discuss problems they experience with raising children.	Identifying specific sources of stress is the first step in problem resolution.	Parents identify problems.
Help parents identify parenting tools other than physical force that are age appropriate for their children.	Lack of parenting skills contributes to increased use of violence within family.	Parents identify alternative skills.
Help parents identify ways to spend time together without children.	Strengthening the marital relationship and time apart from children will decrease stress and tension.	Parents plan times together as a couple.
Refer to community resources (e.g., crisis hot lines, Parents Anonymous, family therapy, or group therapy).	Follow-up with community resources will decrease isolation, improve family relationships, and offer support during times of crisis.	Parents follow through on referrals.

Nursing Diagnosis: 08.01.04 Powerlessness/Powerlessness related to feelings of being dependent on abuser*
Goal: Client will not feel forced to remain in an abusive, dependent relationship

Intervention	Rationale	Expected Outcome
Help client identify past dependency relationships.	Identifying patterns throughout life will help client focus on how she maintains her own feelings of powerlessness.	Client identifies lifelong process of dependency.
Have client formulate a list of ways she is dependent on abuser (e.g., emotional and economic areas of dependency).	High levels of dependency make it difficult for victim to leave abuser without intense support.	Client formulates list.

continued

Nursing Care Plan: The Victim of Family Violence (*Continued*)

Intervention	Rationale	Expected Outcome
Help client identify intrapersonal and interpersonal strengths.	Recognition of strengths will decrease feelings of helplessness.	Client identifies strengths.
Help client identify aspects of her life under her control.	Feelings of control will decrease feelings of powerlessness.	Client identifies situations of control.
Provide assertiveness training.	Continued submission to violence often results in an escalation of the violent behavior.	Client behaves more assertively with abuser.
Refer to community resources for financial aid, legal aid, or job training.	Increasing community support and intervention will decrease high economic dependency on abuser.	Client follows through on referrals.

Nursing Diagnosis: 06.03.04 Altered self esteem/Self-concept; disturbance in: Self-esteem related to feeling guilty and responsible for being a victim*
Goal: Client will not assume responsibility and guilt for the abuse

Intervention	Rationale	Expected Outcome
Help client identify strengths in coping with abusive partner thus far.	Identification of strengths will increase feelings of competency and positive self-esteem.	Client identifies strengths.
Explain theories of violence to client.	Understanding the theories will relieve client of feelings of responsibility for the abuse.	Client acknowledges she is not responsible for abusive behavior.
Help client identify what behavior she will and will not accept from abuser.	Setting limits on inappropriate behavior will reinforce a positive self-respect.	Client establishes limits on abusive behavior she will accept.

Nursing Diagnosis: 06.03.04 Altered self esteem/Self-concept; disturbance in: Role performance related to stereotyped gender roles and use of violence*
Goal: Family will not use violence to maintain stereotyped gender roles

Intervention	Rationale	Expected Outcome
Give family members the opportunity to describe their perceptions of the various roles in the family system.	Individuals may have differing perceptions about roles of family members.	Family describes family roles.
Have family members identify sources of these roles (e.g., tradition, rules, society, religious beliefs).	Family may not be aware of how roles developed. Awareness of source of roles must precede a change in roles.	Family identifies sources of family roles.
Discuss issues of stereotyping role behavior according to gender.	Less stereotyping increases interdependent behavior and decreases acceptance of aggression.	Family discusses beliefs about gender roles.
Help men identify compulsive masculinity and women identify submissive behavior as it relates to the use of violence.	Identification of behaviors that contribute to violence precedes a change in those behaviors.	Family identifies roles that may contribute to the use of violence.

continued

Nursing Care Plan: The Victim of Family Violence (*Continued*)

Intervention	Rationale	Expected Outcome
Discuss with family how gender roles can be expanded.	Expanding the roles will decrease the need to defend stereotypic behavior and thereby decrease stress and tension.	Family formulates changes in role behavior.
Discuss with family in what ways the power base in the family can be more equally distributed.	The more democratic the power base is within the family, the less likely that violence will occur.	Family formulates a more democratic family structure.

Nursing Diagnosis: 05.05.02 Social isolation/Social isolation related to shame about family violence*
Goal: Family will increase interactions with others outside the family system

Intervention	Rationale	Expected Outcome
Help family identify supportive network systems (e.g., family, friends, neighbors, church).	The process of identification may enable family to recognize a wider network of supportive people than was previously known.	Family makes list of people and places available for support.
Discuss with family ways to reach out and ask for help from supportive network.	Being able to ask for outside support during times of tension and crisis will decrease the use of violence as a coping behavior.	Family formulates plan on how to ask for help.
Refer family to self-help groups dealing with the same problem of violence.	Peer groups decrease isolation and provide emotional support and feelings of connectedness.	Family follows through on referral.

Nursing Diagnosis: 05.05.01.02 Violent behaviors toward others/Violence, potential for: directed at others related to a history of the use of physical force within the family*
Goal: Family will not remain violent

Intervention	Rationale	Expected Outcome
Assess the level of danger for the victim.	Homicide may be a realistic potential if previous threats have been made.	Victim identifies likelihood of being seriously hurt.
Assess the level of danger for the abuser.	The severity of the violence is the factor that most contributes to women killing their abusers in self-defense.	Victim identifies likelihood of seriously injuring the abuser.
If level of danger is high, contact protective services or the police for emergency custody placement or removal to a shelter.	Family members may need to be separated until they have greater control over their violent impulses.	Abuser complies with removal from the family system.
Help family use problem solving to determine if the victim will remain within the family system.	Writing out alternatives and making rational choices will increase family's ability to problem solve, which may decrease the use of violence.	Family uses problem-solving approach.
Discuss with family methods to manage anger appropriately:	When clients can use alternative expressions of anger, the use of violence will decrease.	Abuser implements alternative expressions and management of anger.

continued

Nursing Care Plan: The Victim of Family Violence (*Continued*)

Intervention	Rationale	Expected Outcome
• Assume responsibility for own behavior • Talking out anger as it occurs • Relaxation training • Physical exercise • Striking safe, inanimate objects (e.g., pillow, couch, or punching bag)		
Discuss with family the facts about intrafamily violence.	Violence tends to escalate unless the system is changed.	Family identifies potential of increasing violence.
Help family establish limits and definite consequences if violence recurs.	Setting and enforcement of limits will lead to extinction of violence in the family.	Family enforces limits on violence.
Help victims establish a detailed plan of escape if violence should occur.	Exact and careful preplanning will aid escape during a time when anxiety and fear are at high levels.	Victim formulates escape plan.
Refer victims to legal resources.	Victims may be unaware of legal rights to stop family violence.	Family follows through on referral.

*PND-I/NANDA diagnoses.

and Barrett (1984) state that short-term evaluations center on:

- The identification of intrafamily abuse
- The family's ability to recognize that a problem exists
- The family's willingness to accept assistance by the follow-through with referrals
- The removal of the victim from a volatile situation

Nurses in long-term settings or within the community have the opportunity to evaluate the effectiveness of the multidisciplinary treatment plan over an extended period. Sharing in the process of family growth and healthy adaptation in the ceasing of violence can be a tremendous source of professional satisfaction.

All nurses can evaluate their professional obligations and practice in counteracting those aspects of the society that foster violence. Violence is a mental health problem of national importance, and nurses should be leaders in preventing violence in future generations. Questions to guide evaluation of nursing practice are (Campbell 1984c):

- What action have I taken to decrease violence in the media?
- Have I been an advocate for gun control?
- Have I volunteered to teach parenting classes at the grade school and high school level?
- Have I confronted the use of physical punishment in the school system?
- How have I supported programs to assist the elderly?

INTRAFAMILY VIOLENCE—SEXUAL ABUSE

Sexually abused children and adult survivors of incest are crying out for help. A few cry out loudly in protest, but the majority cry inwardly in silence. As many as one in four girls and one in ten boys are abused sexually before age 18 (Burgess 1984). Intrafamily sexual abuse occurs in all racial, religious, economic, and cultural subgroups. The perpetrators are not monsters; they love their children, are steady workers, provide for the family, and are seen as good family men.*

Intrafamily sexual abuse is defined as inappropriate sexual behavior, instigated by an adult family or surrogate family member, whose purpose is to sexually arouse the adult or the child. Behaviors range from exhibitionism, peeping, and explicit sexual talk to touching, caressing, masturbation, and intercourse (Warner 1980, Trepper and Barrett 1986a). The term is often used interchangeably with *incest*.

Incest is defined as the occurrence of sexual relations between blood relatives. A broader definition includes sex between two persons related to one another by some form of kinship tie. Social taboos against incest have roots in psychologic as well as sociologic factors. While accurate figures of the incidence of incest are difficult to obtain because of the shame associated with it, most authorities believe that contemporary social, cultural, physiologic, and psychologic variables have all contributed to a breakdown in the incest taboo. For example, incestuous behavior has been associated with alcoholism, overcrowding, and rural isolation. Major mental disorders and intellectual deficiencies are also associated with cases of incest.

Intrafamily sexual abuse creates problems for the family system different from sexual abuse by neighbors, friends, or strangers. Within the family system, all the participants—that is, victim, perpetrator, and conspirators—must continue to interact and function as a unit. There is no way of avoiding one another or dealing directly with the anger and rage aroused. Strangers must use physical force or threats of physical violence to rape another person, but most typically, physical force is not used in intrafamily sexual abuse. Psychologic coercion by the adult is used to ensure the silence and compliance of the child (Warner 1980). Statements are made such as, "You must not tell anyone what we are doing, or they will take me away, and you won't have a father anymore," or "You are very special to me, and we don't want anyone else to know how special or they might feel bad," or "You know I'll buy you lots of toys and gifts as long as you don't tell anyone about our secret."

Incidence of Sexual Abuse

It is difficult to estimate accurately the incidence of intrafamily sexual abuse. With increased public awareness, there

has been an increase in the reporting of cases. It is believed that the actual rate has not increased but that the secrecy around current and past occurrences is decreasing. In the past, it was thought that intrafamily sexual abuse began when the child was around 10 or 12 years old. Current research has shown that many victims are under the age of 5, and some are as young as 3 to 6 months. The average age for sexual molestation is 4 years, and the average age for intercourse with a family member is 9 years (Lecture notes).

Characteristics of Intrafamily Sexual Abuse

It is difficult to predict which of the following characteristics a given child or family will exhibit in the face of intrafamily sexual abuse. Some will exhibit most of the characteristics, others will exhibit some, and still others will exhibit none. These characteristics should be taken as cues for further investigation since they may also be signs and symptoms of other emotional problems in children and families.

Although it is known that many victims suffer long-term problems such as anxiety disorders, sexual dysfunctions, sleep disorders, and multiple personality, there are also instances where there appear to be no lasting negative consequences. In studies of women who were not in therapy and who had been victims as children, it was found that many had made adequate adjustments to adult life. Again, nurses must find the balance between the extremes of denial of pathology and excessive victimization of the individual and family (Trepper and Traicoff 1983).

Behavioral Characteristics

Children who are victims of intrafamily sexual abuse may exhibit regressive behavior. This may take any form of regression, but the most common is bedwetting. Sleep disturbances are common in children, particularly among those who have been molested during their sleep. Some return to a clinging form of attachment to one or both parents. Children may become extremely affectionate, both within the family and with others outside the family. Other children isolate themselves at school and in the neighborhood and limit the majority of their interpersonal interactions to family members.

Children who are victims may act out sexually with other children or adults. This must be distinguished from the normal childhood behavior of mimicking sexual behavior observed between parents or in the media. Sexual acting out behavior is seen in child victims who initiate genital or oral sex with other children or adults.

Victims of intrafamily sexual abuse may run away from home to escape an intolerable situation. Some of the victims turn to prostitution since they have learned in the family that sexual behavior is the method whereby one

---

*This text uses the male adult–female child configuration, unless otherwise noted, since this is the most frequently reported type of intrafamily sexual abuse.

receives affection, love, and attention. Other victims attempt or commit suicide if they experience the hopelessness of being trapped in a pathologic family system (Warner 1980).

Affective Characteristics

Victims of incest may experience many fears. They fear if they tell another adult, they will not be believed or that they themselves will be blamed, and the nonmolesting parent will side with the molesting parent. They may have fantasies of being thrown out of the family if the molesting behavior becomes known to other family members. Some victims fear loss of parental love. They may fear the family will be separated, especially if this threat was made by the abusing parent. Some fear that if they resist the sexual advances or tell the secret, they will be physically abused, even if the parent has never before used or threatened physical abuse.

The affective responses to sexual abuse are often confusing to the child. Opposing feelings may occur simultaneously, which creates ambivalence within the child. Developmentally, the child may not have the skills to manage the conflict that arises from ambivalent feelings. Victims often experience physical pleasure in the sexual interactions. In addition, they may enjoy being the "special" child within the family and the degree of power they experience over the molesting parent and the other siblings. At the same time, they may feel responsible for the sexual behavior and guilty they have not been able to stop the abuse. Further, because they are emotionally and physically dependent on the abusing parent, they may feel helpless and powerless.

Cognitive Characteristics

Denial of intrafamily sexuality may take several forms. Some victims deny that the abuse ever occurred. Others, acknowledging that sexual activity occurred, deny the impact and say it was not important. This is evidenced by statements such as, "It's not so bad. It only happens once a month," or "It's all right because it stopped when I was 11 years old." Still others acknowledge the sexual activity and the negative consequences but deny the parent's responsibility and assume they are to blame for their parent's behavior. Evidence of denial of parental responsibility is heard in such statements as, "It's my fault, I seduced my grandfather," or "If I had not been running around in my swimming suit it would not have happened" (Barrett et al. 1986). Denial may be used to protect the family system as well as the individual victim. The fear that the family may be separated by the removal of the parent or the removal of the child to a foster home may be so overwhelming that the secret is kept within the family system.

Children molested during the night may experience nightmares in response to the abuse. They may begin to dream they are being molested, and this may lead to their being unable to separate the reality from the dream and the belief the abuse did not happen but was simply a dream.

Sarah, age 19, describes her relationship with her father when she was 12 years old in this way: "I don't remember how it started, but my father conned me into soaping up his stomach, testicles, and erect penis when he was in the bathtub. This took place at his apartment when my brothers and I went there for the weekend. I didn't particularly enjoy it, but my father encouraged it. I got completely turned off by it when he offered to do me. One time, while I was sleeping on the bed, I woke up from a violent shaking of the bed. I was dressed in a shirt and shorts. I realized my father was rubbing his penis between my thighs and feeling on my vagina. I didn't let him know I was awake, and I turned slightly, hoping he would stop. I never wore that tee shirt or shorts again. I've never told anyone. Even my father doesn't know that I know. I think my experiences have had a deep effect on my relationships. Every time I get close to a man, I become afraid. I think what I'm most afraid of is being used. My childhood experiences seem to bother me the most when my friends talk about their childhood with their fathers and how they were 'Daddy's little girl.' Feelings of rage, anger, and total disgust burn deep inside me."

Physiologic Characteristics

The obvious physical signs of sexual abuse in a child are irritated or swollen genitals, rectal tissue, or both; the presence of a sexually transmitted disease; and pregnancy. Chronic vaginal or urinary tract infections, with no known medical cause, may be indicators that the child is being sexually abused. Some children may have sexually transmitted diseases in their mouths and throat. Since oral sex is a frequent behavior in these interactions, the child's throat may be irritated. The child may also exhibit a hyperactive gag reflex and, at times, unexplained vomiting. Younger children may complain of tummy aches with the discomfort located near the diaphragm. The penis is seen as so huge that when penetration is attempted or completed, the child has visions of its reaching up to the chest area.

Some children will, consciously or unconsciously, attempt to abuse their bodies to either prevent or halt the sexual abuse. A great deal of weight may be gained in the hopes of becoming so ugly that the abuser will be appalled and leave the child alone. Anorexia may also be a response to intrafamily sexual abuse. If an older child is being abused, a younger sister may become anorexic in an attempt not to mature and experience the same abuse. This lack of care for the body may continue into adult life in an unconscious attempt to keep distance and avoid intimate relationships (Lecture notes).

Sociocultural Characteristics

A number of sociocultural characteristics may contribute to intrafamily sexual abuse. Rigid or compulsive gender roles increase the vulnerability of the children within the family. It is difficult for a child to protest any type of abusive treatment in a highly structured, authoritarian family system. Rigid gender roles place women and children in a submissive and obedient position. In a culture that has traditionally supported male supremacy and viewed women and children as the property of males, it is not surprising that sexual abuse has been, and even continues to be, tolerated (Burgess 1984, Trepper and Barrett 1986b).

There is a widespread belief that the mother always knows when her husband is sexually involved with one or more of the children. In reality, mothers are rarely aware of intrafamily sexual abuse (Trepper and Traicoff 1983). Some women deny any evidence of the abuse because they feel inadequate to cope with the family problems. Others use denial because they fear their husbands' retaliation against them if the accusation of incest is brought into the open. Denial may be a defense mechanism used by women who fear financial, social, and emotional problems if their husbands are removed from the family (Warner 1980, Barrett et al. 1986). When cues to intrafamily sexual abuse are discovered, some women begin to question their own thinking processes. Believing their husbands are incapable of this type of behavior, they, therefore, believe something must be wrong with themselves.

Cherenia has recently become somewhat suspicious that her husband, Joe, may be sexually abusing their daughter. In response to her fears, she says the following things to herself: "You must really have a dirty mind, Cherenia. How could you possibly think those things about Joe. He's a very good husband. He works hard and loves all of us. He goes to church every week, and everyone knows what a good family man he is. How could you even consider that he might be doing something so awful. You must be really sick, Cherenia."

Chronic stress within the family system may contribute to intrafamily sexual abuse. Families that are socially isolated and have few support systems are more vulnerable to the effects of acute and chronic stress. When internal and external resources are depleted, the family dynamics may become pathologic. In some incestuous families, alcohol abuse may be a factor. That is not to say that alcohol abuse causes incest but rather that intoxication decreases inhibitions and is often used as an excuse for irresponsible behavior (Trepper and Barrett 1986b).

Theoretical Perspectives

There is no single cause of intrafamily sexual abuse. In fact, the abuse is not a primary diagnosis but a symptom of dysfunction in the individual, family, and societal systems. All these systems must be considered if the nurse is to understand the dynamics of a particular family (Warner 1980, Trepper and Barrett 1986b). Individual and family systems theories of incest are presented in this section. (See the section on Physical Abuse for the sociologic theories of causation.)

Intrapersonal Theories

There are many descriptions of the perpetrators and victims involved in intrafamily sexual abuse. Many of these descriptions are contradictory, and there is no agreement on a personality pattern peculiar to all perpetrators or victims (Barrett et al. 1986). Nurses must remember that many people experience these same factors of vulnerability but do not become involved with intrafamily sexual abuse. These theories are guidelines for assessment, not absolute proof of sexual abuse.

The intrapersonal theories view the adult perpetrator as the "sick" or pathologic family member. These people may be insecure and have inadequate self-esteem. They may be fearful of interacting with adults and more secure in interpersonal interactions with children. This fear of failure may contribute to a sexual dysfunction in adult relationships. When the sexual dysfunction does not occur in the sexual relationship with their child, there is positive reinforcement to continue the behavior. Some perpetrators were emotionally deprived as children and thus have a great need for constant, unconditional love, which is more easily obtained from children than from adults. If they were sexually abused themselves as children, they may have learned to associate all feelings of love with sexual behavior (Warner 1980, Trepper and Barrett 1986b).

Some perpetrators are described as lacking impulse control and the inability to experience feelings of guilt. Others have been described as rigid and overcontrolled. They may be dominant and aggressive. Lack of parenting skills or the loss of the mother from the family may result in role confusion among the family members. The father may turn to the daughter for companionship when he feels deprived of it in adult relationships (Warner 1980, Trepper and Barrett 1986a).

The mothers of victims may be emotionally and financially dependent on the marital relationship. Denial may be the major mechanism that allows them to remain in the marriage. They may also have been victims of sexual abuse during their own childhood, which may contribute to an adult dysfunction such as female sexual arousal disorder. The mother's lack of parenting skills may contribute to the daughter's assuming responsibility for the younger children in the family. Along with this parent role, the daughter may be expected to fulfill the role of sexual partner (Warner 1980, Barrett et al. 1986).

Daughters who are victims may feel emotionally deprived and need unconditional love and attention. If they have an inadequate self-esteem, the "special" attention from their fathers may help them feel attractive, desired, and needed. The daughter may exhibit seductive and provocative behavior, a learned response to the father's inappropriate sexual behavior (Warner 1980, Trepper and Barrett 1986a).

Family Systems Theory

The family systems perspective views intrafamily sexual abuse as arising from and being maintained by the interactions of all family members. Rather than looking at *why* the behavior occurs, as the intrapersonal theorists do, family systems theorists look at *how* the behavior occurs.

Family Structure

The structure of the family is organized around hierarchical membership according to age and roles and distribution of power. Typically, the adults, who are older, assume the parental roles and are the most influential members of the family system. The structure of incestuous families, however, is often quite different. An adult may move downward in the structure, or a child may move upward in the structure in terms of roles and influence. If the father moves downward, he assumes a childlike role and is cared for and nurtured by his wife, as are the children in the family. In this position, the father assumes little parental responsibility. He may then turn to the daughter, as a peer, for sexual and emotional gratification. In other family systems, the daughter may move upward and replace the mother in the hierarchical structure. Usually the mother does not move downward in the structure but rather moves out of the structure by distancing herself emotionally or physically from the family. As the daughter assumes the parental roles and responsibilities, the father may turn to her for fulfillment of emotional and sexual needs (Barrett et al. 1986, Trepper and Barrett 1986b).

Family Cohesion

Family cohesion refers to the degree of emotional bonding within a family. At one end of the continuum of cohesion is the family system that is disengaged, that is, the family members are isolated and alienated from one another. At the other end of the continuum is the enmeshed family system in which the members are immersed in and absorbed by one another. The most adaptive family systems function between these two extremes.

Intrafamily sexual abuse usually occurs in an enmeshed family. The need to be overinvolved in one another's lives is accompanied by intense fears of abandonment and family disintegration. The family system is closed to external input and support in an attempt to maintain closeness. If the parent's marital dyad does not provide adequate emotional and sexual fulfillment, the father turns to the daughter for these needs rather than searching outside the family system for a different partner (Warner 1980, Barrett et al. 1986).

Family Adaptability

Family system adaptability to change is also described along a continuum. At one extreme is the rigid family system and, at the other end, the chaotic family system. Incestuous families tend to fall on either end of the continuum. Rigid family systems have strict rules and stereotyped gender role expectations with minimal emotional interaction. Children are given no power and authority, even over their own bodies. They are not allowed to question or protest inappropriate sexual behavior within the family. In contrast, chaotic family systems have either no rules or constantly changing roles. The parents are unable to assume parental roles or leadership positions. Within the chaotic system, there may be no assigned roles or no rules regarding appropriate sexual behavior, which may contribute to the incidence of intrafamily sexual abuse (Warner 1980, Trepper and Barrett 1986b).

Family Communication

Communication patterns within the family system may contribute to the occurrence of intrafamily sexual abuse. Within some families, messages between two persons are communicated through a third family member. This indirect communication perpetuates secrecy and avoidance of conflict (Barrett et al. 1986, Trepper and Barrett 1986b). Intrafamily sexual abuse is dependent on keeping the secret within the family. In family systems that avoid conflict, accusations of sexual abuse are not tolerated. Peace must be kept at all costs, even the cost of abuse.

Box 25–9

NURSING HISTORY TOOL FOR ASSESSMENT OF INDIVIDUALS AND FAMILIES FOR INTRAFAMILY SEXUAL ABUSE

Behavioral Assessment

Individual child

Have there been any signs of regressive behavior in the child?

Is the child having sleeping problems?

Is the child exhibiting clinging behavior to the parents or others?

Does the child have friendships with other children?

Has there been any sexual acting out on the part of the child?

Has the child ever run away or threatened to run away?

Has the child ever attempted suicide?

Perpetrator

Describe how discipline is handled in the family.

Do you see yourself as the dominant person in the family?

At what age do you believe parents should give up control of their children?

How many adult friends do you have?

Describe your relationship with these friends.

Describe your relationship with your spouse.

What kinds of sexual difficulties are you and your spouse experiencing?

When you were young, who was the closest family member with whom you had any sexual activity?

Family system

Describe who has responsibility (mother, father, both parents, or children) in the following areas of home management:

   Caring for the younger children?

   Cooking?

   Cleaning?

   Paying bills?

   Shopping?

   Outside home maintenance?

   Budget planning?

   Decisions about leisure time?

   Supervising children's homework?

   Taking children to activities?

   Putting children to bed?

Who are the best communicators in the family?

Who talks to whom the most?

Who is unable to talk to whom very much?

How are secrets kept from one another within the family?

How are secrets prevented from leaking outside the family?

Affective Assessment

Individual child

How helpless do you feel about changing any of the family's problems?

In what way are you responsible for family problems?

Do you get enough love within the family?

Are you more loved than the other children in the family?

Tell me about the fears you may have if any family secrets are told:

   Fears of not being believed?

   Fears of being blamed for the problems?

   Fears that your parents will not love you?

   Fears that you will be moved to a foster home?

   Fears that your parents will be taken away?

   Fears of physical abuse?

Perpetrator

Who loves you the most within the family?

Who is able to give you unconditional support and affection?

How do you see yourself responsible for family problems?

How does fear of failure affect your life?

Family system

Describe the emotional relationships among family members.

Does everybody know each family member's business?

How is privacy protected within the family?

Do you have any fears of the family unit disintegrating?

What will happen if the family is separated?

Cognitive Assessment

Individual child

Tell me about your nightmares.

How would you describe the family's problems?

What effect do these problems have on you?

What effect do these problems have on the rest of the family?

Who do you believe is responsible for these problems?

Perpetrator

Describe what kind of a person you are.

What are your personal strengths?

What are your personal limitations?

Describe how you handle new situations.

Do you enjoy changing situations?

Family system

Who sets the family rules?

Tell me about the most important family rules.

How do rules get changed within the family?

continued

Box 25–9 (*continued*)

What are the expectations of the males in the family?
What are the expectations of the females in the family?

Sociocultural Assessment

What significant events have occurred for your family in the past year?

What support systems do you have outside the family?
How often do you visit with friends?
Who are the problem drinkers in the family?
How is the issue of drugs managed within the family?

The Nursing Process in Intrafamily Sexual Abuse

Assessment

It is vitally important that nurses acknowledge the reality of intrafamily sexual abuse. Those nurses who deny the existence of the problem miss the individual and family cues and thereby fail to complete a more detailed assessment. Nurses knowledgeable about the incidence and characteristics of the problem at all levels of society are alert for cues that demand an in-depth nursing assessment. A note of caution must be added, however. Families who have not been involved in intrafamily sexual abuse have been torn apart by rumors and false accusations. Nurses need to assess carefully and maintain a balance between denying incest and assuming automatic guilt.

When assessing children, it must be remembered that some will exhibit most of the characteristics presented, others will exhibit only some, and still others will exhibit none of them. It must also be remembered that these same behavioral, affective, and intellectual characteristics may be signs and symptoms of other emotional problems in children. Family dynamics also need to be assessed before an assumption is made of intrafamily sexual abuse. Routine questions on nursing histories such as that in Box 25–9 may provide an opportunity for survivors of incest to share their pain and obtain treatment as adults. Now that intrafamily sexual abuse has been identified as a major health problem, nurses in every clinical setting must be alert to cues from both individuals and families. Guidelines for physical assessment are in Box 25–10.

Nursing Diagnosis

The most common nursing diagnoses for families in which sexual abuse exists are:

NANDA

- Coping, ineffective family: disabled
- Coping, ineffective individual
- Family processes, altered
- Parenting, altered

PND-I

- 05.03.03 Altered parenting role

Additional nursing diagnoses will be determined by the individual needs of family members and by the family system as a whole.

Box 25–10
PHYSICAL ASSESSMENT OF THE SEXUAL ABUSE VICTIM

Complete a head-to-toe physical assessment with emphasis on the following:
Weight and nutritional status
Throat irritation
Gag reflex
Episodes of vomiting
Abdominal pain near diaphragm
Smears of the mouth, throat, vagina, and rectum for sexually transmitted diseases
Genital irritation or trauma
Rectal irritation or trauma
Chronic vaginal infections
Chronic urinary tract infections
Pregnancy

Planning and Implementing Interventions

It is important to identify individual and family system strengths so that they can be reinforced and supported. Because family therapy is critical to the healthy resolution of intrafamily sexual abuse, referral to therapists who specialize in treating incestuous families is a priority in nursing intervention.

Intrafamily sexual abuse is an emotionally laden health problem. Nurses need to identify their personal values and determine if these will interfere with the ability to care for all members of the family system. Beliefs about maintaining or splitting up of the family unit will influence nursing care. Many nurses experience a great deal of anger and hostility toward the perpetrator and the parent who was not able to prevent or stop the abuse. If the nurse is a survivor of childhood sexual abuse, personal issues and feelings may interfere with effective nursing care. Some nurses may need to disqualify themselves from caring for incestuous families because of their personal values and feelings.

See below for a nursing care plan for the family with sexual abuse.

Nursing Care Plan: The Victim with Sexual Abuse

Nursing Diagnosis: Ineffective family coping: disabling, related to child being sexually abused
Goal: Family will no longer engage in inappropriate sexual behavior

Intervention	Rationale	Expected Outcome
Help each family member write list of individual and family goals for treatment.	Writing a list of expected outcomes will increase each member's participation in therapy.	Family formulates lists.
Help family identify individual and family strengths.	If clients are able to identify strengths, they will feel more optimistic about change rather than feel defeated at the onset.	Family identifies strengths; verbalizes hope for the future.
Help family identify how some members cross generational boundaries by discussing roles and role reversals.	Crossing of boundaries is a contributing factor in intrafamily sexual abuse, because parent and child relate to one another as peers.	Family identifies inappropriate roles according to the generation of each family member.
Discuss ways that parents can maintain generational boundaries.	Parents need to assume responsibility for parenting all of their children.	Family makes decisions on ways to change roles.
Help family members communicate directly with one another.	New and more effective communication styles are needed to improve family system functioning.	Family communicates directly.
Discourage secrecy within family.	Secrecy contributes to lack of trust and supports sexual abuse.	Family communicates openly.

Nursing Diagnosis: Ineffective individual coping related to being a perpetrator of sexual abuse
Goal: Client will develop adaptive coping skills

Intervention	Rationale	Expected Outcome
Discuss client's family of origin in regard to sexual abuse and parenting styles.	Many abusers were sexually abused as children. People tend to parent the way in which they were parented.	Client discusses childhood as it relates to present problem.
Help client discuss feelings around being discovered as an abuser.	Client needs to identify and manage feelings of guilt, shame, or anger to regain a positive self-regard.	Client shares feelings.

continued

Nursing Care Plan: The Victim of Sexual Abuse (*Continued*)

Intervention	Rationale	Expected Outcome
Discuss factors client believes contributed to the incidents of abuse.	Examining the multiple factors will help client determine changes that must be made.	Client lists contributing factors.
Help client problem solve to find alternative coping behavior.	Client must be actively involved in assuming responsibility for change.	Client identifies specific changes in behavior.

Nursing Diagnosis: Ineffective individual coping related to being a nonabusing parent
Goal: Client will not become a secondary victim

Intervention	Rationale	Expected Outcome
Help client identify feelings toward self since the abuse was discovered.	Many nonabusing parents experience guilt for not being aware of or stopping the sexual abuse.	Client identifies that she is not responsible for spouse's behavior.
Help client identify feelings toward other family members.	The anger, fear, and anxiety must be identified and managed if the family system is to remain intact.	Client shares feelings.

Nursing Diagnosis: Ineffective individual coping related to being a victim of intrafamily sexual abuse
Goal: Client will adapt to the trauma of being sexually abused

Intervention	Rationale	Expected Outcome
Use play therapy with children under the age of 5.	Play therapy helps young children to express feelings, reduce guilt, and reestablish trust.	Client participates in play therapy.
Help older children to identify and discuss feelings about the abuse.	Feelings of shame, guilt, anxiety, and anger must be normalized as part of the therapeutic process.	Client shares feelings.
Help client learn methods to avoid future abuse such as telling others about advances, saying "No," and refusing to be left alone with the abuser.	Supporting child's alternatives and problem solving for future occurrences may prevent future victimization.	Client lists methods of coping in the future.

Nursing Diagnosis: Alteration in family process related to disruption of family unit when abuse is discovered
Goal: Child will remain safe within old or new family structure

Intervention	Rationale	Expected Outcome
Refer family to protective services who will implement one of four plans:		
1. Family remains intact.	Families who have not used violence, where there is no substance abuse, and who can assure the child's safety may be allowed to live together. This is rarely recommended.	Family acts in accordance with legal decision made by protective services.
2. The abuser is removed from family.	This most frequent option is chosen when the nonabusing parent is able to protect the child, and the abuser must	

continued

Nursing Care Plan: The Victim of Sexual Abuse (*Continued*)

Intervention	Rationale	Expected Outcome
	face the responsibility for own behavior.	
3. The child is removed from family.	This rare choice occurs when it is felt that the nonabusing parent would be unable to protect the child. This may place additional guilt on child.	
4. Both child and abuser are removed from home.	This will maximize safety of child and decrease child's feelings of responsibility when nonabusing parent is unable to protect the child.	

Nursing Diagnosis: 05.03.03 Altered parenting role/Parenting, altered: Actual related to enmeshed family system that is either rigid or chaotic*
Goal: Family will move to a moderate position between the extremes of rigid and chaotic

Intervention	Rationale	Expected Outcome
Discuss ways family can increase flexibility of roles and rules.	Rigid family systems are a contributing factor in intrafamily sexual abuse.	Family increases flexibility of rules and roles.
Discuss ways family can organize appropriate roles and formulate consistent rules.	Chaotic family systems are a contributing factor in intrafamily sexual abuse.	Family formulates consistent rules and roles.
Help family identify appropriate roles and power structure within family.	When parents have increased sense of competency and authority, they will parent more effectively.	Parents function in parental roles and children function in age-appropriate roles.
Teach family the problem-solving process.	Increasing alternative coping skills will decrease incidences of abuse.	Family uses the problem-solving process.
Help family anticipate management of developmental transitions within family.	Anticipatory guidance may prevent the recurrence of intrafamily sexual abuse.	Family verbalizes understanding of developmental phases.

*PND-I/NANDA diagnoses.

Evaluation

Nurses in acute care settings may not have the opportunity for long-term evaluation of the family unit. Short-term evaluations center on:

- The identification of sexual abuse within the family
- The family's ability to recognize that a problem exists
- The willingness of the family to accept assistance by following through with referrals

Nurses in long-term settings or within the community have the opportunity to evaluate the effectiveness of the multidisciplinary treatment plan over an extended period. Sharing in the process of family growth and healthy adaptation in the ceasing of sexual abuse can be a tremendous source of professional satisfaction.

Questions to guide the evaluation of the treatment plan are:

- What are the implications for the family if (a) the family stays intact, (b) the abuser is removed, (c) the child is removed, or (d) the child and the abuser are both removed?
- Have the family members learned to communicate directly?

- Has the family structure become more flexible in terms of gender roles?
- Have the parents demonstrated more effective parenting skills?
- Is the family less socially isolated?
- Is the family able to use support systems?

Part II Highlights

- Rape is a crime of violence perpetrated against victims of all ages.
- Behavioral characteristics of rape victims include agitation, outward calmness, crying, nightmares, sleeping problems, or phobias.
- Affective characteristics of rape victims include shock, anxiety, fear, depression, shame, embarrassment, helplessness, and vulnerability.
- Intellectual characteristics of rape victims include disbelief, depersonalization, dissociation, denial, confusion, self-blame, obsessions, and fears for future safety.
- Causative theories relating to rape involve revenge, dominance, eroticized assault, inadequate interpersonal relationships, rigid gender role expectations, and agism.
- Nurses must function as client advocates for rape victims to prevent additional victimization.
- The family home is a place of danger for many women, children, and elderly people.
- Behavioral characteristics related to intrafamily violence include hitting, kicking, shoving, beating, and use of weapons. The pattern of violence tends to escalate in frequency and severity.
- Affective characteristics related to intrafamily violence include jealousy, hostility, dependency, inadequacy, guilt, helplessness, and depression.
- Intellectual characteristics related to intrafamily violence include self-righteousness, inadequate self-esteem, unrealistic expectations, rationalization, and hope for reform.
- There is a higher risk for intrafamily violence under conditions of rigid gender roles, social isolation, high stress, and highly dependent family members.
- Causative theories relating to intrafamily violence include alterations in the limbic system of the violent person, substance abuse, impulsiveness, learned behavior, poverty, and enmeshed family systems.
- Intrafamily sexual abuse occurs in all racial, religious, economic, and sociocultural subgroups.

- Behavioral cues to victims of sexual abuse include regression, sleep disturbances, isolation, extreme affection, sexual acting out, running away, or suicide.
- Affective cues to victims of sexual abuse include fears, ambivalence, guilt, helplessness, and powerlessness.
- Intellectual cues to victims of sexual abuse include denial and thoughts of responsibility.
- Causative factors related to intrafamily sexual abuse include rigid gender roles, chronic stress, inadequate self-esteem, fear of adult relationships, impulsivity, altered family structure, and low adaptability to change.

References

Barash DA: Dynamics of the pathological family system *Perspect Psychiatr Care* 1979;17:17–25.

Barrett MJ, Sykes C, Byrnes W: A systematic model for the treatment of intrafamily child sexual abuse, in Trepper TS, Barrett MJ (eds): *Treating Incest: A Multiple Systems Perspective.* Hayworth Press, 1986.

Becker JV, et al.: Level of postassault sexual functioning in rape and incest victims. *Arch Sex Behav* 1986;15(2):37–47.

Burgess AW: Intra-family sexual abuse, in Campbell J, Humphreys J (eds): *Nursing Care of Victims of Family Violence.* Reston, 1984.

Burgess AW, Holmstrom LL: *Rape: Crisis and Recovery.* Prentice-Hall, 1979.

Burt MKR: Cultural myths and supports for rape. *J Personality Soc Psychol* 1980;38:217–230.

Campbell J: Abuse of female partners, in Campbell J, Humphreys J (eds): *Nursing Care of Victims of Family Violence.* Reston 1984a, pp 74–108.

Campbell J: Nursing care of abused women, in Campbell J, Humphreys J (eds): *Nursing Care of Victims of Family Violence.* Reston, 1984b, pp 246–280.

Campbell J: Nursing care of families using violence, in Campbell J, Humphreys J (eds): *Nursing Care of Victims of Family Violence.* Reston, 1984c, pp 216–245.

Campbell J: Theories of violence, in Campbell J, Humphreys J (eds): *Nursing Care of Victims of Family Violence.* Reston, 1984d, pp 13–52.

Davis LV: Battered women: The transformation of a social problem. *Social Work* 1987;32(4):306–311.

De Nitto D, et al: After rape: Who should examine rape survivors? . . . Nurse rape examiners? *Am J Nurs* 1986; 86(5):538–542.

Elvik SL: Child sexual abuse: The role of the NP. *Nurs Practice,* 1986;11:15–22.

Father convicted of manslaughter in baby's death. *Chicago Sun-Times,* March 5, 1985.

Finkelhor D, Vllo K: Marital rape. *Women's Day* 1985;48:60.

Foley TS: The client who has been raped, in Lego S (ed): *The American Handbook of Psychiatric Nursing.* Lippincott, 1984, pp 475–491.

Foley TS, Davies MA: *Rape: Nursing Care of Victims.* Mosby, 1983.

Freunk K, et al.: Males disposed to commit rape. *Arch Sex Behav* 1986;15(2):23–27.

Giles-Sims J: *Wife Battering: A Systems Theory Approach.* Guilford, 1983.

Golan N: *Treatment in Crisis Situations.* Free Press, 1978.

Griffith-Kenney J: *Contemporary Women's Health.* Addison-Wesley, 1986.

Groth AN, Birnbaum HJ: The rapist, in McCombie SL (ed): *The Rape Crisis Intervention Handbook.* Plenum, 1980, pp 17–26.

Hafen B, Frandsen K: *Psychological Emergencies and Crisis Intervention.* Morton, 1985.

Hirst S, Miller J: The abused elderly. *J Psychosoc Nurs* 1986;24(10):29–34.

Humphreys J, Campbell J: Introduction: Nursing and family violence, in Campbell J, Humphreys J (eds): *Nursing Care of Victims of Family Violence.* Reston, 1984, pp 1–12.

Humphreys J: Nursing care of abused children, in Campbell J, Humphreys J (eds): *Nursing Care of Victims of Family Violence.* Reston, 1984, pp 281–314.

Jackson B: Storm center. *The Wall Street Journal,* February 25, 1985.

Jaffe P: Critical issues in the assessment of children's adjustment to witnessing family violence. *Can Mental Health* 1985;32:13–17.

Kaufman J, Zigler E: Do abused children become abusive parents? *Am J Orthopsychiatry* 1987;57(2):186–192.

Leatherland J: Do you know child abuse when you see it? *RN* 1986;49(11):28–30.

Lecture notes: The Child Sexual Abuse Treatment and Training Center of Illinois, Inc., Bollingbrook, Illinois 60439.

Ledray LE: *Recovering From Rape.* Henry Holt, 1986.

Limandri BJ: The therapeutic relationship with abused women. *J Psychosoc Nurs* 1987;25(2):9–16.

Lowery M: Adult survivors of childhood incest. *J Psychosoc Nurs* 1987;25(1):27–31.

Margolin G: The multiple forms of aggressiveness between marital partners: How do we identify them? *J Marriage Fam Therapy* 1987;13(1):77–84.

Montague MC: Physiology of aggressive behavior. *J Neurosurg Nurs* 1979;11:10–15.

Munro JU: The nurse and the legal system: Dealing with abused children, in Campbell J, Humphreys J (eds): *Nursing Care of Victims of Family Violence.* Reston, 1984, pp 384–402.

O'Connor PJ: Sitter charged with biting boy to death. *Chicago Sun-Times,* February 24, 1985.

Phelan P: Incest: Socialization within a treatment program. *Am J Orthopsychiatry* 1987;57(1):84–92.

Resick PA: Sex-role stereotypes and violence against women, in Franks V, Rothblum E (eds): *The Stereotyping of Women.* Springer, 1983, pp 230–256.

Resources Against Sexual Assault. Rape Prevention Education Program, University of California, San Francisco, 1987.

Rossi R: Dad convicted of plot to kill son, 17. *Chicago Sun-Times,* February 7, 1985.

Russell DE: *The Politics of Rape: The Victim's Perspective.* Stein and Day, 1975.

Seeley D: Encountering rape: Not for women only. *Chicago Tribune,* February 7, 1985.

Sengstock MC, Barrett S: Domestic abuse of the elderly, in Campbell J, Humphreys J (eds): *Nursing Care of Victims of Family Violence.* Reston, 1984, pp 145–188.

Shapiro S: Self-multilation and self-blame in incest victims. *Am J Psychother* 1987;41(1):46–54.

Solin C: Displacement of affect in families following incest disclosure. *Am J Orthopsychiatry* 1986;56(4):570–576.

Straus MA, Gelles RJ, Steinmetz SK: *Behind Closed Doors: Violence in the American Family.* Anchor Press/Doubleday, 1980.

Straus MA, Hotaling GT: *The Social Causes of Husband-Wife Violence.* University of Minnesota Press, 1980.

Thorman G: *Family Violence.* Charles C Thomas, 1980.

Trepper TS, Barrett MJ: Introduction to a multiple systems approach for the assessment and treatment of intrafamily child sexual abuse, in Trepper TS, Barrett MJ (eds): *Treating Incest: A Multiple Systems Perspective.* Hayworth Press, 1986, pp 5–12.

Trepper TS, Barrett MJ: Vulnerability to incest: A framework for assessment, in Trepper TS, Barrett MJ (eds): *Treating Incest: A Multiple Systems Perspective.* Hayworth Press, 1986b, pp 13–25.

Trepper TS, Traicoff ME: Treatment of intrafamily sexuality: Issues in therapy and research. *J Sex Educ Ther* 1983;9:14–18.

Vanderschaeghe L: Child abuse and community mental health practice. *Can J Psych Nurs* 1986;33:13–17.

Walker LE: Violence against women: Implications for mental health policy, in Walker LE (ed): *Women and Mental Health Policy.* Sage Publications, 1984, pp 121–156.

Warner CG: *Rape and Sexual Assault.* Aspen Systems, 1980.

Yates A: Should young children testify in cases of sexual abuse? *Am J Psychiatry* 1987;144(4):476–480.

Zolanuk JM, Harris CC, Wisian NL: Adolescent pregnancy and incest: The nurse's role as counselor. *JOGNN* 1987;16(2):99–103.

TWENTY-SIX

The Role of the Psychiatric Nurse in the AIDS Epidemic

Carol Ren Kneisl

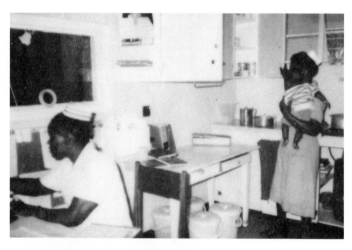

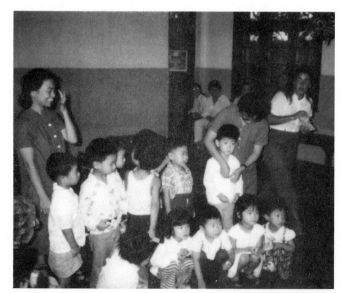

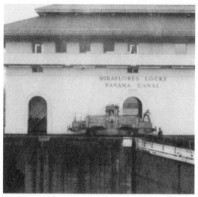

After reading this chapter, students should be able to

- Explain why certain populations are at risk for acquired immune deficiency syndrome (AIDS)

- Discuss the incidence and geographic distribution of AIDS

- Describe the biologic, psychologic, developmental, social and cultural, economic, legal, political, and ethical impact of AIDS

- Provide direct nursing care to persons with AIDS in in-patient psychiatric settings

- Incorporate AIDS risk reduction education and counseling regarding sexual behavior and substance abuse in work with clients and people in the community

- Identify the means by which psychiatric nurses can support AIDS caregivers

- Support the bereaved, such as persons with AIDS and their friends, family, and caregivers

- Suggest avenues of self-help for persons with AIDS and their significant others

- Explain why continued nursing involvement in AIDS research is important

- Engage in advocacy and political activism related to AIDS

Cross References

Other topics relevant to this content are: Caring for clients with organic mental disorder, Chapter 15; Caring for depressed clients, Chapter 18; Caring for substance-abusing clients, Chapter 16; Dying clients and their families, Chapter 37; Visualization and stress management techniques for self-healing and pain and symptom control, Chapter 28.

When the people lead, eventually leaders will follow.

Key Terms

acquired immune deficiency
  syndrome (AIDS)
AIDS-related complex (ARC)
care-partners
fisting
guerrilla AIDS clinics
HIV-seropositive
homophobia

human immunodeficiency
  virus (HIV)
Kaposi's sarcoma
nonoxynol-9
opportunistic diseases
Pneumocystis carinii
  pneumonia
poppers
rimming
works

To Tommy,
Alone with death, the long-awaited scourge—I hope you
  were ready;
Yours was a horrible, helpless dying, full of fear.
Betrayed unceasingly by your body, you wasted away from
  TB, pneumonia, and diarrhea;
Your mind also was ravaged—first mania, then depression.
The man became his parents' child again, though grown;
  dependency and humiliation were enraging;
You tried to keep believing that it wouldn't get you, as did
  your family.
And in the end you were alone when death claimed you;
A new ward, nurses afraid and repulsed, not knowing you,
  seeing only the grotesqueness of your decaying flesh.
Did anyone know your death was near, could someone have
  held your hand?

Jill M. Strawn (1987, p 126)

Acquired immune deficiency syndrome (AIDS), a contagious and fatal condition of immune system depression for which there is no known cure, is a clinical issue of concern to all nurses, including psychiatric nurses. Psychiatric nurses are caregivers who, by the nature of their commitment and responsibility, become involved in human experiences. And AIDS is unquestionably one of the most tragic of human experiences. Clients with AIDS require care that promotes quality existence and personal growth in the face of serious illness, care that psychiatric nurses are the very best at offering.

OVERVIEW OF AIDS

AIDS relentlessly disarms the immune system, preventing it from fighting infection. **Opportunistic diseases** normally warded off by a healthy immune system are given the opportunity to attack the body. Eventually weakened by the persistent and debilitating onslaught, the person with AIDS is vulnerable at any time to a final, all-out attack. Sometimes this happens within a few months, but often the progression of the disease runs for a few years after symptoms appear.

What Causes AIDS

An extremely tiny retrovirus (about 230 *million* would fit on the period at the end of this sentence), the **human immunodeficiency virus (HIV)**, causes AIDS. It consists basically of a double-layered shell or envelope full of proteins, surrounding a bit of ribonucleic acid (RNA). The AIDS virus homes in on helper T-lymphocytes in much the same way that the hepatitis virus invades cells in the liver.

Like Greeks hidden inside the Trojan horse, the HIV enters the body concealed inside a helper T-cell from an infected host. When the foreign T-cell meets a defending T-cell, the virus slips through the cell membrane into the defending cell and disables it. Once inside an inactive T-cell, the virus may remain dormant for months, even years.

Unlike true life forms, a virus cannot metabolize nutrients (in fact does not need them), does not grow, and cannot reproduce unless it has the assistance of a living host cell. Certain events shorten the latency period for the HIV-infected person. Repeated exposure to semen absorbed into the blood, infections such as hepatitis B or tuberculosis, use of drugs that suppress the immune system (such as corticosteroids) and recreational drugs (such as marijuana, cocaine, or amyl nitrate "poppers"), poor nutrition, stress, or lack of sleep weaken the immune system and trigger the division of invaded T-cells. The HIV begins to multiply by inserting its genes into the DNA of the host cell and ordering it to produce carbon copies of itself. The fact that it can clone itself a thousand times faster than any other known virus explains why AIDS is such a rapidly progressive and devastating disease.

Who Is at Risk and Why

The presence of HIV has been documented in blood, blood plasma, bone marrow, semen, cervical secretions, vaginal secretions, saliva, breast milk, lymph nodes, brain tissue, skin, tears, and cerebrospinal fluid. The presence of the virus in so many body fluids and tissues is one reason why the general public fears that AIDS can be transmitted by casual contact. However, the research overwhelmingly indicates that the major modes of transmission of the virus are:

1. Intimate sexual contact with an **HIV-seropositive** person (one who has tested positive for the HIV antibody)

2. Parenteral injection of blood or blood products infected with the HIV virus

3. Transfer of the virus from an HIV-infected mother to a fetus or newborn infant in utero, during labor or delivery, or in the early newborn period

Because of the nature of these major modes of transmission, several groups have been identified as being at *high risk* of developing AIDS:

- Homosexual/bisexual men (and their sexual partners)
- Intravenous drug abusers (and their sexual partners)
- Hemophiliacs (and their sexual partners)
- Children born to parents with AIDS or at risk for AIDS
- Prostitutes

Note that family members and friends in close contact with AIDS victims are not listed among the high-risk categories. In the one instance in which a mother apparently acquired the virus from her infant, she did not follow recommendations for handling her infant's secretions (Centers for Disease Control 1986). Research has confirmed that there is little or no risk to those having long-standing household exposure to persons with AIDS (Friedland et al. 1986).

Health care providers are also not in the high-risk category. In addition to having close contact with persons with AIDS, health care workers may be concerned about contracting AIDS as the result of an accidental needlestick or being cut with a sharp instrument. A study of almost 1000 health care workers that documented parenteral or mucous membrane exposure to the blood or body fluids of persons with AIDS indicated that only two health care workers tested positive for HIV at a fifteen-month follow-up (McCray 1986). Three other health care workers identified in 1987 as infected with the HIV virus had been exposed to large amounts of infected blood (Centers for Disease Control 1987). Although later research is sure to demonstrate other similar instances, the incidence among health care workers is extremely small.

Protection for health care workers and others in close contact with persons with AIDS is discussed in more detail later in this chapter. Counseling others in strategies for preventing AIDS is also discussed later in this chapter.

Homosexual/Bisexual Men

Homosexual/bisexual men continue to account for the highest percentage of reported cases. In San Francisco AIDS is considered the major health problem for gay men (Cohen 1987), and in New York City AIDS is the leading cause of death in men aged 30 to 39 years (Kaplan 1986).

Studies of risk factors for homosexual/bisexual men indicate that having a large number of different male sexual partners appears to be the most significant risk factor. Certain sexual practices such as receptive anal intercourse and fisting (inserting the fingers, a hand, or a fist into the rectum), which cause trauma and injury to rectal tissue, are more frequently associated with increased risk (Jaffe et al. 1985). Other studies have demonstrated the possibility of genetic susceptibility to the development of Kaposi's sarcoma (present in about 48 percent of homosexual men with AIDS) that may relate to an underlying immune defect (Krigel and Friedman-Kien 1985).

Intravenous Drug Abusers

The second largest transmission category for AIDS is intravenous drug abusers. The virus is believed to be transmitted among intravenous drug abusers through the transfer of small amounts of blood in shared needles or syringes. Intravenous drug abusers also constitute a bridge to others—their fetuses, newborns, and sexual partners—putting them at increased risk. It is believed that the category known as "heterosexual cases" is largely composed of the heterosexual partners of intravenous drug abusers.

Hemophiliacs

The risk to hemophiliacs and persons with other coagulation disorders comes from receiving clotting factor concentrates. Pooled plasma that may contain material from between 2500 and 25,000 blood or plasma donors is used to make clotting factor concentrates (Levine 1985). As early as 1984 there was almost a total HIV seroconversion (the development of antibodies in response to infection) linked to the administration of factor concentrates contaminated with HIV. Levine (1985) notes that AIDS may soon surpass hemorrhage as the leading cause of death among hemophiliacs. Hemophiliacs also constitute a bridge (although a much smaller one than intravenous drug abusers) to children and female sexual partners.

Blood Transfusion Recipients

The risk to blood or blood product transfusion recipients comes from receiving blood from an HIV-positive donor. Testing of potential donors by enzyme-linked immunoabsorbent assay (ELISA) and screening of potential donors at risk for AIDS has been instituted to protect the blood supply. Although the number of persons who contract AIDS in this way is low (2 percent), the possibility of contracting AIDS from tainted blood remains. False negative reactions are possible because of the *window* that exists (the period of time between which a person becomes infected and the development of antibodies) or because of errors in testing. Although the window was thought to be 6 to 8 weeks in length, recent findings indicate that it can take up to 14 *months* for HIV seroconversion to occur. Researchers are working to develop new tests with a smaller window.

Incidence and Geographic Distribution

National

By September 14, 1987, 41,825 cases of AIDS had been reported to the Centers for Disease Control (CDC), and the known deaths since records were first kept in early 1981 numbered 24,070, or 58 percent (Centers for Disease Control, September 14, 1987). The current incidence picture is illustrated in Figure 26–1(A) for adults and adolescents age 13 years and over and in Figure 26–1(B) for infants and children.

At the national level, AIDS has been reported in all fifty of the United States. New York, California, Florida,

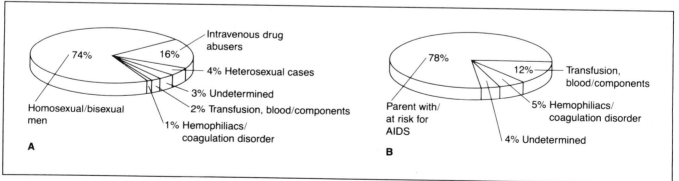

Figure 26–1

A, Incidence of AIDS among adults and adolescents age 13 years and older. (Eight percent of homosexual/bisexual men also reported using intravenous drugs.) B, Incidence of AIDS among infants and children. Note that due to rounding off, the percentages total 99 percent.

Source: Centers for Disease Control: AIDS Weekly Surveillance Report. *Sept. 14, 1987.*

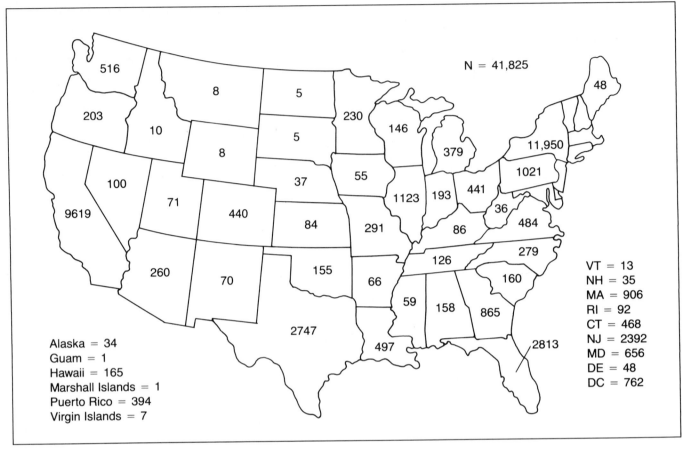

Figure 26–2
Distribution by state of reported cases of AIDS in the United States.
Source: Centers for Disease Control: AIDS Weekly Surveillance Report. *Sept. 14, 1987.*

New Jersey, and Texas have the highest percentage of AIDS cases (Figure 26–2). The metropolitan areas with the largest number of AIDS cases are listed in Box 26–1. The incidence in homosexual men is highest in New York City, San Francisco, and Los Angeles. The incidence of AIDS among intravenous drug abusers is highest in the New York/New Jersey metropolitan area and in neighboring Connecticut. Of heterosexuals whose only known exposure was through sex with a person at risk, approximately two-thirds are female partners of male intravenous drug abusers. In the undetermined category, slightly over half had heterosexual contact with a person with or at risk for AIDS, and slightly under half were born in countries in which heterosexual transmission is thought to play a major role (Haiti or central Africa). Approximately one-third of those who cannot be placed in a high-risk category had sexual contact with female prostitutes (among whom the incidence of AIDS continues to rise).

Estimates of the number of people in this country infected with the AIDS virus range from 2 million to 3 million people. The CDC computer predictions of the increase in AIDS in the five-year period from 1987–1991 are grim:

- About 235,000 new cases will be reported.
- The cumulative total of deaths at the end of 1991 will be 179,000 people.
- The number of children with AIDS will probably increase tenfold.
- By 1991 the medical care of persons with AIDS will require between $8 billion and $16 billion, not including home care given by friends or family or lost income due to illness.
- The number of heterosexual cases will increase to 9 percent.

The epidemic is growing every day, partly because people who may not know they are infected are spreading the virus.

International

At the international level, AIDS has been reported in every continent of the world except for Antarctica. International statistics are not always reliable since there is no international law that requires the reporting of AIDS cases. It is unclear whether the scope of the problem is as well known in the rest of the world as it is in the Americas. In the Americas, the countries with the highest number of reported cases are the United States, Brazil, Canada, and Haiti. The European countries of France, West Germany, Denmark, Switzerland, and Belgium report a high number of cases. Most of the AIDS cases in Africa are from what has become known as the "AIDS belt"—Zaire, Zambia, Rwanda, Burundi, Kenya, Uganda, and Tanzania. It is estimated that one out of every twenty people in these African nations is infected with HIV.

THE BIOPSYCHOSOCIAL IMPACT OF AIDS

AIDS does not discriminate in its effect on the individual or society. It affects the biologic, psychologic, developmental, social, cultural, economic, political, legal, and ethical spheres.

Biologic

The extent of the symptoms and signs associated with HIV infection can vary from none, through nonspecific manifestations, to a variety of opportunistic infections and malignancies. Some people, although infected with HIV, remain healthy and never develop AIDS. They can, however, transmit the virus to others.

Symptoms and Signs of ARC

Some people have a mild immune deficiency but do not have any life-threatening disease. These people are said to have **AIDS-related complex (ARC)**. (For reporting purposes, the Centers for Disease Control uses a classification system that uses more specific and inclusive definitions than those presented here. However, for the purposes of this textbook, we are using the popular definition of ARC.)

Initially the symptoms of ARC and AIDS may be the same as for any of a number of other conditions or illnesses; however, with HIV infection, they tend to be particularly prolonged. Persons with ARC may have symptoms and signs that include any combination of the following:

- Fatigue, possibly combined with headaches or lightheadedness
- Low-grade fever
- Night sweats

Box 26–1
METROPOLITAN AREAS (UNITED STATES) WITH THE HIGHEST REPORTED CASES OF AIDS AS OF SEPTEMBER 14, 1987

New York, New York (10,851)
San Francisco, California (4098)
Los Angeles, California (3553)
Houston, Texas (1346)
Washington, District of Columbia (1222)
Miami, Florida (1149)
Chicago, Illinois (1009)
Newark, New Jersey (973)
Philadelphia, Pennsylvania (818)
Dallas, Texas (796)
Atlanta, Georgia (666)
Boston, Massachusetts (663)
San Diego, California (530)
Fort Lauderdale, Florida (529)
Nassau-Suffolk, New York (514)
Jersey City, New Jersey (467)
Seattle, Washington (408)
Denver, Colorado (369)
New Orleans, Louisiana (360)
Anaheim, California (348)

Source: Centers for Disease Control. AIDS Weekly Surveillance Report. September 14, 1987.

- Cervical, axillary, or femoral lymphadenopathy over several weeks
- Weight loss greater than 10 percent or 15 pounds not related to exercise or dieting
- Easy bruising or unexplained bleeding
- Chronic diarrhea

Symptoms and Signs of AIDS

The formal diagnosis of AIDS depends on whether the person can be diagnosed with one or more of the specific life-threatening opportunistic diseases the CDC has defined as indicative of AIDS (Box 26–2). These individuals are said to have *full-blown AIDS*.

The most serious opportunistic disease is *Pneumocystis carinii* pneumonia, caused by the protozoa *Pneumocystis carinii,* the leading cause of death among persons with AIDS. It has symptoms similar to other severe forms

---

Box 26–2
OPPORTUNISTIC INFECTIONS AND NEOPLASMS ASSOCIATED WITH AIDS

- Monilial infections of the mouth, trachea, esophagus, bronchi, or perineal and perianal areas caused by *Candida albicans*
- Cytomegalovirus infections
- Cryptococcal meningitis
- *Cryptosporidium* enterocolitis
- Herpes simplex virus and herpes zoster virus infections
- Kaposi's sarcoma
- *Pneumocystis carinii* pneumonia
- Primary lymphoma of the central nervous system
- Progressive multifocal leukoencephalopathy
- Toxoplasmosis
- Tuberculosis and other mycobacterial infections caused by *Mycobacterium avium* and *Mycobacterium intracellulare*

---

of pneumonia, such as dry cough, difficulty breathing, and fever. This particular opportunistic disease has been implicated in 58 percent of the deaths from AIDS (Centers for Disease Control, September 14, 1987).

The most common malignancy is **Kaposi's sarcoma.** Usually appearing first on the legs as blue-violet or red-brown nodules or plaques, Kaposi's sarcoma can occur anywhere on the surface of the skin, in the mouth, or in the visceral organs such as the digestive tract and the lungs. Previously a rare malignancy of elderly men who survived for ten or more years after diagnosis, Kaposi's sarcoma is now the second most common cause of death among persons with AIDS. This malignancy was uncommon in North America and Europe until the AIDS epidemic. Currently, Kaposi's sarcoma has been implicated in 46 percent of the deaths from AIDS (Centers for Disease Control, September 14, 1987).

Neuropsychiatric Syndromes in HIV-Infected Persons

Because of the ability of the virus to invade central nervous system (CNS) tissue and because several of the opportunistic infections and neoplasms associated with AIDS also affect the CNS, significant numbers of persons with ARC and AIDS develop acute delirium progressing to chronic dementia. From all indications, neurologic or neuropsychiatric problems are extraordinarily common in HIV-infected persons (even those who are seropositive but asymptomatic), whether or not other symptoms and signs of ARC or AIDS are present. The neurologic disease states (both central and peripheral nervous systems) and clinical manifestations in persons with ARC and AIDS are presented in Table 26–1. Organic mental disorders in AIDS are listed in Box 26–3. Care must be taken to make appropriate distinctions between delirium or dementia and depression and not to mistake one for the other.

Psychologic

AIDS threatens psychologic integrity as well as physiologic integrity. The concept of loss is central to an understanding of the psychologic impact of AIDS and the depression, anxiety, and suicidal ideation that often accompany it. AIDS is irretrievably linked with several different loss experiences. These include loss of:

- Energy, appetite, strength, and physical stamina
- Control of body functions such as elimination, mobility, speech, sight, hearing, and tactile sensations
- Control of body appearance because of dramatic weight loss, oozing wounds, skin breakdown, hair loss, skin lesions, and so on
- Self-worth
- Mental clarity and cognitive ability
- Privacy
- Self-sufficiency and self-determination
- Employment, health insurance, salary
- Personal competency
- Physical intimacy including sexual expression
- Friends and lovers to earlier deaths from AIDS
- Social support
- Hope
- Peace of mind and spirit
- Life itself

These losses or fears of these losses are experienced by persons with AIDS and by their families, friends, and caregivers. One psychiatric nurse (McEnany 1987) is concerned with the mental health effects that such an overwhelming number of losses will have on the increasing numbers of people being touched personally by AIDS as friends, loved ones, or colleagues die from it. McEnany predicts an increase in the numbers of people with the psychiatric diagnosis of post-traumatic stress disorder as more people are faced with such overwhelming losses.

Table 26–1
Neurologic Disease States and Clinical Manifestations in Persons with AIDS and ARC

	Disease Process	Clinical Manifestations
Cerebrum	Acute meningitis	Headache, nausea, vomiting, fever, lethargy, delirium, meningeal irritation, expressive language dysfunction, focal neurologic deficits, seizures
	Acute encephalitis	
	Acute meningoencephalitis	
	Cerebrovascular accident	
	Mass lesions (infections, neoplasms)	Seizures, hydrocephalus, movement disorders, focal neurologic deficits, increased intracranial pressure
	Chronic meningitis	As above, plus cortical atrophy, dementia, organic affective and personality syndromes
	Chronic meningoencephalitis	
	Chronic encephalitis	
Brainstem	Meningitis	Long tract dysfunction (motor, sensory), impaired respiratory and cardiovascular regulation
	Infections	
	Neoplasms	
Cerebellum	Infections, neoplasms	Gait disorders, incoordination
Spinal cord	Posterolateral column	Sensation impairment, motor (flaccid, spastic) incontinence
	Lateral column (ALS)	
	Viral myelitis	
Neuropathies, myopathy	Cranial and peripheral mononeuropathies and neuropathies, radiculitis myopathy, polymyositis	Sensory and motor dysfunction (e.g., distal symmetrical), Bell's palsy, dermatomal pain, muscle pain, tenderness, and wasting

Source: Wolcott DL: Neuropsychiatric syndromes in AIDS and AIDS-related illnesses, in McKusick L: What to do About AIDS: Physicians and Mental Health Professionals Discuss the Issues. University of California Press, 1986, p 34. © University of California Press, 1986.

Developmental

Most persons with AIDS are young adults or adults in their middle years. The period known as young adulthood is normally the healthiest and is characterized by peaks in muscular strength. Cognitive development should be completed and cognitive abilities should be refined at this stage. Recall from Chapter 6 that the psychosocial task of identity consolidation is the major developmental task of young adulthood. AIDS disrupts the person's ability to successfully negotiate this challenge.

Typically, the middle years are very productive in the arenas of work and family. During this period, adults typically consolidate relationships and occupational status and goals. AIDS interferes on all fronts with the individual's ability to accept the responsibilities inherent in such roles as parent, worker, mate or partner, and so on. Questions of dependence and independence, thought to have been resolved previously, are reawakened as illness forces a return to earlier developmental phases.

Children and adolescents with AIDS face delays or changes in skills on all developmental fronts—physical, cognitive, and psychosocial—as they meet acute life-threatening illness and chronic disability. Failure to thrive is a striking feature of this illness in children, some of whom have been diagnosed with AIDS as early as 4 months of age (Boland 1987).

Social and Cultural

The social and cultural environments of most persons with AIDS, at risk for AIDS, or affected by AIDS is generally hostile to them. Several factors seem to account for this sociocultural hostility. Strawn (1987) notes that the majority of persons with AIDS, at risk for AIDS, or affected by AIDS ". . . are members of groups whose skin color, ethnic and cultural background, and/or life-style habits are regarded by many in the mainstream of American life with repugnance, fear, and moral condemnation."

Box 26–3
ORGANIC MENTAL DISORDERS IN AIDS

I. Chronic organic mental disorder (OMD)

A. Dementia (process–agents)

1. Diffuse subacute encephalitis—HIV, cytomegalovirus (CMV), and other infections

2. Meningitis—*Cryptococcus neoformans, Mycobacterium avium* and *intracellulare,* aseptic, other

3. Meningeal lymphoma—B cell

4. Cerebral mass lesion—lymphoma, Kaposi's sarcoma, *Toxoplasma gondii,* other polymicrobial infections

5. Stroke syndrome—cerebral hemorrhage, nonbacterial thrombotic endocarditis, cerebral arteritis

6. Possible nutritional deficiency

B. Organic affective syndrome—subacute encephalitis

C. Organic personality syndrome—subacute encephalitis

II. Acute organic mental disorders—delirium: contributing factors

A. Primary central nervous system disease

1. Infectious, neoplastic, cerebrovascular factors as in chronic organic mental disorder

2. Increased intracranial pressure from cerebral mass lesions

3. Seizure disorder—postictal states

4. CNS effects of treatment (chemotherapy, interferon)

B. Secondary CNS disease

1. Systemic infections

2. Hypoxemia from respiratory insufficiency (e.g., *Pneumocystis carinii* pneumonia)

3. Electrolyte imbalance (diarrhea, inappropriate antidiuretic hormone)

C. Environmental and psychologic factors

1. Visual loss from ophthalmic infections

2. Prolonged sensory understimulation and inactivity

3. Disrupted circadian rhythms (sleep/wake cycle)

4. Psychologic distress (anxiety, fear)

Source: Reprinted by permission of the publisher from "Acquired immune deficiency syndrome (AIDS) and consultant-liaison psychiatry," Wolcott D, Fawzy F, Pasnau R. General Hospital Psychiatry, *7, p 283. Copyright 1985 by Elsevier Science Publishing Co., Inc.*

The majority of persons with AIDS are in two risk categories—homosexual/bisexual men and intravenous drug abusers—that engender fear, anger, and prejudice. **Homophobia** is the term used to describe unrealistic fear of homosexuality and homosexuals based on myths and stereotypes associated with homosexuality. According to Hughes, Martin, and Franks (1987, pp 107–108), homophobia may exist on both overt and covert levels and may be internalized, externalized, or institutional:

• Internalized homophobia is the self-rejection (feelings of shame, fear, guilt, and wrongdoing) that gay people may experience.

• Externalized homophobia is the rejection gay persons experience from others.

• Institutional homophobia is evident in the rules and regulations of hospitals, churches, employers, and other institutions, which invalidate the gay life-style by, for example, restricting hospital visitors in intensive care

units to blood relatives only or denying gay people the right to worship.

Moral indignation is a frequent response to both gay people and to intravenous drug abusers. Many people consider homosexuality, bisexuality, and substance abuse evidence of lack of character, criminal behavior, or a sinful life-style. The two risk groups share other common characteristics (Hughes et al. 1987):

1. Friends and partners (or lovers) are nontraditional support systems. Families of origin may be unaware of, or may reject, the individual's life-style and thus may be unable or unwilling to provide support.

2. Persons in both risk categories may be estranged from institutions, such as organized religion, that view their life-style as sinful or immoral.

3. Both groups may be set apart from the mainstream because of differences in norms, values, and language.

4. The caregivers and support systems of persons in either

of these groups may be members of the same high-risk groups, with which the nurse may not have had much previous contact.

On one hand, children with AIDS or persons who have contracted AIDS from transfusion of blood or a blood product are usually perceived as "innocents" rather than sinners. On the other hand, they may be as feared and subject to discrimination as gays and drug abusers.

In her book *Illness as Metaphor* (1977) Susan Sontag suggests that people with illnesses that arouse feelings of apprehension and vulnerability in others become objects of that dread. This is especially true of AIDS. The well fear contamination by the sick with an illness for which there is no known cure.

Economic

For the individual, AIDS can mean an unstable financial situation. Days lost from work because of illness may cost the person with AIDS his or her job and insurance benefits. Some insurers are avoiding or reducing claims by isolating high-risk applicants with AIDS antibody tests, denying new policies to those at risk, and aggressively fighting existing policyholders' claims in court. Family and friends may be unable or unwilling to assist financially. Young adults, many in their early thirties, find themselves having to seek public assistance such as Medicaid for help in meeting health costs associated with AIDS. The price of azidothymidine (AZT; marketed as Retrovir) is set at $8300 a year wholesale and $10,000 retail (Chase 1987), a cost that by itself places AIDS treatment beyond most persons' means.

Experts predict that by 1991 AIDS care will cost the nation more than kidney dialysis or cancer of the lung, breast, or colon. Only care for cardiac clients and auto accident casualties is expected to cost more. Federal authorities estimate that about 40 percent of all persons with AIDS will eventually be without means or insurance and will need to rely on Medicaid.

Volunteer programs such as San Francisco's Shanti Project, a private organization of 350 volunteers who donate 75,000 hours of their time per year, provides a lifeline for persons with AIDS. Shanti provides emotional support counselors to the dying and their families; sends out workers to clean, cook, shop, and provide transportation; runs several low-cost residences; and shuttles persons with AIDS back and forth to hospital and clinic appointments.

A comprehensive study by the National Academy of Sciences (1986) urged that $2 billion dollars—$1 billion for research and another $1 billion for education—be spent annually by 1990, with half coming from the federal budget. The federal budget request for fiscal 1988 is less than half this amount. Only $400 million has been earmarked for AIDS research, compared with $1.3 billion for cancer research and $900 million for heart research. Unquestionably, AIDS presents an economic problem of severe proportions.

Legal

Law on AIDS is still in the formative stage. Several legal questions have not yet been answered. Some recommend legislation to ban discrimination against people infected with HIV, while others urge legislation to require mandatory testing and quarantine as two measures to protect the general public. Testing will probably not become common until people do not have to worry that they will lose their jobs or insurance if they test positive for HIV. The dilemma has to do with the violation of individual rights (by such activities as mandatory premarital or antepartal testing or mandatory testing of persons at high risk) as opposed to violation of the concept of societal good.

Bompey (1986) has reached the following conclusions on the direction of law related to employment rights and AIDS based on recent court decisions:

- AIDS is a "protected handicap."

- An employer cannot deny employment to an applicant with AIDS unless the disease is far advanced and renders the applicant incapable of performing the duties of the job.

- Segregation of persons with AIDS in the workplace is without medical justification and would probably violate prohibitions against discrimination on the basis of disability.

- Other employees generally cannot refuse to work with people who have AIDS unless a claim can be substantiated that a dangerous work condition exists; such employees, after educational interventions, may be subject to discipline or dismissal if they still refuse to work with affected persons.

- Employers may not discharge an employee with AIDS merely because they believe that individual will soon become incapacitated.

- Employers may not generally ask job applicants if they have AIDS or have been exposed to the disease.

- Employers can probably require blood tests as part of the preemployment physical examination, but the employer would be limited in using the test results. Disclosure of such information to others would be highly inadvisable.

- Employers cannot force employees with AIDS to take a medical leave unless they are unable to perform their jobs.

There are several cases in the courts over denied AIDS-related medical insurance claims and life insurance policy claims. Insurance companies have been accused of using legal tactics to delay the resolution of litigation on the theory that the life of a person with AIDS is shorter than the life of a lawsuit. The wills of people who have died from AIDS and bequeathed their estates to gay partners are also being contested by estranged blood relatives.

Because cognitive impairment is common in persons with AIDS, decision-making regarding treatment, investments, and other financial matters is often transferred to another person with power of attorney.

Political

Leaders in the gay community have been concerned about the slow pace of the Food and Drug Administration (FDA) in approving new drugs for the treatment of AIDS and argue that the FDA should be far more liberal in allowing use of untested drugs by those who have no hope of cure. The lack of easy access to drugs has encouraged the development of **guerrilla AIDS clinics.** These informal clinics, in living rooms and kitchens throughout the United States, provide a variety of medicines. Some are readily available prescription drugs. Others are more exotic mixtures of nutritional additives or items such as Brazilian tree bark and Chinese mushrooms. Still others are chemicals such as DNCB (a photographic solvent readily available at chemical supply houses, and traditionally used to treat warts), which is painted on Kaposi's sarcoma lesions with cotton-tipped applicators. Those who are desperate travel to Mexico and Europe to obtain drugs not yet approved for sale in this country.

The political climate also affects potential legislation to ensure confidentiality and to ban discrimination. For example, it may not be politically feasible for a legislator seeking reelection by a conservative, frightened, or unknowledgeable constituency to advocate measures his or her electorate would see as contrary to their best interests. Some politicians point to the AIDS epidemic as graphically illustrating huge gaps in the health care system and the need for a comprehensive federal medical care program.

Ethical

According to Durham (1987), the mysterious nature of AIDS, the lack of an effective cure, and its highly lethal outcome combine to stigmatize persons with AIDS. Durham also suggests that persons with AIDS are doubly stigmatized because most of them are already members of other stigmatized groups—homosexuals, bisexuals, drug abusers, blacks, and Hispanics. The statistics for homosexuals, bisexuals, and drug abusers have been discussed ear-

lier in this chapter and illustrated in Figure 26–1A. The CDC (September 14, 1987) reports that 38 percent of the reported adult and adolescent cases of AIDS are among blacks (24 percent) and Hispanics (14 percent), and 78 percent of the infant and child cases are also among blacks (54 percent) and Hispanics (24 percent).

Breaches of confidentiality, such as reporting the results of testing to government agencies, employers, and insurance companies, or tattooing individuals who test HIV positive so that potential sex partners would be aware the individual has been exposed to the virus, would further stigmatize persons with AIDS.

The ethical issues surrounding AIDS probably prompt most emotional responses. Some of the ethical questions that have arisen are:

- Should AIDS antibody testing be made mandatory? If so, who should be tested—gay men, intravenous drug abusers, pregnant women, persons admitted to hospitals, prisoners, couples applying for marriage licenses, food handlers, health care workers, child care workers, people applying for health and life insurance, everyone?

- Is it in the public interest to identify, report, and make public the names of persons with AIDS or at risk for AIDS?

- To what extent would the undertaking of preventive health measures be a matter of public health responsibility?

- Should persons infected with the virus be tattooed in order to protect potential sex partners from infection?

- Should persons with AIDS be placed in quarantine for the public good?

- Can or should employers suspend, terminate, or refuse to hire persons with AIDS? If they are teachers? Food handlers? Health care workers?

- Should people who have had sexual contact with persons with AIDS or received infected blood products be traced and informed by public health authorities?

- Do health care workers have a duty to inform those at risk when a person with AIDS does not modify his or her behavior?

- Is it appropriate to make experimental drugs and treatments that are not yet proven safe and effective available to persons with AIDS?

- Should research protocols that call for administering placebos to some persons (who thus remain untreated) and experimental drugs to others be allowed?

- Can nurses or other health care professionals refuse to provide care to persons with AIDS?

Engaging in the process of ethical reflectiveness discussed in Chapter 10 can be used to analyze these and other issues and resolve the ethical dilemmas inherent in them.

In 1985 the American Nurses' Association (ANA) reaffirmed its specific commitment to nursing care for persons with AIDS (ANA 1985b). In addition to this specific commitment to nursing care for persons with AIDS, the first two statements in ANA's code of ethics (ANA 1985a) provide guidance to nurses with respect to these nursing care dilemmas:

1. The nurse provides services with respect for human dignity and the uniqueness of the client unrestricted by considerations of social or economic status, personal attributes, or the nature of health problems.

2. The nurse safeguards the client's right to privacy by judiciously protecting information of a confidential nature.

Both the New York State Nurses Association (1983) and the California Nurses Association (1985) have published statements relative to nursing practice that make clear the professional nurse's responsibility in relation to the care of persons with AIDS. These statements address the need to provide appropriate care (both direct and indirect), health teaching, and advocacy.

ROLES FOR PSYCHIATRIC NURSES

Psychiatric nurses will work with clients all along the continuum of AIDS disability. Schietinger (1986) has proposed the following continuum for describing the impact of AIDS in terms of the person's functional ability. It conceptualizes four levels of disability:

1. *Apparently well.* The apparently well person has either ARC or AIDS but requires little or no medical intervention. An example would be a functionally independent gay man with a skin lesion diagnosed as Kaposi's sarcoma.

2. *Acutely ill.* The acutely ill person may be experiencing an opportunistic infection. Hospitalization may be required for treatment to stabilize the condition.

3. *Chronically ill.* The chronically ill person has experienced a relapse of an opportunistic disease, has received a diagnosis of a new opportunistic disease, or has a progression or deterioration in his or her physical or mental condition.

4. *Terminally ill.* The terminally ill person has a prognosis of six months or less to live.

Psychiatric nurses may be involved in working with persons with AIDS in in-patient settings in psychiatric hospitals, psychiatric units in general hospitals, mental health clinics, community health agencies, hospices or homes, private practice, industry, or schools and as citizens and neighbors. In addition to working with people at the four levels of disability listed above, psychiatric nurses have active roles with well people, with the family and friends of persons with AIDS, and with bereaved survivors.

Direct Nursing Care in In-Patient Psychiatric Settings

Persons with AIDS

Several authorities have predicted that increasing numbers of persons with AIDS will require hospitalization in a psychiatric setting. Psychiatric hospitalization may be needed because the client is depressed, suicidal, or psychotic or has an AIDS-related behavior disturbance, probably because of organic mental disorder.

Psychiatric nurses caring for clients with AIDS on in-patient units encounter a number of issues that are uncommon in psychiatric settings:

- The client has a multitude of physical problems.
- The client has a condition that calls for infection control precautions.
- The quality of the nurse-client relationship is intensified through the additional contact required in giving physical care.
- The psychiatric nurse must confront the issue of caring for clients with life-threatening illnesses.

Nursing care specific to be physical problems of persons with AIDS is outlined in the nursing care plan on pages 703–707. General infection control precautions are listed in Box 26–4.

A necessary modification has to do with the use of touch. The physical care needs of AIDS clients require modifying the usual psychiatric injunction of limiting physical contact with clients. Because AIDS is such an isolating and stigmatizing condition, giving a massage or holding the client's hand has therapeutic value by reducing the isolation so commonly experienced by those with AIDS.

The psychiatric nurse will have to creatively combine and modify the nursing care for clients with a dual diagnosis that includes AIDS. Nursing care for clients with depression, suicidal ideation, psychosis, or organic mental disorder has been discussed in earlier chapters in this text. Care must be taken with persons with AIDS that delirium is not mistakenly diagnosed as depression.

The clinical example below (from Baer et al. 1987) illustrates the complexities involved in caring for a dual diagnosis client in an in-patient psychiatric setting.

John was a 38-year-old gay white man with no psychiatric history except episodic binge drinking and a two-month history of AIDS (*Pneumocystis carinii* pneumonia). He was admitted after he became disruptive

---

Box 26–4
GENERAL INFECTION CONTROL PRECAUTIONS*

1. Handle the blood of *all* clients as potentially infectious.

2. Wash hands before and after all client contact and all specimen contact. (This is the single most important means of preventing infection.)

3. Wear gloves for potential contact with blood and body fluids, including instances when the health care provider has a cut, scratch, or dermatologic lesion on the hands.

4. Wear a gown when contact with blood or body fluids is anticipated.

5. Wear a mask only if tuberculosis is a possibility or the client is coughing or likely to cough.

6. Wear protective eyewear and mask if splatter with blood or body fluids is possible (e.g., bronchoscopy, oral surgery, other invasive procedures).

7. Place used syringes immediately in a nearby specially designated impermeable container; do not recap, bend, clip, or manipulate the needle in any way.

8. Treat all linen soiled with blood or body fluids as infectious.

9. Discard all disposable supplies and equipment in a specially designated container.

10. Label all soiled, reusable equipment and supplies and place them in an impervious bag before sending for decontamination and reprocessing.

11. Process all laboratory specimens as potentially infectious.

12. Place mouth pieces and resuscitation equipment where resuscitation is predictable.

13. Clean all blood and body fluid spills with an appropriate disinfectant (seek advice from your health care facility's infection control practitioner).

Infection control guidelines may change as more is known about AIDS. Be sure to contact an appropriate source for up-to-date guidelines (the infection control practitioner in your health care facility or the Centers for Disease Control in Atlanta, Georgia).

---

caused by HIV infection of his brain or were part of a reactive or "functional" disorder. A negative CT scan and lumbar puncture suggested the latter was the case. John improved moderately after treatment with antipsychotic medication; lithium was not used as John had recent renal complications of AIDS. He was released ten days after admission, following a successful challenge of his mental health hold in Superior Court.

John was readmitted ten days later after increasing fatigue and severely impaired judgment rendered him unable to provide food, clothing, and shelter. Treatment with antipsychotic medication was reinstituted. At first he continued to exhibit manic symptoms. On one occasion he became threatening and required seclusion. He repeatedly abused the telephone, calling 911 so the police would rescue him, badgering friends, and trying to order everything from plane tickets to brass bands.

After a few weeks, John's clinical status began to change. Many of his "manic" symptoms diminished or disappeared; for the most part, he maintained his grandiose denial of his prognosis although this was punctuated by periodic lucidity and acknowledgment of his illness. He began to show signs of dementia: decreased attention to grooming and common etiquette, disorientation, failing short-term memory, wandering, and visual-spatial recognition deficits. He had a number of medication complications, although he was able to tolerate a neuroleptic and gradually required less of this. His dementia progressed rapidly, and he grew weaker and more in need of nursing assistance with basic activities.

John was placed on permanent conservatorship and no longer required acute psychiatric hospitalization after approximately two months, although he remained on the unit for nearly six months until he could be placed in a residential program with twenty-four-hour care. He died ten days after discharge.

Other Clients

The other clients on the unit will need health education to help them understand AIDS and the behavior of persons with AIDS in their midst. In their experience with AIDS clients on an in-patient psychiatric unit, Baer et al. (1987) noted that not all clients react favorably to the presence of persons with AIDS. In their experience clients with paranoid disorders had the greatest difficulty accepting persons with AIDS. Some of the behaviors that arose were hostility, incorporating AIDS into paranoid delusions, insisting on being transferred to another unit, and insisting on the persons with AIDS being transferred to another unit.

Providing education, offering support, allowing the other clients to vent their fears and express their concerns, and emphasizing that the care of ARC and AIDS clients is

in an alcohol treatment program. Clinically, he appeared to be suffering an episode of bipolar disorder (mania) and exhibited insomnia, hyperactivity, pressured speech, flight of ideas, lability, grandiose and religious delusions, auditory and visual hallucinations, markedly impaired judgment, and complete denial of his AIDS diagnosis. It was unclear if his symptoms were directly

Text continued on p. 707.

Nursing Care Plan: Persons with AIDS

Problem or Need	Intervention	Expected Outcome
1. Anxiety, anger, depression, and/or fear due to • Nonspecific diagnosis, prognosis, and/or treatments • Self-image changes and/or disfigurement • Concepts of death and dying	1. Provide an atmosphere of individual acceptance. 2. Provide opportunities for client to express feelings. 3. Involve Shanti,* chaplaincy, and/or psychiatric liaison as appropriate for client, significant others, and family. 4. Encourage honest, consistent communication by all members of caretaking team. 5. Assess need for psychopharmacologic intervention.	1. Client expresses feelings. 2. Client has adequate support. 3. Significant others, family, and friends are integrated into care and support. 4. Caregivers and client are aware of and use community resources.
2. Alterations in mental status due to • Disease process • Opportunistic infections • Medications	1. Clarify baseline mental status. 2. Monitor for changes in neurologic status at least every four hours. 3. Assess possible drug-related causes. 4. Provide safe environment (see Problem 13).	1. Etiology is identified where possible. 2. Further deterioration is minimized.
3. Fatigue and malaise due to • Disease process • Change in nutritional status • Medications	1. (a) Provide restful and quiet environment. (b) Assess need for pharmaceutical intervention. (c) Monitor tolerance for visits and telephone calls; suggest limits as appropriate. (d) Avoid awakening client except as necessary. (e) Encourage frequent naps. 2. (a) Titrate doses of symptom-relieving medications to achieve optimal benefits. (b) Assist with activities of daily living. 3. See interventions for Problem 5.	1. Client feels rested and gets adequate sleep. 2. Side-effects of medications are minimized. 3. Admission weight is maintained or increased.
4. Respiratory distress including shortness of breath, dyspnea on exertion, tachypnea, cough, cyanosis due to • Infiltrates • Effusions • Cavitations • Pneumothorax	1. Assess respiratory status every four hours or more frequently as indicated. 2. Monitor vital signs, chest sounds, color, and nail beds for relevant changes. 3. Assess need for respiratory therapy and evaluate efficacy of therapy administered.	1. Optimal respiratory status is achieved and maintained.

Source: Courtesy of Staff of San Francisco General Hospital's Special Care Unit for Persons with AIDS.

continued

Nursing Care Plan: Persons with AIDS (*continued*)

Problem or Need	Intervention	Expected Outcome
• Anemia • Hypoxemia 5. Anorexia, nausea/vomiting, diarrhea, dehydration due to • Disease process • Gastrointestinal infection and/or masses • Medications	1. Monitor weights, intake and output, and calorie counts as appropriate. 2. Monitor for signs of dehydration. 3. Encourage nutritional supplements as tolerated. 4. Encourage significant others to provide appealing and nutritious foods. 5. Consult dietitian as appropriate.	1. Optimal nutrition is received. 2. Optimal electrolyte balance and hydration are achieved and maintained.
6. Inadequate resistance to infection due to • Disease process • Neutropenia	1. Initiate precautions against neutropenia per hospital protocol. 2. Wash hands before entering room. 3. Monitor vital signs, especially temperature, as appropriate. 4. Monitor white blood cells counts and differentials for changes. 5. Monitor skin integrity every shift, including intravenous line sites, rectum, mouth. 6. Instruct client and significant others regarding infection control.	1. Nosocomial infection is prevented.
7. Fevers due to • Disease process • Infection • Drug reaction	1. Monitor temperature every four hours, or more frequently as needed. 2. Administer antipyretics as ordered and evaluate efficacy. 3. Evaluate need for cooling measures (i.e., cooling blankets, alcohol rubs, ice packs) and institute as needed. 4. Encourage fluid intake.	1. Fevers are optimally controlled.
8. Bleeding due to • Disease process • Medication	1. Monitor vital signs and note tachycardia, hypotension, pallor, anxiety, restlessness at least every four hours. 2. Monitor body surfaces for ecchymosis, petechiae, hematomas every shift. 3. Check urine, stool, vomit for heme. 4. Use safety precautions if platelet count is low (i.e., under 20,000 per cu mm):	1. Bleeding is minimized.

continued

Nursing Care Plan: Persons with AIDS (*continued*)

Problem or Need	Intervention	Expected Outcome
	(a) No tooth brushing; use alternative oral hygiene.	
	(b) Use electric razor.	
	(c) Use side rail and fall precautions.	
	5. Instruct client and significant others about safety precautions.	
9. Alteration in skin integrity due to • Disease process • Immobility • Poor nutritional status • Incontinence	1. Assess skin surfaces at least once per shift, documenting any breakdown and daily changes in breakdown. 2. Assist client with position change as necessary. 3. Encourage mobility within functional limits. 4. Assist with or provide bath and massage with soap, lotions, or oils. 5. Use appropriate beds or appliances for pressure relief. 6. Implement pressure-sore care as indicated. 7. See interventions for Problem 5.	1. Skin integrity is maintained.
10. Pain due to • Disease process • Other (specify)	1. Assess character and intensity of pain. 2. Administer analgesics as ordered and assess efficacy and side-effects. 3. Consider benefits of routine versus as-needed use of analgesics.	1. Client is maximally pain free.
11. Need for intravenous therapy due to • Dehydration • Medication administration • Electrolyte imbalances • Total parenteral nutrition	1. Examine site every shift for infiltration and inflammation. 2. Change site, bag, tubing, and dressing per hospital policy. 3. Teach client and significant others signs and symptoms of inflammation and infiltration.	1. Intravenous line is maintained without inflammation, infiltration, or infection.
12. Local and systemic reactions to medications: • Nausea/vomiting, diarrhea • Fever • Hypotension or hypertension • Orthostasis • Hypoglycemia or hyperglycemia • Rash	1. Monitor appropriate laboratory test values (i.e., complete blood count, serum glucose, liver function tests, renal panel, and so on). 2. Assess need for premedication preparation with antihistamines or antiemetics and evaluate efficacy of those administered. 3. Assess need for antidiarrheals and	1. Reactions are minimized.

continued

Nursing Care Plan: Persons with AIDS (*continued*)

Problem or Need	Intervention	Expected Outcome
• Neutropenia	assess efficacy of those administered.	
	4. Monitor skin and mucous membranes for location and nature of rash.	
	5. Assess hydration status and fluid balance to restrict or encourage fluid as needed.	
13. Injury due to falls	1. Identify risk factors:	
	(a) Weakness	
	(b) Sedation	
	(c) Mental confusion	
	(d) Diarrhea	
	2. For weak clients:	
	(a) Encourage use of call lights.	
	(b) Assist with ambulation.	
	(c) Leave belongings within reach.	
	3. Evaluate client for effects of sedation; check drug interactions.	
	4. For clients with mental confusion:	
	(a) Restrain as appropriate.	
	(b) Reorient frequently and remind to call for assistance.	
	5. For clients with diarrhea, provide bedside commode and/or place bedpan within reach.	
	6. For client with orthostasis:	
	(a) Monitor for side-effects of medications.	
	(b) Encourage use of call light.	
	(c) Assist with standing and walking.	
14. Substance abuse	1. Evaluate client for substance use.	1. Information regarding interrelationship between substance abuse and AIDS is accessible.
	2. Provide information about AIDS Substance Abuse Program (ASAP).	
	3. Refer directly to Alcohol Evaluation and Treatment Center (AETC) if indicated.	2. Client demonstrates knowledge of treatment options and referrals.
	4. Consult with AETC when ASAP is not available.	
15. Need for education of client, significant others, family regarding	1. Teach client and significant others about	1. Client and significant others are knowledgeable, to the extent of

continued

Nursing Care Plan: Persons with AIDS (*continued*)

Problem or Need	Intervention	Expected Outcome
• Disease process • Infection control • Transmissibility of virus • Safe sexual practices • Medication and side-effects • Other (specify)	(a) Disease process (b) Infection control (c) Safe sexual practices (d) Medication and side-effects (e) Other (specify) 2. Assess and document efficacy of teaching in nursing progress notes.	their ability, regarding pertinent information.
16. Need for clarification of resuscitation status	1. Coordinate process of decision making and ensure appropriate documentation. 2. Involve significant others, Shanti, chaplain, and medical and nursing ethicists as appropriate. 3. Assess client's understanding of currently ordered resuscitation status to ensure informed consent. 4. Support client decision.	1. Client makes informed consent with regard to resuscitation status.
17. Need for identification of legal issues: • Wills • Power of attorney	1. Assess knowledge of legal options. 2. Coordinate with Shanti to provide legal aid.	1. Client is given opportunity to complete legal documents as appropriate.
18. Terminal care	1. Use appropriate pharmacologic interventions for pain control, sedation, feelings of air hunger. 2. Bathe, provide oral hygiene, turn, and reposition for comfort. 3. Attend to psychosocial needs of significant others.	1. Client is maximally comfortable. 2. Focus is on palliative care.

*The Shanti Project of San Francisco is a volunteer community project that offers emotional, practical, and residential support to persons with AIDS.

an important and normal part of the unit routine helps other clients tolerate the milieu. The clients most vocal in their protests use the AIDS issue to avoid dealing with some of their own problems (Baer et al. 1987). Psychiatric nurses should keep this in mind when developing individual nursing care plans or dealing with milieu issues.

Risk Reduction Education and Counseling

Taking a leading role in risk reduction education and counseling is a crucial role for all nurses during the AIDS epi-

demic. Risk reduction education is directed toward three broad goals:

1. Educating clients, the public, other professionals, colleagues, friends, and neighbors in strategies to reduce the risk of contracting AIDS
2. Counteracting the myths, stereotypes, and hysteria that surround AIDS
3. Correcting misinformation

General guidelines from the CDC for the prevention of AIDS and HIV infection are reproduced in Box 26–5. These general guidelines can be used as a basis for programs of

Box 26–5

CDC GENERAL GUIDELINES FOR THE PREVENTION OF AIDS AND HIV INFECTION

I. Community health education programs should be aimed at members of high-risk groups to: (a) increase knowledge of AIDS, (b) facilitate behavioral changes to reduce risks of HIV infection, and (c) encourage voluntary testing and counseling.

II. Counseling and voluntary serologic testing for HIV should be routinely offered to all persons at increased risk when they present to health care settings. Such facilities include, but are not limited to, sexually transmitted disease clinics, clinics for treating parenteral drug abusers, and clinics for examining prostitutes.

   a. Persons with a repeatedly reactive test result should receive a thorough medical evaluation, which may include history, physical examination, and appropriate laboratory studies.

   b. High-risk persons with a negative test result should be counseled to reduce their risk of becoming infected by:

     (1) Reducing the number of sex partners. A stable, mutually monogamous relationship with an uninfected person eliminates any new risk of sexually transmitted HIV infection.

     (2) Protecting themselves during sexual activity with any possibly infected person by taking appropriate precautions to prevent contact with the person's blood, semen, urine, feces, saliva, cervical secretions, or vaginal secretions. Although the efficacy of condoms in preventing infections with HIV is still under study, consistent use of condoms should reduce transmission of HIV by preventing exposure to semen and infected lymphocytes.

     (3) For IV drug abusers, enrolling or continuing in programs to eliminate abuse of IV substances. Needles, other apparatus, and drugs must never be shared.

   c. Infected persons should be counseled to prevent the further transmission of HIV infection by:

     (1) Informing prospective sex partners of his/her infection with HIV, so they can take appropriate precautions. Clearly, abstention from sexual activity with another person is one option that would eliminate any risk of sexually transmitted HIV infection.

     (2) Protecting a partner during any sexual activity by taking appropriate precautions to prevent that individual from coming into contact with the infected person's blood, semen, urine, feces, saliva, cervical secretions, or vaginal secretions. Although the efficacy of using condoms to prevent infections with HIV is still under study, consistent use of condoms should reduce transmission of HIV by preventing exposure to semen and infected lymphocytes.

     (3) Informing previous sex partners and any persons with whom needles were shared of their potential exposure to HIV and encouraging them to seek counseling/testing.

     (4) For IV drug abusers, enrolling or continuing in programs to eliminate abuse of IV substances. Needles, other apparatus, and drugs must never be shared.

     (5) Not sharing toothbrushes, razors, or other items that could become contaminated with blood.

     (6) Refraining from donating blood, plasma, body organs, other tissue, or semen.

     (7) Avoiding pregnancy until more is known about the risks of transmitting HIV from mother to fetus or newborn.

     (8) Cleaning and disinfecting surfaces on which blood or other body fluids have spilled, in accordance with previous recommendations.

     (9) Informing physicians, dentists, and other appropriate health professionals of his/her antibody status when seeking medical care so that the patient can be appropriately evaluated.

III. Infected patients should be encouraged to refer sex partners or persons with whom they have shared needles to their health care provider for evaluation and/or testing. If patients prefer, trained health department professionals should be made available to assist in notifying their partners and counseling them regarding evaluation and/or testing.

IV. Persons with a negative test result should be counseled regarding their need for continued evaluation to monitor their infection status if they continue high-risk behavior.

V. State and local health officials should evaluate the implications of requiring the reporting of repeatedly

continued

Box 26–5 (Continued)

reactive HIV antibody test results to the state health department.

VI. State or local action is appropriate on public health grounds to regulate or close establishments where there is evidence that they facilitate high-risk behaviors, such as anonymous sexual contacts and/or intercourse with multiple partners or IV drug abuse

(e.g., bathhouses, houses of prostitution, "shooting galleries").

Source: Additional recommendations to reduce sexual and drug abuse-related transmission of human T-lymphotropic virus type III/lymphadenopathy-associated virus. Morbidity and Mortality Weekly Report *1986;35:153–154.*

---

risk reduction education. Because more is being learned about AIDS and appropriate and effective risk reduction and prevention, *readers should consult current CDC guidelines before implementing programs for persons at risk for contracting AIDS.*

Teaching risk reduction can best be accomplished by listening, informing, and supporting clients in making choices that reduce their risk. Bjorklund (1987) suggests that nurses need to understand the following principles in order to motivate clients to reduce their risks:

- Risk reduction education is important for members of high-risk groups and their sexual contacts since a large percentage of members of high-risk groups have already been exposed to the HIV virus.
- An HIV-positive person is at risk for (1) developing AIDS, and (2) transmitting the virus even if healthy.
- The role of reexposure to HIV or other infectious organisms is not completely understood; reexposure may be implicated in the progression from either an asymptomatic state or ARC to full-blown AIDS.
- The change to low-risk behaviors for high-risk individuals may necessitate lifelong change. Lifelong change can be more effectively maintained if sexual activities that incorporate risk reduction techniques are also satisfying.
- Clients need support to maintain low-risk behavior in an environment that reinforces high-risk behavior.

Sexual Behavior

Many AIDS experts fear that educating persons about "safe sex" generates a false sense of security. In this AIDS era, these experts say, the only safe sex is no sex. Realistically, however, abstinence is not a lifelong change that will be

maintained by many. Counseling persons about safer sex, or about high-risk sexual behaviors, low-risk sexual behaviors, and risk-free sexual behaviors makes more sense especially in terms of the principles outlined in the list above. High-risk sexual behaviors are those in which there is an exchange of blood or body fluids. Receptive anal intercourse is thought to be of highest risk because of the trauma that can be caused to the mucous membranes of the rectum. *Fisting* (inserting a finger or fingers, hand, or fist into the rectum) can also cause trauma and bleeding. **Rimming** (oral-anal contact) can bring people into contact with contaminated blood or feces. Guidelines for counseling in terms of safer sex are given in Box 26–6.

It is evident that the use of condoms is important in decreasing risk. However, condoms must be used effectively to decrease risk. Remember to include the following information about condoms in any risk reduction program:

- Latex condoms are probably safer to use than natural condoms since the HIV may be small enough to be able to pass through the pores in natural condoms.
- Condom packages should not be opened until use. Packages should be opened carefully. (This helps prevent damage that might result from rough handling or jagged fingernails.)
- Condoms should be stored at room temperature. (Excessive heat or cold can damage the latex.)
- The condom should be applied in advance of sexual intercourse. (Semen and seminal fluid may be discharged in advance of ejaculation.)
- The condom should be held at the tip and rolled down over the entire erect penis. Uncircumcised men should pull back the foreskin before applying the condom. (This provides a more effective seal.)
- The air should be gently pressed out of the condom tip to leave an airless space at the tip, and the condom

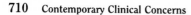

should be smoothed over the entire penis to eliminate air bubbles. (Air bubbles can cause condoms to break.)

- A water-based product such as lubricating jelly or spermicidal jelly should be added before penetration. (Insufficient lubrication can cause condoms to tear or pull off. Oil-based lubricants such as petroleum jelly, vegetable oil, mineral oil, cold cream, or lotion may cause the latex to disintegrate.)

- Spermicidal foams, creams, or jellies containing **nonoxynol-9** can be used in conjunction with condoms. (Nonoxynol-9 may inactivate the virus if the condom should break.)

- After sex, the base of the condom should be held firmly while the penis is gently withdrawn. (This prevents the escape of semen from the condom.) The used condom should be safely discarded and never reused.

Since AIDS is most commonly transmitted through sex, being sexually active without taking proper precautions is definitely high-risk behavior. In this AIDS era, a person does not simply go to bed with one other person. When one calculates the possible length of the HIV latency period, a person goes to bed with the other person's entire sex history for approximately the past ten years.

Substance Abuse

The transmission of HIV and intravenous drug use are linked in the following ways:

- Direct transmission of the virus through the sharing of intravenous drugs and equipment for injecting drugs (the most obvious link)

- Sexual transmission by infected intravenous drug users to their sexual partners

- Neonatal transmission by infected women who are themselves intravenous drug users or the sexual partners of intravenous drug users

While these modes of transmission address intravenous drug users, there are other less well known links to nonintravenous substance use and AIDS. The use of **poppers** (volatile amyl and butyl nitrates in breakable glass capsules inhaled to enhance sexual pleasure) may be a cofactor in the development of AIDS and Kaposi's sarcoma because they are thought to lead to a generalized suppression of the immune system. Alcohol, as well as drugs such as amphetamines, cocaine, and marijuana are also thought to damage the immune system. Another factor is disinhibition. That is, with loss of inhibition, a person under the influence of alcohol or drugs is more likely to engage in high-risk behaviors.

Box 26–6
AIDS RISK REDUCTION GUIDELINES: SEXUAL BEHAVIOR

Risk-Free Behaviors

Most of these behaviors involve skin-to-skin contact only. The virus is unlikely to be transmitted from one person to another unless breaks in the skin exist.

- Mutual masturbation (male or female)
- Body massage, hugging
- Frottage (body-to-body rubbing without penetration)
- Dry (social) kissing
- Using one's own sex toys (dildos or vibrators) that are not shared
- Light S and M (sadism and masochism) activities (without bruising or bleeding)

Low-Risk Behaviors (Possibly Safe)

Small amounts of some body fluids may be exchanged during these activities. The risk of transmitting the virus is thought to be increased in proportion to the number of contacts.

- Anal intercourse with condom (if used properly)
- Vaginal intercourse with condom (if used properly)
- Fellatio (oral sex) without ingestion of seminal fluid or semen
- Wet kissing (also called French kissing)
- Cunnilingus (oral-vaginal contact; risk is probably enhanced during menstruation)
- Using shared sex toys that are cleaned between uses and covered with a condom
- Urine contact (also called watersports) when skin is unbroken and urine is not taken by mouth or by rectum

High-Risk Behaviors (Unsafe)

These activities involve tissue trauma or exchange of blood or body fluids that may transmit HIV or other microbes.

- Anal intercourse without condom (both receptive and insertive)
- Vaginal intercourse without condom
- Fisting (manual-anal contact)
- Fellatio with ingestion of semen
- Rimming (oral-anal contact)
- Using unclean, unprotected sex toys
- Piercing or drawing blood

Realistic approaches to AIDS risk reduction education for intravenous drug users consist of more than informa-

Box 26–7
AIDS RISK REDUCTION GUIDELINES: SUBSTANCE ABUSE

- Remember that people who look healthy can carry the AIDS virus.

- Never share intravenous drugs or works (equipment).

- If a new needle and syringe are not available or equipment must be shared, remember to clean the works (refer to Figure 26–3).

- Prevent sexual transmission (refer to Box 26–6).

- Avoid alcohol, marijuana, amphetamines, cocaine, and poppers.

- If you want to have children but have shared needles or may have been exposed to AIDS through sexual contact with someone who has, get medical advice.

syringes, or other drug paraphernalia with others. If a new needle and syringe are not available, it is important that clients clean their **works** (syringe and needle) as recommended in Figure 26–3. Bleach kills the AIDS virus.

Risks to sexual partners are the same as those discussed earlier in this chapter. Prevention of risk to sexual partners is important because intravenous drug users serve as a bridge for transmitting AIDS to their sexual partners or to fetuses and newborns. Women who are intravenous drug users or the sexual partners of intravenous drug users are urged to postpone pregnancy until more is known about the significance of a positive antibody test for a pregnant woman, the relationship between pregnancy and the onset of symptoms associated with HIV infection, and the risk of transmission to fetuses and infants (Centers for Disease Control 1985a).

tion about, and encouragement to obtain treatment for, substance abuse. Those who are not ready for treatment must be counseled on how to reduce the risk to themselves and to others. Risk reduction guidelines for intravenous drug users are given in Box 26–7. A counseling plan for clients with a dual diagnosis of AIDS/ARC and substance abuse is given in Box 26–8.

Clients' risks to themselves derive from the practice of sharing drug use equipment with others. Clients should be instructed to never share intravenous drugs, needles,

Support for Caregivers

Psychiatric nurses can be a vital support link for the wide spectrum of people who are caregivers of persons with AIDS. This spectrum includes nurses and other health care professionals; the family members, friends, and **care-partners** (those to whom gay persons are committed in a long-term relationship) of persons with AIDS; firefighters, police officers, and correction officers; and community volunteers.

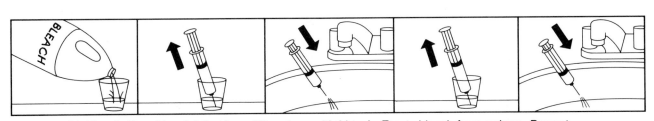

1. *Flush with bleach.* Pour bleach into glass. Fill syringe with bleach. Empty bleach from syringe. *Repeat.*

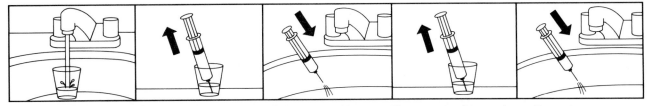

2. *Flush with water.* Fill a glass with clean water. Fill syringe with water. Empty water from syringe. *Repeat.* (Caution: Be sure the client knows not to omit this important step.)

Figure 26–3
Cleaning the works.
Source: Reprinted with permission from the San Francisco AIDS Foundation.

Box 26–8
COUNSELING PLAN FOR CLIENTS WITH A DUAL DIAGNOSIS OF AIDS/ARC AND SUBSTANCE ABUSE

- Check the level of understanding of basic AIDS information and develop an education plan based on client needs.

- Confront denial or lack of commitment to minimize risk behavior.

- Offer hope for stabilization of health through positive health care measures.

- Check the need for and depth of motivation for referral to chemical dependency or alcohol treatment programs.

- Encourage joining or continuing commitment to the recovery process in treatment for chemical or alcohol dependency.

- Check the need for and refer to medical follow-up, emotional or sexual counseling, support groups, and other self-help programs.

- Help client verbalize feelings of anger, grief, and loss generated by the diagnosis; the need for change in sexual and drug use behavior; or possible delay in child bearing.

- Reinforce the fact that taking action now may help stabilize the client's health and slow further deterioration.

- Discuss "contagion' issues with client and family members to allay fears of spread by casual contact.

- Encourage and support client verbalization of such feelings as:

1. Fear of dying of AIDS
2. Fear of having exposed others to AIDS or doing so through continued risk behavior
3. Feelings of guilt over risk behavior in the past
4. Feelings of loss over necessary behavior changes and possible postponement of childbearing
5. Fear of what others will think or do, or fear of being isolated and/or rejected

- Compile and distribute a list of community resources to serve people with AIDS concerns or AIDS/ARC diagnosis.

- Stress the use of tools learned in recovering from chemical dependency and alcoholism in coping with this life crisis.

- Continue to confront the drug abuse as you would with other clients not diagnosed with AIDS.

- Emphasize positive things the client can do to maximize health.

- Extend hope that, with continued attention to health matters, the client may live longer, possibly extending life until more effective treatments become available.

Source: O'Neil M: AIDS and Bereavement: Partners, Families, Friends, in Hughes AM, Martin JP, Franks P: AIDS Home Care and Hospice Manual, 1987, p 137. By permission of the Visiting Nurses Association of San Francisco.

Nurses are now and will continue to be the health care professionals who are the frontline workers in providing health care to increasing numbers of persons with AIDS.

Special emotional stamina is needed to care for persons with AIDS. Not only must nurses and other caregivers care for and comfort those who face great suffering and death, they also care for those infected with the virus who fear they will develop the disease. At the same time they provide help, nurses must cope with their fears for their own and their family's health (especially if the nurses themselves are members of a risk group) and their own pain in caring for persons who do not get well or whose future is an uncertain one.

Specifically, the skills and knowledge of psychiatric nurses make them particularly appropriate people to:

- Facilitate caregivers' expression of fears and concerns

- Help caregivers acknowledge their susceptibility to increased stress and burnout in AIDS work

- Instruct caregivers in stress management strategies and relaxation techniques

- Identify what needs to be reorganized and renegotiated in the work milieu to maintain the health of caregivers and clients such as (1) staff support groups, (2) networking with AIDS providers in other agencies and communities, (3) respite time for staff, (4) time off to attend funerals or memorial services, (5) rearranging staff assignments to avoid overloading or overburdening particular staff members, (6) creating getaway space for staff in the work setting

- Provide help to caregivers unused to dealing with delirium and dementia, who may have unrealistic expectations about the client's ability to adhere to procedures and treatment as mental capacities diminish
- Encourage administration to arrange time off and fund attendance at conferences and meetings that provide support and facilitate networking among people engaged in AIDS work

Successful stress management is particularly important because neither a cure nor a vaccine is in sight. This means that increased numbers of people (those who are currently infected with the virus and have yet to develop ARC or AIDS) will need nursing care in the coming years.

Bereavement Support

There are several groups of people to whom the psychiatric nurse can provide bereavement support. The most obvious is the person with AIDS who grieves over a fatal diagnosis,

the loss of other friends or family to the disease, or any of the several other losses discussed earlier in this chapter in the section on the biopsychosocial impact of AIDS.

Bereavement support to family, friends, and caregivers should continue after death has occurred. Home visits to friends, lovers, and family members demonstrate the nurse's continuing interest and concern for the survivor's well-being. Bereavement support groups and individual and family counseling can all be helpful, depending on individual situations and the availability of volunteers and professionals. Unresolved family issues or conflicting feelings about the deceased person can hinder or delay the mourning process. The grieving of spouses and lovers at risk for developing AIDS is complicated by fear for their own health (Strawn 1987) and perhaps by anger at being left by the deceased or having been put at risk. The variables unique to AIDS and grief for partner, family, and friends are discussed in Table 26–2.

RESEARCH NOTE

Citation

Andre BC: Nurses' attitudes toward patients requiring isolation precautions. Presented at Nursing Transitions' AIDS: The National Nursing Conference, Hilton Head, South Carolina, November 20, 1987.

Study Problem/Purpose

The diagnosis of acquired immune deficiency syndrome (AIDS) can produce severe stress in both client and nurse. Myths, ignorance, and misconceptions about AIDS contribute to the development of fear, anxiety, prejudice, and excessive physical and psychosocial isolation of the person with AIDS. This descriptive study was designed to explore nurses' attitudes toward clients requiring isolation precautions.

Methods

A researcher-designed care study vignette and a questionnaire with opportunity for open-ended commentary were administered to a sample of 42 registered nurses preregistered for an AIDS nursing in-service program.

Findings

The majority of nurses surveyed (64 percent) would begin cardiopulmonary resuscitation (CPR) on the AIDS client in the case study questionnaire, although some nurses (58 percent) would delay CPR until a protective airway device became available. Nurses (67 percent) would not

refuse to provide care to an AIDS client; however, nurses (67 percent) fear AIDS contagion from caring for AIDS clients. Almost three-quarters of the nurses (74 percent) judge the client to be personally responsible for contracting AIDS, but 60 percent stated that they would not discriminate between an AIDS client and any other client requiring isolation. A greater number of nurses (79 percent) stated that they would not differentiate the treatment of an AIDS client from other clients not requiring isolation. A high number of nurses (86 percent) felt unsure about the transmission of AIDS and how best to protect themselves.

Implications

The nurse's attitude toward isolation clients (such as persons with AIDS), and the nurse's behavior as a reflection of attitude, may affect the quality of nursing care delivered to the client in isolation. Fear of AIDS contagion, the belief that persons with AIDS are personally responsible for their illness, and lack of knowledge of how AIDS is transmitted and what can be done to protect themselves are attitudes that may adversely affect the care AIDS clients receive. In-service education programs or client care conferences would help to promote knowledgeable and humane care to people requiring isolation precautions. A psychiatric liaison nurse would be an appropriate person to encourage the discussion of personal biases, preconceptions, and value judgments that can impede client care and to participate in the planning of holistic care to people in isolation.

Table 26–2
Variables Unique to AIDS and Grief

Variable	Partner	Family	Friends
Homophobia	Fear of homosexuals because it may lead to AIDS. Leads to isolation.	Blaming homosexual partner for AIDS diagnosis.	May be similar to partner and/or family.
Internalized homophobia	Self-hate, shame in being homosexual—AIDS is seen as punishment for being homosexual. Leads to depression.	May be operant in one or more family member(s) if he/she is homosexual and identity is not solidified.	May be similar to partner and/or family.
Absence of institutional sanctioning for homosexual partnerships	Lack of permission to participate in funeral, lack of claim to property of deceased. Leads to invalidation of grief experience. Dispute over wills, life insurance. Not granted bereavement leave from work.	Risk for lack of validation of grieving experiences of partner.	May be similar to partner and/or family.
Secrecy regarding cause of death	Leads to an inability to disclose cause of death and isolation. May be fearful of talking about the death to employers and own family. Leads to denial of death.	Friends won't "understand" shame of disease and implications—i.e., deceased is associated with high-risk group(s). Leads to delayed grief, isolation.	May be similar to partner and/or family.
Fatigue resulting from caregiving responsibilities	Low level of physical and emotional reserve after the death.	May be similar to partner if participated in care. May not understand fully the cause of illness/death.	May be similar to partner and/or family.
Multiple losses	Deceased partner may be one of many loved ones who have died of AIDS—particularly true for homosexuals and drug abusers. May lead to grief overload.	May have multiple family members who have died of AIDS and/or other illnesses.	May be similar to partner and/or family.
Fear/worry about own health status	Worry about contracting AIDS as result of relationship.	Lack of information about AIDS transmission may result in fear of contagion.	May be similar to partner and/or family.
Positive HIV test results	May occur prior to or shortly after the death. May lead to delayed grief.	May occur if family member(s) also belong to risk group.	May be similar to partner and/or family.
ARC/AIDS diagnosis	May occur prior to or after the death.	May occur if family member(s) also belong to risk group.	May be similar to partner and/or family.

Source: O'Neil M: AIDS and Bereavement: Partners, Families, Friends, in Hughes AM, Martin JP, Franks P: AIDS Home Care and Hospice Manual, 1987, p 137. By permission of the Visiting Nurses Association of San Francisco.

Self-Help Support

Self-help is one way in which persons with AIDS can move to reestablish a sense of self-control and reduce feelings of helplessness and powerlessness. Self-help can occur on several levels depending on the client's physical and mental abilities and motivation. Clients should participate as much as possible in their own care and in decision making that affects them. Nurses can encourage clients to join peer support groups and engage in AIDS advocacy activities in their communities.

Clients may benefit from such activities as nutritional counseling and psychologic counseling. Boosting the immune system also helps keep people healthy. Stress management techniques and visualization and imagery for self-healing and pain and symptom control (such as those discussed in Chapter 28) are believed to boost the immune system by reducing stress.

Research

Not enough is known about AIDS as an illness; the common nursing diagnoses in AIDS, ARC, and HIV seropositivity; or the strategies that help people cope when AIDS affects them or their loved ones. Psychiatric nurses have a direct role in research and an indirect role in supporting ongoing research and encouraging the undertaking and funding of new research. Being knowledgeable about the current research and incorporating it into clinical practice enables the psychiatric nurse to act on the basis of what is currently known or supposed.

Advocacy and Political Activism

Persons with AIDS and their loved ones need advocates. Psychiatric nurses can be effective advocates by speaking out against dehumanizing measures that threaten the well-being of persons with AIDS.

A proposition was introduced in California that could have forced public health officials to establish camps to quarantine persons with AIDS, as well as anyone infected by the virus, whether healthy or unhealthy. This measure would also have flatly banned people testing HIV positive from attending or teaching in public schools or holding jobs that involve food handling. The California Nurses Association was among the groups that actively spoke against the proposition and contributed to its failure.

As citizens and as advocates, nurses should be politically aware of pending legislation and move to influence it in a positive direction.

Earlier in this chapter, brief mention was made of state nurses' associations with published statements about the care of persons with AIDS and nursing's role. Other state nurses' associations and national specialty groups are also active in mobilizing the professional and political resources of the nursing community. It is each nurse's responsibility to find out what nursing groups are accomplishing or not accomplishing on local, state, and national levels. Beginning at the local level by becoming involved in local AIDS councils, self-help groups, and nursing organizations is a good way to start. Local involvement is a bridge to state and national involvement. Nurses can and should be part of a nationwide effort to lobby for adequate public and private funding for research, education, prevention, treatment, and cure for AIDS.

Chapter Highlights

- AIDS, a contagious and fatal condition of immune system depression, is a clinical issue of concern to all nurses, including psychiatric nurses.

- Homosexual/bisexual men (and their sexual partners), intravenous drug abusers (and their sexual partners), hemophiliacs (and their sexual partners), children born to parents with AIDS or at risk for AIDS, and prostitutes are groups of people who have been identified as being at high risk of developing AIDS.

- AIDS threatens the biopsychosocial integrity of individuals and of society.

- Persons with AIDS experience several different losses, may have neurologic or neuropsychiatric involvement because the virus invades the central and peripheral nervous systems, and find that their ability to successfully negotiate age-appropriate developmental tasks is disrupted.

- Persons with AIDS may experience social and familial rejection; discrimination in employment, housing, and health insurance; estrangement from institutions such as organized religion; and financial losses.

- Several ethical issues surround AIDS. Many of them revolve around questions of individual rights versus the public good.

- Psychiatric nurses can anticipate the need to care for increasing numbers of persons with AIDS in psychiatric settings and in other community settings.

- Psychiatric hospitalization may be needed if the client is depressed, suicidal, psychotic, or has an AIDS-related behavior disturbance, probably because of organic mental disorder. The psychiatric nurse will have to creatively combine and modify the nursing care for clients with a dual diagnosis that includes AIDS.

- Taking a leading role in risk reduction education and counseling is a crucial role for all nurses during the AIDS epidemic.

- Psychiatric nurses can be a vital support link for the wide spectrum of people who are caregivers of persons with AIDS.

- Psychiatric nurses have direct roles in AIDS research and indirect roles in supporting ongoing research and encouraging the undertaking and funding of new research.

- Psychiatric nurses can be effective advocates by speaking out against dehumanizing measures that threaten the well-being of persons with AIDS; influencing legislation in a positive direction; and becoming part of a nationwide effort to lobby for adequate private and public funding for research, education, prevention, treatment, and cure.

- Nurses are now and will continue to be the health care professionals who are the frontline workers in providing health care to increasing numbers of persons with AIDS.

References

Amchin J, Polan J: A longitudinal account of staff adaptation to AIDS patients on a psychiatric unit. *Hosp Community Psychiatry* 1986;37(12):1235–1238.

American Nurses' Association. *Code for nurses*. ANA, 1985a.

American Nurses' Association. *Nursing profession urges health care community to step up efforts on AIDS (News release)*. ANA, 1985b.

Baer J, Holm K, Lewitter-Koehler S: Treatment of AIDS/ARC patients on an inpatient psychiatric unit. *Focus: A Review of AIDS Research* 1987;2(2):1–3.

Binder R: AIDS antibody test on inpatient psychiatric units. *Am J Psychiatry* 1987;144(2):176–180.

Bjorklund E: Prevention: Reducing the risk of AIDS, in Durham JD, Cohen FL: *The Person With AIDS: Nursing Perspectives*. Springer, 1987, pp 178–191.

Boland MG: The child with AIDS: Special concerns, in Durham JD, Cohen FL: *The Person With AIDS: Nursing Perspectives*. Springer, 1987, pp 192–210.

Bompey S: AIDS—An employment issue for the eighties. *Digest Publication of International Foundation of Employee Benefit Plan* 1986;23(2):6–10.

California Nurses Association. *Resolution on mobilization of nurses for care of AIDS patients*. CNA, 1985.

Centers for Disease Control: Recommendations for assisting in the prevention of perinatal transmission of human T-lymphotropic virus type III/lymphadenopathy-associated virus and acquired immunodeficiency syndrome. *Morbidity and Mortality Weekly Report* 1985a;34:721–732.

Centers for Disease Control: Recommendations for preventing transmission of infection with HTLV-III/LAV in the workplace. *Morbidity and Mortality Weekly Report* 1985b;34(45):681–695.

Centers for Disease Control: Revision of the CDC surveillance case definition for acquired immunodeficiency syndrome. *Morbidity and Mortality Weekly Report* 1985c;36(1S):3S–15S.

Centers for Disease Control: Apparent transmission of human T-lymphotropic virus type III/lymphadenopathy-associated virus from a child to a mother providing health care. *Morbidity and Mortality Weekly Report* 1986;35:76–79.

Centers for Disease Control: *AIDS Weekly Surveillance Report*. September 14, 1987. Department of Health and Human Services.

Chase M: *AIDS drug comes to a market worried about its cost. Wall Street Journal*, March 23, 1987.

Cohen FL: The epidemiology and etiology of AIDS, in Durham JD, Cohen FL: *The Person With AIDS: Nursing Perspectives*, Springer, 1987, pp 9–51.

Dilley JW: Diagnosis and treatment of major depression in AIDS. *AIDSfile* 1987;2(1):6–7.

Durham JD: The ethical dimensions of AIDS, in Durham JD, Cohen FL: *The Person With AIDS: Nursing Perspectives*. Springer, 1987, pp 229–252.

Faltz B, Rinaldi G: *AIDS and Substance Abuse: A Training Manual for Health Care Professionals*. University of California, 1987.

Faultisch M: Psychiatric aspects of AIDS. *Am J Psychiatry* 1987;144(5):551–556.

Flavin DK, Franklin JE, Frances RJ: The acquired immune deficiency syndrome (AIDS) and suicidal behavior in alcohol dependent homosexual men. *Am J Psychiatry* 1986;143(11):1440–1442.

Friedland GH, et al: Lack of transmission of HTLV-III/LAV infection to household contacts of patients with AIDS or AIDS-related complex with oral candidiasis. *N Engl J Med* 1986;314:344–349.

Frierson RL, Lippmann SB, Johnson J: AIDS: Psychosocial stresses on the family. *Psychosom* 1987;28(2):65–68.

Gottlieb M, et al.: *AMFAR Directory of Experimental Treatments for AIDS and ARC*. Mary Ann Liebert, Inc., 1987.

Herman PA: Neurologic effects of HTLV-III infection in adults: An overview. *Mount Sinai J Med* 1986;53(8):616–620.

Holland JC, Tross S: The psychosocial and neuropsychiatric sequelae of the acquired immunodeficiency syndrome and related disorders. *Ann Intern Med* 1985;103:760–764.

Hughes A, Martin JP, Franks P: *AIDS Home Care and Hospice Manual.* AIDS Home Care and Hospice Program, VNA of San Francisco, 1987.

Jaffe HW, et al.: The acquired immunodeficiency syndrome in gay men. *Ann Intern Med* 1985;103:662–664.

Kaplan JE: A modern-day plague. *Natural History* 1986;95(2):28–33.

Kneisl CR, Ames SW: *Adult Health Nursing: A Biopsychosocial Approach.* Addison-Wesley, 1986.

Krigel RL, Friedman-Kien AE: Kaposi's sarcoma in AIDS, in DeVita VT Jr, Hellman S, Rosenberg SA (eds): *AIDS: Etiology, Diagnosis, Treatment, and Prevention.* Lippincott, 1985, pp 185–211.

Lederman MM: Transmission of the acquired immunodeficiency syndrome through heterosexual activity. *Ann Intern Med* 1986;104:115–117.

Leibowitz RE: Infection control measures in institutional settings. *The Person With AIDS: Nursing Perspectives.* Springer, 1987, pp 81–94.

Levine PH: The acquired immunodeficiency syndrome in persons with hemophilia. *Ann Int Med* 1985;103:723–726.

McCray E: Occupational risk of the acquired immunodeficiency syndrome among health care workers. *N Engl J Med* 1986;314:1127–1132.

McEnany G: Personal communication, September 25, 1987.

Menenberg S: Somatopsychology and AIDS victims. *J Psychosoc Nurs* 1987;25(5):18–22.

National Academy of Sciences. *Confronting AIDS: Directions for Public Health, Health Care and Research.* National Academy Press, 1986.

Navia RA, Price RW: The acquired immunodeficiency syndrome dementia complex as the presenting or sole manifestation of human immunodeficiency virus infection. *Arch Neurol* 1987;44:65–69.

Nelson WJ: Nursing care of acutely ill persons with AIDS, in *The Person With AIDS: Nursing Perspectives.* Springer, 1987, pp 95–109.

New York State Nurses Association. *The Role of the Nursing Practitioner Re: Acquired Immunodeficiency Syndrome (AIDS).* NYSNA, 1983.

Nursing care plan for persons with AIDS. *QRB* October, 1986, 361–365.

Perry S, Markowitz J: Psychiatric interventions for AIDS-spectrum disorders. *Hosp Community Psychiatry* 1986;37(10):1001–1006.

Rich CL, Fowler RC, Young D, Blenkush M: San Diego suicide study: Comparison of gay to straight males. *Suicide and Life-Threatening Behavior* 1986;16(4):448–457.

Salisbury D: AIDS, psychosocial implications. *J Psychosoc Nurs* 1986;24(12):13–16.

Saunders JM, Valente SM: Gay and lesbian suicide: A review. *Death Studies* 1987;11:1–23.

Schietinger H: A home care plan for AIDS. *Am J Nurs* 1986;86:1021–1028.

Serinus J: *Psychoimmunity and the Healing Process.* Celestial Arts, 1986.

Shapira J, Schlesinger R, Cummings JL: Distinguishing dementias. *Am J Nurs* 1986;86(6):698–702.

Shilts R: *And the Band Played On.* St. Martin's Press, 1987.

Sontag S: *Illness as Metaphor.* Vintage Books, 1977.

Strawn J: The psychosocial consequences of AIDS, in Durham JD, Cohen FL: *The Person with AIDS: Nursing Perspectives.* Springer, 1987, pp 126–149.

Wolcott DL, et al.: Illness concerns, attitudes toward homosexuality, and social support in gay men with AIDS. *Gen Hosp Psychiatry* 1986;8:395–403.

PART FIVE

Intervention Modes

TWENTY-SEVEN

The One-to-One Relationship

Beth Moscato

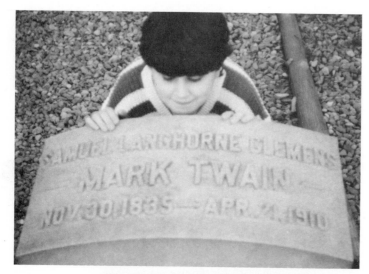

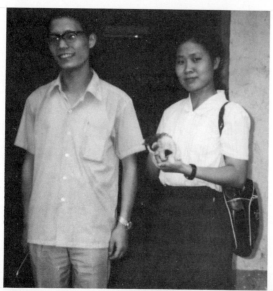

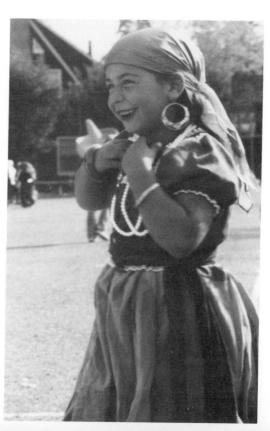

After reading this chapter, students should be able to

- Identify common characteristics of one-to-one relationships

- Recognize humanistic interactionist aspects of one-to-one relationships

- Describe the interpersonal skills of the nurse that facilitate one-to-one relationships, including therapeutic use of self

- Delineate the client abilities and behaviors most often associated with growth-producing outcomes

- Analyze the following special concerns as these relate to psychiatric nurses: critical distance, self-disclosure, gifts, use of touch, and values

- Discuss the concept of resistance in one-to-one relationships, including its definition, possible manifestations, and general intervention strategies

- Specify the normal and troublesome aspects of transference and countertransference in one-to-one relationships

- Explain the three phases of therapeutic relationships, highlighting main objectives and therapeutic tasks of each phase

- Apply the nursing process in establishing and maintaining one-to-one relationships

Cross References

Other topics relevant to this content are: Assessment, Chapter 12; Communication skills, Chapter 11; Cultural considerations in one-to-one work, Chapters 11 and 38; Facilitative personal characteristics of the nurse, Chapter 3; Historical aspects, Chapter 2; Self-disclosure, Chapter 3; Therapeutic use of self, Chapter 3; Values, Chapters 3 and 11.

You are but one, but still you are one. You cannot do everything, but you can do something. Because you cannot do everything, you cannot refuse to do the something that you can.

Key Terms

acting out
confidentiality
countertransference
learned helplessness
negative transference
one-to-one relationship
orientation phase
positive transference
problem-solving strategies
psychotic transference

resistance
self-disclosure
termination phase
therapeutic alliance
therapeutic contract
therapeutic use of self
transference
working phase
working relationship

The psychiatric nurse who enters into a one-to-one relationship with a client finds that the invitation to any individual relationship is at once intriguing, challenging, and anxiety provoking.

A one-to-one relationship may evolve in any nursing situation: between a nurse who makes home visits and an ailing client, between a hospital nurse and a child intermittently hospitalized with leukemia, or between a nurse-counselor and a high-risk pregnant woman. Of particular relevance is the one-to-one relationship that evolves between the psychiatric nurse and the client. This may occur in medical facilities, psychiatric institutions, community mental health centers, and private practice settings. The individual psychiatric nurse-client relationship is the cornerstone of psychiatric nursing theory and practice.

How is it possible to define, initiate, and effectively use a one-to-one relationship? This chapter demystifies the characteristics, processes, phases, and problems of one-to-one relationships so that beginning psychiatric nurses can approach these relationships with increased awareness of their own interpersonal effectiveness. Practical guidelines on how to facilitate interpersonal effectiveness with clients are included. The principles, processes, and phases discussed in this chapter also apply to family, group, and community interventions or therapies.

COMMON CHARACTERISTICS OF ONE-TO-ONE RELATIONSHIPS

The **one-to-one relationship** between psychiatric nurse and client is a mutually defined, collaborative, and goal-oriented professional relationship.

Professional

One-to-one relationships reflect a professional, rather than social, relationship. Psychiatric nurses use their personalities, interpersonal skills and techniques, and theoretical knowledge of psychiatric nursing practice in a purposeful, goal-directed manner to facilitate a useful change in their clients' lives. This professional relationship differs from a social relationship in several significant ways. A social relationship is generally structured for companionship and pleasure, while a one-to-one relationship generally involves the systematic working through of troublesome thoughts, feelings, or behaviors. A social relationship does not usually involve a delineation of roles. In the one-to-one relationship between psychiatric nurse and client, the nurse intends to play a specific role, using professional psychiatric nursing skills and interventions. The focus of the one-to-one relationship is on the client's identifying, developing, and assessing ways to meet personal needs effectively, rather than on meeting the personal needs of the nurse. Table 27–1 summarizes the major differences between professional and social relationships.

The one-to-one relationship may also be differentiated from the nurse-client interaction. An interaction is some segment of actual behavior that takes place between the psychiatric nurse and the client. The one-to-one relationship may be viewed as a planned series of sequential nurse-client interactions with the following additional elements:

- The interactions occur over a designated period of time (daily, weekly, monthly).
- The interactions take place within a structure in which specific phases, processes, and problems evolve that are unique to the developing relationship between psychiatric nurse and client.

- The interactions occur in a designated setting that tends to remain stable over time (home, private-practice office, mental health clinic, in-patient psychiatric unit, medical unit).

A professional one-to-one relationship can be either informal or formal. Spontaneous, informal nurse-client relationships may occur at one end of the continuum, with more formalized relationships in individual counseling or psychotherapy at the other end.

Informal

Informal nurse-client relationships may be prearranged and planned, but more often they occur spontaneously. They consist of a set of interactions limited in time. There is minimum structure and a sense of immediacy. These relationships occur in numerous medical and nonmedical settings and are particularly common in psychiatric institutions and community mental health settings.

Formal

The more formalized one-to-one relationship is used in crisis intervention, counseling, or individual psychotherapy. It requires more planning, structure, consistency, nursing expertise, and time. It occurs in various psychiatric settings, including psychiatric institutions, community mental health centers, and private practice.

The choice and effectiveness of informal or formal relationships depend upon:

- The client's level of functioning
- The psychiatric nurse's current abilities and skills
- To some degree, the time available to both participants

Table 27–1
Differences Between Professional and Social Relationships

Characteristic	Professional Relationship	Social Relationship
Purpose	Systematic working-through of troublesome thoughts, feelings, and behaviors Planned evaluation (through stages)	Companionship, pleasure, sharing of interests Evolves spontaneously
Role delineation	Roles for psychiatric nurse and client with explicit use of psychiatric nursing skills and interventions	Generally not present, except for broad social norms governing the particular type of relationship (friend versus lover)
Satisfaction of needs	Client encouraged to identify, develop, and assess ways to met own needs more effectively Does not address personal needs of psychiatric nurse	Mutual sharing and satisfaction of personal and interpersonal needs
Time frame	Usually time-limited interactions with an expected termination	Usually not time limited, either in duration or frequency of contact No planned termination is planned

It is crucial to note that the principles, phases, processes, and problems of an *informal* relationship parallel those of a formal one. A comprehensive overview of all aspects of therapeutic relationships guides the nurse in applying principles to practice, even if the nurse is not directly involved in individual psychotherapy.

Table 27–2 highlights the similarities and differences of informal and formal relationship work. The differences between informal and formal relationships are discussed throughout this chapter.

Mutually Defined

A one-to-one relationship is mutually defined by the two participants. Both psychiatric nurse and client voluntarily enter the relationship and specify the conditions under which it is to evolve. For example, the client may seek immediate alleviation of symptoms rather than long-term individual psychotherapy. Nurse and client identify together where and when they will meet and other conditions of their participation. This contractual aspect of the one-to-one relationship is explored further in the discussion of the beginning (orientation) phase of therapy later in this chapter. Once the relationship is established, its maintenance depends on the commitment of both participants.

Collaborative

Both participants enter a relationship in which goals, strategies, and outcomes evolve within the context of the therapeutic work together (see Figure 27–1). Mutual collaboration implies that each participant brings personal abilities, capabilities, and power to the relationship. Thus, the psychiatric nurse does not assume responsibility for client behaviors but actively works with the client to assess the self-defeating and growth-promoting aspects of specific behaviors. Mutual collaboration also means that the psychiatric nurse assesses and is accountable for her or his own behavior with the client. Ongoing supervision often helps the nurse meet these particular goals.

Goal Directed

A one-to-one relationship is always goal-directed. The client is expected to identify and achieve specific physical, emotional, and social goals within the context of the relation-

	Table 27–2	
	Similarities and Differences of Informal and Formal One-to-One Relationships	
	Nature of Relationship	
Characteristic	Informal	Formal
Setting	Varied	Generally psychiatric settings
Frequency and duration of contact	Flexible depending on client need or tolerance. Example: short, frequent intervals on daily basis	Structured. Example: once weekly, with possible crisis sessions. Duration usually set at thirty minutes or one hour
Duration of relationship	May or may not involve time commitment. Generally a few days to a few weeks	Involves time commitment. Weeks to months, for short-term work. Months to years, for long-term work
Type of dysfunction	In general, more effective with severe dysfunction	In severe dysfunction, may be useful after client is stabilized on medication
Use of therapeutic contract	May involve simple therapeutic contract	Utilizes therapeutic contract; the more specific, the better
Fees	Usually not relevant	May be relevant. May be part of therapeutic contract
Degree of skill required	Nursing student or psychiatric nurse	Advanced degree beneficial, but not essential
Degree of supervision	Some degree and type of supervision is always necessary	Consistent supervision or consultation usually necessary
Degree of effectiveness	For both, depends on client's level of functioning, skills of the psychiatric nurse, and time allotment	

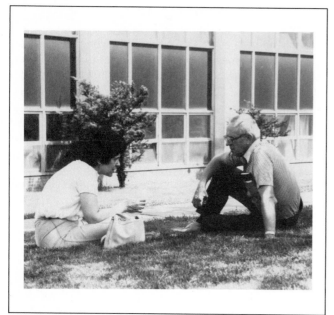

Figure 27–1
The essence of the one-to-one client-nurse relationship is mutual collaboration. In this interaction the nurse is attending to both *content* and *process*.

ship. Client goals vary widely in type and depth. For example, in informal relationship work, a client's goal may be to initiate one peer relationship within an in-patient psychiatric unit. Other examples include resolution of a divorce involving children and shared personal possessions, or coming to terms with the client's impending death from acute, terminal physical illness. Often the client's initial goal is to solve an immediate problem, and this serves as a basis for establishing more extensive psychosocial goals. The psychiatric nurse also formulates personal therapeutic goals to enhance the growth-producing elements of the relationship.

HISTORICAL AND THEORETICAL FOUNDATIONS

The one-to-one relationship between psychiatric nurse and client has evolved as the cornerstone of psychiatric nursing theory and practice. In this century, nurses have moved from being primarily responsible for observing, reporting, and maintaining ward order to functioning members of an interdisciplinary treatment team. Although psychiatric nursing has expanded to include group, family, milieu, and a host of other therapies, one-to-one relationships remain the cornerstone.

Sound theoretical foundations are of critical importance. Peplau contends that psychiatric nursing is in a state of transition, moving from medical to nursing models for practice (Fitzpatrick et al. 1982, p vii). Nurses are no longer required to rely solely upon theoretical foundations from outside sources (medicine, psychology, sociology, and communication sciences) as they participate in therapeutic relationships. Nursing conceptual models have emerged that characterize the psychiatric-mental health nursing approach.

Humanistic Interactionist Framework

Humanistic philosophy in one-to-one relationships involves viewing humanness not as a static condition, but as an evolving, active process unique to each person.

Openness

Humanistic interactionist philosophy stresses openness and honesty in human relations. Within a humanistic framework, the one-to-one relationship between nurse and client may be viewed as an experience in *shared dignity*. The psychiatric nurse adapts to the client to allow the client to reveal his or her humanness freely and openly to the nurse. Each aspect of the nurse's verbal and nonverbal behavior encourages or inhibits the client from further revealing humanness.

Negotiation

The humanistic interactionist views the client as exercising free will, as an active decision maker. In addition, humanism stresses the client's uniqueness and the subjectiveness of the experiences underlying personal actions. The one-to-one relationship relies on the client to determine the type and length of involvement and to be personally accountable for the work. The atmosphere of give and take within the relationship emphasizes mutuality, reciprocity, and interpersonal fairness. Establishment of a clearly defined, mutually agreed-on therapeutic contract represents a prime example of negotiation in one-to-one work. (The therapeutic contract is covered in this chapter.)

Commitment

Commitment is based on the therapeutic contract between nurse and client. The contract establishes the limits of the relationship, as well as the time and energy that will be allotted to it. At some point in the relationship, the psychiatric nurse will be confronted by the reality of the client's dysfunction. The beginning psychiatric nurse may respond by actively colluding with the client to deny or ignore the dysfunction and remain on a superficial, social level of communication. This collusion protects the nurse from having to address the client's helplessness, desperation, hostility, or raw grief. The nurse who does not let the client express these feelings is not sufficiently committed to the client. The opposite is also nontherapeutic. The overcommitted psychiatric nurse may assume an omnipotent or rescuer role to "cure" the client. This role robs the client of active decision-making power and accountability. The client will test the nurse's commitment in some phase of the relationship. This test needs to be dealt with explicitly on verbal and nonverbal levels by both nurse and client.

Responsibility

Personal responsibility for the one-to-one relationship is also based on the therapeutic contract between nurse and client, and it, too, will be tested by the client in some phase of the relationship. Beginning psychiatric nurses usually encounter responsibility problems as they begin to perceive unattractive, dysfunctional, or blatantly offending interpersonal behavioral patterns or habits in their clients. Both nurse and client must deal explicitly with "who is responsible for what." In addition, the nurse should avoid making any agreements with a client that the nurse may be unable to fulfill.

Authenticity

The appreciation of spontaneity and authenticity is another aspect of humanistic interactionist philosophy that applies particularly to one-to-one relationships. Psychiatric nurses need to create an atmosphere that conveys permission to express pain and pleasure. Expressions of joy and assessments of client abilities, talents, and capabilities are an often-neglected, yet essential, aspect of relationship work.

Search for Meaning

Within the humanistic interactionist philosophy, personal identity is not considered a fixed product. Personal identity is constantly confirmed through interaction with others. The nurse-client interaction is subject to continuous reassessment of the client by the nurse and the nurse by the client. This process is called *identity confirmation*. Meanings of individual words, gestures, events, and situations must be explored to determine the exact significance that the client assigns to them.

In a more general way, psychiatric nurses are working with clients in a search for meaning in their lives. It is essential that nurses establish their own personal meaning and integration of self, for these are key resources in treatment. For psychiatric nurses to be effective, they must already possess the personal skills to deal with the client's symptoms. They must have personally worked through any

problems that resembled those of the client. For example, a nurse who cannot cope with her own depressed feelings will not be effective with a severely depressed client.

Overview of Current Therapies

Psychotherapeutic treatment in recent years has moved from intensive psychoanalysis to diversified techniques and systems of psychotherapy.

Recent systems of psychotherapy include transactional analysis, reality therapy, rational-emotive therapy, gestalt therapy, primal therapy, and logotherapy. A critical discussion of these popular approaches is beyond the scope of this chapter. The development of a new approach to one-to-one work, namely, short-term dynamic psychotherapy (STDP), is highlighted here. Concerns regarding a decrease in the availability of long-term psychotherapy are discussed. Other systems of psychotherapy are addressed elsewhere in this text (see Chapters 5 and 28–32).

Short-Term Dynamic Psychotherapy

Short-term dynamic psychotherapy (STDP) is the synthesis of several approaches. STDP has evolved to treat a maximum number of clients with numerous issues in a minimum amount of time. Characteristics of STDP include brief duration (usually sixteen to twenty hour-long sessions), a very active therapist role, identification of a central issue or "core conflict," limited goals that address the specific problems for which the client seeks treatment, and a wide range of therapeutic techniques. Transference is a concept basic to STDP.

Prospective clients are carefully assessed for their potential to benefit from STDP. The following clients would generally be excluded from participation in STDP (Davanbo 1985; Heber et al. 1984):

- Persons with chronic obsessions or phobias
- Persons with organic or functional psychoses
- Persons with poor impulse control
- Persons with a history of substance abuse
- Persons who are highly self-destructive
- Persons who seek symptom relief rather than change
- Persons who cannot choose a major life problem and maintain this focus throughout treatment
- Persons who cannot tolerate the very active role of the therapist
- Persons who need extensive long-term psychotherapy

A high degree of motivation for change on the part of the client is critical for selection.

Long-Term Psychotherapy

The recent emphasis on efficiency in client selection and therapeutic outcome has decreased the emphasis on long-term psychotherapy. The extensive exclusion criteria for STDP may leave the severely dysfunctional client with minimal programs in today's mental health care delivery system. As we discuss in Chapters 22 and 40, the staggering increase in the number of street people across the United States is a symptom of our nation's inefficiency in providing comprehensive programs to meet the needs of people with chronic and complex problems.

In addition to formal long-term psychotherapy, specific skill training can address the chronic problems of long-term psychiatric clients. Such training may include communication skills, skills needed in activities of daily life, community living skills, stress-management skills, problem-solving skills, and medication education. The nurse-client relationship is just as crucial in these approaches as in STDP with more acutely ill clients.

Phenomena Occurring in One-to-One Relationships

Sometimes in therapeutic relationships the nurse may initially sense confusion regarding what is happening in the nurse-client relationship. This uneasiness may be difficult for the nurse to identify, describe, and explore. Keep the following phenomena in mind when attempting to "make sense" of a one-to-one relationship.

Resistance

Resistance inevitably surfaces in the course of one-to-one work. It most often occurs as the client begins to address self-defeating thoughts, feelings, and behaviors.

Definition

Resistance refers to all the phenomena that interfere with and disrupt the smooth flow of feelings, memories, and thoughts. Resistance in the traditional psychoanalytic sense means anything that inhibits the client from producing material from the unconscious. Conscious phenomena (feelings, memories, thoughts) may be forceful or weak, significant or unimportant. The same is true of uncon-

scious material. However, in the psychoanalytic view, some unconscious productions may be intense forces under pressure to be discharged (archaic sexual and aggressive impulses), regardless of whether they are unrealistic, inappropriately timed, or illogical. These intense forces can be controlled only by another force equal in strength, which is labeled resistance.

Resistance is often mistakenly seen as the client's struggle against the nurse. Instead, the client is struggling against change, against self-awareness, and against responsibility for actions. Although the client's behavior patterns may have self-defeating aspects, they have also provided some satisfaction or prevented some discomfort. The client may also resist giving up a defense that offered protection from the anxiety associated with unbearable thoughts and impulses. Thus, resistance in therapeutic relationships is best understood as the client's struggle against change.

Resistance occurs in varied situations and settings. It may surface as a primary concern in the following examples: during therapeutic work of any kind (one-to-one, group, family) in community liaison services, home visitation programs, or consultative activities.

Manifestations

In general, the nurse may suspect resistance when the client's behavior appears to block the progress of the relationship. There are innumerable ways to express resistance. The following may be examples of resistance:

- Forgetting events
- Focusing on the past to avoid talking about the present (or vice versa)
- Consistently avoiding certain topics or inquiries
- Expressing antagonism toward the nurse
- Falling in love with the nurse
- Acting out (discussed later in this chapter)

Some manifestations of resistance may be more subtle. For example, a client may introduce an abrupt crisis, an alarming childhood memory, or an intense new relationship whenever a certain topic is approached. Likewise, a client may use flirtatious or seductive behaviors that embarrass the nurse to avoid working on a particular problem. Silence may indicate resistance, and so may an invigorating clinical discussion intended as a filibuster or "smoke screen" to avoid emotive expression or problem resolution.

The nurse must exercise caution in evaluating a client's behavior as resistive. The client's silence may indicate pensiveness, a pause before emotive expression, or a sense of completion. The client who is habitually late may have real difficulties adjusting a full personal schedule to accommodate the sessions. Resistance to specific topics or concerns may indicate that the client is not ready for investigative work at the time. Likewise, the client may resist giving up a defense that is desperately needed in order to keep anxiety about a present situation at manageable levels.

The humanistic stance is that the client has a right to assume a genuine and legitimate position of resisting one aspect of or the entire therapeutic process, as a matter of choice. The client's resistive behavior should be openly discussed, rather than ignored. The humanistic nurse views the client as exercising free will—as an active participant in decisions that shape the client's well-being, including the one-to-one relationship.

Acting Out

Acting out is a particularly destructive form of resistance in which the client puts into action (that is, "acts out") a memory that has been forgotten or repressed. It is important to recognize that the client is externalizing his or her inner conflict to people in the immediate environment. Rather than verbalizing conflicts or feelings, the client displays inappropriate behaviors. Examples of acting out may include forcefully slamming a door, dressing provocatively, or slapping someone. In acting out, the client acts toward a mate, friend, relative, or other person those feelings and attitudes that he or she does not express toward the nurse. An example of acting out is the development of third person relationships to absorb the emotions and fantasies that belong within the therapeutic relationship. Exaggerated feelings of intense hostility toward the nurse may lead to violence or physical harm to the client, nurse, or the third person. Intense feelings of love for the nurse or therapist may precipitate an affair or marriage with the third person.

Acting out is difficult to deal with because the client does not talk about the feelings that precipitate the behavior and later tends to conceal or rationalize the behavior. Acting out can abruptly break up treatment, unless it is identified and dealt with explicitly. Specific nursing interventions regarding acting out include:

- Bring acting out to the attention of the client.
- Encourage the client to *talk about* impulses rather than to act them out.
- Encourage identification of feelings *before* putting them into action.
- Increase frequency of contact.
- Look for evidence of transference phenomena toward the nurse.
- With repeated dangerous acting out, consider withdrawing from the relationship unless the client sets limits on these personal behaviors.

The following clinical example illustrates acting out in a clinical setting:

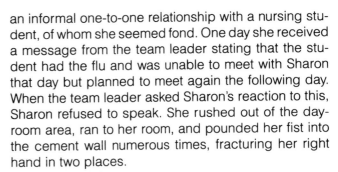

Sharon is a 15-year-old with a history of self-abusive behavior. She had been the victim of repeated incestuous experiences with her stepfather over several years, despite her mother's knowledge of such activity. On an in-patient adolescent evaluation unit, she met daily in an informal one-to-one relationship with a nursing student, of whom she seemed fond. One day she received a message from the team leader stating that the student had the flu and was unable to meet with Sharon that day but planned to meet again the following day. When the team leader asked Sharon's reaction to this, Sharon refused to speak. She rushed out of the day-room area, ran to her room, and pounded her fist into the cement wall numerous times, fracturing her right hand in two places.

The next day, the nursing student approached Sharon. Sharon offered no comment. The student's inquiry regarding the previous day's message also met with no comment. The student stated her concern for Sharon's welfare and her confusion regarding Sharon's injury. Sharon remained silent. The student stated her wish to sort things out together as they had done in the past and then sat quietly with Sharon. After two minutes, Sharon began crying, and talked about feeling alone.

The nonverbal behaviors of nurses affect clients. Acting out can be demonstrated by the nurse who manifests parental, erotic, sexual, or hostile behaviors. Examples of acting out by the nurse may include:

- Placing the hands on hips or pointing a finger while setting limits on a client's behavior (parental)
- Patting a client on the shoulder and offering reassurance (parental)
- Blushing and giggling when a client makes a sexual remark (sexual)

These behaviors by the nurse encourage gross acting out by the client.

Parental or caretaker behaviors are the most common among beginning psychiatric nurses. They express the nurse's need to nurture and feed the client. These behaviors may indicate a countertransference problem for the nurse and discount the client's ability to ensure his or her well-being. Recognition of acting out by the psychiatric nurse is essential and reinforces the need for formal supervision.

General Intervention Strategies

Several consecutive approaches are used as general nursing intervention strategies for resistance. They begin with the psychiatric nurse's awareness of the resistance. Helpful intervention strategies may include:

- Labeling the resistant behavior with the client. The psychiatric nurse may allow the resistance to occur several times to demonstrate its presence to the client. It is as if the psychiatric nurse were holding up a mirror for the client, reflecting and clarifying the specific resistant behavior.

- Exploring the accompanying emotion and history of its development.
- Exploring what function the resistance may serve, especially any self-defeating aspects.
- Facilitating working through the resistance by fully understanding and appreciating its implications in the client's life.

This sequence may occur repeatedly before a resistant behavior is resolved. Many examples of specific interventions are presented later in this chapter.

Transference

Transference is a normal phenomenon that may surface and inhibit effectiveness in any phase of one-to-one relationship work. The term *transference* originated in psychoanalytic theory. **Transference** occurs when a client has unresolved childhood experiences with significant others. Instead of remembering the past, the client "transfers" these unresolved feelings, attitudes, and wishes into present significant relationships in an attempt to resolve these in a more satisfying manner. Thus, the client misunderstands the present based on the unresolved problems of his or her past. The client is unaware of the nature of this action.

It is important to understand that transference is a form of resistance. The client unknowingly resists any recollection of childhood conflicts. Instead, the client transfers these conflicts to present relationships, including the nurse-client relationship.

A humanistic interactionist may view transference phenomena as distortions of meaning between psychiatric nurse and client in one-to-one relationship work. The nurse may suspect that a client is in transference when the client repeatedly assigns meanings to the nurse-client relationship that belong to one or more of the client's past relationships. It is as if the client's ability to assess the nurse-client interactions becomes confused and thwarted by the unfinished conflicts belonging to past interactions with significant others. Thus, the psychiatric nurse may be viewed as parent, sibling, lover, or friend.

The development of transference offers the psychiatric nurse an opportunity, by direct observation, to understand the development of the client's past conflicts. The appearance of highly emotional responses that do not "fit" the current therapeutic situation may indicate client transfer-

ence. In traditional psychoanalytic work, handling the transference becomes the core of treatment. In the humanistic interactionist approach to transference, the psychiatric nurse explores the meaning of individual words, gestures, events, and situations in the current one-to-one relationship to determine how these reflect or replay distortions in past relationships. The therapeutic task is to separate feelings, thoughts, and behaviors that belong to the current one-to-one relationship from those that represent unresolved conflicts in past relationships. Increasing awareness of the transference process often frees the client to work through past conflicts and explore the more creative, self-actualizing aspects of personal identity as they evolve in the current relationship. The psychiatric nurse must not behave as the client's parent or other transference figure has behaved. Rather, the nurse helps the client bring an unconscious event into consciousness, to examine its cause and meaning. The following example illustrates how transference may surface in a clinical setting:

Conrad Wilson is a 40-year-old married man hospitalized with moderate depression, which is manifested by restless agitation, inability to complete tasks, and subjective feelings of hopelessness. Conrad was assigned to a primary counselor, a male psychiatric nurse. Over the course of several meetings with his counselor, Conrad assumed a cowering, ingratiating manner. He seemed to resemble a little boy awaiting punishment from an intimidating, punitive father. This interpersonal orientation was observed by other male staff who informally initiated interaction with Conrad on the unit. In this instance, the transference figure appeared to be a father figure.

The counselor chose not to explore Conrad's past relationships. The aim of short-term work was to focus on concrete ways to decrease depressed feelings in Conrad's present life situation. The counselor addressed ingratiating behaviors in the nurse-client relationship only when they appeared to have an adverse effect on their short-term work together.

In the clinical example, the primary counselor chose to focus on present rather than past relationships in an effort to stabilize the hospitalized client. Transference may be dealt with in many ways, depending upon the client's functioning, the counselor's theoretical orientation, and the type of therapy.

Transference may be positive or negative. **Positive transference**, that is, positive feelings for the therapist, occurs when the client generally has had satisfying past relationships with significant others in his or her childhood. The therapeutic relationship is usually able to progress in this instance. **Negative transference** is a source of problems; it is discussed later in this chapter.

Countertransference

While transference involves the client's reactions to the psychiatric nurse, **countertransference** involves the nurse's reactions to the client. The psychiatric nurse may develop powerful counterproductive fantasies, feelings, and attitudes in response to the client's transference or personality. A humanistic interactionist may also view countertransference as a distortion of meaning between psychiatric nurse and client in one-to-one relationship work. A clinical instructor or supervisor may suspect countertransference when the psychiatric nurse repeatedly assigns meaning to the nurse-client relationship that belongs to the nurse's other past relationships. In countertransference the psychiatric nurse's ability to assess the nurse-client interactions becomes confused or thwarted by unresolved past conflicts. Thus, the nurse may unconsciously employ behaviors (as parent, sibling, lover, or friend) that attempt to replay in the current situation some past identity with significant others. Countertransference indicates unresolved conflict in the psychiatric nurse. This conflict may be expressed in acts of omission or commission and in irrational friendliness or annoyance. These expressions may be covert or overt.

Countertransference is a normal occurrence, requiring supervision or consultation to prevent degeneration of the one-to-one relationship. Supervision may enable the psychiatric nurse to separate feelings, thoughts, and behaviors that belong to the current relationship from those that represent unfinished conflicts in past relationships. Awareness of the existence of countertransference is crucial. Unrecognized countertransference may be acted out and may inhibit client understanding. Unrecognized countertransference can undermine the entire psychotherapeutic process. A later section of this chapter briefly explores specific problems and appropriate interventions in troublesome cases of transference and countertransference.

INTERPERSONAL SKILLS IN THERAPEUTIC RELATIONSHIPS

Therapeutic Effectiveness of Psychiatric Nurses

The effectiveness of psychiatric nurses has often been subjectively assumed, unquestioned, or discounted without a scientific data base for evaluation. This discussion of their therapeutic effectiveness includes a brief exploration of current research, of the conflict between caretaker and therapist roles, and of personal characteristics known to facilitate therapeutic effectiveness.

Fagin (1983) believes that the 1980s are a challenging time in the health care environment. Reimbursement for professional services is a prime focus. As health care providers become increasingly competitive, Fagin encourages

nurses to participate openly in the marketplace. She reviews studies documenting the cost effectiveness of nurse therapists and endorses nurses' movement into private practice. According to Fagin, nurse specialists do psychotherapy effectively and inexpensively. Research by Hardin and Durham (1985) reinforces Fagin's belief in the effectiveness of nurse therapists. In this research, both nurse therapists and clients viewed psychotherapy as a satisfying and successful experience. (See the Research Note.)

Pelletier (1984) conducted a similar survey aimed at assessing types of clients treated by nurse therapists. In contrast to Hardin and Durham, Pelletier found that most clients were of lower to lower-middle occupational status. Two similarities between studies were the reason for seeking treatment and clients' age range. The majority of clients in Pelletier's study suffered from depression and anxiety neurosis. They were between 33 and 39 years of age. Pelletier found a predominance of women as therapists and clients, suggesting that a female caseload might reflect the therapist's focus on contemporary women's experience.

The therapeutic effectiveness of psychiatric nurses is also an international psychiatric nursing issue. A major theme in recent publications is the mental health nurse as therapist. Several authors suggest that greater use of nurses as therapists may ease therapist shortages and help prevent the "revolving door" syndrome—repeated psychiatric hospitalizations (Horsfall 1983, Quinn 1985).

Scott and Philip (1985) researched attitudes of psychiatric nurses toward clients and treatment in a British long-term in-patient setting. The study sample incorporated psychiatric nurses and nursing assistants on all shifts. Significant attitudinal differences were found between psychiatric nurses and nursing attendants in relation to professional preparation, age, and sex. Staff with more professional preparation were less authoritarian and more personal toward clients. Staff under the age of 30 were less authoritarian and more personal toward clients than staff over the age of 45. Female staff were significantly more authoritarian and formal than male staff in the study sample. They were also more inclined toward physical methods of treatment (Scott and Philip 1985). Whether stereotyped sex-role nursing behaviors are evident in American in-patient settings is a topic for further research.

Conflict between Caretaker and Therapist Roles

Traditional nursing education may keep the psychiatric nurse from developing therapeutic effectiveness if it stresses the denial of personal feelings and the need for a caretaker role. Nurses may erect rigid defenses aimed at denying their feelings because of the emotional demands of nursing. For example, some procedures actually require the nurse to violate a client's emotional or physical state (injections, dressings). Defending against feelings becomes one way for the nurse to cope with inflicting pain on another person. Yet psychiatric nurses can deal effectively with the feelings of clients only to the extent that they explore their own personal feelings.

Continued assumption of the caretaker role also undermines the therapeutic effectiveness of psychiatric nurses. The caretaker role tends to involve sympathy rather than empathy. The difference between these two responses is significant to therapeutic outcomes.

A one-to-one relationship requires the psychiatric nurse to help the client actively explore the meaning underlying the client's personal pain, distress, or discomfort. Nurses must avoid the caretaker role in which they alleviate pain. Rather, they must encourage clients to develop ways to do so for themselves. Similarly, the caretaker role requires nurses to make decisions for clients. It does not encourage clients to be accountable for their own decisions.

Facilitative Personal Characteristics

Psychiatric nurses may increase their therapeutic effectiveness by knowledge and practice of specific interpersonal skills in therapeutic relationships. Schuable and Pierce (1974) demonstrated that clients who were successful in therapy had therapists who functioned with more empathy, warmth, genuineness, and concreteness than the therapists of clients who were unsuccessful in therapy. Research repeatedly indicates that interpersonal skills may be acquired, increased, and refined through education, workshops, and human relations laboratories.

Therapeutic Use of Self

Therapeutic use of self involves a pulling together of several important personal elements to bring to any one-to-one relationship work.

- Development of healthy self-awareness
- Exploration of the growth-facilitating, humanistic self and personal impact on others
- Thorough use of theoretical and experiential knowledge in mental health

Therapeutic use of self is discussed in Chapter 3.

Within the humanistic framework, the psychiatric nurse adapts to the client to allow the client to reveal his or her humanness freely and openly to the nurse. The goal is to develop commitment, therapeutic processes, and a thera-

peutic relationship between client and nurse. Sometimes the nurse may feel uneasy, awkward, or offended if the client unexpectedly asks personal questions, presents a gift, discusses values such as religion, or seeks physical contact. Although these experiences may happen during any phase of therapeutic work, they frequently occur during the working phase. During this phase, the client slowly gets to know the psychiatric nurse as a separate, concerned person. Critical distance is an additional concern for the nurse from the moment that she or he attempts interpersonal contact. Each of these concerns requires ongoing nursing assessment and evaluation so that positive therapeutic outcome may be maximized.

Critical Distance

It is important for the nurse to observe how the client uses physical space. Hall (1966) asserts that people need to keep a critical distance between themselves and others to maintain their well-being. That specific distance depends on the relationship between the individuals. In the 1960s, Parks (1966) suggested that nurses interpose physical distance between themselves and clients, especially early in therapy. This distance promotes verbal communication and reduces any existing anxiety and hostility. Parks's suggestion is still valid today. Moving rapidly toward closeness, especially in establishing the nurse-client relationship, may overwhelm the client and increase anxiety.

The physical distance between the psychiatric nurse and the client can be indicative of other therapeutic processes. For example, a client may sit in a chair at a great distance from the nurse during initial meetings but move closer and closer as the working relationship is established. The psychiatric nurse needs to assess the possible interpersonal implications of proximity (nearness) for each client. As the relationship progresses, the nurse must assess whether physical distance or proximity reduces client anxiety. The client's need for distance usually increases as the client experiences panic or near-panic levels of anxiety.

Self-Disclosure

Self-disclosure means being open to personal feelings and experiences, being "real" as opposed to hiding behind a professional facade or being a technician of various communication skills. If the nurse reveals personal feelings when appropriate, the client learns that it is OK to explore feelings in the therapeutic setting. How much should a nurse share with a client? Under what circumstances?

It may be helpful to view self-disclosure on a continuum. One end represents underdisclosure; the other, overdisclosure. When evaluating any self-disclosure at a given time, nurses should ask themselves two essential questions. First, what is the purpose of the revelation, i.e., who is this self-disclosure for? Does this self-disclosure meet the client's therapeutic goals or does it meet the nurse's needs? Second, does this self-disclosure foster the development of a more productive therapeutic relationship?

Facilitative self-disclosure must be used within the context of the therapeutic relationship, where attention is given to its timing, appropriateness, and degree. For example, self-disclosure must be cautiously used with a severely dysfunctional client with poor ego boundaries. This client may not be able to separate thoughts and feelings that belong to the client from those that belong to the nurse. The client might misinterpret the nurse's self-disclosure or might not be able to make sense of the disclosure. The client may also fear engulfment by the nurse, i.e., the nurse's feelings might be perceived as so threatening that they overwhelm the client. Facilitative self-disclosure fosters the development of the therapeutic relationship rather than threatening its continuance. Auvil and Silver (1984, p 60) consider the client's feelings toward helping persons when assessing self-disclosure:

It has been our experience that patients ask questions as to our religion, nationality, age, marital status, and family background. Before disclosing any personal data, we make an assessment of our patients' diagnosis and our perceptions of the patients' feelings toward us. If they are positive, and the patients' needs would be served by knowing about us as real people, we accede to their requests. However, if we are unsure of the patients' feelings, or we perceive them as negative, we avoid disclosing personal information to prevent any negative acting out behavior provoked by the data disclosed. For example, from the first week of a chronic schizophrenic patient's confinement to

RESEARCH NOTE

Citation

Hardin SB, Durham JD: First rate: Exploring the structure, process, and effectiveness of nurse psychotherapy. J Psychosoc Nurs Ment Health Serv 1985;23:9–15.

Study Problem/Purpose

This descriptive study was designed to explore nurse psychotherapy as perceived by nurse therapists and their clients. Purposes of the study were to determine the structural parameters of therapy, characteristics of the nurse-client relationship, and therapeutic effectiveness of treatment.

Methods

The study included eighty-two nurse therapists throughout the United States. Each was a psychiatric nurse prepared at the master's level and was a primary psychotherapist for individual clients. Thirty-eight nurse therapists (46%) agreed to send questionnaires to former clients. The ninety-five clients in the study had been treated for at least six sessions in the previous year by a nurse therapist cooperating in the study. A major limitation of the study was that nurse therapists selected the client sample.

The measure utilized by nurse therapists was a nurse psychotherapist questionnaire. Measures for clients were a client attitude scale and a client questionnaire to measure general satisfaction with psychotherapy. These questionnaires from both groups provided demographic, quantitative, and qualitative data. Measures were based on previously used research tools.

Findings

Nurse therapists were predominantly female, had extensive psychotherapy experience, and were highly educated (some held doctorates or were enrolled in doctoral

programs). Fifty-four percent worked alone, while others identified psychiatrists, psychologists, social workers, and other nurses as their co-workers. Clients were generally unmarried, well-educated females between 20 and 40 years of age. They most often sought treatment for depression or for problems in coping with separation and divorce. Nurse therapists tended to screen acting out, psychotic, and chemically addicted clients from their practices.

The structure of practice typically consisted of verbal psychotherapy on a weekly basis. The average duration of treatment was fourteen months at an average charge of $37 per session.

Nurse therapists rated highest as empathic, warm, and excellent listeners. Other helping actions with clients included increasing insight, imparting skill in problem solving, improving self-esteem, validating feelings, and increasing independence.

Both nurse therapists and clients viewed psychotherapy as a satisfying and successful experience. Ninety percent of clients expressed satisfaction regarding an overall evaluation of their psychotherapy experience. Seventy percent of clients claimed extreme satisfaction. Ten percent of clients reported dissatisfaction with therapy.

Implications

This descriptive study is noteworthy, since there is little systematic research regarding nurse therapists, i.e., whom they treat, how they conduct treatment, and how desirable this treatment is. The authors view the study sample as effective, self-directed therapists. They further suggest that nurse therapists will probably not attain true autonomy without additional powers. These powers may include hospital privileges and prescriptive authority. The authors also urge nurses to continue their organized efforts to bring about third-party payment, based upon the findings of this study.

the unit, it was apparent to the staff that he was obsessed around religious ideation. He would approach the nurses to ask what religion each professed. When they unwisely shared their religious preferences with him, he would sweep around the unit, loudly informing one and all that "they were gonna' burn in hell . . ."

When the nurse chooses to disclose personal information in a given instance, nursing evaluation must follow. If the "flow" of the work together was enhanced, then the nurse suspects that the self-revelation was facilitative. If the psychiatric nurse is unsure of the outcome, a frank inquiry may be in order. For example, "How did you feel when I told you my age?" The client's reaction and subsequent exploration together can be a gauge for measuring how this client perceives and responds to self-disclosures by the nurse. As the nurse expresses feelings about the evolving relationship, the client may feel free to reciprocate. At times, the psychiatric nurse may choose to role model emotive expression.

When the psychiatric nurse chooses to avoid self-disclosure in a given instance, several communication techniques may be helpful. For instance, a client might ask the nurse to disclose her or his marital status, home address, religious affiliation, or most pressing personal problem. Auvil and Silver (1984) offer the following ways to deflect a request for self-disclosure:

- *Use honesty.* "I don't want to share my home address with you."

- *Use benign curiosity.* "I wonder why you're asking me this today?"

- *Use refocusing.* "You were talking about how your father treats you. I wonder why you changed the topic? You were saying that . . ."

- *Use interpretation.* "I notice that every time you talk about your father, you change the subject and ask me a question." (pause)

- *Seek clarification.* "You keep asking me my home address. I wonder what concerns you might have about me today and as we work together?"

- *Respond with feedback and limit-setting.* "I'm really uncomfortable when you ask me who pays my tuition. Talking about my finances isn't part of our agreement to work together." Adding "the last time we met, you were deciding if you were going to call your boss on the phone . . ." helps to restructure the situation.

These communication techniques are used within the context of the therapeutic relationship, where client response is assessed and evaluated by the responsible nurse in an ongoing manner.

The giving of gifts may be a special concern in therapeutic relationships. Gift giving may take various forms: a fleeting social amenity (e.g., the purchase of a cup of coffee), a gesture (e.g., the loan of a favorite book), or the present of a valued object (e.g., the giving of an original painting). Like self-disclosure, gift giving in any instance must be met with ongoing nursing assessment and evaluation to determine its form, intent, appropriateness, and meaning within the context of the therapeutic relationship. No rule covers all instances of gift giving. Rather, several broad guidelines can help the nurse evaluate the particular situation.

The Client as Gift Giver   During the orientation phase of a therapeutic relationship, the client may overtly offer or ask for a gift. This gesture may be as incidental as offering the nurse (or asking for) a cigarette. The psychiatric nurse examines this overture, keeping in mind several possible motivations. The client may seek to bribe or manipulate the nurse, thereby seeking to control the direction of the therapeutic relationship. The client may seek to "buy" the nurse's time and attention. The client may ask for small gifts to reinforce a helpless, "take-care-of-me" interpersonal stance. Of course, the client may have no covert intent and may simply need a cigarette. In the orientation phase, it may be helpful for nurses not to accept or give any gift they feel uncomfortable giving. Rather the nurse should explore the client's intent. Often this mutual exploration not only clarifies the client's intent but also helps to define the parameters of the evolving relationship and models the exploratory process for the client.

During the working phase, particularly after the client has implemented positive growth, the client may offer a gift in the form of a craft or skill. As in the orientation phase, the intent of the gift needs to be made explicit. Such exploration may be encouraged by such statements as "How is it that you're sharing this gift with me?" or "What feelings might you want to share with this gift?" A client might give a gift during the working phase for several reasons. The client may wish to acknowledge the mutual work that has taken place. The client may wish to show appreciation for being allowed to share his or her concerns with another person. A gift may be given as a "smoke screen" to block further exploration of a major dynamic. A gift may be given outwardly to cover up anger or frustration felt inwardly. Finally, a gift may indicate that the client perceives that the therapeutic work is finished and feels ready to terminate. In every instance, the nurse must assess the intent of the gift, as well as its timing and appropriateness, within the context of the therapeutic relationship.

Gifts are most often given during the termination phase of one-to-one relationships. In this phase, a gift may have several overt and covert meanings. The client may wish to give a token of appreciation for any positive personal growth that occurred in this mutual learning endeavor. The client may desire to change the therapeutic relationship into a social one. The client may wish to prolong sessions to avoid the final good-bye. Some nurses accept a small gift from a client at the time of termination if feelings regarding the gift have been explored and clarified. (The gift may be an appropriate remembrance of a mutual and positive growth experience.) The nurse may find receiving a gift at times to be awkward and "artificial." Yet such a situation gives the nurse the opportunity to help the client toward further self-expression and self-knowledge.

The Nurse as Gift Giver The nurse is an infrequent and judicious gift giver. Most often, the psychiatric nurse relates to the client by therapeutic use of self rather than through objects, such as gifts. There are possible exceptions. For instance a psychiatric nurse may give a gift to establish initial contact with a severely dysfunctional client in a ward setting. During the working phase, the nurse may share a resource (e.g., a book or article) about some facet of the client's therapy or growth. During termination, the nurse may give the client a small gift to acknowledge mutual growth during therapeutic work. In every instance, the psychiatric nurse evaluates the client's response and the meaning assigned to this gift. The nurse also evaluates her or his own motives and the personal meaning the giving has to the nurse.

Use of Touch

Physical contact is used cautiously in therapeutic work. It is best to avoid unplanned physical contact without therapeutic rationale. Clients with poor ego boundaries may become intensely threatened and feel overwhelmed by physical contact. For example, a client may lose the ability to distinguish self from the nurse during simple hand contact. Such contact may be perceived as a hostile or sexual gesture, although not intended as such by the nurse. In contrast, an acutely grief-stricken client, too distraught to focus on words, might receive needed support from being held.

The psychiatric nurse employs the nursing process when considering any use of touch in one-to-one relationships. The nurse must ask: First, does touch meet the client's therapeutic goals or does it meet the nurse's needs? Second, does touch foster a more productive therapeutic relationship? As with self-disclosure, the use of touch must be evaluated within the context of the therapeutic relationship, paying attention to its timing, appropriateness, and type. For example, a client is thrilled to achieve an employment goal that has taken much personal time and effort. The psychiatric nurse determines that a firm handshake and a statement of congratulations are facilitative in this instance and at this working phase of the relationship. If the nurse is unsure of the effect of such a gesture, a frank inquiry may be in order: "How did you feel when I shook your hand a few moments ago?" Again, the client's reaction and subsequent exploration can be a gauge for measuring how the client perceives and responds to the use of touch. A later section of this chapter concerning manipulation

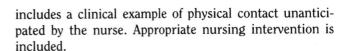

includes a clinical example of physical contact unanticipated by the nurse. Appropriate nursing intervention is included.

Values

Psychiatric nurses may need to consider values (both of the client and of the nurse) as these arise in the therapeutic relationship. Personal value systems, which include an individual's beliefs and attitudes, are often difficult to grasp and examine. Yet value systems determine much of our day-to-day behaviors. Black (1983, p 41) stresses the importance of recognizing and owning one's personal values:

> Equally desirable for both helper and client is a recognition, however limited, of their own personal values, those meanings to which they attach merit or approval. . . . When one is able to get close to one's feelings, they can serve as an immediate clue to one's values. The things, events, actions, and people that we feel completely and consistently right, or OK, about are in keeping with our values. Those that we feel definitely not OK about, we may be sure, contradict our values in some sense.

Black views the client's sense of values as central to the helping encounter. The psychiatric nurse should not expect the client to adopt the nurse's values during this encounter. Black further challenges humanistic helpers to investigate their own motivating values as a significant part of increasing personal self-awareness (Black 1983).

Other authors also stress the importance of identifying personal value systems. This process may be enhanced by introspection, by feedback, and by determining the place of individual culture and religion in the nurse's orientation.

It is crucial for psychiatric nurses to be aware of their personal value system, since the therapeutic relationship may be a vehicle for value transmission. In this process, the client may change cultural, religious, and personal values, usually in the direction of the nurse's value system. Such transmission may be helpful or detrimental, and it requires consistent nursing assessment and evaluation (Herron and Rouslin 1982).

Nurses must also address client values and beliefs that interfere with adaptive functioning. The following people hold cultural values and beliefs that may interfere with constructive change:

- The abusive spouse who believes the partner should be subservient and, conversely, the partner who defers personal needs to preserve the relationship

- The abusive parent who believes that to "spare the rod" is to "spoil the child"

- The child, raised with the family injunction that family

problems should not be discussed outside the home, who may view the nurse as invading his or her privacy

Religious beliefs, too, may become delusions or at least interfere with change:

- The client who believes that God takes care of His people, and so there is no need to solve personal problems
- The client who believes that divorce is a sin and therefore will never be forgiven (or forgive self)

Initially, the nurse should become aware of the specific values and beliefs that influence the immediate relationship work. It is often useful to label the value or belief with the client, exploring its history, importance, and impact. Nonjudgmental, alternative values may be discussed if the client initiates such an exploration. Competent and consistent supervision is useful to the nurse regarding the issue of values. The humanistic nurse respects the client's values and beliefs, and the client's ultimate choices regarding his or her personal value systems.

Client Abilities

The psychiatric nurse can increase the chances of success by knowing the client's abilities. Schuable and Pierce (1974) have demonstrated that the following client characteristics are conducive to effective relationship work:

- The nurse-client relationship will be more effective if clients are aware of and show willingness to assume responsibility for their feelings and actions. In contrast, some clients act as if their problems are entirely external and beyond their control.
- Clients must admit their feelings and show awareness that the feelings are tied to specific behaviors. This contrasts with clients who avoid accepting their personal feelings and view them as belonging to others or as situational and outside themselves.
- Clients need to express a clear desire to change and cooperate with the nurse as opposed to resisting involvement.
- Clients must show willingness to learn how to differentiate feelings, concerns, and problems and must recognize their unique reactions and individuality.

Only an ideal client has all these abilities. Such a client is not typically found in the long-term public facilities in which many psychiatric nurses have their clinical experi-

ences. Nurses who work with chronic, resistant, long-term clients may learn that clients can make concrete improvements if both the client and nurse work specifically with one client ability over time. Awareness of client abilities conducive to one-to-one relationships is essential regardless of the setting.

The Therapeutic Alliance

The **therapeutic alliance** is a conscious relationship between a helping person and a client. In this process, the nurse forms a mature alliance with the growth-facilitating aspects of the client. Each implicitly agrees that they need to work together to help the client with personal problems and concerns. More specifically, the nurse identifies and provides feedback regarding the client's patterns of reaction, abilities, and potentials. The client can use these assets to handle unresolved problems constructively. The establishment of the therapeutic alliance enhances informal one-to-one relationships. It is essential in formal one-to-one relationships. Such a binding alliance between nurse and client enables the one-to-one relationship to continue, especially when the client experiences increased anxiety and resistance to change.

PHASES OF THERAPEUTIC RELATIONSHIPS

A one-to-one relationship has three distinct phases:

1. The **orientation** (beginning) **phase**, characterized by the establishment of contact with the client
2. The **working** (middle) **phase**, characterized by maintenance and analysis of contact
3. The **termination** (end) **phase**, characterized by the termination of contact with the client

Each phase of a one-to-one relationship is distinguished by important goals and therapeutic tasks.

The time required for each phase depends on the severity of client dysfunction, the psychiatric nurse's skills, the number and types of problems surfacing during treatment, and the type of therapeutic contract negotiated between psychiatric nurse and client. Although these phases are presented here in their entirety to develop a comprehensive theoretical framework, nurses rarely experience them in such detail and sequence. Nurses are more likely to experience the development of several short-term goals and to experiment with several subsequent interventions in any phase of relationship work. Nevertheless, an exploration of each phase will increase the nurse's familiarity with the flow—that is, "what comes next"—and may also provide a framework in which the psychiatric nurse can see client and nurse behaviors as partial expressions of a specific phase. Finally, an understanding of each phase of a one-to-one relationship may help the nurse select interventions appropriate to that phase. Nursing interventions appropriate in the beginning phase may be very different from those appropriate in the working phase.

In addition to needing familiarity with significant phases of one-to-one relationships, the psychiatric nurse needs to develop awareness of and effectiveness in using numerous processes that occur in any one-to-one relationship work. The beginning nurse often attends carefully to the *content* of the client sessions—i.e., what the client says—and only after considerable experience becomes actively attuned to *processes. Process* here does not mean nursing process but rather a complex communication skill that allows the nurse to focus on several aspects of the nurse-client relationship at the same time. Process involves attention to all nonverbal and verbal client behaviors. It involves responding to client "themes," e.g., anger, hopelessness, and powerlessness. The experienced nurse is simultaneously aware of both content and process, interweaving both for maximum therapeutic effectiveness. Process is discussed further in Chapters 11 and 29.

Orientation (Beginning) Phase: Establishing Contact

The primary goal of the beginning phase is to establish contact, or a working relationship with the client. The phase of establishing contact includes the initial encounters between psychiatric nurse and client—how they approach and interact with each other, both verbally and nonverbally. The nurse and the client meet to discuss how they will work together toward a common goal. The nurse is aware of having impact on the client and acknowledges the client's personal impact as a unique individual.

In informal relationships, contact usually begins when the psychiatric nurse seeks out the client in an in-patient psychiatric setting. Establishment of contact may involve developing client awareness of the nurse's presence, followed by working to communicate with the client on a verbal level.

In formal relationships, contact may begin when the client inquires about services or when the psychiatric nurse contacts the client following referral. Settings may include an in-patient unit, an outpatient clinic, or community settings, including home visits and private practice facilities. In formal relationships, the sense of working together in a therapeutic alliance enables the client to endure anxiety and deal with resistance to change, which inevitably surface during the course of one-to-one relationships. This phase of the therapeutic relationship concludes with mutual agreement on a therapeutic contract, which may be verbal and quite simple. The contract spells out the client's goals for treatment and the nurse's professional responsibilities.

Issues of trust and confidentiality arise during the orientation phase, both for the client and the nurse. Another concern for the nurse is how best to develop a verbal contract with the client. Initial verbal therapeutic contracts are discussed below. More formal (sometimes written) therapeutic contracts are explored in the section on the working phase of one-to-one relationships.

Issues During the Orientation Phase

Trust

Concerns about trust surface in this first phase of the relationship. Trust between psychiatric nurse and client evolves over time as the client tests the emotional climate of sessions, risks self-disclosure, and observes nurse follow-through on responsibilities delineated in the therapeutic contract. The nurse can promote trust by responding to all the client's feeling states without being judgmental or attempting to control emotive expression. The following interventions enhance initial trust:

- Listen attentively to client feelings
- Respond to client feelings
- Exhibit consistency, especially regarding appointment times
- View situations from the client's world view

Self-awareness of personal feeling states on the part of the nurse also enhances trust. It allows the client to disclose uncomfortable, even forbidden, feelings in safety. A common failing among those learning relationship skills is focusing on technique. This produces mechanical, unfeeling responses. It is also important to avoid giving premature reassurances about trust, which may inhibit exploration of this vital therapeutic issue and create distance between therapist and client. The verbatim example in Table 27–3 illustrates the emergence of trust as an initial therapeutic issue.

Confidentiality

Client concerns about the level of **confidentiality** also surface in this first phase of the therapeutic relationship. Like the issue of trust, the issue of confidentiality must be explicitly addressed when the client makes even vague reference to it. The psychiatric nurse should state explicitly which persons will have access to client revelations (clinical instructor, case supervisor, consultant, colleague) and explore how the client feels in response to this information.

Table 27–3 Verbatim Example, Orientation Phase		
Verbatim Interaction	**Nursing Intervention**	**Rationale**
Client: It's so difficult for me to talk . . . to let you know about me.		
(Thirty-second pause.)	None	To allow client space to proceed at own pace; if silence is uncomfortably long to client in first few contacts, nurse may use reflection, e.g.: "I sense how difficult talking is for you."
Client: Every time I start to tell anybody about myself, they usually end up laughing at me.		
Nurse: Can you give an example of this?	Encourage elaboration	To explore meaning of this statement to client
Client: Well, just last week I started talking to my neighbor. I told him that I was laid off from work again. Next thing you know, he's laughing, slapping my back, and saying "Hey, hard times, eh?"		
(Shifts in chair, poor eye contact.)		
Nurse: What was this like for you?	Explore client's personal reaction, especially accompanying feelings	To further explore meaning of this specific incident as perceived by the client
Client: Awful . . . lousy . . . that's all.		
(Pause.)		
Nurse: I wonder if you're concerned that the same might happen here—that you'll be laughed at?	To apply concern regarding "external" issue to here-and-now, i.e., one-to-one relationship	Issues concerning client's immediate life situations often reflect parallel issues in nurse-client relationship
Client: Well, maybe. . . . I don't know you, so how do I know what you might do? You don't look like the type, but then again—how do I know?		
Nurse: It sounds like you're wondering if it's safe to trust me.	Move to what appears to be the *metamessage* or underlying central concern (theme)	Reflection of what appears to be the central concern (theme) encourages client assessment by validation or correction
Client: Yeah . . . no offense, though.		
Nurse: Let's talk about how safe you feel today and as we continue to work together.	Underline trust as an issue for further exploration; stress evolving working relationship	Avoid premature reassurances so that trust can evolve and be assessed periodically

Initial Therapeutic Contract

A simple verbal therapeutic contract between client and nurse is helpful at the beginning of the orientation phase. It may simply involve the client's definition of goals to work on (however simple), some determination of time and place for meeting together, and a delineation of the nurse's responsibilities.

In informal relationships, the nurse may begin by saying: "I'd like to talk with you to get to know you better" or "I'd like to talk with you to see if there is anything we can discuss together." An initial verbal contract helps to build trust, convey empathy, and develop rapport. This contract is crucial in an in-patient setting, where clients may be suspicious or withdrawn.

Even a simple therapeutic contract may take several meetings to formulate. For example, an elderly in-patient with organic mental disorder agrees to meet with a nursing student every Wednesday when she visits his unit. He wants to learn ways to deal with isolation after his discharge. The nursing student agrees to telephone the client if she is unable to meet with him on any specific Wednesday.

Carefully and thoroughly attending to a mutual agreement on an initial verbal contract precedes, and has priority over, data collection. Comprehensive client assessment is not possible unless the client at least agrees to talk with the nurse regularly for a definite purpose. Even in formal relationships, the agreement to meet the first time can be viewed as an initial contract. Provisions for the contract can be flexible and dynamic. These provisions may be renegotiated according to changing needs or circumstances. The contract is redefined, i.e., more formal goals and responsibilities are established, as the orientation phase progresses. Other concerns (critical distance, self-disclosure, gifts, use of touch, and values) that may surface during the course of treatment were dealt with in previous discussion.

Assessment

Client assessment begins at the first moment of contact. Assessment continues throughout the therapeutic relationship but is particularly important during the orientation phase. The client is the primary source of data. It is very important to repeat or "replay" important data for the client. This replay gives the client ample time to identify, articulate, and adjust data so that the nurse gets the closest approximation to the "real picture" of the client's world. Also, it is essential to note any factors that may influence data collection, such as cultural or language differences.

The degree of collaboration depends upon client ability. Ideally, the client is able and willing to participate fully with the psychiatric nurse in all aspects of data collection. Realistically, depending upon the functioning ability of the client at initial assessment, part of the assessment data may come from significant others who have known the client for some time. For example, a very suspicious client may not tolerate a comprehensive assessment during the initial interview. Family may be asked to help the nurse develop a "beginning picture" of the client's overall level of functioning. After the client stabilizes, the psychiatric nurse may choose to validate important data with the client. In long-term in-patient settings, data collection may be incomplete due to client dysfunction and lack of other data sources.

Observation

Observation, a process long regarded as essential to clinical nursing practice, is of particular importance in one-to-one relationship work. Peplau (1952, p 263) emphasizes the interpersonal function of observation:

> The aim in observation in nursing, when it is viewed as an interpersonal process, is the identification, clarification, and verification of impressions about the interactive drama, of the pushes and pulls in the relationship between nurse and patient, as they occur.

Peplau maps out the following steps in the process of observation:

- Observation generally begins on a subjective, sensory level.
- The observer conceives of a generalization or "hunch" about what is occurring in a particular situation. This observation is accurate when the psychiatric nurse attends only to what is observable in the situation.
- The observer collects data to analyze whether or not personal observations are accurate in this particular setting.
- The observer elaborates on the first whole impression. The psychiatric nurse must note many minute details to gain an overview of what is occurring.
- The observer, as participant in the observing process, refines the intuitive abilities that can then be applied to other situations.

Observation is an intensive process requiring concentration and practice to gather data through the use of all the senses. It includes attention to verbal, nonverbal, and environmental cues. The observer strives to develop simultaneous sensitivity to vision, hearing, smell, taste, and touch in nurse-client interactions. The observer also needs to check out personal distortions, biases, or unreality. In addition to observing what elements are present, the nurse notes elements in the nurse-client interaction that are missing, distorted, or imbalanced. What the client avoids discussing is often more crucial than what is shared. Observation is discussed in more detail in Chapter 12 of this text.

Examination

Data collection by examination ideally includes the following: mental status examination, complete physical examination, nursing history, and psychologic testing, as needed. Which examinations are done and by whom are generally determined by the particular agency or institution utilizing the psychiatric nurse, and by the psychiatric nurse's expertise in these specific areas. Robitaille-Tremblay (1984) offers a data collection tool for nurses seeking to take nursing histories. She incorporates the following helpful suggestions:

- Respect the client's pace. When questions appear threatening, do not insist. Return to them later.
- Rearrange the order of questions if the client appears defensive or distrustful.
- Take into consideration all of the information given by the client.
- Avoid an inquisitive attitude so that the client does not feel interrogated.
- Adapt questions to the client's abilities, using examples as necessary.

Interview

Interviewing is a process that generally occurs in the beginning (orientation) phase of one-to-one relationships. Although a psychiatric nurse may use the structured initial interview in formal one-to-one work, it is rarely used in informal relationships. Nevertheless, it is important for beginning nurses to familiarize themselves with the kinds of background data collection useful in mental health work. They can incorporate various elements of the initial interview as appropriate for specific clients over an extended time span. The initial interview has the following purposes:

- To initiate trust building
- To establish rapport with the client
- To obtain pertinent client data
- To initiate client assessment
- To make practical arrangements for treatment

The initial interview is crucial because it sets the stage for subsequent therapeutic contact.

Amount of Structuring The psychiatric nurse must structure the initial interview to establish rapport, decrease anxiety, and convey willingness to address the client's suffering. The psychiatric nurse may begin the interview by introducing herself or himself, inviting the client to be seated, and making a statement about information thus far known about the client's seeking of services. An open-ended question, such as "How is it that you are here today?" provides an opportunity for the client to talk about concerns. The psychiatric nurse may inform the client that the purpose of the initial interview is to get an overview of the client's current situation and then determine the availability of appropriate services.

Essential Data One primary purpose of structuring the initial interview is to collect essential data. The presenting problem or chief complaint is a concise statement of the most distressing current problem, recorded in the client's own words. After gathering the client's personal, descriptive account, the nurse begins to obtain specific information about the presenting problem in a directive manner: its history, development, manifestation, effect on present physical functioning (appetite, sleep, sexual expression), and effect on present social functioning (family, employment, friends). It is important to pinpoint the event that caused the client to seek services. The client should also describe any other current problems. Additional areas of brief exploration at the initial interview include: family constellation, physical health status, psychosocial development, history of previous emotional difficulties, history of therapy, drug and alcohol use/abuse, coping skills and methods of resolving conflict, and present level of motivation. One final relevant area of data collection involves the client's identifying characteristics: name, age, sex, address, telephone number, marital status, education, occupation, employment record, and cultural and ethnic origins. The Initial Contact Sheet used by the Erie County Department of Mental Health at Buffalo, New York, shows the data collected in the initial interview process (see Figure 12–1).

In in-patient settings, it is unusual for students to collect all data from the hospitalized client. Students may rely on chart data more than independent practitioners do.

The psychiatric nurse needs to address client resistance if it surfaces during the initial interview. This resistance may occur when the client has initiated services at someone else's request or insistence, has fears and misconceptions about therapy, or has had an unsatisfactory therapeutic experience in the past. Nursing intervention calls for explicit exploration of the specific resistance before further data collection. Refer to the earlier discussion regarding general intervention strategies for resistance. If the client is confused about or misinterprets information given during the initial interview, he or she may have a moderate to high anxiety level. Most clients experience such anxiety at the beginning of therapy. Manifestations of anxiety must be differentiated from manifestations of resistance. The nurse may need to repeat information several times or in subsequent meetings.

Areas to Avoid Wolberg (1977, pp 455–457) offers the following list of practices for the psychiatric nurse to avoid during the initial interview. These apply to informal, as well as more formal, one-to-one relationships.

- Do not argue with, minimize, or challenge the client.
- Do not praise the client or give false reassurance.

- Do not make false promises.
- Do not interpret to the client or speculate on the dynamics of the client's problem.
- Do not offer the client a diagnosis even if he or she insists on it.
- Do not question the client on sensitive areas.
- Do not try to "sell" the client on accepting treatment.
- Do not join in attacks the client launches on parents, mate, friends, or associates.
- Do not participate in criticism of another therapist.

Remember that shortcuts taken in assessment procedures almost always jeopardize the ultimate quality of care. Crucial areas of concern may go unaddressed or be treated superficially.

Nursing Diagnosis

Following a comprehensive assessment of the client in one-to-one relationships, the psychiatric nurse gathers and organizes all the data collected during the assessment phase in order to formulate preliminary nursing diagnoses. The word *preliminary* is used to imply the ongoing potential for revision as client behaviors unfold during the course of the relationship.

The goal in organizing the data is to attempt to understand the data as they reflect the client's unique, private world. Data are scientifically and systematically grouped into categories that reflect the client's potential problems, actual problems, strengths, and abilities. The nurse attempts to look for dominant themes or central issues in the client's response to his or her environment.

When the assessment in the beginning phase is comprehensive, organized, and analyzed, then the nursing diagnoses seem to "flow" from the data. Nursing diagnoses should be prioritized, with the most pressing and detrimental pattern listed first, followed by others of decreasing significance. It is then easier for the nurse to identify goals and determine appropriate intervention strategies.

Planning and Implementing Interventions

Making a Therapeutic Contract

Client assessment and nursing diagnosis are the basis on which the psychiatric nurse formulates a plan of action. This plan is a **therapeutic contract** negotiated in a one-to-one relationship. The therapeutic contract evolves to become the client's definition of personal goals for treatment plus the nurse's professional responsibilities. The goal of the beginning phase of one-to-one work is to establish contact and begin a working relationship with the client. The therapeutic contract is a concrete, detailed, and mutually nego-

tiated expression of this working relationship. The therapeutic contract may be modified over time but always serves as a tool for evaluating the benefit to the client and the effectiveness of the nurse.

Planning is achieved by arriving at client-centered therapeutic goals, which represent the client's personal goals for treatment. These may be long-term or short-term goals, but they always specify detailed, observable outcomes. The nurse strives for the most concise, detailed, and accurate description of client goals in the beginning phase. Clearly stated goals facilitate subsequent mutual evaluation during the middle and end phases of one-to-one work. Goals may focus on:

- Decreasing or eliminating troublesome behaviors
- Increasing socialization
- Increasing living skills

A frequently overlooked area of goal formation is preventive health education. For example, the psychiatric nurse may provide a client with information or literature regarding health precautions against AIDS when the client has indicated concern or fear.

In an informal therapeutic relationship, the therapeutic contract differs from the usual care plan often developed in in-patient settings. In in-patient settings, the client participates in the formation of a therapeutic contract by determining his or her personal goals. At times, client goals may be long term or even inappropriate. In this situation, the psychiatric nurse may help the client define initial steps toward the long-term goal. For example, a readmitted chronic client may pinpoint discharge as an important goal. The nurse may then work with this client to determine the steps needed to achieve this goal. One step may be to maintain self-care in the area of bathing/hygiene. When severe dysfunction limits client input into planning, the nursing staff may supplement goals that are determined to be beneficial to the client.

In a formal therapeutic relationship, as in individual psychotherapy, the therapeutic contract is more detailed and generally includes three practical matters:

1. Determination of the place, duration, and time of therapy
2. Establishment of fees and payment intervals, if any
3. Consideration of optional referral sources, should the client be unable to negotiate an agreement on the first two matters

The most essential aspect of the therapeutic contract is the client's definition of goals for treatment. Client goals most often contribute to the establishment of a working relationship when they are specific, address intrapersonal or interpersonal behavior patterns, and delineate the degree of change necessary for client self-satisfaction.

In formal therapeutic relationships, the therapeutic contract may not reflect client problems and strengths in their entirety. At that moment, the client may not determine that an area is, in fact, a problem for him or her. Thus, the therapeutic contract in formal relationship work reflects the *client's* definition of personal goals at one moment in time. The psychiatric nurse, in this instance, remains aware of other probable problem areas and assesses these areas with the client in an on-going manner, as appropriate.

Some nurses advocate the use of immediate, intermediate, and ultimate objectives in delineation of therapeutic goals. The nurse and client mutually determine the ultimate therapeutic goal and then work backward, determining the intermediate and finally the immediate goals (Ward 1984).

Regardless of the form that goal delineation takes, the therapeutic contract serves the following functions:

- Facilitates humanistic involvement with the client as an individual
- Involves the client as a full partner in the therapeutic process
- Serves as a basis for communication in the therapeutic process
- Provides continuity for the client and everyone involved with the client

The initial goals of the therapeutic contract may be modified or deleted in subsequent phases of the one-to-one relationship as appropriate or necessary.

The therapeutic contract should also reflect the nurse's professional responsibilities, i.e., independent, interdependent, or dependent nursing functions. Psychiatric nursing students are most likely to be limited by institution policies to concrete independent functions, such as problem solving, skill training, and teaching. Although students may attend team meetings and collaborate with staff in designing plans, they are not likely to take over nursing functions, such as conducting an intake interview by themselves.

At the independent level, the nurse and client work together in assessment, diagnosis, planning of care, and its full implementation. At the interdependent level, the nurse is part of a health team. At the dependent level, the nurse carries out direct orders of a physician or follows a treatment protocol, e.g., giving emergency treatment for a drug overdose, as defined in a specific setting.

Nurses need to develop a working knowledge of therapeutic contracts and to learn appreciation for their versatility. A contract can be designed to meet specific client needs. Figure 27–2 shows a sample mental health contract suggested by Ralph Nader's health research group. This contract addresses three important areas: specific practical arrangements for meetings, intrapersonal and interpersonal behavioral patterns, and degree of confidentiality.

Addressing the Client's Suffering

Interventions during the orientation phase are valid and important, even if the nurse does not reach the working phase of a one-to-one relationship with a particular client (e.g., because of time limitations or because the client is unable to agree upon goals). The psychiatric nurse intervenes by directly addressing the client's suffering. This intervention allows the client to share how he or she perceives, experiences, and manifests the problem. The following verbatim example illustrates how the nurse encourages a client to "move outside himself" and begin to assess the interpersonal impact as one aspect of his suffering. Assessment has already occurred regarding the severity of the client's depression on the "inside," i.e., how it feels to the client in relation to sleep, appetite, and activity level.

Client: This depression is like a big log weighing on my chest.

Nurse: How might I, or someone else, know that you are suffering in this way?

Client: Well . . . I sigh a lot . . . I don't move a lot, only when I have to . . . I wouldn't look at you, or bother to talk to you. I guess when I feel like this, I close people out. Yeah, I close everyone out, even my wife.

Nurse: So when you suffer in this way, you "close people out." And what is this like for you?

Client: I'm alone and lonely. Not a soul on earth cares for me.

Clarifying Purpose, Roles, and Responsibilities

An additional therapeutic task is for the nurse to directly intervene to clarify the purpose of the relationship work, the role of the nurse, and the responsibilities of the client. When this preliminary exploration of purpose, roles, and responsibilities is explicit and detailed, each participant better understands how to move within the one-to-one relationship. Such a task also decreases anxiety and the chance that a client may use the relationship to obtain special privileges. From the first meeting the nurse also intervenes to reinforce effective coping skills and increase client self-esteem. Table 27–4 summarizes the important goal, therapeutic tasks, and subsequent nursing interventions in the orientation phase of one-to-one relationships.

SAMPLE CONTRACT

① I, *Mr. Client,* agree to join with *Ms Nurse* each Thursday after-
② noon from May 1, 1988, until June 5, 1988, at 3 p.m. until 3:50
③ p.m. During these six 50-minute sessions we will direct our
mutual efforts towards three goals:

④ 1. Enabling me to fly in airplanes without fear
   2. Explaining to my satisfaction why I always lose my temper
      when I visit my parents
   3. Discussing whether it would be better for me to give up
      my full-time job and start working part-time

⑤ I agree to pay $45 per session for the use of her resources,
⑥ training, and experience as a psychiatric nurse. This amount
is payable within 30 days of the session.

⑦ If I am not satisfied with the progress made on the goals
here set forth, I may cancel any and all subsequent appointments for these sessions, provided that I give Ms Nurse 3
days warning of my intention to cancel. In that event I am not
required to pay for sessions not met. However, in the event
that I miss a session without forewarning, I am financially
responsible for that missed session. The one exception to this
arrangement being unforeseen and unavoidable accident or
illness.

⑧ At the end of the six sessions Ms Nurse and I agree to
renegotiate this contract. We include the possibility that the

⑨ stated goals will have changed during the six-week period. I
⑩ understand that this agreement does not guarantee that I will
have attained those goals; however, it does constitute an offer
on my part to pay Ms Nurse for access to her resources as a
nurse and her acceptance to apply all those resources as a
nurse in good faith.

⑪ I further stipulate that this agreement become a part of the
medical record, which is accessible to both parties at will, but
to no other person without my written consent. The nurse will
respect my right to maintain the confidentiality of any information communicated by me to the nurse during the course
of therapy. In particular, the nurse will not publish, communicate, or otherwise disclose, without my written consent, any
such information that, if disclosed, would injure me in any way.

_____

Date

_____

Name

_____

Name of Professional

Figure 27–2

Elements of a contract. A contract cannot by itself guarantee results. It does represent an attempt to define the nature of services to be provided by the psychiatric nurse and fosters accountability on the parts of both the therapist and the client while providing ongoing documentation of those services. To give the consumer an idea of what a contract might look like, a sample is shown here. This form should not be considered definitive or restrictive—indeed, the flexibility of the contract is one of its most valuable characteristics. It is intended only as a fictitious example.

1. Name of each party
2. Date of beginning and end of agreement
3. Length of each session
4. Goals of sessions stated as specifically as possible
5. Cost per session and when payable
6. Definition of services provided by psychiatric nurse stated as clearly as possible
7. Provisions for cancellation:
   a. No penalty for termination
   b. Amount of time necessary for warning nurse of cancellation
   c. Protection for nurse against willful no-show on part of client
   d. Provision for unavoidable and unforeseen events causing client to be unable to meet session
8. Renegotiation at end of stipulated period
9. Allowance for changing goals within stipulated period
10. Definition of nature of services; no guaranteed results; guarantee of intention and good faith
11. Establishment of access by client and nurse to document that becomes part of medical record; guarantee of confidentiality and control by client over medical record and its contents and use of any information therein.

Source: Adapted and excerpted from Adams S, Orgel M: Through the Mental Health Maze, Health Research Group, 2000 P Street, N.W., Washington, D.C. 20036. © Copyright 1975 by Public Citizen's Health Research Group. Reprinted here by permission. Copies of the entire book are available from the Health Research Group for $4.00.

Table 27–4 Summary of Orientation (Beginning) Phase		
Goal	**Therapeutic Tasks**	**Nursing Interventions**
Establishment of contact in the form of a working relationship with the client	Clarification of purpose of relationship work, role of nurse, and responsibilities of client	Educative. Provide information regarding purpose, roles, and responsibilities in relationship work to alleviate initial client anxiety
		Immediately and explicitly address any misconceptions, fantasies, and fears regarding relationship work and/or nurse
	Addressing client suffering directly, and offering to work with the client toward its alleviation	Use facilitative characteristics, especially empathic understanding
		Avoid premature reassurance (allow trust to evolve)
		Be explicit about who has access to client's revelations (degree of confidentiality)
	Negotiation of therapeutic contract (client's definition of personal goals for treatment and nurse's professional responsibilities)	Whenever possible, encourage delineation of goals that: • Are specific • Address intrapersonal and interpersonal behavioral patterns • Designate degree of change necessary for client self-satisfaction
		In informal relationship work, contract generally includes determination of time and place for working together to the extent that client function permits
		In formal relationship work, the contract generally includes: • Place, duration, and time of therapy • Fees and payment intervals, if any • Optional referral sources

Evaluation

In the orientation phase, evaluation includes the nurse's initial comprehensive evaluation of client behaviors, any initial steps toward the development of client self-evaluation, and the psychiatric nurse's ongoing self-evaluation. The more specific and goal-oriented the therapeutic contract, the easier it is for the client and nurse to evaluate the effectiveness of the therapeutic relationship.

In addition to evaluating the effectiveness of each therapeutic task, the psychiatric nurse needs to evaluate the important goal of the orientation phase: Has a working relationship evolved between the client and nurse, and, if so, to what degree? The **working relationship** in this initial phase is the framework upon which the client constructs behavioral change in the next phase. Table 27–5 highlights common signs of a working relationship. These signs are predicated on trust and a sense that the nurse can be helpful.

Evaluation of specific goals and outcome criteria generally occurs in the working and resolution phases of one-to-one relationships. Crucial to any evaluation is the need for the nurse to engage in consistent clinical supervision to maximize therapeutic use of self and constructive outcomes. Clinical supervision is addressed later in this chapter.

Table 27–5 Signs of a Working Relationship	
For Nurse	**For Client**
Sense of making contact with the client	Nonverbal and verbal evidences of liking the nurse
Sense that client is responding well to the relationship	Sense of relaxation with nurse
Sense that nurse can facilitate client growth regardless of severity of client dysfunction	Sense of confidence in nurse
Sense of commitment to address client problems	Nonsuperficial (in nature and depth) problems addressed

Assessment

Assessment is continued, detailed, and expanded upon. The nurse builds on the data obtained during the orientation phase of one-to-one work. The nurse's observations of nonverbal, verbal, and environmental responses continue to have vital importance as the client begins to address personal response patterns. In addition, the nurse continues to assess emotive, cognitive, and behavioral aspects. The nurse seeks to fill gaps of information not obtained in the orientation phase. The nurse may just now acquire a detailed assessment about a subject that the client was unable to share or ignored in the orientation phase. The following clinical example illustrates that what was not said (that is, what was avoided, blocked, rejected) by the client may have more significance than what the client shared.

During initial sessions, 18-year-old Maureen avoided any inquiries about her parents, other than to say that she lived alone. She negotiated to work on fear associated with recent, short-term employment.

After several sessions, the nurse again asked about the parents. Maureen replied softly with tears welling in her eyes. "They're dead. They died in a car crash two years ago." She slowly related how, since their deaths, she has spent so much energy trying to survive that she has barely felt much of anything. Subsequent sessions dealt with her apparent delayed grief reaction.

Working (Middle) Phase: Maintenance and Analysis of Contact

Once contact is established, attention turns to maintenance and analysis of contact in the working or middle phase of one-to-one relationships. *Analysis of contact* refers to an in-depth exploration of how the client relates to others as manifested in the nurse-client relationship. In this working phase, the client may address developmental and situational problems, as well as interpersonal problems. This phase is called the working phase because it is during this phase that the nurse and client actively and systematically identify, explore, link, modify, and evaluate specific behaviors, especially those determined to be dysfunctional for the client.

The client's clearly stated goals in the therapeutic contract are now explored with the nurse. The nurse has the following two therapeutic goals in this working phase:

- *Behavioral analysis.* The nurse and client determine the dynamics of the client's response patterns, especially those considered to be dysfunctional. Such analysis also addresses dysfunctional thought and emotive patterns, as these inevitably alter the client's behavior. This analysis flows from the therapeutic contract, in which the client identified specific goals for the one-to-one relationship.

- *Constructive change in behavior,* especially in dysfunctional response patterns.

Thus, the psychiatric nurse and client work together to analyze behavior and institute behavioral change in this most essential phase of the one-to-one relationship.

The new data caused the nurse to revise and update the tentative nursing diagnoses and make a marked change in the direction of the sessions. Such shifting is not uncommon in one-to-one relationships. When a change in direction occurs, the nurse assesses if the sudden change indicates the need to avoid a certain topic, or indicates a move toward a deeper level of emotive expression.

In the working phase, the nurse facilitates many aspects of assessment with the client. First, the psychiatric nurse collaborates with the client in identifying important behavioral trends and patterns. Once a pattern is identified, it is explored in elaborate detail to determine its origin, causes, operation, and effects on the client and those who populate his or her world. Environmental factors (familial, political, economic, or cultural) are separated from intrapersonal factors (e.g., depression or anxiety) contributing to the pattern. The client figuratively holds the pattern to the light to examine and make sense of its every aspect. The elements of one pattern will inevitably link with others, so

Table 27–6
Verbatim Example, Working Phase

Verbatim Interaction	Nursing Intervention	Rationale
Client: My nosy relatives are at it again. Since my mother died and I'm living alone, they keep phoning me to see if I'm all right.		
Nurse: You sound irritated. . . .	Reflection of feeling tone to explore client's reaction to this situation	Reflection of feeling tone encourages client to validate or clarify emotive response to situation
Client: Not irritated—mad! Those phonies don't care about me. Why should they? Why should they?!? They don't.		
Nurse: What do you think motivates them to call?	Seeking clarification about how client perceives the immediate situation	Clarifying statements help explore the meaning of this specific situation as perceived by the client
Client: To pester me. People do it all the time. That one woman at work that I told you about last week—she does the same thing. She smiles and says good morning. She's concerned . . . but I don't want anything to do with her either.		
Nurse: You're talking about two situations where you don't want to deal with people: your relatives and the woman at work. I remember your description of how you wanted to avoid an old classmate last month. Is there something common to all these situations?	Actively linking elements of several behavioral patterns accumulated over time (current session, last session, last month) to search for commonality	Elements of one pattern may link to others with a gradual unfolding of central life patterns
Client: I can't see anything—except that I go out of my way to avoid people. I avoid everyone. I live alone and want to stay alone.		

that the major life patterns gradually unfold. The verbatim example in Table 27–6 from the middle (working) phase demonstrates how elements of one behavioral pattern are linked to others and gradually reveal central life patterns. In this case the client's initial anger in reaction to concerned relatives led to awareness of the need to avoid contact in several additional situations. The nurse may now help the client explore what appears to be a central life pattern of interpersonal isolation devoid of intimacy. The first part of Table 27–7 summarizes the therapeutic tasks undertaken to achieve this objective and offers specific nursing approaches to helping the client.

There are two noteworthy considerations regarding therapeutic tasks of the first objective:

1. As clients begin to describe and reexperience conflict, they will consciously or unconsciously use defenses to ward off the anxiety this awakens. The development of a good working relationship enables clients to tolerate increased anxiety in the working phase of the one-to-one relationship.

2. As clients become familiar with self-assessment, they may modify original personal goals, or develop additional goals, in keeping with what they have learned.

<table>
<tr><td colspan="3">Table 26–7
Summary of Working (Middle) Phase</td></tr>
</table>

Goals	Therapeutic Tasks	Nursing Interventions
Behavioral analysis (mutual determination of dynamics of response patterns identified by client, especially those considered dysfunctional)	Identification and detailed exploration of important response patterns	Explore response pattern in depth, including origin, causes, operation, and effect of pattern (intrapersonally and interpersonally)
		Separate environmental factors (familial, political, economic, cultural) from intrapersonal factors
		Link elements of one response pattern to other patterns as appropriate, for a gradual unfolding of central life patterns
	Analysis of client's mode of conflict resolution	Encourage detailed exploration of how client reacts to reduce anxiety associated with conflict
		Increase awareness of defenses employed to ward off anxiety awakened by such exploration
	Facilitation of client self-assessment of growth-producing and growth-inhibiting response patterns	Encourage client to evaluate each response pattern to determine which are self-defeating and/or thwart gratification of basic needs
Constructive change in behavior, especially in dysfunctional response patterns identified by client	Address forces that inhibit desired change (troublesome thoughts, feelings, and behaviors)	Assist client in challenging client's personal resistance to change
		Use problem-solving strategies, active decision making, and personal accountability
		Assist client to learn and apply problem-solving strategies
		Encourage client to assert own needs when external environmental conditions (group, agency, institution) are an inhibiting force
	Create an atmosphere offering permission for active experimentation to test and assess effectiveness of new behaviors	Allow freedom to make and assess mistakes and blunders
		Avoid parental judgment of any behavioral experimentation—encourage client self-assessment instead
	Facilitate development of coping skills to deal with anxiety associated with constructive changes in behavior	Address, rather than avoid, anxiety and its manifestations
		Strengthen existing growth-promoting coping skills, especially regarding unalterable conditions (e.g., terminal illness, physical deformity, loss of significant other by death)
		Encourage development of new coping skills and their application to actual life experiences

It is important in the working phase for the psychiatric nurse to encourage client self-assessment of growth-facilitating and growth-inhibiting behaviors. Often as the client assesses one specific response, he or she is able to transfer this skill to begin assessing other aspects of life as well. A realistic self-assessment process is perhaps the most valuable skill that the client can "take home." It is often thrilling for the nurse to experience the client "taking over"

and further applying realistic assessment skills developed in one-to-one work. As the above discussion indicates, assessment is an ongoing process for both the client and the nurse in the working phase of one-to-one relationships.

The initial goal of behavioral analysis of client's response patterns continues throughout the working phase. The goal is achieved when the client has awareness of, understanding of, and insight into the causes and manifestations of patterns in his or her current personality structure and can assess these major trends.

Nursing Diagnosis

In the working phase, nursing diagnoses may be revised, expanded upon, or deleted to more accurately reflect a central pattern of concern in the evolving one-to-one relationship. In the previous clinical example, the nurse made a tentative diagnosis of fear related to employment. An additional nursing diagnosis of dysfunctional grieving was added later. This second diagnosis was given higher priority because, as the client indicates, it is related to difficulty in overall functioning ability.

As the working phase proceeds, the priority assigned to a nursing diagnosis may change, e.g., when the client is able to implement positive change in some areas. Those nursing diagnoses designated as "potential problems" may move up or down on the priority list, depending on what interventions, if any, have been effective. A "potential" diagnosis may decrease in priority after preventive health education, if both the client and the nurse evaluate this intervention as beneficial.

Planning and Implementing Interventions

In the working phase of one-to-one relationships, planning is ideally done collaboratively between client and nurse. Such planning involves frequent consideration of the client's initial goals. When planning has been systematic and thorough, there is hardly a moment to worry about "what to do." The short-term and long-term treatment goals in the form of the therapeutic contract are a map indicating the direction, momentum, and steps needed to reach a designated point.

There is, however, a potential danger in the implementation of the planning component: moving too quickly and incompletely through an exploration of the client's feelings and thoughts in an attempt to fulfill a designated goal. *Slowness* and *thoroughness* are all-important here. Change needs to take place in the client's feelings, thoughts, and behaviors. If change does not occur in all aspects, then it is destined to be short-lived and ineffectual in the long run and may contribute to client discouragement.

When the client is working on an issue that is unresolved at the end of a meeting, it is often helpful to summarize the unfinished work for the next meeting. This technique may help the client anticipate, plan, or prepare to tackle this area of concern again. "Homework assignments," e.g., listing the pros and cons of potential solu-

tions, may be given between sessions. Some clients may be able to continue working through a problem on their own between meetings.

As short-term and long-term goals are achieved, they are noted in the therapeutic contract. Thus, the therapeutic contract represents an accurate, current statement of the client's perceived treatment goals. Concise, detailed planning in the first two phases of a therapeutic relationship contributes to smooth, efficient evaluative procedures in the resolution phase of that relationship.

Active intervention is especially important to achieve the second goal of the working phase. This goal is the initiation of constructive changes in behavior, particularly in self-defeating, growth-inhibiting behavior patterns. Establishing behavioral change flows from the first goal of behavioral analysis. The objectives are interrelated and essential for successful therapeutic work. Understanding and insight need to be complemented by behavioral implementation. This statement deserves much attention, since particular clients may consistently generate and thrive on sophisticated insights while continuing to assume a powerless stance about implementing constructive change in their condition. Table 27–7 also highlights therapeutic tasks and specific nursing interventions for the second goal.

The psychiatric nurse also uses active experimentation to test the effect of new behaviors. The introverted male client who resolved to establish relationships with women may assume various postures (cavalier, paternal, seductive) with a female psychiatric nurse to determine the appropriateness of these behaviors before displaying them outside of sessions. Permission to "try on" or role play new ways of being must also include freedom to make mistakes. Errors and blunders are rich sources of additional learning and occasional fun. A client who is able to see humor in errors in a nondefeatist manner has acquired a new skill. The client can be encouraged to apply this skill, and any other coping skills learned in relationship work, to normal maturational and situational crises encountered throughout life.

In in-patient settings, the nurse must work with other members of the staff to make all members of the team aware of the meaning of the client's behavior as positive actions that may be exaggerated at first. For example, a depressed client may be encouraged by some staff members to verbalize anger and begin by shouting. If there is no staff collaboration, the client may receive negative feedback (e.g., room restrictions) for testing out new coping skills.

Problem-Solving Strategies

Problem-solving strategies, as a mode of intervention, are particularly important in the working phase. Problem-solving strategies are essential after the client has identified, explored, and assessed important behavioral patterns. The psychiatric nurse can help the client use the sequential problem-solving strategies discussed below.

Observation Observation as a problem-solving strategy involves gathering and analyzing facts about a potential problem area. It eliminates opinions and impressions and emphasizes facts. Observation, as an aspect of assessment, is discussed earlier in this chapter.

Definition Definition is perhaps the most significant and far-reaching problem-solving strategy. It involves an initial specification of a problem, followed by a question. Starting a problem-solving exploration with the word "How" (for example, How is it? How does it manifest itself? How has this come about?) focuses on the process regarding a specific problem. It is generally more useful than asking "Why," which emphasizes rationale. ("Why" questions are explored in Chapter 11.) For example, an adolescent girl finds herself repeatedly tense in the presence of her middle-aged male employer despite his kind manner. The question "How is it?" is asked to determine if the problem has been defined in its most basic form. The answer may be that the client senses tension because her employer is a middle-aged male, and she usually experiences anxiety with this age group. As the same inquiry is repeated, this second definition may appear as a subproblem in a more basic definition of the problem. Thus, the client may redefine her problem: "In what ways can I deal with the anxiety associated with paternal figures?" Note that the statement of the problem begins with "in what ways," rather than "how," to allow for numerous approaches.

Next, it is helpful to determine whether the problem involves fact finding (calling for data answers), judgment or decision, or creative exploration. In dealing with problems requiring creative exploration, all the ideas that imagination can produce may be helpful. Thus, evaluation is temporarily deferred or suspended to allow for the consideration of numerous alternatives.

The following clinical material illustrates definition of the most basic form of a problem:

Fern is a 19-year-old, single female seeking individual counseling at a local university counseling center. She was referred because she felt depressed following a split with her boyfriend over the summer. Emotional concerns included a marked feeling of depression, plus verbalized feelings of guilt, loneliness, and confusion. Physical concerns involved sleep disturbance (difficulty falling asleep with resultant sense of fatigue), eating disturbance (increased compulsive eating when under stress, with subsequent sudden weight gain), and minor self-mutilation (picking skin around fingernails and scratching face). Fern denied suicidal ideation and appeared to be a minimal suicide risk. She showed a general flatness of affect, characterized by very slow and monotonous speech, minimal facial or

body gestures, and periodic silences and quiet weeping. She lives in an apartment with three female roommates and maintains a 3.8 academic average as a junior student majoring in biology. She negotiated for weekly one-hour sessions of individual psychotherapy for the duration of the school year. The following exchanges occurred in the final ten minutes of the third session:

Fern: This weekend will be a long weekend. I don't know what to do.

Nurse: I'd like to hear more about this long weekend.

Fern: Well, Marc might want to go out with someone else, so I don't want to take up his time. My three roommates are busy. . . . I don't want to call Marty. . . . My friend Judy won't be home. . . .

Nurse: Which of these is most troublesome for you?

Fern: Well, I don't care about Marc anymore. . . . My roommates are always busy. . . . Sometimes Judy gets on my nerves. . . .

Nurse: What do you suppose is the problem about all this?

Fern: I feel that I'm not going to have a good time. I won't study. Usually no one is home, and I'll be lonely. Yeah, . . . I'll be lonely again.

Nurse: The problem with this long weekend seems to be more loneliness for you.

Fern (Sighs): That sums it up.

In the previous verbatim example, the client moved from identifying several subproblems to the more basic problem of loneliness. The nurse assisted the client by encouraging definition and reflecting the probable central theme back to the client.

Preparation Preparation involves collecting additional pertinent data related to the basic problem that may prove useful in later stages of problem-solving strategies. This aspect of problem-solving enables one to "anticipate" which data might be most useful.

Analysis Analysis as a problem-solving strategy involves breaking down the relevant material into subproblems so that each subproblem may be assessed separately.

Ideation Ideation involves accumulating alternative ideas on how to resolve the basic problem. The following clinical material illustrates Fern's initial use of ideation as a problem-solving strategy in the beginning of the fourth session:

Fern: My weekend wasn't that bad. (Laughs mildly.)

Nurse: Let's hear about it.

Fern: Well, Saturday night I went out to dinner with my roommate, and Friday night I went to the movies.

Nurse: I wonder what were the "good" and "bad" parts of this.

Fern: Well, I can honestly say that I enjoyed the movie, and dinner with Sara (roommate) was OK, too.

Nurse: What did you do to make your weekend "not that bad"?

Fern: Well, I planned my time, so I wasn't always alone. I had some studying to do for one exam.

Fern changed the topic to discuss one teacher who added requirements to his course. When she mentioned the weekend again, the nurse tried to refocus.

Nurse: Fern, are you aware of any steps involved in dealing with loneliness over the weekend?

Fern: Yeah. I actively sought out doing things. I made sure that I was doing things.

Nurse: Can you be more specific?

Fern: I kept busy. I had to study. I went to the library on Saturday so I wasn't home alone. I told you about going out to dinner and the movie.

Incubation   Incubation is used when the problem-solving process or one aspect of it is set aside for a period of time to allow for illumination.

Synthesis   Synthesis as a problem-solving strategy involves putting all elements of the basic problem, subproblems, and possible alternatives together.

Evaluation   Evaluation consists of making judgments about the resultant ideas.

Development   Development as a final problem-solving strategy involves planning the implementation of these ideas.

Problem-solving abilities may improve with time and experience. During the eighth session, Fern and the nurse were skilled enough to piece together the "map" in Figure 27–3. It concerns Fern's definition of her current problem: how to handle angry feelings without feeling trapped by them. The map is not complete, but it represents a sorting of the known dynamics.

The situation precipitating that exploration was that Fern's roommate repeatedly left dishes in the sink for days, after having agreed to clean them nightly. Fern identified

two problem-solving alternatives in this session. First, Fern could set the dirty dishes aside for her roommate to see. She evaluated this activity to be a less satisfactory solution, since her roommate might then avoid the kitchen area. Second, Fern might directly share her anger with the roommate. Fern previously avoided sharing anger directly with anyone. She anticipated that she could maintain her assertive position by justifying that everyone has to help with housework. Fern judged that if her roommate washed the dishes, then the outcome would be satisfactory for her. Table 27–8 summarizes Fern's possible problem-solving outcomes.

Fern used preparation and incubation as problem-solving strategies, since Fern had determined many pieces of the "map" in the interim between the seventh and eighth sessions. Synthesis was apparent in Fern's integration of known subproblems of an identified problem and active seeking of alternatives. She used ideation and evaluation in her identification of problem-solving alternatives and evaluation of the potential outcome of each. In informal relationship work, some or all elements may be used in a similar manner.

Challenging the Client's Resistance to Change

The nurse also assists the client by challenging the client's resistance to change. There are two major categories of forces that inhibit desired change:

1. Intrapersonal forces, which may arise from troublesome thoughts, feelings, or behaviors. Examples include: thoughts that hamper the client's sense of worth; the client's inability to control and express emotion appropriately; or the client's inability to relate to others in a meaningful manner.

2. The client's personal resistance to change, which is the greatest inhibiting force. In fact, the client's challenge to this resistance constitutes the major work in one-to-one relationships.

Problems of resistance and general intervention strategies are discussed earlier in this chapter. Of equal significance is the previous discussion of transference and countertransference phenomena, as these may require careful, planned nursing interventions. Sometimes transference and countertransference are so intense that they become a problem for the beginning psychiatric nurse. Problems in transference and countertransference are explored later in this section.

Intervening in Interpersonal Withdrawal

Withdrawal is the behavior pattern characterized by avoidance of contact. Clients may avoid interpersonal relationships and/or a sense of reality. Withdrawal as a behavior pattern may be functional or dysfunctional. Temporary withdrawal as a response to crisis is an important coping

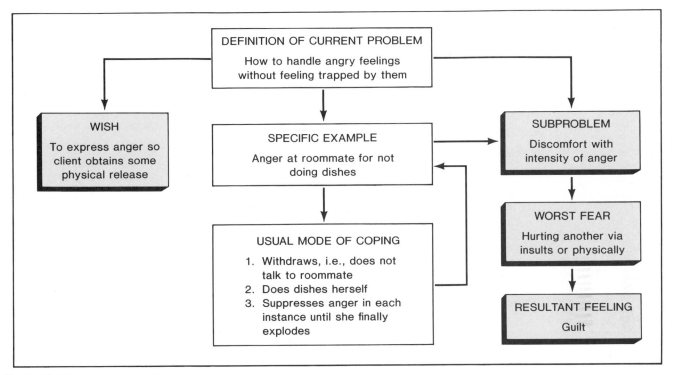

Figure 27–3
Client's "map" of current problem.

skill for particular individuals. Severe or permanent withdrawal from interpersonal or reality-based contact is dysfunctional and requires nursing intervention. The primary goal in nursing intervention is to enhance the client's self-esteem and therefore increase the client's willingness to satisfy emotional needs through interpersonal contact.

Physical Withdrawal Physical withdrawal, in its extreme form, is manifested by suicide attempts, gestures, or threats. Suggested interventions include:

- Avoid punishment of the client.
- Encourage ventilation of feelings.
- Accept any expressions of anger.
- Explore the source of present distress and the history of past distressing experiences.
- Decrease isolation.
- Provide crisis contact with the nurse, other therapist, or a crisis service.
- Assess what the client values.

In in-patient settings, the client may manifest physical withdrawal by sitting or standing apart from others, retreating to another room, purposely hiding, or assuming

catatonic postures. In severe withdrawal, the emphasis is on the establishment of contact through physical proximity. Suggestions for intervention include:

- Move into the client's visual field (same eye level).
- Identify self.
- Make a general introductory inquiry.
- Invite the client to speak.
- State how much time you are willing to stay with the client, whether the client chooses to speak or not.

Attention to physical needs may be an effective intervention to establish some initial bond of contact. Withdrawal by preoccupation with hallucinations, ritualistic compulsions, obsessional thinking, and the like is discussed in Chapters 17–19.

When the client misses sessions in in-patient, one-to-one relationship work, the nurse may use the following strategies:

- Follow through by locating the client.
- Explore the absence in a concerned manner.
- State the necessity for the client to share responsibility for the continuance of the relationship.

**Table 27–8
Evaluation of Client's Problem-Solving Alternatives**

Alternative	Evaluation
Set aside dirty dishes for roommate to see	Anticipates that roommate might avoid kitchen area
	Probable unsatisfactory outcome
Tell roommate directly about anger regarding dirty dishes	Never shared anger with anyone
	Anticipates following sequence:
	Shares anger regarding dirty dishes
	Roommate gives excuses
	Maintains assertive position that everyone help with housework
	Roommate agrees to do task
	Outcome judged satisfactory if task is done by roommate

- Change the context of the contact (for example, go for a walk together).

The following clinical example shows how one psychiatric nurse intervened when the client physically withdrew in an in-patient setting.

Jason is a 40-year-old, single male who was hospitalized following his second suicide attempt (drug overdose). Both attempts were preceded by gradual social isolation, i.e., withdrawal from friends and neighbors. In addition, Jason lived alone in a small apartment. He hesitantly negotiated for daily one-to-one relationship work with a female psychiatric nurse. The first two sessions were characterized by silence and a few superficial interactions. He did not attend the third session. The psychiatric nurse waited the thirty minutes, then sought Jason out on the ward. The following exchanges occurred:

Nurse (Sitting in chair to be at eye level with client): Hi, Jason. I'd like to talk with you for a few minutes, if it's OK with you.

Jason: (Forty-five-second silence)

Nurse: I'm not sure what your silence means.

Jason (After thirty-second silence): Go ahead. . . .

(Gestures in what appears to be an agreeable manner, as if to indicate to continue.)

Nurse: I waited for you in the conference room today and was concerned when you didn't come.

Jason (Winces eyes in what appears to be a questioning manner, after twenty-second silence): I didn't want to.

Nurse: I respect your choice not to meet together today. Can you fill me in on how it was that you chose not to come?

Jason (In monotone voice seemingly devoid of feeling): I don't want to talk anymore now.

Nurse: I hear you. I'll be available between four and five o'clock today, and I'll be in the conference room tomorrow at the time that we agreed on together, Jason.

In this example, the psychiatric nurse used the following intervention techniques: She sought to explore the meaning of the client's silence, stated her concern, and affirmed Jason's option not to participate. Yet she sought out his rationale, stressed her availability, and emphasized her expectation of mutual continued contact rather than mutual withdrawal.

In outpatient settings, physical withdrawal may necessitate outreach by telephone and changing the setting in terms of time, place, or persons. For example, the client may respond better to home visits than to an office with a crowded waiting room. One client brought his dog to initial sessions since he viewed the dog as his only support system and contact.

Verbal Withdrawal Verbal withdrawal represents avoidance of contact through silence or, in its extreme form, mutism. When periodic silence occurs in the therapeutic relationship, it is important to explore its significance. But the nurse must learn to tolerate silences without verbalizing unnecessarily. Silence may indicate that the client is resistant, pensive, or simply has nothing more to say. Strategies for intervention include:

- Explore "what is said" by silence.
- Take an attitude of continued interest.
- Accept the client's self-expression at present through silence.

In cases of mutism, Gruber (1977) recommends the no-demand, third-person interview in which the client is referred to in the third person, yet given the freedom to comment. The nurse may also say to the client: "This is your time. It's been set aside for you. I'll sit with you and I'm ready to listen when you're ready to speak." In this instance, it is important for the nurse to state that the client will not be left because he or she is mute. The following clinical example demonstrates how one nurse began to work with a nonverbal client.

Karen is a 14-year-old, single female referred by her parents to an outpatient adolescent unit because of gradual withdrawal from family and peers during the past six months. She has refused to go to school, staying in her bedroom for the last two weeks. Although Karen was mute during the entire initial interview, she consented (by shaking her head) to meet with a psychiatric nurse for one-hour sessions weekly. During the initial two sessions, Karen sat in a chair, avoided eye contact, and said nothing. Two strategies for the third session were: (a) to decrease sessions to a half hour to decrease discomfort, and (b) to invite the client to use the available blackboard, paper and pencil, or sketch pad if she chose. Although Karen remained motionless during the session, a handwritten note was found on the nurse's desk that same day. It read: "I don't want to talk right now, but I like you." Similar notes continued until the ninth session, when Karen began talking.

Intervening in Hostility-Aggression

Hostility is the behavioral pattern characterized by actual or threatened aggressive contact. Hostility is differentiated from anger in that anger may be constructive, whereas hostility is destructive in intent. The operational steps in direct expression of hostility are:

- The client experiences a frustration or threat.
- Anxiety surfaces, associated with feelings of helplessness and inadequacy.
- Verbal or motor aggressive action alleviates the increased anxiety.

The aggressive action in this case is directed toward destruction of the object perceived as the source of the frustration or threat. This object may be self, others, or an inanimate object. When forces inhibit the direct expression of hostility, the client may cope with the hostility by using various defense mechanisms. Examples include displacement and projection.

Basque and Merhige (1980) researched the type and frequency of dangerous behaviors encountered in psychiatric facilities. They found that nurses encountered these behaviors at least once a week:

- Three-fourths of the nurses encountered verbally abusive clients.
- One-third of the nurses encountered clients who were physically abusive to other clients.
- One-fifth of the nurses encountered clients who physically abused staff.
- One-third of the nurses encountered clients who endangered themselves.

Although Lathrop (1978) believes that prevention is the most successful form of intervention when dealing with aggressive behaviors, three-fourths of the nurses in the Basque and Merhige study reported no training in the prevention and management of aggressive behaviors.

Verbal Threats   The psychiatric nurse may receive hostile threats, comments, or insults from clients. When any of these occur, suggested strategies for intervention include:

- Continue client contact rather than avoid it.
- Allow the client to verbalize feelings associated with the threat or frustration (helplessness, inadequacy, anger, etc.).
- Defuse the situation by "talking the client down."

A further possible intervention for hostile threats is to explore the client's need for extreme controls. These may consist of medication, exercise, and assessment of the degree of closeness the client tolerates. In addition, the nurse may provide a consistent set of expectations and guidance toward client self-control. These latter strategies are used in the following dialogue:

Client: Look out for me today.
Nurse: How come?
Client: I feel like breaking bones. (Moves closer.)
Nurse: You and I can talk about this feeling "like breaking bones."

In this dialogue, the psychiatric nurse demonstrates regard for the client while clearly stating the expectation that further self-expression will be verbal rather than physical.

Exploration is antitherapeutic when the client is about to lose control. When the client is in control, the following strategies may be helpful:

- Explore the threat or frustration that preceded the indication of hostility.
- Encourage the client to make the connection between the specific threat or frustration, the subsequent feelings, and the specific manifestation of hostility.

Physical Aggression   The nurse may also have to deal with physical aggression by clients. Physical aggression may vary in degree (from irritation to global rage) and target (inanimate objects, self, others). For example, the client may break his or her cigarette, a chair, or another client's nose. In addition to the intervention strategies described above for verbal threats, the following may prove helpful:

- Address, rather than avoid, the client and the specific behavior.
- Avoid any retaliatory actions.
- Approach the client in a calm, firm manner.
- Clearly indicate what the client is or is not to do, e.g., "put down the chair."
- Attempt to talk with the client.
- Convey acceptance of the client, but not of the aggressive behavior.
- Encourage an alternative expression of aggression, such as use of Bataccas (cylindrical clubs of a soft, padded material so that injury is avoided), pillows, paper or foam balls, or punching bags.
- Intervene early when the client first gives verbal and nonverbal signs of aggression (frowns, threats, clenching of fists).
- Remove the client from the immediate environment and/or use restraints when necessary, to help reestablish self-control. This may involve an organized team approach to be practiced in mock situations before use with clients.

Lenefsky et al. (1978) elaborate on safe intervention of violent behaviors via physical restraint. Steward (1978) illustrates specific physical techniques to restrain a weapon-wielding client. He emphasizes, however, that other approaches, plus an increased number of visible staff, usually suffice to maintain control and prevent injury.

Intervening in Manipulation

Manipulation occurs in one-to-one relationship work when the client maneuvers to have the therapist meet the client's immediate needs. Table 27–9 analyzes examples of manipulative maneuvers used by a client to avoid accountability for personal problems, create nurse discomfort, and control interactions. This table also illustrates how the nurse may shift the focus of interactions from an emphasis on content (what is said) to an emphasis on process (what is happening in the nurse-client relationship at that moment). This is particularly useful when the client uses behaviors intended to disturb, confuse, or anger the nurse. (Manipulation is thoroughly discussed in Chapter 21.)

Seduction as a form of manipulation is characterized by verbal or physical advances toward sexual contact. Seductive behaviors (comments, suggestions, or physical contact) from clients of the same or opposite sex may cause

---

Table 27–9
Analysis of Verbatim Example of Attempted Manipulation

Verbatim Interaction	Analysis of Responses
Client: Sometimes I feel uncomfortable about you. You meet with me every week and listen to my problems. I wonder if you're bored sometimes	Manipulative maneuver: suggests that nurse has a problem regarding boredom
Nurse: I don't know how to respond. Has this happened before—that someone listens to you and you wonder if they're bored?	Nursing interventions: avoids angry or defensive response; suspects projection, and gives client option to work on boredom as client's own problem
Client: Once in a while, but not here. It's probably not boredom—maybe you're just nervous. Sometimes I see you shifting back and forth in your chair. Maybe you're new at this and not sure of yourself yet	Manipulative maneuvers: discounts boredom as own problem; abruptly switches to other problems—suggests nurse has problems with nervousness and inexperience
Nurse: You seem to have a lot of questions about me today	Nursing interventions: avoids angry or defensive responses; moves to focus on *process* rather than *content* of session, i.e., client's focus on nurse's behavior

---

discomfort to the nurse. Seductive behavior needs to be explicitly discussed rather than avoided, by client and nurse together. The following clinical material illustrates this point:

Sandra began employment as a psychiatric nurse in an institution for the treatment of drug abuse. The female clients could opt for a daily walk outside if accompanied by staff. Sandra saw this as an opportunity to establish rapport. While she was walking with five female clients, one walked very close to her and started to stroke Sandra's arm in a consistently teasing, sexual manner. The following interaction occurred:

Sandra (In a very firm voice): Stop stroking my arm.

Client (Discontinuing stroking): Simmer down, sweetheart. You have no idea what it's like here without men!

Sandra: I'd like you to tell me about your predicament in words, and I'll listen.

Discussion of the meaning of the seductive behavior can follow.

Intervening in Detachment

Detachment is the behavioral pattern characterized by a generalized aloofness in interpersonal contact. Detachment, as a form of resistance, can retard relationship work and discourage the nurse. Types of detachment include intellectualization, denial, and superficiality. Intellectualization and denial are discussed in Chapter 7.

Superficiality is a form of resistance characterized by shallowness of contact. It is used by clients to avoid interpersonal intimacy. The client may be superficial in the definition and exploration of problem areas or in the implementation of behavioral change.

Interventions for detachment and any of its manifestations (intellectualization, denial, superficiality) emphasize making the client aware of the process of detachment—i.e., what the client does to detach from or remain aloof in interpersonal contact. The psychiatric nurse may encourage the client to assess how this response serves the client, including delineating any self-defeating aspects. Finally, the nurse may explore any fears and fantasies that inhibit emotional expression and actively emphasize emotive content in subsequent work. The following verbatim exchange illustrates how a problem behavior pattern of detachment was handled:

Client: I keep exploring this inner realm of my consciousness between sessions, in an effort to determine the type of existence I'm seeking.

Nurse: I don't understand. Can you be more specific about what you want for yourself?

Client: Oh, it's an existential dilemma of sorts. I'm searching, constantly searching. . . .

Nurse: And how do you feel as you search?

Client: Feel? Unsettled? Is it unsettled? I guess so.

Nurse: Can you describe how "unsettled" feels to you?

Client: Sort of sad. . . .

The nursing interventions used included seeking clarification of unclear responses, encouraging the client to move from global generalities to specific personal comments, and emphasizing awareness and exploration of feelings.

Intervening in Excessive Dependence (Learned Helplessness)

Excessive dependence is characterized by attempts to establish and maintain contact by adopting a helpless, powerless stance. Learned helplessness may be expressed by maneuvers to have the nurse make decisions about, guide, or otherwise assume responsibility for the client's behavior. Exclusiveness may also characterize this behavior pattern, manifested by the message "No one understands me but you." Thus, the client uses a stance of helplessness that was learned in previous relationships and avoids growth toward self-awareness, mutuality, and autonomy. This common behavior pattern deserves emphasis, since clients who adopt it frequently view nurses as mother substitutes and since the nurse may readily assume a caretaker role.

Specific nursing interventions regarding excessive dependence include the following:

- Set clear, firm, and consistent limits on the various forms of excessive dependency.
- Avoid any retaliatory actions, including withdrawal.
- Emphasize the client's determination and accountability for personal feelings, thoughts, and behaviors.
- Avoid making decisions about, guiding, or otherwise assuming responsibility for the client's behavior.
- Give positive reinforcement for development of more independent, growth-facilitating behaviors over time.

The following clinical material shows how these principles can be applied:

Terry is a 27-year-old, single female with an extensive history of psychotherapy and one psychiatric hospitalization. The precipitating event for hospitalization was a suicide gesture by overdose. The result was that Terry's mother slept by her bedside for several subsequent months. Presenting problems at the initial interview were depression, boredom, obesity, and an inability to initiate peer relationships. Terry was unemployed and lived at home with her mother but did not participate in any household tasks. Terry's mother drove her two blocks to attend sessions, regardless of weather conditions.

Terry negotiated for weekly half-hour sessions of individual psychotherapy. Her behavior in the sessions was characterized by emphasis on the exclusivity of the therapeutic relationship, thus attempting to duplicate this aspect of the mother-daughter relationship. After several sessions, Terry began requesting, and later demanding, that the nurse physically hug her several times during the course of each session. At the close of one session, Terry took out a bottle of tranquilizers and screamed, "If you don't hug me, I'll take these! Here! Keep these from me!" She threw herself on the floor and sobbed. The nurse verbally reflected Terry's apparent desperation and discomfort, acknowledged that Terry had the power to make a choice regarding the tranquilizers, and reinforced the use of crisis contact by telephone. Terry chose not to take the pills and continued with individual psychotherapy.

Intervening in Problems with Transference and Countertransference

Negative Transference   In negative transference, the client shows a number of reactions based on forms of hate (hostility, loathing, bitterness, contempt, annoyance). Although there are both positive and negative aspects to every transference, a predominantly negative transference is uncomfortable for client and nurse alike. The client does not like to be aware of and express this hate, and the nurse does not like to be the target of it. When negative transference appears unresolvable, it may be advisable to terminate relationship work rather than run the risk of further client dysfunction.

It is important to note that negative transference responses that seem related to deep-seated depression or paranoia are usually not dealt with in relationship work. The reason is that exploration may stir up issues and intense emotions that cannot be dealt with in a limited time span (Arieti 1975).

Psychotic Transference   In psychotic transference, or transference psychosis, the relationship with the psychiatric nurse supersedes all other relationships, although the client has no insight into the existence of the transference and denies its presence. Psychotic transference requires repetitive, concrete reality testing to separate the nurse from significant others in the client's life. In addition, psychotic transference may be minimized by decreasing the frequency and/or duration of contact with the client. Both negative transference and psychotic transference problems require consistent supervision and cautious management.

Unanalyzed Countertransference   Unanalyzed countertransference is almost always a problem, because it inhibits client understanding and may be acted out. One purpose of clinical supervision is to help the mental health professional develop awareness of individual countertransference reactions. Chessick (1974) highlights the following signs of countertransference in waking life or while dreaming:

- Anxiety reactions
- Reactions of irrational concern about and irrational kindness toward the client
- Reactions of irrational hostility toward the client

More specific signals that countertransference may be a problem include:

- Uneasy feelings during or after meetings
- Being late or extending the agreed-upon duration of meetings for no apparent reason
- Dreaming about the client
- Preoccupation with the client during the nurse's leisure time

It is reassuring that most countertransference problems can be resolved by self-assessment with professional supervision. Once the countertransference process is identified, the nurse can consciously develop therapeutic, goal-directed responses. In rare instances, however, referral to another nurse is appropriate when the first nurse remains unable to control her or his disturbed attitudes and emotions.

Evaluation

Several levels of evaluation occur simultaneously in the working phase of one-to-one relationships. First, the nurse does an ongoing evaluation of the client's various levels of intrapersonal and interpersonal functioning. Feedback from family, community agencies, or the client's employer may enhance any current comprehensive evaluation. For example, does the client seem to be facing an impending crisis? If so, the nurse may choose to switch from intrapersonal exploration to a crisis intervention strategy. Second, the nurse encourages the client to evaluate himself or herself, as explored in previous discussion. Finally, the nurse constantly evaluates herself or himself as a helping person growing in skill and experience. This evaluation is done by informal discussions with staff and other mental health personnel and by formal clinical supervision. (The functions of supervision are highlighted later in this chapter.)

"On-the-spot" evaluations of relevant short-term and long-term goals can occur during any meeting with the client. For example, as the client talks about increasing socialization skills, the nurse may reflect: "Let's look at our contract together. You originally wanted to date a girl of your choice for two hours during an evening without leaving the situation. How do you think this compares with what you're now saying has happened?" The nurse supports any effort at evaluation on the part of the client and explores what else needs to happen for the client to achieve the short-term goal. An additional area of evaluation involves the client's "trying on" alternative behaviors to determine if these new behaviors may work for the client.

The client and nurse should mutually evaluate the appropriateness of goals in any one of the following areas in the light of current functioning: degree of client success in achieving specific goals, client's growth-producing and growth-inhibiting behavior patterns, and unfinished business that must be resolved to achieve a desired goal. In addition, the working phase may also involve ongoing evaluations of the status, characteristics, and depth of the nurse-client relationship. The client may view the nurse in different ways (parent, sibling, friend) at various times. It is only when these views are made explicit that the nurse may intervene to clarify roles and responsibilities in a facilitative manner.

The psychiatric nurse and the client have moved through the first two phases of therapeutic relationships when:

- They have established a working relationship
- They have analyzed the dynamics of the client's behavioral patterns
- The client has effectively instituted behavioral changes in keeping with the therapeutic contract

In informal relationship work, the nurse may touch upon only one or two aspects of the middle (working) phase of one-to-one relationship work. Even the advanced psychiatric nurse rarely addresses all therapeutic tasks in this phase of relationship work.

Termination (End) Phase

During the termination (end) phase of one-to-one relationships, the psychiatric nurse and client discontinue contact. This phase is as important as the previous two phases, although it is frequently avoided by the nurse and client alike because of past difficulties with separation.

The goal of the end phase is termination of the one-to-one relationship in a mutually planned, satisfying manner. The nurse should remind the client that termination was first addressed in the orientation phase, when the duration of the relationship was discussed. The nurse also needs to emphasize the growth and positive aspects of the relationship, rather than focus exclusively upon separation.

A smooth and complete termination sometimes occurs in actual practice. In informal relationship work in inpatient settings, termination more often occurs with the client's abrupt departure or planned medical discharge. Even in formal relationship work in community settings, contact often ceases without explanation after a series of missed appointments, or with a phone call by the client to inform the therapist of the client's decision to terminate, or with the client abruptly leaving a session and failing to resume subsequent contact. In these instances, the nurse can call or write the client and suggest an additional session to deal with either the therapeutic good-bye or a willingness to continue the relationship work. Termination requires careful preparation, adequate time for the client to work through the feelings about ending, and an opportunity for the psychiatric nurse to explore personal reactions with a clinical instructor, colleague, supervisor, or consultant.

Assessment

Assessment as a component of the nursing process in the resolution phase deals primarily with determining when the client may be ready to terminate, how the client deals with termination, and how the nurse deals with termination. The following criteria may be useful to determine whether the client is ready to terminate:

- *Relief from the presenting problem.* Symptoms no longer interfere with the client's comfort.
- *Achievement of treatment goals.* These ideally are planned goals included in the therapeutic contract between the nurse and client.
- *Improvement in social functioning.* The client experiences increased satisfaction in interpersonal relationships.
- *Acquisition of adaptive coping strategies.* Ideally, these strategies include the client's use of effective problem-solving strategies on a daily basis.
- *Acquisition of more effective defense mechanisms.* If the client cannot achieve adaptive coping strategies, he or she should develop more effective defense mechanisms to ensure stabilization.
- *Attainment of identity.* The client experiences self-satisfaction and no longer needs to depend on the nurse for a sense of well-being.
- *Disruption due to a major impasse in the one-to-one relationship.* Stubborn resistances may surface and persist on the part of the client. Uncontrollable countertransference may develop on the part of the nurse.

Many factors influence how the client reacts to termination. These factors include:

- *Degree of client involvement.* The greater the involvement, the more intense the client's reaction to termination.
- *Length of treatment.* In general, the longer the nurse-client relationship lasts, the more time should be spent in exploring all aspects of termination.
- *Client's past history of significant losses.* A client who has lost significant others may reexperience past conflicts and emotional responses.
- *Ability to separate from others.* The client's reaction to termination is influenced by how well he or she has mastered the early separation-individuation phase of development.
- *Degree of success achieved.* Reaction to termination

depends on how successful and satisfying the relationship has been for the client.

- *Degree of transference in the relationship.* The greater the transference in the nurse-client relationship, the more intense the client's reaction to termination.

The psychiatric nurse must be alert to client responses during termination. Any number of client responses (e.g., repression, regression, anger, denial, sadness, withdrawal, avoidance, acceptance, or joy) may surface. It is not unusual for several to surface at once. When repressing, the client shows no emotional response. Regression on the part of the client is an extremely common response to termination. Regressive behavior may range from statements of abandonment and hopelessness to inability to tend to personal hygiene. The central message conveyed is: "See? I can't make it without you!"

Finally, assessment involves how the nurse personally manages separation in the one-to-one relationship. Like the client, the nurse can have any number of responses. Some common responses are:

- Regret that the client did not achieve more than the client actually did

- Hesitation to give up the dependency elements of the relationship

- Collusion with the client to prolong sessions to avoid the inevitability of separation

Nursing Diagnosis

Nursing diagnoses during termination should reflect the termination behaviors manifested by the client. A wide variety of nursing diagnoses may be relevant. Potential nursing diagnoses that stem from regression during the termination phase may be: self-care deficit, hopelessness, powerlessness, and ineffective individual coping. These and other nursing diagnoses should be modified as necessary as the client moves through the termination experience.

Planning and Implementing Interventions

Planning involves the preparing for the final good-bye and making any needed referrals (to another nurse or therapist, self-help group, community agency, or job-training program). When a referral is made, it is often wise for the client to have an initial contact with the referred person or agency before termination. In this way, the nurse can immediately deal with any initial misconceptions. Termination should include planning with the client where he

or she may seek future help if the need arises. Options most frequently include returning to the nurse, referral to crisis services, or referral to other community agencies. The shift to dependence on other support systems (referrals, family, friends) is a therapeutic task requiring the psychiatric nurse's awareness of planning and intervention strategy.

Intervention strategies depend upon the behaviors manifested by the client. The nurse may respond to the client who is repressing the reality of termination by repeatedly observing that the client is not addressing the issue of the impending separation. The nurse may then attempt to explore this avoidance with the client. Useful interventions for clients who are regressing in response to termination include:

- Address the possible underlying fears of abandonment
- Emphasize the growth achieved by the client
- Continue to focus on the realities of separation

The acting-out client may protest termination in numerous ways (suicide gestures or attempts, psychiatric hospitalization, terminating employment, rejection of therapist) before the termination date. In general, the underlying feelings, fears, and fantasies need ventilation, exploration, and working through. The client reactions of anger, depression, or grief require the same. An exception to this general guideline is the client who uses distraction maneuvers, such as introducing explosive new material in final sessions. The following clinical example illustrates a client's manipulative attempts to prevent termination by using acting-out behaviors. Limit setting, rather than exploration, was used by the psychiatric nurse because of time constraints specific to this one-to-one work. The example also illustrates that there may be "unfinished business" despite planning and effort.

Kim was a 19-year-old, single female who was self-referred to a local university student counseling center. Her chief complaint was an inability to maintain relationships with both female and male peers. Her history included excessive drug experimentation and frequent superficial sexual encounters with males who subsequently mistreated and left her.

Kim negotiated for two semesters of individual psychotherapy and was informed that the psychiatric nurse was not available beyond this time due to relocation. Kim's behavior in the sessions was characterized by attempts to trap the nurse, displace and project anger onto others, and avoid accountability for her presenting problem. Although termination was carefully planned and referral sources considered, Kim resisted by offering money, crying, and leaving sessions early. She resisted exploration of any thoughts or feelings regarding termination and refused to consider referral.

During the last session, she eagerly reported having her first homosexual experience with a woman who resembled the nurse. She then asked how the one-to-one relationship could end without exploring this new behavior. The nurse was aware of the far-reaching implications of this final issue in terms of Kim's psychodynamics as well as its impact on the one-to-one work. The nurse was also aware of Kim's challenging attitude associated with another attempt, this time regarding sexual acting out, to prolong sessions. The nurse emphasized that this explosive issue needed further exploration, again discussed and encouraged use of referrals, and addressed the issue of good-bye. Both nurse and client were dissatisfied with the time limitation in this case. A sense of mutual termination was not realized.

The nurse has the final task of participating in an explicit and therapeutic good-bye with the client. Nursing responsibilities in this final phase of one-to-one relationship work include anticipating the nurse's personal reaction to separation and optionally, expressing this reaction in a manner that does not burden the client. In addition, the nurse may share a special wish for the client, based on the client's particular assets within the therapeutic relationship. A therapeutic good-bye gives the client a sense of freedom to move on to other relationships. The end phase may take from one meeting to several months of meetings, depending on the duration of the one-to-one relationship. In gen-

eral, the longer the duration of the relationship, the longer the time needed to deal explicitly with termination of contact. Table 27–10 summarizes the goal, therapeutic tasks, and specific nursing interventions of the end phase of one-to-one relationship work. Ideally, the client can completely work through feelings regarding separation so that there is no unfinished business between the psychiatric nurse and client. The nurse-client relationship has given the client the opportunity to depend on another in a realistic and mature manner. Assessment of the experience helps the client practice self-assessment skills and may help set the stage for additional relationship work in the future. Participating in a direct, explicit good-bye is frequently the first such experience for the client. It is usually a moment of unique humanness for both the psychiatric nurse and client.

Evaluation

Evaluation is a vital component of the nursing process during the resolution phase of one-to-one relationships. The psychiatric nurse has the task of helping the client evaluate the therapeutic contract. The criteria for evaluation are the goals formulated in the orientation and work-

---

Table 27–10 Summary of Termination (End) Phase		
Goal	**Therapeutic Tasks**	**Nursing Interventions**
Termination of contact in a mutually planned, satisfying manner	Assist client evaluation of therapeutic contract and of therapeutic experience in general	Encourage client's realistic appraisal of personal therapeutic goals (motivation, effort, progress, outcome) as these evolved in treatment
		Provide appropriate feedback regarding appraisal of goals
		Review client's assets and therapeutic gains
		Review areas for further therapeutic work
	Encourage transference of dependence to other support systems	Encourage client to develop reliance on others in client's immediate environment (spouse, relative, employer, neighbor, friend) for empathic, emotional support
	Participate in explicit therapeutic good-bye with client	Be alert to surfacing of any behavior arising on termination (repression, regression, acting out, anger, withdrawal, acceptance)
		Assist client in working through feelings associated with these behaviors
		Anticipate own reaction to separation and share in a manner that does not burden client
		Allow "time" and "space" for termination; the longer the duration of the one-to-one relationship, the more time is needed for the termination phase

ing phases of the one-to-one relationship. Each goal is evaluated in terms of measurable, observable behavior. Were the goals appropriate, practical, and specific to the client? Did the goals actually help evaluate motivation and effort? Did the goals enable the client and nurse to evaluate progress and outcome? What are the therapeutic gains? What are the areas for possible further therapeutic work? How does the client evaluate his or her motivation, effort, progress, and outcome?

The psychiatric nurse also assists client evaluation of the therapeutic experience in general. Evaluation of the experience may help set the stage for future psychotherapeutic work. Would the client seek a similar experience in the future, if deemed necessary? The nurse may also invite feedback from the client in relation to her or his impact on the client. In certain clinical settings, the nurse also has the therapeutic task of evaluating the effectiveness of the psychiatric treatment service in relation to this particular client (Stanley 1984).

The nurse's personal ongoing self-evaluation also warrants emphasis here. It is essential that the psychiatric nurse continuously evaluate which personal behaviors consciously or unconsciously promote, inhibit, and actively block growth-producing client abilities.

Supervision is essential if the one-to-one relationship is to be effective. Professional supervision helps the psychiatric nurse use transference effectively and recognize countertransference phenomena. Mellow (1968) identifies the following functions of a supervisor in relation to the supervised psychiatric nurse:

- A teaching function for the transmission of learnable techniques and attitudes

- A supportive function for difficulties that are inherent in or imposed on the therapeutic relationship

- An analytic function to increase the awareness of how he or she affects the therapeutic relationship and outcome

More recently, Benfer (1979) used the supportive function of supervision to monitor the personal needs of the nurse and decrease the likelihood of severe clinical stress and burnout. There are various methods of evaluation: interpersonal process recordings, videotapes, client evaluations, audiotapes, didactic instruction, and referral to specific clinical readings. There are several kinds of supervision available, such as intradisciplinary supervision with a psychiatric clinical nurse specialist, or interdisciplinary supervision by another mental health professional (psychologist, psychiatrist, psychiatric social worker). All can be helpful, depending on the skills and availability of supervisors or

consultants. Supervision helps the psychiatric nurse effectively define, initiate, use, and evaluate client and self in any therapeutic relationship.

Chapter Highlights

- A therapeutic one-to-one relationship may evolve in any nursing situation.

- The one-to-one relationship between psychiatric nurse and client is a mutually defined, mutually collaborative, goal-oriented professional relationship.

- Characteristics of a humanistic one-to-one relationship include openness, negotiation, commitment, responsibility, and authenticity.

- Client abilities that tend toward successful therapy outcomes include awareness and ownership of feelings, desire to change, and ability to differentiate feelings, concerns, and problems.

- The establishment of a therapeutic alliance is an essential ingredient of formal one-to-one relationship work.

- Psychiatric nurses need to be aware of both content and process in a one-to-one relationship.

- Resistance is best understood as the client's struggle against change; the humanistic stance is that the client has a right to resist the therapeutic process.

- One-to-one relationships may be organized around the nursing process.

- Phases of a therapeutic relationship include the orientation (beginning), working (middle), and termination (end).

- The orientation (beginning) phase of therapeutic relationships is characterized by the establishment of contact and the formation of a working relationship. This phase focuses on establishing rapport, obtaining pertinent information, initiating client assessment, developing a therapeutic contract between the client and nurse, and making practical arrangements for treatment.

- The working (middle) phase of the relationship is characterized by behavioral analysis and constructive behavioral change.

- Counterproductive behavioral patterns frequently occurring in therapeutic relationships include interpersonal withdrawal, hostility-aggression, manipulation, detachment, excessive dependency, and untherapeutic transference and countertransference phenomena.

- The termination (end) phase of the therapeutic relationship is characterized by the termination of the relationship in a mutually planned, satisfying manner.

- Evaluation is an ongoing psychotherapeutic process as well as a step in the nursing process, and includes continuous evaluation of client behaviors, development of client self-evaluation, mutual evaluation of the relationship, and the nurse's self-evaluation in each one-to-one relationship.

References

Arieti S (ed): *American Handbook of Psychiatry,* ed 2. Basic Books, 1975, vol 5.

Auvil CA, Silver BW: Therapist self-disclosure: When is it appropriate? *Perspect Psychiatr Care* 1984;22:57–61.

Basque L, Merhige J: Nurses' experiences with dangerous behavior: Implications for training. *J Continuing Educ Nurs* 1980;11:47–51.

Benfer B: Clinical supervision as a support system for the care-giver. *Perspect Psychiatr Care* 1979;17:13–17.

Black K: *Short-Term Counseling: A Humanistic Approach for the Helping Professions.* Addison-Wesley, 1983.

Carter EW: Psychiatric nursing, in Kaplan HI, Sadock BJ: *Comprehensive Textbook of Psychiatry,* ed 4. Williams and Wilkins, 1985, pp 1936–1939.

Chessick R: *The Technique and Practice of Intensive Psychotherapy.* Jason Aronson, 1974.

Cronbach L: Beyond two disciplines of scientific psychology. *Am Psychol* 1975;30:116–127.

Davanloo H: Short-term dynamic psychotherapy, in Kaplan HI, Sadock BJ: *Comprehensive Textbook of Psychiatry,* ed 4. Williams and Wilkins, 1985, pp 1460–1467.

Diener C, Dweck C: An analysis of learned helplessness: Continuous changes in performance, strategy, and achievement cognitions following failure. *J Pers Soc Psychol* 1978;36:451–462.

Fagin CM: Concepts for the future: Competition and substitution. *J Psychosoc Nurs Ment Health Serv* 1983;21:36–40.

Fagin CM: Psychotherapeutic nursing. *Am J Nurs* 1967; 67:298–304.

Fitzpatrick J, et al: *Nursing Models and Their Psychiatric Mental Health Applications.* Brady, 1982.

Flaskerud JH: The distinctive character of nursing psychotherapy. *Issues Ment Health Nurs* 1984;6:1–19.

Gruber L: The no-demand, third person interview of the non-verbal patient. *Perspect Psychiatr Care* 1977;15:38–39.

Hall E: *The Hidden Dimension.* Doubleday Anchor Books, 1966.

Hardin SB, Durham JD: First rate: Exploring the structure, process, and effectiveness of nurse psychotherapy. *J Psychosoc Nurs Ment Health Serv* 1985;23:9–15.

Heber S, Levin S, Sookram S: The nurse as short-term psychotherapist. *Can Nurse* 1984;80:32–35.

Herron WG, Rouslin S: *Issues in Psychotherapy.* Brady, 1982.

Hoeffer B, Murphy S: The unfinished task: Development of nursing theory for psychiatric and mental health nursing practice. *J Psychosoc Nurs Ment Health Serv* 1982;20:9–14.

Horsfall J: The mental health nurse as therapist. *Aust Nurs J* 1983;12:45–48.

Johnston J: *Nursing Mirror* Mental Health Forum. The nursing process and psychiatry. *Nurs Mirror* 1984;158:i–ii.

Johnson MN: Theoretical basis for nursing diagnosis in mental health nursing. *Issues Ment Health Nurs* 1984;6:53–71.

Kaplan HI, Sadock BJ: *Comprehensive Textbook of Psychiatry,* ed 4. Williams and Wilkins, 1985.

Lakovics M: Classification of countertransference for utilization in supervision. *Am J Psychotherapy* 1983; 37:245–256.

Lathrop V: Aggression as a response. *Perspect Psychiatr Care* 1978;16:202–205.

Lego S: The one-to-one nurse-patient relationship, in Huey F (ed): *Psychiatric Nursing 1946–1974: A Report on the State of the Art.* American Journal of Nursing, 1975.

Lego S: Point/counterpoint: A psychotherapist is a psychotherapist . . ." *Perspect Psychiatr Care* 1980;18:27,39.

Leibenluft E, Goldberg R: Guidelines for short-term inpatient psychotherapies. *Am J Psychiatr* 1986;143(12): 1507–1517.

Lenefsky B, de Palma T, Locicero D: Management of violent behaviors. *Perspect Psychiatr Care* 1978;16:212–217.

Loomis M: Levels of contracting. *J Psychosoc Nurs* 1985;23(3):8–14.

Mellow J: Nursing therapy. *Am J Nurs* 1968;68:2365–2369.

Milne D: "The more things change the more they stay the same": Factors affecting the implementation of the nursing process. *J Adv Nurs* 1985;10:39–45.

Parks S: Allowing physical distance as a nursing approach. *Perspect Psychiatr Care* 1966;4:31–35.

Pelletier LR: Nurse-psychotherapists: Whom do they treat? *Hosp Community Psychiatry* 1984;35:1149–1150.

Peplau H: *Interpersonal Relations in Nursing.* Putnam, 1952.

Peplau H: Interpersonal techniques: The crux of psychiatric nursing. *Am J Nurs* 1962;62:50–54.

Quinn P: The new psychotherapists. *Nurs Times* 1985; 81:28–30.

Robitaille-Tremblay M: A data collection tool for the psychiatric nurse. *Can Nurse* 1984;81:26–31.

Scott DJ, Philip AE: Attitudes of psychiatric nurses to treatment and patients. *Br J Med Psychol* 1985;58:169–173.

Schuable P, Pierce R: Client in-therapy behavior: A therapist guide to progress. *Psychotherapy* 1974;11:229–234.

Spunt JP, Durham JD, Hardin SB: Theoretical models and interventions used by nurse psychotherapists. *Issues Ment Health Nurs* 1984;6:35–51.

Stanly R: Evaluation of treatment goals: The use of goal attainment scaling. *J Adv Nurs* 1984;9(4):351–356.

Steward A: Handling the aggressive patient. *Perspect Psychiatr Care* 1978;16:228–232.

Strupp HH, Blackwood GL: Recent methods of psychotherapy, in Kaplan HI, Sadock BJ: *Comprehensive Textbook of Psychiatry,* ed 4. Williams and Wilkins, 1985.

Trotter CMT: I never promised you a rose garden . . . but I must remember to tell you about the thorns. *J Psychosoc Nurs* 1985;23(3):15–17.

Ursano R, Hales R: A review of brief individual psychotherapies. *Am J Psychiatry* 1986;143(12):1507–1517.

Ward M: The nursing process in psychiatry. I. The teachers' dilemma. *Nurs Times* 1985;80(24):37–39.

Witherspoon V: Using Lakovic's system. Countertransference classifications. *J Psychosoc Nurs Ment Health Serv* 1985;23:30–34.

Wolberg L: *The Technique of Psychotherapy,* vols 1 and 2. Grune and Stratton, 1977.

TWENTY-EIGHT

Stress Management

Carol Ren Kneisl

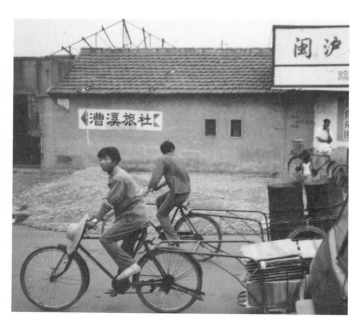

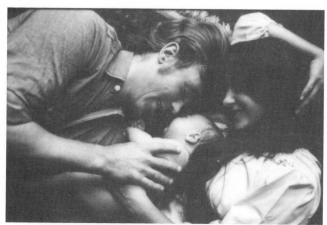

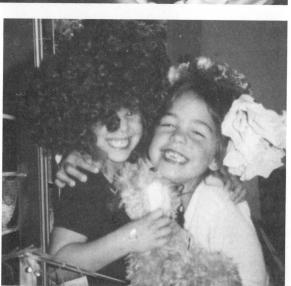

After reading this chapter, students should be able to

- Discuss the bases on which stress management techniques appear to be effective

- Enumerate the therapeutic uses of each of the stress management techniques discussed in this chapter

- Describe the stress management techniques discussed in this chapter

- Practice stress management strategies before using them with clients

- Apply stress management strategies to the care of clients in psychiatric settings

- Apply stress management strategies to the care of clients in other health care settings

- Apply stress management techniques at a personal level to enhance personal and professional functioning

- Teach clients and their families how to use stress management techniques to promote, maintain, and restore emotional well-being.

Cross References

Other topics relevant to this content are: Anxiety disorders, Chapter 19; Psychophysiologic disorders, Chapter 23; Psychotropic medications that may cause hypotension during stress reduction exercises, Chapter 32; Role of stress, anxiety, and coping, Chapter 7.

Nurses' Alliance for Prevention of Nuclear War, Amnesty International, Physicians for Social Responsibility, and Beyond War are some of the organizations that are concerned with the danger of increasing militarization of the world and are committed to nonviolent methods of solving conflicts.

active progressive relaxation
alternate-nostril breathing
autogenic training
bioenergetics
biofeedback
body scanning
deep breathing
irrational self-talk
mantra

meditation
passive progressive relaxation
rolfing
self-hypnosis
therapeutic touch
thought stopping
visualization

Helping clients to manage stress creatively and helping nurses to manage their own stress creatively are the subjects of this chapter. Although no one can escape all the stresses of life completely, one can learn to counteract habitual counterproductive responses to them. Being able to relax decreases the alarm response to stress and returns the body to a more normal or balanced state.

Although we do not know exactly how stress-reduction techniques work, research shows that most persons find them helpful. These techniques help people gain control of their lives and ease tension before it becomes unmanageable. As a result, the quality of their lives is enhanced.

The techniques described in this chapter can be used by nurses in any setting. Other techniques such as autogenic training, self-hypnosis, and biofeedback require additional training or equipment and are discussed only briefly in this chapter. To learn more about them, refer to the references at the end of this chapter. This chapter explores stress-reduction techniques that go beyond the everyday ways to cope with stress discussed in Chapter 7.

THE NURSING ROLE IN THE CREATIVE MANAGEMENT OF STRESS

Stress management is a creative and powerful tool as long as clients learn to use the methods properly. Unfortunately, many clients do not reduce the stresses in their lives because they do not realize that they are at the mercy of involuntary *fight-or-flight* responses. Many fail to identify environmental, physiologic, or cognitive sources of stress.

Like clients in any other health care setting, psychiatric clients must endure time pressures, weather, noise, crowds, interpersonal demands, job performance demands, and various threats to security and self-esteem. Genetics,

Portions of this chapter appeared in Kneisl CR, Ames SW: *Adult Health Nursing: A Biopsychosocial Approach.* Addison-Wesley, 1986.

developmental changes, biochemical makeup, aging, illness, nutrition, and sleep patterns are some of the physiologic factors influencing how well people cope with stress. And, perhaps more than clients in many of the other settings in which nurses practice, psychiatric clients experience cognitive stress because of how they interpret and label their experiences. For instance, a client might interpret the boss's facial expression as amused rather than pleased or as disgruntled rather than quizzical. This interpretation is likely to provoke anxiety. Dwelling on one's concerns and anxieties causes physical tension in the body, which in turn creates the subjective feeling of uneasiness and leads to more anxious thoughts.

The nurse should begin with the assessment phase of the nursing process to identify clients who might benefit from stress-management techniques. Assessment of stress and anxiety are discussed in Chapter 7. Once assessment has been accomplished, nurses can play a significant role in making clients aware of these methods and facilitating their effective use. Of course, if planning to use these techniques to help others who are experiencing stress, nurses must first develop personal familiarity with them.

Monitoring Physical Problems

Anyone undergoing a stress-reduction program should first discuss the program with the health care provider monitoring any physical problems. Because these techniques lower the blood pressure, decrease the heart rate, and reduce pain and anxiety, persons beginning a stress-reduction program should have their medications closely monitored. Monitoring is particularly important for psychiatric clients receiving psychotropic medications that may cause hypotension.

Experimenting with What Works

It is not necessary to use every suggestion or technique in this chapter. If a particular technique for stress reduction or relaxation doesn't seem to help, move on to another one. What is important is to give each a fair trial and experiment to find out what works in each person's individual situation.

Enhancing Chances of Success

Stress management is not magical; one has to work at it and enhance chances of success through regular practice.

It is unrealistic to expect that simply reading about these techniques is all that is required to use them in times of stress or that everyone will be able to make a commitment to daily practice. Nurses can make it easier for clients to make the commitment and to follow through by:

- Recommending stress-reduction strategies to clients and their families.

- Providing information about stress-reduction strategies that are likely to meet the client's specific needs.

- Encouraging the client to make the decision to practice relaxation.

- Encouraging the client to take this time for himself or herself alone.

- Enlisting the support of family members, fellow workers, and friends in meeting the client's need for uninterrupted time in a quiet setting.

- Encouraging family members, fellow workers, and friends to lend verbal support to the client.

- Reminding family members, fellow workers, and friends that because they are also under stress, they too may find relaxation techniques helpful.

Enhancing Relaxation with Music

Many persons find that listening to certain kinds of music is relaxing. Dentists have used music to help their clients relax and to mask the sounds of the drill. Several health care facilities use soothing music in conjunction with guided visualizations on audiotape or videotape as a substitute for pain medication and tranquilizers when the client chooses. Sometimes the tapes are prescribed before or during surgery, during chemotherapy or kidney dialysis, and during recovery from spinal injury or burns.

The therapeutic use of music has led to a new health-related career. Music therapists use a combination of visual imagery and music to teach clients to lower their blood pressure ten to twenty points. Music with sixty beats per minute can help those with cardiac dysrhythmias achieve a more relaxed heart rate.

How does music achieve its relaxing effect? One theory is that music produces endorphins in the brain—the same "feel-good" chemicals that running and meditation produce. These natural opiates, secreted by the hypothalamus, reduce the intensity with which pain is felt.

Because persons vary in their response to music, encourage clients to experiment with different kinds of music to discover which has positive effects and then to develop their own personal library. Tapes and records specifically for stress reduction are sold in bookstores and through catalogs. They are often available through the public library. Recommend that clients pay attention to their breathing as they listen to music. Slow and deep breathing enhances the relaxing effect of music.

Assessing Body Tension

Many persons fail to recognize stress in themselves. They direct their attention externally rather than internally. Because stress and body tension are simultaneous, one of the first steps in recognizing stress is to recognize tension in the body. Recognizing body tension helps people recognize stress and anxiety. **Body scanning** helps increase awareness of muscular tension.

Make sure that the spine is straight before beginning body scanning or any of the other exercises described in this chapter. Stand, sit, or lie on the floor—whichever is most comfortable—while maintaining good posture (Figure 28–1).

Begin by closing your eyes and turning your attention to your own internal world by focusing on your body. Focus on your toes and move up slowly. As you do this, ask yourself: Where am I tense? Become aware of all of the muscles in your body and especially of the parts of your body that feel tense or tight. Note the location of the tenseness and talk to yourself about it, reminding yourself that muscular tension is self-produced. Perhaps you might say: "The muscles in the back of my neck feel tight. This means that I'm creating tension in my body. Tension causes me problems."

Body scanning should be a prelude to the stress-reduction techniques that follow. Use the body-scanning method to determine where tension collects in your body.

The importance of body states and their relationship to stress have been emphasized by eastern philosophies

such as yoga and zen. In this century, Western psychiatrists were persuaded to study this interaction by Wilhelm Reich, originally a student of Freud. Two contemporary therapies that focus on the body and its relationship to emotional stress are the bioenergetic therapy of Alexander Lowen and the gestalt therapy of Fritz Perls. Both emphasize the notion that the body registers stress long before the conscious mind does.

According to Lowen, body tension is an inevitable response to stress. Once stress is removed, tension goes away. In Lowen's theory, specific muscle groups are tightened by specific attitudes. For example, chronic neck tension and pain can occur in a person who believes that it is bad to express anger.

According to Perls, it is important to differentiate between external awareness (stimulation of the five senses from the outside world) and internal awareness (physical sensations or emotional discomfort or comfort within the body). This distinction helps people separate the world from one's physical reaction to it. Perls believes that we fail to feel the tension in our bodies because we direct most of our awareness to the outside world. Recognizing the tension in our bodies is the first step in reducing stress.

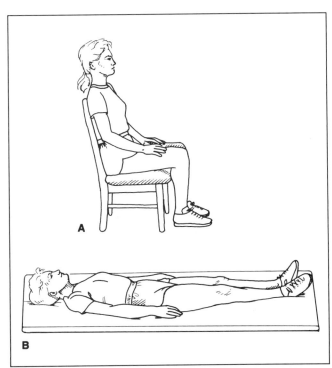

Figure 28–1
Body postures for stress-reduction exercises. A, Sitting. B, Lying.
Source: Kneisl CR, Ames SW: Adult Health Nursing: A Biopsychosocial Approach. Addison-Wesley, 1986, p 67.

Keeping a Stress-Awareness Diary

Most people find that some parts of the day are more stressful than others and that some events produce more physical and emotional symptoms than others. Keeping a stress-awareness diary helps people identify how particular stresses result in predictable symptoms. Some persons react to interpersonal confrontations with a stomach upset or with diarrhea. Feeling rushed or overloaded with tasks or responsibilities may result in vasoconstriction and cause a headache or hypertension.

Clients can keep a stress-awareness diary to discover and chart their own personal stressful events and characteristic reactions. In the sample stress-awareness diary in Figure 28–2, a gasoline station manager records the events of a Friday. Note that it indicates the time that a stressful event took place as well as any physical or emotional reactions that could be related to the stressful event. Clients should keep a stress-awareness diary for at least two weeks, tracking this information daily.

STRESS-MANAGEMENT TECHNIQUES

The stress-management techniques that follow are based on the belief that mind and body are interrelated and that

Stress Awareness Diary

Date ___5/6/88___ Day of the week _Friday_

Time	Stressful Event	Physical and Emotional Reactions
6⁵⁰ AM	Alarm didn't go off; rushing to get to work	
7⁴⁵ AM	Late to relieve night clerk; he threatened to quit	
9³⁰		Slight headache; took aspirin
10⁰⁰		Headache pounding; aspirin not helping
11⁰⁰	Customer backs into gas pump & dents pump	Anger
2³⁰	Teenager drives away without paying for gas	Anger
3³⁰		Headache back
4⁰⁰	Employee calls in sick; have to call in relief worker	
5³⁰	Commute traffic heavy; twice as long to get home	Indigestion
7⁰⁰	Argument with son	
7⁰⁵	Wife defends son	
7¹⁰	Argument with wife	
7³⁰		Indigestion worse
8³⁰		Went to bed

Figure 28–2
Stress-awareness diary.

the condition of one will eventually affect the condition of the other. A relaxed body is incompatible with anxiety. If the body is relaxed, the mind will feel relaxed as well. These stress-management techniques teach you how to relax in order to enhance your personal life and your professional life as a nurse. You can then teach these relaxation techniques to clients in any type of health care setting.

Breathing Exercises

Under most circumstances, people take breathing for granted as an automatic body function. They usually become aware of their pattern of breathing only when it has gone awry, such as when they are out of breath. Nurses notice the apneic client or the client with Cheyne-Stokes respirations because they know something has gone wrong and that breathing is essential to life. Breathing properly can, by itself, reduce stress. Psychiatric nurses and maternal health nurses who prepare expectant women for labor have long recognized that breathing exercises can reduce tension. Unfortunately, breathing techniques are virtually ignored in other clinical areas.

Breathing calmly and deeply keeps the blood well oxygenated and purified. It helps to remove waste materials from the blood and clears thinking. Poorly oxygenated blood may contribute to fatigue, mental confusion, anxiety, muscular tension, and feelings of depression. The following exercises are designed to facilitate proper breathing.

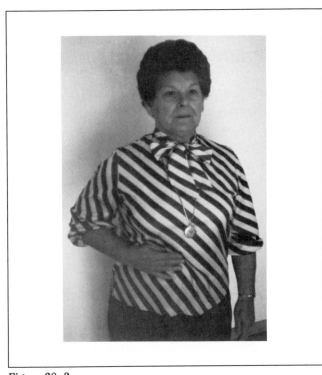

Figure 28–3
Breathing awareness.
Source: Kneisl CR, Ames SW: Adult Health Nursing: A Biopsychosocial Approach. *Addison-Wesley, 1986, p 68.*

Awareness of Breathing

Do you breathe properly or does your breathing actually deprive you of oxygen? Take time to pay attention to your own breathing, just as the person in Figure 28–3 is doing. Begin by placing one hand just below your rib cage and taking a deep breath. Note what happened when you inhaled. Did your hand move in? Did your hand move out? Did your hand move at all? If your hand moved out, you were breathing properly. But if your hand moved in or didn't move at all it was probably because you learned, as most did, to hold your stomach in and push your chest out while breathing. People who breathe this way do not fill the lungs to full capacity; they fill only the top third or top half.

Deep Breathing

During deep breathing, you move the diaphragm downward and fill the lower part of the lungs with air. The chest expands as the middle part fills with air, and the shoulders move upward as the upper part fills. To teach yourself or a client how to take deep, healthful breaths follow the directions in Box 28–1.

Deep breathing becomes easier with practice. It may become almost automatic. This is an exercise few resist— it is easy to do, it is inconspicuous, and it gives fast results.

Ten-to-One Count

This exercise is also quick and simple. Inhale, taking a deep breath, while saying the number 10 to yourself. Then exhale slowly, letting out all the air in your lungs. Inhale again saying the number 9 to yourself. As you exhale, tell yourself: "I feel more relaxed than I did at number 10." With your next breath, say the number 8 to yourself. As you exhale remind yourself: "I feel more relaxed than I did at number 9." Continue counting down and experience increasing calmness as you approach the number 1. Some persons use an abbreviated version and begin counting at the number 5; others require the full count of 10 to feel calm.

Alternate-Nostril Breathing

Although somewhat more difficult, **alternate-nostril breathing** also helps to reduce tension and sinus head-

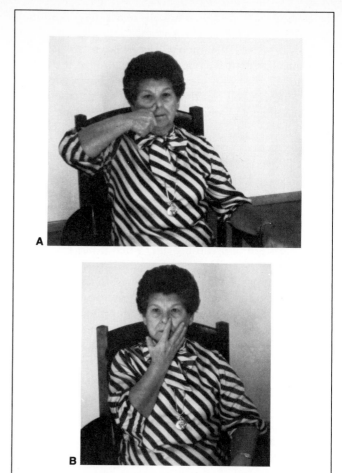

Box 28–1
DEEP-BREATHING GUIDELINES

1. Sit, stand, or lie with your spine straight.

2. Scan for body tension.

3. Place one hand on your chest and the other on your abdomen.

4. Inhale slowly and deeply so that your abdomen pushes up your hand.

5. Visualize your lungs slowly filling with air. Your chest should move only slightly as you inhale, but you should be aware of the movement of your abdomen.

6. Exhale through your mouth, making a soft, whooshing sound by blowing gently. Keep your face, mouth, and jaw relaxed.

7. Be aware of what it feels like and what you sound like when you breathe properly.

8. Continue to take long, slow, deep breaths for at least 10 minutes at a time, once or twice a day.

9. Increase the frequency if you wish once you have mastered the technique.

10. Scan your body for tension again, comparing the tension to what it was like before you began the deep-breathing exercise.

Source: Kneisl CR, Ames SW: Adult Health Nursing: A Biopsychosocial Approach. Addison-Wesley, 1986, p 68.

Figure 28–4
Alternate-nostril breathing. A, Inhale through the left nostril slowly and quietly while using the thumb to keep the right nostril tightly closed. B, Use the index finger to close the left nostril, and exhale through the right nostril. Then inhale through the right nostril and repeat A and B.
Source: Kneisl CR, Ames SW: Adult Health Nursing: A Biopsychosocial Approach. Addison-Wesley, 1986, p 69.

aches. First, close off your right nostril by lightly pressing it with your right thumb. Now inhale through your left nostril as slowly and quietly as possible, as the woman in Figure 28–4 is doing. Remove your thumb from the right nostril and use your forefinger to close off the left nostril. Now exhale slowly through your right nostril. Inhale through your right nostril as slowly and quietly as possible and follow the same procedure outlined above, closing your right nostril with your right thumb while simultaneously exhaling through your left nostril.

The basic cycle for alternate-nostril breathing should begin with ten breaths and can be increased up to twenty-five breaths. It may be easier to breathe through the right nostril at certain times of the day and through the left nostril at other times. The reason is that people breathe primarily through one nostril for approximately four hours, then breathe primarily through the other for the next four hours.

Progressive Relaxation

Progressive relaxation is based on a theory developed in 1929 by Chicago physician Edmund Jacobsen. The technique of progressive relaxation is based on the premise that muscle tension is the body's physiologic response to anxiety-provoking thoughts. Muscular tension increases the feeling of anxiety and reinforces it. Deep muscle relaxation, by contrast, decreases physiologic tension and blocks anxiety.

Progressive relaxation decreases pulse and respiratory rates, blood pressure, and perspiration. In addition, it helps to reduce anxiety. Clients with muscle spasms, low back pain, tension headaches, insomnia, anxiety, depression, fatigue, irritable bowel, hypertension, or mild phobias are among those who can achieve positive results using this technique.

It may take longer to master progressive relaxation than the deep breathing stress-reduction techniques discussed earlier in this chapter. With practice, one can learn to relax faster and easier.

Active Progressive Relaxation

Active progressive relaxation helps people identify which muscles or muscle groups are chronically tense by distinguishing between sensations of tension (purposeful muscle tensing) and deep relaxation (a conscious relaxing of the muscles). Each muscle or muscle grouping is tensed for five to seven seconds and then relaxed for twenty to thirty seconds. This cycle is repeated. Four major muscle groups are covered—hands, forearms, and biceps; head, face, throat, and shoulders; chest, abdomen, and lower back; thighs, buttocks, calves, and feet. Use the instructions in Box 28–2 as a guide to a typical exercise. This guide was written by a nurse (Flynn 1980) who uses these principles in her clinical practice.

Counsel clients to observe some cautions while carrying out this technique. The muscles of the neck and back should not be excessively tightened to avoid soft-tissue and spinal injury. Tightening the muscles of the toes and feet too vigorously could also result in uncomfortable muscle cramps.

Practice progressive relaxation while lying down or seated in a chair with a head support. Remember to check for muscle groups that are only partially relaxed and return to them to bring about deeper relaxation.

Passive Progressive Relaxation

In passive progressive relaxation, the muscles are not tensed. The goal is to relax the muscles without first tightening them. The sequence in which body parts are relaxed differs from that of the active progressive method. Begin with muscles easiest to relax (in the toes) and progress to muscles most difficult to relax (in the head). The sequence is:

- Feet
- Lower legs
- Knees and upper legs
- Hips and buttocks
- Lower back
- Lower arms and hands
- Chest and diaphragm
- Abdomen
- Pelvis and genitals
- Neck
- Forehead and upper face
- Mouth and jaw

Some report feeling less alert after either active or passive progressive relaxation. When alertness is important, one of the other exercises is probably better.

Visualization

A French pharmacist, Emil Coue, began to use the power of imagination with clients around the turn of the century. Carl Jung used it in his psychiatric practice in the early part of the century. Most recently, Carl Simonton and Stephanie Matthews Simonton have had remarkable success in treating cancer clients with visualization. Author Norman Cousins has written of his control over serious illness by using the healing power of his own imagination.

Positive visualizations use a person's own imagination and positive thinking to reduce stress or promote healing. It was Coue who asked his clients to repeat this now-famous phrase twenty times to themselves on awakening: *"Every day in every way I am getting better and better."* He believed that predicting failure or success in advance was bound to make it happen. Thus, positive visualizations anticipating success reduce stress. Visualization should be used in conjunction with the body-scanning and deep-breathing exercises discussed earlier.

Not everyone finds using the imagination in this way easy, and the technique may not work for everyone. Constructing a detailed, effective visualization requires time, patience, and practice.

Visualization for Relaxation

Relaxing through visualizing is enhanced by constructing in one's own mind a relaxing environment. Some find the soothing sounds of a seashore calming; others prefer to imagine themselves floating above the world on a soft cloud or a magic carpet. Still others relax as they imagine themselves descending on a slow-moving escalator into a calmer and more relaxed state.

If visualization seems difficult (and if a warm bath, hot tub, or swimming pool is relaxing) try constructing a visualization while in warm water, combining the physiologic effects of the warm water with the products of the imagination (see Box 28–3).

Visualization for Symptom Control or Healing

Although visualization techniques for symptom control or healing are practiced in a variety of health care settings

Box 28–2
ACTIVE PROGRESSIVE RELAXATION EXERCISE

Sit or lie in a comfortable position and let your eyes close.

I take a moment to be here (allow time).

I focus my attention on my right hand, and I make a fist.

Slowly and steadily, I clench my fist and study the tension.

Now I let go and feel the difference.

I repeat that.

I clench my fist, tightly, feeling the tension.

I let go and enjoy the contrast in my feelings.

Now I tense my right forearm.

Studying the tension.

And let go and notice the difference.

Now I tense my biceps—tighten.

And let go.

I stretch my arm straight out and feel the tension in my arm and shoulder.

I let go and appreciate the difference.

Now I focus my attention on my left hand, and I make a fist.

Slowly and steadily, I clench my fist and study the tension.

Now I let go and feel the difference.

I do that again.

Clenching my fist, tightly, feeling the tension.

And let go and enjoy the contrast in my feelings.

Now I tense my left forearm.

Studying the tension.

And let go and notice the difference.

Now I tense my biceps—tighten.

And let go.

I stretch my arm straight out and feel the tension in my arm and shoulder.

I let go and appreciate the difference.

I focus my attention on my scalp.

I tighten it.

And now I smooth it out.

I pay attention to the muscles of my forehead—I frown.

And study the tension as I frown.

I let go and notice the difference.

(continued next column)

I raise my eyebrows and hold them for a few seconds.

And let go.

Now the muscles around my eyes—I tense and tighten them.

And let go.

The muscles of my cheeks, I tighten them.

And release, acknowledging the difference.

Now I tighten my jaw muscles, tighter—

And let go.

I bring my tongue to the roof of my mouth and tighten it.

And let go.

I let it relax.

And now the muscles in the back of my neck—I tighten those.

I feel the tension, and now I let it go.

I pull my shoulders back and up and tighten the muscles between my shoulders.

Tighten and notice the tension.

And let go.

Now I tighten the muscles of my upper back.

Tighten—and let go.

I focus my attention now on the muscles of my lower back.

I tighten them and notice the tension and

Let go.

Now the muscles of my buttocks.

Tighten—feel the tension.

And let go.

Breathing easily and calmly, deeply and efficiently.

I bring my attention to the muscles of the front of my neck.

I tighten them, bringing my chin up.

And let go.

Now I tighten my chest muscles—tighten.

And let go.

I let myself take in a good deep breath and hold it, feeling all my muscles expand.

And now I let go—letting all the breath out.

continued

Box 28–2 (continued)

I repeat this and notice my feelings.

I tense the muscles of my abdomen.

I tighten them and notice the tension.

And let go and appreciate the relaxation.

And my pelvic muscles—I tighten them—tight.

And let go.

My thighs—I tighten those muscles.

And let go noticing the difference.

Now the muscles of my calves and lower legs.

I tense them tighter and note the tension.

And let go.

(continued next column)

And the muscles of my feet—tighten them.

Letting go and appreciating the difference.

And now I take a moment to scan my body—noticing any part of my body that still needs relaxation.

And I tense that part and let go.

Any other muscles—I take a moment to tense them.

And let go.

And now feeling the pleasure of this relaxation, I take a few moments to bring my attention back to this time and this place, and filled with energy and peace I open my eyes, stretch, and get up.

Source: Flynn PAR: Holistic Health: The Art and Science of Care. Brady, 1980, pp. 165–167. By permission of Appleton & Lange.

around the country, they should be part of a well-rounded health program. For example, visualization can be used with conventional medical treatment for cancer clients and with preoperative clients to control postoperative pain and enhance tissue healing. Persons with vascular problems—migraine headache, hypertension, or Raynaud's disease—benefit from visualization. Allergies, asthma, rheumatoid arthritis, gastritis, colitis, peptic ulcer, insomnia, depression, and chronic pain all respond to visualization. Two sample visualizations for the reduction of pain are in Table 28–1.

Meditation

Meditation is a kind of self-discipline that helps one to achieve inner peace and harmony by focusing uncritically on one thing at a time. Meditation has been associated with various religious doctrines and philosophies for thousands of years. It is seen as a way of becoming one with God or the universe, finding enlightenment, and achieving such virtues as selflessness. However, the person who practices meditation need not associate it with religion or philosophy. It can be practiced as a means of reducing inner discord and increasing self-knowledge.

The state of meditation is equivalent to a state of deep rest. The heart rate slows, the body uses less oxygen, and blood lactate—a waste product of metabolism—decreases sharply. Alpha waves, which characterize brain activity during states of calm alertness, increase.

Meditation seems to have long-standing effects as well. Stress-related problems such as insomnia and asthma diminish. It has been used successfully in the prevention and treatment of hypertension, heart disease, and stroke. Meditation has also helped people decrease their consumption of food, alcohol, tobacco, and drugs and curtail obsessive thinking, anxiety, depression, and hostility. It also improves concentration and attention.

Some theorists believe that meditation quiets the brain, as the person makes contact with more orderly and coherent levels of the mind. The left hemisphere, thought to be responsible for rational and logical thinking, comes into electrical balance with the underdeveloped right hemisphere, thought to modulate intuition, holistic comprehension, and artistic qualities.

Meditation exercises can be relatively easy to learn. Some people experience immediate relief and pleasure in only one session. To experience deeper effects, the person needs to practice meditation regularly for at least a month.

The four major requirements of meditation are:

1. A quiet place
2. A comfortable position
3. An object or thought to dwell on
4. A passive attitude

Box 28–3
VISUALIZATION FOR THE BATH

In a warm bath, it is difficult to worry or to sustain an anxiety attack. The body feels lighter, muscles are relaxed by the heat and movement of the water, and circulation is increased. Being in warm water for a half hour will lower the blood pressure and slow down your breathing. Though the effects will be the opposite for the first two minutes and you may feel stimulated, the calming properties of warm water will soon soothe you.

This visualization can be used in a bathtub, hot tub, heated swimming pool, or any warm body of water. The temperature should not be over 103°F, and you should not stay in the water for longer than thirty minutes. If you are alone, ask someone to call you on the phone after one-half hour or set a music alarm to rouse you. Turn out the lights and light a candle or use a small night light.

Get into a comfortable position, either reclining or sitting. Be sure that your back is supported and your breathing unconstricted. Take a full, deep breath and exhale fully and completely. Slowly close your eyes and feel your heart beating strongly and then begin to slow down. Let your thoughts just drift through your consciousness, as you allow them to leave with the warm air. Imagine that with each and every breath, you can breathe away tension or anxiety, as you allow yourself to relax more and more. All the day's burdens, worries, and expectations are leaving your consciousness and evaporating with the hot, moist steam. Feel your arms floating on the water, and the warm, soothing water gently lifting and caressing your body. As you continue to breathe slowly and naturally, let go of any thoughts still remaining in your mind. Watch as your thoughts flow through you and out of you, and see them disappear into the air, leaving your mind clear and calm.

Gently turn your attention to your body, and scan your body for any tension that you might still be holding. Allow it to leave with the next exhalation, as the warm water evaporates into steam. As you continue to breathe slowly and calmly, turn your awareness to your feet and to your legs. The water tenderly massages your legs and your feet, as the tension flows through you and out of you. With your next breath, breathe away any tightness still remaining in your feet. Move your attention to your abdomen and your chest, allowing the muscles to just let go, and the tension to melt away from your body. Feel your abdomen and your chest relax, as you gently loosen all the muscles and just breathe away any remaining tension. Focus on relaxing your arms and your hands, letting the muscles go completely loose and limp. Relax your fingers, and your hands, and let the feeling of deep relaxation spread up into your arms. Breathe away any tension still remaining.

Now, relax the muscles of your shoulders and your neck, and feel the heaviness gradually increase throughout your musculature, as all your muscles just let go. The muscles in your back go loose and limp, as the water gently supports your whole body. Allow the relaxation to spread to your head and your face, and the muscles around your eyes, in your jaw, your tongue, and in your forehead. Let yourself drift deeper into a dreamlike state of calm relaxation.

Imagine that the blue water becomes the sky, and the soft clouds gently support you as you drift up above the trees. You no longer feel the weight of your head upon your shoulders, and gravity no longer ties you to the earth. The warm, soft, billowy, pink clouds support you as the sun's gentle heat penetrates through any remaining tension. As you peacefully float through the warm air, the golden sun fills your body with warming heat and light. This golden light penetrates through any tension still remaining in your body. As you free-float in space, your body is becoming lighter and lighter.

When you have floated as high as you wish, you become still, and the clouds gently cradle you in the warmth of the sun's golden rays. The golden sun finds any tension still remaining in your body, and dissolves it in the warm, glowing light. Whenever you are ready, you may return. Feel the warm, pink clouds transform into water, and become aware of the water gently cradling you. Take a few, deep breaths, becoming more and more aware of your surroundings. When you are ready to become fully alert, take a full, deep breath and gently open your eyes on the exhalation. Take a few more deep breaths, and slowly get out of the water, gently drying yourself and feeling the relaxation throughout your body.

Source: Reprinted with permission from Mason JL: Guide to Stress Reduction. *Celestial Arts, 1986, pp 61–63. © 1980, 1986, Celestial Arts, Box 7327, Berkeley, CA 94707.*

The environment for meditation should be one that minimizes distractions—a quiet place set aside as a haven from the urgencies of everyday life. A comfortable position that can be held for twenty minutes without stress facilitates meditation. Some possible positions are illustrated in Figure 28–5. Avoid meditating within two hours of a heavy meal since digestion interferes with the ability to relax. Something to dwell on—e.g., a repeated word, an object

Table 28–1
Visualization for Relief from Pain

Alternative I	Alternative II
Imagine that your body is filled with orange and blue lights.	Concentrate on the part of your body where the pain exists.
The orange lights signify areas of pain or tension.	Attach a symbolic visual image to the pain (a knot in your stomach, a hammer pounding your head).
The blue lights signify pain-free or calm areas.	
Imagine changing the orange lights to blue lights.	Imagine the symbol being relaxed, becoming looser, getting smaller or weaker as you feel your pain becoming less and less.
Note that the pain is going away and that you're feeling more and more relaxed.	

Source: Kneisl CR, Ames SW: Adult Health Nursing: A Biopsychosocial Approach. *Addison-Wesley, 1986, p 71.*

or symbol to look at or think about, or a specific thought or feeling—helps keep distracting thoughts from entering the mind. A passive attitude requires understanding that thoughts and distractions will occur and can be cleared from the mind. If they occur, they should be noted and let go without concern about their interference. It is counterproductive to worry about how well you are doing at meditating.

Some of the stress-management techniques discussed earlier—body scanning, the breathing ten-to-one count, and visualization—can satisfy the requirement of an object

to dwell on. Many people who meditate prefer to use a **mantra**, a syllable, word, or name that is repeatedly chanted aloud. Some teachers of meditation insist that each person have a special mantra with a specific meaning and vibration to achieve individual effects. Others recommend the use of any word or phrase the individual is drawn to, e.g., *peace, love,* or *calm.* Some popular eastern mantras are *om* (I am), *so-ham* (I am he), and *sa-ham* (I am she). Avoid chanting too loudly or too vigorously. After about five minutes, shift to whispering the mantra as you relax more deeply. When it is not possible to chant aloud, some people chant silently.

The best results from meditation are achieved by persons who meditate for fifteen minutes a day, five to seven days a week for two weeks. After this period of time, the length of the sessions may be increased to thirty minutes if desired.

Therapeutic Touch

Therapeutic touch was developed by Dolores Krieger (1979) as a nursing activity, although the "laying on of hands" to help or heal is as old as history. It is defined as the specific transfer of energy in a therapeutic manner in which some of the excess energies of the healer are directed to the client, or energy is transferred from one place to another within the body of the client. This technique is based on

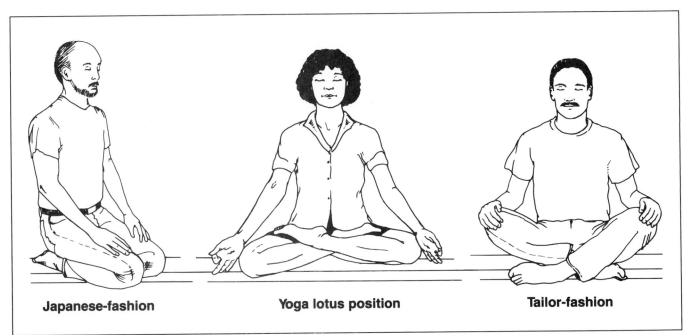

Japanese-fashion **Yoga lotus position** **Tailor-fashion**

Figure 28–5
Meditation postures.

the concept of illness as an imbalance of energies in the body. *Prana* is the subsystem of energy which Krieger believes is the basis of the energy transfer in therapeutic touch. Normally healthy people have an excess of prana, and since each person is an open system, energy can be transferred to another person. This transfer of energy is not a cure but provides an infusion of energy for people depleted by struggles with illness until their own healing processes take over.

Therapeutic touch is a conscious, deliberate act composed of three steps called centering, scanning, and rebalancing. The healer first prepares for the procedure through *centering,* the discovery of an inner physical and psychologic stability in which the healer achieves a sense that all faculties are under command. This gathers and focuses the healer's energies on the client and excludes extraneous thoughts from the mind, a process akin to meditation.

The healer then *scans* the client from head to foot without actually touching his or her body, attempting to sense temperature changes or feelings of pressure. These areas indicate a static condition, an imbalance, or congestion in the client's energy field.

Intervention consists of mobilizing or *rebalancing* these congested areas. The healer places his or her hands, with palms facing away from the client, in the area where pressure is felt and moves the hands away from the client's body in a sweeping gesture while consciously directing a flow of energy to the client, a process called *unruffling the field.* Therapists report relief of the sense of pressure they feel in problematic areas of the client's body and consider the treatment complete when they no longer perceive an imbalance in the person's symmetry.

Clients report a sense of relaxation and relief from pain. Krieger (1979) has demonstrated experimentally that therapeutic touch has produced a significant change in the hemoglobin component of red blood cells. Advocates of therapeutic touch have found that the freeing of bound energy is not long lasting but that it does seem to facilitate the repatterning of energy necessary for healing. However, the published research literature indicates that empirical support for the practice of therapeutic touch is, at best, weak (Clark and Clark 1984).

Rolfing

Rolfing, or structural integration, is based on the belief that psychologic conflicts are recorded and perpetuated in the body. Ida Rolf (1977), the founder of this therapy, viewed the body as an area of energy within the earth's gravitational field. To function properly, a person must be in correct alignment with the forces of gravity. When the body is in an incorrect position, the myofascia or connective tissue that supports the body weight shortens and undergoes metabolic changes that decrease its energy and interfere with free movement.

Many people are not in proper relationship to the field of gravity because they have become alienated from their own bodily sensations. At different points in their development, they have responded to inner and outer threats by turning off their responses. They have inhibited those responses by contracting the muscles that are related to the impulse that is being blocked. For example, if the impulse is aggressive, they may contract arm muscles. Repeated inhibition and the resulting muscular contractions produce chronically spastic muscles that inhibit motility. The musculature acts as a repository of stored feelings. Energy that would otherwise be available for conscious use is expended internally to keep these muscles tense.

As people age, their posture becomes a reflection of accumulated unresolved feelings. When people become aware of how they contract their muscles in traumatic situations, they can begin to take responsibility for their own physical structure by experimenting with alternative responses. Gracefulness and unitary movement are signs of personal integration. When a body is coordinated and balanced physically, there is a corresponding emotional balance.

Rolfing is a method of working with the body to achieve a realignment of the body structure. The basic therapy consists of ten one-hour sessions. The rolfer massages and manipulates the client's deep connective tissue. Once this tissue is freed, the body is able to realign itself with gravitational forces. The emotional release and physical healing that often accompany rolfing are not the major goal of therapy. However, they are proof that emotional and physical problems are related to the body's misalignment. Many clients who have been rolfed report they have changed so much that they have difficulty relating to their past environment and must alter their work, interpersonal relationships, and values.

Bioenergetics

Alexander Lowen (1967, 1972), founder of the Institute for Bioenergetics, also emphasizes body work. **Bioenergetics** offers techniques for reducing muscular tension through the release of feelings. It makes less use of direct body contact (between client and therapist) than other body therapies, guiding the client instead through a series of exercises and verbal techniques. Stressor and releasor exercises are used to increase the client's awareness of body defenses. The exercises begin with deep breathing and progress to stretching and kicking the limbs. This enables the client to break through muscular rigidity and express feelings previously trapped in habitual postural modes. These modes, which are called *muscular armoring,* prevent the free flow of energy. The theory is comparable to that of other body-mind therapists.

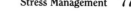
If the body is relatively unalive, perceptions and responses are diminished. People in this situation are often depressed. According to Lowen, depressed people were denied the mother love they needed. Now they have no faith in themselves or in life. They cannot pursue the goals they really wish to achieve, and they are usually unaware of the reasons for their lifelessness. During bioenergetic therapy, these people are encouraged to make deep contact with their feelings of sadness. Lowen discusses a client with chronic depression who benefited by a session of screaming and kicking. Her depression lifted as she went through this series of exercises and was able to release her emotional controls. The intense energy that had previously been immobilized in depression became available to her. Lowen emphasizes that clients must break through frozen emotions by themselves and thus become able to care for themselves in the way their parents failed to do.

Lowen also thinks that the study of *auras,* or energy fields around the body, can be used to diagnose disturbances in body functioning. In the energy field of a person with schizophrenia, for example, a trained observer can see characteristic alterations, such as interruptions of energy flow or color changes. Different parts of each person's body radiate different kinds of feelings. When chronic muscle tension blocks energy, negative feelings result. The head, neck, and shoulders can radiate openness and affirmation or express hostility and holding back. The belly can radiate pleasure and laughter or suffering. The legs can radiate security and balance or instability. When there are no constrictions that disturb energy flow, the feeling is positive, the personality is integrated, and the aura is bright and intense.

People excite and depress each other through their energy fields. People with strong energy fields influence others in a positive way. We are in touch with others only when our energy contacts and excites their energy. Bioenergetics attempts to facilitate this free flow of energy through exercises.

Autogenic Training

Autogenic training is used across the country in stress-reduction and holistic health centers to teach self-regulation of the autonomic nervous system. It has its origins in the research done by Oskar Vogt, a brain physiologist who worked in Berlin in the last decade of the nineteenth century. Johannes Schutz, a Berlin psychiatrist, combined Vogt's research into the effects of hypnosis on the brain with some yoga techniques and published his first work on autogenic training in 1932. Wolfgang Luthe brought autogenic training to the United States in 1969. In its contemporary form, autogenic training does not require a hypnotist. Most individuals can learn autogenic exercises in four to ten months through a systematic training program or a written course of study.

Autogenic training is based on the achievement of six physiologic outcomes:

1. Heaviness in the extremities
2. Warmth in the extremities
3. Regulation of the heartbeat

RESEARCH NOTE

Citation

Carter MA: An experimental trial of therapeutic touch in the treatment of arthritis. West J Nurs Res *1983; 5(3):56–64.*

Study Problem/Purpose

The purpose of this study was to see if the use of therapeutic touch by nurses would increase the range of motion of joints and decrease pain in persons with arthritis.

Methods

This study used an experimental design. Subjects were drawn from a convenience group of clients from an ambulatory, senior citizen practice of nurse faculty. Twenty-eight subjects (14 control and 14 experimental) were selected from subjects who volunteered for the study. All subjects had a diagnosis of arthritis and were taking at least one drug for arthritis daily. The range of motion of shoulders, knees, and hips was measured for each subject. Level of pain was assessed by a linear scale from $0 =$ no pain to $10 =$ the worst pain ever experienced. The experimental group then received 15 minutes of therapeutic touch from a nurse experienced in this modality. The pulses of the control group were taken in their wrists, ankles, and knees by the same nurse who performed therapeutic touch for the experimental group. The pulse-taking procedures also took 15 minutes. All subjects were remeasured for range of motion and level of pain. Data were analyzed by use of repeated measures ANOVA.

Findings

No significant differences were found between pretest and posttest or between experimental and control groups for range of motion or level of pain.

Conclusions and Implications

Therapeutic touch did not produce an immediate effect measured by changes in range of motion or levels of pain. Of interest were subjects who said that therapeutic touch made them "feel better" and yet showed no changed in range of motion or pain levels.

4. Regulation of breathing
5. Abdominal warmth
6. Cooling of the forehead

Once clients learn to perform the six standard exercises designed to achieve these results, they may go on to learn meditative exercises specifically developed for each client or neutralization exercises to promote abreaction and verbalization.

Autogenic training has proved helpful for the following problems:

- Hyperventilation and asthma
- Gastrointestinal problems, e.g., constipation, diarrhea, gastritis, ulcer, and gastrointestinal spasm
- Cardiovascular problems, e.g., cardiac dysrhythmias and hypertension
- Some thyroid conditions
- Headaches and insufficient circulation to the extremities
- Anxiety, irritability, and fatigue
- Pain
- Sleep disorders

It is not recommended for children under five years of age or for psychotic persons. Persons with serious physical health problems should be under the supervision of a health care provider while in autogenic training. Any trainees who experience distress, uncomfortable symptoms, or changes in blood pressure during autogenic training should continue only under the supervision of a qualified instructor.

Self-Hypnosis

Milton Erickson is generally recognized as a leading proponent of the use of hypnosis in medical and psychotherapeutic contexts (Bandler and Grinder 1975). Erickson redefined hypnosis as an experience originating in the client in order to cope with a problem overwhelming to the conscious mind.

People practice **self-hypnosis** to achieve significant relaxation, to make positive suggestions for change (e.g., to lose weight, to stop smoking, to overcome fear of the dark, or insomnia), to increase learning and remembering, and to uncover significant but forgotten events. Table 28–2 gives examples of some life problems and hypnotic suggestions that can be used to overcome them. Contrary to popular belief, even the most inexperienced of self-hypnosis practitioners cannot harm themselves.

Most people can achieve significant relaxation within two days with self-hypnosis. Self-hypnosis can be self-taught through books on the subject (see the references at the end of this chapter). Community adult education programs or holistic health centers often offer courses on self-hypnosis. Self-hypnosis is clinically effective in relieving insomnia, low to moderate levels of chronic pain, tics and tremors, and low to moderate levels of anxiety. It is a well-established treatment for chronic fatigue.

Thought Stopping

Thought stopping is a behavior therapy technique that is particularly useful in helping a person control obsessive and phobic thoughts (Wolpe 1969). It involves concentrating on the unwanted thoughts and, after a short time, suddenly interrupting the thought and emptying the mind. Thought stopping is based on the belief that negative and frightening thoughts invariably precede negative and frightening emotions. Controlling these thoughts can reduce stress. Some of the obsessive and phobic thought processes that can be interrupted by thought stopping are color naming, counting, rechecking, hypochondriasis, sexual preoccupation, recurring thoughts of failure, and simple phobias among others. Thought stopping is more successful with phobias than it is with compulsive ritualistic behavior.

Thought stopping begins by using the command "stop," a loud noise, or a distracter such as pinching oneself or pressing the fingernails into the palm of the hand to interrupt the unpleasant thoughts. Once the individual has mastered interrupting the unpleasant thought, the next step involves *thought substitution* (replacing the obsessive or phobic thought with a positive assertive statement that is appropriate to the situation). For example, the person who is afraid to drive across a bridge might say to himself or herself, "This is a gorgeous view from up here."

To be effective, thought stopping should be practiced conscientiously throughout the day for three days to one week. At first the thought will return, but with practice it returns less frequently, and in many instances, eventually ceases to recur.

Refuting Irrational Self-Talk

Self-talk is intrapersonal communication, the thoughts with which we describe and interpret the world to ourselves. Irrational or untrue self-talk causes stress and mental disorder. Two common forms of **irrational self-talk** are statements that "awfulize" (catastrophic, nightmarish interpretations of an event or experience) or "absolutize" (words such as *should, must, always,* etc. that imply the need to live up to a standard). These ideas are based on the rational-emotive therapy formulated by Albert Ellis (1975).

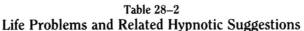

Table 28–2 Life Problems and Related Hypnotic Suggestions	
Life Problem	**Hypnotic Suggestion**
1. Fear of coming into the dark house at night	1. I can come in tonight feeling relaxed and glad to be home.
2. Anxiety that prevents working or studying to meet deadlines	2. I can work steadily and calmly. My concentration is improving as I become more relaxed.
3. Insomnia	3. I will gradually become more and more drowsy. In just a few minutes I will be able to fall asleep, and sleep peacefully all night.
4. Chronic fatigue	4. I can waken feeling refreshed and rested.
5. Obsessive and fearful thoughts about death	5. I am full of life now. I will enjoy today.
6. Minor chronic headache or backache	6. As I become more relaxed, my headache (backache) lessens. In just a few minutes, it will go away. Soon my head will be cool and relaxed. Gradually I will feel the muscles in my back loosen. In an hour, they will be completely relaxed. Whenever these symptoms come back, I will simply turn my ring a quarter of a turn to the right and the pain will relax away.
7. Feelings of inferiority	7. The next time I see _____, I can feel secure in myself. I can feel relaxed and at ease because I am perfectly all right.
8. Anxiety about an upcoming evaluation or test	8. Whenever I feel nervous, I can say to myself . . . (insert your own special key word or phrase here) . . . and relax.
9. Chronic anger (or chronic guilt)	9. I can turn off anger (guilt) because I am the one who turns it on. I will relax my body and breathe deeply.
10. Worry about interpersonal rejection	10. Whenever I lace my fingers together, I will feel confidence flowing through me.
11. Chronic tension in a particular part of the body	11. I will think about my _____ every hour and let it relax.

According to Ellis, emotional reactions are not caused by events or by our emotional reaction to events but by belief systems. Being insulted, for instance, does not cause us to withdraw from others. Our *beliefs* about being insulted are what cause us to withdraw. Though it is rational to feel angry about insults, since they are destructive, withdrawal is irrational because it indicates that an individual has defined being insulted as a frightening event to be avoided. Ellis defines beliefs as rational when they help the individual accept reality, live in intimate relationships with others, work productively, and enjoy recreational pursuits. Irrationality is self-destructive behavior.

Rational-emotive therapy emphasizes human values as the important component of personality. Healthy functioning is possible only when the values we believe in are rational ones. Absolutist, perfectionist attitudes are irrational. Ten basic irrational ideas described by Ellis are discussed in Box 28–4.

Both emotions and behavior depend on the cognitive mediating process that occurs in relation to every experience. Rational-emotive therapy helps people dispel their disturbing beliefs by explaining what irrational beliefs are and how they cause emotional difficulty. After they have logically analyzed their irrational beliefs, clients see how unnecessary they are and eliminate them.

Rational-emotive therapy frequently uses reinforcing techniques to help people change. Clients are taught to reward themselves for working on self-defeating ideas and to penalize themselves if they do not. Clients are also shown how to speak and think more objectively and give up the use of vague terms and overgeneralizations in order to define their own problems in specific terms. For example, the client is shown that the statement "I have some characteristics that are irritating to others" is more precise than "I am an irritating person."

Rational-emotive therapy narrows the focus for change to specific traits and behavior. Since people create most of their own psychologic symptoms, they can eliminate these symptoms by changing their values.

Biofeedback

Biofeedback, or visceral learning, is a technique for gaining conscious control over such involuntary body functions as blood pressure and heartbeat, which are mediated by the autonomic nervous system. The clinical application of biofeedback was pioneered by Alyce and Elmer Green of the Menninger Foundation in the late 1960s. Many other researchers have followed them in exploring this method of treatment. Certified biofeedback practitioners can be found in almost any large city, and training is available at most large universities.

Biofeedback treatment is based on the ability to voluntarily control some autonomic functions to a degree once thought impossible. It has been shown, for instance, that migraine headaches can be relieved by increasing blood flow to the hands.

The technique is based on giving continuous feedback about the results of each consecutive attempt at control. In a typical session, a person might be given this feedback by equipment that amplifies body signals and translates them into a flashing light or a steady tone. Once people can "see" a heartbeat, for instance, and observe when it slows down or speeds up, they have the information they need to control their heart rate. They are instructed to change the signal as they observe it. They are not told to slow the heartbeat, but to slow the flashing light. If they can do this, their heart rate will be modified.

Inexpensive monitoring equipment for home use has been developed within the past few years (Figure 28–6). The drawback is that these systems usually measure only temperature, heart rate, or the alpha activity of the brain, thus giving feedback on only a single system. Single-system feedback often isn't enough to achieve total relaxation.

Biofeedback has been found useful in treating a variety of problems, e.g., tension or migraine headaches, insomnia, muscle or colon spasm, pain, hypertension, anxiety, phobias, asthma, stuttering, bruxism (grinding of the teeth), and epilepsy. The psychologic states achieved through biofeedback can be beneficial in decreasing tension and reactions to unpleasant stimuli.

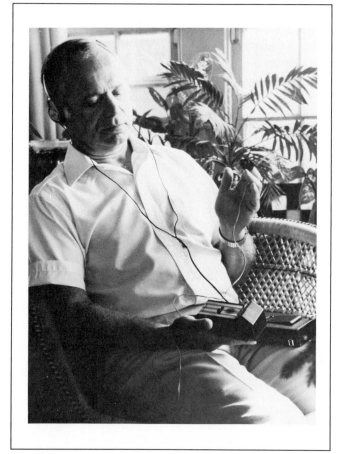

Figure 28–6
Biofeedback is a popular alternative healing therapy that represents a shift toward independence and away from professional control. This man uses biofeedback to reduce job-related stress and to improve his racquetball game.

Box 28–4
ALBERT ELLIS' TEN BASIC IRRATIONAL IDEAS

1. **It is an absolute necessity for an adult to have love and approval from peers, family, and friends.** In fact, it is impossible to please all the people in your life. Even those who basically like and approve of you will be turned off by some behaviors and qualities. This irrational belief is probably the single greatest cause of unhappiness.

2. **You must be unfailingly competent and almost perfect in all you undertake.** The results of believing you must behave perfectly are self-blame for inevitable failure, lowered self-esteem, perfectionistic standards applied to mate and friends, and paralysis and fear at attempting anything.

3. **Certain people are evil, wicked, and villainous, and should be punished.** A more realistic position is that they are behaving in ways that are antisocial or inappropriate. They are perhaps stupid, ignorant, or neurotic, and it would be well if their behavior could be changed.

4. **It is horrible when people and things are not the way you would like them to be.** This might be described as the spoiled-child syndrome. As soon as the tire goes flat the self-talk starts: "Why does this happen to me? Damn, I can't take this. It's awful, I'll get all filthy." Any inconvenience, problem, or failure to get your way is likely to be met with such awfulizing self-statements. The result is intense irritation and stress.

5. **External events cause most human misery—people simply react as events trigger their emotions.** A logical extension of this belief is that you must control the external events in order to create happiness or avoid sorrow. Since such control has limitations and we are at a loss to completely manipulate the wills of others, there results a sense of helplessness and chronic anxiety. Ascribing unhappiness to events is a way of avoiding reality. Self-statements *interpreting* the event caused the unhappiness. While you may have only limited control over others, you have enormous control over your emotions.

6. **You should feel fear or anxiety about anything that is unknown, uncertain, or potentially dangerous.** Many describe this as, "a little bell that goes off and I think I ought to start worrying." They begin to rehearse their scenarios of catastrophe. Increasing the fear or anxiety in the face of uncertainty makes coping more difficult and adds to stress. Saving the fear response for actual, perceived danger allows you to enjoy uncertainty as a novel and exciting experience.

7. **It is easier to avoid than to face life's difficulties and responsibilities.** There are many ways of ducking responsibilities: "I should tell him/her I'm no longer interested—but not tonight . . . I'd like to get another job, but I'm just too tired on my days off to look . . . A leaky faucet won't hurt anything . . . We could shop today, but the car is making a sort of funny sound."

8. **You need something other or stronger or greater than yourself to rely on.** This belief becomes a psychologic trap in which your independent judgment, and the awareness of your particular needs are undermined by a reliance on higher authority.

9. **The past has a lot to do with determining the present.** Just because you were once strongly affected by something, that does not mean that you must continue the habits you formed to cope with the original situation. Those old patterns and ways of responding are just decisions made so many times they have become nearly automatic. You can identify those old decisions and start changing them *right now*. You can learn from past experience, but you don't have to be overly attached to it.

10. **Happiness can be achieved by inaction, passivity, and endless leisure.** This is called the Elysian Fields syndrome. There is more to happiness than perfect relaxation.

Source: Adapted from Davis M, Eshelman ER, McKay M: The Relaxation and Stress Reduction Workbook. *ed. 2. New Harbinger Publications, 1982, pp 106–107.*

Chapter Highlights

- There are environmental, physiologic, and cognitive sources of stress. Psychiatric clients may experience more cognitive stress than most other persons do because of how they interpret and label their experiences.

- Most persons, including clients and nurses, find stress-reduction techniques helpful in counteracting habitual counterproductive responses to the stresses of life.

- Nurses who plan to use stress-management techniques with clients must first develop personal familiarity with them.

- Anyone participating in a stress-reduction program should be sure that any physical problems and medications are closely monitored by a health care provider.

- Psychiatric clients taking psychotropic medications that may cause hypotension should be closely monitored when they do stress-reduction exercises.

- Regular practice enhances the chances of successfully using stress-management techniques.

- People should use the relaxation and stress-management techniques that work best in their individual situations.

- Body tension is an inevitable response to stress; once stress is removed, tension goes away.

- Keeping a stress-awareness diary helps people identify how particular stresses result in predictable symptoms.

- Breathing calmly and deeply keeps the blood well oxygenated and purified. Breathing properly can, by itself, reduce stress.

- Progressive relaxation teaches clients to decrease physiologic tension and block anxiety by achieving deep muscle relaxation.

- Positive visualizations use a person's own imagination and positive thinking to reduce stress or promote healing.

- The state of meditation is equivalent to a state of deep rest. It helps a person to focus uncritically on one thing at a time in order to achieve inner peace and harmony.

- Biofeedback is a technique for gaining conscious control over unconscious body functions.

- Therapeutic touch is the "laying on of hands" to help or heal. It is based on the ability of a healer to transfer excess energy to a client, or to transfer energy from one part of the client's body to another.

- In rolfing, the structural realignment of the body to the field of gravity is accompanied by a corresponding emotional balance.

- Bioenergetics offers techniques for reducing muscular tension by releasing feelings through physical exercises and verbal techniques.

- Autogenic training is a structured program of exercises that have been found to be effective in the treatment of numerous physical symptoms. It is also used to reduce anxiety, irritability, and fatigue; to modify the reaction to pain; and to reduce or eliminate sleep disorders.

- Self-hypnosis is clinically effective in relieving insomnia, low to moderate levels of chronic pain, tics and tremors, and low to moderate levels of anxiety. It is a well-established treatment for chronic fatigue.

- A behavior therapy technique, thought stopping helps to control phobic and obsessional thoughts.

- Irrational self-talk creates stress and mental disorder. Changing irrational beliefs can reduce or eliminate emotional difficulty.

- People can learn to control involuntary body functions through biofeedback and reduce or eliminate stress-related conditions.

References

Bandler R, Grinder J: *Patterns of the Hypnotic Techniques of Milton H. Erickson,* vol 1. Meta Publications, 1975.

Borysenko J: *Minding the Body, Mending the Mind.* Addison-Wesley, 1987.

Bramson RM, Bramson S: *The Stressless Home: A Step-by-Step Guide to Turning Your Home into the Haven You Desire.* Doubleday, 1985.

Brown B: *Stress and the Art of Biofeedback.* Harper & Row, 1977.

Clark PE, Clark MJ: Therapeutic touch: Is there a scientific basis for the practice? *Nurs Res* 1984;33(1):37–41.

Dawkins JE, Depp FC, Selzer NE: Stress and the psychiatric nurse. *J Psychosoc Nurs* 1985;23:8–15.

Ellis A: *A New Guide to Rational Living.* Prentice-Hall, 1975.

Flynn PAR: *Holistic Health: The Art and Science of Care.* Brady, 1980.

Goldberger L, Breznitz S (eds): *Handbook of Stress: Theoretical and Clinical Aspects.* Free Press, 1982.

Hamilton JM: Effective ways to relieve stress. *Nurs Life* 1984;4:24–27.

Hoover RM, Parnell PK: An inpatient education group on stress and coping. *J Psychosoc Nurs* 1984;22(6):16–23.

Jacobson E: *Progressive Relaxation.* University of Chicago Press, Midway Reprint, 1974.

Kreiger D: *The Therapeutic Touch.* Prentice-Hall, 1979.

Kinzel SL: What's your stress level? *Nurs Life* 1982;2:54–55.

Lachman VD: *Stress Management: A Manual for Nurses.* Grune and Stratton, 1983.

Larson D: Helper secrets: Internal stressors in nursing. *J Psychosoc Nurs* 1987;25(4):20–27.

LeCron L (ed): *Techniques of Hypnotherapy.* Julian Press, 1961.

LeShan L: *How to Meditate.* Bantam Books, 1974.

Lowen A: *The Betrayal of the Body.* Macmillan, 1967.

Lowen A: *Depression and the Body.* Macmillan, 1967.

Lowen A; *Bioenergetics.* Penquin Books, 1976.

Luthe W (ed): *Autogenic Therapy,* 6 vols. New York: Grune and Stratton, 1969.

Mason LJ: *Guide to Stress Reduction.* Peace Press, 1980.

Meichenbaum D, Jaremko M (eds): *Stress Reduction and Prevention.* Plenum Press, 1983.

Miller J: *States of Mind.* Pantheon Books, 1983.

Miller NE: Rx: Biofeedback. *Psychol Today* 1985: 19:54–59.

Morris F: *Self-Hypnosis in Two Days.* Intergalactic, 1974.

Pelletier KR: *Mind As Healer, Mind As Slayer.* Dell, 1977.

Randolph GL: Therapeutic and physical touch: Physiological response to stressful stimuli. *Nurs Res* 1984;33(1):33–36.

Rolf I: *Rolfing: The Structural Integration of Human Structure.* Rolf Institute, 1977.

Sawaswati, SJ: *Yoga, Tantra, and Meditation.* Ballantine, 1976.

Scully R: Stress in the nurse. *Am J Nurs* 1980;80:912–914.

Shaffer M: *Life after Stress.* Plenum Press, 1982.

Spreads C: *Breathing—The ABC's.* Harper & Row, 1978.

Sterman MB: Biofeedback and epilepsy. *Hum Nature* 1978;23:50–57.

Stokols D: A congruence analysis of human stress. *Issues Ment Health Nurs* 1985:7:35–41.

Stroebel CF: *The Quieting Reflex: A Six-Second Technique for Coping with Stress Anytime, Anywhere.* G. P. Putnam's Sons, 1982.

Stroebel CF: Biofeedback and behavioral medicine, in Kaplan HI, Sadock BJ (eds): *Comprehensive Textbook of Psychiatry,* ed 4. Williams and Wilkins, 1985.

Sutterley DC, Donnelley GF (eds): *Coping with Stress: A Nursing Perspective.* Aspen, 1982.

Tache J, Selye J: On stress and coping mechanisms. *Issues Ment Health Nurs* 1985;7:3–24.

Tolman R, Rose SD: Coping with stress: A multimodal approach. *Social Work* 1985;30:151–158.

Turin AC: *No More Headaches! Practical, Effective Methods for Relief.* Houghton Mifflin, 1981.

Vandereycken W, et al: Body-oriented therapy for anorexia nervosa patients. *Amer J Psychother* 1987; 41(2):252–259.

Wilson LK: High-gear nursing: How it can run you down and what you can do about it. *Nurs Life* 1986;6:44–47.

Wollert R, Levy L, Knight B: Help-giving in behavioral control and stress coping self-help groups. *Small Group Behav* 1982;13:204–218.

Wolpe J: *The Practice of Behavior Therapy.* Pergamon Press, 1969.

TWENTY-NINE

Crisis Intervention

Carol Ren Kneisl
Mary-Eve Zangari

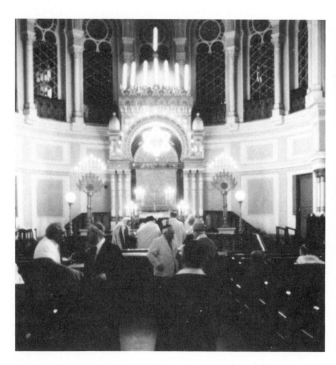

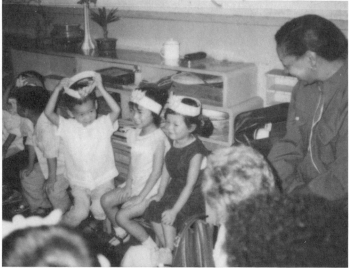

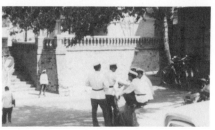

After reading this chapter, students should be able to

- Trace the crisis sequence and relate its significance for nursing care of clients in crisis
- Define the types of crisis a person may encounter
- Identify the social, demographic, and clinical variables that influence suicidal behavior
- Explain the process of lethality assessment
- Develop a plan for nursing intervention with suicidal clients
- Discuss the major crisis intervention modes

Cross References

Other topics relevant to this content are: Adolescent suicide, Chapter 35; Anxiety, stress, and coping, Chapter 7; Child suicide, Chapter 34; Depression, Chapter 18; Elderly suicide, Chapter 36; Ethics, Chapter 10; Grieving, Chapter 37; Growth and development, Chapter 6; Nursing intervention in anxiety and panic, Chapter 19; Post-traumatic stress disorder, Chapter 19; Stress management, Chapter 28; Violence and abuse, Chapter 25.

Key Terms

crisis	suicidal attempt
crisis counseling	suicidal gesture
hot line	suicidal threat
lethality assessment	suicide

This chapter explores those extremely difficult points in a person's life when circumstances produce an unbearable situation. Under such pressure, a person may make unsound decisions, may become mentally disordered, or may commit or attempt suicide. It is an intriguing puzzle to understand what constitutes a crisis for an individual and how that individual behaves in response to it. This inquiry into the cause and effect of crisis is the focus of crisis theory.

Humanism is the basis of crisis theory in that individuals are recognized as having their own unique view of the word. Crisis points are as unique as the individual's responses to the crisis. Humanism also promotes the individual's ability to reason and choose freely. In accordance with these concepts, the task of the person who intervenes in the crisis is (a) to help the individual understand what combination of events led to the crisis and (b) to guide the individual toward a resolution that will meet the client's unique needs and foster future growth and strength.

Early writers have described crises in Western culture since writing about Adam and Eve leaving the Garden of Eden. In finding ways to cope with this first crisis, Adam and Eve engaged in what must have been the first example of crisis intervention. We have since come to a better understanding of just what a crisis is, why people behave the way they do in crisis situations, and how to help people in crisis.

Nurses are in a unique position to intervene in crises. Clients and families in crisis come to their attention in the multitude of health care settings in which nurses work. However, crisis intervention is not the speciality of any one professional group. Crisis intervenors come from the fields of nursing, medicine, psychology, social work, and theology. Police officers, teachers, school guidance counselors, rescue workers, and bartenders, among others, are often on the spot in moments of crisis. Crisis intervention can be the business of many different persons.

CRISIS DEFINED

The word *crisis* stems from the Greek *krinein,* "to decide." In Chinese two characters are used to write the word *crisis*—one is the character for *danger* and the other the character for *opportunity.* A **crisis** is a situation in which

As nurses, we believe that every human being is unique and irreplaceable and has a right to live in peace and good health.

customary problem-solving or decision-making methods are not adequate. Crisis situations are life turning points or junctures. Successful negotiation of a crisis leads either to a return to the precrisis state or to psychologic growth and increased competence. Unsuccessful negotiation leaves the person undergoing a crisis feeling anxious, threatened, and ineffective. Persons may also respond to a crisis event with disturbed personal coping or frankly psychotic behavior.

Because a state of disequilibrium is so uncomfortable to bear, a crisis is self-limiting. It lasts a few days to a few weeks and eventually runs its course with or without intervention. However, the person who experiences a crisis alone is more vulnerable to unsuccessful negotiation than the person who works through a crisis with help. Working with a helping person increases the likelihood that a crisis will be resolved in a positive way.

Basically, there are two types of crises.

1. Internal or developmental crises are the anticipated crises of human maturation.

2. External or situational crises are stressful life events that may or may not be anticipated.

Table 29–1 defines and gives examples of each type. Natural, accidental, and man-made disasters and suicide are discussed later in this chapter. Other kinds of crisis are covered in appropriate chapters.

Two events in the 1940s can be said to have provided the starting point for contemporary crisis theory and intervention. One was the report by psychiatrist Erich Lindemann (see Lindemann 1944; Cobb and Lindemann 1943) of the crisis response many people had in their direct or indirect experience with the tragic Cocoanut Grove nightclub fire in Boston, in which hundreds of people lost their lives. Lindemann's observations and theoretical developments formed a landmark in understanding the behavior of people facing emergency situations and the grieving behavior of people whose relatives or friends died in the fire or its aftermath.

The other event was the observation and treatment by military psychiatrists of battle-weary and emotionally upset military men. In most instances, men who received immediate help at the front lines were able to return to duty rather than being sent to in-patient psychiatric facilities. This immediate front-line treatment was therefore the preferred mode. Later studies and observations during the Korean War added to the knowledge of the behavior of people under stress.

James Tyhurst (1957) contributed further to the understanding of people's responses to natural disasters. He also studied transition states such as parenthood and retirement. Gerald Caplan (1965), who is best known for his work in preventive psychiatry and anticipatory guidance, had similar interests. Many of his methods were tested in the early days of the Peace Corps.

Table 29–1 The Typology of Crisis		
Type	**Definition**	**Examples**
Developmental	Crisis that occurs in response to stresses common to all (or most) persons in periods of human maturation and transition	
Common to all		Birth, early childhood, preschool, puberty, young adulthood, adulthood, old age
Common to many		Beginning school, birth of siblings, divorce of parents, dating, marriage, birth of children, death of significant others, imprisonment, hospitalization, severe illness
Situational	Crisis that occurs in response to stressful or traumatic event	
Victim	Traumatic event involving physically aggressive and forced act by another person	War, rape, riot, murder, assault, incest
Man-made or natural disasters		Tornado, hurricane, earthquake, flood, fire, plane crash

The report of the Joint Commission on Mental Illness and Health (1961) was an important development in crisis work. Its far-reaching mental health recommendations have been discussed in other chapters. Conclusions of the Joint Commission specific to this chapter are:

- People in crisis did not receive immediate help but instead were put on lengthy waiting lists.

- When they did receive attention, it was often through lengthy and expensive psychotherapy.

- Extended and/or late psychotherapy is often not helpful to people in crisis.

- When people in crisis needed help, almost 50 percent sought out their clergyman, family physician, or other non-mental-health professional.

- Interested persons with minimal training could be helpful to people in trouble.

- A large group of interested persons in the community had been neglected as a resource for helping people in crisis.

Soon after publication of the Joint Commission report, large amounts of federal funding were made available for community-based mental health programs. One result was the establishment of suicide prevention and crisis services throughout the country. These were spearheaded by the efforts of mental health professionals on the West Coast. Crisis telephone counseling services, known popularly as **hot lines**, became common. So did the use of both paid and volunteer nonprofessional crisis workers. As community-based mental health programs became more firmly established and organized, many of them took on these crisis intervention functions.

Norris Hansell (1976) has developed a contemporary approach to people in crisis. Hansell's work with those in distress is based on findings of the theorists and researchers discussed earlier. In Hansell's social framework approach, the reestablishment of severed social attachments is necessary for successful crisis resolution. In this view, the emphasis is on social factors as the sources of problems. Other individuals whose work has influenced modern-day crisis intervention are Abraham Maslow (1970) and Erik Erikson (1963).

The Crisis Sequence

Howard Parad and Harvey Resnik (1975) have identified a crisis sequence that involves three time periods—precrisis, crisis, and postcrisis.

An individual in the precrisis period is operating in a way to ensure that most of his or her needs get met. The person in crisis experiences a period of disorganization. This period is characterized by trial-and-error disequilibrium responses, in which the person attempts to reduce

the feelings of discomfort. The resolution of the crisis or postcrisis period can result in either an increase or a decrease in the person's level of functioning or a return to the level of functioning evident in the precrisis period.

The three periods of the crisis sequence are shown in Figure 29–1. They are distinguishable in the following case example:

Mike was relatively free of emotional and physical stresses for most of his early adult life, and he was able to handle those that he did experience. On his thirty-fifth birthday, Mike was offered the opportunity to purchase a deteriorating bar and restaurant on prime urban property near a large university. He went into debt to revamp the bar and restaurant into Dante's Disco, a discotheque Mike hoped would bring him financial success. After the first two years of its existence, it became apparent that Dante's Disco would not return Mike's investment. Early one Sunday morning, Dante's Disco burned to the ground, a total loss.

A year later, Mike was arrested and charged with arson for setting the fire. He had collected a quarter of a million dollars from the company that insured Dante's Disco, but the insurance company investigator considered the fire suspicious and had continued to investigate even after the claim was paid. The breakthrough in the case came when Mike's 15-year-old daughter provided the arson investigator with the evidence needed to arrest her father.

Mike was unable to handle this stressful event. His business prospects seemed to be ruined, and he faced a jail term if convicted. On top of it all he perceived his daughter's behavior as a betrayal. His current coping mechanisms were overtaxed, and he experienced a crisis state. Mike's lawyer obtained bail, and Mike was able to go home, but he became highly anxious and felt hopeless. He also began to experience severe migraine headaches. Three days after his release Mike shot himself and died in the ambulance on the way to the hospital.

Crisis Intervention as a Therapeutic Strategy

Crisis intervention as a therapeutic strategy is strongly humanistic. People are viewed as capable of personal growth and able to control their own lives. According to the

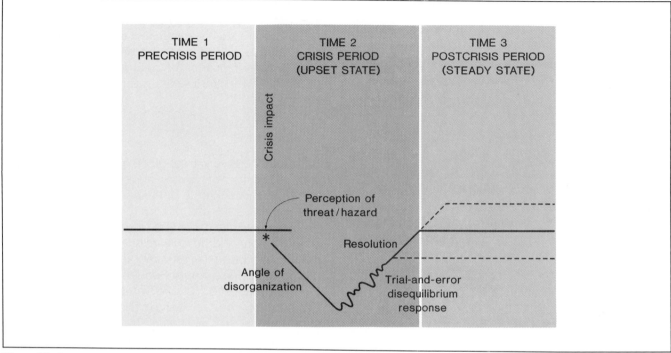

Figure 29–1
Crisis sequence diagram. The asterisk indicates the onset of a crisis period, which occurs directly after the crisis impact. An angle of disorganization develops during the crisis period and may vary from steep to gradual. This variance also occurs during the resolution (recovery or reorganization) phase. During time 3 (postcrisis period) the level of functioning may be about the same as during time 1 (precrisis period), or it may be higher or lower, depending on the nature of the stress, available resources, and whether the crisis resolution is adaptive or maladaptive.
Source: Parad HJ, Resnick HLP: A crisis intervention framework, in Resnick HLP, Ruben HL (eds): Emergency Psychiatric Care. Charles Press, 1975, p 4.

humanistic orientation, effective planning for crisis resolution must be:

- Based on careful assessment
- Developed in active collaboration with the person in crisis and the significant others in that person's life
- Focused on immediate, concrete, contributing problems
- Based on an understanding of human dependence needs
- Appropriate to the crisis-ridden person's level of thinking, feeling, and behaving
- Consistent with the person's life-style and culture
- Time limited, concrete, and realistic
- Mutually negotiated and renegotiated
- Organized to provide for follow-up

A crisis resolution plan with these components demon-

strates respect for the crisis-ridden person's self, values, culture, and abilities.

SUICIDE

Suicide is destructive aggression turned inward. Although statistical reports indicate that suicide is the eleventh most common cause of death in the United States and that 25,000 people are known to commit suicide per year, it is conservatively estimated that 250,000 people will *attempt* suicide each year. These estimates are really only guesses—no one knows for sure how many deaths labeled accidental are suicides. Some are called accidents because the determination is difficult to make. Other suicides are called accidents for social or economic reasons—to avoid stigmatizing a family in a community or to collect on insurance policies that do not pay when the cause of death is suicide.

Suicide is a behavior fraught with mystery. It is the subject of some age-old tales and myths. Myths that continue to surround it include those presented in Table 29–2. Self-destructive people are those who harm themselves in any of a variety of ways: nail biting, head banging, wrist cutting, cigarette smoking, drug and alcohol abuse, failing to take insulin or necessary medications, and reckless driving. The ultimate form of self-destruction is suicide. Four broad groups of self-destructive people are:

1. Those who actually do commit suicide
2. Those who threaten to commit suicide
3. Those who attempt suicide
4. Those who are chronically self-destructive in more indirect ways (the substance abuser, the bulimic person, etc.)

The varying levels of suicidal behavior are defined and described in Box 29–1. A number of social, demographic, and clinical variables affect suicidal behavior. They are outlined in the following section.

Box 29–1
VARYING LEVELS OF SUICIDAL BEHAVIOR

- **Suicidal threat:** More serious than a casual statement of suicidal intent and is accompanied by other behavior changes. These may include mood swings, temper outbursts, a decline in school or work performance, characterologic changes, sudden or gradual withdrawal from friends, or other significant changes in attitude.

- **Suicidal gesture:** A more serious warning signal than a statement and may be followed by a suicidal act that is carefully planned to attract attention without seriously injuring the subject. A superficial scratch across the wrist, if it goes unheeded, may be followed by a more dramatic display.

- **Suicidal attempt:** A strong and desperate call for help. It is often the final call, for unlike the suicidal gesture it involves a definite risk. The outcome frequently depends on the circumstances and is not under the person's control. For example, someone who takes a heavy overdose of sleeping pills may or may not be discovered in time.

Table 29–2
Suicide Myths and Realities

Myth	Reality
A suicide threat is just a bid for attention and should not be taken seriously.	All suicidal behavior should be taken seriously; a bid for attention may be a cry for help.
It is harmful for a person to talk about suicidal thoughts. The person's attention should be diverted when this occurs.	Of prime importance in planning nursing care is an accurate assessment of the lethality of the person's suicide plan.
Only psychotic persons commit suicide.	The majority of successful suicides are committed by persons who are not psychotic.
People who talk about suicide won't do it.	Most people do talk about their suicide intention before making a suicide attempt.
A nice home, good job, or an intact family prevents suicide.	Persons of all emotional, social, and economic backgrounds may commit suicide.
A failed suicide attempt should be treated as manipulative behavior.	Failed suicide attempts are more likely to be evidence of a person's ambivalence toward killing himself or herself.

Assessment

Social Variables

Low suicide rates are noted among the following:

- Developing communities and groups in which hope and optimism are high
- Cultures that are warm and nurturing, such as the Irish, Italians, and Norwegians
- Communities in which there is strong disapproval of suicide as an act, such as in Italy, Spain, and Ireland, where the Catholic Church is highly influential

High suicide rates are associated with the following:

- Societies in which social unrest, internal governmental problems, or pessimistic outlooks for the future predominate

- Subcultures that are uncaring and cold and lack concern for people in trouble, such as skid rows and disorganized inner-city areas
- Societies, such as the United States, Japan, Russia, and Germany, that value independence and individual performance
- Social roles, occupations, and professions in which people exhibit high concern and nurturance toward others (e.g., physicians and police)

Demographic Variables

Suicide rates are higher among the following:

- Single people and married people without children
- Men in general, although rates for white women have increased 49 percent and for black women have increased 80 percent in the past twenty years
- White people, although the rate for young, urban black persons between 20 and 35 years of age is twice that of white persons in the same age group
- Persons above the age of 40, although rates for adolescents are rising (persons over 65 account for 25 percent of the total number of reported suicides)

Clinical Variables

Suicide rates are higher among the following:

- People who have attempted suicide before
- People who have experienced the loss of an important person at some time in the past or the loss of both parents early in life, or the loss of or threat of loss of their spouse, job, money, or social position
- People who are depressed or recovering from depression or a psychotic episode
- People with physical illness, particularly when the illness involves an alteration of body image or life-style
- People who abuse alcohol and drugs, thus decreasing their impulse control

Clues or Cries for Help

People bent on suicide almost always give either verbal or nonverbal clues of their intent. Suicidologists and crisis workers who work with suicidal people believe that people bent on self-destruction actually make a powerful attempt to communicate to others their hurt and desperation. They are crying out for help.

Sixty-five percent of persons who commit suicide signal their need for help by making contact with the health care system three to six months before the suicide because of various physical complaints (Rose-Grippa 1984). But, when questioned, many will express feelings of depression and thoughts of suicide. The nurse should be alert to patterns that may at first seem coincidental.

A single woman, age 22, visited an orthopedist for back pain. The office nurse noted that her history included five major automobile accidents in the past two years. The client related that four of these accidents had occurred while her boyfriend was drunk and driving. The last incident was a suicide attempt after the client's boyfriend had beaten her during another drinking bout.

The cry for help may be indirect or subtle. A person may say: "I just can't take it anymore," "There's no reason to go on," "Sometimes I think I'd be better off dead," "I won't be seeing you anymore," "Take care of my dog and cat," "Too bad I won't get to see my little brother grow up," "Will you be sorry when I'm gone?" Sometimes their behavior provides the clue. They may:

- Give away prized possessions
- Make out or change a will
- Take out or add to an insurance policy
- Cancel all social engagements
- Be despondent or behave in unusual ways
- Be unable to sleep
- Feel hopeless
- Have trouble concentrating at school or on the job
- Suddenly lose interest in friends, organizations, and activities.

An assessment for suicide should *always* be done whenever the nurse suspects suicidal thought or intent.

Because a Korean nursing student had failed the same major clinical course twice, she was asked to leave the BSN program. She desperately fought to be allowed to continue even though the faculty had deemed her unsafe in the clinical area. The faculty could not understand her refusal to accept failure until they considered her cultural and family background, in which personal defeat is strongly condemned. They decided to have the student speak with the psychiatric nursing instructor who assessed the student's emotional state and found that she had no intentions of self-harm.

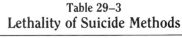

Nurses and others who may have contact with potentially suicidal people must be alert to both clear and veiled communications about suicide. Once clues have been identified, the next step is to undertake an accurate lethality assessment.

Assessing Lethality

A **lethality assessment** is an attempt to predict the likelihood of suicide. An accurate lethality assessment is essential in formulating a plan for helping a suicidal person. It also gives the nurse cues about the client's possible need for hospitalization. Carrying out a lethality assessment requires direct communication between client and nurse concerning the client's intent.

The elements to be considered in a lethality assessment are listed below in order of decreasing importance.

1. Suicide plan. Does the person have suicidal ideas? Is the person considering a highly lethal method, or one of low lethality? (The lethality of various suicide methods according to Hoff [1984] is categorized in Table 29–3.) Are the means for carrying out suicide available—that is, does the person have access to a gun, pills, ammunition? Has a specific plan been worked out?

2. History of suicide attempts. Has the person attempted suicide before? Is the method the same, or is it more or less lethal? What was the outcome of the previous suicide attempt? Was the person rescued accidentally? Has the person been hospitalized for attempting suicide in the past?

3. Resources and communication with significant others. What are the person's internal and external resources? Is the person alienated from others?

4. Isolation. Is the person physically alone or emotionally isolated? Are significant others rejecting? Do others fail to approve of the person's role performance?

5. Hostility directed toward caregivers or others.

6. Mental disorder, disorientation, or disorganization. If a person has hallucinations in which he or she is commanded to commit suicide, risk is increased. However, the belief that only the mentally disordered commit suicide is inaccurate.

7. Drinking and drug abuse. (See the clinical variables identified earlier.)

8. Age, sex, and race. (See the demographic variables identified earlier.)

9. Recent loss. (See the clinical variables identified earlier.)

Table 29–3
Lethality of Suicide Methods

Low Lethal Methods	High Lethal Methods
Wrist cutting	Gun
House gas	Jumping
Nonprescription drugs (excluding aspirin and Tylenol)	Hanging
	Drowning
Tranquilizers, e.g., diazepam (Valium), flurazepam (Dalmane)	Carbon monoxide poisoning
	Barbiturates and prescribed sleeping pills
	Aspirin and Tylenol (high doses)
	Car crash
	Exposure to extreme cold
	Antidepressants, e.g., amitriptyline (Elavil)

10. Physical illness. (See the clinical variables identified earlier.)

11. Unexplained change in behavior. Change in behavior from careful to careless or impulsive may indicate suicide risk.

12. Depression. A significant number of suicide victims are depressed.

13. Social factors. A broken home, delinquency and truancy, family discord, unemployment, forced retirement, or a move to another residence may increase a person's risk of suicide.

14. Biologic markers. An abnormal dexamethasone suppression test may indicate clients at increased risk.

Assessment of suicide risk is not easily accomplished. One barrier is the nurse's fear of asking the appropriate questions. It is not possible to "cause" a person's suicide by assessing feelings and thoughts. The nurse who is not comfortable with this kind of interview needs to seek assistance from an experienced clinician.

Question the client gently and directly; do not use euphemisms. Some sample phrases might be: Do you have any thoughts of harming yourself? Have you ever thought of taking your own life? Have you ever been so sad that you wanted to end it all, maybe by dying?

Another problem in assessment occurs when the client asks the nurse to promise not to tell anyone about a suicide plan. A nurse should never promise to keep clinical infor-

---

Table 29–4
Signs That Help Predict Suicide Risk: Comparing People Who Complete or Attempt Suicide
with the General Population

Signs	Suicide	Suicide Attempt	General Population
Suicide plan*	Specific with available, relatively lethal method; does not include rescue	Less lethal method, including plan for rescue; risk increases if lethality of method increases	None, or vague ideas only
History of suicide attempts*	Sixty-five percent have history of relatively lethal attempts; if rescued it was probably accidental	Previous attempts are usually less lethal; rescue plan included; risk increases if there is a change from many less lethal attempts to a relatively lethal one	None or less lethal with definite rescue plan
Resources* • Psychologic • Social	Very limited or nonexistent; *or,* person *perceives* self with no resources	Moderate, or in psychologic and/or social turmoil	Either intact or able to restore them through nonsuicidal means
Communication*	Feels cut off from resources and unable to communicate effectively	Ambiguously attached to resources; may use self-injury as a method of communicating with significant others when other methods fail	Able to communicate directly and nondestructively for need fulfillment
Recent loss	Increases risk	May increase risk	Is widespread but is resolved nonsuicidally through grief work, etc.

If all four of these signs exist in a particular person, the risk for suicide is very high regardless of all other factors. If other signs also apply, the risk is further increased.

Source: Adapted from Hoff LA: People in Crisis, ed 2. Addison-Wesley, 1984, pp 192–193.

continued

---

mation a secret and should explain to the client that information is shared with the treatment team. The nurse will probably need to discuss the issue of confidentiality further and to explore the dynamics of the nurse-client relationship.

Many institutions and crisis centers use structured protocols for assessing suicide risk and have published these forms in the literature. However, research efforts to *predict* suicide by testing, use of scales, or clinical judgments have not been successful (Capodanno 1983). Table 29–4 identifies the signs that are thought to help predict suicide risk and compares persons who complete or attempt suicide with the general population.

Nursing Diagnosis

The core nursing diagnoses given to suicidal persons are:

• Violence, potential for, self-directed (NANDA)

• 05.02.01.03 Aggressive/violent behaviors toward self (PND-I)

Planning and Implementing Interventions

Do people have the right to commit suicide, and can or should nurses intervene when people try to kill themselves? Nurses should know that, ethical concerns aside, they may be prosecuted under state laws, making it a crime to aid or abet a suicide, under any circumstance, even when a terminally ill person decides to end his or her life. Questions about a client's right to suicide and society's right to control suicide have not been answered. The nursing interventions discussed below are based on the traditional belief that mental health professionals should do everything possible to prevent suicide. Engaging in the process of ethical reflectiveness suggested in Chapter 10 will help nurses in their search for a personal position.

Table 29–4 *(Continued)*
Signs That Help Predict Suicide Risk: Comparing People Who Complete or Attempt Suicide with the General Population

Signs	Suicide	Suicide Attempt	General Population
Physical illness	Increases risk	May increase risk	Is common but responded to through effective crisis management (natural or formal)
Drinking and other drug abuse	Increases risk	May increase risk	Is widespread but does not lead to suicide of itself
Physical isolation	Increases risk	May increase risk	Many well-adjusted people live alone; handle physical isolation through satisfactory *social* contacts
Unexplained change in behavior	A possible clue to suicidal intent, especially in teenagers	A cry for help and possible clue to suicidal ideas	Not applicable in absence of other predictive signs
Depression	Sixty-five percent have a history of depression	A large percentage are depressed	A large percentage are depressed
Social factors or problems	May be present	Often are present	Widespread but do not of themselves lead to suicide
Mental illness	May be present	May be present	May be present
Age, sex, race, marital status	*Statistical* predictors that are most useful for identifying whether an individual belongs to a high-risk *group,* not for clinical assessment of individuals	May be present	May be present

The nature of the interventions depends, in part, on the setting in which the nurse encounters the suicidal client. Here, in approximately chronologic order, is a general approach for all settings and specific suggestions for emergency rooms and in-patient units.

- Remove the client from immediate danger by confiscating pills or other harmful objects in the client's possession, or by moving the client to a physically safe environment.
- Relieve the client's obvious immediate distress. Does the client need bathing, clean clothing, food, sleep?
- Find out what the client sees as his or her most pressing need. This may be a wish to see a friend or family member or to arrange for someone to pick up the children from school.
- Assume a nonjudgmental, caring attitude that does not engender self-pity in the client.
- Ask the client why he or she chose to attempt suicide at this particular moment. The answer may provide information that can lead to other helpful interventions.

- Organize a plan with the client. Discuss all important problems, prioritize them, and list several approaches to each problem. *Write down* this plan, noting who is responsible for which actions.
- Do not make unrealistic promises or remarks. Remain honest but hopeful.
- Have the client continue daily activities as much as possible. The nurse can assign tasks for the client that are distracting but not taxing.
- Decide with the client which family members and friends are to be contacted and by whom.
- The nurse should be prepared to deal with a family that may be confused, angry, or uninterested. Strive to remain neutral and not make assumptions about the family's behavior.
- Evaluate the need for medication.
- It is crucial to evaluate the plan developed above with the client and arrange for appropriate follow-up.
- The nurse must monitor personal feelings about the client and decide how they may be influencing the nurse's clinical work.

Box 29–2
BASIC SUICIDE PRECAUTIONS: SAMPLE PROTOCOL

1. The client is to remain in his or her room with the door open unless he or she is accompanied by staff or a family member. The client may use the bathroom alone.

2. Check the client's whereabouts and safety every 15 minutes. Have a check-off sheet on client's door to document safety checks.

3. Stay with the client while all medications are taken.

4. Search the client's belongings with him or her for potentially harmful objects.

5. Allow the client to have regular food tray but check whether the glass or any utensils are missing when collecting the tray.

6. Allow the client to have visitors and telephone calls unless the client wishes otherwise.

7. Check that visitors do not leave potentially dangerous objects in the client's room.

8. The plan may be started without a physician's order, but a psychiatric consultation must be arranged as soon as possible.

9. Maintain protocol until it is canceled by a psychiatrist.

10. Inform the client of reasons for and details of precautionary measures. This explanation must be made by nurses and physician and documented in the chart.

In the emergency department, the main thrust of treatment is toward saving the person's life. Although the ER staff may be excellent at technical interventions, the staff may voice or feel contempt for the client who is a "repeater," especially if the attempt is not a serious one. The client needs a professional, nonpunitive approach and a smooth transition to other caretakers or agencies. Leaving the person alone or with access to harmful objects is obviously a hazard to be avoided in a busy emergency department.

Most in-patient psychiatric units have written policies for suicide precautions. General hospital units often do not have written policies. Lack of a plan may lead to anxiety and confusion when a client becomes suicidal and requires a suitable care plan. In all units, it is advisable to be prepared by developing a unit philosophy and matching care plan for the suicidal client. Two sample protocols, one for basic suicide precautions and one for maximum suicide precautions, are in Boxes 29–2 and 29–3. Note that an important precaution in both of these sample guidelines is *not to isolate* the suicidal client.

Evaluation

Suicide, like all crisis situations, calls for ongoing evaluation of the plan made by the nurse and client. Because events often occur rapidly, a care plan may initially need changing almost daily. In addition to evaluating individual care plans, a staff who deals with suicidal clients needs to evaluate its overall approach and philosophy periodically.

Pediatric Suicide

Suicide by children, while relatively rare, occurs often enough to cause alarm. In 1985, for example, there were 311 suicides among children aged 1–14 (*Monthly Vital Statistics Reports,* September 1986). Children commit suicide by simple but highly lethal methods, e.g., poisoning, firearms, hanging, jumping, and darting into the path of a moving car. Pediatric suicide may not be "intentional" because a child (unlike an adult) may view death as reversible or like a peaceful sleep. Teachers and school nurses can practice prevention by being alert to self-destructive behavior, aggression, and depression in children and by encouraging psychiatric evaluation of children with suspected problems. Pfeffer (1985) found that 12 percent of a group of school children with no psychiatric history had suicidal impulses. She suggests that all suicidal fantasies and actions in children be taken seriously and be closely evaluated.

Adolescent Suicide

Adolescent suicide is a serious problem. There has been a two- to three-fold increase in suicide rates for this group in the last twenty-five years (Sudak et al. 1984). In 1985, for example, there were 4734 reported adolescent suicides (ages 15–24), making it the third leading cause of death, after accidents and homicides, among this age group (*Monthly Vital Statistics Report,* September 1986). Some indicators of a troubled youth are:

- Tendency to spend lots of time alone
- Difficulty communicating with others
- Alcohol and drug abuse
- Lack of hope for the future
- Feelings of unhappiness, frustration, and failure and of having disappointed one's parents

One way that schools can intervene is to foster discussion of suicide as an adolescent issue along with sexuality, drugs, and alcohol.

The Elderly

Of all age groups, the elderly are at greatest risk for suicide. They are less likely to make gestures, use more lethal methods, and have less recuperative strength to survive a suicide attempt. The elderly as a group frequently experience serious illness, death of a spouse, status changes, and other losses and changes that make them likely candidates for mental health intervention. However, the elderly tend to underutilize these services and thus are often difficult to reach (McIntosh 1985). Better assessment and follow-up are essential when these clients are in contact with the health care system in non-mental-health situations.

Psychiatric Clients

There is a serious risk of suicide among those persons diagnosed with a psychiatric illness. Roy (1985) suggests that the risk of suicide among this group is three to twelve times greater than the risk among the general population and that 10 percent of all persons labeled schizophrenic die by suicide.

Among psychiatric clients in general, factors that indicate increased suicidal risk are:

- Female sex
- Young age
- Diagnosis of depression or schizophrenia (Black 1982)
- History of past attempt, living alone, unemployment, and being unmarried and recently admitted to psychiatric care (Roy 1985)

The suicide rate for schizophrenics may be increasing because of stress from community living and frequent brief hospitalizations. The schizophrenic client most at suicide risk is a young white male who is in remission. He is well educated (several years of college) and has high expectations of himself. He feels hopeless, depressed, inadequate, and unable to cope with the chronicity of his illness. Other factors are previous suicide attempts and current threats or ideation. Suicide occurs most often early during hospitalization or soon after discharge (Drake 1984).

Survivors of Suicide

A 27-year-old woman called her former boyfriend and told him to look out of his window so that he could watch her die. He hung up on her. Only minutes later

---

Box 29–3

MAXIMUM SUICIDE PRECAUTIONS: SAMPLE PROTOCOL

The following is a protocol for maximum suicide precaution. These measures can be instituted without a physician's order under emergency conditions. However, a psychiatric consultation must be obtained as soon as possible.

1. Provide one-to-one nursing supervision. The nurse must be in the room with the client at *all* times. When the client uses the bathroom, the bathroom door must remain open.

2. Use no restraints on general hospital floors.

3. Do not allow the client to leave the unit for tests or procedures.

4. Allow the client to have visitors and telephone calls unless he or she wishes otherwise. The nurse maintains one-to-one supervision during visits.

5. Look through the client's belongings *with* the client and remove any potentially harmful objects, e.g., pills, matches, belts, razors, glass, tweezers.

6. Check that visitors do not leave potentially harmful objects in the client's room.

7. Serve the client's meals in an isolation meal tray that contains no glass or metal silverware.

8. Prior to instituting these measures, explain to the client what you will be doing and why. A physician must also explain this to the client. Document this explanation in the chart.

9. Do not discontinue these measures without an order from a psychiatrist.

---

he heard a crash. She had driven her car into a tree in front of his apartment building. The impact killed her instantly.

A 17-year-old high school student killed himself in his home after holding his mother hostage for three hours and forcing her to type his suicide notes. The young man tied his mother to a chair and forced her to type four suicide notes. When she finished, he shot himself in the head.

After a suicide, friends, spouses, children, nurses, and others who are left behind have painful feelings. It is not unusual for them to feel sadness, anger toward the lost person, or a sense of failed responsibility for allowing the suicide to occur. If the relationship was very difficult, with the deceased constantly refusing help, the survivor may feel a sense of relief. In contrast, some survivors do not accept the death as a suicide, choosing to believe it was an accident.

Problems survivors may face are depression, serious personality disturbances, and preoccupation with suicidal thoughts, especially on significant dates or anniversaries. After a parent's suicide, a child may exhibit learning disabilities, sleepwalking, delinquence, or fire-setting.

To prevent such reactions, nurses must make special outreach efforts to offer services to these clients. The nurse can remember to get names and telephone numbers of relatives and friends of suicide victims. Information can be collected from the coroner's office, emergency department, police, clergy, or funeral director.

When a client commits suicide as an in-patient, the staff needs help to reduce pain and develop coping skills. They will feel many of the emotions described above. Cotton et al. (1983) suggest the following interventions to help staff deal with their own and the other clients' experience of a client's suicide:

- Immediately after the suicide, hold a staff meeting to provide accurate information and make necessary decisions.

- Assign one person the duty of dealing with police and reporters.

- Hold ward meetings to inform other clients, answer questions, and assure clients of staff availability.

- Assess clients individually and decide on changes in treatment plans.

- Unit leadership should meet with the treatment team to review their work with the deceased client.

- Encourage all to seek peer support and to attend funeral services.

- Some months after the event, hold a conference to review the suicide.

Those staff members who have little medical training or experience suffer more than those who have previously encountered illness and death. These workers need extra attention.

NATURAL AND ACCIDENTAL DISASTERS

We have only recently begun to understand crisis intervention in disaster situations. Although federal aid for reconstruction of communities devastated by natural disasters has been available for many years, the provision of crisis intervention services through the National Institute of Mental Health (NIMH) was organized only as recently as 1972. Before then, a community in crisis depended on the voluntary help of social service and religious groups.

Nurses are often at the scene of natural disasters.

A number of nurses were in the Hyatt Regency Hotel—Kansas City, Missouri's newest hotel—in July 1981 when two skywalks in the four-story lobby collapsed, killing 111 and injuring 188 persons. These nurses, along with others who responded to calls for emergency personnel, assisted the injured and provided crisis intervention services. Some of the same nurses provided counseling services for people in the community, such as a fireman who was terrified to go on the next emergency call and 200 people from the community who attended a session to understand their responses and reactions. Some of the nurses themselves reported that since the disaster they have experienced shock, helplessness, nightmares, and difficulty in relaxing and concentrating.

The Dunlap article (1981) about the Kansas City disaster makes it clear that helpers on the scene may have many of the same responses to a disaster as its victims do. These responses are delineated more specifically below.

Assessment

James Tyhurst (1951, 1957) identifies three overlapping phases in response to disaster. The first stage, *impact,* is stimulated by the catastrophe. The victims recognize what is happening to them and are concerned mainly with the present. During this acute phase the victim's major concern may be staying alive. According to Tyhurst, about 75 percent of the victims experience shock and confusion. Although they appear dazed, they also exhibit the physical signs of fear. Another group of people, up to 25 percent, are "together." They logically and rationally assess the situation and develop and implement a plan for dealing with the immediate problems brought on by the catastrophe. A third group, also up to 25 percent, may panic or become immobilized with fear. They may behave hysterically, or they may be overlooked because they sit and silently stare into space.

In *recoil,* the second stage, the initial stress of the disaster has passed, and victims may no longer find their lives in immediate danger, although injuries and other discomforts come to their awareness. Emergency shelter, food, and clothing become available. Behavior of victims is usually dependent—they want to be taken care of. Weeping is common as survivors begin to realize all that has happened to them.

The full impact of the losses the victims have experienced comes in the third, or *posttrauma* period. Grief is a predominant response as persons mourn the losses in their lives. Disturbed and psychotic responses may occur.

Many people essentially "relive" the experience in their dreams by having recurrent nightmares. Other sleep disturbances, including insomnia, often occur. Victims may feel a psychic numbing or emotional anesthesia in relationship to other people; previously enjoyed activities; and feelings of intimacy, tenderness, and sexuality. They may have difficulty in concentrating and remembering. The survivors of mass trauma may also feel guilty about having survived or about behavior they undertook in order to survive. When victims are exposed to situations that resemble or in some way symbolize the traumatic event, their symptoms may increase and they may feel even greater distress.

The brief examples below illustrate the posttrauma experience.

On December 3, 1984, 2000 people were killed and 200,000 were injured because of a lethal gas leaking

from a Union Carbide pesticide plant. Twenty-five percent of all babies born during January and February of 1985 to mothers affected by the gas died soon after birth. On the one-year anniversary, a general strike paralyzed the city and effigies of Union Carbide officials were burned.

At the Dallas/Fort Worth Airport, Delta flight 191 crashed on August 7, 1985, while attempting to land during a thunderstorm. The dead numbered 137; survivors numbered 27. A survivor pays a daily visit to his wife, who has been comatose since the accident. Another survivor lost his high-paying job because of worry about his recovering wife and children.

At Cape Canaveral, Florida, on January 28, 1986, the space shuttle *Challenger* exploded seventy-five seconds after launching, killing all seven astronauts aboard. The entire nation grieved. Each subsequent discovery (finding the remains of the astronauts, finding parts of the spacecraft) renewed their families' torment.

RESEARCH NOTE

Citation

Murphy SA: After Mount St. Helens: Disaster stress research. J Psychosoc Nurs 1984;22:9–18.

Study Problem/Purpose

This investigator asked the following questions about the victims of a volcanic eruption:

1. Is there a relationship between illness and the loss of a significant other or of one's property?

2. Do social supports and self-efficacy lessen the negative effects of stress on health?

3. How do the media affect one's coping with loss following a disaster?

Methods

Four different victim groups were compared with a matched control group. The victim groups consisted of surviving relatives of persons confirmed or presumed dead and of persons whose recreational or permanent housing had been completely destroyed. Subjects were interviewed and given tests that assessed their life stress, physical health, and mental health.

Findings

1. High-stress levels were connected with lowered levels of health in both the bereaved groups and groups of people who had lost property.

2. Self-efficacy and social support were found to reduce depression.

3. The bereaved groups perceived the media as a hindrance to recovery.

Implications

This study supports the idea that crisis intervention can lessen the impact of a disaster. Those likely to come into contact with disaster victims should be trained in crisis management. These persons include nurses, clergy, teachers, physicians, and social workers as well as nonprofessional workers. Crisis intervention should be provided at temporary morgues and shelters where victims may express their experience to a trained listener. These victims should be assessed for such high-risk factors as multiple deaths, lack of resources, and number of moves to temporary housing. The media may be useful in providing people with some ideas of what responses they expect of themselves and in giving information about available services.

Nursing Diagnosis

The nursing diagnoses determined for these persons depend on their individual responses. Table 29–5 lists possible diagnoses according to DSM-IIIR, PND-I, and NANDA.

Planning and Implementing Interventions

The type of help needed by disaster victims changes as the disaster unfolds. Initially, people need information about evacuation plans, rescue efforts, locations of food, shelter, and medical care. The media can provide this information, especially when there is time to plan and anticipate need (as with floods or hurricanes).

After acute needs are met at the disaster scene, in makeshift hospitals, or in emergency rooms, morgues, and shelters, more far-reaching interventions are necessary. People need housing, jobs, and help in reconstructing their emotional lives. The following guidelines address the psychologic needs of victims both during and after a disaster (Hoff 1984, p 289):

- Talk out the experience and express their feelings of fear, panic, loss, and grief.

- Become fully aware and accepting of what has happened to them.

- Resume concrete activity and reconstruct their lives with the social, physical, and emotional resources available.

To assist victims through the crisis, the crisis worker should:

- Listen with concern and sympathy and ease the way for the victims to tell their tragic story, weep, express feelings of anger, loss, frustration, and despair.

- Help the victims of disaster accept in small doses the tragic reality of what has happened. This means staying with them during the initial stages of shock and denial. It also may mean accompanying them back to the scene of the tragedy and being available for support when they are faced with the full impact of their loss.

- Assist them to make contact with relatives, friends, and other resources needed to begin the process of social and physical reconstruction. This could mean making telephone calls to locate relatives, accompanying someone to apply for financial aid, giving information about social and mental health agencies for follow-up services.

People who are hysterical or panicked should receive prompt attention to avoid the contagion of panic that sometimes occurs in large groups. It sometimes helps hysterical or panic-stricken persons to perform a small but structured task that focuses their energies constructively. Nurses should remember, however, that assigning tasks beyond the person's capabilities at that time will add to the person's anxiety and feeling of helplessness.

Nurses will also find that in disaster situations they will be incorporating concepts and intervention strategies related to death and loss described in Chapter 37.

Immediate and effective community responses to disaster or crisis situations help victims and survivors resolve their experiences satisfactorily. The two examples below demonstrate how a community crisis or disaster can be managed.

On November 4, 1985, ten persons were killed in Roanoke, Virginia, in a flood that left hundreds homeless and caused an estimated $750 million in damages. The Mental Health Services of the Roanoke Valley immediately launched plans to help. Pamphlets were distributed that explained normal emotional reactions after a disaster and encouraged people to come and seek help. A specially trained team of counselors organized programs for flood victims, and for rescue and medical personnel.

At the one-year anniversary of the flood, newspaper stories and fliers asked people to assess their recovery and to prepare for possible future disasters. A community get-together commemorated the "human success stories, trials, and triumphs" of the first year.

On June 11, 1987, three graduating high school seniors and a popular driving education instructor in a small upstate New York community were killed by a drunken driver who was estimated to be going over seventy miles per hour. Despite several phone calls from concerned citizens who observed the erratic driving, the police arrived about twenty seconds too late. A team of forty grief and crisis counselors from a nearby metropolitan area arrived at the school the next morning to hold small group and large group sessions for students and teachers. Several clergy were on hand in the parking lots to meet arriving school buses and private cars, to keep reporters away from students and teachers, and to provide spiritual counseling. A memorial service was attended by the students, faculty, friends, family, and the community. The crisis and grief counselors continued to meet with those involved, many of whom expressed sadness over the deaths of the students and the teacher and anger over the survival of the drunk driver and his companion.

Table 29–5
Comparison of DSM-IIIR and Psychiatric Nursing Diagnoses

DSM-IIIR Diagnoses	PND-I Diagnoses		NANDA Diagnoses
309.89 Post-traumatic stress disorder	01.04.03	Insomnia	Adjustment, impaired
	01.04.04	Nightmares	Coping, ineffective individual or family
	02.01	Altered decision making	
	02.02	Altered judgment	Anxiety
	02.05.01	Amnesia	Fear
	02.08.02	Altered concentration	Social isolation
	04.01.01	Rape-trauma syndrome*	Hopelessness
	04.02.01	Anger	Spiritual distress
	04.02.02	Anxiety*	Self-concept, disturbance in
	04.02.05	Fear*	
	04.02.06	Grief*	Grieving, dysfunctional
	04.02.07	Guilt	Sleep pattern disturbance
	05.05.02	Social isolation/withdrawal*	
	05.99.01	Potential for violence*	Social interaction, impaired
	06.04.03	Hallucinations	
	06.04.04	Illusions	Posttrauma response
	06.03	Altered self-concept*	Rape-trauma syndrome
	06.01.02	Hyperalertness	
	08.02.01	Spiritual distress*	Violence, potential for
	08.01.02	Helplessness	Thought processes, altered

*PND-I diagnoses also in NANDA list.

Evaluation

It is difficult to evaluate the effectiveness of disaster intervention because of the large numbers of people involved and the innately disruptive nature of a disaster. Evaluation can take place at many different levels: Nurses can evaluate their work with individual clients; mental health agencies can monitor statistics on groups of clients; government agencies can assess the numbers of unemployed and homeless; public health departments can measure the extent of disease and disability. The most important aspect of evaluation is the opportunity it gives for reflection on the nature of the disaster. Some catastrophes are accidents, some are clearly avoidable, some are caused by human greed and insensitivity. All afford the survivors the chance to be better prepared for future crises.

CRISIS INTERVENTION MODES

Telephone Counseling

Suicide prevention and crisis intervention centers rely heavily on telephone counseling by volunteers who have professional consultation available to them. Sometimes called *hot lines* and often available round-the-clock, they allow the caller to remain anonymous and test what it is like to

Text continues on p. 800

CASE STUDY: A Client Requiring Crisis Intervention

This client came to the city's free clinic for a pregnancy test. A psychiatric nurse was the mental health counselor that evening. The nurse was asked to give the client the test results (positive) and assess her reaction to the news.

Identifying Information

Ms M, age 16, single, white, lives in a lower-middle-class section of the city in an apartment building. She is a public high school student (grade 10), self-referred to the free clinic.

Client's Definition of Present Problem, Precipitative Stresses, Coping Strategies, Goals for Care

Ms M came to clinic because she missed her period and felt "sick to her stomach" for the past three mornings. She complains of headache and lethargy. She fears she is pregnant.

History of Present Problem

N/A

Psychiatric History

None

Family History

The client's mother died of cancer two years ago. Ms M lives with her mother's sister (Aunt Claire). The client's father lives in Moneta (thirty minutes away) with the client's two teenage brothers. She feels close to her aunt and sees her father and brothers on weekends and vacations. Aunt Claire works as a secretary. The father repairs machinery at a fabric mill.

Social History

Ms M describes herself as an average student. She works after school at a fast-food restaurant. She has a few girlfriends and is especially close to one. She has been sexually active with her boyfriend (her first partner) for two months. They were using a "rhythm" method of birth control, but intermittently. She does not smoke, drink, or use recreational drugs.

Significant Health History

Ms M was diagnosed with epilepsy three years ago. She takes anticonvulsants daily. She recently has had fainting spells during which she becomes cold, weak, and dizzy. These pass after she eats and rests. She has not had a checkup in three years.

Current Mental Status (After Receiving News of Positive Pregnancy Test)

Well-groomed, mildly obese, alert, tearful. Oriented in all spheres; fund of knowledge adequate for age; memory, recall, and calculations satisfactory; judgment satisfactory. Client crying softly but able to converse easily and openly. Motor behavior is awkward and clumsy. No hallucinations, delusions, or suicidal ideation. Thought processes intact. No inappropriate defenses evident. Adequate insight into problem pregnancy; realistic view of problem.

Other Significant Data

Currently taking phenytoin (Dilantin) 50 mg three times daily. No history of suicide attempt and no present suicidal ideation. Client is uncertain about pregnancy; wishes to discuss options with her aunt and counselor.

continued

Diagnostic Impression *Nursing Diagnosis (PND-I/ NANDA)*		
	02.01	Altered decision making (associated with unplanned pregnancy) /Anxiety
	07.99	Potential for altered physiologic processes /Potential for injury to fetus related to phenytoin.
	02.03.03	Knowledge deficit* (related to birth control) /Knowledge deficit

DSM-IIIR Multiaxial Diagnosis

Axis I: V.62.89 Phase of Life Problem: Unplanned pregnancy
Axis II: None
Axis III: Epilepsy, pregnancy
Axis IV: 4 Severe (death of parent)
Axis V: Current GAF: 80 Transient and expectable symptoms

PND-Idiagnosis also in NANDA list.

Nursing Care Plan

Nursing Diagnosis (PND-I/NANDA)	Client Care Goals	Nursing Planning/ Interventions	Evaluation
02.01 Altered decision making (associated with unplanned pregnancy)	1. Client will discuss options with significant other and professional counselor. 2. Client will verbalize satisfaction with choice. 3. Client will take decisive action.	1. Explore with client her feelings about pregnancy. 2. Explain options and give information about counseling centers available. 3. Provide acceptance and support and hopefulness that a satisfactory solution can be found. 4. Give client a written plan to take home: a. Go home by bus; tell Aunt Claire about pregnancy. b. Decide with her whether to tell boyfriend and father. c. Call Planned Parenthood in morning (has telephone number) and get appointment with counselor. d. Call physician (has telephone number)	Client to call "free clinic" should plan prove unsatisfactory. Ask client to call clinic, if possible, and report outcome to nurse on duty.

continued

Case Study (continued)

Nursing Diagnosis (PND-I/NANDA)	Client Care Goals	Nursing Planning/ Interventions	Evaluation
		and make appointment for reevaluation of epilepsy medication. Client knows to tell the nurse that she is pregnant and needs an appointment as soon as possible. e. Arrange for time off from work if necessary to keep appointments. f. Call the clinic and ask for clinic director (has name and number) if she needs further assistance.	
07.99 Potential for altered physiologic processes /Potential for injury to fetus related to phenytoin	Client will consult private physician.	Inform client about need for physician supervision in cases of pregnancy during phenytoin therapy.	Client to contact clinic if unable to get appointment.
02.03.03 Knowledge deficit (birth control)* /Knowledge Deficit	Client will discuss birth control options with counselor.	Provide information on counseling centers available.	Client to contact clinic if more information necessary.

PND-I diagnosis also in NANDA list.

ask for help. No appointment, travel, or money is necessary, and help of some kind is immediate. The volunteers usually work within a protocol that indicates what information they need from the client to assess the crisis. Their goal is to plan steps to provide immediate relief and then long-term follow-up, if necessary.

Just as in person-to-person contact, the nurse who provides telephone counseling must do a lethality assessment. This is accomplished by asking the caller direct questions, as described earlier in this chapter. Other interventions important in telephone counseling are (Neville 1985):

- If the caller is reluctant to give a name and location, do not press for this information. The caller may feel threatened and hang up.

- Listen for background noises that may give clues to the caller's location.

- Use a note pad to write messages to co-workers so that the conversation is not interrupted.

- Keep the caller talking. This gives the nurse time to begin to develop a relationship, to trace the call, or to contact relatives or police if necessary.

- Allow the caller to ventilate all feelings. The nurse should accept anger, manipulation, etc., in order to keep contact.

- Emphasize that the nurse is available to talk as long as the caller needs to do so.

- Reinforce positive responses and actions, such as the fact that the caller is talking instead of acting out hopeless feelings.

- Acknowledge that the caller feels distress but explain that the caller does not need to harm himself or herself in order to emphasize it.

- Do not overuse reflection of feelings, which, in this

setting, may sound uncaring or superficial. Instead, offer direction and solutions to problems.

- If the nurse is knowledgeable about making a no-suicide contract, this can ease the transition from telephone to in-person treatment (Twiname 1981).

This type of intervention can be very stressful for the nurse/counselor. It is helpful to remember that despite our efforts to communicate concern, the ultimate decision maker is the caller.

Home Crisis Visits

Home visits are made when telephone counseling does not suffice or when the intervenors need to obtain additional information by direct observation or to reach a client who is unobtainable by telephone. Home visits are appropriate when the intervenors need to initiate contacts rather than waiting for clients to come to them—e.g., when a telephone caller is assessed to be highly suicidal or when a concerned neighbor, physician, or clergyman informs the agency of clients in potential crisis.

Often these clients are too disorganized or distraught to seek help by themselves. The police may arrange for a home crisis visit to avoid imprisoning or hospitalizing a client. Problems commonly encountered are spouse battering, child abuse, and psychiatric emergencies.

The crisis intervenors are usually a male-female team who are highly skilled and experienced in crisis intervention. The male-female team might be perceived as less threatening than two men, two women, or a single person. Their goal is to defuse the situation with as little disruption and violence as possible and to engage the clients in longer-term treatment.

Crisis Counseling

Crisis counseling is a type of brief therapy. As opposed to therapies that focus on bringing about major personality changes, crisis counseling focuses on solving immediate problems. It lasts from five to six sessions and involves individuals, groups, or families. The following techniques are used:

- Listen actively and with concern
- Encourage the open expression of feelings
- Help the client gain an understanding of the crisis
- Help the client gradually accept reality
- Help the client explore new ways of coping with problems
- Link the client to a social network

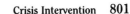
- Engage in decision counseling or problem solving with the client
- Reinforce newly learned coping devices
- Follow up the case after resolution of the crisis

Chapter Highlights

- Everyday living brings desirable and undesirable changes that result in stresses and tensions with the potential for becoming crises.

- A crisis is a self-limiting situation in which usual problem-solving or decision-making methods are not adequate.

- A crisis offers the opportunity for renewal and growth.

- Working with a helping person increases the likelihood that a crisis will be resolved in a positive way.

- Nurses are often in key positions to help clients grow through the crisis experience.

- Crises may be classified into two types: internal or developmental (the anticipated crises of maturation), and external or situational (stressful life events that are usually not anticipated).

- The crisis episode may be understood as a sequence that involves three time periods—precrisis, crisis, and postcrisis.

- Crisis intervention as a therapeutic strategy is strongly humanistic in that people are viewed as capable of personal growth and able to control their own lives.

- Intervention strategies such as individual crisis counseling, crisis groups, family crisis counseling, telephone counseling, and home crisis visits are appropriate modes for dealing with either internal or external crisis.

- Suicide is a maladaptive response to crisis.

- Suicidal behavior is affected by a number of social, demographic, and clinical variables.

- A lethality assessment is the first step in helping self-destructive persons and is the basis on which the nurse formulates subsequent responses.

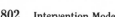

References

Aguilera DC, Messick JM: *Crisis Intervention: Theory and Methodology,* ed 5. Mosby, 1986.

Bartelo S: The aftermath of suicide on the psychiatric inpatient unit. *Gen Hosp Psychiatry* 1987; 9(3):189–197.

Black D, Warrack G, Winokur G: The Iowa Record-Linkage Study: Suicides and accidental deaths among psychiatric patients. *Arch Gen Psychiatry* 1985;42:71–75.

Britton JG, Mattson-Melcher DM: The crisis home: Sheltering patients in emotional crisis. *J Psychosoc Nurs* 1985;23(12):18–23.

Busteed EL, Johnstone C: The development of suicide precautions for an inpatient psychiatric unit. *J Psychosoc Nurs* 1983;21:15–19.

Caplan G: *Principles of Preventive Psychiatry.* Basic Books, 1965.

Capodanno AE, Targum SD: Assessment of suicide risk: Some limitations in the prediction of infrequent events. *J Psychosoc Nurs* 1983;21:11–13.

Cobb S, Lindemann E: Neuropsychiatric observations after the Cocoanut Grove fire. *Ann Surg* 1943;117:814.

Cotton PG, et al: Dealing with suicide on a psychiatric inpatient unit. *Hosp Community Psychiatry* 1983;34:55–59.

Crisis intervention. *Adv Nurs Sci* 1984;6:entire issue.

Disasters and Mental Health. National Institute of Mental Health. American Psychiatric Press, 1986.

Drake RE, et al: Suicide among schizophrenics. Who is at risk? *J Ment Nerv Dis* 1984;172:613–617.

Dunlap MJ: Nurses assist injured at Hyatt disaster. *Am Nurse* 1981;13:1.

Erikson E: *Childhood and Society,* ed 2. W. W. Norton, 1963.

Everstine DL, Everstine L: *People in Crisis: Strategic Therapeutic Interventions.* Brunner/Mazel, 1983.

Friesen M: Self-inflicted injury: Breaking a tragic cycle. *Nurs Life* 1985;5(3):22–25.

Hansell N: *The Person in Distress.* Human Services Press, 1976.

Hatten CL, Valente SM, Rink A: *Suicide Assessment and Intervention.* Appleton-Century-Crofts, 1977.

Hoff LA: *People in Crisis: Understanding and Helping,* ed 2. Addison-Wesley, 1984.

Janosik EH: *Crisis Counseling: A Contemporary Approach.* Wadsworth, 1984.

Joint Commission on Mental Illness and Health. *Action for Mental Health.* Basic Books, 1961.

Klerman GL: *Suicide and Depression Among Young Adults.* American Psychiatric Press, 1986.

Kolk BA: *Psychological Trauma.* American Psychiatric Press, 1986.

Lewis S, et al: Saving the suicidal patient from himself. *RN* 1986;49(12):26–28.

Lindemann, E: Symptomatology and management of acute grief. *Am J Psychiatry* 1944;101:101–148.

Maslow A: *Motivation and Personality,* ed 2. Harper & Row, 1970.

Merker MS: Psychiatric emergency evaluation. *Nurs Clin North Am* 1986;21:387–396.

McIntosh, JL: Suicide among the elderly: Levels and trends. *Am J Orthopsychiatry* 1985;55:288–293.

Michael S, et al: Rapid response mutual aid groups: A new response to social crises and natural disasters. *Social Work* 1985;30(3):245–252.

Minrath M: Breaking the race barrier. *J Psychosoc Nurs* 1985;23(8):19–24.

Mullis M: Vietnam: The human fallout. *J Psychosoc Nurs* 1984:22(2):27–32.

Mullis M, Byers P: Social support in suicidal inpatients. *J Psychosoc Nurs* 1987;25(4):16–19.

Murphy SA: Perceptions of stress, coping, and recovery one and three years after a natural disaster. *Iss Ment Health Nurs* 1986;8:63–77.

Neville D, Barnes S: The suicidal phone call. *J Psychosoc Nurs* 1985;23:14–18.

Parad HJ, Resnick HLP: A crisis intervention framework, in Resnick HLP, Ruben HL (eds): *Emergency Psychiatric Care.* Charles Press, 1975, pp 3–7.

Pfeffer CR: Suicidal fantasies in normal children. *J Nerv Ment Dis* 1985;173:78–83.

Post JM, Oteri EM: Sign-out rounds. *J Psychosoc Nurs* 1983;21(9):11–17.

Rose-Grippa MK: Psychiatric Emergencies, in Cosgriff JH, Anderson DL (eds): *The Practice of Emergency Care.* Lippincott, 1984, pp 55 + .

Roy A: Suicide and psychiatric patients. *Psychiatr Clin North Am* 1985;8:227–241.

Sudak HS, Ford A, Rushforth NB: Adolescent suicide: An overview. *Am J Psychotherapy* 1984;38:350–363.

Sullivan-Taylor L: Policemen and nursing students: Crisis intervention team. *J Psychosoc Nur* 1985;23:31–33.

Tyhurst JS: Individual reactions to community disaster. *Am J Psychiatry* 1951;107:764–769.

Tyhurst JS: The role of transition states—including disasters—in mental illness. Paper read at the Symposium on Preventive and Social Psychiatry, Walter Reed Army Institute of Research and the National Research Council, Washington, D.C., April 15–17, 1957.

Twiname BG: No-suicide contract for nurses. *J Psychosoc Nurs* 1981;19:11–12.

Using Crisis Intervention Wisely, Nursing Skillbook, Nursing 81 books. Intermed Communications, 1980.

Victoroff VM: *The Suicidal Patient: Recognition and Intervention.* Medical Economics Books, 1983.

Walker JI: *Psychiatric Emergencies: Intervention and Resolution.* Lippincott, 1983.

THIRTY

Group Therapy

Carol Ren Kneisl

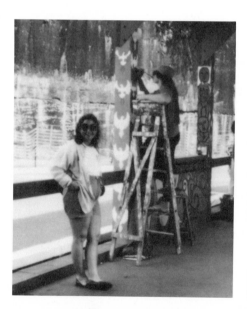

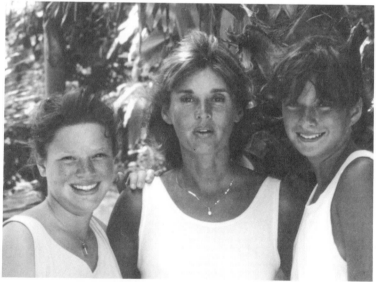

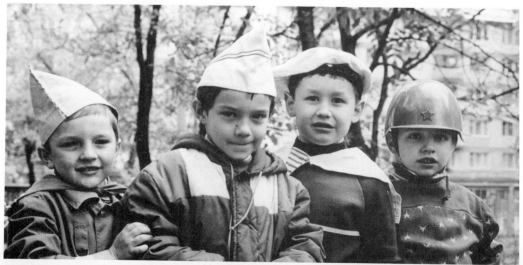

After reading this chapter, students should be able to

- Describe four frameworks for the assessment and understanding of therapy groups
- Assess small groups in terms of their functional, structural, and interactional characteristics
- Relate the egalitarian cotherapy approach to humanistic psychiatric nursing practice in interactional group therapy
- Describe the process of creating and maintaining a group
- Identify the stages in therapy group development
- Discuss the application of here-and-now activation and process illumination to psychotherapy groups
- Describe other related group therapies and therapeutic groups

Cross References

Other topics related to this content are: Group dynamics, Chapter 13; Influence of the milieu, Chapter 31; Mutual self-help groups as social support, Chapter 8.

Key Terms

affection need
catalyst
conflicted member
cotherapy
control need

group therapy
inclusion need
psychodrama
unconflicted member

Groups influence a person's psychologic well-being. Mental well-being can be preserved, maintained, and restored through interaction with others in productive groups. Group intervention is one way that psychiatric nurses can provide humanistic care for their clients. Therapy through the group process gives clients the opportunity to seek validation, give and receive interpersonal feedback, and test new and different ways of being that may improve quality of life.

The psychiatric nurse, in the role of group leader/facilitator/therapist, may function autonomously or in collaboration with other members of the mental health team. Effectiveness depends not on the helping person's background discipline but rather on the match between the abilities and characteristics of the helper and the needs of clients.

This chapter discusses four frameworks for assessment of group processes (based on Chapter 13) and various methods of group intervention. It emphasizes the strategies in freely interactive verbal group therapy.

HISTORICAL PERSPECTIVES

Joseph Hersey Pratt, a Boston physician, began to work with tubercular persons in groups in the United States in 1906. His learning groups were organized as weekly classes of twenty to twenty-five people to whom he lectured on the importance of strict hygiene, diet, and rest in the treatment of tuberculosis. Pratt also offered support and encouragement to his clients, whose long course of illness was discouraging at best. By 1930 he had established a clinic at the Boston Dispensary in which the group method was the central therapeutic focus. His writings throughout more than fifty years of work with groups of tubercular clients demonstrate his increasing awareness of the group dynamics of this style of treatment. He is usually credited with being the founder of group psychotherapy.

Just before World War I, some physicians in the United States began to use group approaches in the treatment of psychiatric clients. E. W. Lazell (1921), one of the better-known physicians, published the first contribution to the literature on use of group treatment with psychotic (spe-

We join with others in search of a peaceful world.

cially schizophrenic) individuals. Like Pratt, he used the lecture method. During this period, the emphasis was on encouraging, inspiring, and persuading group members, while providing information designed to educate and influence them. At about the same time, a minister named L. C. Marsh (1935), who became a psychiatrist, began to use other techniques such as art and dance classes in his work with groups.

Joshua Bierer (1942) began his work in 1939 in Great Britain, where he established social clubs for the treatment of the mentally disordered. His methods included discussion, writing, painting, and entertainment. Bierer believed that it was best to discuss individual problems in an impersonal way. He often disguised the problems for discussion to keep members of the group from realizing that their particular problems were under consideration. Bierer attempted to help persons solve their problems of daily living and change their attitudes toward life to more positive ones. His methods were based on those of Alfred Adler, who was using group psychotherapy in his child guidance work. Adler, a socialist and one of Sigmund Freud's first students, had established clinics to provide a variety of services and resource persons to large groups of working-class people with emotional problems. Social clubs like Bierer's gained importance in the United States over the years. Social clubs for the rehabilitation of "nervous persons" are still popular and can now be found throughout the United States. Perhaps the best known is Recovery, Inc. (see the Resources in Appendix C).

A Viennese psychiatrist, Jacob L. Moreno (1946), introduced the term **group therapy** into the clinical literature in 1932. His interest in drama led him to formulate a particular kind of group psychotherapy called **psychodrama**. He used dramatic techniques and the language and settings of theatrical productions to achieve psychotherapeutic goals. Moreno founded the first professional journal concerned with group psychotherapy and the first professional organization of group psychotherapists—known today as the American Society of Group Psychotherapy and Psychodrama.

During the late 1920s and early 1930s, Trigent Burrows (1927), another pupil of Freud, became interested in applying psychoanalytic principles of treatment within group settings. An American psychoanalyst, Alexander Wolff (1949, 1950), began to apply these principles in groups. In his psychoanalytic group, Wolff analyzed the individual in interaction with other individuals instead of treating a group. He took the position that it is not valuable, and may be detrimental, to attend to group dynamics in group analysis. At about the same time that Wolff was establishing psychoanalytic groups in the United States, S. H. Foulkes began a similar practice in Great Britain (Foulkes and Anthony 1957). Both Wolff and Foulkes implemented their techniques with the armed forces in the United States and Great Britain.

Samuel R. Slavson, who is best known for developing activity group therapy for children, was also active in using psychoanalytic concepts in therapy groups (Slavson 1947). He was a prime mover in establishing the American Group Psychotherapy Association and was the first editor of the *International Journal of Group Psychotherapy.*

During World War II, group psychotherapy grew extensively in the United States. It was hailed for its economic advantages, since a large number of clients could be treated by the relatively few available psychotherapists. It was also popular among military psychiatric personnel, who found themselves overwhelmed with the number of soldiers experiencing post-traumatic stress disorder and needing some form of psychotherapy.

Nurses have long been involved in working with clients and their families in small groups brought together for health teaching or supportive purposes. The role of the psychiatric nurse as group therapist, however, is relatively recent. It first received professional endorsement by the American Nurses' Association (ANA) in 1967. Qualifications of the group therapist are identified later in this chapter.

THEORETICAL PERSPECTIVES

Operational frameworks for group analysis provide the means for understanding the dynamic processes that go on in groups. Frameworks help the group leader know where the group is, predict in what direction it might move, and identify the potentials within the group that might be facilitated or developed. The four models discussed below are useful guides against which to compare a group. Perceptions of a group should not be forced to fit any model but should emerge through the process of comparison.

The Johari Awareness Model

There are many ways to think about self-awareness. Some theorists have used the image of multiple masks that people wear under various circumstances. Others have written about the "true self" versus "the false self" or the "good me," the "bad me," and the "real me." Common to all these concepts is the idea that self-awareness is a complex, multidimensional phenomenon, often contradictory and partly undiscovered. The Johari Awareness Model, often called the Johari Window, is a theoretical tool used to represent self-awareness in relation to other people.

Joseph Luft and Harry Ingham (1955), the creators of the Johari Awareness Model, maintain that interpersonal interaction, in a group setting, for example, is facilitated when people have sufficient knowledge about one another's actions, motivations, and feelings. Group members can use this knowledge to understand the significant events in a group more clearly.

Johari Window

The Johari Window is Luft and Ingham's graphic representation of their self-awareness model. It is described here and illustrated in Figure 30–1.

- **Johari Window Quadrant 1—Open Activity** The first quadrant of the window represents aspects of the self known about oneself and readily available or known to others as well. This is the part of the self that engages in daily social conversation.

- **Johari Window Quadrant 2—Risk** Quadrant 2 contains characteristics known to others but not to oneself. In this quadrant is information about how the person affects others intentionally or unintentionally. It is an aspect of self about which a person may get honest, genuine, uncensored feedback from others. It is also an area that influences reactions from others that may surprise and shock the individual.

- **Johari Window Quadrant 3—Private Life Space** Quadrant 3 represents the knowledge one has about oneself that is not known to others. These are the secrets, the personal and private feelings.

- **Johari Window Quadrant 4—the Unknown** Quadrant 4 contains knowledge about the self that is unconscious for the individual and unknown to others. This quadrant may be brought into awareness through free association, hypnosis, or dream analysis with special guidance.

Intragroup Relations

Major elements in this awareness model are its assumptions that humans respond to groups and that change or learning can follow opportunities for new interaction. The primary principle of change in relation to the Johari Window is: A change in one quadrant will affect all other quadrants. Certain other general principles of change that derive from the Johari Window are particularly suited to the understanding of small group behavior. These principles are:

- A large open quadrant (Q1) facilitates working with others. Therefore, more of the resources and abilities of group members can be brought to bear on the group task when members have large Q1 areas.

- The open quadrant can be enlarged, and awareness increased, by learning about group processes as they are being experienced.

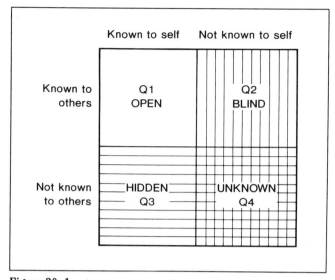

Figure 30–1
The Johari Awareness Model.
Source: Adapted from Group Processes: An Introduction to Group Dynamics *by Joseph Luft by permission of Mayfield Publishing Company (formerly National Press Books). Copyright 1963, 1970 by Joseph Luft.*

- How a group confronts the unknown quadrant is influenced by the group's value system.

In a new and immature group, Q1 is small, because free and spontaneous interaction does not occur in new groups. As the group matures, Q1 expands and Q3 shrinks accordingly. This means that members are becoming freer to be themselves and to perceive others as they really are. An atmosphere of increasing trust, risk taking, and self-disclosure begins to form. An enlarged area of free activity means that the group uses more energy to work on the group task than to maintain or defend the hidden or avoided area of Q3. Q2 also diminishes as members learn more about themselves. Q4 changes more slowly and to a lesser degree, because it represents an area in which unknown behaviors and motives reside. Figure 30–2 compares the degrees of openness in immature and mature groups.

A group can also be understood and diagrammed according to the Johari Windows of the individual members.

Sam was a person with limited freedom. Although he was polite, he appeared to be superficial and constricted. He devoted large amounts of energy to walling off the behavior and motivations of Q2, Q3, and Q4 by intellectualizing. Laura was a group member whose great inner resources allowed her to develop a very

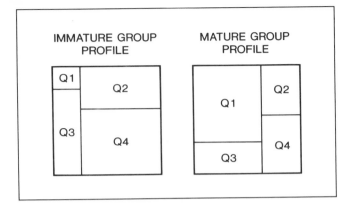

Figure 30–2
The immature versus mature group.
Source: Adapted from Group Processes: An Introduction to Group Dynamics *by Joseph Luft by permission of Mayfield Publishing Company (formerly National Press Books). Copyright 1963, 1970 by Joseph Luft.*

large area of free activity. In contrast, Debbie was what Luft has termed a plunger. Debbie's spontaneity and "openness" lacked discretion and created distance in her relationships with other group members. Van and Maria, the other two members of this group, tended not to take many risks in their interactions with others, although their moderate openness indicated flexibility.

The Johari Window configurations of this group are illustrated in Figure 30–3. Sam's Johari Window shows a greatly reduced and constricted open quadrant. His behavior and feelings are likely to be limited in range, variety, and scope. His interactions tend to be conventional, and he is likely to be threatened by group behaviors that go beyond the bounds of convention. Laura's Johari Window represents a person whose interactions are characterized by great openness to the world. Much of her potential has been developed and realized. Debbie's Johari Window is that of the inappropriately transparent person who deals with others by disclosing too much. The Johari Windows of Maria and Van show moderately large open areas although Q2, Q3, and Q4 are equally large.

The awareness configurations raise an interesting question: What behaviors might be predicted in a group with members such as these? Obviously this group needs to resolve several problems. An "underdiscloser" like Sam reveals too little, thus reserving control for himself. He tends to quell spontaneous reactions in order to double-check. He may be one of the last to acknowledge the development of trust. Debbie's failure to control her overdisclosures means that her relationships with others in the group will be either too smothering (because of being too close)

or too demanding (because she imposes herself on others without considering their intimacy needs). She may trust everyone because she has not learned to discriminate among relationships. Her behavior forces others to take responsibility for defining the nature of the relationship. Group members are likely to feel threatened by her early spontaneous disclosures, which they may experience as overwhelming. Problems of trust, intimacy, and risk taking may arise in her interactions with these members.

Laura, because of her high degree of self-awareness, will be less preoccupied with defensiveness and distortion than other members. She will be able to accept the differences in others and serve as a model for them. Maria and Van, whose awareness configurations demonstrate they have progressed to moderate openness, should continue to grow in this direction with minimal discomfort to themselves and other group members.

Intergroup Relations

A group can also be viewed as a whole entity in interactions with other groups. Q1 includes the open, available information that is known to the group as well as to others. Q2 is the area that others outside the group see but the group itself does not. Q3 has to to with the secret, hidden things that the group keeps to itself. Knowledge may be hidden purposefully to enable the group to manipulate other groups. A group of business people who hide the flaws in a property they put up for sale illustrate this. Groups keep things hidden for other reasons as well, such as being ashamed of some activity or attitude or finding an event or belief hard to explain because it refers to idiosyncratic occurrences known only to the members. Hidden things form the *lore* of the group. Q4 includes behavior and motives that are unknown to the group and to outsiders as well. A covert and unrecognized split among the members with regard to the group goals would be one example. Difficulties in effective group functioning could result from such an unrecognized split.

FIRO: The Interpersonal Needs Approach

The Fundamental Interpersonal Relationship Orientation (FIRO) is a popular approach developed by William Schutz (1958a, 1958b). Some of his ideas were generated during his work for the Department of the Navy. The Navy was concerned with interpersonal problems experienced by the crews of nuclear submarines during their long-term cruises beneath the polar ice cap. While some crews functioned effectively and were satisfied with one another, others performed ineffectively and voiced their dissatisfactions. Schutz set out to learn how to predict which people were compatible with which other people. Theoretically, nuclear submarine crews could be composed of compatible individuals who would be more likely to perform effectively

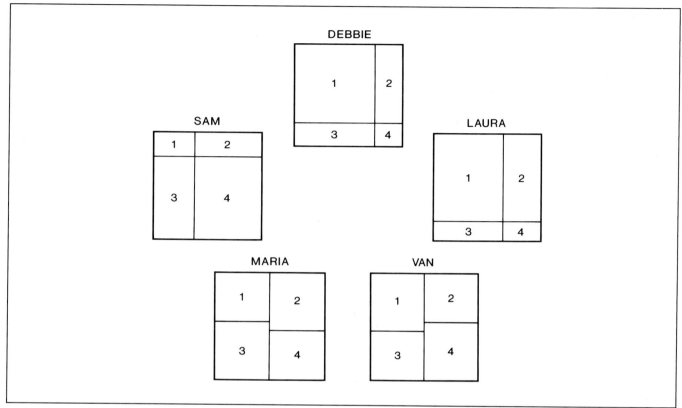

Figure 30–3
Awareness configurations in a specific group.

together and would find their lengthy enforced togetherness, if not totally pleasurable, at least tolerable.

The basic assumption of Schutz's theory is that people need people. In addition, people need to establish some equilibrium between themselves and the people in their environment. This equilibrium is determined by the interaction of certain interpersonal needs, and it appears to be synonymous with interpersonal compatibility.

Three Basic Interpersonal Needs

An interpersonal need is one that can be satisfied only through relationships with people. Schutz reasoned that every individual has three interpersonal needs: inclusion, control, and affection.

Inclusion

The interpersonal **need for inclusion** may be defined as the need to establish and maintain relationships with others that offer interactions and associations satisfying to the individual. A satisfying position in terms of inclusion includes:

- A psychologically comfortable relation with people somewhere on a continuum that ranges from initiating or originating interaction with all people to not initiating interaction with anyone. In other words, this dimension is *expressed* toward others.

- A psychologically comfortable relation with people in regard to wanting others to initiate interaction somewhere on a continuum that ranges from always initiating interaction with you to never initiating interaction with you. In other words, this dimension is *wanted* from others.

To put this another way, *expressed inclusion* is the ability to take an interest in others to a satisfactory degree, and *wanted inclusion* is the ability to allow other people to take an interest in you to a satisfying degree to yourself.

Connotative terms that point to a positive inclusion relation are: *associate, interact, mingle, communicate, belong, companion, comrade, attend to, member, togetherness, join, extrovert.* At the other end of the scale are terms that connote lack of inclusion, such as: *exclusion, isolate, outsider, outcast, lonely, detached, withdrawn, abandoned, ignored.* This need determines whether a person is outgoing or prefers privacy.

Control

The interpersonal **need for control** may be defined as the need to establish and maintain a satisfactory relation between oneself and other people with regard to power and influence. A satisfactory position in terms of control includes:

- A psychologically comfortable relation with people somewhere on a continuum that ranges from controlling all the behavior of other people to not controlling any behavior of others
- A psychologically comfortable relation with people in regard to their control behavior on a continuum that ranges from always wanting to be controlled by them to never wanting to be controlled by them

To put this another way, *expressed control* is the ability to take charge to a satisfactory degree, and *wanted control* is the ability to establish and maintain a feeling of respect for the competence and responsibleness of others to a satisfying degree to yourself.

Connotative terms for primarily positive control are: *power, authority, dominance, influence, control, ruler, superior officer, leader.* At the other end of the scale are terms that connote lack of control, or negative control: *rebellion, resistance, follower, anarchy, submissive, henpecked, Milquetoast.*

Affection

The interpersonal **need for affection** may be defined as the need to establish and maintain a satisfactory relation between the self and other people with regard to love and affection. A satisfactory position in terms of affection includes:

- A psychologically comfortable relation with others somewhere on a continuum that ranges from initiating close, personal relations with everyone to originating close, personal relations with no one
- A psychologically comfortable relation with people in regard to their affection behavior on a continuum that ranges from wanting everyone to originate close, personal relations toward you, to wanting no one to originate close, personal relations toward you

To put this another way, *expressed affection* is being able to love other people or to be close and intimate to a sat-

isfactory degree, and *wanted affection* is having others love you or to be close and intimate with you to a satisfactory degree.

Connotative terms for an affection relation that is primarily positive are: *love, like, emotionally close, positive feelings, personal, friendship.* At the other end of the scale are terms that connote lack of affection or negative affection: *hate, dislike, cool, emotionally distant.*

The dimensions of the FIRO theory are illustrated in Figure 30–4.

Group Development

The interpersonal needs theory asserts that any group, given enough time, moves through three interpersonal phases—inclusion, control, and affection, in that order—that correspond to the three basic interpersonal needs.

Inclusion Phase

The first or inclusion phase is concerned with the problem of *in or out.* People attempt to find their place within the group and are concerned with learning whether they will be acknowledged as individuals or left behind and ignored. Because these concerns give rise to anxiety, this phase is dominated by behavior centered around the self. Overtalking, withdrawal, exhibitionism, and sharing other group experiences and biographies are some examples.

Frequently, *goblet issues* predominate. These are issues of minor importance to the group that help people get to know one another and test each other. They are a vehicle for sizing up people. Goblet issues may resolve around the weather, the World Series, rules of procedure, and so on.

Control Phase

The second or control phase is concerned with the problem of *top or bottom,* which becomes salient after problems of inclusion have been resolved. Concern about decision-making procedures predominates, and the problems that emerge involve the sharing of responsibility and the distribution of power and influence. This phase is dominated by competitive behavior. There are struggles for leadership and about the structure, rules of procedure, and methods of decision making. Members are attempting to establish comfortable positions for themselves in terms of responsibility and influence.

Affection Phase

The third or affection phase is concerned with the problem of *near or far,* and it follows satisfactory resolution of the preceding two phases. Individual members are now faced with the problem of becoming emotionally integrated. Concerns about not being liked by, being too close to, or not being close enough to others become relevant. The

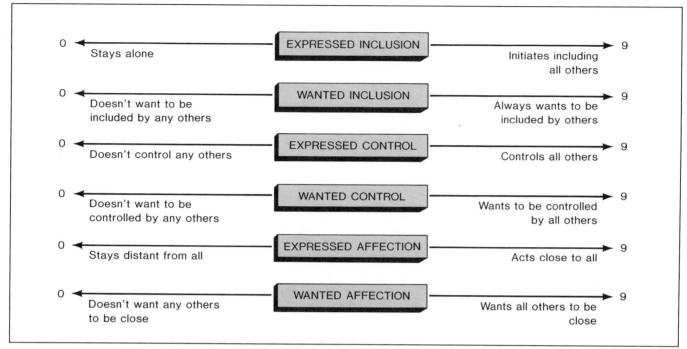

Figure 30-4
Dimensions of the FIRO theory.

behavior in this phase is generally characterized by high emotion—positive feelings, jealousy, hostility, and pairing are some examples. Schutz (1958a) describes this phase as one in which, like porcupines, people attempt to get close enough to receive warmth, yet avoid the pain of sharp quills.

Interweaving of Phases

None of these phases is distinct, since all three problem areas are present at all times, even though only one predominates. Schutz (1958a, p 130) uses a tire-changing analogy, what he calls *tightening the bolts,* to describe the sequence of the phases:

> When a person changes a tire and replaces the wheel, he first sets the wheel in place and secures it by tightening the bolts one after another just so the wheel is in place and the next step can be taken. Then the bolts are tightened further, usually in the same sequence, until the wheel is firmly in place. Finally each bolt is gone over separately to secure it.

The leader helps the group work on all three interpersonal need areas in similar fashion, returning to and working over each area to a more satisfactory level than was reached the last time.

Applying the Theory

Clearing the air by making covert interpersonal difficulties overt is a major step in applying the FIRO theory. Although this step is initially uncomfortable, the final result is rewarding. Interpersonal difficulties that can be made overt are:

- Withdrawal or silence by members
- Inactivity and unintegrated behavior by members
- Overactivity and destructive behavior by members
- Power struggles between members
- Battles for attention among members
- Dissatisfaction with the leadership
- Dissatisfaction with the amount of recognition a member receives for contributions
- Dissatisfaction with the amount of affection and warmth demonstrated in the group

A group that is relatively compatible can function smoothly with minimal discussion of its problems. Groups in which the interpersonal problems are extremely minor can usually ignore them (or, if problems exist between two members, work them out outside the group) without hampering group effectiveness. A group that is basically incompatible has to spend much time and energy resolving its interpersonal problems so that it can function effectively.

The interpersonal needs approach of Schutz is based on the belief that the way to attack problems within groups is by investigating what is going on among the individuals in the group and attempting to improve their interpersonal relations.

The Authority Relations/Personal Relations Approach

Two major areas of internal uncertainty or stress in groups, according to the theory developed by Warren Bennis and Herbert A. Shepard (1956), are dependence (authority relations) and interdependence (personal relations). The first area has to do with group members' orientations toward authority—the handling and distribution of power within the group. The second area has to do with group members' orientations toward one another. A central assumption in this theory is that the principal obstacles to a valid group communication (and hence to group effectiveness) derive from the members' orientations toward authority and intimacy.

A new group is highly concerned with authority and power. Earlier experiences with authority influence and partially determine members' orientations toward other members. Bennis and Shepard have called this Phase I. As the group develops, it moves away from its preoccupation with authority toward a preoccupation with personal relations. This constitutes the second major phase in group development, called Phase II. These major phases, and their subphases, are summarized in Box 30–1.

Relevant Aspects of Member Personality

Bennis and Shepard view members as either conflicted or unconflicted around the dependence and personal aspects of group life. A **conflicted member** is one whose posture toward dependence or intimacy may be viewed as inflexible, rigid, or compulsive. These members insist on adopting certain roles despite the situation. Conflicted members are responsible for confused communication within groups. An **unconflicted member**, also called an *independent*, is better able to assess situations and alter roles or behavior as appropriate.

There are two ways in which persons can be conflicted around authority relations. Members who are comforted by rules of procedure and agendas and rely on the decisions of others (who are viewed as experts) are said to be *dependent*. Members who are uncomfortable with structure and

---

Box 30–1
THE BENNIS AND SHEPARD MODEL

Phase I (Dependence-Power Relations)

Subphase 1: Dependence-Submission This subphase is characterized by dependency and flight. Members discuss problems external to the group. Assertive or aggressive members play dominant roles. Self-oriented behavior and subgrouping are evident.

Subphase 2: Counterdependence This subphase is characterized by counterdependence and fight. Members discuss the organization and structure of the group. Assertive counterdependent and dependent members play dominant roles. Group searches for what to talk about and how to make decisions. Uncertainty causes anxiety.

Subphase 3: Resolution This subphase is characterized by involvement in the group tasks. Assertive independents play dominant roles. The group unifies to pursue the task and members take over some leadership roles.

Phase II (Interdependence-Personal Relations)

Subphase 4: Enchantment This subphase is characterized by a high level of solidarity, fusion, camaraderie, and suggestibility. Members talk about the positive aspects of the group and its members. For the first time in its history, there is general distribution of participation. Overpersonals play dominant roles. Laughter and joking are common as is planning social events outside of the group.

Subphase 5: Disenchantment This subphase is characterized by fight-flight evidenced in distrust and suspicion of various group members. The content themes in Subphase 1 are revived. The most assertive counterpersonal members play dominant roles; overpersonal members are also active. The group may divide on the basis of shared attitudes toward intimacy. The group may be disparaged by the members in a variety of ways.

Subphase 6: Consensual Validation This subphase is characterized by understanding and acceptance. Assertive independents play dominant roles. The group views itself and its accomplishments in realistic terms. Consensus on important issues is easier to achieve.

---

authority are *counterdependent.* Counterdependents manifest their dissatisfaction with authority by opposing it regardless of its style or intent. Nothing the authority or leader does is acceptable. Failure to design an agenda is viewed by the counterdependent as evidence of the authority's lack of ability. Paradoxically, designing an agenda may be viewed as too controlling. The counterdependent takes a "damned if you do, and damned if you don't" stance toward authority.

Members can be conflicted around personal relations in two ways as well. People who direct uninterrupted efforts toward reaching a high degree of intimacy with all other group members are termed *overpersonal*. Members who expend great amounts of energy in avoiding intimacy and maintaining distance are said to be *counterpersonal*.

Persons unconflicted in terms of either the authority relations or the personal relations in the group are responsible for major movements in the group's development toward valid communication. These unconflicted members who move the group on to the next phase are called catalysts. They reduce the internal uncertainty or stress in the group. Actions of these unconflicted members that move the group forward into the next phase are called *barometric events*. Figure 30–5 presents a grid of these aspects of member personality.

Relationship to Group Strategies

The Bennis and Shepard model demonstrates group development along a continuum from the emphasis on power to the emphasis on affection. The activities of Phase I are concerned with such things as social class, ethnic background, and personal and professional interests. Concern with personality and reaction to feelings, such as warmth, anger, love, and anxiety, arise in Phase II. Bennis and Shepard believe that group therapies should be based on an adequate understanding of the group dynamic barriers to communication.

The Therapeutic Problem Approach

The final approach to the analysis of groups that is considered in this chapter is one that describes group development—specifically, therapy group development—in six discrete phases. E. A. Martin and William F. Hill (1957) formulated this theory of group development from the basic assumption that distinct and common growth patterns exist in therapy groups and can be described, observed, and predicted. The major therapeutic problem encountered is the focal point for describing each phase. In this model, transitional stages between the developmental plateaus indicate potentials for movement from one phase to another. The six phases of therapy group development, according to Martin and Hill, are:

- *Phase I.* Individual unshared behavior in an imposed structure
- *Phase II.* Reactivation of fixed interpersonal stereotypes
- *Phase III.* Exploration of interpersonal potential within the group
- *Phase IV.* Awareness of interrelationships, subgrouping, and power structure
- *Phase V.* Responsiveness to group dynamic and group process problems

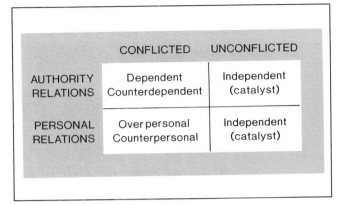

Figure 30–5
Member personality categories.

- *Phase VI.* The group as an integrative-creative social instrument

Like the other theorists discussed above, Martin and Hill see groups as passing along a developmental continuum from minimal to optimal effectiveness. Groups differ in the time they spend in any phase and the problems they face. Most groups disband before reaching the sixth, or ultimate, phase of development.

Phase I—Individual Behavior

The group in Phase I is best described as an aggregate of social isolates held together loosely by vague perceptions of the therapist and his or her role. Imposed structure, such as regularity of meeting time and place, consistency of membership, and a group seating arrangement, encourage "groupness," slight though it may be. Because of a lack of interpersonal, group-relevant structure, esprit de corps and cooperative ventures are latent but not yet realized. There is little justification for calling the aggregate of individuals in Phase I a group.

Transition from Phase I to Phase II

The major characteristic of the first transitional phase is that the therapist emerges as the leader of the group and is publicly acknowledged by the members. Autistic behavior diminishes. It is replaced by an *asyndetic* mode of interaction, a form of interpersonal interaction in which elements in a statement by one speaker function as a cue for the next speaker. A third, fourth, or fifth speaker may similarly be cued by the preceding speaker. It is a chain reaction that seems highly autistic, in that the material evoked by the cues is highly personal and does not enhance or elaborate the productions of the earlier speaker. There is some group relevance, however, in that the remarks indicate that members have paid at least some attention to each other. They thus establish indirect social contacts. The therapist can help the group move on to the next phase through modeling behavior that is not asyndetic but rather recognizes the members as social beings.

Phase II—Fixed Stereotypes

In the second phase, members' perceptions of one another are based on previously learned stereotypes. Although members publicly acknowledge one another's existence, the acknowledgment is in terms of "ghosts" of earlier interpersonal experiences. These stereotyped perceptions or ghosts fail to acknowledge the uniqueness of each member. A member may be called a "redneck," "sweet," or "macho," based not on how the person really is but rather on the stereotype assigned to that individual. The leader is frequently typecast in some sort of omniscient role, and dependence on the leader emerges. It is the socialization aspects of this phase that provide therapeutic value.

Transition from Phase II to Phase III

Social stereotypes break down during this transition period. Members openly express resentment of being stereotyped and insist on their own rights and views. Appraisals of one another become more realistic. The members' idiosyncratic perceptions of the leader begin to give way to a group view. The therapist assists the group by helping members become more aware of the discrepancies in their views of the therapist.

Phase III—Exploration of Potential

This phase is characterized by active emotional exchange geared to giving group members recognition as individuals. Although many asyndetic processes and autisms still occur, the group begins to deal with the here-and-now events in the group and with their perceptions of one another. A group norm appears that places high value on individual importance. It may be demonstrated by the devotion of one or more entire sessions to the problems or personality of one member or by a rapidly shifting give-and-take. Because the individual is of paramount importance, membership is valued, and absences, tardiness, or dropping out are grave concerns. In this phase, members learn to give emotional feedback to one another and become more aware of their

effects on one another. The experience of being valued gives one a sense of purpose and facilitates self-worth.

Transition from Phase III to Phase IV

At the third transition point, the group becomes restless, finding the detailed analysis of one another's personalities boring and repetitious. The excitement and novelty of exploration diminish, and group discussions turn to consideration of the relationships that have developed among group members. The therapist can help the group transcend this feeling of "same old faces and same old problems" by making members aware of their boredom and encouraging their exploration of the relationships among members.

Phase IV—Awareness of Interrelationships

Growing awareness of certain relationships between and among members surfaces during Phase IV. Pairing relationships and hierarchical relationships are among those that emerge. Member skill at identifying relationship dynamics encourages them to consider their attempts to structure specific relationships with the therapist. "Teacher's pets" and "junior therapists" may be identified at this time. The group becomes divided, as opinion leaders and emotional attitude leaders begin to surface and subgroups are established around them. Consequently, rivalries also develop, and subgroups struggle for power. The therapist's task is to help the members identify subgroup leaders and supporters and consider the potential consequences of a power struggle.

Transition from Phase IV to Phase V

A high state of tension exists within the group, and there is decreasing tolerance for the tension in the transition stage. Members may attempt, usually unsuccessfully, to replace subgroup operation with a total group orientation. To help the group attain a level of total group orientation, the therapist should make the group aware of the source of its dissatisfaction and provide helpful techniques, such as role playing, to identify and highlight the subgroup problems that have emerged.

Phase V—Responsiveness to Group Dynamics

Individual and subgroup problems become reinterpreted as group problems in the fifth phase. The group becomes process oriented and attuned to the group dynamics. It demonstrates its awareness of silences, difficulty in getting started, taboo topics, and similar phenomena. The group seems to be concerned about learning how it functions. The therapist can help by providing expertise in the description and comprehension of dynamics and processes. Because it is difficult for a group to remain for long at this sophisticated level of operation, regression to earlier behaviors is common.

Transition from Phase V to Phase VI

After experiencing process analysis as a rewarding endeavor, the group attempts to remedy or take care of unwanted or undesirable features that came to light in the analysis. However, the desire to remedy does not always ensure the ability to remedy. The group finds itself frustrated in its problem-solving attempts and may need to rely on the skills of the therapist.

Phase VI—The Group as Social Instrument

The sixth phase constitutes the ideal phase of group life. The group becomes superbly effective at engaging in cooperative problem solving, diagnosing process and dynamics, making acceptable and appropriate decisions. In short, this group is characterized by competence. Leadership is fully distributed among the members, and the therapist becomes a resource person. Martin and Hill (1957, p 28) describe the members of such groups as "masters of their fate."

INTERACTIONAL GROUP THERAPY

There is a great diversity and flux in the field of group therapy. Many types of groups are found in mental health settings or in communities at large. Persons may be members of encounter groups, sensitivity training groups, gestalt groups, transactional analysis groups, psychodrama groups, psychoanalytic groups, nonverbal groups, body movement groups, nude swimming therapy groups, etc. This list is certainly incomplete—a wide and bewildering array of group approaches is available to the willing.

Certain common principles seem to apply to all therapeutic groups, although specific methods and techniques may vary according to the purpose of the group or the skills and theoretical orientation of the therapist. Irvin Yalom (1985) uses the term *interactional group therapy* to describe a process of group therapy in which member interaction plays a crucial role. The common principles that apply to interactional group therapy are discussed below.

Advantages of Group over Individual Therapy

The advantages of group therapy stem from one major factor—the presence of many people, rather than a solitary

therapist, who participate in the therapeutic experience. Specifically, group therapy provides:

- Stimuli from multiple sources, enabling distortions in interpersonal relationships to be revealed so that they can be examined and resolved
- Multiple sources of feedback
- An interpersonal testing ground that enables members to try out old and new ways of being in an environment specifically structured for that purpose

Qualified Group Therapists

Mental health professionals may believe, in error, that group therapy is less complex and therefore "easier" than individual therapy, for example, because the presence of more people makes interactions between therapist and client less intense. While it is true that the intensity of interactions between any one member and the therapist may be less intense because interactions are dispersed among others, it *does not follow* that anyone can be an effective group therapist.

To be effective, the group therapist should have the following special preparation:

- Education in small group dynamics
- Education in group therapy theory
- Clinical practice with groups
- Expert supervision of the clinical practice (with ongoing supervision and/or consultation, depending on level of expertise)

The ANA Standards (see Chapter 3) identify the group psychotherapy role as appropriate for clinical specialists prepared at the master's level. Competent therapists report that it is also valuable to be a member of a therapy or sensitivity training group, before becoming a group leader.

The Curative Factors

Yalom (1985) contends that eleven interdependent curative factors or mechanisms of change in group therapy help people. These factors are the framework for an effective approach to therapy, because they constitute a rational basis for the therapist's choices of tactics and strategies. They are identified and defined in Table 30–1.

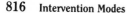

Table 30–1
Curative Factors of Group Therapy

Factor	Definition
Therapist:	
Instilling of hope	Imbuing the client with optimism for the success of the group therapy experience
Universality	Disconfirming the client's sense of aloneness or uniqueness in misery or hurt
Imparting of information	Giving instruction, advice, or suggestions
Altruism	Finding that the client can be of importance to others; having something of value to give
Client:	
Corrective recapitulation of the primary family group	Reviewing and correctively reliving early familial conflicts and growth-inhibiting relationships
Development of socializing techniques	Acquiring sophisticated social skills, e.g., being attuned to process, resolving conflicts, and being facilitative toward others
Imitative behavior	Trying out bits and pieces of the behavior of others and experimenting with those that fit well
Interpersonal learning	Learning that one authors his or her interpersonal world and moving to alter it
Group cohesiveness	Being attracted to the group and the other members with a sense of "we"-ness rather than "I"-ness
Catharsis	Being able to express feelings
Existential factors	Being able to "be" with others; to be a part of a group

Types of Group Leadership

Groups can be led by a therapist working alone or by cotherapists working together in a variety of ways. Leaderless groups are another possibility. Each approach is described and evaluated in the sections that follow.

The Single Therapist Approach

Groups led by a single therapist are common. They have an economic advantage in that only one therapist need be involved. A disadvantage is that the therapist cannot compare analyses of the group process with a cotherapist or get instant feedback or validation from a peer. Therapists working alone, however, do not have to direct their energies toward creating and maintaining a relationship with a colleague.

Recorders or observers may be used to help the solitary therapist be aware of the multiple complexities of any one group session. Nonparticipant observer/recorders are especially useful when they give the therapist feedback and focus on the nonverbal aspects of the session. If they are truly to be nonparticipants, recorder/observers must be very careful not to react on a nonverbal level to the content or process of the session.

The Cotherapy Approach

It is becoming more common to see groups led by two therapists who share responsibility for leadership of the group to varying degrees. The two models seen most often are the junior-senior and the egalitarian styles of cotherapy.

The Junior-Senior Position

In the junior-senior approach, the therapists have unequal responsibilities toward the group. The senior member of the team is usually the more experienced or more highly educated of the two. Besides having major responsibility for the success of the group, the senior therapist is responsible for training the junior member of the team. This approach is commonly used in agency settings, because it provides in-service training of new personnel and non-professionals under the guidance and watchful eye of an experienced group leader. However, relationship problems frequently surface when the roles of the leaders are not clear, or when one or both leaders are unable, or unwilling, to remain in the designated roles. The members of the group may also be unclear about the subordinate/superordinate roles and unsure of how to deal with and respond to leaders of unequal abilities and responsibilities.

The Egalitarian Position

In the egalitarian approach to cotherapy, two therapists of relatively equal skill, ability, and status share equally in responsibility for the group. This method is also used for training, with both cotherapists working under clinical supervision. It is preferable to the junior-senior approach for many reasons, which are set forth in Table 30–2. The egalitarian position is not without certain potential disadvantages, however. These are listed in Table 30–3. Overall, the advantages of the egalitarian approach outweigh its

Table 30–2
Advantages of Egalitarian Cotherapist Approach

Advantage	Rationale
Facilitates group development	Two therapists of similar abilities can monitor and facilitate group development better than one alone.
Facilitates dealing with heightened affect	One therapist can relate more directly to the member experiencing heightened affect, while the other therapist assumes responsibility for assisting the group members with their responses. When one therapist is involved in an interaction with a member or members, the other can take an observer stance, helping those involved to become more aware of the interaction and their participation in it.
Enhances therapists' personal and professional development	Egalitarian cotherapists can provide one another with corrective feedback and help one another analyze group process and plan intervention strategies.
Provides a synergistic effect	This is another way of saying "two heads are better than one." It is likely that two persons working together will make better decisions than one person working alone. The synergistic effect is similar to that of making decisions by consensus.
Provides an opportunity for modeling	Group members observe the acceptance and respect for one another that egalitarian cotherapists demonstrate. The therapists tolerate differences and disagreement between them in an atmosphere of mutual trust.
Reduces dependence	Because leadership is shared, the problem of dependence is somewhat dissipated.
Promotes appropriate pacing	Cotherapists check one another's timing, thus allowing the process to emerge. The presence of a cotherapist provides a respite from being continually "on guard" in relation to group process.

Table 30–3
Potential Disadvantages of Egalitarian Cotherapist Approach

Potential Disadvantage	Rationale
Creates conflict if therapists have different orientations	Although there is room for uniqueness and difference, radically different styles or beliefs about group therapy between cotherapists may hinder therapeutic work within the group.
Requires extra energy and time	Each therapist must spend time and energy maintaining an effective working relationship with the other, since the quality of the relationship between them determines their effectiveness in the group setting.
May make members feel overloaded	If the style of the therapists turns out to be "two-on-one" (both working at once with one group member), members may feel overwhelmed or "overtherapized."
May suffer from the fact that the therapists share blind spots	Therapists who are very similar in style and personality may have the same blind spots and fail to give one another corrective feedback.
May provide the opportunity for misleading modeling	The model the therapists provide may be negative if their relationship is tense, mistrustful, closed, competitive, or threatening.

potential disadvantages. Cotherapists who arrange for supervision or consultation for themselves find that potential disadvantages can be turned in their favor. Identification and analysis of disadvantages that arise can lead to learning and behavior change in the cotherapists.

Nurses considering an egalitarian cotherapy relationship with one another need to engage in preliminary work to determine whether such a relationship is feasible for them. Exploration should include a discussion of each therapist's theoretical approaches, intervention styles, past experiences with groups, background, and personality characteristics. The therapists should consider and resolve such issues as how and when feedback is to be given, how disagreements between them are to be handled in the session, and the general conditions under which they will work together.

Decisions on client selection, length and number of sessions, time, and place are made together. Decisions of an emergency nature made by one therapist in the absence of the other should be based on mutually agreed procedures for just such situations.

Obviously, egalitarian cotherapists must establish and maintain clear channels of communication. Not only must they expend a great deal of time and energy in preparation for the group experience, but they must also plan for presession and postsession meetings, joint analysis of data, and joint supervision or consultation.

The Leaderless Approach

There is increasing interest in leaderless groups in two common forms—the occasional or regularly scheduled leaderless meeting as part of the structure of a group that is basically led by a therapist, and the leaderless group structured in some programmed format, usually through audiotapes.

Leaderless meetings in a therapist-led group should not be scheduled until the group has become cohesive and has established productive norms. Then the process can foster a sense of autonomy and responsibility. However, therapists should identify and examine their rationale for planning leaderless meetings. The repercussions of leaderless meetings are varied and complex and require an experienced group therapist to deal with them.

Other leaderless groups may be structured totally around following directions in a booklet and on tape. Encounter group or sensitivity training tapes are common. For example, members listen to a tape explaining the exercises assigned for that session. The members participate as instructed on the tape and spend the remainder of the session discussing the exercise and their reactions to it.

Creating the Group

The effectiveness of a group depends heavily on the conditions under which it is created. Much as architects design buildings, therapists design groups with certain functions and characteristics in mind.

Selecting Members

Selecting the members is one of the most important functions of the therapists, since the quality of the interpersonal relationships among the members constitutes the core of successful group treatment. This is one of the major differences between group and individual therapy.

Inclusion Criteria

It is more difficult to identify the characteristics of people who make good candidates for group therapy than those of people who do not make good candidates. We know that a person's motivation for therapy in general, and group therapy in particular, is of primary importance. Inclusion in a therapy group should also be at least partially determined by the effect a prospective member will have on the others, in terms of the prospective member's ability to bring the curative factors into play. Inclusion is also determined by the balance, in terms of behavior or characteristics, a prospective member will bring to the group. Will the person's subdued presentation prevent a member with similar behavior from being marginal and alone in the group? Does the person's age, occupation, or sex match another's so that the member will not feel singled out as different or deviant? The factor that appears to be most important, however, is that members be homogeneous in terms of their vulnerability or ego strength. Highly vulnerable members retard the progress of the less vulnerable, and vice versa.

Exclusion Criteria

There have been a number of studies of group therapy dropouts. Dropouts significantly reduce the effectiveness of a group. They tend to have a demoralizing effect on the remaining group members. Group members see the act of dropping out as a comment on the worth of the group. For this reason, therapists should gear selection to avoid taking on members who are likely to terminate prematurely. Irvin Yalom (1985) identified several reasons given for premature termination. They are detailed in Table 30–4. Yalom's research has also demonstrated that people who drop out are likely to have some of the following characteristics:

- They use denial to a significant extent.
- They somatize frequently.
- They are less well motivated than those who continue.
- They are less psychologically oriented than those who continue.
- They have more severe psychiatric pathology.
- They are less likable (by group therapists).
- They are lower in socioeconomic status than those who continue.

- They are less effective socially than those who continue.
- They have lower IQs than those who continue.

It is also not uncommon to find that group therapy drop-outs are persons who used the group for crisis resolution. They drop out once the crisis has passed.

The Selection Interview

The pregroup interview session has two major purposes: selecting the members and establishing the initial contract. Cotherapists should always interview potential members jointly, and both should make all decisions regarding membership. The interview session gives members and therapists the opportunity to be exposed to one another. The therapists should accomplish the following tasks in the selection interview:

- Determine the motivation of the potential member
- Determine the presence and extent of any exclusion criteria
- Identify the presence of any external crisis that may have propelled the person into treatment
- Encourage the client to ask questions about the group
- Correct erroneous prejudgments or misinformation the client has about group therapy
- Inquire about any major pending life changes that may prevent the client's full and continued participation in the group
- Inquire about what hurts; what the client sees as a need to work on
- Establish and clarify the initial group contract

During this period, therapists and members have a chance to decide whether they can work together in the specific group under consideration. Clients as well as therapists can choose whether they will participate or not.

The Group Contract

The group contract identifies the shared rights and responsibilities of therapists and members. It is a negotiated set of rules or arrangements for the structure and functioning of the group. It may be written or verbal, and it should cover the following elements:

- Goals and purposes of the group
- Time and length of meetings
- Place of meetings
- Starting and ending dates

Table 30–4
Client Reasons for Premature Termination of Group Therapy

Reason	Rationale
External factors	
Physical reasons	Distance, commuting, transportation, or scheduling problems may arise.
High external stress	An extremely stressful life may make it difficult or impossible for a client to expend energy participating in the group.
Group deviance	Members who differ significantly from others may wish to terminate; however, deviance that is unrelated to the group task is irrelevant.
Problems of intimacy	Isolated and withdrawn persons, or those with a pervasive dread of self-disclosure, are threatened by group therapy.
Fear of emotional contagion	Members may find they become highly upset on hearing the problems of others.
Early provocateurs	Members may create a nonviable role for themselves in the group; they plunge in with behavior that provides the main focus, are furiously active, then wish to withdraw.
Problems in orientation to group therapy	If pretherapy tasks have not been properly undertaken, the member may not be realistically prepared for the group.
Complications arising from subgrouping	Subunits that split up the group may disrupt therapeutic work if not understood and handled appropriately.
Complications arising from concurrent individual and group therapy	The member's two therapies may work at cross-purposes; members may "save" their affect and experiences in the group for exploration in an individual session.

- Addition of new members
- Attendance
- Confidentiality
- Roles of members and therapists
- Fees

Goals and Purposes

The purpose of the group must be clear to all persons involved. In interactive group psychotherapy, the purpose is to bring about enduring behavioral and character change. The interactive group psychotherapy experience takes place largely in the here-and-now.

Goals may be long term or short term and are both group oriented and individualized. Some goals may be identified as early as the selection interview, and others may be added as they emerge during the life of the group. Goals may be altered as appropriate.

Time, Length, and Frequency of Meetings

Time of meetings may be mutually determined by the participants. The length and frequency of meetings should be determined by the therapists after consideration of the clients' needs. Most out-patient clients find one eighty- to ninety-minute session per week useful. Shorter periods may not allow adequate time for discussion. Longer periods are generally beyond the endurance and alertness levels of both members and therapists. In-patient groups are generally held more than once per week and frequently last for fifty to sixty minutes, although they may be longer or shorter depending on the anxiety and tolerance levels of the particular clients.

Place of Meetings

The physical environment is important and influences the interaction among members. It is best to choose a pleasant room with comfortable chairs, preferably placed in a circle. The room should be private and free from external distractions.

Starting and Ending Dates

If the group has a predetermined life span and the inclusive dates are known, members should be told the dates. Groups without fixed termination dates usually plan termination individually as each member is ready to move away from the group.

Addition of New Members

Open groups accept members after the first session; closed groups begin with a certain number of members and do not add new members. Open groups maintain their size by replacing members who leave the group. They may continue indefinitely or have a predetermined life span. Closed groups are more common in settings where stability of membership is likely. Such settings include residential facilities of various types, long-term psychiatric in-patient settings, and prisons. A major problem with the closed group is that it runs the risk of extinction as members leave the group for various reasons.

Attendance

It is important that members make a commitment to attend every session. Absences hinder the establishment of cohesion and have a demoralizing effect, especially when perceived as evidence that a member lacks interest or that the group is not attractive and valuable to its members. Stability of membership and high attendance have been demonstrated to be critical factors in the successful outcome of group therapy.

Confidentiality

Some rules regarding confidentiality should be established, and clients' concerns about which people will have access to information concerning them should be explored. Many therapists like to use tape recorders in order to have their work evaluated afterward by supervisors. They must obtain the clients' agreement to use of a tape recorder.

Rules about confidentiality and access may be determined by the therapists' employing agency. In some instances, therapists may be required to make regular notes concerning each member's participation. Therapists may also wish to establish with group members guidelines on confidentiality that allow the therapists to share content with professionals when clients are dangerous to themselves or others. A good rule of thumb is: *Promise only what you can safely deliver.* Members should also be held accountable to maintain the confidentiality of the group.

Roles of Members and Therapists

Therapists and clients should reach an understanding about the responsibilities of participants. Humanistic psychotherapy involves the full and informed participation of the client in the therapeutic process. Participants should share their expectations about the behavior and functions of clients and therapists and should clearly understand the modes for participation.

Fees

Fees should be determined in advance and arrangements for payment made. Most mental health agencies have a sliding fee scale determined by the client's income and ability to pay. Clients should know whether fees will be charged for missed sessions.

Stages in Therapy Group Development

There is comfort in being able to predict, to some extent, the behavior of members at specific points in the group's life. Therapists organize predictions around stages or phases in the therapeutic experience, hoping to be prepared for expressions of behavior. They must bear in mind, however, that human experiences are dynamic and fluid and do not always progress as neatly as predicted.

The Schutz, Bennis and Shepard, and Martin and Hill frameworks, presented earlier in this chapter, give clear indications of how group life develops. This section focuses on the characteristics of member behavior and therapist interventions in the beginning, middle, and termination phases of interactional group therapy. As members' problems in living are revealed, the group life becomes richer and more complex. Therefore, there is no "cookbook" method that a therapist can follow to respond to every situation. Table 30–5 is presented simply as a guide for identifying some common member behaviors and therapist interventions at various points in the life of the group.

RESEARCH NOTE

Citation

Gordon VC, Gordon EM: Short-term group treatment of depressed women: A replication study in Great Britain. Arch Psychiatric Nurs 1987;1(2):111–124.

Study Problem/Purpose

The purpose of this study was to replicate a group therapy nursing intervention developed in the United States to evaluate it for its effectiveness in relieving symptoms of depression, hopelessness, loneliness, and anxiety in depressed women in Great Britain.

Methods

Twenty women between 40 and 60 years of age who tested out as being mild to moderately depressed on the Beck Depression Inventory (self-report form) and within the normal range on the SCL-90-R Inventory (to screen out women who were psychotic or had suicidal tendencies) were randomly selected and randomly assigned to a control (n = 10) and a treatment group (n = 10). Two professional nurses with group experience functioned as facilitators for the cognitive-behavioral intervention treatment group, which met in 2-hour sessions for 14 weeks. The control group received no intervention between pretesting and posttesting. The pretreatment and posttreatment measures were the Beck Depression Inventory (self-report form), the Beck Depression Inventory (significant other form), the Young Loneliness Inventory, Beck Hopelessness Scale, Beck Anxiety Checklist, Coopersmith Self-Esteem Inventory, and the Social Adjustment Self-Report Questionnaire. The first hour of each session was devoted to lecture, education, and discussion. The second hour was spent in activities that reinforced the application of skills (such as conflict management, relaxation, building relationships, and so on). A step-by-step structure was identified for each of the 14 sessions. The nurse group facilitators also kept observation notebooks.

Findings

Significant improvement in self-esteem and reduction in expressed feelings of depression and hopelessness were found for the subjects in the treatment group. However, they were still mildly depressed and expressed mild levels of hopelessness. They also experienced significant improvement in self-esteem when compared with the control group. Feelings of loneliness and anxiety did not show improvement in the treatment group. The level of social adjustment also did not show significant improvement.

Implications

Nurse-facilitated group intervention is an effective means of helping to alleviate symptoms of depression and hopelessness in depressed women. The structured nursing intervention developed by Gordon can be effective in elevating self-esteem in depressed women. The results suggest that perhaps a 14-week interval is insufficient to reduce depression and hopelessness to the normal range as measured by Beck's scale. The failure of the study to demonstrate improvement in loneliness and anxiety might also be due to the short time period. Gordon's cognitive-behavior approach may provide an alternative way for nurses to engage in health promotion and illness prevention with depressed women.

822   Intervention Modes

Table 30–5			
Characteristic Member Behaviors and Nursing Interventions in Phases of Group Therapy			
Member Behavior	Nursing Interventions	Member Behavior	Nursing Interventions
Beginning Phase		Self-disclosure increases	Encourage exploration and move to problem solving
Anxiety is high	Move to reduce anxiety; avoid making demands until group anxiety has abated	Members are more aware of interpersonal interactions in the here-and-now	Encourage members to participate in observing and commenting on here-and-now; make process comments
Members unsure of what to do or say; need to be included	Be active and provide some structure and direction; suggest members introduce themselves; work to sustain therapeutic rather than social role; include all members and encourage sharing but limit monopolizing	Additions and losses of members evoke strong reactions	Prepare members for additions and losses where possible; provide opportunity to talk about addition and loss experience
Members unclear about contract	Clarify contract; give information to dispel confusion or misunderstandings	Ability to maintain focus on one topic increases	Encourage exploration of topic area in depth
Members test therapists and other members in terms of trustworthiness, value stances, etc., often through goblet issues	Capitalize on opportunity to "pass" tests by proving trustworthy and by being open to and accepting the values of others	**Termination Phase**	
		Feelings about separation may run gamut (anger, sadness, indifference, joy, etc.)	Provide adequate time in as many sessions as necessary to work through affective responses; be sure members know termination date in advance; help members leave with positive feelings by identifying positive changes that have occurred in individual members and in group
Beginning attempts at self-disclosure and problem identification are made	Focus on related themes; begin exploration; begin to focus on here-and-now experiences in session		
Members have sense of "I"-ness, little sense of "we"-ness	Encourage involvement with others through curative factor of *universality*	Members may feel lost and rudderless	Explore support systems available to individual members; bridge gap where possible (to another agency, another therapist, etc.); keep in focus task of resolving loss
Middle Phase			
Sense of "I"-ness is replaced by "we"-ness	Encourage cohesion; provide opportunity for expression of warm feelings		

The Here-and-Now Emphasis

The core of interactional group therapy is the here-and-now. According to Irvin Yalom (1985, p 136), the here-and-now work of the interactional group therapist occurs on two levels:

1. Focusing attention on the member's feelings toward other group members, the therapists, and the group

2. Illuminating the process (the relationship implications of interpersonal transactions)

Thus, group members need to become aware of the here-and-now events—i.e., *what* happened—and then reflect back on them—i.e., *why* it happened. Yalom has called this the *self-reflective loop*.

The first task of the therapist is to steer the group into the here-and-now. As the group progresses and becomes comfortable with awareness of the here-and-now, much of the work is taken on by the members. Initially, however, the therapist actively steers group discourse in an *ahistoric* direction. In other words, events in the session take precedence over those that occur outside or have occurred outside.

If the group is to engage in interpersonal learning, the therapist must illuminate process. This is the second task of prime importance. The group must move beyond a focus on content toward a focus on process—the how and the why of an interaction. The process can be considered from any number of perspectives. The perspective chosen should be determined by the mood and needs of the group at that particular time. The group must recognize, examine, and understand process. The task of illuminating it belongs mainly to the therapist.

Process commentary is anxiety-producing, because there are so many injunctions against it in social situations. For example, commenting on someone's nervousness at a cocktail party is generally taboo. It not only makes the nervous person uncomfortable but also puts the process commentator in a high-risk situation. The comment may well be taken as criticism or viewed as inappropriate to the social context, and the commentator is then vulnerable to retaliation from others.

Focus on the here-and-now experience differentiates interactive group psychotherapy from many other group therapies or therapeutic groups. The following section discusses some of these other approaches.

OTHER GROUP THERAPIES AND THERAPEUTIC GROUPS

Analytic Group Psychotherapy

Analytic group psychotherapy stems from psychoanalysis and shares its goal of personality reconstruction. In this process, there is an intensive analytic focus on the individuals within the group. It is sometimes described as treatment of one person in front of an audience of many. Dream material and fantasies are explored within the group, and the technique of free association is used. The interpersonal interactions of the members are of secondary importance and are explored in terms of how they demonstrate unresolved conflicts in the individual members' earlier relationships.

Psychodrama

Psychodrama is chiefly concerned with problems unique to the individual. It provides a medium through which catharsis can be achieved on both the nonverbal action and gesture level and the verbal level. In psychodrama groups, members act out real or imagined situations, while alter egos (other members) attempt to add what they think the actor may be feeling or thinking. The participants are encouraged to change roles. The practice of role reversal offers them the opportunity to "get into the other person's skin." The psychodramatist (therapist) is called a "direc-

tor" whose responsibility is to direct the drama toward the goal of achieving catharsis and reaching for insight.

The psychodramatic stage may be quite complex. It sometimes consists of a series of tiers where different parts of the drama are acted out. Complex lighting and mood music may also be used to achieve the desired effect.

Self-Help Groups

Self-help groups are sometimes called self-directed groups or lay groups in the literature. The major operating principle in self-help groups is that the help given to members comes from members. A professional mental health worker is viewed as unnecessary. In fact, many of these groups were developed because of the failure of programs planned and implemented by professionals. In most, leaders are former members. Alcoholics Anonymous is a relatively well-known example.

There are a wide variety of self-help groups. Some are:

- Recovery Incorporated, Schizophrenics Anonymous, and Neurotics Anonymous, concerned with mental illness
- TOPS, Weight Watchers, Diet Workshop, and Overeater's Anonymous, concerned with obesity
- Gamblers Anonymous and Gam-Anon, concerned with compulsive gambling
- Five-Day Plan and Smoke Watchers Anonymous, concerned with smoking
- Child Abuse Listening Mediation, Inc. (CALM) and Parents Anonymous, concerned with child abuse
- La Leche League, concerned with breast-feeding
- Al-anon and Al-a-teen, concerned with the families of alcoholics
- Daytop and Phoenix House, concerned with drug addiction

Self-help groups are proliferating rapidly. Groups for divorced, widowed, or single persons, for parents of runaways and troubled adolescents, for parents who abuse their children, and for the recently bereaved are becoming a common part of the scene in most major cities throughout the world. Client clubs for persons having had a colostomy, ileostomy, laryngectomy, mastectomy, or amputation are also popular.

The role of the nurse in self-help groups is that of a resource person. Nurses need to be informed about such groups so that they can refer potential members to groups appropriate to their needs or to provide consultation when invited to do so. For this reason, self-help groups are included in the Resources appendix.

Remotivation and Reeducation Groups

Remotivation and reeducation groups were developed to help persons who had undergone long-term institutionalization become less isolated and more socially adept. Long-term institutionalization produces apathy and isolation. Clients ready for release are often unaware of accepted norms or socially appropriate behavior and therefore ill equipped to live outside a totally protected environment. Remotivation and reeducation groups help prepare these people to live beyond the confines of the institution. The groups bring members up to date with contemporary society. They can be led effectively by people with minimal preparation in group work. In many psychiatric hospitals, this role falls to the psychiatric aide. Nurses are more likely to supervise than to lead remotivation groups.

Client Government Groups

Most therapeutic milieus have numerous group activities. One common activity is some form of client government. Client governments take many forms, but in most cases staff and clients meet together once or twice a week to discuss and resolve day-to-day issues on the ward. Generally, these are key principles in client government.

- The client government should actually make and enforce most of the ward rules.
- The client government should organize and execute most of the routine ward tasks.
- No staff member should attempt to solve a problem if it can be delegated to the client government.

Among the problems the client government considers are the tidiness of the unit, late-night use of the television, the decision to have or not to have a Christmas tree, and individual clients' disruptive behavior. To make client government work, staff members must consciously refrain from making unilateral decisions that override client prerogatives. Needless to say, this strategy produces power relationships unlike those in the traditional medical model, in which it is believed that doctors and nurses are the experts and clients do not know what is best for them. Client government does not require that staff sit silently by, however. Rather, staff members should offer their perspective while agreeing to abide by the group's decision. Obviously, client

government raises many thorny issues. Decisions about the granting of leave or the issuing of medications have legal implications that sometimes make client government impractical. In many cases the real decisions on these subjects are made in a substructure of separate staff meetings. It is often preferable for staff members to discuss issues that present problems for them in the open forum of the client government meeting. Otherwise, clients have no way of knowing how the system really operates, how decisions are made, or what their place is in the overall structure. A client government usually:

- Has a constitution with bylaws, holds regular meetings, and elects officers
- Votes on complaints and suggestions and presents the outcome to hospital authorities as the collective wishes of the group rather than of one individual
- Organizes ward rules
- Recommends changes in ward rules
- Arranges, organizes, conducts, and assumes responsibility for social activities
- Originates, plans, and carries through a variety of special activity programs, such as mural painting or writing and editing a newspaper

Proponents of client government as a strategy of milieu therapy argue that it is a logical and effective way of permitting clients to provide themselves with a more creative and wholesome hospital life. Ideally, instead of experiencing hospitalization as a combination of idleness, inactivity, boredom, and regimentation, they will learn democratic living and acquire more versatile social skills. The success of this approach, however, depends on the willingness of hospital administrators and psychiatric professionals to be receptive to clients' ideas and suggestions. If they do not accept as valid the client's definitions of their hospital experience, nothing can be accomplished.

Client government has many advantages. It offers:

- A way of making life in a mental hospital resemble life in the external community
- A way of controlling deviant behavior with group pressure
- Group support for very disturbed clients
- A way of increasing recreational activities
- An opportunity for clients to understand administrative policy and help formulate it
- A way of increasing clients' self-esteem
- An opportunity for clients to express annoyances and resentments
- A channel of communication between clients and staff members
- A way to improve morale through the free interchange of ideas and feelings

- A way to uncover and work out tensions between staff and clients

The psychiatric staff nurse often serves as a resource person to client government groups, attending meetings to discuss issues of concern to clients and staff.

Activity Therapy Groups

Activity therapies are manual, recreational, and creative techniques to facilitate personal experiences and increase social responses and self-esteem. Although nurses may participate, activity therapies are generally the province of health and recreation specialists specifically educated to perform these roles.

Some activity therapies, such as the creative arts therapies discussed below, are organized and conducted in groups. Although there are specifically educated creative arts therapists, their numbers are small. Nurses may participate in these groups or use their principles to reach beyond the ordinary realm of verbal communication with clients.

Poetry Therapy Groups

The goal of poetry therapy groups is to help members get in touch with feelings and emotions through the use of poetry. Poems that are read aloud provide the stimulus for understanding and catharsis. They are selected as the therapeutic medium because they are powerful but not explicit avenues of communication. It is not necessary to be able to write poetry to be a member or leader of a poetry therapy group, although some members or leaders may be stimulated to write poems of their own.

Art Therapy Groups

Painting offers many people a comfortable opportunity for social exchange. In art therapy groups, the art produced by each member gives the art therapist a personal insight into the artist's personality. The art is produced during the session and is used as the basis for discussion and for exploring the members' feelings.

Music Therapy Groups

Music therapy consists of singing, rhythm, body movement, and listening. It is designed to increase the group members' concentration, memory retention, conceptual development, rhythmic behavior, movement behavior, verbal and nonverbal retention, and auditory discrimination. It is also used to stimulate the member's expression and discussion of affect.

Dance Therapy Groups

Dance as a therapeutic mode combines movement and verbal modes. In dance, members find it easier to express nonverbally the feelings and emotions that are a part of them but have been difficult to realize and communicate by other means. The person's inner sense is often reflected in body movements, and dance therapists work to help members integrate their experiences on the verbal level as well as the nonverbal one.

Bibliotherapy Groups

In bibliotherapy, literature is the means for achieving a therapeutic goal. The purpose of a bibliotherapy group is to assimilate the psychologic, sociologic, and aesthetic insights books give into human character, personality, and behavior. Literature provides the stimulus for the members to compare events and characters with their own interpersonal and intrapsychic experiences.

Groups of Medical-Surgical Clients and Their Families

Groups composed of medical-surgical clients are increasingly common, as psychiatric nurses move into general hospital settings offering liaison and consultation services to clients and hospital staff. Group work is useful for chronically ill or disabled persons, preoperative and postoperative clients, clients with regulative medical problems (such as diabetes, cardiac disease, or kidney disease), dying clients, the aged, and clients with psychophysiologic disorders, among others.

Such groups generally focus on the stress of hospitalization and illness and have as their goal the reduction of stress. Groups may be composed of clients alone, family members alone, or a combination.

Community Client Groups

Psychiatric nurses in community settings are involved with different kinds of community groups. These settings include schools, youth centers, industries, neighborhood centers, churches, prisons, summer camps, single-room occupancy boarding houses, transitional facilities (halfway houses), apartments for the elderly, and residential facilities for delinquent youths, runaways, and unwed mothers. The clients may also be persons who have direct contact with these groups, such as teachers, youth counselors, prison guards, police officers, and camp counselors.

Groups with Nurse Colleagues

There is increasing interest among nurses who work together in forming discussion and counseling groups to help reduce their job-related stress and to help them deal with problems of interpersonal relationships in more satisfying ways. Nurses in various intensive care and other high-pressure settings identify with increasing frequency the need for group work services that the psychiatric nurse can provide. The psychiatric nurse may also identify the need and offer this opportunity to colleagues.

Chapter Highlights

- Nurses can provide humanistic care to clients in a variety of settings through the mode of group intervention by offering them opportunities to seek validation, give and receive interpersonal feedback, and test new and different ways of being that may increase their quality of life.

- According to the Johari Awareness Model, people can use knowledge about one another's actions, motivations, and feelings to understand the significant events in a group.

- According to Schutz's FIRO approach, groups move through three interpersonal phases: inclusion, control, and affection.

- According to the Bennis and Shepard theory (authority relations/personal relations), obstacles to communication in groups stem from the orientations of the group members toward authority and intimacy.

- The theory of Martin and Hill (therapeutic problem approach) is that therapy groups have distinct and common growth patterns that can be described, observed, and predicted.

- A commonality among all four frameworks is the notion that group development occurs in identifiable stages and has implications for member behavior and therapist intervention.

- Curative factors, or mechanisms of change that constitute a rational basis for the therapist's choices of tactics and strategies, are unique to the group therapy process.

- The most advantageous leadership style in interactional therapy groups is the egalitarian cotherapy approach in which leadership is shared by two therapists of relatively equal skill, ability, and status.

- The egalitarian style also provides an important opportunity for the group leader's personal and professional development.

- The early design and construction of a group has the most significant impact on its future success and effectiveness.

- Critical considerations in designing a group are the selection of members and the establishment of a group contract.

- In interactive groups, member interaction plays a crucial role in change, which is achieved through the use of the here-and-now to illuminate group process.

References

Alfonso DD: Therapeutic support during inpatient group therapy. *J Psychosoc Nurs* 1985;23(11):21–25.

Amdur MA, Cohen M: Medication groups for psychiatric patients. *Am J Nurs* 1981;81:343–345.

Beeber LS, Schmitt MH: Cohesiveness in groups: A concept in search of a definition. *Adv Nurs Sci* 1986;9:1–11.

Bennis W, Shepard HA: A theory of group development. *Hum Relations* 1956;9:415–437.

Benton DW: The significance of the absent member in milieu therapy. *Perspect Psychiatr Care* 1980;18:21–25.

Bierer J: Group psychotherapy. *Bri Med J* 1942;1:214–217.

Birckhead LM: The nurse as leader: Group psychotherapy with psychotic patients. *J Psychosoc Nurs* 1984;22:6–11.

Bloch S, Crouch E: *Therapeutic Factors in Group Psychotherapy.* Oxford University Press, 1985.

Bogdanoff M, Elbaum P: Role lock: Dealing with monopolizers, mistrusters, isolaters, helpful hannahs, and other assorted characters in group psychotherapy. *Int J Group Psychother* 1978;28:247–261.

Burrows T: The group method of analysis. *Psychoanal Rev* 1927;19:268–280.

Collison CR: Grappling with group resistance. *J Psychosoc Nurs* 1984;22(8):6–12.

Corbin DE: Self-help groups: What the health educator should know. *Health Values* 1983;7:10–14.

Davis LE: Racial composition of groups. *Soc Work* 24(1979):208–213.

Echternacht MR: Day treatment transition groups. *J Psychosoc Nurs* 1984;22(10):11–16.

Eklof M: The termination phase in group therapy: Implications for geriatric groups. *Small Group Behav* 1984; 15:4–9.

Erickson RC: *Inpatient Small Group Psychotherapy: A Pragmatic Approach.* Charles C Thomas, 1984.

Farhood L: Choosing a partner for cotherapy. *Perspect Psychiatr Care* 1975;13:177–179.

Foulkes SH, Anthony EJ: *Group Psychotherapy.* Penguin Books, 1957.

Hellwig K, et al: Partners in therapy: Using the cotherapy relationship in a group. *J Psychiatr Nurs* 1978;16:42–44.

Hierholzer R, Liberman R: Successful living: A social skills and problem-solving group for the chronically mentally ill. *Hosp Community Psychiatry* 1986;37(9):913–918.

Hunka CD, O'Toole AW, O'Toole RW: Self-help therapy in parents anonymous. *J Psychosoc Nurs* 1985;23(7):24–32.

Jacobs BC, Rosenthal TT: Managing effective meetings. *Nurs Econ* 1984;2:137–141.

Kahn EM: The choice of therapist self-disclosure in psychotherapy groups: Contextural considerations. *Arch Psychiatr Nurs* 1987;1(1):62–67.

Kanas N: Inpatient and outpatient group therapy for schizophrenic patients. *Am J Psychother* 1985;39:212–218.

Lazell EW: The group treatment of dementia praecox. *Psychoanal Rev* 1921;8:168–179.

Loomis ME: *Group Process for Nurses.* Mosby, 1979.

Luft J: The Johari Window: A graphic model of awareness in interpersonal relations, in *Group Processes,* ed 2. National Press Books, 1970, pp 11–20.

Luft J, Ingham H: The Johari Window: A graphic model of interpersonal awareness. *Proceedings of the Western Training Laboratory in Group Development.* University of California, Los Angeles, Extension Office, August 1955.

Marsh LC: Group therapy and the psychiatric clinic. *J Nerv Ment Dis* 1935;32:381–390.

Martin EA Jr, Hill WF: Toward a theory of group development. *Int J Group Psychother* 1957;7:20–30.

Maves PA, Schulz JW: Inpatient group treatment on short-term acute care units. *Hosp Community Psychiatry* 1985;36:27–34.

Moreno JL: *Psychodrama.* Beacon press, 1946.

Newton G: Self-help groups: Can they help? *J Psychosoc Nurs* 1984;22(7):27–31.

Pelletier LR: Interpersonal communications task group. *J Psychosoc Nurs* 1983;21(9):33–36.

Reed G, Sech ES: Bulimia: A conceptual model for group treatment. *J Psychosoc Nurs* 1985;23(5):16–22.

Rose L, Finestone K, Bass J: Group support for families of psychiatric patients. *J Psychosoc Nurs* 1985;23(12):24–29.

Roback H, Smith M: Patient attrition in dynamically oriented treatment groups. *Am J Psychiatry* 1987;144(4):426–431.

Sadock BJ: Group psychotherapy, combined individual and group psychotherapy, and psychodrama, in Kaplan HI, Sadock BJ: *Comprehensive Textbook of Psychiatry,* ed 4. Williams and Wilkins, 1985, pp 1403–1427.

Schutz WC: Interpersonal underworld. *Harvard Business Review* 1958a;36:123–135.

Schutz WC: *The Interpersonal Underworld: FIRO.* Science and Behavior Books, 1958b.

Selander JM, Miller WC: Prolixin group: Can nursing intervention groups lower recidivism rates? *J Psychosoc Nurs* 1985;23(11):16–20.

Shoham H, Neuschatz S: Group therapy with senile patients. *Soc Work* 1985;30:69–72.

Shotman L: *The Skills of Helping Individuals and Groups,* ed 2. Peacock, 1984.

Slavson SR: *The Practice of Group Psychotherapy.* International Universities Press, 1947.

Small LL: Finding your leadership style in groups. *Am J Nurs* 1980;80:1301–1303.

Spitz HI: Contemporary trends in group psychotherapy: A literature survey. *Hosp Community Psychiatry* 1984;35:132–142.

Tozman S, Hanks T, Minkowitz HB: The rap group: A milieu treatment model for the chronically mentally ill in an outpatient setting. *Int J Group Psychother* 1981;31:233–238.

White E, Kahn E: Use and modifications in group psychotherapy with chronic schizophrenic outpatients. *J Psychoc Nurs* 1982;20(2):14–19.

Wolff A: The psychoanalysis of groups. *Am J Psychother* 1949;3:525–558 and 1950;4:16–50.

Yalom ID: *Inpatient Group Psychotherapy.* Basic Books, 1983.

Yalom ID: *The Theory and Practice of Group Psychotherapy,* ed 3. Basic Books, 1985.

THIRTY-ONE

Milieu Therapy

Susan Hunn Garritson

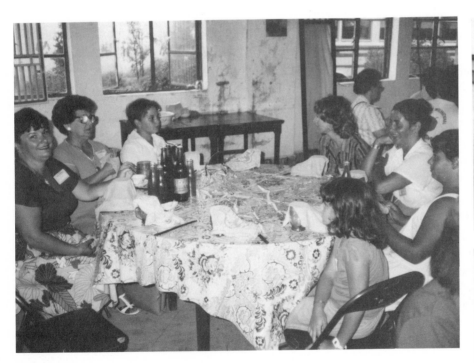

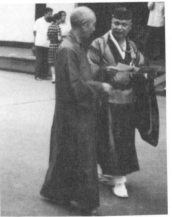

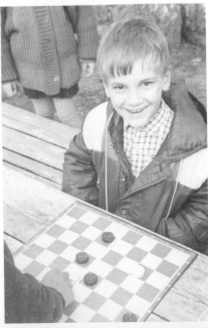

After reading this chapter, students should be able to

- Define milieu therapy
- Describe three historical events that have affected the current status of milieu therapy
- Discuss Wiedenbach's nursing theory and its application to humanistic psychiatric nursing practice
- Describe two physical structure and two social issues that influence the characteristics of the milieu
- Apply the nursing process to intervention techniques based on manipulation of inanimate qualities of the environment
- Identify three social interaction therapy principles
- Apply the nursing process to intervention techniques based on social interaction
- Identify three behavior modification principles
- Apply the nursing process to intervention techniques based on behavior modification principles

Cross References

Other topics related to this chapter are: Behaviorism, Chapter 5; Community mental health and deinstitutionalization, Chapter 40; Era of moral treatment, Chapter 2; Ethics, Chapter 10; Group therapy, Chapter 30; Legal issues, Chapter 39

We need to discover the shared humanity of all people.

Key Terms

custodial care
client government
dehumanizing
deinstitutionalization
institutionalization

least restrictive alternative
milieu therapy
moral treatment
therapeutic community

In this chapter **milieu therapy** is defined as the purposeful use of people, resources, and events in the client's immediate environment to promote optimal functioning in the activities of daily living, development or improvement of interpersonal skills, and ability to manage outside the institutional setting.

This definition of milieu therapy incorporates the important concepts of social influences (people) and physical setting (resources) considered so essential during the revolutionary changes in psychiatric care of the 1800s. This definition has also been influenced by more recent events in the history of psychiatry, including:

- The decline of the state mental hospital
- The emergence of psychiatric theories that emphasize the significance of disturbed interpersonal relations and the curative potential of therapeutic interpersonal encounters
- The influence of legal concepts and decisions on clinical management techniques and philosophy
- Deinstitutionalization

These historical influences and the importance of the external environment to psychiatric care are discussed in the "Historical Overview" section of this chapter. Wiedenbach's nursing model is presented in the "Theoretical Foundations" section as a framework to implement milieu therapy in humanistic psychiatric nursing. Physical structure and social issues that affect the milieu are described in the section on "Context for Nursing Practice." Assessment and manipulation of these factors can indirectly influence client behavior. Interaction and behavior modification principles and techniques are described in the section on "Professional Treatment Techniques." Case examples and nurse-client dialogues are used throughout the chapter to illustrate specific issues.

HISTORICAL OVERVIEW

Ideas about mental illness and human nature have always influenced approaches to client care and management. During the 1600s, madness was thought to be caused by man's "animal nature" because the insane acted like wild beasts. Men and women were chained in their cells, as one might chain a dog, when they were violent. Blankets, clothes, and food were withheld since the lunatic was considered to be insensitive to cold and hunger. People were burned at the stake or confined to dungeons to remove their evil nature. The external environment was used cruelly and harshly to manage the behavior of the mentally ill.

During the 1800s, ideas about human nature began to emphasize the importance of the individual. This focus on the individual, combined with a growing spirit of social reform, drew attention to the inhumanity of the lunatic's surroundings. Philippe Pinel (1745–1826) released the inmates of the Bicêtre and Salpêtrière from their chains and provided food, clothing, fresh air, and kind treatment. William Tuke (1732–1822) established the York Retreat in England as a refuge for those suffering from lunacy, "the greatest of human afflictions" (Rosenblatt 1984, p 246). Tuke considered bleedings and purges—then common medical treatment for the insane—inadequate to relieve human suffering. The philosophy of the retreat emphasized hearty meals; warm and clean clothes; beautiful countryside; and the distractions of walks, readings, music, and conversation.

Moral Treatment

Humanitarian approaches to the care of the mentally ill ushered in the era of moral treatment. During the 1800s, the term *moral* was equivalent to *emotional* or *psychological*. The word *moral* was associated with *morale* and implied hope, spirit, and confidence. **Moral treatment** was considered to be a mandate on those more fortunate to provide compassionate and understanding care to sufferers.

Benjamin Rush (1746–1813) stimulated the interest of American physicians in humanitarian treatment of the mentally ill. Moral treatment became a principal technique in the growing number of mental institutions in America during the 1800s. Although the physician-client relationship was gaining importance, the greatest asset of moral treatment was the attention it gave to the value of the physical setting and social influences of hospital life as curative agents (Bockoven 1963). The philosophy and techniques of moral treatment were the forerunners of modern day milieu therapy.

Decline of State Mental Hospitals

The early success of moral treatment led to continued expansion of state mental facilities. Vast numbers of people were hospitalized despite the original tenet of moral therapy to treat no more clients than the psychiatrist could know intimately. During the second half of the nineteenth century, major population shifts from rural to urban lifestyles and the influx of poverty-stricken immigrants resulted in a tremendous demand for mental hospital services. Day rooms were converted to dormitories to meet requirements for more beds, but nothing replaced dwindling recreational rooms. Ethnic prejudice obscured clinical judgment and human kindness, and insane immigrants were assumed to be incapable of appreciating comfortable surroundings. The standard of living in mental hospitals and the ratio of attendants and physicians to clients severely deteriorated. Finally, the original proponents of moral treatment failed to train sufficient successors, and by 1870 most moral treatment leaders had died or retired.

Public Concern for Conditions in Mental Hospitals

As early as 1900, professional reports documented the miserable state of mental hospitals. In 1908 Clifford Beers published *A Mind That Found Itself,* in which he described the abuses and suffering experienced by clients in mental institutions. While critics questioned any form of institutional care, numerous social factors hindered early efforts to close mental institutions. These factors included lingering influence of the belief in humanistic care, investment of great sums of money in the asylum system, strong public opposition to community treatment, lack of any other social structure to provide for the indigent, and growing professionalization of medicine and efforts by institutional superintendents to identify themselves as a medical specialty, thereby limiting public interference with their professional domain (Schull 1977). Finally, the public's opinion that mental illness was incurable made organizational change and improved treatment seem futile.

Therapeutic Potential of Interpersonal Relations

Following World War II, several factors contributed to renewed interest in mental health services. Large numbers of men had been rejected from military service due to psychiatric symptoms, and other veterans developed psychiatric problems during military duty. Traditional psychiatric treatment in the context of a one-to-one relationship was inadequate to deal with the volume of new clients, and further institutional expansion was incomprehensible.

At the same time psychodynamic perspectives were increasingly influenced by the social sciences. Treatment approaches shifted from attention to forces within the individual to interest in interpersonal relations and events in the social context. In 1931 Harry Stack Sullivan reported on an intensive interpersonal treatment approach with a small group of schizophrenic clients and a variety of hospital personnel. Others extended interpersonal techniques to *prescribe attitudes* specific to each client's symptoms and to define clients as responsible participants in the recovery process. Bettleheim applied therapeutic environment approaches in a facility for severely disturbed children. Maxwell Jones applied similar ideas to launch the **therapeutic community** movement in England. "The concept of the therapeutic community draws attention to the need to make optimal use of the potential in trained staff, volunteers, clients, their relatives, and any other people with a contribution to make to mental health" (Devine 1981, p 20). As Maxwell Jones refined his techniques and ideas of therapeutic community, traditional roles among staff members and between staff and clients became blurred. His ideas emphasized a decline in hierarchical organizational structures, shared decision making, and equal distribution of authority (APA 1984). The recognized interaction between environment and mental illness added a new dimension to psychiatric thinking.

Impact on Nursing

Therapeutic concepts were applied in numerous settings and were incorporated into the professional roles of various disciplines. Nurses described both the theoretical relevance and the practical significance of interpersonal and environmental perspectives in nursing practice. In her 1952 book, *Interpersonal Relations in Nursing,* Hildegard Peplau described nursing as a "significant therapeutic interpersonal process." She discussed various roles the nurse assumes, including teacher, resource, counselor, leader, technical expert, and surrogate (Belcher and Fish 1980). She noted that both the nurse's and client's culture, religion, race, education, past experiences, and preconceived ideas influenced their interpersonal interaction (Belcher and Fish 1980).

The interactive nurse-client relationship was critically analyzed by Gwen Tudor in her 1952 discussion of mutual withdrawal. The problem of mutual withdrawal involves reciprocal avoidance between staff and client, resulting in a limited and stable though stagnant pattern of interaction. Staff may rationalize their avoidance through labels such as "hopeless," "unresponsive," or "assaultive" and thereby discourage new approaches to interaction. Such labeling and routinized staff behaviors reinforce the client's behavior, and the interaction cycle is perpetuated.

Influence of Legal Concepts

Legal involvement in commitment hearings was informal during the first half of the 1900s. Court involvement in social welfare cases gradually increased during the 1960s and 1970s, and the momentum of the Civil Rights movement carried over to psychiatric clients. Concern was focused

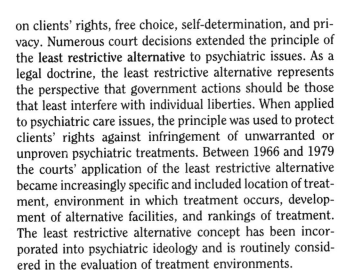

on clients' rights, free choice, self-determination, and privacy. Numerous court decisions extended the principle of the **least restrictive alternative** to psychiatric issues. As a legal doctrine, the least restrictive alternative represents the perspective that government actions should be those that least interfere with individual liberties. When applied to psychiatric care issues, the principle was used to protect clients' rights against infringement of unwarranted or unproven psychiatric treatments. Between 1966 and 1979 the courts' application of the least restrictive alternative became increasingly specific and included location of treatment, environment in which treatment occurs, development of alternative facilities, and rankings of treatment. The least restrictive alternative concept has been incorporated into psychiatric ideology and is routinely considered in the evaluation of treatment environments.

Deinstitutionalization

Deinstitutionalization refers to the closing of state mental hospitals and discharge of thousands of mentally ill inmates. Proponents of deinstitutionalization were motivated by a humanitarian philosophy and were committed to the notion that clients should receive treatment in their own communities. Many social, economic, and psychiatric treatment factors influenced the public's receptiveness to community care.

Custodial Care in State Hospitals

The concept of the therapeutic potential of the environment was slow to reach state mental hospitals. Clients continued to receive minimal attention to their basic needs. This **custodial care** contrasted sharply with advances in psychiatric treatment outside the state hospitals.

Numerous discussions and critiques of state hospital treatment have been published. Stanton and Schwartz (1954) contrasted the low prestige of the twenty-three hours of the day devoted to daily living activities with the status of the psychotherapy hour. They also described the impact of the hospital environment and staff actions (i.e., staff conflict and poor communication) on client behavior.

A study by Strauss et al. (1981) contrasted three treatment environments: (1) the chronic services of a state hospital, (2) the treatment services of a state hospital, and (3) a private psychiatric research and training hospital. They identified that staff lacked psychotherapy knowledge on the chronic services and provided hydrotherapy, work therapy, good food, and medical care—techniques consistent with a belief that mental illness has a physical origin. The treatment services at both the state and private hospitals pro-

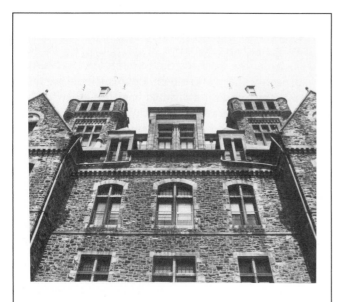

Figure 31–1
Confinement in imposing structures such as this public mental hospital often meant condemning a person to life within the walls of an asylum. Wrongful confinement and loss of personal liberty play a significant part in the history of legal issues that concern psychiatric nurses.

vided psychodynamic treatments. The psychotherapeutic treatment was individually oriented at the private hospital. However, since the treatment services at the state hospital dealt with large numbers of clients with fewer staff, milieu therapy was the principal psychodynamic treatment. The study concluded that treatment philosophy, professional identity, and type of institution are critical determinants of psychiatric treatment.

Goffman (1961) was influential in raising awareness about institutional environments. He described the restrictive institutional atmosphere as derived from regulations and judgments by staff and from sanctions for activities from outside the client group (Figure 31–1). Staff move clients in blocks to manage large groups of people in the institution. Free movement is restricted because it increases the difficulty of overall surveillance. Contact with the outside becomes a privilege. Patients are separated from their outside roles and identities via limitations on visitors, confiscation of personal property, and lack of private space. Contact is largely confined to other inmates. Telephone use, cigarette smoking, and communication with a physician may be controlled by staff. Goffman described clients as "institutionalized" when they exhibit dependence on the institution, apathy about discharge, lack of interest and competence in outside activities, and resignation toward institutional life.

Gruenberg (1974) used *social breakdown syndrome* to refer to behavior that was once thought to stem from psychosis but that seems to resolve when environmental restrictions are removed. Social breakdown syndrome may be caused by conflict between what the client is capable of doing and what the institution demands or requires. It is manifested by danger of self-damage and self-destructive acts, disturbing noisiness, and inability to manage daily living activities such as eating, dressing, toileting, and going to bed (Gruenberg 1974, p 702).

Cost of Institutional Care

In addition to legal challenges and criticisms about institutional care, other social and economic forces increased public receptivity to the closing of state mental hospital systems. The rate of institutional hospitalization was growing at a rate disproportionate to general population growth. The original asylums needed massive repair, and construction of new facilities was tremendously costly. Other sources of expense stemmed from the unionization of state hospital employees, the forty-hour week, and the results of class action suits, which had limited the use of clients as unpaid employees and established the client's legal right to treatment. The growing welfare system provided a way to support clients in the community more cheaply than in an institution. There was less opposition from organized psychiatry since new areas of specialization could be developed in community care. Other events that supported and accelerated this process included availability of social security (at federal expense) to noninstitutionalized clients, financial inducements to the counties to avoid sending clients to state hospitals, growth of privately owned and community-based "institutions," and tightening of the eligibility for involuntary commitment (Schull 1977, p 140). By 1975 approximately two-thirds of state hospital clients had been discharged back to their communities.

Current Ideas about Milieu Therapy

The deinstitutionalization movement and continued decline in length of acute psychiatric hospitalization have shifted attention to environmental issues in community-based settings and decreased the emphasis on the in-patient therapeutic environment as a technique for resolution of long-standing conflicts. The therapeutic use of the hospital environment remains significant, however. The environment reflects professionals' concerns for human values such as privacy, autonomy, and dignity; it provides a "here and now" focus for staff assessment of client functioning and intervention related to self-care and interpersonal relations; and it can be used as a resource to support positive behavior through *limit setting,* expectations, and material resources (Maxmen et al. 1974).

Various terms such as *therapeutic milieu, therapeutic environment, therapeutic community,* and *milieu therapy* have been applied to discussions of the treatment environment. While some argue that each term has distinguishing strategies and theoretical perspectives, these labels are frequently used interchangeably and are based on the general premise that resources in the environment can be used therapeutically on behalf of the client. The term *milieu therapy* was defined in the introduction to this chapter and will be used throughout the remaining sections to refer to the therapeutic potential of the hospital setting. By addressing the entire context within which the management and care of the client takes place, milieu therapy incorporates an endless array of human and inanimate variables. Specific techniques have evolved from the manipulation of environmental factors, and these are equally linked to milieu therapy. The remaining sections provide further theoretical development of milieu therapy and demonstrate how the nurse employs the milieu to accomplish the nursing process.

THEORETICAL FOUNDATIONS

Nurse-Client-Environment Interactive Model

In 1969 Ernestine Wiedenbach published a theory of nursing based on three factors (Bennett and Foster 1980):

1. Central purpose of the discipline
2. Activities to fulfill the central purpose
3. Realities in the immediate situation

These key factors provide a useful framework for understanding and implementing milieu therapy in humanistic psychiatric nursing practice.

Wiedenbach describes the central purpose of nursing as reverence for the gift of life; respect for the dignity, value, autonomy, and individuality of each human being; and resolution to act on these beliefs. Using this humanistic philosophy, the nurse works with the client to develop a plan for care (Box 31–1). The care plan is mutually understood and agreed on. The client directs how actions are carried out. The nurse recognizes and deals with the realities of the situation in which nursing care is provided (Box 31–2).

The central purpose, care plan activities, and realities are interdependent and interactive. The nurse's beliefs about human beings influence the selection of nursing interventions. The facility within which the nurse and client find themselves further limits and guides potential nursing actions. Finally, the nurse's interventions are specific to the client's unique behavior.

Box 31–1
PHILOSOPHIC CONCEPTS INFLUENCING NURSING CARE

Privacy

Individuals routinely vary their contact and withdrawal from others as well as the information they share about themselves. The very nature of psychiatric hospitalization clashes with the need for privacy. Intimate personal details are examined and discussed and there may be no opportunities to remove oneself from staff surveillance or social contact. Nurses respect clients' privacy by limiting surveillance and monitoring to situations necessary for client safety, respecting the confidentiality of personal information, and maintaining routine social practices such as knocking on doors and waiting for an answer before entering bedrooms or bathrooms.

Autonomy

The rules and schedules that characterize psychiatric treatment settings usually promote the management of groups of people and may interfere with the personal decision making and self-control exercised by the individual client. While mentally ill clients may be significantly impaired in their ability to carry out age-appropriate roles, the therapeutic milieu provides opportunities for normal functioning according to each client's abilities.

Safety

Mentally ill clients may pose significant safety hazards to themselves or others due to suicidal or assaultive behaviors, poor judgment, or confusion. Nurses' efforts to maintain clients' safety may clash with the privacy and autonomy concepts. For example, clients requiring close surveillance have little or no privacy; nurses may intervene to override decisions made by clients whose judgment is impaired.

Group Well-Being

A client's behavior may be disruptive or detrimental to the overall well-being of other clients. Some clients may require monitoring or management to maximize the common good. As with the concept of safety, the individual's privacy and autonomy may be violated when group well-being is considered primary. (Some philosophers, however, consider that the group's well-being enhances the individual's autonomy.) Since issues of individual autonomy, individual well-being, and group well-being usually cannot predominate simultaneously, nurses must be sensitive to situations in which clashes occur.

Box 31–2

REALITIES INFLUENCING NURSING CARE

1. Nurse (or delegate): personal characteristics, competence, capabilities

2. Client: personal characteristics, problems, capacities, and ability to cope with current experiences

3. Goal: the desired result to be attained through nursing care

4. Means: method (based on application of knowledge and spiritual and material resources)

5. Framework: human, environmental, professional, and organizational facilities that make up the context (and provide limits) within which nursing is practiced

Source: Adapted from Bennett AM, Foster PC: Ernestine Weidenbach, in Nursing Theories: A Base for Professional Nursing Practice. *Prentice-Hall, 1980, p 141.*

These interacting beliefs, interventions, and realities impact the individual's capacity to think, plan, relate to others, and experience a sense of self apart from others. "An environment that subverts, interferes with, or prevents the use of these qualities threatens human dignity" (Proshansky 1973, p 2). Nurses' philosophies about client autonomy and the growth-enhancing potential of the environment also influence the more informal expectations and operational procedures that involve both staff and clients. Rules, routines, and procedures that negate client input and are controlled by staff also control staff and increasingly restrict the milieu.

Nursing Process

The nurse uses the nursing process to assess the client's behavior within the context of the treatment environment and to assess characteristics of the environment that may influence the client's behavior. Thus the familiar components of the nursing process—assessment, planning, intervention, and evaluation—are also performed on aspects of the milieu. For example, the nurse considers subjective and objective data about a client and develops a nursing diagnosis (see Box 31–3 for examples). Next the nurse considers behaviors of staff and other clients and characteristics of the environment to determine whether any of these contextual areas contribute to the client's diagnosed problem. The nurse implements a milieu-therapy–based inter-

---

Box 31–3

NURSING DIAGNOSES USED IN CASE EXAMPLES

Psychiatric Nursing Diagnosis (PND)

01.03.05	Altered participation in health care
02.06.01	Confusion
02.06.03	Disorientation
05.02.02.05	Unpredictable behaviors
02.02	Altered judgment
01.04.01	Difficult transition to and from sleep
06.03.03	Altered personal identity
01.97	Undeveloped activity processes
06.03.01	Altered body image
01.03.01	Altered eating
05.05.02	Social isolation/withdrawal
06.02.01	Discomfort
05.98	Altered interpersonal processes not otherwise specified
05.02.01.01	Aggressive/violent behaviors toward environment

North American Nursing Diagnosis Association (NANDA)

Injury, potential for
Health maintenance, altered
Thought processes, altered
Sleep pattern disturbance
Social interaction, impaired
Violence, potential for: self-directed or directed at others
Social isolation
Self-concept, disturbance in: personal identity
Coping, ineffective individual
Self-concept, disturbance in: body image
Self-care deficit: feeding

---

vention by manipulating the aspect of the environment that seems to contribute (by either its presence or its absence) to the client's behavior. The nurse evaluates the results by reassessing the client's behavior and assessing the overall environment for unanticipated or unintended changes. In this interactive model, the nurse considers the impact of environmental interventions on the behavior of other clients and staff. The therapeutic environment must maintain basic safety and group well-being, which sometimes conflicts with efforts to promote an individual's autonomy. A central task in creating and managing milieu therapy is to achieve a balance between attention to the needs of the group and promotion of individuality. Thus many philosophical, technical, and situational forces influence the nursing process.

Humanistic Interactionist Implications

In this chapter milieu therapy is broadly interpreted to reflect the therapeutic potential of people, resources, and events. Wiedenbach's nursing framework provides the humanistic and interactionist perspectives that make milieu therapy an effective and versatile technique in psychiatric nursing practice. Nurses' twenty-four-hour-a-day contact with clients affords a unique opportunity to claim the creation and management of the therapeutic milieu as a special domain for nursing. No other discipline literally shares with clients the living space of the ward. Nurses individually influence the milieu through their presence, by providing human contact, support, and direction and by sharing philosophy and values, establishing collaborative work relationships, and exhibiting professionalism.

Using the nurse-client interaction process as a medium, nurses introduce various techniques such as lists of activities, expectations, or contracts to help clients learn new behaviors. Group activities are also successful media in which to learn new behavior. Groups provide opportunities to experience membership, cooperation, compromise, and leadership. These here-and-now nursing interventions provide opportunities for immediate observation, feedback, and learning (see Box 31–4). When these new experiences occur within a comfortable, humane setting, clients may experience a new sense of self-worth and dignity.

Legal and regulatory agencies have established criteria for the structural environment, yet staff often become insensitive to simple environmental impediments that they could change. Locked doors to bedrooms, bathrooms, kitchen, or laundry interfere with normal aspects of daily living. Simple readjustments of staffing assignments, improved client-staff communication, or use of behavior contracts may accomplish necessary monitoring and behavior management without restricting the environment. These alternative interventions are based on the therapeutic use of individuals, communication, and client participation to create an environment that promotes human achievement.

The therapeutic milieu is more than locker space, square footage requirements, and assorted group experiences, although these are important components. The therapeutic milieu includes the belief in the dignity of all people, and this philosophy pervades the structure, interactions, and interventions that in turn reinforce the therapeutic atmosphere.

CONTEXT FOR NURSING PRACTICE

Physical Environment

Psychiatric treatment takes place in a variety of settings, and these settings have been ranked according to their restrictiveness or interference with the client's independence (Krauss and Slavinsky 1982):

1. Total institutions (e.g., state hospitals)—*most restrictive*
2. Nearly total institutions (e.g., nursing homes)

> ### Box 31–4
> # NURSING INTERVENTION HIGHLIGHTS
>
> 1. Make resources necessary for self-care available to clients.
> 2. Enhance the normality of the environment through use of clocks, calendars, ramps, railings, furniture, and other resources.
> 3. Maintain visibility and availability (i.e., presence) to guide and supervise clients' activities.
> 4. Maintain open communication with nurses, other professionals, and staff.
> 5. Include clients in decisions about their own care.
> 6. When appropriate, write behavioral expectations and agreements for the clients' and other staff's reference.
> 7. Support formal and informal group activities to promote sharing, cooperation, compromise, and leadership.
> 8. Examine personal attitudes toward issues of clients' rights, self-determination, social control, and deviancy.

---

3. Institutions with partially independent residents (e.g., halfway homes)
4. Institutions with independent but isolated residents (e.g., single-room-occupancy hotels)
5. Family of origin, friends, other relatives
6. Family of orientation (i.e., family resulting from marriage or other relationship)—*least restrictive*

The physical structure of many institutions interferes with clients' freedom of movement and individuality through locked doors, communal living arrangements, and limited access to community resources. Thus facilities located in huge hospital complexes, which do not interface with the community's shopping, religious, or entertainment activities or provide for clients' privacy, have a more restrictive milieu than community-based settings.

The physical structure of mental institutions has been linked to the problem of **institutionalization** in which the client's ability to function declines. "Institutionalized" patients become apathetic about discharge, resigned toward institutional life, and dependent on the setting for their total care. Goffman (1961) theorized that clients grew unable to negotiate and manage daily living activities outside the setting when institutions provided for all aspects of their lives and prevented access to the community by high walls, barred windows, or geographic isolation.

Physical structure also has an immediate impact on the milieu. Structural characteristics influence social interaction and clients' opportunities to carry out activities associated with adult roles. Removal of personal property, lack of personal space, and regulation of adult activities such as smoking, telephone use, and visitors diminish privacy and self-control and thereby decrease individuality and autonomy.

Acutely psychotic and chronically mentally ill men and women are admitted to a twenty-bed locked unit in a large county hospital. Nurses on this unit seem rushed and complain of having no time to discuss nursing care issues or write nursing care plans. A nurse consultant observed work patterns for several days and noted that the staff were involved (frequently unnecessarily) in intimate details of the clients' daily activities. This involvement extended to lighting matches for cigarettes and squeezing toothpaste onto toothbrushes. Simple routines that interfered with client autonomy also controlled staff by preventing professional performance and relationships.

Nursing Process

Assessment: Staff complaints of excessive workload
Staff control of clients' daily activities

Nursing diagnosis: 01.03.05 Altered participation in health care
/Health maintenance, altered

Intervention: Increase client self-care according to actual abilities

Evaluation: Improved professional performance and relationships of nurses
Increased client self-care

Changes in the security of the environment, such as unlocking the door of a normally locked unit or locking the door of a normally unlocked unit, have been noted to increase client agitation.

Mrs. A is a 72-year-old woman hospitalized for evaluation of a sudden onset of confusion and forgetfulness.

Nurses locked the unit's main door to keep Mrs. A from inadvertently wandering off the ward. Other clients were free to come and go but were inconvenienced by relying on staff to unlock the door.

Staff noticed an increase in irritability and demanding behavior of several clients soon after the door was locked. Small cliques of clients collected near the door, while others paced nearby.

Staff decided that the impact of the locked door on the overall milieu was detrimental. A nurse was assigned to keep Mrs. A within eye contact at all times to ensure her safety, and the unit door was unlocked. The ward atmosphere soon returned to normal.

Nursing Process

Assessment: Client is confused and forgetful

Nursing diagnosis: 02.06.01 Confusion
02.06.03 Disorientation

Plan and intervention: Lock main door to protect client safety

Evaluation: Client safety maintained though other clients show increased irritability and demanding behavior

Intervention: One-to-one nursing care of Mrs. A

Wilson (1982) studied "infracontrol" phenomena at Soteria House, an experimental personal growth community for schizophrenics. Conventional control mechanisms such as locked doors, medications, and strict regulation of activity or property are avoided in this setting. Soteria's ideology emphasizes self-regulation, tolerance for deviance, and group cohesiveness. However, an ideology of eliminating structural control does not eliminate the need to maintain safety or the problem of social control of psychotic clients' behavior. Wilson studied how problems of social control are solved in the absence of conventional psychiatric control structures. The process of *presencing* was identified as a key mechanism to manage resident behavior. Staff and residents spend a great deal of daily living time together, and the basic *presence* of people with individual tolerance and interaction patterns guides and limits behavior. Such a milieu might well be characterized as "low EE" or low *expressed emotion* (see Chapters 8 and 17). Nurses frequently use the presencing technique by sitting with or listening to clients, although they are apt to describe it as "providing support" or "the therapeutic use of self." The last example illustrated how the use of presencing not only kept Mrs. A safe but also improved the environment by allowing the unit door to remain unlocked.

Structural controls may not always be obvious, of course, and staff can become oblivious over time to controls that were instituted for a specific purpose that no longer applies.

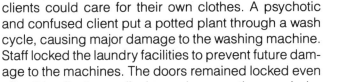

A fifteen-bed unlocked ward had laundry facilities so clients could care for their own clothes. A psychotic and confused client put a potted plant through a wash cycle, causing major damage to the washing machine. Staff locked the laundry facilities to prevent future damage to the machines. The doors remained locked even after this client was discharged, preventing any independent client access to the facilities. Preventing possible future damage to machines became a predominant staff concern.

Nursing Process

Assessment: Client is psychotic and confused

Nursing diagnosis: 02.02 Altered judgment /Thought processes, altered 05.02.02.05 Unpredictable behaviors

Plan: Maintain client safety and avoid damage to environment

Intervention: Lock laundry facilities

Evaluation: Damage avoided though independence and self-care of other clients declined

Intervention: Unlock doors

A voluntary, unlocked unit has a progressive nursing philosophy emphasizing client self-care, autonomy, and independence. The clients' dining room has a small kitchenette, and clients frequently prepare their own snacks. The clients' refrigerator had always been located in the locked medication room. Thus, any independent meal preparation or simple decision to have a glass of juice required the client to request access to the refrigerator. Despite the inconvenience of having to unlock the door, staff were initially reluctant to move the refrigerator. They rationalized that they could better monitor clients' intake by controlling access to the refrigerator. Once the refrigerator was moved to the kitchenette, however, staff were more likely to discuss food and fluid intake with their clients. This elimination of a structural control provided an opportunity for client-staff communication and improved staff's counseling and education related to clients' diets.

Nursing Process

Assessment: Clients frequently approach staff for juice and snacks

Nursing diagnosis: 01.03.05 Altered participation in health care /Health maintenance, altered

Plan and intervention: Move refrigerator to community area

RESEARCH NOTE

Citation

Whitehead CC, Polsky RH, Crookshank C, Fik E: Objective and subjective evaluation of psychiatric ward redesign. Am J Psychiatry 1984;141(May):639–644.

Study Problem/Purpose

The study was directed at two areas:

- Does physical and environmental design of a psychiatric unit correlate with: social behavior? spatial distribution of behavior? psychopathology?

- Can architectural design be used therapeutically to encourage social interaction?

Methods

A 30-bed psychiatric unit was redesigned from a plan with large open dormitories, long drab corridors, and dayroom lacking in privacy to a plan that emphasized flexible use of group and dayroom areas, subdivided dormitories, and elimination of the long narrow hallway. Behavioral, demographic, and attitudinal data were gathered from two samples: clients and staff on the original unit and clients and staff on the remodeled unit.

Findings

The location of social interactions shifted from the hallways of the original unit to visiting room, dayroom, and cafeteria of the redesigned unit. A significant decrease in bizarre behavior in the remodeled dayroom was identified. Staff's location shifted from the nursing station to the dayroom following redesign. Subjective staff and client responses to the changes were strong and positive. Clients specifically noted that they felt better in the new surroundings.

Implications

A strong relationship between environment and social behavior was identified in this study. Attractive furnishings and comfortable visiting areas promoted a sense of normalcy and encouraged general functioning. Opportunities for therapeutic staff-client contact were also enhanced. The decline in clients' psychopathologic behavior may have resulted from the combination of increased staff contact and response to the improved surroundings.

Evaluation: Improved access to necessary resources for self-care and enhanced staff-client communication

The structural environment should not only avoid **dehumanizing** its inhabitants but also should actively contribute to their improved functioning and comfort. Reality-orientation techniques such as the following contribute to a sense of normality:

- Clocks and calendars to promote time orientation
- Newspapers to encourage awareness of social events
- Ramps and rails to promote movement
- Furniture arranged to promote interaction

These techniques may be taken for granted by healthy individuals, yet they provide critical resources to the impaired client.

Mrs. T is a 47-year-old woman with severe depression. She is very agitated and is having trouble sleeping. Although sleep medication has been ordered, Mrs. T has been in and out of bed and is pacing. As a result of her restlessness, the sheets and blankets are strewn about and the plastic mattress cover is exposed. The rumpled bedding and cold mattress further contribute to Mrs. T's discomfort. Nurses order a mattress pad and contoured sheets to promote Mrs. T's comfort until her symptoms respond to medication.

Nursing Process

Assessment: Client is agitated, restless, and not able to stay in bed

Nursing diagnosis: 01.04.01 Difficult transition to and from sleep
/Sleep pattern disturbance

Plan and intervention: Decrease discomfort caused by loose bedding by providing padding and contoured sheets and thereby promote client's rest

Evaluation: Distractions and discomfort created by the environment (e.g., bedding) removed

---

Deinstitutionalization has changed the location of psychiatric treatment, and walled institutions with barred windows are less common today than they were forty years ago. However, structural controls remain in community psychiatric settings. Lack of access to rooms, equipment, or pleasantries of normal life perpetuate the restricted atmosphere of institutions. The previous examples demonstrate how staff may justify structural controls, structural controls interfere with client autonomy, and elimination of structural controls can improve client-staff communication and the ward atmosphere.

Social Environment

Social norms affect the environment by creating both overt and covert rules governing actions and relations to others. Social norms are derived from:

- Public influences such as clients' rights groups, regulatory agencies, or court decisions
- Styles of interaction among staff (Schatzman and Strauss 1966)

Public Influences

Wyatt v Stickney, 1972, a landmark mental health court case, upheld clients' rights to treatment as opposed to mere custodial care (see Box 31–5). The decision also established

---

Box 31–5
WYATT v STICKNEY, 1972: AN OVERVIEW

Bryce State Hospital, the first public institution for the mentally ill in Alabama, opened in 1861 in response to the efforts of Dorothea Dix to have the mentally ill hospitalized rather than left to wander the streets. Over the next 100 years the buildings were inadequately maintained and overcrowded with patients. Treatment for the mentally ill stagnated.

In 1970 the Alabama State Department of Mental Health faced a tremendous budget deficit due to a decline in tobacco tax revenues and an across-the-board salary increase. The department decided to lay off 120 professional staff at Bryce, both to manage the fiscal crisis and to dramatize to the legislature the need for more funding. Several employees and a patient, Ricky Wyatt, filed a complaint in federal court charging that the layoffs would effectively end all treatment programs and only custodial care would be provided. The federal court agreed to hear the portion of the case concerned with patients' rights to treatment and ordered the state to produce an adequate treatment program. Without treatment, the court said, involuntary hospitalization would result in confinement without due process of law.

The state produced a vague program found inadequate by the court. The court ultimately adopted staffing and physical plant standards deemed to provide a humane physical and psychological environment.

standards for the treatment environment. The standards specified minimum square footage per client in bedrooms, dayrooms, and dining facilities; maximum number of clients per bedroom, toilet, and shower; and requirements for personal storage space, basic furniture, dayrooms with outside windows, and bathroom facilities with curtains and doors.

The Joint Commission on Accreditation of Hospitals (1987) has also specified criteria for the therapeutic environment (see Box 31–6). These standards address requirements for lighting; ventilation; furnishings; storage; general aesthetic appeal of clients' living area; and eating, bathing, and toileting facilities. (These standards currently apply only to nonhospital-based psychiatric facilities and are no longer requirements for hospital-based psychiatric services.)

The Joint Commission and *Wyatt v Stickney* criteria are similar, and both illustrate the impact of social norms and expectations for care of the mentally ill on the physical features of the hospital setting. While the court's standards applied only to Bryce State Hospital in Alabama, the court's willingness to hear the *Wyatt v Stickney* case demonstrated concern for the plight and rights of the mentally ill. The Joint Commission's regulatory authority extends these standards to multiple facilities. Furthermore, enforcement of environmental requirements by the Joint Commission has legislative support since reimbursement for Medicare clients depends on accreditation status.

In addition to requirements related to physical characteristics, Joint Commission standards deal with the recreational and social aspects of the therapeutic milieu. These standards specify availability of books, crafts, games, outdoor access, and recreational equipment. The importance of these resources to the therapeutic environment is confirmed by the National Association of Private Psychiatric Hospitals (1985), whose guidelines for psychiatric hospital programs are used by some insurance companies to define medical necessity for treatment and quality interventions. Again, financial reimbursement is linked to the therapeutic environment.

Staff Interaction: Communication

Staff interaction patterns influence the ward milieu and may mirror client interaction patterns.

A consulting clinical nurse specialist met with a group of staff nurses from an adolescent treatment unit to discuss an increase in staff absences due to illness. Several staff complained that administrators' rules limited their ability to make independent decisions. The next day in a group meeting, clients discussed their anger about not receiving weekend passes. That evening two clients left the unit without passes.

Nursing Process

Assessment: Increased staff absences and complaints about limited independence
Client angry about pass restrictions followed by two AWOLs

Nursing diagnosis: 05.98 Altered interpersonal processes not otherwise specified
/Social interaction, impaired

Plan: Decrease avoidance behavior of staff and clients

Intervention: Discuss perceptions of decreased autonomy with all involved
Increase opportunities for independent decision making for both staff and clients

Evaluation: Decline in parallel avoidance behavior

In this example, the parallel issues for staff and clients are related to self-control and autonomous decision making. Both groups acted out tension through avoidance (use of sick leave and AWOL).

Mrs. L is 48 years old with a history of bipolar mood disorder. She is demanding, loud, argumentative, and irritable and has been admitted to an unlocked unit. There has been a recent change in the unit's chief physician administrator. The previous chief recommended rapid medication to calm agitated clients and maintain a quiet environment. The replacement chief physician prefers several medication-free days to evaluate clients' behaviors. Staff are not completely comfortable with managing unmedicated clients, and the ward has been hectic with several psychotic clients under evaluation. In addition, the head nurse has been on vacation for several weeks and her replacement is much less experienced with staff conflict management. Mrs. L's admission triggered bitter staff complaints about the new chief physician and the ward philosophy. Several individuals inquired into transfers to other units and others joked about career changes. Absenteeism increased and several medication errors were made. Two clients became embroiled in an altercation and others expressed concern about their care. When the head nurse returned from vacation the ward milieu was tense and the signs of disintegration were obvious. The head nurse met with both staff and the chief to identify their concerns. The chief believed clients were being medicated too quickly and a period of reconsideration of their symptoms might lead to alternative approaches.

Box 31–6
CRITERIA FOR THE
THERAPEUTIC ENVIRONMENT

1. The facility establishes an environment that enhances the positive self-image of patients and preserves their human dignity.

2. The grounds of the facility have adequate space for the facility to carry out its stated goals.
   2.1. When patient needs or facility goals involve outdoor activities, areas appropriate to the ages and clinical needs of the patients are provided.

3. The facility is accessible to handicapped individuals or the facility has written policies and procedures that describe how handicapped individuals can gain access to the facility for necessary services.

4. Waiting or reception areas are comfortable, and their design, location, and furnishings accommodate the characteristics of patients and visitors, the anticipated waiting time, the need for privacy and/or support from staff, and the goals of the facility.
   4.1. Appropriate staff are available in waiting or reception areas to address the needs of patients and visitors.
   4.2. Rest rooms are available for patients and visitors.
   4.3. A telephone is available for private conversations.
   4.4. An adequate number of drinking units are accessible at appropriate heights.
      4.4.1. If drinking units employ cups, only single-use, disposable cups are used.

5. Facilities that do not have emergency medical care resources have first-aid kits available in appropriate places.
   5.1. All supervisory staff are familiar with the locations, contents, and use of the first-aid kits.

6. Programs providing partial-hospital or 24-hour care services provide an environment appropriate to the needs of patients.
   6.1. The design, structure, furnishing, and lighting of the patient environment promote clear perceptions of people and functions.
   6.2. When appropriate, lighting is controlled by patients.
   6.3. Where possible, the environment provides views of the outdoors.
   6.4. Areas that are used primarily by patients have windows or skylights.
   6.5. Appropriate types of mirrors that distort as little as possible are placed at reasonable heights in appropriate places to aid in grooming and to enhance patients' self-awareness.
   6.6. Clocks and calendars are provided in at least major use areas to promote awareness of time and season.

7. Ventilation contributes to the habitability of the environment.
   7.1. Direct outside air ventilation is provided to each patient's room by air-conditioning or operable windows.
   7.2. Ventilation is sufficient to remove undesirable odors.

8. All areas and surfaces shall be free of undesirable odors.

9. Door locks and other structural restraints are used minimally.
   9.1. The use of door locks or closed sections is approved by the professional staff and the governing body.

10. The facility has written policies and procedures to facilitate staff-patient interaction, particularly when structural barriers in the therapeutic environment separate staff from patients.
    10.1. Staff respect a patient's right to privacy by knocking on the door of the patient's room before entering.

11. Areas with the following characteristics are available to meet the needs of patients:
    11.1. Areas that accommodate a full range of social activities, from two-person conversations to group activities.
    11.2. Attractively furnished areas in which a patient can be alone, when appropriate.
    11.3. Attractively furnished areas for private conversations with other patients, family members, or friends.

12. Appropriate furnishings and equipment are available.
    12.1. Furnishings are clean and in good repair.
    12.2. Furnishings are appropriate to the ages and physical conditions of the patients.
    12.3. All furnishings, equipment, and appliances are maintained in good operating order.
    12.4. Broken furnishings and equipment are repaired promptly.

13. Dining areas are comfortable, attractive, and conducive to pleasant living.
    13.1. Dining arrangements are based on a logical plan that meets the needs of the patients and the requirements of the facility.
    13.2. Dining tables seat small groups of patients, unless other arrangements are justified on the basis of patient needs.
    13.3. When staff members do not eat with the patients, the dining rooms are adequately supervised and staffed to provide assistance to patients when needed and to assure that each patient receives an adequate amount and variety of food.

14. Sleeping areas have doors for privacy.
    14.1. In rooms containing more than four patients, privacy is provided by partitioning or the placement of furniture.
    14.2. The number of patients in a room is appropriate to the goals of the facility and to the ages, developmental levels, and clinical needs of the patients.
    14.3. Except when clinically justified in writing on the basis of program requirements, no more than eight patients sleep in a room.

14.4. Sleeping areas are assigned on the basis of the patient's need for group support, privacy, or independence.

    14.4.1. Patients who need extra sleep, whose sleep is easily disturbed, or who need greater privacy because of age, emotional disturbance, or adjustment problems are assigned to bedrooms in which no more than two persons sleep.

15. Areas are provided for personal hygiene.

    15.1. The areas for personal hygiene provide privacy.

    15.2. Bathrooms and toilets have partitions and doors.

    15.3. Toilets have seats.

16. Good standards of personal hygiene and grooming are taught and maintained, particularly in regard to bathing, brushing teeth, caring for hair and nails, and using the toilet.

    16.1. Patients have the personal help needed to perform these activities and, when indicated, to assume responsibility for self-care.

    16.2. Incontinent patients are cleaned and/or bathed immediately upon voiding or soiling, with due regard for privacy.

    16.3. The services of a barber and/or beautician are available to patients either in the facility or in the community.

17. Articles for grooming and personal hygiene that are appropriate to the patient's age, developmental level, and clinical status are readily available in a space reserved near the patient's sleeping area.

    17.1. If clinically indicated, a patient's personal articles may be kept under lock and key by staff.

18. Ample closet and drawer space are provided for storing personal property and property provided for patients' use.

    18.1. Lockable storage space is provided.

19. Patients are allowed to keep and display personal belongings and to add personal touches to the decoration of their rooms.

    19.1. The facility has written rules to govern the appropriateness of such decorative display.

    19.2. If access to potentially dangerous grooming aids or other personal articles is contraindicated for clinical reasons, a member of the professional staff explains to the patient the conditions under which the articles may be used.

        19.2.1. The clinical rationale for these conditions is documented in the patient record.

    19.3. If the hanging of pictures on walls and similar activities are privileges to be earned for treatment purposes, a member of the professional staff explains to the patient the conditions under which the privileges may be granted.

        19.3.1. The treatment and granting of privileges are documented in the patient record.

20. Patients are encouraged to take responsibility for maintaining their own living quarters and for day-to-day housekeeping activities of the program, as appropriate to their clinical status.

    20.1. Such responsibilities are clearly defined in writing, and staff assistance and equipment are provided as needed.

    20.2. Descriptions of such responsibilities are included in the patient's orientation program.

    20.3. Documentation that these responsibilities have been incorporated in the patient's treatment plan is provided.

21. Patients are allowed to wear their own clothing.

    21.1. If clothing is provided by the program, it is appropriate and is not dehumanizing.

    21.2. Training and help in the selection and proper care of clothing are available as appropriate.

    21.3. Clothing is suited to the climate.

    21.4. Clothing is becoming, in good repair, of proper size, and similar to the clothing worn by patients' peers in the community

    21.5. An adequate amount of clothing is available to permit laundering, cleaning, and repair.

22. A laundry room is accessible so patients may wash their clothing.

23. The use and location of noise-producing equipment and appliances, such as television sets, radios, and record players, do not interfere with other therapeutic activities.

24. A place and equipment are provided for table games and individual hobbies.

    24.1. Toys, equipment, and games are stored on shelves that are accessible to patients as appropriate.

25. Books, magazines, and arts and crafts materials are available in accordance with patients' recreational, cultural, and educational backgrounds and needs.

26. The facility formulates its own policy regarding the availability and care of pets and other animals, consistent with the goals of the facility and the requirements of good health and sanitation.

27. Depending on the size of the program, facilities are available for serving snacks and preparing meals for special occasions and for recreational activities.

    27.1. The facilities permit patient participation.

28. Unless contraindicated for therapeutic reasons, the facility accommodates patients' need to be outdoors through the use of nearby parks and playgrounds, adjacent countryside, and facility grounds.

    28.1. Recreational facilities and equipment are available, consistent with patients' needs and the therapeutic program.

    28.2. Recreational equipment is maintained in working order.

Source: Joint Commission on Accreditation of Hospitals: Consolidated Standards Manual for Child, Adolescent, and Adult Psychiatric, Alcoholism, and Drug Abuse Facilities and Facilities Serving the Mentally Retarded/Developmentally Disabled, *1987, pp 177–182.*

The nurses were concerned about safety. The head nurse suggested the following approach, which was acceptable to both the nurse and physician staff:

1. Teach assaultiveness management theory and skills to all staff
2. Teach staff alternative interventions to use before medication
3. Limit the number of unmedicated psychotic clients at any time through controlled admissions and varying lengths of medication-free trials.

Staff also agreed to discuss the ward milieu specifically during their treatment planning meetings. The overall social environment improved when the head nurse's plan was carried out.

Nursing Process

Assessment: Staff complaints, absenteeism, medication errors
Client assaultiveness and complaints

Nursing diagnosis: 05.98 Altered interpersonal processes not otherwise specified
/Social interaction, impaired
05.02.01.01 Aggressive/violent behaviors toward environment
/Violence, potential for: self-directed or directed at others

Plan: Decrease tension and increase milieu stability

Intervention: Discuss concerns with all group members
In-service education to enhance nurses' skills with unmedicated clients
Milieu management achieved through controlled admissions and varied lengths of medication-free trials
Improved communication through ward milieu discussions

Evaluation: Improved quality of milieu

PROFESSIONAL TREATMENT TECHNIQUES

Interaction Methods

A variety of interaction techniques have been developed from efforts to control the environment and prescribe therapeutic activities. Some techniques, such as community

---

Box 31–7
SOCIAL INTERACTION PRINCIPLES

1. *Expectations* for behavior are clearly communicated in order to maintain or change behavior.

2. The acquisition and maintenance of new behaviors depends on the degree of *personal participation* and *involvement* in learning the necessary new skills.

3. The occurrence of a behavior depends on the *sense of being a member* of the group. Group expectations and sanctions have significant influence on behavior. (Paul and Lentz 1977, pp 49–51)

Source: Adapted from Paul GL, Lentz RJ: Psychosocial Treatment of Chronic Mental Patients: Milieu versus Social Learning Programs. *Harvard University Press, 1977.*

meetings, client government, and specialty theme groups (e.g., movement or work groups), use social interaction, group activities, group pressure, and peer expectations to promote normal functioning. Clients are considered to be responsible people able to take action and adjust their behavior in a purposeful manner (see Box 31–7).

Community Meeting

Groups provide an opportunity for clients to solve problems of conflicting interests, experience cooperation with others, share responsibility, and experience leadership in the group. The most common milieu-oriented group is the community meeting. Its functions include:

- Welcoming new members
- Identifying and discussing unit rules (i.e., expectations)
- Discussing aspects of the unit environment such as cleanliness, privacy, radio and television use, or other interpersonal problems that may interfere with the quality of life for the group
- Planning activities

Patients usually chair the community meeting and report on assignments, such as checking for cleanliness of areas of responsibility (e.g., kitchen or bedrooms).

Unit Rules

All clients should be given the regulations of the setting either before or as soon after admission as possible. While written expectations do not automatically ensure acceptable behavior or prevent harmful behavior, they provide a clear baseline and serve as reminders and structure for clients.

The No Harm Contract (Figure 31–2) and Basic Expec-

I agree that I am in control of my behavior. I understand that intended injury to myself, others, or property is grounds for discharge from this unit or commitment to another psychiatric setting as an involuntary patient.

If I have impulses to harm myself or others, I agree to talk with a staff member, whom I can expect to assist me in controlling my own behavior.

_____   _____
Date   Client

                     _____
                     Witness

Figure 31–2

An example of a "no harm" contract.

Source: Langley Porter Psychiatric Hospital and Clinics, 1985. Nursing Staff, Behavioral Neurosciences Unit.

tations (Box 31–8) establish behavioral requirements for all clients. These rules reinforce staff's commitment to basic safety and specify obligations for all members of the setting. Written expectations may be presented to clients at the time of admission, discussed in community meetings, and used as a reference should a client violate any rule.

A 45-year-old depressed and suicidal man is admitted to a voluntary unit. The nurse greets the client at the time of admission and the following dialogue ensues:

Nurse: Dr. K informed me that you have been very depressed. Have you thought about harming yourself?

Mr. L: Sometimes I wake up in the middle of the night and I think I can't go on. I just want to sleep, but I am tormented by my thoughts.

Nurse: Do you want to kill yourself now?

Mr. L: Not this minute. The middle of the night is the hardest time for me.

Nurse: Nursing staff can sit with you or talk to you when you want to hurt yourself—even during the night. It is important that you tell your nurse when you feel suicidal. You are in control of your behavior even though life seems bleak right now.

Mr. L: All right.

Nurse: Nursing staff have a written agreement to be available to keep you, and all other clients here, safe. (Hands Mr. L the No Harm Contract) Do you feel able to make this commitment to control your behavior?

Mr. L: Yes. (Signs contract)

(Later, in a community meeting)

Nurse: I would like to introduce and welcome Mr. L. (Group members introduce themselves)

Nurse: Since several new members have come to the unit this week, this might be a good time to discuss the unit's rules.

Mrs. A: We all came here for help, but sometimes that means we have to take charge of ourselves.

Nurse: What does "take charge" mean?

Mrs. A: I am ultimately responsible for what I do to myself. I know I can't stay here if I cut myself like I did at home. I asked my nurse to sit with me when I first came in.

Group Living

The community meeting is also used to solve problems related to living with a large group of people or living in the hospital unit.

Patients on a 25-bed unlocked unit had access to two pay telephones. Both were located near the nurses' station, however, and conversations could be overheard easily. Patients complained in community meeting of the lack of privacy and a nurse intervened to help them write a letter to the hospital administration. A new cordless telephone provided a solution by allowing clients to make and receive calls in any area of the unit.

Client Government

Some client community groups also address clients' privileges as consequences of completion of ward jobs or general behavior in the community living groups. Clients are expected to take responsibility for themselves and each other and to learn the consequences of their actions. Client involvement in management of the unit and therapy with other clients provides opportunities for participation, corrective learning experiences, and development of new behavior patterns. Feedback is an essential technique to increase insight and promote learning. This type of community group, known as **client government,** may be most suitable to intermediate and long-term care settings, where the client group is stable and a group culture evolves over time.

The community meeting group of a 20-bed adolescent program makes recommendations for weekend passes based on members' requests and consideration of the individual's functioning in the client community. Lisa, 14 years old, has a history of running away from home, lying, drug and alcohol abuse, prostitution, and suicide threats. She requested a Saturday day pass although she did not have specific plans for how the time would be spent. Other clients commented that Lisa had not completed her ward job of checking the cleanliness of the kitchen, and staff noted that she continued to withdraw from social contacts. The group agreed that Lisa should not take a pass off the unit until she could demonstrate some improved ability to structure her time and interact with others.

Nursing Process

Assessment: Lisa is withdrawn and has failed to complete her ward job.

Nursing diagnosis: 05.05.02 Social isolation/Withdrawal /Social isolation

---

Box 31–8
BASIC EXPECTATIONS

1. Food and Fluid
   I agree to:
   A. Eat all meals in the dining room with the patient group.
      Exception:

   B. Report problems with food/fluid intake to primary care nurse.

2. Elimination
   I agree to:
   A. Maintain positive elimination habits.
   B. Report problems with elimination promptly to assigned nurse.

3. Personal Hygiene and Body Temperature
   I agree to:
   A. Keep myself and my room area clean (including laundry and linen).
   B. Complete my assigned ward job.
   C. Report problems with body temperature or hygiene to assigned nurse.

4. Rest/Activity
   A. Rest
      I agree to:
      1. Arise from bed by 8:00 A.M. and remain up during the daytime.
         Exception: Scheduled nap time after lunch from _____ P.M. to _____ P.M.
      2. Retire to bed no sooner than 9:00 P.M. or later than 12:00 (midnight).
         Exception:
      3. Remain in bed until 7:00 A.M. "wake-up" except to get water or use the bathroom.
      4. Notify staff if unable to sleep and work with them, according to the care plan, to attempt sleep.
   B. Activity
      I agree to:

1. Attend all scheduled R.T. activities, group therapy meetings, Thursday R.T. outings, community meetings, and weekend outings.
2. Accept nursing staff referral to my personal schedule if I have a question about my participation in activities.
3. Use no alcohol or nonprescribed drugs while on the unit or on passes.

5. Solitude/Socialization
   I agree to:
   A. Accept reminders from nursing staff that I have signed the No Harm Contract if I have harmful thoughts, feelings, or impulses.
   B. Accept the offer of the nurse to help me if I have harmful thoughts, feelings, or impulses by: 1) going to my room with me and sitting with me quietly for five to ten minutes, and 2) then assisting me to get involved in a game (cards, pool) or with other patients in a group situation (television, living room).
   C. Accept an option to develop new coping behaviors when I get upset. These may include relaxation techniques, deep-breathing exercises, or writing down my thoughts. I can expect the nurse assigned to my care to assist me by:
   D. Accept a referral to my assigned or primary care nurse when I become upset or distressed. I can expect that nurse to problem solve with me or refer me to my primary therapist.
   E. Discuss my suicidal or self-destructive ideas, feelings, or behaviors only in designated therapy sessions (individual, group, family) or with my primary care nurse and not with other patients.
   F. Discuss other problems including medications only in designated group therapy situations.

Source: Adapted from Langley Porter Psychiatric Hospital and Clinics, 1985. Nursing Staff, Behavioral Neurosciences Unit.

Plan: Help Lisa improve her ability to structure her time and interact with others

Intervention: Client group and staff provide feedback to Lisa regarding her behavior and group expectations for performance responsibilities

Evaluation: Lisa's pass privileges are withheld.

Basic Expectations

Basic Expectations (Box 31–8) have been developed by nurses to assist clients to take care of themselves. When Lisa complained about not receiving a pass, the following conversation ensued:

Nurse: Perhaps we should review the expectations for how you should act so you can earn a pass. Do you have your copy? (Lisa found her Basic Expectations in the back of her nightstand drawer)

Nurse: The expectations are like directions. They explain what you should do to earn pass privileges.

Lisa: I act OK. I should have gotten a pass. I didn't know I was supposed to check the kitchen to get a pass.

Nurse: The directions say you are expected to complete your ward job. The directions also tell you to participate in the activity program.

Lisa: I lost my schedule for the activities.

Nurse: Let's write a new schedule out together so we can talk about what activities you enjoy doing.

Individualized Written Expectations

McEnany and Tescher (1985) described the use of individualized written expectations for clients. They recommended careful selection of clients for written contracting. Clients must have the intellectual capacity to follow through with the contract negotiation process and the motivation to remain with a plan that works toward specific goals. The nurse should be knowledgeable about the client's disorder and its behavioral manifestations, change theory, and teaching-learning principles.

The goals of individualized contracting are to:

- Provide a consistent behavioral approach to the client by all staff
- Give the client an opportunity to use personality strengths by making decisions related to hospital care and discharge

- Give the client an opportunity to learn behaviors that enhance coping skills and ability to function

The following case example illustrates an intervention using individualized behavioral contracting.

Beverly is a 30-year-old white female admitted to an in-patient psychiatric unit following an overdose of trifluoperazine. This twice-married, twice-divorced woman has two children in foster homes. She has a long history of alcohol, marijuana, and cocaine use; multiple psychiatric hospitalizations; and treatment with antipsychotic drugs. On admission Beverly was poorly groomed, pale, and thin. She denied hallucinations, delusions, or dramatic mood shifts, and her reality testing was intact. She said that after her boyfriend left her alone recently, she experienced her body as disjointed and "falling apart" and she feared leaving her hotel room. She described feeling "suffocated" by her relationships, yet she also described her sense of emptiness. She had no long-term relationships. During hospitalization Beverly was emotionally labile, had difficulty following her schedule, and was easily frustrated by the limits and compromises of living in the hospital. She demanded medication, threatened suicide, and complained of paranoia and various somatic symptoms. Beverly's primary nurse proposed that they work together to identify goals and behaviors for improved personal and interpersonal functioning. Beverly identified problems of emptiness, poor relationships, and anger and chose to focus on the goal of improved social skills. Beverly agreed to the following expectations:

- I will participate in group therapy and psychodrama to express my feelings verbally.
- I will participate in movement therapy to express my feelings physically and learn to control my body.
- I will identify uncomfortable situations with other people and discuss the interactions with my nurse at appointed times.
- I will continue my routine activities until the appropriate time to meet with my nurse.

Nursing Process

Assessment: Client's behaviors are labile and manipulative
Client has difficulty maintaining a routine and has poor interpersonal relationships.

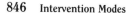

Nursing diagnosis: 06.03.03 Altered personal identity
/Self-concept, disturbance in: personal identity
05.02.02.05 Unpredictable behaviors
/Social interaction, impaired
01.97 Undeveloped activity processes
/Coping, ineffective individual

Plan: Improve personal and interpersonal functioning

Intervention: Individual behavioral contracting

Evaluation: Increased participation and decreased manipulative behavior, resulting in improved social relationships

Behavior Modification

Behavior modification also uses the environment to create behavior change; however, emphasis is on consequences for actions rather than group pressure and encouragement. Key principles of behavior modification are summarized in Box 31–9.

Positive Reinforcement

Positive reinforcement is an environmental consequence that encourages a behavior. For example, praising a client who expresses knowledge about his or her medication encourages the client to demonstrate this knowledge. Praise is positive reinforcement. Sometimes staff actions may also inadvertently encourage a client's symptomatic behavior.

Box 31–9
BEHAVIOR MODIFICATION PRINCIPLES

1. The frequency of a behavior depends on positive or negative *consequences.*

2. Events that occur together will come to be *associated.*

3. New behaviors are developed through others' *teaching and role modeling.*

Source: Adapted from Paul GL, Lentz RJ: Psychosocial Treatment of Chronic Mental Patients: Milieu versus Social Learning Programs. Harvard University Press, 1977.

A client becomes increasingly anxious about discharge. As the date approaches, his ability to follow the ward routine and take care of himself declines. Staff decide he is not ready for discharge. The client's ability to care for himself then improves. A new discharge date is set and, again, the client's behavior deteriorates as the date approaches. Staff again delay the discharge date. The staff's decision to delay discharge positively reinforces the client's anxious behavior as discharge approaches.

Tokens have also been used in behavior modification programs as positive reinforcement. Through acceptable behavior the client earns tokens that can be exchanged for cigarettes, food, or other desirable items.

Negative Reinforcement

Negative reinforcement is used to decrease or eliminate behavior. Examples of negative consequences include:

- No response to undesirable behavior
- Removing something of value for undesirable behavior
- Remove the client from the situation in which undesirable behavior takes place (called "time out")

A young woman with no organic illness repeatedly collapses in front of the nurses' station. Initially staff rushed to her assistance. Over time this reaction positively reinforced an undesirable behavior. Nursing staff agreed to implement a behavior modification plan based on "no response to undesirable behavior." Subsequently when the client fell to the floor at the nurses' station, all staff continued with their work.

In some token-based behavior modification programs, the client may not only earn tokens for desirable behavior but also lose tokens for unacceptable behavior. "Loss of tokens" illustrates a negative reinforcement technique based on removal of a valued item.

Negative reinforcement can also inadvertently discourage acceptable behavior. If, for example, the nurse made no response to the client exhibiting medication knowledge, the client could be discouraged from discussing his or her understanding of medication.

An 18-year-old woman with food gorging and vomiting behaviors was admitted voluntarily to an in-patient psychiatric unit. Karen was 5'7" and weighed 90 pounds. She stated that she was fat and that she could not control her eating patterns. She had agreed to hospitalization only on the insistence of her family. The nurse's diagnoses were:

06.03.01 Altered body image*
/Disturbance in: body image

01.03.01 Altered eating*
/Self-care deficit: feeding

The nursing team agreed that Karen's physical status required stabilization and a behavior modification plan was developed.

Intervention

1. Karen would receive a nutritionally balanced meal on a tray.

2. She would eat the entire meal under supervision of the nurse.

3. Failure to eat the entire meal would require tube feeding of the remaining food.

4. Karen would be supervised by the nurse for 30 minutes following the meal to prevent vomiting.

5. Karen would receive nursing supervision during toileting or showering to prevent vomiting.

Karen was weighed three times per week to determine if she was steadily gaining weight. The desired goal was 110 pounds, and an increase of 2 pounds per week was determined to be acceptable progress. Failure to maintain progress resulted in a loss of privileges to attend group outings and leisure activities. Progressive weight gain would result in increased privileges such as toileting, showering, and eating without nurse supervision.

This behavior modification ploy uses both positive and negative consequences. For example, the possibility of tube feeding reinforced the adaptive behavior of eating the well-balanced meal. Increased independence (i.e., removal of nursing supervision at meals and toileting) was a reward (positive reinforcement) for progressive weight gain. Continued supervision and loss of privileges were negative reinforcers designed to discourage and eliminate continued low weight.

Evaluation

The nurse and Karen reviewed her progress toward gaining weight on a weekly basis. Karen gained 3

pounds the first week, 2 pounds the second week, but nothing the third week. The nurse explored this lack of progress with Karen in the following dialog:

Nurse: You accomplished the expected weight goals the first two weeks, but there was no progress this third week.

Karen: (Crying) I don't want to gain any more weight.

Nurse: Are you concerned about being fat?

Karen: No. I enjoy having you sit with me and I know you will stop when I have gained enough weight.

The nurse realized that close supervision, originally intended to eliminate low weight, actually reinforced it since Karen enjoyed the personal attention.

The nurse, with Karen's agreement, revised the treatment plan.

Intervention

1. Other staff would supervise Karen's eating and toileting but would not engage in any discussion. This would allow staff to monitor Karen's eating and possible vomiting, but the "no response" technique would negatively reinforce (or eliminate) Karen's efforts to initiate a social relationship.

2. Karen's primary nurse would meet with Karen three times a week, contingent upon successful weight gain. This meeting would act as additional positive reinforcement to gain weight since Karen enjoyed meetings with her nurse.

Reevaluation: Karen resumed her pattern of progressive weight gain, thus indicating that the revised intervention was successful.

In this example, the treatment-planning process was similar to the earlier example of individualized behavior contracting. In both cases the expected behaviors were identified and the client participated in the plan development. Karen's example illustrates selected principles of positive and negative reinforcement. Social interaction or no response might also be interpreted as components of a therapeutic interpersonal relation approach. This blurring of the boundaries between behavior modification and interpersonal techniques highlights the underlying principle common to both approaches: Milieu therapy is based on the purposeful use of people, resources, and events in the client's immediate environment to achieve optimal functioning.

Ethics

Despite successful results, strict behavior modification programs are controversial since they frequently use as rewards access to activities, pleasurable items, or privacy, at least some of which are considered rights. Some programs have used aversive techniques, such as mild electric shock, as negative consequences to discourage behavior. Extraordinary care must be taken to protect the client's rights and human dignity when such negative reinforcements are used. Finally, Skinner's (1971) "science of behavior," based on the control of human functioning through environmental manipulation, creates doubt about the existence of free will and the notion of the autonomous person. These ideas contrast sharply with a humanistic emphasis on rights to privacy, choice, autonomy, and self-determination.

Chapter Highlights

- The therapeutic nature of the milieu is derived from the purposeful use of people, resources, and events in the immediate environment to promote optimal functioning in daily activities, development or improvement of interpersonal skills, and capacity to manage outside the institutional setting.

- The humanistic interactionist perspective of milieu therapy stems from belief in the importance of the individual and human/environment interaction theories.

- Beliefs in the importance of humane physical surroundings proposed during the moral therapy era continue to be reflected in modern legal and regulatory standards.

- Milieu therapy provides a therapeutic (rather than custodial) role unique to psychiatric nursing.

- The nursing process is used to assess client behavior within the context of the treatment environment and to plan interventions that draw on the therapeutic potential of the individual nurse, other people, and environmental facilities.

- The nursing process can also be used to assess and intervene in characteristics of the environment that influence a client's behavior.

References

American Psychiatric Association: *The Psychiatric Therapies.* APA, 1984.

Belcher JR, Fish LJB: Hildegard Peplau, in *Nursing Theories: A Base for Professional Nursing Practice.* Prentice-Hall, 1980.

Bennett AM, Foster PC: Ernestine Wiedenbach, in *Nursing Theories: A Base for Professional Nursing Practice.* Prentice-Hall, 1980.

Bockoven JS: *Moral Treatment in American Psychiatry.* Springer Publishing, 1963.

Devine BA: Therapeutic milieu/milieu therapy: An overview. *J Psychosoc Nurs Ment Health Serv* 1981;20–24.

Gerlock A, Solomons HC: Factors associated with the seclusion of psychiatric patients. *Perspect Psychiatr Care* 1984;21(April–June):46–53.

Goffman E: *Asylums.* Aldine Publishing, 1961.

Gruenberg E: The social breakdown syndrome and its prevention, in Arieti S (ed): *American Handbook of Psychiatry,* ed 2. Basic Books, 1974.

Joint Commission on Accreditation of Hospitals: Therapeutic environment, in *Consolidated Standards Manual for Child, Adolescent, and Adult Psychiatric, Alcoholism, and Drug Abuse Facilities and Facilities Serving the Mentally Retarded/Developmentally Disabled.* Joint Commission on Accreditation of Hospitals, 1987, pp 177–182.

Krauss J, Slavinsky A: *The Chronically Ill Psychiatric Patient and the Community.* Blackwell Scientific Publications, 1982.

Maxmen JS, Tucker GJ, LeBow MD: *Rational Hospital Psychiatry: The Reactive Environment.* Brunner/Mazel, 1974.

McEnany G, Tescher B: Contracting for care. *J Psychosoc Nurs Ment Health Serv* 1985;23:11–18.

National Association of Private Psychiatric Hospitals: *Requirements for NAPPH Membership.* NAPPH, 1985.

Paul GL, Lentz RJ: *Psychosocial Treatment of Chronic Mental Patients: Milieu versus Social Learning Programs.* Harvard University Press, 1977.

Proshansky HM: The environmental crisis in human dignity. *J Soc Issues* 1973;29:1–20.

Richardson B: Psychiatric inpatients' perceptions of the seclusion room experience. *Nurs Res* 1987; 36(4):234–238.

Rosenblatt A: Concepts of the asylum in the care of the mentally ill. *Hosp Community Psychiatry* 1984;35:244–250.

Schatzman L, Strauss A: A sociology of psychiatry: A perspective and some organizing foci. *Social Problems* 1966;14:3–16.

Schull AT: *Decarceration: Community Treatment and the Deviant: A Radical View.* Prentice-Hall, 1977.

Skinner BF: *Beyond Freedom and Dignity.* Alfred A. Knopf, 1971.

Stanton A, Schwartz M: *The Mental Hospital.* Basic Books, 1954.

Strauss A, Schatzman L, Bucher R, Ehrlich D, Sabshin M: *Psychiatric Ideologies and Institutions,* rev ed. Free Press of Glencoe, 1981.

Tudor GE: A sociopsychiatric nursing approach to intervention in a problem of mutual withdrawal on a mental hospital ward. *Perspect Psychiatr Care* 1970;8:11–35. (Reprinted from *Psychiatry: Journal for the Study of Interpersonal Processes* 1952;(May):15.)

Whitehead CC, Polsky RH, Crookshank C, Fik E: Objective and subjective evaluation of psychiatric ward redesign. *Am J Psychiatry* 1984;141(May):639–644.

Wilson HS: *Deinstitutionalized Residential Care for the Mentally Disabled—The Soteria House Approach.* Grune & Stratton, 1982.

THIRTY-TWO

Biologic Therapies

Geoffry McEnany

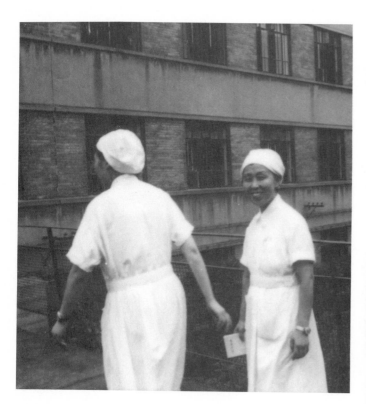

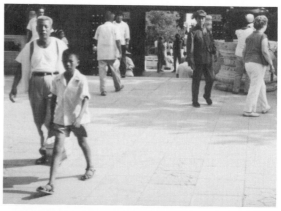

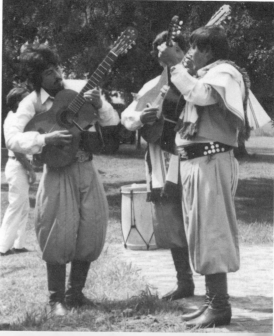

After reading this chapter, students should be able to

- Outline the historical foundations of biologic therapies

- Discuss two reasons for interest by psychiatric nurses in the biologic model of illness

- List and describe the classes, properties, uses, and side-effects of the major psychotropic medications

- Identify four pieces of information concerning clients' drugs that must be included in client teaching

- Develop a teaching plan appropriate to clients being discharged from a hospital setting with psychotropic medications

- Discuss two indications for the use of electroconvulsive therapy

- Describe three different visual-imaging techniques used in psychiatry

- Discuss one appropriate indication for the use of psychosurgery

- List and describe two humanistic interactionist implications for biologic therapies in psychiatry

Other topics related to this chapter are: Mood disorders, Chapter 18; Anxiety disorders, Chapter 19; Historical perspectives, Chapter 2; Philosophic perspectives, Chapter 13; Psychology, Chapter 9; Recidivism among the chronically mental ill, Chapter 22; Schizophrenia, Chapter 17.

akathisia
anticholinergic side-effects
antidepressant medication
antipsychotic medication
anxiolytic medication
catatonic
decanoate
disinhibition
drug holidays
extrapyramidal side-effects
hypertensive crisis
neuroleptic
neuroleptic malignant syndrome (NMS)
occulogyric crisis
opisthotonos
phenothiazines
postural hypotension
recidivism
tardive dyskinesia
torticollis

HISTORICAL FOUNDATIONS OF BIOLOGIC THERAPIES

In Chapters 2 and 9 you read about the historical underpinnings of contemporary psychiatry and psychobiologic thought. Biologic therapies have been interwoven into the evolutionary fabric of psychiatry and, more recently, psychiatric nursing. Over time the philosophic pendulum has swung between fully biologic explanations of mental disorders to etiologic beliefs based fully on demonological, magical, or spiritual reasoning. Treatment has largely depended on the philosophic and socially accepted attitudes of a given society during a specific era. For example, the ancient Greek and Roman civilizations maintained strong beliefs about the biologic substrates of mental disorders. A similar psychobiologic understanding of behavior and illness is emerging today in Western societies. However, the period between early civilizations and the twentieth century was characterized by a potpourri of approaches to and interventions for mental disorders that were mainly spiritual, moralistic, or psychodynamic in origin.

Exploring the Biologic/Psychologic Linkage

From a biologic perspective all behavior is the result of neurochemical actions and reactions in the central nervous system. Of course, the systematized chemical reactions are influenced by many factors, such as the environment, interpersonal social exchanges, stress, and the idiosyncratic responses of one's body systems (endocrine, neurologic, immunologic, etc.). So behavior is the holistic response of a set of body systems to a given stimulus.

As nurses we are challenged with the responsibility of protecting the health of present and future generations.

Portions of the material in this chapter were contributed to the second edition of this text by Andrew E. Skodol, M.D.

Psychobiology and the biologic understanding of human behavior may eliminate dualism and a fragmented approach to client care. But if this is true, why have the nursing and medical sciences not revolutionized approaches to client care by fully adopting a psychobiologic framework in understanding illness? To answer that question, one must appreciate the influences of time, tradition, and the dominant philosophic viewpoints of caregivers today. The biological approach to mental disorders is not new, but it *is* undergoing a renewed interest by clinicians and researchers in different parts of the world. However, many professionals in nursing, psychiatry, and collaborative disciplines know little or nothing of psychobiologic mediation of behavior. Their training and philosophies may not support the perception of mental disorder as a psychobiologic entity. Such dissonance between learned philosophies and advances in the biology of behavior make it difficult to take a fully unified approach to care for the mentally disordered.

Trends in Biologic Therapies Over Time

Chapter 2 addresses many of the biologic therapies used from preliterate times through to the twentieth century. In this chapter the goal is to review advancements in biologic therapies over the last 100 years, which have produced the most scientific and precise psychobiologic discoveries known to psychiatric care and have witnessed a revolution in the assessment of, and traditional approaches to, behavioral problems and mental disorders.

Perhaps a reasonable way to conceptualize the current changes in understanding the biologic underpinnings of behavior called mental disorder is to frame the biologic approaches as molecular rather than "psychologic," "social," or "cultural." In other words, biologic therapies often yield healing because they produce changes in the function of cells in the central nervous system, which permits the emergence of new behavior.

ECT

Probably the earliest "new" biologic intervention in the twentieth century was electroconvulsive therapy (ECT). Introduced in 1938, the then unrefined treatment was used for clients with unremitting or recurrent severe depression, some forms of schizophrenia, or bipolar disorder. Of course, lack of standardized nomenclature for diagnostic labeling during the first half of the twentieth century made it difficult to know *who* was being treated with ECT; what one diagnostician called "schizophrenia" may have been considered "depression with psychotic features" by another. This raised the unanswered question of whether schizophrenia and various forms of mood disorders might be part of the same continuum—a blasphemous thought in the opinion of some clinicians today! ECT will be more thoroughly discussed later in this chapter.

Drugs

Other biologic therapies that have revolutionized psychiatry include the various drugs developed and applied to clinical practice since the late 1940s. The earliest medication discovery was made in 1949 by an Australian physician, John Cade. Dr. Cade found that lithium worked to subdue wild behavior in animals. To the astonishment of his colleagues, Cade went one step further and gave lithium to humans. Since then of course lithium has become the drug of choice for the treatment of bipolar affective disorder.

This century has witnessed many other great pharmacologic discoveries, including most of the drugs used in psychiatry today. In the 1950s antipsychotic, antidepressant, and some anxijolytic medications were discovered. Until then the care of psychiatric clients had consisted mainly of behavioral interventions, seclusion, and various forms of restraint. Suddenly many clients were suffering less, getting better, and returning to the mainstream of life. However, for a variety of complex reasons, some clients found themselves lodged in the psychiatric system, unable to do much more than become permanent residents of the psychiatric community.

Interest in the Biologic Model by Psychiatric Nurses

Other biologic therapies continue to unfold as time passes. While physicians continue to look for biologic markers or clear physical indices of mental illness, some nurses are trying to understand how select nursing interventions affect the psychobiology of clients. Subjects of such nursing research include:

- Specific types of dietary influences on behavior
- Ways in which clients' normal circadian rhythms can be assessed and "harnessed" to improve the specificity of nursing interventions and overall care to clients
- Effects of exposure to full-spectrum light during winter months as a preventive measure against seasonal cyclic depressive disorders
- Effects of limited sleep deprivation to reduce the response time of depressed clients to antidepressant medications
- Biologic effects of relaxation techniques
- Biologic effects of seclusion or restraint

Nurses and Psychobiology

Psychiatric-mental health nurses need to understand and remain abreast of current advances in psychobiology. By doing so nurses can maintain an updated knowledge base for clinical work with clients and therefore develop accurate and effective nursing interventions.

The biologic model is of particular interest to any nurse who administers medications and is involved in client teaching. The biologic model supports the fact that *the mind is not separate from the brain,* and that there are underlying biologic reasons for all behavior. An understanding of biologic reasoning allows nurses to adopt a truly holistic approach to mental disorder while working with and teaching clients.

PSYCHOTROPIC MEDICATIONS AND NURSING RESPONSIBILITIES

The word *drugs* conjures a variety of powerful positive and negative images. A recent weekly news magazine illustrated one set of images on its cover, which showed a line of cocaine, an empty hypodermic needle, and a "joint" of marijuana. Above the picture was the headline, "The Drug Crisis—*Saying No!*" Another image leaps from the pages of nursing and medical journals; pharmaceutical advertisements show people leading productive lives or smiling nurses, allegedly grateful for a medication that controls psychiatric symptoms. Still another drug-related image is that of school children being inoculated against diphtheria, polio, and pertussis. All these images are powerful, and each is backed by truth.

Nurses' responsibilities to clients receiving psychotropic medications are very different from the responsibilities of nurses in other settings. A nurse working with clients having cardiac difficulties, for example, may have clear physiologic indices for the administration of certain drugs like isosorbide dinitrate or nitroglycerin, but psychiatric nurses rarely have comparable consistent complexes of symptoms on which to base clinical judgments. In psychiatric work, nurses must often observe client behaviors closely to be aware of the sometimes subtle nature of the presenting symptom. Pacing, mild diaphoresis, slight increases in blood pressure or pulse, a heightened muscle tone, and hypervigilant posture may be indicative of escalating anxiety, but they may also point to other problems such as caffeine toxicity or excessive use of tobacco. Accurate nursing assessment of client behavior is crucial if medications are to be given effectively and appropriately (Figure 32–1). For example, over the last two or three years there has been an increasing trend among hospital psychiatrists to prescribe a class of drugs known as *benzodiazepines* (the diazepam/Valium family) more liberally in conjunction with low-dose antipsychotic drugs (also known as *neuroleptic drugs*). This minimizes the use of the neu-

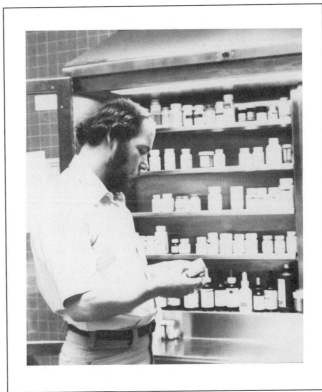

Figure 32–1
The nurse's role is crucial in the use of the most widely prescribed of all biologic therapies, psychotropic drugs—medicines that literally act upon the mind.

roleptics and possibly diminishes the potential for tardive dyskinesia, an extreme side-effect of neuroleptic use among some clients receiving this class of drugs. In light of this trend, nurses must be able to assess the finer differences between anxious and psychotic behavior. Sometimes the two are difficult to differentiate, especially when the client's anxiety is high and the psychotic behavior is "covered" or "masked" by the client.

Medication Teaching

In addition to assessment, nurses have the major responsibility of planning for client learning about medication. Compliance with medication regimens is often an issue for psychiatric clients, and nurses have explored the efficacy of teaching as a means to improve adherence to medication regimens after discharge. In exploring factors related to compliance with lithium regimens, Kucera-Bozarth, Beck, and Lyss (1982) reviewed the literature and identified several variables related to compliance: socioeconomic class, marital status, number of concurrent medications, diagnosis, side-effects, health benefits, and health values. While the research data vary on the degree of influence of these variables, there was better compliance among people who were upper middle class, married, taking more than four types of medication, and carrying a diagnosis of bipolar disorder with reported mild or nonexistent side-effects from medications. Since the authors do not indicate whether their subjects were randomly selected or voluntary, it is difficult to determine if these findings can be generalized. However, the issue is noteworthy: Clients' individual differences must be addressed in the course of the teaching-learning process.

An issue of great concern to many nurses involves the planning of teaching-learning experiences for clients who suffer from chronic mental illness. While this population has learning needs concerning care and treatments, teaching is often difficult, depending on the severity and chronicity of the client's illness. Selander and Miller (1985) express concern over clients' recidivism and the learning needs of chronically mentally disordered people. Specific to the work of Selander and Miller, the term recidivism refers to a tendency to relapse into a previous mode of behavior. The target population of these authors included clients who predominantly carried a schizophrenic diagnosis and received fluphenazine decanoate (Prolixin Decanoate) as part of their treatment. The authors hypothesized that recidivism rates would decline for the clients who were involved in the fluphenazine groups. Nurses organized the groups, incorporating group therapy, teaching, medication surveillance, and medication administration into a regular format. Selander and Miller found that admission rates dropped significantly and length of stay was significantly briefer.

Other areas of concern for nurses working with mentally disordered clients involve the need to assess the learning capacity of clients at different points in their disorders. For example, when clients are first admitted to an in-patient unit, they may be too disorganized to focus on specific learning tasks. Looking at clinical situations from a psychobiologic perspective, the depressed client may be so psychomotorally slowed, due to hormonal shifts and dysfunctional neurotransmitter activity at the synapses, that learning is impossible. Given appropriate treatment and care, however, the clients' psychobiologic disequilibrium may become balanced and learning will then be possible.

When a nurse perceives a client is ready to learn (i.e., cognitive abilities are intact), it does not necessarily mean that learning will occur. Neizo and Murphy (1983) discuss medication groups on an acute psychiatric unit and address the importance of not only assessing cognitive abilities but also exploring affective and social issues that may contribute to effective learning experiences. Clients are no different in many ways from other learners. When presented with material that is clearly beneficial to them, they are likely to be more interested in the learning process.

Evaluation of teaching efforts is essential to complete the teaching-learning process. This part of the process can be as informal or formal as the nurse chooses or deems necessary to check the client's knowledge of information taught. Evaluation of a client's understanding of information usually requires at least an accurate verbal reiteration of information or a return demonstration of the skill. A nurse desiring a more extensive evaluation may consider using a paper and pencil "pretest/posttest" format. With such an approach, the nurse develops a written test to cover the content of the teaching and has the client complete the test before the nurse begins teaching. This provides a written measure of the client's learning needs. After the nurse implements the teaching plan, the client completes the same examination (a posttest). Comparison of the pretest and posttest results yields a documented measure of how much learning has occurred as a result of the nurse's teaching intervention.

Antipsychotic Drugs

Background

The discovery of the first antipsychotic drug, chlorpromazine (Thorazine), is a prime example of the role chance has played in the history of psychopharmacology. Chlorpromazine was initially synthesized as an antihistamine and was not tried as a tranquilizer for schizophrenic persons until 1952. Its effects on the behavior, thinking, affect, and perception of schizophrenic persons were so profound that knowledge of its properties was rapidly disseminated and it became widely used within three or four years. Chlorpromazine's effects on the hospital practice of psychiatry were staggering. Its use reversed a steadily increasing census in United States mental institutions, and the mental hospital population has progressively decreased ever since. One might say that chlorpromazine gave birth to the modern notions of psychiatric treatment—unlocked wards, milieu treatment, occupational and recreational therapy, and halfway houses. The entire field of community mental health is ultimately linked to its discovery, because it enabled clients to return to their homes.

Major Effects

The beneficial effects of antipsychotic medications in all psychotic states have been demonstrated beyond question, using multiple and varied criteria to measure improvement. The manifestations of disintegrative patterns affected by these drugs include delusional thinking, confusion, motor agitation, and motor retardation. Antipsychotic drug treatment also decreases formal thought disorder, blunted affect, bizarre behavior, social withdrawal, hallucinations, belligerence, and uncooperativeness.

The most common disintegrative condition treated with antipsychotic drugs is the group of symptoms traditionally labeled schizophrenia. (The proper manner for evaluating the schizophrenic client and the diagnostic criteria in DSM-IIIR appear in Chapter 17.) The problem of assessment is complicated by the fact that many diseases can cause organic brain syndromes with features like those of schizophrenia. For example, clients suffering from either schizophrenia or an organic brain syndrome may experience auditory hallucinations. Such hallucinations may indicate a variety of DSM-IIIR conditions, including schizophrenia and organic brain syndrome. The finer points of differentiation between these two conditions include assessments of cognitive functioning and the client's presenting history. Chapter 9 offers a more detailed delineation of organic brain syndrome and related disorders. Suffice it to say that all clients manifesting psychotic symptoms should have a thorough medical history and physical examination to rule out treatable "medical" illnesses, many of which present behaviors considered to be psychotic or "psychobiologic" in nature.

Choice of Specific Drug

Although there are a great many antipsychotic medications on the market and claims are made for the greater effectiveness of one over another, especially by the respective drug companies, controlled studies have failed to demonstrate substantial differences in antipsychotic effects among the drugs. The choice of a particular medication, then,

depends on knowledge of the various pharmacologic properties and side-effects, the client's or a family member's history of drug response, and the psychiatrist's experience with various compounds. Important client variables are past successes with specific drugs, history of allergies, and history of serious or intolerable side-effects. Certain side-effects can often be used beneficially with clients, as we will discuss below. A certain amount of trial and error is expected in each clinical application.

Table 32–1 summarizes the characteristics of the major antipsychotic drugs. As the list of these drugs is extensive and growing, it makes sense for each member of the treatment team to become familiar with just a few representative drugs, their predictable effects, and their common side-effects. The characteristics covered in the table are discussed in sequence in the sections that follow.

There are now five distinct chemical classes of antipsychotic medications commonly used in the United States. One class, the **phenothiazines**, can be broken down into three different types of medications. This provides a broad choice in terms of side-effects and potential client responsiveness. A client who is unresponsive to one class may well respond to another that circumvents a problem in absorption, accumulation at neurotransmitter receptor sites, or metabolism.

Table 32–1 indicates that there is a wide variety among these medications in milligram-per-milligram potency. This

| | | | | | | Side-Effects | |
Class	Generic Name	Trade Name	Potency (mg equivalent to 100 mg Chlorpromazine)	Usual Dosage Range (Mg/Day)	Sedative	Extra-pyramidal*	Anti-cholinergic*
Phenothiazines							
Aliphatic	Chlorpromazine	Thorazine	100	150–1500	Very strong	Moderate	Strong
Piperadine	Thioridazine	Mellaril	100	150–800	Moderate	Minimal	Moderate
Piperazine	Trifluoperazine	Stelazine	5	10–60	Weak	Strong	Weak
	Fluphenazine	Prolixin	2	3–45	Weak	Strong	Weak
	Perphenazine	Trilafon	10	12–60	Weak	Strong	Weak
Butyrophenones	Haloperidol	Haldol	2.5	2–40	Weak	Strong	Weak
Thioxanthenes	Thiothixene	Navane	5	10–60	Weak	Strong	Weak
	Chlorprothixene	Taractan	100	40–600	Strong	Moderate	Strong
Dihydroindolones	Molindone	Moban	10	15–225	Weak	Moderate	Weak
Dibenzoxazepines	Loxapine	Loxitane	20	10–100	Moderate	Strong	Moderate

Table 32–1
Antipsychotic Drugs

Extrapyramidal and anticholinergic side-effects are discussed later in this chapter.

fact has most relevance when treating clients who require large doses. In such cases a potent medication is best.

Dosage

Dosage ranges vary widely among clients. Medications must be titrated against the psychotic target symptoms and the appearance of side-effects. Most approaches to management start with a relatively low dose (e.g., 25 to 50 mg orally or 25 mg intramuscularly [IM] of chlorpromazine) to test for adverse effects for one to two hours. Then the medication is typically given in a starting dose of 300 to 400 mg (or IM equivalent) per day, and gradually increased by 25 to 50 percent a day until maximum improvement is noted or intolerable side-effects are encountered.

The treatment setting frequently influences the drug regimen. In a crowded hospital emergency room, for example, hourly doses of medication may be given until a client is sedated. In more completely staffed, private in-patient units, a client may be observed drug-free for a couple of days before medication is instituted. It is interesting to note, however, that in terms of long-term outcome and length of eventual remission, neither approach can claim documented superiority.

Clients who are extremely agitated, violent, severely withdrawn, or **catatonic** require significant doses during the first few days of treatment, delivered by injection to ensure rapid relief. Chlorpromazine, 50 to 100 mg IM, may be used, particularly if sedation is required. The nurse must be aware that this is an irritating drug; injections must be deeply intramuscular in either the buttocks or upper arms, and sites must be rotated. Substantial IM doses of the more potent antipsychotics, such as haloperidol 10 mg or trifluoperazine 10 mg, may be given to agitated clients. This approach frequently avoids some of the more troublesome side-effects while bringing behavior and cognitive processes into control.

Because the antipsychotic medications have a rather long biologic half-life, and many have significant sedative effects, there is little reason to give divided doses of medication after the initial days of treatment. It is recommended that the drugs, particularly the sedative ones such as chlorpromazine, be given in substantial doses at bedtime. In addition to promoting sleep, decreasing the chances the client will forget to take a dose after discharge, and saving nursing time in the hospital, this method saves money since large-dose capsules or tablets cost less than an equivalent amount of medication prepared in smaller doses.

After maximum clinical improvement has been obtained, antipsychotic drugs are generally reduced gradually. Continuing to give a client modest doses of an antipsychotic medication following a psychotic episode lowers the chances of relapse and rehospitalization. Psychotherapy with schizophrenic clients may not be particularly effective without maintenance medications in conventional treatment settings, but it does improve psychosocial functioning in clients who are also taking maintenance medications. It is generally believed that clients should be kept on doses of antipsychotics sufficient to suppress symptoms for three months to one year following an acute episode. After such an interval, the particular client's course and life situation must be considered and treatment individualized. Some clients will recover from a psychotic episode completely within six months. These clients, with schizophreniform disorder, should not receive long-term maintenance drug treatment. For individuals who have already experienced recurrent episodes and demonstrate a deteriorating course, it is clearly advantageous to prevent relapses with drugs if possible.

Because of the long-term toxic effects of antipsychotics, **drug holidays** are generally recommended as part of maintenance treatment. This might mean that medications are taken every other day or five days a week with weekends off. No significant increases in relapse rates have been observed with these intermittent schedules.

Decision to Use a Drug

The general principles that govern antipsychotic drug use today are:

- Drugs are given to treat target symptoms of schizophrenia or other psychotic disorders.

- Initial treatment may require parenteral doses. These are changed to oral pill or concentrate forms as the behavior disturbance subsides.

- Total dosages are tailored to individual needs; wide variations exist among clients.

- As soon as practical, divided doses are changed to a single dose given at bedtime to maximize use of the drugs' sedative properties.

- Most clients with a chronic course require maintenance doses for sustained improvement.

Special Considerations

There are three special considerations involving the use of antipsychotic medication.

1. *A unique route of administration.* The phenothiazines fluphenazine (Prolixin) and haloperidol (Haldol) are available in long-acting intramuscular injectable forms that behave like sustained-release capsules. These medications are gradually released over a long period of time—two to three weeks. Long-acting fluphenazine and haloperidol are available in **decanoate** (long-acting depot injection) preparations. The main advantage of the long-acting injectable forms are that they circumvent a client's ambivalence about taking med-

ication and eliminate the need for constant pill taking. The treatment team must also honor the client's civil liberties; truly involuntary treatment can be performed only according to due process, as required by a particular state's mental hygiene laws.

The psychiatric nurse in a community setting may frequently have occasion to administer the long-acting fluphenazine or haloperidol. A dose of regular fluphenazine or haloperidol is usually taken first to rule out the possibility of allergic reactions. Such reactions can be devastating if discovered after a two- or three-week supply of medicine has been given. If no adverse reactions are noted within one hour, the long-acting form is injected, usually in the upper, outer quadrant of the buttocks.

2. *The medication requirements of certain age groups, specifically the elderly and children.* In elderly persons the agitation often associated with organic mental syndromes is markedly responsive to phenothiazines. Other sedatives, such as the barbiturates and the benzodiazepines, may further compromise cerebral functioning (further depress the level of awareness and concentration) and thus worsen such syndromes. Doses of phenothiazines are generally reduced for the geriatric population. Trifluoperazine (Stelazine) 5–20 mg per day, or haloperidol, 1–6 mg per day, might constitute adequate treatment.

Antipsychotic medications are effective in treating childhood psychoses and in managing the behavior problems associated with mental retardation. The general principle of reduced dosage is again applicable. The upper limit of the usual daily dosage for children under twelve might be 200 mg per day of chlorpromazine (Thorazine) or thioridazine (Mellaril) or 20 mg per day of trifluoperazine. Amounts of individual intramuscular injections must also be kept at 25 to 50 mg.

3. *Evaluating the potential side-effects of the antipsychotic medications.* Their continuous contact with clients gives nurses an advantage over physicians, who may be seeing a client only every other day or, at best, once every day at the same time. Both the dangerous and the more uncomfortable side-effects frequently have a rapid onset and need attention promptly.

The side-effects of antipsychotic medications that nurses must recognize can be divided into the following general classes:

- Autonomic nervous system
- Extrapyramidal
- Other central nervous system
- Allergic
- Blood
- Skin
- Eye
- Endocrine

Refer to Table 32–2 for a listing of side-effects from various antipsychotic medications.

Autonomic Nervous System Effects

The antipsychotics all possess **anticholinergic** and **antiadrenergic** side-effects. That is, they interfere with the usual transmission of nerve impulses by acetylcholine and epinephrine, in both central and peripheral nerves. The most common side-effects encountered are the anticholinergic effects. These include dry mouth, blurred vision, constipation, urinary hesitance or retention, and, under rarer circumstances, paralytic ileus.

Postural hypotension is a common antiadrenergic effect. The primary danger here is injury from a fall. Clients receiving parenteral medications, such as chlorpromazine intramuscularly, must have their blood pressure monitored lying and standing before and a half hour after each dose. Clients should be advised to rise from a supine position gradually and to sit back down if they feel faint. Support stockings and a large intake of fluids may be indicated. This problem is much less significant with oral administration of the drugs. However, nurses working with clients receiving oral antipsychotic medications should take both baseline and routine measures of vital sign readings at regular intervals. Such a practice establishes the client's tolerance for medications without the untoward side-effects of orthostatic hypotension and subsequent falls.

Extrapyramidal Effects

Another common and sometimes frightening group of adverse reactions results from the effects of antipsychotics on the extrapyramidal tracts of the central nervous system, which are involved in the production and control of involuntary movements. These **extrapyramidal side-effects** can be broken down into four types, each with distinguishing clinical characteristics and times of onset after the initiation of drug therapy.

The earliest and most dramatic reactions are the *acute dystonic reactions.* These occur in the first days of treatment, sometimes after a single dose of medication. They involve bizarre and severe muscle contractions usually of the tongue, face, or extraocular muscles, producing **torticollis, opisthotonos,** and **occulogyric crisis.** These reactions can be physically painful and are almost always frightening to the individual. They are readily reversible with one of the antiparkinsonian agents—benztropine, 1 to 2 mg, or diphenhydramine, 25 to 50 mg, intravenously (for immediate relief), intramuscularly (for rapid action), or orally (for relief within hours). Table 32–3 summarizes useful information about the antiparkinsonian agents.

Table 32–2
Side-Effects of Antipsychotic Medication

Effect	Chlorpromazine (Thorazine)	Haloperidol (Haldol)	Loxapine (Loxitane)	Molindone (Moban)	Thioridazine (Mellaril)	Thiothixene (Navane)	Trifluoperazine (Stelazine)	Fluphenazine (Prolixin)
Akathisia	Occasional	Frequent	Occasional	Frequent	Occasional	Occasional	Frequent	Frequent
Allergic skin reactions	Occasional	Rare	Rare	Rare	Not reported	Rare	Rare	Rare
Anticholinergic effects	Frequent	Not reported	Rare	Occasional	Frequent	Occasional	Frequent	Frequent
Blood dyscrasia	Occasional	Occasional	Not reported	Rare	Rare	Rare	Rare	Rare
Cholestatic jaundice	Occasional	Rare	Not reported	Not reported	Rare	Rare	Rare	Rare
Dystonias	Occasional	Frequent	Rare	Occasional	Occasional	Occasional	Frequent	Frequent
Impotence	Occasional	Not reported	Not reported	Not reported	Occasional	Not reported	Occasional	Occasional
Parkinsonism	Occasional	Frequent	Frequent	Occasional	Occasional	Occasional	Frequent	Frequent
Photosensitivity	Occasional	Rare	Not reported	Not reported	Occasional	Rare	Occasional	Occasional
Postural hypotension	Frequent	Occasional	Rare	Rare	Frequent	Occasional	Rare	Rare
Retinitis pigmentosa	Not reported	Not reported	Not reported	Not reported	Occasional	Not reported	Not reported	Not reported
Sedation	Frequent	Not reported	Occasional	Rare	Frequent	Frequent	Not reported	Occasional

Table 32–3
Antiparkinsonian Agents

Trade Name	Generic Name	Maximum Daily Dosage	Available in Injectable Form
Symmetrel	Amantadine	300 mg	No
Cogentin	Benztropine	8 mg	Yes
Benadryl	Diphen-hydramine	100 mg	Yes
Kemadrin	Procyclidine	15 mg	No
Artane	Trihexyphenidyl	15 mg	No
Akineton	Biperiden	8 mg	Yes

Sources: Derogatis L: Clinical Psychopharmacology. *Addison-Wesley, 1986;* Appleton WS, Davis JM: Practical Clinical Psychopharmacology. *MedCom, 1973.*

The *parkinsonian syndrome,* named because of its striking resemblance to true Parkinson's disease, commonly occurs after a week or two of the therapy. The hallmark signs include masklike facies, resting tremor, general rigidity of posture with slow voluntary movement, and a shuffling gait. This syndrome is treatable with the antiparkinsonian agents listed in Table 32–3. Oral medication is usually sufficient, since urgency is seldom a consideration in the management of this syndrome.

A third reversible extrapyramidal syndrome is known as **akathisia.** This characteristically is a motor restlessness perceived subjectively by the client and experienced as an urge to pace, a need to shift weight from one foot to another, or an inability to sit or stand still. Akathisia is generally a later complication of drug treatment, occurring weeks to months into the course of therapy. Nonetheless it responds to oral antiparkinsonian agents as well.

Accurate observation of the course of therapy by the psychiatric nurse can promote prompt recognition and proper interpretation of these syndromes. If care is not taken, the health care provider may misinterpret the increasing withdrawal, emotional blunting, apathy, and lack of spontaneity as a deterioration in schizophrenic behavior. This error in interpretation may lead to a mistaken increase in dosage of antipsychotic medication, which will aggravate the syndrome. Akathisia can also be confused with psychotic agitation, and this error also prompts an increase in medication. For a comparison of the two conditions, see Table 32–4. Clients with akathisia require a reduction in the dosage of phenothiazines or other offending agents and/or treatment with an antiparkinsonian drug. The nurse can save the client many uncomfortable and worrisome days by being aware of the frequency with which these syndromes complicate treatment and by reporting any suspicious sign or symptom to the physician, while reassuring the client of the reversibility of the syndrome in almost all cases.

Whether clients should be treated prophylactically with antparkinsonian agents, in view of the relatively high incidence of these syndromes, is open to debate. Some argue that the use of antiparkinsonian agents eventually leads to relatively higher antipsychotic doses and thus increases the probability of serious side-effects. Another argument is that antiparkinsonian agents have their own toxicity and thus should be used only to counteract extrapyramidal syndromes, not to guard against their possible emergence. Moreover, a great many clients never develop the syndromes. Suffice it to say that, if the likelihood of an extrapyramidal reaction is high (if, for example, the client has a history of them) and the possible consequences signifi-

Table 32–4
Comparison of Akathisia and Agitation or Psychotic Relapse

Akathisia	Agitation or Relapse
Relieved by reducing phenothiazine dosage	Worsened by reducing phenothiazine dosage
Worsened by increasing phenothiazine dosage	Improved by increasing phenothiazine dosage
Outside voluntary control	Controllable
Responsive to antiparkinsonian agents	Unresponsive to antiparkinsonian agents
Motor restlessness predominant	Verbalization predominant

cant (that is, the client may discontinue medication or drop out of treatment altogether), antipsychotic and antiparkinsonian agents are frequently initiated simultaneously.

The last extrapyramidal syndrome to emerge in the course of treatment is also the severest, since it can be largely irreversible. This is tardive dyskinesia, a disorder characterized by involuntary movements of the face, jaw, and tongue that produce bizarre grimaces, lip smacking, and protrusion of the tongue. There may also be jerky choreiform movements of the upper extremities, slow writhing athetoid movements of the arms and the legs, and tense, tonic contractions of the neck and back. The symptoms are categorized in Table 32–5. The syndrome frequently comes on after years of antipsychotic drug treatment, although it can occur earlier. It usually occurs after a maintenance dose is discontinued or reduced, and it can be masked—but not treated—by reinstituting the medication or the dosage or by switching to another drug. There is no known cure for the syndrome. The recommended intervention is to stop all medication to see if the syndrome will spontaneously remit. This course of action must be weighed against the client's need for medication and the likelihood of relapse into psychosis. Reserpine, deanol, and several other drugs have been used experimentally to treat tardive dyskinesia, with equivocal results.

Other Central Nervous System Effects

Other central nervous system side-effects of antipsychotic medications are sedation and reduction of seizure threshold. Since antipsychotic drugs vary in their sedative effects, this side-effect is troublesome, but it can be managed by changing to a less sedative agent. Seizures are not a contraindication for the drugs, but they do require close client observation.

Allergic Effects

The principal allergic manifestation of the antipsychotics is cholestatic jaundice, which arises with chlorpromazine treatment. This occurs much less commonly than in the early days of psychopharmacology, and it is usually a benign and self-limiting condition.

Blood, Skin, and Eye Effects

Among the other side-effects, agranulocytosis (that is, a marked decrease in granulated white blood cells, or leukocytes) is the most serious. It is both potentially fatal and, fortunately, extremely rare. Usually the person gets an infection and deteriorates rapidly or begins to bleed spontaneously. It requires emergency medical attention. Skin eruptions, photosensitivity leading to severe sunburn, blue-

gray metallic discolorations over face and hands, and pigmentary changes in the eyes are all potential side effects from chlorpromazine. Clients are generally advised to avoid prolonged exposure to sunlight or to use a sunscreen agent such as Uval when outdoors. These conditions usually remit. One serious eye change that is permanent is retinitis pigmentosa, which may occur in persons on doses of thioridazine exceeding 800 mg a day. This reaction may lead to blindness. Therefore, doses exceeding 800 mg per day are contraindicated.

Endocrine Effects

Lactation in females and gynecomastia and impotence in males lead a list of endocrine changes that can occur with antipsychotic drug treatments. The nurse should be alert to any changes in body functions reported by clients receiving such drugs.

Psychobiologic Considerations

Why do antipsychotic medications ease the symptoms of a psychotic brain? As discussed in Chapter 9 neurotransmitters are a series of chemicals contained in the presynaptic and postsynaptic neuronal membranes. These chemicals permit the transmission of messages along neurons, allowing for behavior, thought and emotion. Dopamine is a plentiful neurotransmitter, available in many parts of the brain, and considered to be the neurotransmitter on which many antipsychotic drugs work.

Many antipsychotic drugs bind to the postsynaptic neuronal membrane. In such a state, dopamine released by the presynaptic neuron cannot bind to the membrane of the postsynaptic neuron. When this occurs, the neuron is in a state of *dopamine blockade*, and hence the antipsychotic drugs are *dopamine antagonists*. In this explanation lies the basis for the dopamine hypothesis of schizophrenia.

Clinical Implications

Nurses have many responsibilities to clients to whom they are administering neuroleptic drugs. One of their primary responsibilities is to be aware of the incompatibilities between neuroleptics or the problems with administering neuroleptics with certain juices or liquids. Kerr (1986) points out that oral liquid neuroleptics are often mixed with juices or syrups. Because of the acid-base characteristics of the drug, precipitates may form and adhere to the containers or cups from which the medications are administered. The result seems obvious: potential underdosing of the medications. Kerr also points out that neuroleptic effectiveness suffers with the client's consumption of coffee, tea, or cola beverages, due to the tannic acid content of those liquids. Table 32–6 is a chart of compatibilities between different neuroleptics and liquids.

Table 32–5
Extrapyramidal Effects of Antipsychotic Medications

Type	Timing	Symptoms	Treatment	Nursing Implications
Acute dystonic reaction	First days of treatment; possibly after the first dose	Physically painful, bizarre, and frightening symptoms; severe muscle contractions of the face, extraocular muscles, and tongue with torticollis, opisthotonos, and oculogyric crisis (eyes look upward, head is turned to one side).	Antiparkinsonian agents such as benztropine (Cogentin), trihexyphenidyl (Artane), biperiden (Akineton), procyclidine (Kemadrin), diphenhydramine (Benadryl)	Secure order for p.r.n. antiparkinsonian agents when antipsychotic medications are first begun so client discomfort can be treated quickly. Respond immediately to any symptoms and administer antiparkinsonian medication. Reassure client that side-effect is reversible. Remain with client until side-effect abates.
Parkinsonian syndrome	After 1 to 2 weeks of treatment	Similar to Parkinson's disease; mask-like face, shuffling gait, pill-rolling tremor of the hands, rigidity of posture, and slow movement.	Same	Reassure client that side-effect is reversible. Administer antiparkinsonian medication.
Akathisia	Weeks to months into the course of treatment	Characterized by motor restlessness; pacing, shifting weight from one foot to another, foot tapping, inability to sit or stand still or rest. Results from injury to basal ganglion areas.	Same	Careful assessment is necessary to prevent confusing this extrapyramidal response with anxiety or agitation. Confusion may result in increasing the client's dose, thus worsening the extrapyramidal effects. Reassure client that side-effect is reversible. Administer antiparkinsonian medication.
Tardive dyskinesia	Often after years of treatment when a maintenance dose is reduced or discontinued	Involuntary bizarre grimacing, lip smacking, and protrusion of the tongue; jerky choreiform movements of the upper extremities; slow, writhing athetoid movements of the arms and legs; tonic contractions of the neck and back.	No known cure. Medication may be discontinued. Otherwise, the symptoms can only be masked by reinstituting treatment.	Contact physician immediately for medical evaluation. Do not give antiparkinsonian medications—they only worsen the symptoms. Informed consent for continued treatment with antipsychotic medication should be obtained.

Source: Kneisl CR: Wadsworth's Review of Nursing. Reprinted by permission of Jones and Bartlett Publishers, 1983, p 131.

Neuroleptic Malignant Syndrome

Derogatis (1986) addresses the issue of an infrequently noted complication of high-potency drugs (e.g., fluphenazine, thiothixene, haloperidol) known as neuroleptic malignant syndrome. This extreme condition occurs in clients who are severely ill, and is believed to be the result of dopamine blockade in the hypothalamus. Nurses are in the best position to assess for this condition as it manifests itself with symptoms of diaphoresis, muscle rigidity, and hyperpyrexia. Hollister (1984) also reports mutism as a prominent symptom of this condition and warns that if cooling and rehydration are not achieved quickly, the client may die.

As for any other medication, client teaching is essential for clients receiving neuroleptic medication. A medication teaching plan for neuroleptics is presented in Box 32–1.

Antidepressant Drugs

Background

Like the antipsychotic drugs, the major antidepressant drugs were discovered accidentally. Two classes of antidepressants currently exist: tricyclic antidepressants and monoamine oxidase inhibitor antidepressants. In the case of imipramine (Tofranil), the first of the tricyclic antidepressants, investigators were actually searching for effective antip-

---

Table 32–6
Compatible Liquid Vehicles for the Common Neuroleptic Agents and Lithium Citrate

C = Generally compatible together

X = Incompatible: DO NOT MIX

Blank = No information available—choose "C" liquid to dilute

Oral Liquid Neuroleptics	Water	Saline	Milk	Coffee	Tea	Apple juice or cider	Apricot	Cranberry	Grape juice or drink	Grapefruit	Lemonade, reconst. frozen	Orange juice	Pineapple	Prune	Tang	Tomato	V-8	Cola (Coke, Pepsi, etc.)	Mellow-Yellow	Orange	7-Up, Sprite	Soups, Pudding	Chlorpromazine	Haloperidol	Lithium citrate	Thioridazine	Trifluoperazine
Chlorpromazine (generics, Thorazine)	C		C	C*	C*			X		C		C			X	X	C		C		C	C	C		X		
Fluphenazine (Prolixin)	C	C	C	X	X	X	C			C		C	C	C				C	C	X			C	C			
Haloperidol (Haldol)	C	X		X	X	C						C						C			C				X		
Lithium citrate (generic)	C	C	C	C	C	C	C	C	C	C	C	C	C	C	C	C	C	C	C	C	C	C	C	X	X	X	X
Loxapine (Loxitane)										C		C			C			C							C		
Mesoridazine (Serentil)								C	C	C		C															
Perphenazine (Trilafon)	C	C	C	X	X	X	C			C		C	C	C				C	C	X			C	C			
Thioridazine 30 mg/mL (Mellaril)	X		X	X	X	X	X	C	X	C	C	C†	X	X				X	X	X	C		C		X		
Thioridazine 100 mg/mL (Mellaril)	X		X	X	X		C	X	C‡	C	C**							X	X	X	C		C		X		
Thiothixene (Navane)	C		C			X	C	C		C		C	C	C				C	C	X							
Trifluoperazine (generic, Stelazine)	C		C	C						C		C	C	C				C	C	C	C	C	C		X		

* Data differs with brand—avoid if using generics.
† incompatible with orange "drink."
‡ Canned only, not frozen concentrate.
**Canned OJ only.

Source: From "Oral Liquid Neuroleptics" by Lisa E. Kerr as appeared in the Journal of Psychosocial Nursing and Mental Health Services, *March, 1986.*

Box 32–1
MEDICATION TEACHING PLAN: NEUROLEPTICS

Brand Name: _____

Generic Name: _____

Administration: Your medication is taken by mouth or by injection.

Purpose: Your medication provides relief from your symptoms so you are able to participate in activities, use therapy more effectively, and take better care of yourself.

Target Symptoms: Your medication will decrease some symptoms you are having, such as: _____

_____

Report any sore throat, fever, increased fatigue, vomiting, diarrhea, skin rash, or unusual body movements to your nurse and doctor. If you are pregnant, or think you may be pregnant, discuss this with your doctor. Sudden stoppage of your medication may result in a return of symptoms or other side-effects. Discuss any decision about stopping medications with your doctor.

Other special instructions (if any): _____

_____

_____

_____

The material, on both sides of this form, has been presented to me and discussed with me by: _____

Client's Signature _____ Date _____

Air, Food, Fluid

Dry mouth	Rinse mouth with water. Brush teeth more frequently. Chew sugarless candy/gum. Apply Chapstick to your lips and nostrils.
Nasal stuffiness	Avoid use of over-the-counter nasal sprays/drops.
Weight gain	Eat less sugar, starch, and fats. Increase protein intake. Exercise daily. Follow a diet prescribed by your doctor.

Elimination

Difficulty urinating	Drink 6–8 glasses of fluid each day. Notify your nurse and doctor. Do relaxation exercises to promote urination. Apply warm water to genital area. Take warm shower. Listen to running water.
Constipation	Drink 6–8 glasses of fluid each day.

Eat green vegetables and bran each day.
Exercise daily.
Eat prunes or raisins.
Take laxative medication only with your doctor's advice.
Notify your nurse and doctor.

Personal Hygiene and Body Temperature

Decrease of normal bacteria in mouth may result in infection	Avoid foods high in sugar. Observe your tongue for signs of thick white coating. Increase mouth care including brushing tongue and gargling with mouthwash.
Increased sensitivity to the heat and decreased sweating	Shower in lukewarm water. Avoid exertion in hot weather. Dress appropriately for environmental conditions. Take own oral temperature. Avoid temperature extremes such as hot tubs.
Greater chance of a bad sunburn	Use sunscreen and Chapstick when out in the sun.

continued

Box 32–1 (continued)

Personal Hygiene and Body Temperature

	Wear clothes that protect skin, including a hat.
	Wear sunglasses.
Vaginal dryness	Use lubricant such as K-Y jelly.
Menstrual period may stop	Notify your nurse and doctor. Continue to use birth control.
General changes in interest in sex	Notify your nurse and doctor.
Decreased moisture around eyes	Use extra caution if you wear contact lenses to avoid eye irritation.

Rest/Activity

Dizziness	Lie down and rest.
	Get up slowly from lying position; dangle legs over edge of bed.
	Have nurse check blood pressure.
Drowsiness	Drive your car or other vehicles with extra care.
	Avoid alcoholic beverages or street drugs.
	Plan for extra rest time.
	Avoid other medications unless approved by your doctor.

Muscle tightness/ cramping in arms, legs, neck, or face	Notify your nurse and doctor. Take medications for side-effects.
Compulsion to keep moving and inability to sit down; restlessness	Notify your nurse and doctor. Take medication for side-effects.
Blurred vision	Use a magnifying glass for reading.
Eye pain in sunlight	Wear sunglasses out of doors.

Solitude/Socialization

Understanding of illness and medications	Talk with your nurse and doctor to identify symptoms that are part of your illness or side-effects from your medication.
Decreased interest in surroundings and usual activities	Discuss this feeling with your nurse and doctor.

Source: Adapted from Langley Porter Psychiatric Institute Hospital and Clinics, 1984. University of California, San Francisco.

sychotics similar to chlorpromazine. Iproniazid, a monoamine oxidase inhibitor (MAOI), was discovered when tuberculous clients became less depressed when regularly treated with a similar drug, isoniazid. The antidepressants have shed considerable light on the biochemical mechanisms of the brain in both normal and abnormal emotional expression.

The initial distinction to be understood in the psychopharmacology of depression is between true antidepressants and stimulants or euphoriants. The tricyclic antidepressants (TCA) and the MAOI are not stimulants and will not induce euphoria in normal persons but, in a single dose, have a sedative effect. Amphetamines and methylphenidate (Ritalin), on the other hand, are stimulants but not antidepressants in the pharmacologic sense. They can induce an increased sense of well-being in certain individuals, but they do nothing to combat depression on a lasting basis.

MAOI are considered the "first generation" of antidepressant medications; that is, they were among the first medications identified as effective in the treatment of depression. Since these drugs appeared on the psychopharmacologic treatment horizon, yet another generation of antidepressant medications has become available (see Table 32–7). While one of these drugs, nonifensine, is no longer available in the United States (due to documented, serious side-effects), another, buproprion (Wellbutrin) has just been released. Buproprion is a nonsedating drug (Massachusetts General Hospital 1985a). It also has few anticholinergic side-effects and essentially no important cardiovascular effects and has not so far seemed to cause postural hypotension. While this drug has not yet had the "test of time," it seems likely to be helpful for clients who are unable to tolerate other antidepressant medications.

Alprazolam, a benzodiazepine, has recently been found to be helpful in alleviating nonendogenous or unipolar

Table 32–7 Antidepressant "Generations"	
First Generation	**Second Generation**
Imipramine (Tofranil)	Maprotiline (Ludiomil)
Amitriptyline (Elavil)	Amoxapine (Asendin)
Desipramine (Norpramin)	Trazadone (Desyrel)
Nortriptyline (Aventyl)	Buproprion (Wellbutrin)
Protriptyline (Vivactil)	Nonifensine* (Merital)

Nonifensine, while still available in Europe and Canada, was completely recalled in the United States by the Food and Drug Administration. The reasons cited for the recall involved the reporting of untoward side-effects related to the use of Nonifensine.

depression in clients who also experience anxiety, agitation, or insomnia. With recommended dosages up to 4 mg a day to achieve antidepressant effects, Anath (1983) recommends further research before accepting this medication as a drug of choice for treating depression.

Nursing Responsibilities When Clients Receive Uncommon Drug Combinations

In the early 1980s, physicians began to prescribe combinations of antidepressants for clients who had received no relief of depressive symptoms with a single antidepressant medication. Unfortunately, some clients still did not respond, and these treatment-resistant clients received either TCA/MAOI combinations, antidepressant and stimulants, or combinations of all three classes of drugs, with predominant improvement (Massachusetts General Hospital 1985b). However, some clients experienced elevated blood pressure, while others experienced orthostatic hypotension. While no clients in this group experienced a hypertensive crisis, the possibility existed. Other clinically significant side-effects included dizziness, nausea, impaired memory, insomnia, confusion, and hypomania. As drug combinations and innovative psychobiologic therapies become more commonplace in the practice of psychiatry, psychiatric nurses are going to need to be more observant for idiosyncratic responses among clients. Planning and implementing care for this specialized subpopulation of clients is likely to be challenging, and nurses need to be aware of the underlying psychobiology to be aware of potential drug-related behaviors among clients on multiple drug regimens.

Clinical Considerations in Use

The most important clinical consideration in the use of medications to treat depression is that antidepressant drugs are not effective in all cases of depressed mood. Evidence from research and clinical practice indicates that only a portion of depressive disorders respond to this class of drugs.

For example, TCA, MAOI, and amphetamines are generally contraindicated in depression resulting from what commonly has been referred to as grief reaction or pathologic grief. Other types of depression, described in the DSM-IIIR, may be more amenable to psychopharmacologic intervention. Thus, accurate diagnosis is necessary to ensure maximum effectiveness. Persons for whom antidepressants are indicated usually suffer from characteristic symptoms: a severely depressed mood, loss of interests, inability to respond to normally pleasurable events or situations, a depression that is worst in the morning and lessens slightly as the day goes by, early morning awakening (and inability to fall asleep again), marked psychomotor retardation or agitation, significant anorexia and weight loss, and excessive or inappropriate guilt. DSM-IIIR calls this melancholia. In fact, the symptoms of melancholia are the features that most reliably predict response to drug therapy. A significant, and commonly overlooked, clinical consideration is that antidepressants have a delayed reaction onset. A client will not show lessening of depressed mood until a week to ten days after the institution of an adequate dose of tricyclics, for example.

Tricyclics

By far the most important and most commonly used class of antidepressant drugs is the tricyclics. These compounds are close in chemical structure to the phenothiazines and have many similar side-effects, but they have profoundly different effects on mood, behavior, and cognition. Tricyclic antidepressants are not antipsychotic agents when given to schizophrenic persons and may in fact aggravate a disintegrative pattern or precipitate overt symptoms in a client with latent disintegrative behavior. Imipramine (Tofranil) and amitriptyline (Elavil) are the two prime representatives of tricyclic antidepressants. Desipramine (Norpramin, Pertofrane), nortriptyline (Aventyl), and protriptyline (Vivactil) are compounds prepared in simpler forms (similar to the conversions made in normal metabolism) that are reported to reduce the incidence of side-effects.

Dosage

What constitutes an adequate dose of tricyclics is a matter of debate, but most clinicians agree that the bulk of responsive clients with a major depression need doses of 150 to 250 mg per day. Some may respond to as little as 75 mg and some require 400 mg, but these are exceptional doses.

A client is ordinarily started on 25 mg of a tricyclic three times a day for two days, and the dosage is increased by 25 to 50 percent every other day, until 200 or 250 mg is reached or intolerable side-effects are encountered.

Common clinical practice is to use imipramine in the presence of motor retardation and amitriptyline with agitated clients because it has a more sedative effect. Once the client's dosage is established, it can be converted to a single bedtime dose. This practice frequently precludes the need for insomnia medication. The onset of action takes seven to ten days. Although full improvement may take as long as four weeks, a gradual lessening of the symptoms will become apparent in those who are going to respond.

After remission of the symptoms, clients who are put on a reduced maintenance dose (perhaps 50 percent of the acute dosage) show less likelihood of relapse. Therefore most clients are continued on treatment for six months to one year following a major depressive episode. Clients who have had repeated episodes may require longer drug maintenance or should be considered for lithium carbonate treatment because of its prophylactic effects on recurrent major depression and the depressive episodes of bipolar disorder.

Most depressive clients who do not respond to tricyclic antidepressants suffer from a form of illness that is not of the melancholic type. These may include so-called neurotic or characterologic depressions, termed *dysthymic disorder* in DSM-IIIR. Other clients do not reach or maintain effective blood levels of the drugs even when given adequate daily doses because of idiosyncrasies in their metabolic processes. However, tricyclic blood levels can be measured and doses increased until an effective blood level is obtained.

Side-Effects

Many of the common side-effects of the tricyclic drugs are autonomic due to the anticholinergic characteristics of the medications. These side-effects include dry mouth, blurred vision, constipation, palpitations, and urinary retention. Clients with glaucoma must be treated with caution. Some allergic skin reactions have been observed. Tricyclics also cause changes in the normal electrical conduction of the heart, which is particularly significant in treating persons with a history of cardiovascular disease, especially heart block. Sudden death has occurred during tricyclic treatment. Clients with known heart disease and most elderly clients require electrocardiograms before, and periodically during, the course of tricyclic therapy. Several other central nervous system effects may occur, including tremor, twitching, paresthesias, ataxia, and convulsions. Table 32–8 presents the common side-effects of antidepressant medications, along with suggested nursing interventions.

Overdose Effects

One aspect of tricyclic treatment that deserves attention is the consequences of an overdose. Significant overdoses may cause delirium; hyperthermia; convulsions; and even coma, shock, and respiratory failure. A lethal dose of an antidepressant such as amitriptyline is estimated at between ten and thirty times the usual daily therapeutic dose. Drug intake deserves close attention, since many of the clients treated with these drugs are severely suicidal. Serious overdosage is a medical emergency and may require heroic resuscitative measures. When the nurse reports delirium and peripheral autonomic symptoms of anticholinergic poisoning due to mild overdose, the psychiatrist can intervene with intravenous or intramuscular physostigmine (0.2 or 0.4 mg), an anticholinesterase that will reverse the delirium and other symptoms at least transiently.

Client Teaching

Refer to Box 32–2 for a teaching plan that outlines the main side-effects of tricyclic antidepressants and self-care measures to counteract side-effects experienced by the client.

Monoamine Oxidase Inhibitors

Clients who do not respond to tricyclic antidepressants may respond to the other major class, MAOI. These drugs generally are not as effective as tricyclics and are somewhat slower to act, sometimes requiring a month of treatment before improvement shows. Iproniazid (Marsilid) is considered the most effective, with phenelzine (Nardil) and tranylcypromine (Parnate) slightly behind. What complicates the decision to use MAOI is that they are associated with several very severe side-effects. Hepatic necrosis, commonly fatal, and hypertensive crisis leading to intracranial bleeding are among the most threatening. The latter reaction, heralded by severe headache, stiff neck, nausea, vomiting, and sharply increased blood pressure, follows the ingestion of foods that contain the amino acid tyramine and of sympathomimetic medications.

Client Teaching

The MAOI antidepressants require an especially strong, concerted teaching effort from nurses. These medications have many drawbacks that directly affect nursing intervention. For example, clients on MAOI antidepressants *must* avoid foods that contain even moderate amounts of tyramine; failure to do so results in hypertensive crisis. Refer to Box 32–3 for a complete listing of the low-tyramine diet and a teaching plan for the client receiving MAOI antidepressants.

The principles guiding the use of MAOI and TCA medications are as follows:

- Drug treatment does not preclude psychotherapy, electroconvulsive therapy, or behavioral treatments if they are also indicated.

- Tricyclic treatment should be given first unless there are contraindications, clinical indications for MAOI,

Table 32–8
Some Common Side-Effects of Antidepressant Medications

Side-Effect	Intervention	Side-Effect	Intervention
Anticholinergic		**Psychiatric**	
Dry mouth	Encourage frequent sips of water. Suggest lemon juice and glycerine mouth swabs, dietetic or nonsucrose sour ball candies, or a commercial oral lubricant.	Anxiety, restlessness, irritability	Advise physician, as dose may need to be decreased or increased or time of administration changed; medication may need to be changed to one that produces more sedation, such as amitriptyline; sedatives and/or antipsychotics may be required.
Constipation	Encourage intake of bran, fresh fruits and vegetables, and prunes. Maintain adequate fluid intake. Suggest stool softeners or laxatives. Withhold medication and advise physician, as urecholine may be needed to prevent paralytic ileus when constipation is severe.	Hypomania	Withhold medication and inform physician, as antidepressant may be unmasking a bipolar disorder.
Urinary retention and delayed micturition	Monitor intake and output. Check for abdominal distention. Withhold medication and advise physician if client unable to void; catheterization and/or urecholine may be required.	Mental confusion, psychotic behavior	Discontinue drug; administer physostigimine (antidote for severe anticholinergic side effects).
		Neurologic	
Blurred vision	Assure client this is temporary. Suggest eye consult if this persists beyond medication adjustment (about 3 weeks).	Drowsiness	Advise client initially not to operate hazardous machinery. Administer medication at bedtime. If persistent, advise physician, as medication may need to be changed to a less sedative antidepressant.
Diaphoresis	Encourage adequate fluid intake (preferably noncaloric) to replace lost fluid. Observe for symptoms of electrolyte imbalance.	Lowering of seizure threshold	Observe seizure precautions during initial treatment. Advise physician if seizure occurs, as adjustment of anticonvulsant in clients with seizure disorders and/or discontinuation of antidepressant may be warranted.
Atropine psychosis	Withhold medication and advise physician, as medication must be discontinued.	Fine tremor and/or ataxia	If severe, stop medication and advise physician, as change in dose or medication may be needed.
Cardiovascular		**Endocrinologic/ Metabolic**	
Tachycardia	Monitor pulse for rate and arrhythmias. Withhold medication and notify physician if resting pulse rate is faster than 120.	Decreased or increased libido	Assure client that this is usually transitory. If persistent or interfering with compliance, advise physician, as change in medication and/or dose may be indicated.
Orthostatic hypotension	Record blood pressure with client sitting and standing; withhold medication and notify physician if systolic blood pressure drops more than 20 to 30 mm.	Ejaculatory and erection disturbances	Advise physician if this interferes with compliance, as medication or dose may need changing.
Arrhythmias and T-wave abnormalities	Monitor pulse for irregularities. Provide for routine electrocardiogram (ECG) and serial ECGs if client has history of conduction defects.	Weight gain	Monitor weight. Counsel client to eat nutritionally balanced adequate diet.

Source: Adapted from "Antidepressant Drug Therapy," by M. D. DeGennaro et al., copyright © 1981, American Journal of Nursing Company. Reproduced, with permission, from American Journal of Nursing, Vol. 81, No. 7 (July 1981), pp. 1306–1307.

Box 32–2

MEDICATION TEACHING PLAN: TRICYCLIC ANTIDEPRESSANTS

Brand Name: _____

Generic Name: _____

Administration: Your medication is taken by mouth.

Purpose: Your medication provides relief from your symptoms so you are able to participate in activities, use therapy more effectively, and take better care of yourself. Initially you may experience some sedation. The antidepressant effects occur in about 7–28 days.

Target Symptoms: Your medication will decrease some symptoms you are having, such as: _____

_____

Report any sore throat, fever, increased fatigue, vomiting, diarrhea, skin rash, or unusual body movements to your nurse and doctor. If you are pregnant, or think you may be pregnant, discuss this with your doctor. Sudden stoppage of your medication may result in a return of symptoms or other side-effects. Discuss any decision about stopping medications with your doctor.

Other special instructions (if any): _____

_____

_____

_____

_____

The material, on both sides of this form, has been presented to me and discussed with me by: _____

Client's Signature _____ Date _____

Air, Food, Fluid

Dry mouth	Rinse mouth with water. Brush teeth more frequently. Chew sugarless candy/gum. Apply Chapstick to your lips and nostrils.
Nausea, vomiting, poor appetite	Eat crackers, toast, drink tea. Drink protein supplement to maintain weight.
Weight gain	Eat less sugar, starch, and fats. Increase protein intake. Exercise daily. Follow a diet prescribed by your doctor.

Elimination

Difficulty urinating	Drink 6–8 glasses of fluid each day. Notify your nurse and doctor. Do relaxation exercises to promote urination. Apply warm water to genital area. Take warm shower. Listen to running water.

Constipation	Drink 6–8 glasses of fluid each day. Eat green vegetables and bran each day. Exercise daily. Eat prunes or raisins. Take laxative medication only with your doctor's advice. Notify your nurse and doctor.

Personal Hygiene and Body Temperature

Decrease of normal bacteria in mouth may result in infection	Avoid foods high in sugar. Observe your tongue for signs of thick white coating. Increase mouth care including brushing tongue and gargling with mouthwash.
Increased sensitivity to the heat and decreased sweating	Shower in lukewarm water. Avoid exertion in hot weather. Dress appropriately for environmental conditions. Take own oral temperature.

continued

Box 32–2 (continued)

Personal Hygiene and Body Temperature

	Avoid temperature extremes such as hot tubs.
Greater chance of a bad sunburn	Use sunscreen and Chapstick when out in the sun. Wear clothes that protect skin, including a hat. Wear sunglasses.
Vaginal dryness	Use lubricant such as K-Y jelly.
Menstrual period may stop	Notify your nurse and doctor. Continue to use birth control.
General changes in interest in sex	Notify your nurse and doctor.
Decreased moisture around eyes	Use extra caution if you wear contact lenses to avoid eye irritation.

Rest/Activity

Dizziness	Lie down and rest. Get up slowly from lying position; dangle legs over edge of bed. Have nurse check blood pressure.
Drowsiness	Drive your car or other vehicles with extra care. Avoid alcoholic beverages or street drugs.

	Plan for extra rest time. Avoid other medications unless approved by your doctor.
Muscle tightness/ cramping in arms, legs, neck, or face	Notify your nurse and doctor. Take medications for side-effects.
Compulsion to keep moving and inability to sit down; restlessness	Notify your nurse and doctor. Take medication for side-effects.
Blurred vision	Use a magnifying glass for reading.
Eye pain in sunlight	Wear sunglasses out of doors.

Solitude/Socialization

Understanding of illness and medications	Talk with your nurse and doctor to identify symptoms that are part of your illness or side-effects from your medication.
Decreased interest in surroundings and usual activities	Discuss this feeling with your nurse and doctor.

Source: Adapted from Langley Porter Psychiatric Institute Hospital and Clinics, 1984. University of California, San Francisco.

or a past history of unresponsiveness to tricyclic antidepressants.

- The usual therapeutic range is 150 to 300 mg per day. Dosage may vary and may be limited by significant side-effects.

- A response is seen two or three weeks after the therapeutic dose is reached.

- Clients with recurrent major depressive episodes with melancholia may require long-term maintenance treatment, although doses are usually lower than those needed in acute episodes.

Nursing Considerations with "Second Generation" Antidepressants

The second generation antidepressants were the result of a scientific search for drugs with fewer toxic side-effects and greater biologic predictability in the treatment of depression (Coccaro and Siever 1985). They are believed to be more neurotransmitter specific and better able to treat conditions related to dopamine, serotonin, or nonadrenergic dysfunctions. The following medications on p. 872 exemplify the new drug classifications.

Box 32–3
MEDICATION TEACHING PLAN: MAO INHIBITORS

Brand Name: _____

Generic Name: _____

Administration: Your medication is taken by mouth.

Purpose: Your medication provides relief from your symptoms so you are able to participate in activities, use therapy more effectively, and take better care of yourself. It may take several days to a few weeks for you to feel less anxious, more optimistic, and more in control.

Target Symptoms: Your medication will decrease some symptoms you are having, such as: _____
_____

Report the following symptoms to your doctor: rapid heart beat, frequent headaches, yellowing of eyes or skin, severe increases or decreases in blood pressure. If you are pregnant or think you may become pregnant, report this to your doctor.

In general, tell any doctor who is prescribing medication for you that you are taking this medication and check over-the-counter medications with your therapist. If a severe, sudden, or unusual headache develops, it may be a symptom of a rise in blood pressure. Notify your doctor immediately.

Other special instructions (if any): _____
_____

The material, on both sides of this form, has been presented to me and discussed with me by: _____

Client's Signature _____ Date _____

Air, Food, Fluid

Dry mouth	Rinse mouth with water. Brush teeth more frequently. Chew sugarless candy/gum. Apply Chapstick to your lips and nostrils.	Limitations on certain foods	Discuss diet limitations with nurse or doctor. Refer to the low-tyramine diet for foods to avoid. Determine substitute food choices. Continue food and drug limits for 10 days after stopping the medication.
Nausea, vomiting, poor appetite	Eat crackers, toast, drink tea. Drink protein supplement to maintain weight.		
Weight gain	Eat less sugar, starch, and fats. Increase protein intake. Exercise daily. Avoid over-the-counter reducing pills. Follow a diet prescribed by your doctor.	**Elimination**	
		Constipation	Drink 6–8 glasses fluid each day. Eat green leafy vegetables and bran every day. Exercise every day. Take laxative medications only with your doctor's advice. Notify your nurse and doctor.
Limitations on over-the-counter drug use	Avoid cold/hay fever medications. Avoid weight-reducing medications.		
Severe, sudden, or unusual headache due to increased blood pressure	Follow attached diet to prevent problem. Report headache to your doctor immediately.	**Personal Hygiene and Body Temperature**	
		Flushing/sweating	Take lukewarm showers.

continued

Box 32-3 (continued)

Rest/Activity

Dizziness	Lie down and rest. Get up slowly from lying position; dangle legs over edge of bed. Have nurse check blood pressure.
Drowsiness	Drive your car or other vehicles with extra care. Avoid alcoholic beverages or street drugs. Plan for extra rest time. Take medication at bedtime.

Swelling in legs or feet	Eat less salt, salty foods. Sit with feet raised. Practice careful skin care.

Solitude/Socialization

Confusion/poor memory	Discuss this with your doctor or nurse.
Understanding of your illness and medication	Talk with your nurse and doctor to identify symptoms that are part of your illness or side-effects from your medication.

Low-Tyramine Diet

The MAO inhibitors combine with certain foods and medications to produce a significant increase in your blood pressure, which can be a health problem. In general, foods that can cause this reaction are ones that have been pickled, fermented, smoked, or aged. The list below includes the main foods and medications to avoid while you are taking this medication and for two weeks after discontinuing this medication.

Food and beverages to avoid completely:

Meats and fish:
  Pickled herring
  Dried fish
  Unrefrigerated fermented fish
  Liver
  Caviar
  Fermented sausages (bologna, salami, pepperoni, summer sausage)
  Hoisin (fermented oyster sauce used in Oriental dishes)
Vegetables:
  English broad beans
  Chinese pea pods
  Fava beans
Dairy products:
  Most cheeses (exceptions listed below)
  Yogurt
Beverages:
  Chianti, aged red wines
  Imported, aged beers
Combination foods:
  Pizza
  Lasagna
  Souffles
  Macaroni and cheese
  Quiche
  Pate (liver)
  Caesar salad
  Eggplant parmesan

Also:
  All yeast extracts (e.g., Marmite) and all yeast preparations (e.g., brewers' yeast)

Food and beverages to avoid taking in large amounts:

Dairy products:
  Processed American cheese
Fruits:
  Raisins
  Prunes
  Bananas
  Avocados
  Plums
  Canned figs
Caffeine sources:
  Coffee
  Chocolate
  Colas
Beverages:
  Domestic jug red wines
  Domestic beers, ales, and stouts
  Sherry

Food and beverages that may be taken without problems:

Dairy products:
  Cottage cheese
  Cream cheese
  Milk, cream, and ice cream

continued

Box 32–3 (continued)

Food and beverages that may be taken without problems:	Medications to avoid:

Beverages:
    White wines
Also:
    Any baked goods raised with yeast
	Cold medications
	Nasal decongestants (tablets, drops, or sprays)
	Hay fever medications
	Weight-reducing preparations, "pep pills"
	Antiappetite medications
	Asthma inhalants

Source: Adapted from Langley Porter Psychiatric Institute Hospital and Clinics, 1984. University of California, San Francisco.

- Trazadone (Desyrel)—triazolopyridine derivative
- Maprotiline (Ludiomil)—tetracyclic
- Amoxapine (Asendin)—tricyclic dibenzoxazepine

Coccaro and Siever (1985) point out that the second generation antidepressants are as efficient in decreasing depressive symptoms as imipramine or amitriptyline. The side-effects of these medications are generally less than those of the first generation antidepressants. However, nurses need to continue assessing signs of anticholinergic activity, cardiovascular effects, and effects on a given individual to perform psychomotor tasks.

Other Drugs

Stimulants, such as amphetamines and methylphenidate (Ritalin), and the phenothiazines are less commonly used antidepressants. Stimulants are not a proven treatment. Phenothiazines may be particularly useful in the presence of agitation. Some clinicians and researchers believe that major depressive episodes with psychotic features (delusional depressions) respond better to a combination of an antidepressant and an antipsychotic agent or to electroconvulsive therapy (ECT) than to antidepressants alone. Others simply recommend higher-than-usual doses of antidepressants.

Psychobiology of Depression

Chapter 9 gives an overview of the current psychobiologic theories of depression. Studying the pharmacology of the antidepressants has led to a theory of the biochemistry of depression. Basically, all the true antidepressants make the neurotransmitter substances norepinephrine (NE) and serotonin (5-HT) more available to the synaptic receptors in the central nervous system. Tricyclics block the reuptake of these substances into the neuron after their release, thereby postponing their degradation. The MAOI interfere with the enzymes responsible for the actual breakdown of the neurotransmitters. Since both are antidepressants, these observations have led to the theory that NE and 5-HT shortages in the brain cause depression, at least the type of depression that responds to drug therapy. Refer to Chapter 9 for a more detailed discussion of this topic. Box 32–4 details a teaching plan to be used with clients undergoing the dexamethasone suppression test, an examination of psychoendocrine function in light of depressive behavior.

The Antimania Drug (Lithium)

Background

The psychopharmacologic treatment of conditions labeled mania has become virtually synonymous with lithium carbonate therapy in the United States in the past ten years. Many well-controlled clinical studies indicate unequivocally that lithium is the most effective agent for treating the vast majority of acute manic and hypomanic episodes. In addition, due to the absence of sedative side-effects, the client feels much more related to the environment and able to function normally while under the influence of lithium.

In the last few years, several additional drugs have been added to the list of pharmacologic treatments for bipolar disorder. Of special current interest is the use of carbamazepine (Tegretol) as a treatment to control bipolar symptoms in people who either *cannot* take lithium or do not respond therapeutically to lithium. Approximately 30 percent of clients with bipolar disorders do not respond to

---

Box 32–4
DEXAMETHASONE SUPPRESSION TEST INFORMATION

For: _____ Date: _____

Therapists often order a test called the *Dexamethasone Suppression Test* (DST). The results of this test are useful to staff in making decisions about medications to control depressive symptoms. Some forms of depression are associated with a hormonal imbalance in the body that may respond favorably to certain antidepressant medications. Your therapist has ordered the DST for you. This sheet tells you what you can expect during the two-day period required to complete the test.

On the first day of the test, a technician will draw a small amount of your blood at 4:00 PM. The purpose of this test is to measure a hormone in your blood known as *cortisol*. On the evening of the first day at 11:30 PM, you will receive a very small dose (1 mg) of *dexamethasone*. The 1 mg of dexamethasone should not cause any side-effects, but may cause a *decrease* in your blood level of *cortisol*. On the day after you receive the dexamethasone, your blood level of cortisol will be measured two separate times—once at 4:00 PM and again at 11:00 PM. The results of this test will be used, along with other information about you, by your therapist and the treatment team to plan your treatment with you.

If you have further questions about the DST or depression, ask your primary care nurse or primary therapist. Your primary therapist will let you know the results of your test.

1. *Cortisol test:* Blood drawn at 4:00 PM on (date) _____

2. *Dexamethasone:* 1 mg at 11:30 PM on (date) _____

3. *Cortisol test:* Blood drawn at 4:00 PM on (date) _____

4. *Cortisol test:* Blood drawn at 11:00 PM on (date) _____

This was explained to me by _____

Source: Adapted from Langley Porter Psychiatric Institute and Clinics, 1985. University of California, San Francisco.

---

blocks the return of select neurotransmitters (norepinephrine). Such action may be the psychobiologic reason that carbamazepine has the potential effect on behaviors of the bipolar spectrum. Derogatis (1986) also points out that carbamazepine is used in the treatment of such conditions as alcohol withdrawal syndrome, explosive personality, and impulse disorders and in pain management and seizure control. One can only speculate on the underlying psychobiology of these disorders, and wonder if the etiologies are similar and possibly involve a phenomenon such as limbic kindling.

Recognizing the potential effectiveness of carbamazepine in select mood disorders, Puzynski and Klosiewicz (1984) used another seizure medication, valproic acid amide, to treat clients who carried diagnoses of bipolar affective disorder or schizoaffective disorder. The authors observed a 45.6 percent decrease in overt depressed or manic episodes among the clients treated with valproic acid amide. Valproic acid and verapamil, both calcium channel blockers, currently are in use in similar fashions to control affective symptoms. Possibly such innovative uses of various medications will yield valuable information concerning the underlying psychobiology of behavioral disturbances, especially affectively related conditions.

Despite these advances, lithium continues to be the first line pharmacologic intervention for the treatment of bipolar affective disorder and, more recently, cyclic unipolar depressions or "rapid cycling," a condition in which bipolar cycles occur at unusually brief intervals.

Dosage

The management of an acute manic episode involves rapid initiation of lithium, increased to substantial doses during the first week of treatment. Usually between 1500 and 2100 mg per day are needed by the average-size client in an acute period. Lithium is available only in oral form in 250, 300, and 450 mg capsules and time-released tablets or as a liquid known as lithium citrate. Since lithium is an ion, its concentration can be measured in the blood. In the acute phase the blood level usually must attain a concentration of 1.0 to 1.5 mEq/L. After a week to ten days, as the bipolar symptoms subside, the dose can be decreased to 900 to 1200 mg per day, with the blood level maintained in the range of 1.0 to 1.2 mEq/L for continuing control.

The basic principles for antimania drug therapy are as follows:

- Lithium is indicated and effective in the treatment of acute manic episodes and in the prevention of recur-

lithium and up to 50 percent of responders may experience bipolar symptom relapses while taking maintenance doses of lithium (Massachusetts General Hospital 1985b).

Post et al. (1982) discuss a psychobiologic phenomenon known as kindling, and relate this process to aberrant activity in the limbic system, which is often called the emotional brain. Some psychobiologists believe that the characteristic behaviors of bipolar disorder are reflective of underlying limbic system dysfunction. Carbamazepine is chemically similar to the tricyclic imipramine, and it rent manic or depressive episodes, cyclic unipolar depression, or "rapid cycling."

- Lithium is usually given in divided doses with increases in daily dose until the blood level reaches 1.0–1.5 mEq/L in acute stages of the disorder. Blood levels must be monitored after each increase.

- Antipsychotic medications may be necessary early in the course of treatment for behavior control.

- Blood levels are checked every two to three months or when there is a behaviorally indicative reason to suspect a change.

The following clinical example demonstrates the appropriate use of lithium in the case of a client suffering from bipolar disorder.

Walt, a 23-year-old musician, came for treatment after losing his job in a Broadway show. His producer had fired him because he was irritable and argumentative and seemed to refuse to concentrate on his pieces during rehearsals, instead roaming around the stage giving unsolicited advice to others. His wife had called the mental health center in desperation, claiming that Walt was pacing the apartment talking out of his head and that he seemed totally unconcerned about losing his job. The previous day he had been admitted and discharged against medical advice from a local hospital, where he had received chlorpromazine.

On observation, Walt exhibited pressured speech with grandiose ideas, an irritable mood, and inability to sit in the chair in the interviewing room. His family history revealed that his father had lost many jobs and had been taking lithium for the past five years. It was explained to the client that he had bipolar disorder with a genetic basis, and he was started on lithium carbonate 300 mg BID. This was raised by 300 mg every third day, with a blood level sample drawn and tested after each increase, until Walt was on 1500 mg per day and showed a level of 1.3 mEq/L. The client was asymptomatic one week later, without hospitalization, and returned to work.

Side-Effects

Lithium has a significant number of side-effects that can be troublesome and, in some cases, quite dangerous. Significant side-effects are usually correlated with blood levels of lithium above 1.5 mEq/L. Common side-effects include tremor, nausea, thirst, and polyuria. Thyroid goiter has also been seen as a side-effect. Severe lithium poisoning presents a potential medical emergency. Early signs include vomiting and diarrhea, lethargy, and muscle twitching. These may progress to ataxia and slurred speech. The client may become semiconscious or comatose; seizures may occur; and electrolyte imbalances may lead to cardiac arrest. This syndrome of severe toxicity ordinarily occurs only when the client has a lithium level of 2 or 3 mEq/L. The client may have overdosed or severely restricted food or salt intake (or taken diuretics) to induce this state.

Occasionally very violent, agitated, or paranoid individuals with mania will require phenothiazines or phenothiazine/benzodiazepine combinations at the beginning of their treatment. These can be started simultaneously with the lithium, raised to whatever level is required to control the disintegrative behavior, then gradually reduced, and eliminated after therapeutic lithium levels have been effective for approximately one week.

Client Teaching and Nursing Considerations

Refer to Box 32–5 for a teaching plan for the client receiving lithium therapy. Box 32–6 offers an additional medication teaching plan for the client who is undergoing a trial of carbamazepine to control affective symptoms. The nursing care plan on p. 880 offers guidelines for the care of clients receiving lithium therapy.

In a review article on the uses of lithium in clients without major affective illness, Van der Kolk (1986) points out the effective treatment of the following disorders with lithium:

- Impulsive aggressive disorder
- Post-traumatic stress disorder
- Cyclothymia
- Alcoholism
- Bulimia
- Premenstrual tension
- Obsessive-compulsive disorder
- Borderline personality disorder
- Schizoaffective disorder

Perhaps the extensive list of uses for lithium is destined to increase as more is known about the psychobiologic effects of this drug, as well as the underlying biologic substrates for behavior.

Psychobiology of Lithium

While the specifics of bipolar disorder are difficult to delineate, much can be said about the psychobiology of lithium. Lickey and Gordon (1983) point out that lithium, not unlike the antidepressants, affects neurotransmitters, especially

Box 32–5
MEDICATION TEACHING PLAN: LITHIUM CARBONATE

Brand Name: _____

Generic Name: _____

Administration: This medication is taken by mouth.

Purpose: This medication should provide relief from symptoms so that you are able to participate in activities, use therapy more effectively, take better care of yourself and work more productively. It may take 1–3 weeks before improvement is felt.

Target Symptoms: This medication should decrease some symptoms you have, such as: _____

_____

Report the following symptoms to your physician or nurse: diarrhea, vomiting, chills, fever, infection, dizziness, slurred speech, weak muscles, unsteadiness when walking, twitching muscles, sleepiness and/or blurred vision. If you are pregnant, or think you may be, report this to your physician. Follow up with appointments for blood tests to check lithium levels. Do not discontinue taking this medication without the assistance and advice of your physician.

Other special instructions: _____

_____

_____

The material on both sides of this form has been presented to me and discussed with me by: _____

Client's Signature _____ **Date** _____

Air, Food, Fluid

Initial symptoms of nausea	Take lithium with meals or with food in the stomach
	Drink tea or broth and eat soda crackers
Worsening of symptoms of nausea or vomiting	Notify nurse and physician
	Do not take your next dose of lithium until you speak with your nurse and physician
Dry mouth	Rinse mouth with water.
	Brush teeth more frequently.
	Chew sugarless candy/gum.
	Apply Chapstick to lips and nostrils.
Maintain food/fluid intake	Drink 6–8 glasses fluid each day
	Eat usual foods including foods containing salt (ie., ham, pickles, tomato juice)
	Do not diet unless specifically prescribed by your physician

Elimination

Increased urination	Drink 6–8 glasses of fluid each day.

	Notify nurse and/or physician
Diarrhea	Maintain fluid intake
	Notify nurse and/or physician

Personal Hygiene and Body Temperature

Skin breakdown due to swelling	Elevate legs when swelling is present
	Maintain good personal hygiene
Sweating may affect the lithium level	Avoid exposure to changes in temperature
	Wear clothes appropriate to the temperature
	Maintain fluid and salt intake

Rest/Activity

Increased sweating due to exercise	Wear clothes appropriate to the temperature
	Maintain fluid and salt intake
	Do not change exercise habits without discussion with nurse and physician
Muscle weakness	Operate your car and other vehicles with care
	Plan for extra rest time
	Do not use alcoholic beverages or street drugs

continued

Box 32–5 (continued)

Rest/Activity

Tremor/shakiness	Notify nurse and/or physician Lie down and rest Get up slowly from lying position and dangle legs over edge of bed

Solitude/Socialization

Understanding your illness and medication	Talk with nurse and physician to separate symptoms that are part of your

illness from side effects of medication
Learn the material presented in this Teaching Plan
Take medication correctly/as prescribed
Report response to medication accurately and promptly.

Source: Adapted from Langley Porter Psychiatric Institute Hospital and Clinics, 1984. University of California, San Francisco.

Box 32–6
MEDICATION TEACHING PLAN: CARBAMAZEPINE

Brand Name: _____

Generic Name: _____

Administration: Your medication is taken by mouth.

Purpose: Your medication provides relief from symptoms so that you are able to participate in activities, use therapy more effectively, and take better care of yourself.

Target Symptoms: Your medication should decrease some symptoms you are having, such as: _____

_____

Other special instructions: The following drugs may cause increases or decreases in your blood level of carbamazepine: Troleandomycin (Tao), warfarin (Coumadin), erythromycin (Robimycin), phenytoin (Dilantin), isoniazid (INH), propoxyphene (Darvon, Wygesic, Unigesic), and nicotinic acid (Nicobid, Nicolar). Before taking any of these medications, be sure that the prescribing physician is aware that you are taking carbamazepine!

Do *NOT* stop taking this drug without the assistance or advice of your doctor. Carbamazepine is a medicine that must be slowly withdrawn.

If any of the following symptoms occur, report them immediately to your nurse or physician: fever, sore throat, mouth ulcers, easy bruising.

The material on both sides of this form has been presented to me and discussed with me by: _____

Client's Signature _____ Date _____

Air, Food, Fluid

Dry mouth	Rinse mouth with water. Brush teeth more frequently. Chew sugarless candy/gum. Apply Vaseline or Chapstick to your lips and nostrils.
Nausea/vomiting, poor appetite	Eat soda crackers, toast; drink tea. Notify your nurse or physician.

Elimination

Difficulty urinating or increase in frequency of urination	Notify your nurse or doctor. Drink 6–8 glasses of fluid each day. If you are having difficulty urinating, try the following: Apply warm water to genital area.

continued

Box 32–6 (continued)

<table>
<tr><td>Diarrhea</td><td>Take a warm shower.
Listen to running water.
Maintain fluid intake.
Notify your physician and
nurse.</td><td>Drowsiness</td><td>position; dangle legs over
edge of bed for 5 minutes
before standing up.
Have nurse check your blood
pressure.
Drive car or other vehicles with
extra care.
Avoid alcoholic beverages or
street drugs.
Plan for extra rest time.</td></tr>
</table>

Personal Hygiene and Body Temperature

Possible inflammation of the tongue and lining of the mouth	Notify your physician or nurse immediately. Use a soft bristle toothbrush. Rinse mouth frequently. Avoid foods that contain spices such as pepper, nutmeg, or vinegar.
Possible rash/itching skin	Notify your nurse or doctor. Apply lotions to skin. Do not use soaps that dry the skin.

Blurred vision	Notify your nurse or physician. Use a magnifying glass for reading.

Solitude/Socialization

Understanding your illness and medication	Talk with your nurse or physician to identify symptoms that are part of your illness or side-effects of your medication.

Rest/Activity

Dizziness	Lie down and rest. Get up slowly from a lying

Source: Adapted from Langley Porter Psychiatric Institute Hospital and Clinics, 1984. University of California, San Francisco.

norepinephrine and serotonin. In short, lithium aids in the reduction of neurotransmitter release into the synapse and enhances its return, yielding a lower overall amount of the neurotransmitter in the synapse. Behaviorally, these biologic changes can be observed as an absence of mania or depression. What is unclear at this time is why lithium takes up to a few weeks to be fully effective, when the drug's effects can be observed on synaptic activity almost immediately. Or why do some people with bipolar disorder *not* respond at all to lithium therapy? Lickey and Gordon (1983) believe that lithium's effects are likely to be based on neurocellular changes that occur over weeks or months after a client begins lithium therapy. A similar explanation may hold true for the effectiveness of carbamazepine.

Anxiolytic Drugs

Effects

The antianxiety agents—sedatives and hypnotics—have very similar pharmacologic attributes. All can be used in small or modest doses to relieve anxiety and in larger doses to induce sleep. Although they share the major clinical effect of tranquilization or **disinhibition** of fear-induced behavior, their side-effects, including their addictive potentials and overdose sequelae, make certain representations of this class more suitable for routine use and others better to reserve for limited, special circumstances.

The antianxiety agents are sometimes called "minor tranquilizers," but this is a misleading term, since their effects on anxiety are qualitatively, not quantitatively, different from those of the "major tranquilizers" or antipsychotic agents.

Drug Classification

Meprobamate

Meprobamate (Miltown, Equanil) was the first antianxiety agent to gain popularity in the early 1960s. The result of controlled studies of the effects of meprobamate compared to placebos are generally favorable but not overwhelmingly convincing. This, and the addictive and fatal overdose potentials of the drug, prompted investigators to develop more effective and safer medications that have all but made meprobamate obsolete.

Benzodiazepines

The major class of drugs today in the management of anxiety is the benzodiazepines. This group, represented by chlordiazepoxide (Librium) and diazepam (Valium), accounts for a very high percentage of all the psychoactive medications prescribed in the United States by psychiatrists and medical practitioners alike. This fact usually evokes a mixed response in professional circles. The easy distribution of drugs for such a ubiquitous human phenomenon as anxiety fosters the development of a pill-oriented and pill-dependent society, say critics. Sympathizers focus on the proved effectiveness of the drugs, which help people achieve higher levels of functioning, more pleasurable experiences, and even more productive psychotherapies in some instances.

New Drugs

In the last few years, the arena of anxiety-related research has expanded tremendously, and several new anxiolytic drugs have been introduced. Lorazepam (Ativan), alprazolam (Xanax), and clonazepam (Clonopin) are the newest introductions to the benzodiazepine family, but prozepam (Vestran) is a relatively new drug as well. The newer benzodiazepines give prescribers a wider range of therapies to target the often idiosyncratic manifestations of anxiety manifested by clients. Some of the new drugs have more rapid onsets and shorter half-lives (lorazepam, alprazolam), while others have a usual benzodiazepine onset time and an extended half-life (clonazepam).

With the psychobiologic knowledge explosion, a great variety of drugs has been used in the treatment of anxiety disorders. According to Derogatis (1986), the psychopharmacologic treatments of anxiety-related conditions include:

- Benzodiazepines (the Valium family)
- Antidepressants (especially for panic disorders)
- Beta blockers (e.g., propranolol)
- Antihistamine sedatives (e.g., hydroxyzine)
- Major tranquilizers (e.g., neuroleptics)
- Sedatives with hypnotic effects (e.g., barbiturates)
- Propanediols (e.g., meprobamate)
- New drugs (e.g., investigational compounds)

Researchers are asking questions about the psychobiologic connections between conditions such as phobias and anxiety. For example, social phobia is not a well-studied behavioral complex, but its manifestations usually include fearfulness and anxiety. In a recent study, atenolol, a beta-adrenergic blocking agent was given to a group of clients with a diagnosis of social phobia (Gorman et al 1985). The majority of clients in the study improved. This finding indicates autonomic nervous system innervation in social phobia, since atenolol affects that part of the central nervous system.

New drugs and new uses for existing drugs are accompanied by new side-effects and the need for new teaching plans developed by nurses for use in client education. In a recent article, three case reports demonstrated acute paroxysmal excitement (disinhibition) in conjunction with alprazolam treatment (Strahan et al. 1985). Across the United States, hundreds of thousands of doses of alprazolam are probably being administered on a routine basis to anxious clients. The assessment skills of nurses must be finely tuned to detect unusual behaviors in relation to benzodiazepine therapy. The following symptoms are characteristic behaviors of paroxysmal excitement (disinhibition) associated with alprazolam treatment (Strahan et al. 1985):

- Insomnia
- Racing thoughts/persistent thoughts
- Increased energy
- Irritability/hostility
- Impulsiveness
- A feeling similar to that of amphetamines
- Acute onset

Use in Reducing Anxiety

There is no question that the benzodiazepine family offers a rapid, effective, and safe treatment for the emotional state commonly known as anxiety. In contrast to all other sedatives with proved effectiveness, the benzodiazepines have a low physiologic addiction potential and do not interfere with or accelerate the metabolism of medications taken concurrently. Caffeine, however, interferes with the effectiveness of these drugs.

The effects are evident within the first days of treatment. These medications are absorbed much more rapidly and completely from the gastrointestinal tract than from intramuscular injection and are almost always administered orally. An exception is the use of intravenous diazepam to induce sleep before anesthesia or to manage status epilepticus. Peak levels of chlordiazepoxide are reached in the bloodstream two to four hours after oral ingestion and peak levels of diazepam are reached in one to two hours.

The major side-effects of the benzodiazepines are related to their sedative qualities. Clients may complain of excessive drowsiness and must be cautioned against driving a car or operating other machinery in this state.

Other drugs used to treat anxiety but generally less effective include the antihistamines diphenhydramine

(Benadryl) and hydroxyzine (Vistaril, Atarax), the beta blocker propranolol (Inderal), and methaqualone (Quāālude), a synthetic nonbarbiturate sedative. Methaqualone has been a leading drug of abuse, probably due to the intense feeling associated with peak blood levels.

Another common use of benzodiazepines, especially librium, is in the detoxification of individuals addicted to

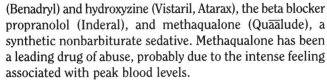

alcohol. Given adequate doses of benzodiazepines to induce sedation (usually starting at 150 to 350 mg per day of

---

RESEARCH NOTE

Citation

Garvey MJ, Tollefson GD: Prevalence of misuse of prescribed benzodiazepines in patients with primary anxiety disorder or major depression. Am J Psychiatry 1986; 143(12):1601–1603.

Study Problem/Purpose

Misuse and abuse of benzodiazepines by psychiatric clients has been consistently documented in the professional literature and in clinical work. The authors of this study attempted to determine the prevalence of benzodiazepine misuse or abuse in specific psychiatric diagnostic groups. In addition to the above stated purpose, the investigators examined potential predictors of benzodiazepine misuse and abuse among study participants.

Methods

Participants in the study were seen in a psychiatric outpatient clinic over the course of 18 months. Any clinic client who received benzodiazepines was given a structured psychiatric interview that explored symptoms, course of illness, history of alcohol use, demographic characteristics, and family history of psychiatric illness. Clients were studied prospectively at one- and four-week intervals.

Three groups of clients who met DSM-III criteria for major depression received benzodiazepines: (1) those who switched to alprazolam (Xanax) after one or more failed trial(s) on tricyclic antidepressants; (2) those who received benzodiazepines (in addition to tricyclic antidepressants) to control symptoms of residual anxiety; and (3) those who received a benzodiazepine hypnotic for severe insomnia. Clients with drug or alcohol abuse or dependence were excluded from the study. Abuse was defined according to DSM-III definition. Benzodiazepine misuse occurred if: (1) the benzodiazepine was used in therapeutically inappropriate ways, e.g., taking more than the prescribed dose; (2) the client reported the medications as lost or stolen; (3) the client's pharmacist reported client requests for additional benzodiazepines; (4) other prescribers reported the client seeking benzodiazepines from them; (5) a client's significant other reported benzodiazepine misuse; (6) a client self-reported misuse; and (7) evidence existed of benzodiazepine intoxication. Clients identified as misusers or abusers were compared to nonmisusers on twenty predetermined variables gathered from the index interview.

Findings

Seventy-one clients received benzodiazepines during the 18-month study period. Diagnostic categories of study participants were as follows: major depression (75%); primary anxiety disorder (24%); and one patient received benzodiazepines for primary insomnia with no associated psychiatric disorder. The mean ± SD dose in diazepam (Valium) equivalents was 24 ± 8 mg/day. The mean follow-up duration was approximately eight months, with mean duration of benzodiazepine use for the entire sample being about five months. Upon termination of the study, thirty-nine of the seventy-one participants were still using some form of benzodiazepine. No benzodiazepine abuse was detected in any subject, but 7 percent of the study group misused benzodiazepines.

Implications

The investigators of this study point out that, *with proper precautions,* benzodiazepines can be used for clients with primary anxiety disorder or major depressive disorder. It is essential to bear in mind that these study participants had no previous history of drug or alcohol abuse or dependence outside a major affective episode.

The implications for nursing from a study such as this one are significant. For example, nurses working with clients on an in-patient unit cannot only observe for the signs of potential benzodiazepine misuse/abuse, but must also use knowledge of those signs within the context of client teaching. When family or significant others are available, discussion of benzodiazepine misuse or abuse will alert family or significant others to *early* signs of difficulty, allowing for early intervention.

The data from this study also has direct implications for nurses who administer p.r.n. dosages of benzodiazepines to clients. It is essential that close and thorough assessment be completed before administering p.r.n. dosages. Such assessment is likely to include severity and quality of presenting symptoms, precipitating factors, and effectiveness of alternative means of symptoms abatement. If alternative methods fail to reduce the severity of the symptom, the p.r.n. dosage may be a reasonable intervention. Once the medication is given, effectiveness in symptom relief needs to be assessed and documented as does any emergent pattern of drug-seeking behavior. Such data are likely to provide nurses with valuable information for the interdisciplinary team, as well as for the teaching efforts of nursing staff.

Nursing Care Plan: Clients on Lithium

Nursing Diagnosis (PND-I/NANDA)	Client Care Goals	Intervention	Evaluation
07.06.02.02 Altered systemic process:* less than body requirements /Nutrition altered: less than body requirements	1. To maintain balanced food and fluid intake	1. Obtain diet history to determine usual intake. 2. Monitor intake of foods containing sodium. 3. Teach clients to avoid fluctuations of sodium intake. 4. Monitor fluid intake. 5. Encourage at least 6–8 glasses fluid per day.	Primary care nurse to evaluate effectiveness of this plan each week by monitoring client's report of side-effects, and their effect on the client's weight and nutritional status.
	2. To support clients when they experience unavoidable side-effects	1. Administer lithium spaced through the day (TID or QID). 2. Give with meals or with food in the stomach. 3. Give tea and crackers for nausea. 4. Teach clients to rinse mouth frequently and practice oral hygiene when they experience dryness of the mouth. 5. Observe for persistence and exacerbations of GI side-effects.	
07.02.02 Altered urinary elimination* /Urinary elimination, altered patterns	1. To maintain balanced intake and output 2. To support clients when they experience unavoidable side-effects	1. Monitor bowel and bladder output. 2. Observe for persistence and exacerbations of GI side-effects. 3. Assess for signs of diabetes insipidus.	Document in progress notes any evidence of urinary elimination difficulties, on a daily basis.
07.08.02 Altered tissue integrity /Skin integrity, impaired, potential	1. To promote and maintain physical hygiene and skin integrity	1. Assess skin condition and hygiene needs. 2. Monitor symptoms of edema through measuring extremities with a tape measure. 3. Teach clients to elevate legs when edema is present. 4. Teach and assist clients to perform routine personal hygiene. 5. Monitor skin condition and observe for signs of dehydration, pruritus, or hypothyroidism.	Primary care nurse will evaluate for signs of altered tissue integrity on a daily basis.

*PND-I diagnosis also in NANDA list.

continued

Nursing Care Plan: Clients on Lithium

Nursing Diagnosis (PND-I/NANDA)	Client Care Goals	Intervention	Evaluation
01.04 Altered sleep/arousal patterns	1. To promote a balance of rest and activity 2. To support the client when he or she experiences unavoidable side-effects	1. Assess rest/activity pattern. 2. Identify activity that may result in excessive perspiration. 3. Protect clients from exhaustion due to overactivity by providing a quiet room and limited stimulation. 4. Promote safety through teaching clients to avoid operating an automobile or smoking alone if they experience lethargy. 5. Assist clients to plan schedule for rest and activity.	Document effectiveness of plan each day, including an evaluation of the client's tolerance for activity and quality/quantity of sleep.
05.02.02.05 Unpredictable behaviors /Social interaction, impaired	1. To develop a balance of solitude/socialization patterns and skills	1. Assist clients to learn the effects and side-effects of lithium carbonate. 2. Assist clients to learn difference between effects, side-effects, and symptoms of their illness.	Document course of assessment/intervention/ evaluation in progress notes.

Source: Adapted from "Nursing Care of Patients on Lithium," by Susan Hunn, Cecile Miranda, Vivian Molyneaux, and Catherine Warshaw, *Perspectives in Psychiatric Care* Vol. 18, No. 5 (Sept.–Oct., 1980), pp. 218–19.

chlordiazepoxide), alcoholic clients can be smoothly withdrawn by stepwise reductions in chlordiazepoxide dose over a one- to two-week period, without encountering alcohol withdrawal delirium or grand mal seizures.

Client Teaching and Nursing Considerations

Client teaching is an especially important element in the care of clients receiving antianxiety agents. As most people know, anxiety is a generally uncomfortable experience. Self-medication often becomes the relief-seeking behavior used by many people who suffer severe anxiety. Such a psycho-pharmacologic approach is *temporarily* helpful in the restoration of a person's capacities and internal comfort. When the client is able and ready to learn, however, other means of anxiety control *must* be taught. Many of the anxiolytic drugs carry a potential for dependence and tolerance (espe-

cially benzodiazepines). Hence, nurses working with anxious clients have a responsibility to assist clients to control anxiety in the most effective and safest way possible. Refer to Box 32–7 for a teaching plan for clients receiving benzodiazepines.

Psychobiology of Anxiolytic Drugs

A common explanation of how antianxiety drugs work rests with synaptic activity involving a neurotransmitter called gamma aminobutyric acid (GABA), a common neurochemical in the brain and spinal cord. Benzodiazepines most likely potentiate GABA, producing muscle relaxation. This mechanism involves a complex process of presynaptic and postsynaptic receptor activity. Recent research has yielded information about the presence of a postsynaptic receptor commonly called the *benzodiazepine receptor*. As the term

Box 32–7

MEDICATION TEACHING PLAN: BENZODIAZEPINES

Brand Name: _____

Generic Name: _____

Administration: Your medication is taken by mouth.

Purpose: Your medication provides relief from your symptoms of anxiety so you are able to participate in activities, use therapy more effectively, and take better care of yourself.

Target Symptoms: Your medication should decrease some symptoms you are having such as: _____

_____

Other special instructions: Do not stop taking this drug without the assistance and advice of your physician. _____ is a medicine that must be slowly withdrawn. Drugs in this category are not intended for long-term use as physical and psychologic dependencies are possible.

Report the following symptoms to your therapist or primary care nurse: marked drowsiness, weakness, staggering gait, tremor, feeling of drunkenness.

The material, on both sides of this form, has been presented to me and discussed with me by: _____

Client's Signature _____ Date _____

Air, Food, Fluid

Food in your stomach will slow the absorption of this medicine.

Do not take medication with meals.
If stomach upset is present, drink tea and broth and take soda crackers.
Notify your nurse or physician if other stomach problems arise.

Effectiveness of this drug is lessened with excessive intake of caffeine or heavy tobacco smoking.

Drink decaffeinated beverages; avoid caffeinated colas, chocolate, or tea.
Keep smoking to a minimum, if possible.

Alcohol increases the sedating effects of this drug.

Alcohol intake is not permitted during your hospitalization on this unit.
Do not use alcohol after discharge, if you continue with this medication.

Personal Hygiene and Body Temperature

Possible rash/itching skin

Notify your nurse or physician.
Apply lotions to skin.
Do not use soap that dries skin.

Rest/Activity

Dizziness

Lie down and rest.
Get up slowly from lying position; dangle legs over edge of bed.
Have your nurse check your blood pressure.
Notify your physician or nurse.

Drowsiness

Drive your car or other vehicles with extra care.
Plan for extra rest time.
Do not take other medications unless approved by your physician.

Blurred vision

Notify your nurse or doctor.
Use a magnifying glass for reading.

Solitude/Socialization

Unusual irritability or nervousness

Notify your physician or nurse.
Ask your nurse for assistance in selecting an appropriate relaxation exercise.

Understanding your illness and medications

Talk with your nurse and physician to identify symptoms that are part of your illness or side-effects from your medication.

Source: Adapted from Langley Porter Psychiatric Institute Hospital and Clinics, 1984. University of California, San Francisco.

implies, benzodiazepines bind perfectly and with great specificity to this membrane, allowing for the sensation of relaxation.

Sedative-Hypnotic Drugs
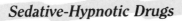

The pharmacologic management of insomnia presents an interesting and challenging clinical problem. Many of the truly hypnotic drugs tend to have undesirable effects, including physiologic addiction, fatal overdose potential, and dangerous interactions with other medications because of liver enzyme induction. The first principle of treatment is to assess whether the insomnia is related to one of the major mental disorders, such as schizophrenia or major depression. If so, the insomnia can and should be treated as part of the larger problem, and sedative antipsychotics or antidepressants may be given at bedtime to accomplish this purpose.

Benzodiazepines

In the management of simple insomnia without an associated major mental disorder, the benzodiazepine compound flurazepam (Dalmane), 15 or 30 mg at bedtime, is the drug of choice. This drug is as free of toxicity as others in its class and therefore is both effective and safe. It is the one sleeping medication that does not seem to interfere with REM (rapid eye movement) sleep and therefore can be used on consecutive nights for approximately a month. Other benzodiazepine compounds that are used for their hypnotic qualities include triazolam (Halcion) and lorazepam (Ativan).

Barbiturates

Barbiturates are less commonly prescribed for their hypnotic effects. Their only advantage over the benzodiazepines is their low cost. Barbiturates, especially the short-acting types, such as secobarbital (Seconal), are powerfully addicting substances. They are frequently used in successful suicide attempts, since overdoses can cause severe central nervous system and respiratory depression. Barbiturates suppress REM sleep, leading to the phenomenon of REM deprivation and REM rebound—that is, after a week or two of treatment, they help create the insomnia they were intended to control. Barbiturates also speed up the metabolism of anticoagulant and other drugs because they induce liver enzyme synthesis. This effect can be fatal. Long-acting barbiturates (phenobarbital) are very useful, however, in the detoxification of barbiturate addicts and the management of epilepsy.

The following groups of hypnotic preparations are commonly prescribed:

- Chloral derivatives (e.g., chloral hydrate)
- Piperidinediones (e.g., Doriden, Noludar)
- Alphatic alcohols (e.g., Placidyl)
- Antihistamines (e.g., Benedryl)

Client Teaching and Nursing Considerations

As with the benzodiazepines, sedative-hypnotic preparations are generally intended for either occasional or short-term use. These medications are appropriate for clients newly admitted to a psychiatric in-patient unit or for clients in out-patient therapy who develop sleep disorders. As other medications start to yield a therapeutic effect (e.g., antidepressants, lithium, neuroleptics), however, the need for sedative-hypnotic medication should almost, if not completely, abate.

Nurses working with clients in the aforementioned situations need to assist these people in the regulation of sleep patterns. Possible ways to help in the reinstitution of regular sleep patterns include:

- Avoidance of caffeine and nicotine
- Exercise several hours before bedtime
- Relaxation techniques, including white noise
- Avoidance of alcoholic beverages before bed
- Warm bath
- Tryptophan-rich foods (see Chapter 9)
- Use of routine hours for retiring and rising
- Avoidance of light during sleep induction

It is essential that the nurse teaching relaxation techniques assess the client's sleep patterns and presleep routines to prescribe the correct technique to meet the client's needs (see Chapter 9). Evaluation of the effectiveness of the relaxation intervention must also be ongoing to allow for a change in approach if necessary.

ELECTROCONVULSIVE THERAPY

The topic of electroconvulsive therapy, more commonly known as ECT, almost always produces some discussion among health care providers. People rarely maintain a neutral stance in relation to ECT; to this day, the subject and procedure remain extremely controversial.

On the side of conservatism, many people refute the benefits of ECT, arguing that there is little scientific basis for the treatment and that producing deliberate seizure activity in the brain could *never* be therapeutic. Such arguments have an element of truth but often fail to consider the many people who have benefited from ECT. The liberal perspective often errs on the side of overenthusiasm for ECT, recommending its application in situations that are basically inappropriate.

A middle road does exist for the application of ECT in psychiatry today. Although it is reserved as a second-line therapy today because of the variety of psychopharmacologic interventions available, it remains a useful and therapeutic biologic alternative. The National Institute of Mental Health (NIMH) and the office of the medical applications of research of the National Institutes of Health (NIH) recently held a conference to explore issues of ECT's uses and to discuss areas of controversy related to ECT. According to a report of the proceedings (Runck 1985), the conference explored the following issues: effectiveness, risks and adverse effects, appropriate uses of ECT, informed consent, proper administration of ECT, and research.

Electroconvulsive therapy was considered effective in the following clinical situations:

- Severe delusional/endogenous depression
- Acute mania
- A subgroup of schizophrenics whose illness is of short duration and who demonstrate concurrent affective symptoms

ECT is unlikely to be effective for the following illnesses:

- Dysthymic disorder
- "Neurotic" depression
- Adjustment disorder with depressed mood
- Chronic schizophrenia

In discussing risks and adverse effects, Runck's report (1985) discussed a death rate of 2.9 deaths per 10,000 clients. Other risks are comparable to the risks of using brief anesthesia with muscle relaxants and the transient application of mechanical respiratory assistance. Possible adverse effects include:

- Transient confusion, memory loss, headache
- Transient hypotension, sinus tachycardia
- Negative perceptions, social stigma of clients receiving ECT

The procedure for the administration of ECT is relatively simple and routine today, but nonetheless requires close assessment and observation of prepared staff. The procedure includes the following steps:

- Give no food/fluid before the treatment.
- Remove dentures, hairpins.
- Encourage the client to void before the procedure.
- Take vital signs.
- Give a methohexital (Brevital) injection to induce anesthesia.
- Give succinylcholine (muscle relaxant).
- Apply electrodes, using electrojelly.
- Give 1 to 130 volts for 0.1 to 0.5 seconds.
- Use mechanical means of respiration during the period following electrical impulse.
- Monitor seizure activity.
- Observe (postprocedure) for signs of respiratory difficulty.
- Reorient the client as she or he becomes alert and able to resume activities.

In the immediate postprocedure period, the client's memory will probably be affected by the procedure; most clients fail to remember the trip into the ECT procedure room. Other nursing concerns involve teaching the client and family or significant others what behavior to expect from the client after the procedure. Nurses may also work with clients, families, and significant others to discuss their concerns and provide accurate information about the procedure while attempting to allay anxiety.

LOOKING FOR BIOLOGIC MARKERS— VISUAL IMAGING TECHNIQUES

Techniques and technology are available today that enable us to visualize the brain and its metabolic activities. The discussion that follows offers a synopsis of these techniques. While all of them are in use, some have more clinical significance than others. In any event, the emergence of new technologies often directly affects nursing actions. If nothing else, nurses have a responsibility to teach clients about the examinations, much as medical-surgical nurses do with clients undergoing fluoroscopy or barium studies, for example.

Computed Tomography (CT Scanning)

Because the mind is not separate from the brain, assessment of behaviors must entail an examination of the biologic substrate for behavior. Weinberger (1984) points out that, more often than not, classic symptoms of neurologic dysfunction (e.g., headache, visual symptoms, seizures) do not yield psychiatric assessment, and until recently, psychiatric symptoms did not routinely receive neurologic assessment. However, mood changes are often the earliest signs of neurologic dysfunction and merit close biologic assessment.

The CT scan is one means of visualizing gross pathology in the brain by taking very fine "photographs" of designated areas of the brain. The capacity of the CT scan is such that it reveals "slices" or "cuts" of the brain, allowing for a very precise and thorough examination of the structures comprising the brain. More specifically, the CT scan examines the densities of given brain structures and compares these findings with those of normal controls.

In 1985 Brown and Kneeland reviewed a variety of studies involving the use of CT scans in psychiatry. They reported biologically observable changes via CT scanning in the following clinical entities:

- *Schizophrenia*—findings included ventricular enlargement, density changes in different parts of the brain, and cortical atrophy.

- *Affective disorders*—findings included ventricular changes and decreased cerebellar mass in some alcoholic bipolar clients.

- *Dementia*—findings demonstrated a lowered brain density.

While these findings are of interest, they remain mainly academic at this time. Enlarged ventricles are not by themselves diagnostic of schizophrenia. However, the CT scan is an important examination in psychiatry because it allows for a clear assessment of the gross anatomy of the brain to determine potential causes for behavioral change.

In preparing clients for the procedure, nurses need to know whether the client's examination is to be done with or without injection of a contrast (dye) material. The contrast injection, used in situations where a more defining and precise scan is desirable, adds the discomfort of an intravenous injection to the procedure.

Facts that the client needs to know concerning the CT scan include:

- The scan lasts approximately 45 minutes.

- During the scan, the client will be lying on a movable stretcher.

- The CT scanner looks something like a huge doughnut, and the client's head is placed in the center or "hole of the doughnut."

- The machine will move to accommodate the electronic requests of the scanner's operator.

- It is essential that the client remain still throughout the procedure; medication sometimes helps the agitated client achieve that end.

- If an injection of contrast is used, the client may expect to feel transient "hot flashes" or experience an unusual taste; other, more severe symptoms may indicate an allergic reaction to the contrast.

- There are no restrictions on food or fluid intake prior to the examination.

Positron Emission Tomography (PET Scanning)

According to Brown and Kneeland (1985), PET scanning is a noninvasive way to measure physiologic and biochemical functions as they occur in live tissue. Scientists can watch brain metabolism through the use of a compound that is inhaled or injected and contains a radioactive "tag." Using a "tagged" glucose compound, for example, one can observe glucose use in the brain. Brown and Kneeland point out that glucose use is directly related to functional activity in regions of the brain. In some of the studies reviewed by the aforementioned authors, PET scans have demonstrated the following:

- Decreased use of glucose in the frontal lobes of unmedicated schizophrenics

- Less use of glucose in the entire left cortex of select schizophrenics

- Less glucose use on the left side of the basal ganglia (see Chapter 9) than on the right

- Diminished glucose uptake in frontal and temporo-parietal cortex (bilateral) in clients with Alzheimer's disease

Currently, PET scanning is reserved for use in research and is not yet available as a clinical diagnostic tool. However, as this technique evolves and becomes more commonplace in the practice of psychiatry, it is likely to assist in significant knowledge gains concerning the psychobiology of mental illness.

Magnetic Resonance Imaging (MRI)

The MRI is a revolutionary technique introduced to clinical work in the recent past. What is new and innovative about this type of imaging is that it does *not* use ionizing radiation but yields pictures of superior quality to those of computed tomography.

According to Brown and Kneeland (1985), the principle is fairly straightforward. Atomic nuclei with an odd number of neutrons or protons act like magnets. Brown and Kneeland describe the process as follows: "MRI images are formed by placing the appropriate part of the client's body within a stationary magnetic field, which causes the nuclei to align in the direction of the field. A radiofrequency pulse . . . is then applied." The result of the radiofrequency pulse is an electric signal that yields an image (see Figure 32–2). The intensity of the image depends on the density of the nuclei being examined; pathologic lesions look different from normal tissue.

In preparing the client for an examination using MRI technology, the nurse may use the following guidelines:

- The MRI equipment is similar in appearance to that of the CT scanner.

- If the client is having MRI imaging of the head, explain that the head will be placed in the magnetic field, while the rest of the client's body remains on a stretcher outside the magnetic field.

- The client must remove all hairpins and jewelry, lest they be drawn into the magnetic field.

- Clients with metallic implants or metallic artificial joints may not be suitable for MRI as the magnetic field is likely to respond to the presence of metal in a way that could be detrimental to the client.

- The examination usually takes about 45 minutes, during which the client must remain still to prevent blurring of the images.

The MRI has great potential for clinical work. Physicians have already been able to apply its refined technology to the presenting psychiatric difficulties of clients, and to translate its results into interventions aimed at relief of incapacity and suffering.

Other visual-imaging techniques continue to evolve, such as *brain electrical activity mapping* (BEAM) and *cerebral bloodflow techniques* (CBF). While BEAM aims to enhance the clinical usefulness of the EEG, CBF explores the relationship between disturbed brain function, cerebral bloodflow, and metabolism of oxygen and glucose in the brain (Brown and Kneeland 1985). Current opinion is that while BEAM may be of use clinically in the near future, the likelihood of the same occurring with CBF is not as probable.

PSYCHOSURGERY

Like electroconvulsive therapy, *psychosurgery* conjures some very strong images in many people's minds. Since the inception of frontal lobotomies for the treatment of schizophrenia starting in 1936, psychosurgery has undergone major changes. Today, frontal lobotomies are mainly a thing of the past and essentially nonexistent in the United States. Modern psychosurgery continues in Western Europe, and consists of stereotaxic operations, performed at various locations in the limbic system (see Figure 32–3).

The desired effect of all psychosurgery is to diminish unpleasant affects. It has little impact on disintegrative

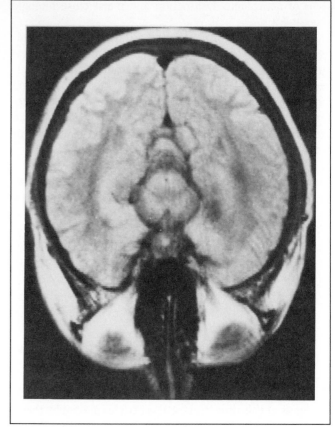

Figure 32–2
Nuclear magnetic resonance scan showing the central portion of the human brain.
Source: Courtesy Alan Jay Cohen, M.D. Clinical Instructor, Department of Psychiatry, University of California at San Francisco/San Francisco General Hospital.

symptoms such as hallucinations or delusions, but the client clearly is no longer threatened, frightened, or distressed by them. Postoperatively clients have little feeling for members of their families, their personal appearance, socially unacceptable behaviors, and their general future. These side-effects are much diminished by the newer stereotaxic methods, however.

In the United States today, psychosurgery has been replaced with other biologic therapies, mainly psychopharmacologic interventions. With the current upsurge in psychobiologic knowledge, the concept of psychosurgery seems outdated, but arguments continue over whether psychosurgery is an appropriate measure for those labeled criminal or sexual psychopaths.

HUMANISTIC INTERACTIONIST IMPLICATIONS

"Humanistic psychiatric nursing practice is enhanced when scientific knowledge is delicately blended with an imagination that is sensitive, aware, and liberally educated" (Wil-

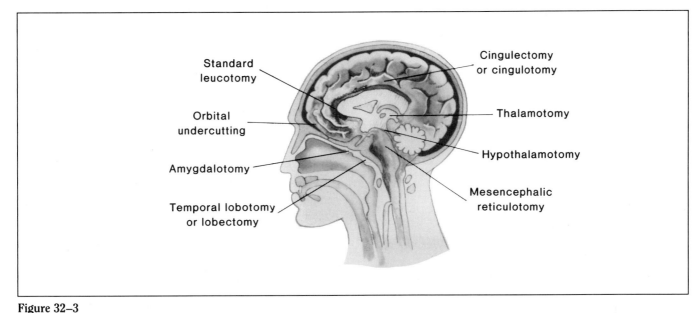

Figure 32–3
Psychosurgery sites
Source: Black P, The rationale for psychosurgery. The Humanist, *July/August 1977, p. 7. Reprinted by permission.*

son and Kneisl 1983). Nothing could be closer to the truth of the nursing profession's relation to the psychobiologic therapies emerging today. Nurses will need to be cautious to maintain the *art* of nursing, as the *science* of nursing's professional work in psychiatry thrusts us onto the threshold of the twenty-first century.

Chapter Highlights

- Biologic therapies have been in existence since ancient times, have taken various forms over the centuries, and are of extreme importance in psychiatric intervention today.

- Through a biologic perspective, any given individual's psychology is the result of neurochemical actions and reactions in the central nervous system.

- Biologic therapies work because of the changes they produce on cells of the central nervous system, permitting the emergence of new behaviors.

- Psychiatric nurses need to understand and remain abreast of current advances in psychobiology.

- *Psychotropic* drugs are drugs that primarily affect the mind by exerting an effect on the cells of the central nervous system.

- In relation to psychotropic medication administration, nurses have responsibilities in the areas of assessment, intervention, and evaluation.

- Medication compliance is a complex phenomenon; nurses have used various teaching strategies in an attempt to improve client compliance.

- The major classes of psychotropic medications include antipsychotics (neuroleptics), antidepressants (TCA, MAOI), anxiolytics (benzodiazepines, etc.), antimania drugs (lithium, carbamazepine, valproic acid), and sedative-hypnotic medications (chloral derivatives, barbiturates, etc.).

- Electroconvulsive therapy is effective for several clinical entities; nursing care is essential for clients receiving this biologic therapy.

- Among the contemporary visual-imaging techniques, the ones that are most clinically useful are computed tomography and nuclear magnetic resonance.

- While psychosurgery is still used in parts of Europe, it is rare in the United States; psychopharmacologic interventions are more commonly used in the United States.

References

Anath J: Choosing the right antidepressant. *Psychiatr J Ottawa* 1983;8(1):20–26.

Appleton WS, Davis JM: *Practical Clinical Psychopharmacology.* MedCom, 1973.

Battle EH, Halliburton A, Wallston KA: Self medication among psychiatric patients and adherence after discharge. *Psychosocial Nurs Men Health Serv* 1982;20(5):21–28.

Brown RP, Kneeland B: Visual imaging in psychiatry. *Hosp Community Psychiatry* 1985;36(5):489–495.

Coccaro EJ, Siever LJ: Second generation antidepressants: A comparative review. *Clinical Pharmacol* 1985;25:241–260.

Derogatis LR: *Clinical Psychopharmacology.* Addison-Wesley, 1986.

Garvey MJ, Tollefson GD: Prevalence of misuse of prescribed benzodiazepines in patients with primary anxiety disorder or major depression. *Am J Psychiatry* 1986; 143(12):1601–1603.

Gorman JM, Liebowitz MR, Fyer AJ, Compeas R, Klein DJ: Treatment of social phobia with atenolol. *J Clin Psychopharmacol* 1985;5(5):298–301.

Hollister L: Antipsychotics and antimanic drugs, in HH Goldman (ed): *Review of General Psychiatry.* Lange Medical Publications, 1984.

Kerr LE: Oral liquid neuroleptics: Administer with care. *Psychosocial Nurs Ment Health Serv* 1986;24(3):33–38.

Kneisl CR: *Wadsworth's Review of Nursing.* Wadsworth, 1985.

Kucera-Bozarth K, Beck NC, Lyss L: Compliance with lithium regimens. *Psychosocial Nurs Ment Health Serv* 1982; 20(7):11–15.

Lickey ME, Gordon B: *Drugs for Mental Illness.* W. H. Freeman, 1983.

Massachusetts General Hospital: Buproprion: The second generation continues. *Biol Ther Psychiatry* 1985a;8(5):17–20.

Massachusetts General Hospital: Treating treatment-resistant depression: Antidepressants and stimulants? *Biol Ther Psychiatry* 1985b;8(6):13–18.

Neizo B, Murphy MK: Medication groups on an acute psychiatric unit. *Perspect Psychiatr Care* 1983;21(2):70–73.

Post RM, Uhde TW, Putman FW, Ballenger JC, Berrettini WH. Kindling and carbamazepine in affective illness. *J Nerv Ment Disorders* 1982;170:717–731.

Puzynski S, Klosiewicz L: Valproic acid amide in the treatment of affective and schizoaffective disorders. *J Affect Disorders* 1984;6:115–121.

Runck B: NIMH report: Concensus panel backs cautious use of ECT for severe disorders. *Hosp Community Psychiatry* 1985;36(9):943–946.

Selander JM, Miller WC: Prolixin group: Can nursing intervention groups lower recidivism rates? *J Psychosocial Nurs Ment Health Services* 1985;23(11):16–20.

Strahan A, Rosenthal J, Kaswan M, Winston A: Three case reports of acute paroxysmal excitement associated with alprazolam treatment. *Am J Psychiatry* 1985;142(7):859–861.

Van der Kolk BA: Psychopharmacology: Uses of lithium in patients without major affective illness. *Hosp Community Psychiatry* 1986;37(7):675.

Van Putten T, May PRA, Marder SR: Response to antipsychotic medication: The doctor's and the consumer's view. *Am J Psychiatry* 1984;141(1):16–19.

Weinberger DR: Brain disease and psychiatric illness: When should a psychiatrist order a CAT scan? *Am J Psychiatry* 1984;141(12):1521–1526.

Wilson HS, Kneisl C: *Psychiatric Nursing,* ed 2. Addison-Wesley, 1983.

PART SIX

Applying the Nursing Process across the Life Span

THIRTY-THREE

Applying the Nursing Process with Families

Carol Ren Kneisl
Marilynn Petit

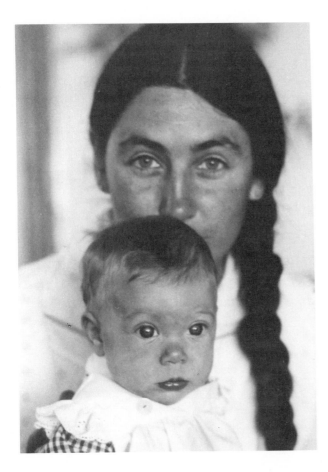

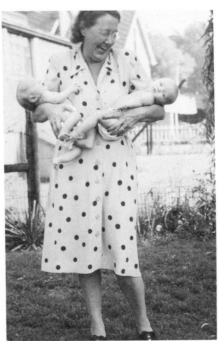

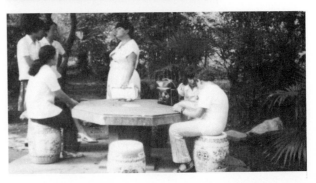

After reading this chapter, students should be able to

- Identify the existing diverse forms of family life
- Identify the developmental tasks that confront couples and families
- Describe the family completely in terms of the relationships, associations, and connections that occur in a dynamic, interacting whole
- Describe the relational and communicational complexities in families as they relate to functional families and families in difficulty
- Relate the major components of family therapy to humanistic psychiatric nursing practice
- Identify primary, secondary, and tertiary prevention approaches that may be used to provide for family mental health
- Describe some of the important factors in the counseling of couples

Cross References

Other topics relevant to this content are: Communication skills, Chapter 11; Developmental stressors in parenting, Chapter 6 (Tables 6–6, 6–7, and 6–9); Family as a social support system, Chapter 8; Family development tasks through the family life cycle, Chapter 6; Intrafamily physical and sexual abuse, Chapter 25, Part II; Negative expressed emotion of families, Chapter 8 (Figure 8–6).

The current proliferation of nuclear arms throughout the world creates the greatest threat to human health in our history.

Key Terms

blended family	feedback
circularity	life script
communal family	nuclear family
couples therapy	paradox
disengagement	pseudohostility
double bind	pseudomutuality
enmeshment	schismatic family
extended family	self-fulfilling prophecy
family life-style	skewed family
family myths	subsystem
family of origin	synergy
family theme	triangulation

The family is the context in which people develop their first relationships with other people. How they view the larger social world outside the family is molded by the events that happen within families and that influence the development of the individual.

Nurses encounter families in many areas of their practice—in the emergency room, the intensive care unit, the school, the cancer hospital, the community health setting, and the mental health setting, among others. Assessment of families in trouble, and intervention on their behalf, must be based on an understanding of how families grow and interact and how family coping patterns develop. This chapter describes those processes and offers strategies for intervention into dysfunctional marital dyads or family systems.

HISTORICAL FOUNDATIONS

Today's family is:

- Mom, dad, and 2.4 kids
- A couple with eight kids—three of hers, three of his, and two of theirs
- A thirty-two-year-old electrical engineer and his three foster children
- A divorced woman and her infant child
- A widowed man, his two children, and his parents
- A grandmother raising her two grandchildren
- Two lesbian mothers and their children
- Two couples sharing an apartment neither could afford alone

- Three gay men who live and work together on a collaboratively owned vegetable farm
- Four couples and their children in a remote commune

Identifying the "real" family has become an issue because of arguments over whether the family is suddenly changing or even dying. Professional meetings have such titles as "The Family—Can It Be Saved?"

Is it true that the family is dying out? Actually, constant transformation or change is the one permanent quality of the family. Many family forms have appeared, disappeared, reappeared, and coexisted within and across cultures. Families have been defined by blood relationships, tribes, households, kinship systems, clans, and language alliances. They have been called *blended, extended, conjugal,* and *communal.* The American family is changing, but not dying: It is simply becoming different.

The Traditional Nuclear Family

The traditional **nuclear family** is a two-parent, time-limited, two-generation family consisting of a married couple and their children by birth or adoption. Despite its name, it is a relatively recent development in human history. It evolved as societies became more urban and industrialized in the move away from agrarianism. It is time-limited because, in most instances, the members of the younger generation begin their own families soon after they are 20 years of age.

Soon after its development, the traditional nuclear family became known as the *isolated nuclear family.* Ties to the **extended family**—all persons related by birth, marriage, or adoption to the nuclear family—were weakened. This diminished the basic support system that formerly surrounded families. The isolated nuclear family had less contact with the adults' **families of origin** (the families from which they came).

The nuclear family is the family structure about which people speak when they are concerned with "strengthening the family." This narrow definition of family, however, does not recognize and consider the wide variety of family constellations that exist in contemporary society.

The Single Parent Family

A *single parent family* is also two-generational and occurs when a lone parent and offspring live together as a nucleus. It is a more common family form than most people believe. The United States Census Bureau reported a 79 percent increase in the number of single parent families between

1970–1980, making the current prevalence one in five (U.S. Census Bureau 1980). It has been estimated that by 1990, fully a third of all children in the United States will see their parents divorce before they reach the age of 18 (Glick 1979). The traditional image of the mother as a woman who stays at home to look after her children will apply to one-quarter of all married mothers (Pitzer 1982). Although it is common knowledge that numerous single parent families exist in the inner-city areas of large, metropolitan centers, their existence in well-to-do suburban communities is acknowledged less often.

After two months of third grade in a large suburban school, 9-year-old Joshua told his father of feeling strange and different because he was from a single parent family. A review of the class list sent home by the teacher surprised both Joshua and his dad. They found that nineteen of the thirty-two children in Joshua's class also lived in single parent homes. The community in which Joshua lived had a 75 percent divorce rate, and most of his classmates in single parent families lived with their mothers.

While most single parent families result from death or divorce, increasing numbers of women are bearing children with the intention of rearing them alone. Single women and men are also adopting children with increasing frequency, something that was not done or even permitted only a few years ago. And more often than ever before, single parent families, like Joshua's, are being headed by men.

Paul Glick, a senior demographer with the U.S. Census Bureau, reports that fully 45 percent of the children born in 1977 will live in single parent families at some time before they reach eighteen years of age (Levine 1978).

The Blended Family

The **blended family**, an increasingly common phenomenon, is one in which one or both marital partners have previously been divorced or widowed, and bring with them their children from a former relationship. Various types of blended families exist. The loosest structure is a weekend blending that occurs when the children from one parent's previous marriage visit that parent's later family for a brief time. In a more permanent blend, the children from a previous marriage live with one parent and a later spouse, forming the new nucleus. A third type of blended family is one in which the children from previous marriages of both spouses are included in the same household. A "mine, yours, and ours" variety also includes children who are the offspring of the new marriage.

Alternative Family Forms

Alternative families consist of persons with or without blood or conjugal (marriage) ties who live and interact together to achieve common goals. Two or more adults, of the same or opposite sexes, and their children, or adults without children, may choose to live together. Unlike the family constellations described earlier, alternative families may be one-generational, consisting of adult members of a single generation.

Communal families, in which many people band together, are found both in sophisticated metropolitan centers and in more remote agricultural areas. The commune is further defined by how members have negotiated the privileges and responsibilities associated with their roles, material possessions, economic concerns, sexual expressions, and parenting activities. The Israeli kibbutzim are among the best known of the communes. Another type of communal arrangement is that of the religious cult.

Households of homosexual (gay) people are another alternative family form. Gay people who live together in the same household are choosing to be open about their life-style. This life-style is not yet recognized as an acceptable alternative by all segments of society, and gays still face restrictions that often prevent them from adopting children or gaining custody of children from their previous heterosexual marriages that ended in divorce.

Even the well-known phrase, "You can choose your friends but you can't choose your relatives," is becoming obsolete according to Lindsey (1982), who has written a book on chosen kin. In her view, two factors in contemporary life are important. The first is economics. Because many singles and the elderly can no longer afford to live alone, there is a trend toward communal, familial living among these groups. The second is geography. Because the average American moves once every three years, an individual who lives in the East may have family on the West Coast. Friends become kin chosen to recreate the extended family. Figure 33–1 illustrates how American family life-styles are changing.

THEORETICAL FOUNDATIONS

Developmental Tasks Confronting Families

Families, like individuals and groups, are confronted with developmental tasks. The family sociologist Evelyn Duvall (1985) lists the following developmental tasks of American families:

- *Physical maintenance*—providing food, shelter, clothing, health care.
- *Resource allocation (both physical and emotional)*— meeting family expenses; apportioning material goods, space, and facilities; and apportioning emotional goods, such as affection, respect, and authority.

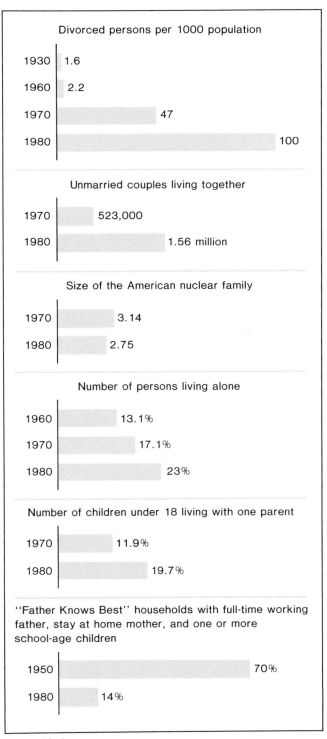

Figure 33–1
Changing family life-styles in America.

- *Division of labor*—deciding who does what in relation to earning money, managing the household, caring for family members, and so on.
- *Socialization of family members*—guiding members

in mature patterns of controlling aggression, elimination, food intake, sexual drives, sleep, etc.

- *Reproduction, recruitment, and release of family members*—giving birth to or adopting children, rearing them for release from the family at maturity, incorporating new members, and establishing policies for including others, such as in-laws, stepparents, and friends.

- *Maintenance of order*—ensuring conformity to family and/or societal norms.

- *Placement of members in the larger society*—interacting with the community, school, church, and economic and political systems to protect family members from undesirable outside influences.

- *Maintenance of motivation and morale*—rewarding members for achievements; developing a life philosophy and sense of family loyalty through rituals and celebrations; satisfying personal needs for acceptance, encouragement, and affection; meeting personal and family crises.

These developmental tasks are a considerable undertaking. It is the families who do not succeed very well at accomplishing them who come to the psychiatric nurse's attention most often.

The Family as a System

In a general systems theory framework, a family can be seen as a system of interrelated parts forming a whole. A family system includes not only the family members but also their relationships, their communication with one another, and their interactions with the environment.

Because a system functions as a whole, its parts are interdependent, and a change or movement in any part of the system affects all other parts. For example, an accomplishment by one member of the family affects all the other members in the family system. Dysfunction in one member also changes the whole system. This concept of *wholeness* is important in understanding families. It means that counseling one family member will change all members in some way.

Another important characteristic of a system is that it strives to maintain a dynamic equilibrium, or balance, among the various forces that operate within and on it. This process is referred to as *homeostasis*. All systems need to balance themselves within a range of functioning in which the work of the system can be accomplished. The mental image of a seesaw may help show what happens in the attempt to

achieve balance. Too much weight on one end will bring it to the ground. It is no longer in balance. However, before that point, balance can be achieved at any of several points, even though the seesaw is not perfectly horizontal. When a family member behaves in a way not prescribed within the family system, other members will react with attempts to minimize the disruption, always trying to maintain a steady state. Don D. Jackson (1957) introduced the concept of *family homeostasis* based on his observations that the families of psychiatric clients often experienced depression or psychophysiologic disorders when the client improved. He postulated that these behaviors of family members and the psychologic disruptions of the client were homeostatic mechanisms that operated to bring the disturbed system back into its delicate balance. When a family has to use most of its energy to maintain balance, little energy is left for the growth of the family or its individual members.

Elements in the system may also be parts of another system. Billy may be simultaneously the oldest child in the family, a catcher for the Little League baseball team, and a member of the debate team. Billy's family is a member of other larger systems as well—the extended family, the city, the nation, etc. The family itself has **subsystems**, such as dyads (Billy and his father), triads (Billy, his brother, and his sister), or other groups of members who are linked together in some special association.

Systems can also be viewed as *open* or *closed,* although these are actually the extremes of a continuum. Some family systems are more open than others, while some are more closed. Openness requires that a system be flexible in adapting to the changes demanded by the environment. Adaptation takes energy to maintain homeostasis in the face of outside information or new input. Families whose systems are more closed tend to shut out or distort information from the environment in order not to upset their balance.

Family systems have *boundaries* as well. Boundaries define who participates in the system. They also tell family members the extent of differentiation permitted (among members and between members and outsiders), the amount or intensity of emotional investment in the system, the amount and kind of experiences available outside the system, and particular ways to evaluate experiences in terms of the family system (Hess and Handel 1967, p 21). Boundaries may be clear, rigid, diffuse, or conflicting. These critical factors in family systems will be referred to throughout this chapter.

Swanson and Hurley (1983) propose a systems model of relationship strains or conflicts (Figure 33–2), which, when applied to clinical work, helps the nurse understand dysfunctional situations in context. This model suggests the systems that can be used to bring about resolution. A strain in "C" between the family and a community reflects the fact that the family's priorities differ from the community's priorities. Intervention needs to take place between these two systems, not in one system alone.

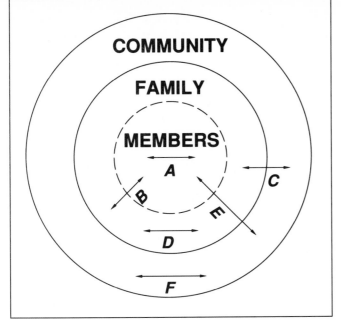

Figure 33–2

A Systems Model of Relationship Strains (Conflicts): A, between individuals in a family; B, between a member of a family and his/her family; C, between a family and community; and other possible lines of strain.

A signifies strain within a family between individual members of a family, as between spouses, where views differ on an issue. If the family as a whole has had a "family solution" to the problem against which one member now "strains," such a strain is represented not by A but by B below.

B signifies strain within a family between one member or a minority of members of a family and the other members. In this strain, the family view on an issue once shared by all members is now opposed by one or more members.

C signifies strain within a community between family and the community at large on one or more issues. The family view differs from the priorities of the community.

D signifies strain within a community between families, or between a family and a community agency. There is no community-wide solution to the problem.

E signifies strain within a community between an individual and the community with which the individual interacts. The individual's view differs from the dominant view of the community.

F signifies strain within society between communities where there exists no shared view of the best solution to the problem.

Source: Swanson A, Hurley P: Family systems: Values and value conflicts. Journal of Psychosocial Nursing and Mental Health Services 1983;21(July):27. Charles B. Slack, Inc.

Family Characteristics and Dynamics

Whether they are functional or dysfunctional, families have certain specific characteristics and dynamics in operation. The functional family is distinguished from the dysfunc-

tional one by the amount and quality of the energy used to maintain the family system.

Roles

Members of a family must determine how to accomplish the family developmental tasks listed earlier in this chapter. They do so by establishing roles, patterns of behavior sanctioned by the culture. Don D. Jackson (1965) believes that families set roles by operating as a rule-governed system—an ordered format designed so that members may be aware of their positions in relation to one another. Although a family system engages in a multitude of behaviors, a relatively small set of rules is sufficient to govern family life. Roles are assigned according to family rules. Families decide which roles will exist within the system, socialize members into the roles, and then expend energy maintaining members within their roles.

When members are unable or unwilling to perform assigned roles, the family experiences stress. For example, the roles of mother and father have long been stereotyped in American society. Mothers were the family nurturers and caretakers, while fathers were the family decision makers and wage earners. These roles are not completely satisfying to all American families, and many women and men have moved to negotiate their roles differently. The trend in society is now toward families with two working parents and families in which fathers share, or assume, the nurturing role. In 1980, dual-earner families accounted for slightly over half of all married couples, and 45 percent of the children under the age of six had working mothers (Hayghe 1982). Even more recently, the Bureau of Labor Statistics reported in 1985 that fully half of the women with children under the age of 2 were in the labor force (*Newsweek* 1985). For the health of the family system, roles often must be negotiated in other than stereotyped ways. When the roles are not negotiated satisfactorily, family disequilibrium results.

Power

Most families have a hierarchical power structure in which the adults wield power, usually in an authoritarian manner. The power structure is often developed in this way because it creates a safe environment in which young children can grow and develop, and because it is easy to operate. However, stress develops when disagreements exist about who holds the power.

Tom, the 17-year-old son in the M family, continually used the family car without permission. Although some serious arguments ensued between Tom and his father, no restrictions were placed on Tom's behavior, and the car keys continued to hang on a key rack in the front hall. Tom's paternal grandfather, who lived with the M family, took Tom's side in his arguments with his father. Grandfather M adopted a fond "boys will be boys" stance. One evening when the family car was in an auto repair shop for some minor work, Tom "borrowed" his grandfather's new car. Tom was involved in a collision about an hour later. Although no one was injured, Grandfather M's car had to be towed away, extensively damaged. Later that night, the adults of the M family managed to come together to agree on a stance that they could mutually support.

Once the adults in the M family were able to openly acknowledge their internal power struggle and come to an agreement on what rules were to be set and by whom, the system was less stressed.

Grandparents residing with a family are not the only causes of disagreements. Disagreements between husband and wife about who holds the power are also common. In some dysfunctional families, there is chronic discord about power.

When children mature and become capable of assuming greater responsibility for their own functioning, power is often diffused among all members of a family system in a more democratic fashion. Certain families do not allow power to be redistributed, however, thus interfering with the individual development of the members who have less power.

Behavior

In the systems view of a family, the family interaction system has four important qualities. The first, *wholeness,* was discussed earlier in this chapter. It refers to the interrelationship of all the elements in the system.

Synergy, the second characteristic, refers to the fact that the whole is greater than the sum of its parts. In other words, combined efforts produce a greater effect than the sum of individual actions. Two young children at play in their mother's cosmetics exemplify the effects of synergy. They encourage one another gleefully and enthusiastically to open and use the various jars, pots, and tubes they have discovered. Before long, the children and the environment have been thoroughly decorated. To their angry mother,

each child blames the other, believing that without the other they would not have been in trouble. The effects of synergy can also be seen in families distinguished by open affection. Open affection stimulates more open affection, which cycles back into the system to stimulate even more of this particular distinguishing characteristic.

Circularity and feedback also characterize family system behavior. Each member engages in behavior that influences the other members. The process has been characterized as an uninterrupted sequence of interchanges (Watzlawick et al. 1967). The usual way people think about relationships does not allow for circularity. In a teenage daughter's view, for example, if her mother would only trust her, they would get along better. The mother's view is that the problem lies with the teen's uncooperativeness. Both mother and daughter are stopping the circular process by seeing one behavior as a cause and the other as an effect. The circular view is that each person's behavior is both cause and effect at the same time. Mother and daughter are caught up in a cycle, as they monitor and influence one another.

FAMILY THERAPY

Nurses in the past have worked with families and family problems in many different settings. Most often nurses encountered family members while in a health teaching role. While caring for the diabetic client, the client who has undergone major surgery, or the client who has had a myocardial infarction, the nurse taught the client's family how to care for that person physically and what life-style changes the illness might impose on the family. The family therapy role, however, is still a relatively new one for nurses.

Family therapy is a different way of viewing problems. In general, family therapists believe that the emotional symptoms or problems of an individual are an expression of emotional symptoms or problems in a family. Therefore, family therapists view the family system as the unit of treatment. Their concerns are basically with the relationships between the family members, not with the intrapsychic functioning of Mom, Dad, Kevin, or Susan.

Various therapeutic strategies have emerged from these shared beliefs. Family therapists do not have as fixed a set of procedures for intervention as psychoanalysts do. However, certain intervention strategies and therapeutic postures seem to flow naturally from the basic beliefs family therapists hold.

Evolution of Family Therapy

Professionals doing psychotherapy were bound by commitment and theoretical orientation to the practice of one-to-one work with clients until the early 1940s. In those early years, Freud's psychoanalytic theory was the dominating force in psychotherapeutic work with clients. The child guidance movement, which began in the 1940s, is credited with including the client's family in the thinking and activities of therapists. However, family thinking at this time was an extension of psychoanalytic theory. Generally, the child was seen by the psychiatrist and the family by the social worker. Child guidance workers saw no reason to work with the child and the parents or other family members together.

The psychoanalytic theory of personality development continued to be tremendously influential in the 1940s. While most theorists and clinicians were aware of the effects of family relationships, they resisted active involvement of the family in treatment. To do so would have been viewed as a violation of the sacred analyst-client relationship.

In the early 1950s, some therapists began to experiment somewhat secretly with family therapy. Many therapists who were seeing families did not talk or write about their work. They had to refrain from alienating the psychiatric establishment, which considered family members irrelevant to the nature and treatment of psychopathology. Because these therapists earned their living in the mental health field, they cautiously avoided incurring the wrath of their professional groups. When persons develop new ideas that threaten the comfortable status quo, it is not uncommon to find that they are shunned by their colleagues.

The family therapy movement gained momentum and began to be acknowledged openly by the mid-1950s. Some theorists and clinicians began to publish their views, experiences, and research and learn of the work of others.

Since that time, the family therapy movement has flourished. There are now several different schools or approaches, each with its own style.

Approaches to Family Therapy

Rather than identify family therapy approaches by the names of the family therapists who developed them, we will briefly discuss the approaches as Jones (1980) suggests. Jones categorizes the research and literature on family therapy into seven major approaches.

1. The integrative approach is represented by the work of Nathan Ackerman (1958). Ackerman emphasized the need to take individual as well as family dynamics into account. Although his approach is the only one that does not rely heavily on systems concepts, it does bridge the gap between the psychoanalytic approach and the "maverick" approaches of those who focus on interpersonal and transactional phenomena.

2. The psychoanalytic approach is based directly on Freudian psychoanalytic theory and conforms to an illness model of family therapy. According to this model,

one or more disturbed marital partners account for the dysfunctions experienced in the family. An emphasis is placed on the reconstruction of the personality of the disturbed mate(s). The names of Boszormenyi-Nagy and Framo (1965) are linked with the psychoanalytic approach.

3. Bowen thought of the family as a system combining both emotional and social relationships. Bowen (1960, 1978) developed his approach into specifics that can be easily taught. Some of his concepts, such as family triangles and multigenerational transmission processes, are discussed later. This approach is an extremely popular one, probably because it is so specific.

4. The structural approach describes the family as an open system governed by rules or boundaries that define who participates with whom, and how (Minuchin 1974). There are two types of dysfunctional patterns—enmeshment and disengagement—both of which are discussed later. The goal of the family therapist in this approach is to transform the family structure in the interest of creating clear boundaries.

5. The interactional approach is called a communicational approach in some of the literature. The unit of analysis for therapy is the behavior and communication among and between family members. These concepts were developed in the 1950s and 1960s through research on the possible relationship between the double-bind concept and schizophrenia and on dysfunctional communication in families (see Jackson 1968a, 1968b, 1957; Bateson et al. 1956; Lidz et al. 1958; Haley 1971, 1976; and Satir 1967, 1972). Many of these concepts are discussed later in this chapter.

6. The social network approach includes the persons—friends, neighbors, relatives, fellow workers—with whom the family in crisis has a social relationship (Speck 1967). Social network therapy is a sort of extended group therapy with the goal of bringing together as many people of a family's social network as possible. It takes place in the home and involves large groups of people (from 40 to 100 is not uncommon). It has been found particularly helpful in crisis and disaster situations and has been compared to the tribal meetings for healing purposes that occur in other cultures (Speck and Attneave 1973).

7. The behavioral approach is based on Skinner's theories of learning. It consists of adapting principles and techniques of behavior modification for use with families. One of the most prominent authors and theorists concerned with the behavioral approach to family therapy is Gerald Patterson (1976).

Qualifications of Family Therapists

Family therapists should be specially educated in the practice of family therapy and strongly committed to a belief in the importance of the family. Increasing numbers of psychiatric nursing clinical specialists are being prepared in graduate programs that provide both theory and supervised clinical practice in this specialized area. While undergraduate nursing programs focus on the importance of relating to families in all settings, they (rightfully) do not prepare nurses as family therapists.

Relational and Communicational Intricacies in Families

People negotiate their views of themselves and others on the basis of their perceptions. Perceptions also influence how people interact with one another on both content and relationship levels. In a family system, each person's behavior is contingent on the behavior of the others. This creates some interesting and complex turns in family relationships.

Functional families allow for individuation and growth-producing experiences. Rigidity within a family system makes it difficult for the family to adapt to change and easier for the family to become dysfunctional. Some of the relational complexities described below exist in all families, but dysfunctional families handle them differently from functional families. Other factors arise only in family systems that are dysfunctional.

Although some of the factors discussed below may be easily categorized as communicational, it is important to recognize their relational aspects. Other communication factors (discounting, disconfirming, disqualifying, symmetry, complementarity, congruity, and incongruity) are discussed in Chapter 11.

The Self-Fulfilling Prophecy and Life Scripts

A self-fulfilling prophecy is an idea or expectation that is acted out, largely unconsciously, thus "proving" itself. In families, self-fulfilling prophecies are often seen in the guise of family life scripts. The Jones family is an example. Believing that "all men are unfaithful," Mrs. Jones isolates and distances herself emotionally from her husband, ultimately encouraging him to fill his need for intimacy outside the marriage and thus fulfilling the prophecy. Claude Steiner (1974, p 51) calls a *script* "the blueprint for a life course." It is a plan decided not by the fates, but by experiences early in life. In Steiner's words (p 54), "Human beings are deeply affected by and submissive to the will of the specific divinities of their household—their parents—whose injunctions they are impotent against as they blindly follow them through life, sometimes to their self-destruction." People with life scripts are following forced, premature, early-childhood decisions. Steiner notes that, although not everyone has a script, script-free living is the exception rather than the rule.

There is an endless variety among life scripts. The Miss America script is decided for the 5-year-old girl whose parents enroll her in the Little Miss New York State (or Kansas or Colorado) competition. There are My Son the Doctor, Delinquent, Alcoholic, and Drug Addict scripts. A person with a script, either "good" or "bad," is terribly disadvantaged in terms of autonomy or life potentials. Unless people recognize what the script is and take steps to change it, they are prevented from living to the fullest human potential.

Family Myths, Life-Styles, and Themes

Family myths, life-styles, and themes help families maintain balance by permitting them to resist change. Family myths are well-integrated beliefs, shared by all family members, about each other and their positions in family life. The beliefs are unchallenged, even though family members may have to resort to distortions to maintain the myth. The family myth is related to the family's inner image—how the family appears to its members. For example, one family myth was that the father had the ability to make wise decisions. Individual members in this family participated to maintain the myth of the father as a Solomon by gearing interactions with him in such a way that he appeared to make high-level family decisions single-handedly.

The concepts of family theme (Hess and Handel 1959) and family life-style (Deutsch 1967) are related in their focus on the family's ways of relating to the outside world. The family theme is the family's perception of its development and history. One family had a theme constructed around second-generation grandparents of Austrian descent, who were able to provide their oldest son with a law school education through their hard work. This family conceived of persons on welfare as "lazy," thus reaffirming its view of the value of working hard and becoming educated. Determining the salient themes in a family's life helps us see how the fates of individual members are shaped by those themes and the pressures with which each person must contend.

The family life-style has to do with the family's biased perception of the outside world and its automated means of coping with this world. Family life-styles are designed to uphold particular images of the family—as the most popular, talented, financially successful, nonconformist, or whatever. The life-style is the front or facade the family strives to present to others.

Coalitions, Dyads, and Triangles

Of all the forms of communicative exchange, dyadic communication is the most common. In fact, a family begins with a dyad, the marital couple. The natural alliance, or coalition, of this dyad presents a united front to the world—to deal with one member, people have to deal with them both. However, if one partner does not actively support the other, severe strain results.

The presence of a third person always has an effect on an existing dyad. When the marital couple gives birth to a child, the relationship becomes triadic. A triad is not a stable social situation, since it actually consists of a dyad plus one. Shifting alliances characterize triads—mother and father may unite to discipline the child, mother and child may unite to argue for a family vacation, or father and child may join forces to go fishing together. The process of forming a triad is called **triangulation**. Triangulation becomes dysfunctional when issues are solved in families by shifting the intimacy among members, rather than by

working the actual issue through. Such coalitions always result in someone feeling "left out." Triangulation is a major concept in the Bowen approach to family therapy.

Coalitions arise basically to affect the distribution of power. By joining forces, two persons can increase their influence over a third. A husband and wife frequently pair up to discipline their child better. However, the child may also attempt to pair up with one parent to avoid discipline. In families with a number of children, typical coalitions involve children closest in age, or children of the same sex.

Pseudomutuality and Pseudohostility

A family in which **pseudomutuality** occurs functions as if it were a close, happy family. According to Lyman Wynne

---

RESEARCH NOTE

Citation

Lund K, Ostwald S: Dual-earner families' stress levels and personal and life-style–related variables. Nurs Res 1985(Nov–Dec);34:357–361.

Study Problem/Purpose

Dual-earner families with young children are a steadily growing population. Yet little is known about the effect of dual-earner life-styles on family stress levels or the health of the family. This study examined the relationship between personal and life-style–related factors and family stress levels in dual-earner families with young children.

Method

The study was a cross-sectional survey conducted in six day-care centers operated by a major day-care provider in a large metropolitan area. Subjects were 200 dual-earner families with children 6 years old or younger. The instrument used in the study was a closed-ended questionnaire with 103 items that measured family stress levels and personal and life-style–related variables. Family stress level was measured by the Family Inventory of Life Events and Changes (FILE). Availability of support systems and planning and organizing of family life were measured by adaptation of items from the Dual-Employed Coping Scales (DECS). The investigators developed additional questions to measure personal and life-style–related variables.

Findings

This study found that the majority of dual-earner families (76 percent) had a moderate level of family stress compared to national stress-level norms calculated for

families in the preschool stage of development. This finding contradicts the commonly held belief that dual-earner families have increased stress due to the mothers' employment outside the home. Thus, the study data indicate that the dual-earner life-style may not, in itself, predispose families to a high level of stress. The authors hypothesized that the advantages that result from a dual-earner life-style may serve to mediate stress and help maintain equilibrium within the family.

Variables that correlated significantly with the family stress score included parental age, age of the children, family income, satisfaction with the income, flexibility in vacation, necessity of separate vacations, and satisfaction with child care. The older the couple and the older the average age of the children, the lower the family stress score. The higher the income and the greater the satisfaction with income, the lower the family stress score. The more flexibility parents had in planning vacation, the lower the family stress score, and the more satisfied the parents were with child care, the lower the family stress score.

Implications

The major changes occurring in family and community life due to dual-earner family life-style demand attention from the health care system. Nurses are in a pivotal position to enhance family coping and reduce stress through education, planning, and providing direct service to support these families. Community health and industrial nurses can advocate to increase flexibility in the workplace, thus further reducing stress on the dual-earner family. Preventive health care for children and their families has always been a focus for nurses and can be expanded to include attention to the need for quality day care.

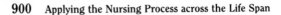

and his associates (1958), who use the interactional approach to family therapy, this pattern of relating has the following characteristics:

- Persistent sameness in the structuring of roles
- Insistence on the desirability and appropriateness of the role structure, despite evidence to the contrary
- Intense concern over deviations from the role structure or emerging autonomy
- Marked absence of spontaneity, enthusiasm, and humor in participating together

In these families, the members do not form intimate bonds with one another as individuals. Instead, an inordinate amount of energy is expended in maintaining ritualized and stereotyped ways of behaving and relating. There is a desperate struggle to maintain harmony. Wynne and associates (1958) give a perfect example in one mother who said: "We are all peaceful. I like peace if I have to kill someone to get it." Such a family requires its members to give up their sense of personal identity.

Pseudohostility exists in families in which there are chronic conflict, alienation, tension, and inappropriate remoteness among the members. As in pseudomutuality, the problems of family life are denied in an attempt to negate the hostility among the members. Family members view their differences as only minor ones. Both pseudomutual and pseudohostile family environments are stifling milieus.

Deviations in the Parental Coalition

In some families, problems develop from the parents' inability to form a satisfying coalition in terms of intimacy and control. Several common deviations are examined in the sections below.

Schism

Theodore Lidz and his associates (1957), who also advocate the interactional approach, have identified two types of families with parental coalition problems. They result from marital schism and marital skew. **Schismatic families** are those in which the children are forced to join one or the other camp of two warring spouses. Lidz et al. (1966) believe that the constant fighting in these families is a defense against intimacy or closeness. In schismatic families, the spouses devalue and undercut one another. This makes it difficult for the children to want to be like either of them. The devaluation thus interferes with the development of a clear sexual identity by the children. Lidz and his associates also believe that marital schism is linked with schizophrenia in female children.

Skew

Skewed families are those in which one spouse is severely dysfunctional. The other spouse, who is usually aware of the dysfunction of the partner, assumes a passive, peacemaking, submissive stance to preserve the marriage. The passive partner is caught between effectively responding to the view of "reality" of the outside world and giving up this view within the home, accepting the dysfunctional mate's view. On the surface, a skewed couple may appear to be complementary. Their relationship is actually lopsided and unsuited to many basic family tasks, however. This pattern has been linked with schizophrenia in male children.

Enmeshment

Other family patterns are enmeshment and disengagement, as described by Salvador Minuchin (1974), who advocates a structural approach to family therapy. **Enmeshed families** are characterized by a fast tempo of interpersonal exchange. Interactions within the family are of high intensity and are directed more toward issues of power than toward issues of affection. In enmeshed families, the mothers are often found to be overcontrolling and become anxious over the possibility of losing control over the children. The mother appears to be trying to prevent herself from becoming helpless. Adult males are often absent in these families, or, if present, are controlled in much the same way the children are.

Disengagement

Disengaged families move to the other extreme from enmeshment—abandonment. Family members seem oblivious to the effects of their actions on one another. They are unresponsive and unconnected to each other. Structure, order, or authority in the family may be weak or nonexistent. Assuming control and guidance increases the mother's anxiety, and she may feel overwhelmed and depressed. In these families, a child often assumes the parental role.

Scapegoating

Scapegoating is a social process that has been written and talked about since the time of the ancient Greeks. A scapegoat is one who is made to bear the blame for others or to suffer in their place. In families, a disturbed member may play the role of family scapegoat, thus acting out the conflicts in the system and stabilizing it. For example, one or both parents may blame the child when things go wrong rather than blame themselves or one another. This enables the parent to declare "our marriage would be fine if it weren't for that kid."

According to Nathan Ackerman (1971) the following constellation of roles occurs:

- The *scapegoat,* or victim, who best symbolizes the conflicts
- The *family persecutor,* who uses a special prejudice as the vehicle of attack
- The *family healer,* who intervenes to neutralize the attack and rescue the victim

Children are not the only persons who are scapegoated. Adults, or whole groups of people, may also be scapegoated.

Paradoxes and Double Binds

A **paradox** is a self-contradictory communication. An example is the paradoxical message that recently appeared on a bumper sticker: "Individualists Unite!" Paradoxes are common in everyday communication. The client who says to the nurse: "Tell me what to do, so I can be independent," creates a paradox for the nurse. The nurse who says: "I think you should find a new job, but it's not my place to say so," creates a paradox for the client.

The **double bind** is a complex series of paradoxes. The example of a double-bind situation classically cited is from Gregory Bateson and his associates (1956, p 259):

A young man who had fairly well recovered from an acute schizophrenic episode was visited in the hospital by his mother. He was glad to see her and impulsively put his arm around her shoulders, whereupon she stiffened. He withdrew his arm and she asked, "Don't you love me anymore?" He then blushed, and she said, "Dear, you must not be so easily embarrassed and afraid of your feelings." The client was able to stay with her only a few minutes more and following her departure he assaulted an aide and was put in the tubs.

The conditions necessary to produce the double bind are present in this example:

- Two persons, one of whom is the victim (the young man)
- A repeated experience, so that the double bind becomes a habitual expectation
- A primary negative injunction, carrying a threat of punishment (mother stiffens)
- A secondary injunction conflicting with the first injunction, but at a more abstract level. Like the primary injunction, the second threatens punishment ("Don't you love me anymore?")

- A tertiary negative injunction prohibiting the victim from escaping from the field ("Dear, you must not be so easily embarrassed and afraid of your feelings.")

It is theorized that repeated exposure to double binds in families produces schizophrenia. The evidence, however, is not totally convincing. While people labeled schizophrenic are victims of double binds, not all victims of double binds are, or become, schizophrenic. Most of the classic and early research on the double bind was carried out by Bateson and his colleagues, now associated in the interactional approach to family therapy.

The Treatment Unit and the Treatment Setting

Most family therapists recommend that all persons in the family constellation participate in the assessment phase of family therapy. Not all agree on what persons comprise the family constellation or the treatment unit. Some include all members of the nuclear family; others include members of the extended family; and still others, large numbers of people in the family's social network. Different coalitions may be seen together at different times to accomplish specific purposes. For example, the mates are often seen together for the first few sessions.

Children four years of age and younger are often omitted from ongoing family therapy sessions. They may misinterpret, or be frightened by, the dialogue. In addition, small children tend to be disruptive. Some therapists, however, make it a point to bring all the children into therapy for at least two sessions to see how the family as a whole operates.

Family therapists often reverse the traditional territorial control of the professional by engaging the family system in therapy in its own milieu—the home. There are several reasons these therapists see families on their own ground:

- The interactions of the family system are more natural in their usual environment.
- Customary roles are more spontaneously played out on home ground.
- Family members reluctant to participate in therapy tend to be less so in the home than in a formal office or mental health agency setting.

While it is common to hold sessions in the home, family therapy may also take place in the professional's office setting.

Family Assessment

Family therapy consists of three major components—assessment, contract or goal negotiation, and intervention. The first phase of a therapeutic process involves the initial assessment of the family. According to Bross (1983), family assessment involves gathering data in the following three areas:

1. Demographic information—data pertaining to gender, age, occupation, religion, ethnicity, and family income
2. Substantive information—data pertaining to past treatment, history, pertinent medical facts, identity of the "identified patient," information regarding sensitive topics or recent events
3. Interactional data—information pertaining to family rules, alignments, coalitions, subsystems (marital, parental, sibling), hierarchy, patterns of behavior, cultural differences

Compton and Galaway (1979, pp 251–252) suggest that a thorough family assessment should consider the following factors:

1. *Family as a social system*
   a. Family as responsive and contributing unit within network of other social units
      (1) Family boundaries—permeability or rigidity
      (2) Nature of input from other social units
      (3) Extent to which family fits into cultural mold and expectations of larger system
      (4) Degree to which family is considered deviant
   b. Roles of family members
      (1) Formal roles and role performance (father, child, etc.)
      (2) Informal roles and role performance (scapegoat, controller, follower, decision maker)
      (3) Degree of family agreement on assignment of roles and their performance
      (4) Interrelationship of various roles—degree of "fit" within total family
   c. Family rules
      (1) Family rules that foster stability and maintenance
      (2) Family rules that foster maladaptation
      (3) Conformity of rules to family's life-style
      (4) How rules are modified; respect for difference

   d. Communication network
      (1) How family communicates and provides information to members
      (2) Channels of communication—who speaks to whom
      (3) Quality of messages—clarity or ambiguity
2. *Developmental stage of family*
   a. Chronologic stage of family
   b. Problems and adaptations of transition
   c. Shifts in role responsibility over time
   d. Ways and means of solving problems at earlier stages
3. *Subsystems operating within family*
   a. Function of family alliances in family stability
   b. Conflict or support of other family subsystems and family as a whole
4. *Physical and emotional needs*
   a. Level at which family meets essential physical needs
   b. Level at which family meets social and emotional needs
   c. Resources within family to meet physical and emotional needs
   d. Disparities between individual needs and family's willingness or ability to meet them
5. *Goals, values, and aspirations*
   a. Extent to which family members' goals and values are articulated and understood by all members
   b. Extent to which family values reflect resignation or compromise
   c. Extent to which family will permit pursuit of individual goals and values
6. *Socioeconomic factors*
   a. Economic factors—level of income, adequacy of subsistence; how this affects life-style, sense of adequacy, self-worth
   b. Employment and attitudes about it
   c. Racial, cultural, and ethnic identification: sense of identity and belonging
   d. Religious identification and link to significant value systems, norms, and practices

Family assessments may be accomplished in a variety of ways. Some suggestions are given below. Others are discussed in the later section on intervention.

Taking a Family Life Chronology

Virginia Satir (1967) suggests that the family therapist should structure at least the first two sessions of therapy by taking a family life chronology. Her rationale is based on the following factors:

- The family therapist enters a session knowing little more than who the "identified patient" (IP) is and what symptoms that person manifests. The therapist does not have clues about the meaning of the symptoms, how the pain that exists in the marital relationship is expressed, how the mates have attempted to cope with their problems, or what models have influenced each mate's expectations about being a mate or parent.

- The therapist knows that the family has a history but does not know what the history is—what events have occurred and which members were influenced (directly or indirectly) by those events.

- Family members are fearful about embarking on family therapy. Structuring early sessions with a family life chronology helps decrease the threat. Members can answer relatively nonthreatening questions, and they tend to relax as the therapist demonstrates ability to take charge and keep things under control.

- Family members are often despairing when they enter therapy. The therapist's structure tells the family that there are specific directions to take in order to accomplish goals. The questions also provide family members with the opportunity to review successes as well as failures.

- The family life chronology is a nonthreatening way to change the focus from a "sick" family member to the family system and marital relationship.

- Taking the chronology gives the family therapist the opportunity to be a model of effective communication and provides the framework within which change can take place.

The structure of the family life chronology recommended by Satir is illustrated in Figure 33–3.

Family Genealogy or Time Line

Walter Toman's family constellation theory (1976), which uses generational transmission concepts, is a useful basis for constructing a family genealogy or time line.

From the study of families in detail, it becomes apparent that patterns are spread over generations. At first Bowen believed that a schizophrenic child could be produced after psychologic impairment in three generations. He now believes that the level of impairment in schizophrenia is not produced until eight to ten generations have passed. An intrinsic difficulty in analyzing generational transmission is that only a minute slice of a family generation— three generations out of at least 4000—can be studied. Few people are able to do what radiation biologist Dr. Joseph K. Gong, of the State University of New York at Buffalo, can. He can trace his paternal ancestry in China back to 2255 B.C.—an incredible 4000 years and 131 generations.

Each generation, according to Laing (1972, p 77), projects onto the next the following elements:

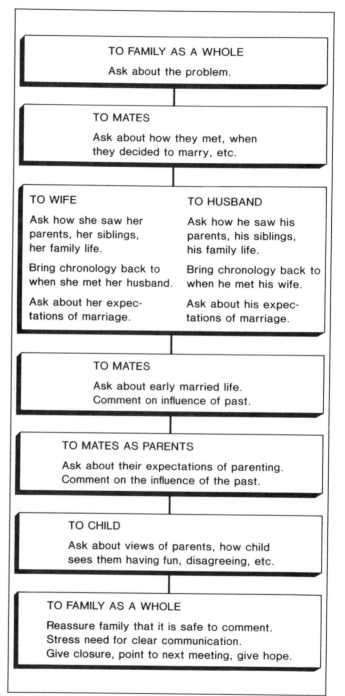

Figure 33–3

Main flow of family life chronology.

Source: Adapted from Satir V: Conjoint Family Therapy, *rev ed. Science and Behavior Books, 1967.*

- What was projected onto it by prior generations
- What was induced in it by prior generations
- Its response to this projection and induction

This process, which Laing calls *mapping,* is endless. Since it is impractical and impossible to understand the effect of 4000 earlier generations on a family, the time line can serve a therapist and a family as a more limited means for understanding the family's roots.

The time line is highly effective as a visual representation. The therapist who draws it on a long, narrow piece of paper that is taped to the wall during the family's sessions can use it time and time again as the family therapy progresses. Colored lines can be used to differentiate individual family members. Colored flags, pins, or asterisks can identify and call attention to significant events in the family history. Births, deaths, marriages, and leavetakings should be noted. The family therapist can use any of several family tree or genealogic tracings for the family time line. One method is illustrated in Figure 33–4.

The Structured Family Interview

A structured family interview (Watzlawick 1966) has elements similar to Satir's family life chronology. In addition, the family members are asked to participate in demonstrating the system's operation. The structured interview is composed of the following segments:

- *The main problems:* Each member is asked separately to identify what he or she considers the main problems in the family. The therapist assures the family member that the answer will not be divulged. Family members are then brought together to discuss this topic. The therapist leaves the room after telling the family members that their conversation will be recorded and they will be observed through a one-way screen. This task undermines the myth that the IP is the only "problem" in the family and paves the way for future work.

- *Planning something together:* The family is asked to plan something together, as a family, in the five minutes during which the therapist leaves the room. The important things in this task are whether and how a decision was reached. The content of the task, while revealing, is of secondary importance.

- *How the mates met:* This task is for the mates only. With the children in another room, the mates are asked how, out of all the millions of people in the world, they got together. The parents share their views of the past and reveal their predominant patterns of interacting in the present.

- *The meaning of a proverb:* The parents are asked to discuss the meaning of the proverb "A rolling stone gathers no moss." At the end of five minutes, they are to call the children in and teach them the meaning of the proverb. This proverb has two valid but mutually exclusive interpretations—that *moss* (roots, stability, friends, etc.) is valuable, or that *rolling* (not stagnat-

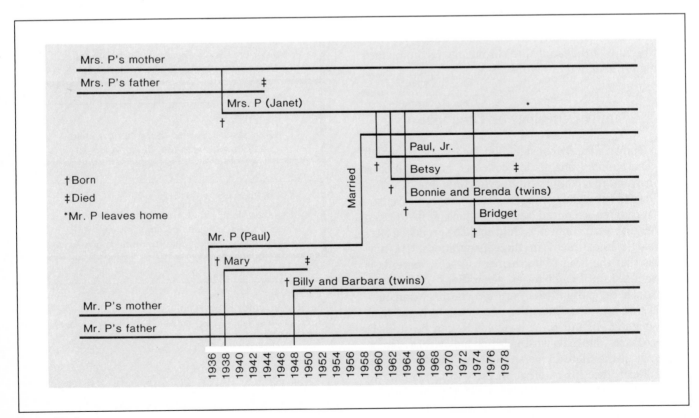

Figure 33–4
Timeline of the P family.

ing, being alert, moving) is desirable. This task reveals how the mates handle disagreements and how they explain things to their offspring.

- *Blaming:* The entire family and the therapist are together for this task. The father sits to the left of the therapist followed at his left by the mother and the children, from the oldest to the youngest, in a clockwise direction around the table. Each family member is asked to write down, on a three-by-five card, the main fault of the person to the left. (The youngest child writes what he or she sees as the main fault of the father.) The therapist writes two cards, which state "too good" and "too weak." The therapist collects the cards and reads them out loud, beginning with the two she or he has written. The therapist then asks to which two family members these cards apply. The other cards are read aloud in random order, and the authors are not revealed. This task reveals such processes as scapegoating, favoritism, and self-blame. This assessment tool may actually serve a therapeutic function and be used as an intervention technique if it helps family members achieve spontaneous understanding of the patterns and relationships in their family.

Contract or Goal Negotiation

The negotiation phase of family therapy is begun by identifying what each member would like changed in the family. When each family member and the therapist have identified what they see as important goals, work begins on negotiating a set of attainable goals that everyone is willing to work on. Compromise is needed to achieve a working goal. At this time, the family therapist may also identify the means—tasks, strategies, etc.—that will be used to reach the negotiated goals.

Written and verbal contracts for work with individuals and groups have been discussed in Chapters 27 and 30. Chapter 27 also illustrates written contracts in current use. They may be adapted for use with families. A structured and specific marriage contract is discussed and illustrated later in this chapter.

Intervention

Therapy for a family system involves understanding and use of the here-and-now, of the basic processes that occur in the system. General guidelines for using the here-and-now process with families are given below. Some of the wide variety of specific strategies and tasks are also discussed.

Role of the Family Therapist

Virginia Satir (1967, pp 160–176) offers the following guidelines for the role of the family therapist:

1. Creating a setting in which members can risk looking at themselves and their actions
   a. Reducing their fears
   b. Giving direction
   c. Helping them feel comfortable and hopeful about the therapy process
   d. Accepting the "expert" label and being comfortable in the role
   e. Structuring questions to gain important data
2. Being unafraid but open
   a. Framing questions to help members be less afraid
   b. Validating members' assumptions and questioning personal assumptions
   c. Eliciting the facts about planning processes, loopholes in planning, perceptions of self and others, perceptions of roles, communication patterns and techniques, sexual feelings and activities
   d. Responding with a belief in the integrity of the members
3. Helping members see how they look to others
   a. Sharing observations of how members manifest themselves
   b. Teaching members how to share their observations with one another
   c. Playing back tape recordings (or video tapes)
4. Asking for and giving information in a matter-of-fact, nonjudgmental, light, congruent way
   a. Verbally recreating situations (with imagination) in order to collect pertinent facts
   b. Being easy about giving and receiving information and thereby making it easier for family members to do so
5. Building self-esteem
   a. Making constant "I value you" comments
   b. Labeling assets
   c. Asking questions that family members can answer
   d. Emphasizing that the therapist and family members are equals in learning from therapy
   e. Responding as a person whose meaning or intent can be checked on
   f. Noting past achievements
   g. Accentuating the family's "good" intentions but "bad" communication
   h. Asking each family member what he or she can do to bring pleasure to another family member
   i. Being human, clear, and direct (and recognizing

that warmth and good intentions are not enough in themselves)

6. Decreasing threat by setting rules for interaction
   a. Seeing to it that all members participate
   b. Making it clear that interruptions are not tolerated
   c. Emphasizing that acting out or making it impossible to converse is not allowed
   d. Making sure that no one speaks for anyone else
   e. Helping everyone speak out clearly so that each can be heard
   f. Using humor appropriately
   g. Connecting silence to covert control

7. Decreasing threat by structuring sessions
   a. Announcing concrete goals and a definite end to the therapy or deadlines for reevaluation
   b. Viewing the family as a family and not taking sides
   c. Seeing units or subsystems of the family alone to accomplish specific work or because this is feasible or practical (e.g., other members are not available), with the knowledge and understanding of all members

8. Decreasing threat by reducing the need for defenses
   a. Discussing anger and hurt openly, thus decreasing fears about showing anger or hurt
   b. Interpreting anger as hurt
   c. Acknowledging anger as a defense and dealing with the hurt
   d. Showing that pain and the "forbidden" are safe to look at
   e. Burlesquing basic fears—painting a picture exaggerated to the point of absurdity—to decrease overprotectiveness and feelings of omnipotence

9. Decreasing threat by handling loaded material with care
   a. Using careful timing
   b. Moving from the least loaded to the most loaded
   c. Switching to less loaded material when things get hot (to another subject or to the past rather than the present)
   d. Generalizing about what a therapist expects to see in families (hurt, anger, fear, fighting, etc.)
   e. Relating feelings to facts (events, circumstances)
   f. Using personal idioms, slang, profanity, or vulgarity when appropriate, and avoiding pedantic words and psychiatric jargon
   g. Preventing closure on episodes or complaints;

assuring that things will become clearer as learning continues

10. Reeducating members to be accountable
    a. Reminding members of their ability to be in charge of themselves
    b. Identifying global pronouns
    c. Dealing openly with tattletales, spokespersons, and acting-out members
    d. Highlighting problems of accountability in the relationship with the therapist

11. Helping members see the influence of past models on their expectations and behavior
    a. Reminding members that they are acting from past models
    b. Openly challenging expectations
    c. Highlighting expectations by helping members verbalize the unspoken
    d. Highlighting expectations by exaggerating them

12. Delineating family roles and functions
    a. Recognizing roles by calling the parents "Mom" and "Dad" when referring to them as parents and "Jane" and "Bill" when addressing them as individuals or as husband and wife
    b. Including members in history taking in the order of their entrance into the family
    c. Questioning members about their roles
    d. Teaching explicitly about role responses and role choices

13. Completing gaps in communication and interpreting messages
    a. Clarifying the content and relationship aspects of messages
    b. Separating comments about the self from comments about others
    c. Pointing out significant discrepancies, incongruities, or double-level messages
    d. Spelling out nonverbal communication

Structured Family Tasks and Therapeutic Techniques

Structured family tasks are used for joint assessment and intervention purposes. They provide historical data and, in some cases, relate the data to present behavior. They offer family members the opportunity to collaborate actively in changing the family system.

Sculpting

Sculpting is a technique in which a client builds a living sculpture, based on his or her perceptions. Family members physically place one another in locations or positions that best represent their perceptions of one another. This live family portrait has the advantage of condensing and projecting into a visual picture the essence of one member's experience in the family (Papp et al. 1973, p 197). Triangles, alliances, and conflicts are choreographed and thus made available for analysis. This often reveals hidden aspects of the family's inner life.

Family Album Photostudy

Rae Sedgwick (1978) suggests photostudy of the family album as a means of providing tangible, longitudinal evidence to raise questions, validate or invalidate hunches, and developmentally examine the individual and the family. Sedgwick suggests that the family picture album is one of the most obvious, and most overlooked, tools for understanding family dynamics. The photographs and the process of selecting them give insights into decision making, themes, interaction patterns, patterns of development, and power and influence relationships within the family. The therapist and family discuss and analyze the photographs together.

Other interesting family tasks suggested by Sedgwick (1976) include: writing a family autobiography; comparing and contrasting family members with one another and with selected families from the neighborhood, the school, or the church; drawing a family picture; writing a family news article or a family epitaph; dispelling a family myth; weaving a family dream; or writing a family play. Such tools are helpful in examining histories, prophecies, scripts, and myths. They are limited only by the imagination and ingenuity of the therapist.

Role Playing, Games, and Simulated Family Experiences

In her practice, Virginia Satir (1967) uses role playing with families. The simulated family experience is used to teach families about themselves. Family members may simulate each other's behavior or their conceptions of it. They may also play themselves in a simulated situation. Videotape feedback helps family members become acquainted with their own behavior. In addition, systems games and communication games (Satir 1967, pp 187–88) are used to help families communicate more effectively and congruently. These role-playing experiences are also effective educational tools in the preparation of family therapists.

Criteria for Terminating Treatment

Reid (1985) suggests that termination in family therapy should occur in a flexible way, helping families achieve realistic goals and end service with a feeling of accomplishment. Satir (1967, p 176) has developed criteria for determining when to terminate family therapy. Termination is appropriate when family members can

- Complete transactions, check, and ask
- Interpret hostility
- See how others see them
- Tell one another how they appear
- Tell one another their hopes, fears, and expectations
- Disagree
- Make choices
- Learn through practice
- Free themselves from the harmful influences of past models
- Give clear messages

THE NURSING PROCESS IN FAMILY COUNSELING

The following case study of the Wilson family (Black 1983) demonstrates a humanistic psychiatric nursing approach to family counseling. It shows how a nurse applied an understanding of family process and dynamics (elaborated on in this chapter) and used the covert rehearsal phase of the symbolic interaction model (illustrated in Figure 11–7) and general communication principles (Chapter 11) along with principles of relationship building (Chapter 27). When you read it keep in mind the nursing process components (Chapter 4).

CASE EXAMPLE*

John, a graduate student in psychiatric-mental health nursing, is assigned to work with the Wilson family during his final clinical placement. The arrangement is made by his instructor in cooperation with the family clinic of the local community mental health center. The family is selected by the staff team that John has joined as a member. The team includes a social worker, a psychiatrist, a psychologist, and a clinical nurse specialist. On each of his clinical days, John attends the daily team meeting in which the group shares their progress in working with their families, exchanges insights, and provides each other with mutual support as family problems are worked through. John's instructor attends several of the meetings on John's clinical days.

*From Black, K., *Short-term Counseling: A Humanistic Approach for the Helping Professions,* pp 200–205. Copyright © 1983 by Addison-Wesley Publishing Co., Inc., Menlo Park, Calif.

The intake report provides the team with information on which to base John's assignment. Mr. and Mrs. Wilson applied to the center as a result of a referral made by a local police official. Ross Wilson, their ten-year-old son, had been brought home by an officer following his fifth runaway episode in as many weeks.

At the request of the team, the intake worker makes a first appointment for John to meet with Ross and his parents at the center. Ross's younger brother and sister are left at home with their aunt. They can be expected to share in the benefits resulting from favorable behavioral and role changes brought about in a significant part of the family system. The assignment of this particular family to John is made mainly because the dysfunction seems to be of recent origin and essentially located within the triangle formed by Ross and his parents. This limits the complexity of the interrelationships that John will be called on to deal with.

Initiating the Relationship

John prepares himself for his first interview with the family by engaging in an inner rehearsal. He anticipates that the parents will be anxious and embarrassed at having to explain their problem to yet another stranger. Their anxiety will be compounded by the prospect of being required to incorporate an outsider into the family's functional system. This, John reasons, might be offset to some extent by the fact that a state of psychologic crisis tends to create an unusual openness in its victims to accepting outside help.

John sees his immediate task as twofold: (a) to build the foundation of a relationship of mutual trust with the client family and (b) to work with them in defining the problem or problems that precipitated the present family crisis. Recognizing that his sensitivity to his clients' feelings will enable him to express genuine concern and a sincere desire to help, he also determines to keep the meetings family centered throughout. He plans to clarify his own role as catalytic but peripheral to the family's identification and implementation of new methods of coping. By these measures he hopes to reinforce the family's potential to function as a complete, interdependent system of mutual support.

Ross proves, on acquaintance, to be the least self-conscious of any in the group. He is an outgoing child, not overtly concerned about his problem behavior, but obviously eager to please his parents in other ways. When John issues a general invitation to all three to fill him in on the details of the problem that brought them to the center, all three participate about equally in the response. The parents tell of their worry over what might happen to Ross during his absence from home. Ross speaks sheepishly, but with a touch of pride, about having been repeatedly picked up in various public places by uniformed police officers late at night. John reflects the parental concern as inevitable under the circumstances, then to Ross his fascination with the police uniform.

Ross responds boastfully that his father also has a uniform and drives a truck. This leads to a description of the family's general life-style and, from that, to the particular events connected with the runaway episodes. The remainder of the first meeting and most of the next is taken up with the family's story. At first, John keeps it moving comfortably with only an occasional continuing response.

It develops that Mr. Wilson, who is employed to drive locally for a department store, is becoming increasingly discontent with the duties the job entails. At this point in the narrative, he and Mrs. Wilson engage in an argument that is a replay of one that, they admit, frequently breaks out at home. The husband says that he wants to transfer to a long-distance assignment, whereupon his wife complains to John that her husband's transfer would leave her with night and day responsibility for the home and family much of the time. Also addressing John, Mr. Wilson raises his voice in angry frustration at not being given an opportunity to explain how much better off the family would be if he could only take a better-paying job.

Mindful of the principles he has studied, John is alert to the danger of being triangled into the family conflict. He reflects Mrs. Wilson's apprehension directly to her and Mr. Wilson's anger to him, and he gently calls their attention to the fact that they are reliving feelings aroused in the past in the midst of the group's present information-gathering task.

With only an occasional outburst centering on the same theme, the sequence of events that typically precedes and follows Ross's leaving home is elicited as follows:

1. The argument about Mr. Wilson's proposed transfer begins in the course of a work-day evening meal.

2. Mr. Wilson shouts in frustration; Mrs. Wilson voices her fears and finally leaves the room in tears with the two younger children to put them to bed.

3. Ross remains with his father, who tells him of the joys of long-distance trucking.

4. On returning, Mrs. Wilson scolds Ross and her husband for lack of consideration for her and sends Ross to do his homework.

5. Mr. and Mrs. Wilson are uncommunicative with each other and with Ross for the next day or two.

6. One evening soon after, Mrs. Wilson prepares her husband's favorite dishes for supper. When Ross is again banished to do his homework, it is obvious to him that his parents are averse to having him present during their reconciliation.

7. Ross wanders off instead of going to school the next morning.

8. The police bring him home late in the evening.

9. His mother cries and scolds Ross, his father whips him with a belt, and he is sent to bed without any supper.

10. At supper the next evening, Mr. Wilson casually asks Ross where he went and what happened on the day that he missed school. He listens to the account with interest. Mrs. Wilson does not participate and, before long, suggests that Mr. Wilson would probably like to run away from the family too.

The argument about the transfer begins again.

John recognizes that Ross, without being fully aware of it, picks up the metacommunicative approval and empathy in his father's questions about his escapades and identifies with his father's desire to see new places. Although Mrs. Wilson has come close to recognizing the command aspect of her husband's transactions, her feedback conveys criticism rather than understanding. With John's help, the three family members are able—the parents grudgingly at first—to identify the meanings that are thinly covered in their pattern of interaction.

Team discussion corroborates John's opinion that the family pattern currently displays a typically dysfunctional family triangle: a repetitive cycle of conflict, distance, and closeness; scapegoating to a minor degree; and the feedback cycle that Weakland describes. These insights are not communicated to the family. The team is in agreement that the maladaptive pattern will be broken up and reassembled as family members move to assume the group task of defining their goals and accepting responsibility for each other in a unified effort at planning and implementation.

Nursing Assessment and Planning

At his third meeting with the family, it is evident to John that Mr. and Mrs. Wilson have done some homework between meetings. Mr. Wilson announces that, although Ross's running away from home is in no way excusable, he and his wife feel that their quarreling has made the child's home too hellish at times for him to want to stay there. Mrs. Wilson adds that the two younger children have been unusually fractious in the worrisome home atmosphere. She perceives her own impatience as both causing and resulting from the family's general state of disorder. Not to be outdone, Mr. Wilson says then that because his job is his own responsibility, he will see what he can do about it without bothering anyone else.

John observes, while Mr. Wilson is speaking, that Mrs. Wilson is becoming flushed and Ross is beginning to squirm. John briefly reinforces the starts the parents have made toward defining their feelings about their present situation. He then points out in matter-of-fact

terms the body language he noted, and he makes the connection between it and Mr. Wilson's statement about solving a significant family problem alone. Mrs. Wilson says emphatically that the problem concerns all of them and that she would like to have some say in how it is solved. Her husband concedes that she has that right, and they begin to discuss the pros and cons of the transfer.

This time, the parents address one another rather than attempting to involve John. Their argument is less heated than at the previous meeting. When they tend to move to positions at extreme ends of the issue, John helps them identify gray areas and calls attention to connections between judgmental opposites. Tendencies to blame or to dwell on the past are diverted into making plans to cope with present and foreseeable circumstances.

Ross's first attempt to contribute to the discussion is disregarded until John breaks in to reflect its underlying feeling. It shows that the boy is beginning to identify more evenly now and is trying to find ways of supporting his mother's point of view as well as his father's. John's response, although directed to Ross, serves to remind the parents that Ross's feelings are a significant factor in the problem as a whole. Thereafter they try, sometimes with John's help, to integrate Ross's comments into their overall assessment.

During the remainder of this meeting and the next, the family group is involved in action planning that is divided between the improvement of family relationships and a solution to the question of Mr. Wilson's transfer. The problem of Mrs. Wilson being left to cope alone while her husband is out of town brings a response from Ross that signifies that, as the man of the house, he is quite able to protect her. It also leads to an assessment of resources outside the immediate family. Grandparents, an uncle, and two aunts who live nearby are identified as being closely concerned with the family's welfare. The parents admit that the relatives' interest in the children has recently been neglected.

As discussion proceeds, John continues to be aware of the importance of modeling clear and accurate communication in his own statements. He also gives and elicits feedback when necessary to clarify the contributions of the other three participants. Generalizations that the parents tend to make on the basis of untested assumptions are exposed and called into question, and interdependent, supportive interactions are strongly reinforced. Frequent summary evaluations of progress serve to reassure, as well as reinforce, the family as an effectively functioning unit.

Implementation

By the fifth meeting, a compromise plan has been reached on the question of the transfer. Implementation of the plan is clearly a family responsibility. The family agrees that Mr. Wilson will postpone making a change until both of the younger children attend school for a full-day session. Mrs. Wilson feels that she will be better able to cope with intercurrent difficulties when they are in someone else's care for a few hours a day. Mr. and Mrs. Wilson resolve to keep in closer touch with the relatives on whom Mrs. Wilson can depend for moral support. Ross promises to stay near his home and to spend some of his free time each day with the younger children.

Evaluation and Termination

John is able to utilize evaluation both as an ongoing impetus to the process of intervention and as a learning experience for himself. The three Wilsons soon participate with pleasure in the reviews, which highlight the steps of their progress in family collaboration as well as in problem solving. At staff team meetings, John reports each day's interaction with as much verbatim content as he can remember, and he joins the other team members in an evaluative exchange of questions, interpretations, and suggestions.

The team discusses the matter of termination midway in the series of six meetings. Progress to date gives every indication that the family will soon be functioning at a somewhat higher level than they achieved before lapsing into dysfunction. The shared prediction is that, if they agree to termination by the sixth meeting, it will be effected at that point without referral or planned follow-up.

Much of the fifth meeting is taken up by the members of the now-functional triangle in telling John how well things are going at home. John periodically expresses his observation of their sensitivity to each other's feelings and their supportiveness of one another. As the meeting ends, he indicates that they are now working together so effectively that there is little need for any help he can give. They assent willingly to his suggestion that the sixth meeting be the last and that it be used as a general windup. When his mother remarks that the children's aunt will be relieved to hear that her babysitting chore is nearly over, Ross suggests that the other two children come along for the last meeting so that John can meet them.

With the two children aged five and six present, the sixth meeting turns out to be a little boisterous. John notes that Ross now identifies with his parents in monitoring the behavior of the younger children in keeping with his parents' commands. When he takes the others to explore a courtyard that can be seen from the window of the meeting room, the parents thank John for all his help, saying that they wish they had known sooner of the work of the family clinic. John uses this opportunity to reinforce their consciousness of new-found strength in their unified approach to problems, adding that there are sure to be more problems as time goes on. He assures them of the continuing availability of the clinic as a community resource. Ross proffers a gruff thank you when the children gather to add their farewells to those of their parents.

FAMILY-ORIENTED PREVENTIVE PSYCHIATRY PROGRAMS

According to William M. Bolman (1972), the family is the most strategic social unit. For this reason, preventive psychiatric services should be oriented toward it. Table 33–1 identifies primary, secondary, and tertiary prevention approaches that may be used to provide for family mental health.

COUPLES THERAPY

Couples therapy is the more contemporary term for what used to be known as *marital therapy*. The later term reflects the existence of interactional dyads not necessarily based on marriage. Couples may seek counseling when difficulties between the couple are specific to their relationship.

Developmental Tasks Confronting Couples

Ellen M. Berman and Harold I. Lief (1975) have added to Erik Erikson's theory of psychosocial development (see Chapter 6) by identifying adult developmental tasks and stages as they relate to the marital life cycle. Their tasks for each stage are outlined in Table 33–2.

Types of Therapy

There are basically four types of therapy for couples. *Collaborative therapy* is individual therapy for each partner by two therapists. *Concurrent therapy* is individual therapy for each partner by the same therapist. Neither one is truly *couples* therapy. Both fit into the one-to-one mode. *Conjoint therapy* occurs when the couple is seen together by a single therapist or by cotherapists. Male and female cotherapists are particularly effective as models in conjoint

Table 33–1 Preventive Approaches for Family Mental Health			
Target Population	**Goals**	**General Approach**	**Specific Examples**
1. Families in crisis due to the loss of a member (death, desertion, chronic hospitalization).	Provision of flexible support according to the event, how perceived and managed, and the resources and the life-style of the surviving family fragment.	Primary and secondary preventive, high-risk and community-wide approaches.	Group meetings in hospital of parents of fatally ill children; expanded emergency room coverage; neighborhood information centers; walk-in clinics for problems of living; some mental health clinics.
2. Families under stress due to a handicapped parent (mental illness, retardation, alcoholism, or other chronic disorder).	Identification and support as needed for these families as in 1, above.	Primary and secondary preventive, high-risk approaches for children; tertiary preventive, community-wide approaches for parents.	Public health nurse makes regular home visits to family of alcoholic; family medical clinics; mental-hospital-based services; homemaker services for mentally ill mothers.
3. Families under stress due to internal imbalance or disorder (schism, double bind, skew, pseudomutuality, and other types of marital discord).	Assistance either in correcting the imbalance or in minimizing the impact on the children.	Primary or secondary preventive, high-risk approaches for children; secondary or tertiary preventive, community-wide approaches for parents.	Marital counseling; family therapy, parents' groups, individual therapy; legal guardian ad litem for children in divorce actions; legal aid for low-income families through neighborhood law offices.
4. Families under stress as a result of vulnerability to normal developmental changes (birth of a child, school entry, puberty, climacteric, retirement).	Sensitivity to the variety of family stresses or crises that may result, leading to earlier recognition and intervention as needed, often via very short-term crisis-oriented therapy.	Primary and secondary preventive, high-risk, community-wide, and milestone approaches.	Many of the above programs, especially neighborhood and/or comprehensive health, mental health, and social welfare services. Awareness of the opportunities for stress and crisis assistance is more important than the specific program setting.
5. Families living in areas lacking necessary biopsychosocial supplies (police protection, housing, quality education, etc.), in areas such as urban slums, depressed rural areas, migrant workers' camps, Indian reservations, and housing projects.	Provision of these basic necessities through community development approaches.	Primary, secondary, and tertiary preventive, high-risk approaches.	Community development approaches originating through schools, churches, social agencies, neighborhood service centers, family life educators, mental health centers, etc.
6. Families caught in the cycle of intergenerational poverty.	Provision of multiple and flexible opportunities for attaining desired personal, social, and economic goals.	Primary, secondary, and tertiary preventive, high-risk approaches.	Same as in 5; also a variety of antipoverty programs, such as Headstart, Upward Bound, and Job Corps, and agencies such as Mobilization for Youth, and Community Progress, Inc.

continued

Table 33–1 *(Continued)*
Preventive Approaches for Family Mental Health

Target Population	Goals	General Approach	Specific Examples
7. Disorganized families characterized by multiple and complex problems (emotional disorder, social dependence, poverty, chronic physical illness, child neglect or abuse, alcoholism and other addictions) and multiple needs (personal, social, medical, economic).	Use of a problem-centered versus a discipline-centered approach to diagnose the total range of causative factors, identify those most accessible to change, and plan a step-by-step program.	Primary, secondary, and tertiary preventive, high-risk approaches for adults and children.	All programs in this section may be relevant. Again, the point of view or approach is more important than the program. Several additional possibilities include twenty-four-hour emergency homemakers, and other emergency care for children needing substitute parenting.
8. Families with potentially stressful role handicaps (childlessness, adoptive parenthood, foster-parenting, working mothers, and student families, such as medical and other graduate students).	Awareness of the potential for stress or crisis so that early recognition and supportive help are available.	Secondary preventive, high-risk, and community-wide approaches.	Groups for adoptive or foster parents, groups for adoptive children; reliable day care centers.

Source: Bolman WM: Preventive psychiatry for the family: Theory, approaches, and programs. Am J Psychiatry 1968;125:464–65. Copyright 1968, the American Psychiatric Association. Reprinted by permission.

Table 33–2
Tasks and Stages in the Marital Life Cycle

Stage	Age	Tasks
I	18 to 21	Pulling up roots; developing autonomy; shifting commitment from family of origin to a new relationship; testing power and intimacy; experiencing conflicts over in-laws; fragile marital boundaries are threatened.
II	22 to 28	Developing intimacy and occupational identification; stresses over parenthood and uncertainty about choice of marital partner; intimacy is deepening but ambivalent; patterns of conflict resolution over power issues are established; work, friends, and potential lovers challenge the marital boundaries.
III	29 to 31	Restlessness; conflicts about work versus marriage, parenthood, and increasing distance from partner; reevaluation; partners vie for power and dominance; compensatory "fortress-building" or extramarital involvement.
IV	32 to 39	Settling down; deepening commitments; long-range goals established; conflicts over productivity of partners; boundaries closed, as dominance and decision-making patterns and powers are firmly established.
V	40 to 42	Mid-life transition; search for a "fit" between aspirations and reality; past is reviewed and new future goals are established; conflicts over individual success, staying in the marriage; increased fantasies about other relationships.
VI	43 to 59	Restabilization and reordering of priorities; "empty nest" syndrome appears; intimacy with partners changes; boundaries are fixed.
VII	60 and over	Aging, illness, and death must be dealt with; marital conflicts and fears center on loneliness and sexual failure; stable plateau of intimacy; marital boundaries solidify; physical environment is critical for maintaining ties with the outside world.

Source: Compiled from Berman EM, Lief HI: Marital therapy from a psychiatric perspective: An overview. Am J Psychiatry 1975;6:583–592. Copyright 1975, The American Psychiatric Association. Reprinted by permission.

therapy. *Couples group therapy* is group therapy engaged in by several couples who meet with a therapist or co-therapists. The latter two modes can be more appropriately termed couples therapy.

Focus of Therapy

Couples therapy focuses on the relationship between the individuals and the similarities and differences between them that comprise the rules and expectations on which the relationship is based.

Couples or marital contracts have existed since the beginning of recorded history. Sager (1983) notes that the term is now used to refer to written contracts as well as to more general "understandings" and assumptions. Norman Sheresky and Marya Mannes suggest in a radical guide to wedlock (1972) that partners explore the rules together *before* marriage occurs. These authors urge that marriage vows be written in the form of a legal contract and that rules be made in the open before trouble occurs.

The following is an example of a premarital contract from their work (1972, pp 36–37)

ARTICLE III
Future Expectations

(a) Donald and Ina have discussed fully where they propose to reside during the course of their marriage. They agree that considerations relating to the location of their respective families should play no part in such determination. They agree their primary consideration shall be proximity to Donald's place of business. That factor should govern regardless of where Ina may be employed and regardless of whose earnings are greater.

(b) Neither party to this Memorandum holds any formal religious beliefs that should in any way interfere with the marriage. Neither insists on, or has even expressed any preference concerning, the other's adherence to any particular religious belief. Neither will, without the consent of the other, impose any religious belief upon any children of the marriage.

(c) It is the parties' present intention that Ina continue to work, health permitting, until such time as she may become pregnant. The parties have no exact intentions concerning the employment of Ina after the birth of any child or children, although Ina has expressed the feeling that simply caring for children would not be sufficiently stimulating to her. Donald's inclination at the present time is that he would prefer for Ina to discontinue any full-time employment if she had a child, but he would not insist upon it.

Both parties agree that any subsequent employment of Ina after the birth of a child should be such that it would permit her to spend reasonable periods of time with the child and that it should not entail any evening or weekend hours.

Sheresky and Mannes believe that such a marriage contract would go a long way toward preventing certain unsuccessful marriages and the resulting crisis of divorce.

In developing a marital contract, Sager (1983) suggests that the contract terms be divided into three categories:

1. Parameters based on expectations of the marriage, e.g., the expectation that the marriage will provide a loyal mate, companionship, sexual intimacy, financial security, future children.

2. Parameters based on intrapsychic and biologic needs, e.g., the amount of closeness or distance preferred by the individual, dominance or submission, use or abuse of power.

3. Parameters based on external foci, e.g., disturbances of transactional behavior patterns such as communication difficulties, child-rearing practices, compatibility of life-style, attitudes toward sex.

HUMANISTIC INTERACTIONIST FOUNDATIONS

By adopting a humanistic interactionist perspective, one recognizes the importance of conceptualizing the individual living in his or her unique family system and environment. Family groups are viewed as critical interacting systems that meet many of the individual's needs. If dysfunctional, this system contributes to ill health. The nurse intervenes in this system to promote and maintain health in a way that is acceptable to the culture and ethics of the client-family group.

Chapter Highlights

• The family is the context in which people develop their first relationships with others. How one views the world is molded by the events that happen within the family.

• Family forms in the United States are changing and becoming more diverse; a wide variety of family constellations exists in contemporary society.

• The family can be viewed as a system in terms of the relationships, associations, and connections that occur in a dynamic, interacting whole.

• The family system includes not only family members but their relationships, communications, and interactions with the environment.

• A change or movement in any part of the family system affects all other parts of the family system.

- The family seeks to maintain a dynamic balance, or "homeostasis," among various forces that operate within and upon it.

- Just as individuals and groups are confronted with developmental tasks, so are families.

- The functional family is distinguished from the dysfunctional one by the amount and quality of energy used to maintain the family system and to achieve the developmental tasks.

- Family therapists believe that emotional symptoms or problems of an individual are an expression of emotional symptoms or problems in a family. In family therapy work, the family system is the unit of treatment.

- Nurses work with families and family problems in many settings. To function as a family therapist, the psychiatric nurse needs graduate level preparation.

- The following affect the functioning of the family and its members: life scripts; family myths, life-styles, and themes; coalitions, dyads, and triangles; pseudomutuality and pseudohostility; marital schism and skew; enmeshment and disengagement; scapegoating; and double binds.

- Contemporary approaches to family therapy include the integrative approach, psychoanalytic approach, Bowen approach, structural approach, interactional approach, social network approach, and the behavioral approach.

- The milieu for family therapy often is the family's own home.

- Major components of family therapy include assessment, contract negotiation, and intervention.

- It is best for all family members to participate in the assessment phase of family therapy.

- The family therapist may use structured family tasks and therapeutic strategies for both assessment and intervention.

- The family therapist helps family members look at themselves in the here-and-now and recognize the influence of past models on their behavior and expectations.

- Preventive approaches toward attaining or maintaining mental health should be oriented toward the family as the basic social unit.

- Couples therapy may be instituted when difficulties between a couple are assessed to be specific to their relationship.

Ackerman NW: *The Psychodynamics of Family Life.* Basic Books, 1958.

Ackerman NW: Prejudicial scapegoating and neutralizing forces in the family group with special reference to the role "family healer," in Howells JG (ed): *Theory and Practice of Family Psychiatry.* Brunner/Mazel, 1971, pp 626–634.

Aponte H: If I don't get simple, I cry. *Family Process* 1986;25(4):531–548.

Bateson G, Jackson DD, Haley J, Weakland, JH: Toward a theory of schizophrenia. *Behav Sci* 1956;1:251–264.

Berman EM, Lief HI: Marital therapy from a psychiatric perspective: An overview. *Am J Psychiatry* 1975;6:583–592.

Black K: *Short-Term Counseling: A Humanistic Approach for the Helping Professions.* Addison-Wesley, 1983.

Bolman WM: Preventive psychiatry for the family: Theory, approaches, and programs, in Erickson GD, Hogan TP (eds): *Family Therapy.* Brooks/Cole, 1972, pp 377–401.

Boszormenyi-Nagy I, Framo J (eds): *Intensive Family Therapy.* Harper and Row, 1965.

Bowen M: A family concept of schizophrenia, in Jackson DD (ed): *The Etiology of Schizophrenia.* Basic Books, 1960, pp 346–372.

Bowen M: *Family Therapy in Clinical Practice.* Jason Aronson, 1978.

Bross A: *Family Therapy.* Guilford Press, 1983.

Compton BR, Galaway B: *Social Work Processes,* ed 2. Dorsey Press, 1979.

Deutsch D: Family therapy and family life-style. *Individual Psychol* 1967;23:217–223.

Doherty W, Burge S: Attending to the context of family treatment: Pitfalls and prospects. *J Marriage Fam Ther* 1987;13(1):37–47.

Drake R, Oscher F: Using family psychoeducation when there is no family. *Hosp Comm Psychiatr* 1987;38(3):274–277.

Duvall E: *Family Development.* Lippincott, 1985.

Glick PC: Children of divorced parents in demographic perspective. *J Soc Issues* 1979;35:112–125.

Griffith J: Employing the God-family relationship in therapy with religious families. *Family Process* 1986;25(4):609–618.

Griffith J, Griffith M: Structural family therapy in chronic illness. *Psychosom* 1987;28(4):202–205.

Haley J: *Problem Solving Therapy.* Jossey-Bass, 1976.

Hayghe H: Dual-earner families: Their economic and demographic characteristics, in Aldous J: *Two Paychecks: Life in Dual-Earner Families.* Sage, 1982, pp 27–40.

Hess RD, Handel G: *Family Worlds: A Psychosocial Approach to Family Life.* University of Chicago Press, 1959.

Jackson DD: The question of family homeostasis. *Psychiatr Q* 1957;[Suppl]:79–90.

Jackson DD: Family rules: Marital quid pro quo. *Arch Gen Psychiatry* 1965;12:589–594.

Jackson DD (ed): *Communication, Family, and Marriage.* Science and Behavior Books, 1968a.

Jackson DD (ed): *Therapy, Communication, and Change.* Science and Behavior Books, 1968b.

Jones SL: *Family Therapy: A Comparison of Approaches.* Robert J. Brady, 1980.

Kanter J, et al.: Expressed emotion in families: A critical review. *Hosp Comm Psychiatr* 1987;38(4):374–380.

Kiecolt-Glaser J, et al.: Marital quality, marital disruption, and immune function. *Psychosom Med* 1987;49(1):13–34.

Koenigsberg H, Handley R: Expressed emotion: From predictive index to clinical construct. *Am J Psychiatr* 1986;143(11):1361–1373.

Kunzer MB: Marital adjustment of headache sufferers and their spouses. *J Psychosoc Nurs* 1987;25(5):12–17.

Laing RD: *The Politics of the Family.* Vintage Books, 1972.

Lesser E, Comet J: Help and hindrance: Parents of divorcing children. *J Marriage Fam Ther* 1987;13(2):197–202.

Levine JA: Real kids vs. the average family. *Psychology Today,* June 1978, pp 14–15.

Lidz T, Cornelison AR, Terry D: The intrafamilial environment of the schizophrenic patient: Marital schism and marital skew. *Am J Psychiatry* 1957;114:241–248.

Lindsey K: *Friends or Family.* Beacon Press, 1982.

McGoldirick K, Rohrbaugh M: Researching ethnic family stereotypes. *Family Process* 1987;26(1):89–99.

Minuchin S: *Families and Family Therapy.* Harvard University Press, 1974.

Newsweek, Bureau of Labor Statistics, Feb. 17, 1985, p 64.

Papp P, Silverstein O, Carter E: Family sculpting in preventive work with "well families." *Family Process* 1973;12:194–204.

Patterson G: *Living with Children: New Methods for Parents and Teachers.* Research Press, 1976.

Pitzer RL: Work and family, in McCubben HI, Pitzer RL: *Stress and Work, Addressing the Needs of Children, Youth, and Parents: Models for Self Reliance (A report of the Min-*

nesota Governor's White House Conference, 1981). University of Minnesota, 1982, pp 38–39.

Reid W: *Family Problem Solving.* Columbia University Press, 1985.

Sager C, et al: *Treating the Remarried Family.* Brunner/Mazel, 1983.

Satir V: *Conjoint Family Therapy,* rev ed. Science and Behavior Books, 1967.

Sedgwick R: Photostudy as a diagnostic tool in working with families," in Kneisl CR, Wilson HS (eds): *Current Perspectives in Psychiatric Nursing: Issues and Trends.* Mosby, 1978, vol 2, pp 60–69.

Sheresky N, Mannes M: *Uncoupling: The Art of Coming Apart.* Viking Press, 1972.

Speck RV: Psychotherapy of the social network of a schizophrenic family. *Family Process* 1967;6:208–214.

Speck RV, Attneave L: *Family Networks.* Pantheon Books, 1973.

Steiner C: *Scripts People Live.* Grove Press, 1974.

Swanson A, Hurley P: Family systems: Values and value conflicts. *J Psychiatr Nurs* 1983;21:24–30.

Toman W: *Family Constellation,* ed 3. Springer Publishing, 1976.

United States Bureau of the Census: Household and Family Characteristics: March 1980, Current Population Reports, series P-20, No. 366, U.S. Government Printing Office, 1981.

Watzlawick P: A structured family interview. *Family Process* 1966;5:256–271.

Watzlawick P, Beavin JH, Jackson DD: *The Pragmatics of Human Communication.* W. W. Norton, 1967.

Worthington E: Treatment of families during life transitions: Matching treatment to family response. *Family Process* 1987;26(2):295–308.

Wynne L, Ryckoff IM, Day J, Hirsch SI: Pseudo-mutuality in the family relationships of schizophrenics. *Psychiatry* 1958;21:205–220.

THIRTY-FOUR

Applying the Nursing Process with Children

Janet Grossman
Kate Mayton

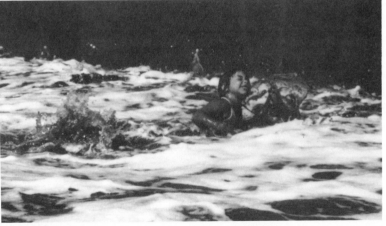

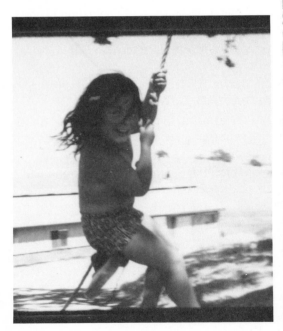

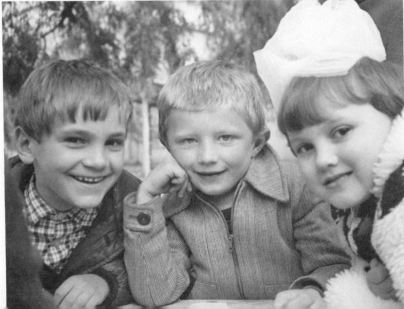

Learning Objectives

After reading this chapter, students should be able to

● Describe the generalist and specialist roles of the nurse in child psychiatry

● Discuss the common child psychiatric disorders

● Apply the nursing process to clinical situations with child psychiatric clients and their families

● Identify the role of the child psychiatric nurse in the various treatment modalities used with children

● Explain the responsibilities of the nurse in caring for children in a milieu

Cross References

Other topics related to this content are: Bulimia and anorexia nervosa, Chapter 35; Family assessment and family therapy, Chapter 33; Growth and development, Chapter 6; Intrafamily physical and sexual abuse of children, Chapter 25, Part II; Milieu therapy, Chapter 31; Severity of psychosocial stressors for children and adolescents (Axis IV of DSM-IIIR), Table 12–3 in Chapter 12.

Key Terms

anhedonia
attention-deficit hyperactivity disorder
autistic disorder
conduct disorder
coprolalia
disruptive behavior disorders
elimination disorders
functional encopresis
functional enuresis
language and speech disorders
life space interview
oppositional defiant disorder
pervasive developmental disorders
play therapy
tic disorders
Tourette syndrome

The plight of the estimated three million children believed to be suffering from serious emotional disorders can be summarized by stating that there are too many children (and families) in need of help, too few services available, and too few child psychiatric specialists to perform the services. This picture is made even bleaker by evidence suggesting that of the specialists available, at least one discipline, child psychiatric nursing, is being underused due to (Pothier et al. 1985):

● Lack of jobs in which nurses provide direct services that take full advantage of their clinical training

● Lack of access to clients due to the existing system of reimbursement for services

● A restricted view of what constitutes treatment and underdevelopment of new roles and models of care

Child psychiatric nursing concerns itself with promotion of mental health in all children as well as treatment of emotionally disturbed children. There is a wide range of psychiatric disturbances in children. Some children are simply overwhelmed by everyday worries; others need constant supervision because they might hurt themselves or others or because their thought processes are disturbed.

Children with severe emotional disorders present a challenge that taxes the knowledge and resources of the psychiatric nurse. Children with these disorders typically experience problems in their families, schools, and communities. They tend to exhibit developmental delays that cause them to lag behind their peers. Their parents or significant others complain about their behavior or are frustrated by their lack of response. These children may also experience somatic problems typical of adults with psychiatric disturbances and may have communication difficulties or confused perceptions of reality.

Not all nurses understand psychiatric disorders, and some find it difficult to plan interventions with these children and their families. But since nurses often encounter these children, particularly those who are undiagnosed or

Psychiatric nurses have a critical role in caring for what has been called our endangered species.

917

essential to coordinate efforts with the parents' therapists, particularly in the area of marital and family treatment.

untreated, knowledge of childhood disorders is important regardless of the nurse's area of clinical practice.

An understanding of childhood disorders also enhances practice in adult psychiatric nursing. Many disturbed adults have children with emotional problems or have difficulty with parenting skills. Psychiatric nurses are typically involved in family-centered care, which may include nursing activities such as conducting family therapy, supervising family visits, planning passes, providing family education, supporting family members in the milieu, and facilitating referrals for services for other family members.

The focus of this chapter is the nursing care of the prepubertal child with emotional problems and the role of the nurse in child psychiatry. Chapter 35 discusses the care of the adolescent with emotional problems.

HISTORICAL AND THEORETICAL PERSPECTIVES

Child psychiatric nursing is a specialty area of psychiatric nursing. The specialty is relatively new, having its inception in the early 1950s when graduate programs opened and training funds became available through the National Institute of Mental Health (NIMH). The early child guidance team did not include the nurse as a team member other than in the milieu. In some residential programs, the majority of milieu staff were from other disciplines, and only one nurse was included for each shift, primarily to attend to the physical needs of the children and administer medications. As the community mental health center movement developed, programs specific for children began to offer appropriate roles for the child psychiatric nurse, including treatment, consultation, education, and medication supervision. However, these programs had great difficulty sustaining themselves. The small number of professional staff in these programs provided few opportunities and low visibility for the child psychiatric nurse. Because positions in child psychiatry were so limited, many of these nurses were also involved in the care of chronically institutionalized adults reentering the community.

The interdisciplinary team in the contemporary milieu consists of child psychiatrists, nurses, social workers, child psychologists, occupational therapists, recreational therapists, special educators, pediatricians, and child care workers. Other specialists are used for consultations as indicated, particularly child neurologists, speech and language specialists, child abuse teams, clergy, and physical therapists. It is not unusual for parents to need psychotherapy themselves. In fact the child may have been referred to the child psychiatrist by the parents' therapist. It is

Emerging Nursing Roles

New nursing roles emerging in child psychiatric specialization underscore the need for a medical-psychiatric approach: focus on biochemical disorders and dual diagnosis. The term *dual diagnosis* is used to describe clients who have a primary medical and psychiatric diagnosis, such as a child who has both diabetes and a conduct disorder. Nurses, who are experienced in working with medically ill people have a knowledge base that is useful in understanding the interaction of medical and psychiatric disorders. Medical conditions tend to be frightening and unfamiliar to members of other disciplines (e.g., social workers, teachers, and psychologists), who are more familiar with children who have a primary psychiatric diagnosis.

Nurses in child psychiatry explain laboratory tests to children, support children during these procedures, and administer antidepressants that require strict and systematic monitoring. These roles capitalize on such characteristics of the child psychiatric nurse as:

- Ability to address the interaction between physical and psychologic symptoms

- Experience in working with chronic populations (tertiary care)

- Knowledge and skills related to pharmacology (educating children and parents, monitoring side-effects)

- Experience in nursing care of medical conditions such as seizure disorders, diabetes, and asthma

Humanistic Interactionism

The development of child psychiatric nursing is congruent with the theme of humanistic interactionism, which recognizes human nature as expressed in childhood and the symbolic meaning of children's behavior. Childhood and adolescence are viewed as stages distinctive from those of adulthood. In the humanistic interactionist view, the essence of nurturing in the nursing process holds special therapeutic value for the child.

Standards of Child and Adolescent Psychiatric and Mental Health Nursing Practice

The Standards of Child and Adolescent Psychiatric and Mental Health Nursing Practice were developed to improve the quality of nursing care given by generalists and specialists in the field (Box 34–1). These standards—devel-

Box 34-1
ANA STANDARDS OF CHILD AND ADOLESCENT PSYCHIATRIC AND MENTAL HEALTH NURSING PRACTICE

Professional Practice Standards

Standard I. Theory   The nurse applies appropriate, scientifically sound theory as a basis for nursing practice decisions.

Standard II. Assessment   The nurse systematically collects, records, and analyzes data that are comprehensive and accurate.

Standard III. Diagnosis   The nurse, in expressing conclusions supported by recorded assessment and current scientific premises, uses nursing diagnoses and/or standard classifications of mental disorders for childhood and adolescence.

Standard IV. Planning   The nurse develops a nursing care plan with specific goals and interventions delineating nursing actions unique to the needs of each child or adolescent, as well as those of the family and other relevant interactive social systems.

Standard V. Intervention   The nurse intervenes as guided by the nursing care plan to implement nursing actions that promote, maintain, or restore physical and mental health, prevent illness, effect rehabilitation in childhood and adolescence, and restore developmental progression.

Standard V-A. Intervention: Therapeutic Environment   The nurse provides, structures, and maintains a therapeutic environment in collaboration with the child or adolescent, the family, and other health care providers.

Standard V-B. Intervention: Activities of Daily Living   The nurse uses the activities of daily living in a goal-directed way to foster the physical and mental well-being of the child or adolescent and family.

Standard V-C. Intervention: Psychotherapeutic Interventions   The nurse uses psychotherapeutic interventions to assist children or adolescents and families to develop, improve, or regain their adaptive functioning, to promote health, prevent illness, and facilitate rehabilitation.

Standard V-D. Intervention: Psychotherapy*   The child and adolescent psychiatric and mental health specialist uses advanced clinical expertise to function as a psychotherapist for the child or adolescent and family and accepts professional accountability for nursing practice.

Standard V-E. Intervention: Health Teaching and Anticipatory Guidance   The nurse assists the child or adolescent and family to achieve more satisfying and productive patterns of living through health teaching and anticipatory guidance.

Standard V-F. Intervention: Somatic Therapies   The nurse uses knowledge of somatic therapies with the child or adolescent and family to enhance therapeutic interventions.

Standard VI. Evaluation   The nurse evaluates the response of the child or adolescent and family to nursing actions in order to revise the data base, nursing diagnoses, and nursing care plan.

Professional Performance Standards

Standard VII. Quality Assurance   The nurse participates in peer review and other means of evaluation to assure quality of nursing care provided for children and adolescents and their families.

Standard VIII. Continuing Education   The nurse assumes responsibility for continuing education and professional development and contributes to the professional growth of others studying children's and adolescents' mental health.

Standard IX. Interdisciplinary Collaboration   The nurse collaborates with other health care providers in assessing, planning, implementing, and evaluating programs and other activities related to child and adolescent psychiatric and mental health nursing.

Standard X. Use of Community Health Systems*   The nurse participates with other members of the community in assessing, planning, implementing, and evaluating mental health services and community systems that attend to primary, secondary, and tertiary prevention of mental disorders in children and adolescents.

Standard XI. Research   The nurse contributes to nursing and the child and adolescent psychiatric and mental health field through innovations in theory and practice and participation in research, and communicates these contributions.

Standards V-D and X apply only to the clinical specialist in child and adolescent psychiatric and mental health nursing.
Source: American Nurses' Association: Standards of Child and Adolescent Psychiatric and Mental Health Nursing Practice. 1985. Reprinted with permission of the American Nurses' Association.

oped by the American Nurses' Association in cooperation with Advocates for Child Psychiatric Nursing, Inc.—pertain to all settings in which child and adolescent psychiatric nurses practice, apply to children and adolescents at all developmental levels, and are relevant in all social systems in which the child or adolescent is involved. A review of the standards reveals the following distinctive interlocking characteristics:

- A preventive approach to intervention
- Consideration of developmental variables
- Attention to interacting social systems
- Focus on nonverbal communication and activity

The standards also describe the specific roles of generalists and specialists in child psychiatric nursing as follow (ANA 1985).

Generalists are nurses who are educated in basic professional nursing programs. Some of the roles that child psychiatric generalists assume include:

- Milieu therapist who shares the responsibility for providing an atmosphere in which all activities and behaviors are focused on the therapeutic care of the child or adolescent
- Counselor or teacher of parents who have an emotionally disturbed or mentally retarded child or adolescent
- Collaborator with other mental health and psychiatric professionals in assessing the needs and planning for the care of a child or adolescent and family
- Responsible citizen and change agent who provides for the mental health needs of children and adolescents
- Promoter of mental health with individuals, families, and groups
- Participant in the research process and consumer of research findings relevant to child and adolescent psychiatric and mental health nursing

Clinical specialists are nurses who hold at least a master's degree in child and adolescent psychiatric nursing; have had supervised clinical practice at the graduate level; and demonstrate breadth and depth of knowledge, skills, and competence in the field. Certification is highly recommended for the specialist. Specialists may assume any of the generalist roles and may also assume, but are not limited to, these additional roles:

- Psychotherapist for individual children, groups of children, and families

- Clinical supervisor of client care staff and graduate nursing students
- Administrator of child and adolescent psychiatric and mental health nursing services
- Educator of nurses and other child care personnel in a variety of academic and clinical settings
- Consultant to professional and nonprofessional individuals or groups concerned with the general welfare, education, and care of children
- Researcher who contributes to the theory and practice of child and adolescent psychiatric and mental health nursing through research in this field or a related field

PSYCHOPATHOLOGY IN CHILDREN

Etiology

Problems that appear in children are not necessarily classified as psychiatric disorders. They may be conditions for which an appropriate diagnosis cannot be determined, for which no psychiatric disorder has been found, or for which a psychiatric diagnosis is not the current focus of treatment. For example, the child's problem might be rooted in parent-child difficulties and therefore is not a psychiatric disorder.

Many factors contribute to the development of psychiatric disorders in children. The variables defined by researchers and clinicians depend on their theoretical framework, but nursing theorists view the etiology of psychiatric disorders as multidimensional. Etiologic factors generally fit the following four categories:

1. Genetic and biophysical factors
2. Social and cultural factors
3. Family system factors
4. Acquired illness and injury

Figure 34–1 shows the etiologic variables that influence the mental health of the child.

Genetic and Biophysical Factors

Genetic and biophysical influences of child psychiatric disorders include heredity, temperament, innate characteristics, congenital disorders, and constitution or health. The child is vulnerable to the strengths and weaknesses of each parent and to the separate effect of their combined genes. Hereditary influences are exemplified by the transmission of recessive genes for phenylketonuria, which causes mental retardation. Constitution or health variables are exemplified by the child's physical appearance and general state

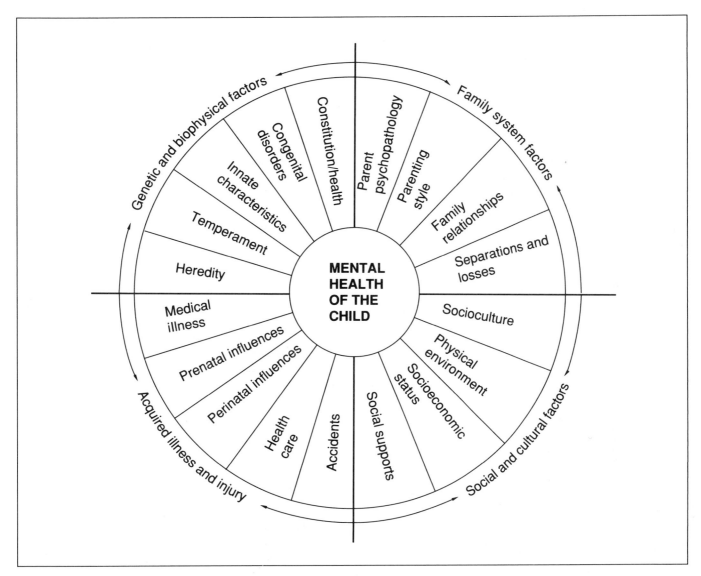

Figure 34–1
Factors that contribute to psychiatric disorders in children.

of health. The child born with fetal alcohol syndrome is an example of how innate factors resulting from mutation and regrouping of genes in the parents are then transferred to the child at conception. Premature birth is one type of congenital disorder that can affect behavior and social adaptation (Achenbach 1982).

Social and Cultural Factors

The role of social and cultural factors in the etiology of psychiatric disorders has been acknowledged in the last twenty years. Gerald Caplan (1961), who has advocated

primary prevention for adults and children, viewed psychiatric disorders as one of a set of social problems that must be handled at the community level.

The social and cultural variables affecting the child's mental health include the physical environment of the home and community, the family's socioeconomic resources, and cultural and social supports. When the child's environment is inadequate, as is the case with poverty or deprivation, the child is at greater risk for developing psychiatric problems. For example, a child from a family with few socioeconomic resources is more likely to develop symptoms of conduct disorder such as stealing, lying, fights, and truancy.

Family System Factors

Family system variables exert influence on the developing child through parenting styles, parent psychopathology, family relationships, and losses and separations. Parents shape their children's behavior by modeling and reinforcement through rewards and punishment. For example, modeling of antisocial behavior by a parent contributes to the child's refusal to follow rules in the school, home, and community.

Frequent moves or early loss of a parent through death or divorce impair the child's ability to form close relationships and make them prone to depression. Parent psychopathology such as depression or psychosis can result in failure to meet the child's basic needs or development of symptoms in the child similar to those of the parents. Physical or sexual abuse of the child by a parent typically results in chronic psychiatric disorders in the child such as self-destructive behavior, depression, or post-traumatic stress disorder. Dysfunctional family relationships, such as severe marital conflict or enmeshed relationships among child, parent, and grandparents, can create anxiety and confusion in the child.

Acquired Illness and Injury

Acquired illness and injury exert powerful influences on the emotional health of the child both through direct influence and through the secondary effect of interference with stages of personality and intellectual development in the child. For example, accidental poisoning can lead to cognitive deterioration. Chronic diseases developed in the perinatal period, such as asthma, can result in severe restriction of the child's physical activity and social experiences.

Mood Disorders

Mood disorders in children have become a popular topic in both professional and lay literature. While there is widespread agreement in child psychiatry that depression exists as both a syndrome and an affect in children, there continues to be confusion about the clinical diagnosis, lack of knowledge about effective treatment, and uncertainty about incidence and etiology. Clinical work and research in the field of childhood depression are far behind the work in adult depression, which was spurred on by findings in psychobiology and psychopharmacology. Despite these questions, mood disorders in children must be viewed as a major mental health problem. Depression is the most com-

mon psychiatric problem in children who attempt suicide, and youth suicide rates continue to rise.

The most common type of depression seen in children is secondary, or reactive, depression. This is the sadness that occurs in response to particular situations, including the trauma of hospitalization, surgery, or separation from a family member. Children might become depressed secondary to medical diseases, such as diabetes mellitus, asthma, and cardiac anomalies, or cognitive and behavioral problems. Children with learning disabilities frequently become depressed because of their frustration with school, particularly if the disorder is not recognized or special academic assistance is not provided. Depression that is not a response to the stress of an event is termed *primary depression.* Primary depression is a depressive syndrome with identifiable symptoms; its etiology is not clearly understood, however.

It is important to distinguish between the child who has depressive feelings and the child who has a depressive syndrome. Many children feel sad at some point during a day, but the sadness does not last all day or for several days. For example, in an interview with a nurse, one 10-year-old girl said that she felt sad but the sadness went away when she talked to her mother or when she woke up the next day. Unlike this child, depressed children have sad feelings that persist for significantly longer periods. One depressed child reported to the nurse that she could not remember the last time she felt happy or had a good time.

Causes of Mood Disorders in Children

Mood disorders may be caused by grief. Grief reactions in most children are not well understood. The timing of extended grief, which is considered pathologic in children, is not defined and may vary across the developmental stages. Children also may rework grief reactions when they enter new developmental stages. Some children with major life changes, such as parental divorce or a move to a new community, fail to make transitions within a reasonable amount of time. In addition to difficulties in adjustment (such as not making friends or a decrease in school performance), the child may be sad. These situations, however, are not usually viewed as primary depression because the sadness is secondary to adjustment problems.

Mood disorders in children have been explained by genetic factors, biochemical factors, drugs, neurologic disorders, psychoanalytic theories, and learning theories (Shaffer and Erhardt 1985). Twin and adoption studies provide genetic evidence for major depressive disorders. Family psychiatric history studies provide evidence for depression occurring throughout families (Grossman et al. 1984). However, these occurrences in families could be related to genetic or environmental influences or both.

The biochemical studies revolve around depletion or elevation of noradrenaline and serotonin. These hypotheses have been tested more extensively in adults and no theory predominates in children. Even the diagnostic usefulness of the dexamethasone suppression test in children is being questioned due to discrepant sensitivity and specificity across studies (Poznanski et al. 1987). Drugs such as stimulants can lead to depressive symptoms in children, as can cerebral hemisphere dysfunction and adrenal hyperplasia (Shaffer and Erhardt 1985).

Psychoanalytic theorists tended to reject the idea of depression in children. This was based on the belief that anger toward a lost object is repressed and results in guilt and loss of self-esteem leading to depression. Since superego development is not developed in the child, psychoanalysts believed guilt could not occur. Interest in children's reactions to maternal separation and loss developed in the 1920s and has continued with Bowlby's (1973) theory that early loss can predispose a child to depression in later years. However, early loss is difficult to research as there are many confounding variables.

Learning theorists discuss how depression in an individual is the result of inadequate reinforcement in the environment. Theorists are beginning to examine the reciprocity of depression in the marital couple, but efforts to develop a family systems model of depression that incorporates children are primitive at best.

Symptoms and Signs of Depression in Children

Children differ from adults in the biologic, developmental, and cognitive manifestations of depression, although depressive symptoms in adolescents are similar to depressive symptoms in adults. Little has been published on the developmental aspects of the clinical manifestations of depression in children. The possibility of a depressive syndrome even in infancy is beginning to be explored by a few researchers.

Children with mood disorders exhibit depressed affect or dysphoria, which generally lasts a minimum of one to four weeks. Poznanski (1982) described nonverbal signs of sadness such as fleeting smiles and a bland, frozen look. Even the most experienced nurses might not be able to identify sadness in the face of a child if they are looking for characteristic adult features. Poznanski also distinguished between verbal and nonverbal sadness, because children might appear sad but verbally deny these feelings. Children use a variety of terms such as *bad, gloomy, blue, empty,* and *not able to stand it* (Puig-Antich et al. 1980) to describe sad feelings. The nurse needs to listen carefully to the child's description.

Anhedonia or the inability to enjoy oneself or have fun, is the most characteristic symptom of depression in children. Play is a primary experience in a child's day. Children who are questioned about their activities typically report several interests, whereas a depressed child might have difficulty thinking of one enjoyable thing. One depressed child, for example, spent many hours watching television but could not remember what he had watched. Children

occasionally experience boredom, but a child who reports being bored 50 to 90 percent of the time is probably anhedonic.

By middle childhood, children with a positive self-concept can describe their appearance, schoolwork, and friendships positively. A child with a poor self-concept is more likely to describe personal characteristics negatively and report the use of derogatory nicknames by other children as if they were accurate.

RESEARCH NOTE

Citation

Stull M, Deatrich J. Measuring parental participation: Part I. Issues Compr Pediatr Nurs *1986;9:157–165.*

Study Problem/Purpose

To identify specific activities pertaining to parental involvement during a child's hospitalization.

Methods

Data were collected from twenty-four parents using a semistructured interview guide and daily diary and then transcribed. A qualitative approach was used to do a content analysis of the data into categories. A panel of nineteen nurse experts was used to assess content validity of the categories.

Findings

Eleven parental involvement activities were identified and were supported through the literature review. The activities included active playing, quiet times, child's schoolwork, general comforting, routine physical needs, spending time with other hospitalized children, spending time with parents/family members, spending time alone for rest and relaxation, parent programs, and conferences with staff. The activities were judged to be appropriate by 82 percent or more of the experts. Three conceptual categories of activities were derived from the experts: direct/child oriented; indirect/child oriented; and refueling/parent oriented.

Implications

This research-based information was applied to nursing practice by developing a reliable, valid, and easily administered questionnaire for staff nurses to use in the assessment of parental participation activities. This is described in a subsequent article. This article is a model for the development of a systematic assessment and program to involve parents in their child's psychiatric hospitalization.

Social withdrawal is also characteristic of depressed children but must be distinguished from the withdrawal of a child who has never developed good peer relationships. Many depressed children had good peer relationships at one time but now report that, "I have no friends," or "The kids don't like me." The withdrawn child might reject opportunities to play with other children or watch other children play.

Schoolwork is often impaired when a child is depressed, even though the child may previously have done well in school. The impaired schoolwork may be the result of the general apathy, an inability to concentrate, or distraction by internal stimuli.

Children who are depressed are often preoccupied with morbid thoughts, typically about themselves or others dying. For example, one child drew himself in a family drawing as if he was thinking of his grandmother who had died 2 years earlier. Suicidal thoughts, plans, or actions are also reported by depressed children. Children are influenced by their parents' suffering and mood. One 7-year-old girl tried to jump out of a car on a busy expressway. Her mother had also been depressed and suicidal following the imprisonment of the child's father, who had committed several violent crimes. Professionals and parents must acknowledge that children do think about suicide and may try to kill themselves.

Associated symptoms of depression include irritability, weeping, and somatic complaints. Irritable children are easily bothered by the smallest event. Some depressed children cry more than their peers, feel like crying frequently, or appear to be about to cry. Depressed children might complain of minor aches and pains that have no organic cause (Poznanski 1982).

Symptoms and Signs of Mania in Children

A depressed child will occasionally have some symptoms of mania. Manic symptoms are difficult to diagnose in children, although in adolescents the symptoms resemble adult symptoms. One study identified the following manic symptoms in children (Puig-Antich et al. 1980):

- Elation, expansive mood: elevated mood and/or optimistic attitude about the future lasting four hours and being out of proportion to the circumstance

- Decreased need for sleep: less need for sleep than usual in order to feel rested

- Unusually energetic: more active than usual without expected fatigue

- Increase in goal-directed activity: more active in scholastic, social, or leisure activities (e.g., new projects, telephone calls, letter writing) compared with usual activity

- Grandiosity: increased self-esteem and approval of own worth, power, or knowledge compared with usual level

- Accelerated, pressured, or increased amount of speech: rapid or continual talking that can't be stopped

- Racing thoughts: thoughts racing through mind, having more ideas than usual or more ideas than can be handled

- Flight of ideas: accelerated speech with abrupt changes from topic to topic usually based on understandable associations, distracting stimuli, or play on words

- Poor judgment: excessive involvement in dangerous activities without recognition of potential for painful consequences

- Distractability: difficulty focusing attention on questions; jumping from one thing to another; failure to keep track of answers; and drawn by irrelevant stimuli that cannot be shut off

- Motor hyperactivity: constant movement, e.g., pacing up and down

Symptoms of depression and mania in children often occur in other psychiatric disorders in children. The diagnosis of a mood disorder is made on the basis of a composite of symptoms.

Suicide

Youth suicide has increased threefold over the last two decades. It continues to rise although there has been a major increase in awareness of the children at risk by both parents and professionals. In addition, it is estimated that the rate is at least four times greater than reported because professionals and families collude to maintain the myth that no child could feel so despairing as to end his or her own life.

Coroners rarely label a child's death suicide even when the child's intent is clear. Parents of a child who has committed suicide may feel too guilty or too concerned about the opinions of family and friends to acknowledge the suicide. The following example illustrates denial and lack of information in parents of a suicidal child.

A 10-year-old boy set up a rope over a door to hang himself. His attempt was stopped by his parents. The door, a second entrance to the room, was painted shut and the subject of suicide was not discussed. His parents failed to recognize the same symptoms in the child two years later. However, at this time, severe behavior problems in school and pressure by school personnel forced the parents to bring the child for a psychiatric evaluation.

The topic of youth suicide is one of the most difficult issues for professionals. Even as they gain more knowledge and clinical expertise, professionals must continue to try to understand how it feels to be so desperate and what intervention can really give the youth hope. Intensive efforts are being undertaken to deal with this problem. During 1985, designated the Year of Youth in America, a group of professionals, the National Committee for Youth Suicide, and the Department of Health and Human Services planned and held the first national conference on youth suicide with a theme of "Choose Life."

Many factors place youth at risk for suicide. These factors include:

- Depression
- Psychosis
- Impulsive traits
- Substance abuse
- Incomplete developmental tasks
- Lack of family cohesion
- Overemphasis on achievement
- Frequent exposure to aggression
- Lack of religious identification
- Losses (e.g., peers, relationships)
- Poor school performance
- Family factors, such as frequent moves, deprivation of love and attention, marital conflict, parental unemployment, parental losses, suicidal behavior in other family members, and poor management of divorce

Disruptive Behavior Disorders

The DSM-IIIR lists three basic categories under the heading of **disruptive behavior disorders.** They are **attention deficit-hyperactivity disorder, oppositional defiant disorder,** and **conduct disorder.** The following criteria for these disorders assist child psychiatric professionals in not only differentiating among the behavior disorders but also in sorting out behavior that may be associated with other primary disorders. Children often act out with disruptive behavior during the course of affective disorders. Also since disruptive behavior is more likely to come to the attention of school and police authorities, it is most often the immediate cause for referral for psychiatric services.

Knowledge of the sets of behaviors specific to each diagnostic category aides the nurse in the assessment phase. Few children will exhibit all the behaviors in a category. More commonly they exhibit behaviors across categories. In addition normal healthy children may at times exhibit individual behaviors within diagnostic categories. The task of the multidisciplinary treatment team in child psychiatry is to sort out from all the behavior of the child the number, extent, and duration of behaviors that have become a problem and find a fit between the behavior and diagnostic category to provide appropriate treatment.

Attention Deficit-Hyperactivity Disorder

Attention deficit-hyperactivity disorder is characterized by three criteria. Onset must occur before the age of 7 years, it must not occur only during the course of autistic disorder, and the episode must be for a period of six months or more in which a set of the following behaviors has been present:

- Has difficulty remaining seated when required
- Fidgets with hands or feet or squirms in seat
- Has difficulty playing quietly and sustaining attention to tasks or play activities
- Talks excessively
- Shifts from one uncompleted activity to another and has difficulty following through on instructions from others (not due to oppositional behavior or failure of comprehension)—e.g., fails to finish chores
- Is easily distracted by extraneous stimuli
- Interrupts or intrudes on others (e.g., butts into other children's games)
- Blurts out answers to questions before they have been completed and has difficulty waiting turn in games or group situations
- Engages in physically dangerous activities without considering possible consequences (not for the purpose of thrill-seeking)—e.g., runs into the street without looking
- Is extremely messy or sloppy
- Loses things necessary for tasks or activities at school or at home (e.g., toys, pencils, books, assignments)
- Doesn't seem to listen when spoken to

Oppositional Defiant Disorder

Oppositional defiant disorder may occur between 3 and 18 years of age, must be of more than 6 months duration, and consist of a combination from a set of behaviors. The behaviors must be present other than during the course of another disorder like conduct disorder, or hypomanic or manic episode. This child frequently argues with adults; loses his or her temper; and is angry, resentful, spiteful, or vindictive. He or she often actively defies or refuses adult requests or rules (e.g., refuses to do chores at home), often deliberately does things that annoy other people (e.g., grabs another child's hat), and is often touchy or easily annoyed by others. The child often swears or uses obscene language, blames others for his or her own mistakes, and bullies or is mean to other children (other than physically cruel).

Conduct Disorder

Conduct disorder is the appropriate diagnosis if the individual is not 18 or older and the following behaviors have been present for a period of six months or more:

- Often is truant, "borrows" other children's possessions without permission in situations in which obtaining permission is expected, cheats in games with other children or in school work, and initiates physical fights
- May have run away from home overnight at least twice while living in parental or parental surrogate home, but not as a direct reaction to physical or sexual abuse, used a weapon in more than one fight, forced someone into sexual activity, or been physically cruel to animals or to other people (e.g., tied another child to a tree)
- May have deliberately destroyed others' property (other than fire-setting), deliberately engaged in fire-setting, and had voluntary sexual intercourse that began unusually early for general subculture
- May have regularly used tobacco, liquor, or other non-prescribed drugs and began regular use unusually early for general subculture
- Often lies (other than to avoid physical or sexual abuse); has broken into someone else's house, building, or car; has stolen outside the home without confrontation of a victim on more than one occasion (including forgery); or has confronted a victim (e.g., mugging, purse-snatching, extortion, armed robbery)

Tic Disorders

Tic disorders, which are often called habit spasms, are rapid, rhythmic, involuntary movements of individual muscle groups. Fifteen percent of all children develop transient tic disorders in the school years. These include such common symptoms as grimacing, eye blinking, nose puckering, and squinting. These disorders are more common in males, may run in families, and may occur in clusters. Stress, such as excitement and fatigue, may accentuate these habits.

Tourette syndrome is the most debilitating tic disorder, being a chronic and usually lifelong disorder, and occurring as early as two years of age. The disorder includes compulsions, meaningful utterances, simple tics, or fast meaningful sounds. The most disturbing symptom is **coprolalia**, a complex phonic tic, which consists of uttering obscene and aggressive words and statements.

Assessment and treatment of these children are difficult and complicated. Cohen et al. (1985) have developed a detailed symptom checklist that nurses and parents can use to record specific simple, phonic, and behavior symptoms. The most effective treatments for the motor and phonic symptoms are pharmacologic treatments such as neuroleptics. These medications have the potential to cause serious side-effects, however, and the children need to be monitored carefully.

Elimination Disorders

The most common type of **elimination disorder** is **functional enuresis**, a chronic, involuntary passage of urine during sleep in children age five or older. Younger enuretic children may also have occasional or regular daytime incontinence or urinary frequency or urgency during the day. This condition, which is most common in males, should be differentiated from nocturnal incontinence caused by medical diseases such as diabetes or bladder infections. About one fifth of enuretic children have psychiatric symptoms. Most enuretic children are distressed by the condition.

The most effective interventions with enuretic children include working with the parents to set up a behavioral program, which may include the use of a bell that wakes the child up when he starts to urinate. Medications are sometimes used to treat this disorder. Small doses of imipramine (Tofranil) have been found to be the most effective in numerous drug studies (Shaffer et al. 1985). The action of imipramine on enuresis is not clear. However, it is known that the action is more than an anticholinergic effect, since anticholinergic drugs do not suppress enuresis.

Functional encopresis is repeated passage of feces of normal or near normal consistency into places not appropriate for that person. The passage may be voluntary or involuntary and the occurrence must be at least once a month for six months. The child must be at least 4 years old and must not have a disorder such as a ganglionic megacolon.

Language and Speech Disorders

Most children achieve language by age 4 years. However, many neurophysical and psychologic disorders can interfere with speech and language. Childhood **language and speech disorders** can be separate, overlap, or coexist.

Speech abnormalities include voice, rhythm, and articulation disorders. These disorders are caused by a physical defect such as cleft palate, functional difficulties, processing difficulties, involuntary movements, and mental retardation. Language allows persons to communicate by putting perceptions and concepts of the world into words. Inadequate language skills can interfere with listening, speaking, reading, and writing in the learning situation. Language disorders include deviations in syntax (grammar), content (semantics), or pragmatics (use) from age-expected behavior. Language disorders can be primary or secondary to other conditions such as mental retardation, psychiatric disorders, hearing impairment, or deprivation.

Intervention for language disorders optimally begins within the first four years of life. Speech and language pathologists and audiologists diagnose and provide treatment, which can include a parent-child program, individual therapy, and group therapy. If children with language disorders are not treated, they are at risk for developing learning problems. The efforts of the specialists should be coordinated with those of schools, which typically offer a broad continuum of possible services. Children with these disorders usually need long-term services and monitoring but do very well with early intervention.

Autistic Disorder

Prior to the development of a classification system for psychiatric disorders in children, autism tended to be viewed as a psychotic disorder. This was related to the difficulty in reality testing and the grossly abnormal behavior displayed by autistic children. More recently, however, an appreciation of the pervasive effects on development of these children led to establishment of a new category, **pervasive developmental disorders. Autistic disorder** is the only subgroup of this category. Autism is a rare disorder and is more frequent in boys. However, a larger number of children with other developmental disorders display autistic-like features. Developmental disorders to a less severe degree are quite common in children.

The diagnosis is based on an extensive developmental history, including prenatal and postnatal factors. Also considered are language, social interaction, play, developmental milestones, aggressiveness, destructiveness, habits, routines, disturbance in conduct, somatic disturbances, affect, and cognitions.

The diagnostic criteria include onset before 30 months of age, deviant social development, deviant language development, stereotyped behavior and routines, and the absence of delusions, hallucinations, and schizophrenic-type thought disorder. Mental retardation is present in about three fourths of the children, and mentally retarded children may show some of the features of this disorder. Neurodevelopmental disorders such as poor coordination are often seen in the children with this disorder (Rutter and Hensov 1985). No child with autism shows all the behaviors.

Deviant social development is most often demonstrated by a lack of emotional responsiveness and social reciprocity along with failure to bond. The parents may describe how the child never differentiated the parent from other adults. The child does not come to the parents for comfort when ill, hurt, or tired. These children tend to treat people as inanimate objects.

Deviant language development is first seen in the child's inability to understand spoken language and lack of response to language. Babble, gesture, or mime may not be present or may be less than usual. Parents describe the child as not greeting them or as failing to mold or stiffening when they pick the child up. These children tend to produce little speech and are unable to carry on a conversation.

Stereotypic behaviors and routines are the third set of characteristics of autistic children. Rocking, hand flicking or twisting, and spinning are examples of stereotypic body movements. The child may insist that the same routine be followed every time he or she is involved in an activity such as shopping. The child may become severely distressed over minor changes in the environment (e.g., a piece of furniture moved out of its usual place).

Schizophrenic Disorder

Schizophrenic disorder can be found in children as young as age 5 years, but it is rare in children before age 6 or 8. Onset in adolescence is more common. Prepubertal onset of schizophrenia is in fact rarer than pervasive developmental disorders. Schizophrenic disorder in childhood is differentiated from pervasive developmental disorders by the presence of hallucinations or delusions. Tanquay and Cantor (1986) describe children at least 6 years of age who have been diagnosed as schizophrenic (using DSM-IIIR criteria). These children have a thought disorder and symptoms including excessive anxiety, constricted affect, speech abnormalities, bizarre ideas and fantasies, morbid thoughts, lack of peer relationships, primitive defense mechanisms, and concrete thinking.

Incidence

The incidence of psychotic disorders in children is difficult to estimate because of the inconsistency of diagnostic measures. Studies agree that the disorder is rare, occurring in fewer than 1 of every 1000 children (Werry 1982). Psychosis in children is rare compared with the adult incidence (Achenbach 1982). Males are more likely to develop schizophrenia prior to puberty. Schizophrenic disorder in children is so rare that the psychiatric nurse is unlikely to come in contact with such a child.

Symptoms and Signs

Schizophrenic disorder is a complex disorder with a variety of severe and bizarre symptoms, and it is difficult to diagnose. Cantor (1982) began to specify the developmental variations of this disorder in children and adolescents and has compiled a comprehensive physical description. However, researchers have not reached a general consensus regarding the associated characteristics and variations. Any child with a schizophrenic disorder exhibits only some of the characteristic symptoms.

Both hallucinations and delusions are rare before adolescence. In addition, research has shown little agreement about what constitutes a childhood hallucination. Hallucinations in children can be confused with other mental phenomena, such as fantasies, obsessions, imaginary play objects and companions, and dreams. Researchers have tried to distinguish between these processes and hallucinations by describing the characteristics of the hallucinations as bizarre and nonvolitional (Rothstein 1981). The following clinical example illustrates hallucinations and delusions as experienced by a child.

Doris, an 11-year-old, described hearing the voice of her mother calling her name and yelling at her, although her mother was not present. At times, she heard her own voice telling her to do things such as chores for her mother. She experienced her mother's voice as coming from outside her head and her own voice as coming from inside her head. She reported seeing a woman who looked like her mother and she thought was her mother. She also believed that her mother was watching her. Doris described going to the bathroom in the morning and "daydreaming" that objects were weapons (e.g., Q-tips were sticks to stab people, and washcloths were used to smother people). All these experiences seemed real to Doris as they happened. Doris also believed that the world was coming to an end. She described hearing on the news that a hole was breaking apart pieces of the earth, and she thought this was going to happen. She also expressed concern that a heat wave might result in there not being enough air to breathe.

Schizophrenic disordered children exhibit developmental delays, particularly in speech. Speech may be monotonous, or the child may speak very little. Afflicted children may have eating and sleeping disturbances, with such behaviors as picky food preferences, taking prolonged periods to complete meals, and wandering around during the night. Mannerisms include activities such as pacing, rocking, and head banging. Repetitive behaviors are more frequently seen in children with schizophrenic disorder than in schizophrenic adults. Many questions about etiology (e.g., contribution of genetics and family social behaviors), manifestations (e.g., neurologic signs), and treatment remain unanswered. These questions continue to be pursued because of the severe disruption of the child's life (Tanquay and Cantor 1986).

THE NURSING PROCESS IN CHILD PSYCHIATRIC NURSING

Child psychiatric nursing may be carried out in the outpatient psychiatric department, day program, or in-patient psychiatric unit of a medical center; a community mental health center or community agency; a therapeutic school; or a private practitioner's office. If the child has a medical card he or she will most likely be treated in a public agency. However, increasing numbers of children are being treated in medical centers because of the limited amount of outpatient reimbursement available from insurance carriers. Families in health maintenance organizations have limited access to psychiatric services, particularly in-patient services.

Schools are required by law to provide special education services for handicapped students including those with psychiatric disorders. However, it is becoming increasingly difficult for school districts to provide tuition reimbursement for children to attend therapeutic schools (other than the services of that district) or to be placed in residential care.

Assessment

Nursing assessment in child psychiatry is a multistep process.

Basic Assessment of Child

The basic assessment of a child includes both psychosocial and physical components and is a necessary first step in initiating the plan of care. During this phase, information is gathered from the parents as well as from the child client. The nurse needs to obtain not only such information as allergies and hygiene habits (about which children are usually poor historians) but also information on the child's and parents' views of the difficulties. A nursing assessment guideline is provided in Box 34–2.

A physical condition may precipitate a behavioral problem, so a complete physical examination is necessary to

---

Box 34–2
CHILD PSYCHIATRIC NURSING ASSESSMENT GUIDELINES

Demographic data: Name, age, date

Past history: Birth history, allergies, illnesses, medication

History of the presenting problem

Child's definition of the problem

Activities of daily living: Nutrition—weight, schedules, preferences; sleep—habits, quality; elimination—habits, problems; handicaps, limitations

Physical assessment: Skin, head, hair, eyes, ears, nose, mouth, respiratory, cardiovascular, musculoskeletal, neurologic

Social assessment: Living arrangement, play activities, family health history, legal status, family visiting plan

Mental status: Mood, thought process, and content; hallucinations, perceptions; speech, orientation; suicidal ideation, homicidal ideation

---

rule out any medical problems. For example, children with chronic physical conditions such as diabetes or asthma often develop disruptive behaviors in an attempt to cope with and regain control of their environment and their symptoms. A physical examination will also establish a baseline in the event psychopharmacologic treatment is indicated. The physical examination may also be used to rule out child abuse. Children with psychiatric disorders are frequently referred for neurologic evaluations to rule out disorders such as seizures.

From this initial assessment the nurse not only sets a care plan in motion but also determines what behaviors need to be assessed in greater depth in the second phase of assessment.

Regular assessments of all children in all settings include evaluation of growth and development, physical health, academic skills, and risk factors. Assessment of these areas are the basis for primary prevention of psychiatric problems in children. Nurses are well prepared to participate in assessment of these areas and to educate others, such as parents, about the growth and development of the child. Nurses frequently are in a position to observe risk factors such as environmental factors, family characteristics, and characteristics of the child that make him or her vulnerable to risk (e.g., of developmental disabilities, accidents, illnesses).

More comprehensive diagnostic assessments are indicated when children are demonstrating symptoms such as acting out, school failure, withdrawal, or inability to cope with tasks. The most comprehensive diagnostics are typically done in multidisciplinary diagnostic programs. A diagnostic evaluation may range from a one-session interview with the child and parents to several sessions. In addi-

tion, in-patient units provide a twenty-four-hour milieu in which to evaluate the child in the entire life space.

Life Space Interview

The second phase of assessment occurs in the milieu in what Redl (1966) referred to as the life space interview. Redl and many others maintain that it may take several interviews to obtain a complete assessment. The child is best assessed during normal daily routines and activities over a period of time. The initial time frame for in-patient care is a week to ten days with revisions based on on-going assessment over the length of stay. Since the routines of most child units mimic the usual daily routines of children, the nurse is able to see in action the child's social skills with peers and adults, self-care abilities, and mental status. The nurse then places this information in the context of the child's developmental stage to assess for age appropriateness. The assessment is done sometimes by observation but more often as part of direct interaction with the child. What appears to the outsider as simple play may be attempts to assess such qualities as creativity, attention span, and frustration tolerance. The nurse is then able to develop a more individualized nursing treatment plan and to contribute to the multidisciplinary plan by verifying the type, amount, and extent of the behaviors present.

Family Assessment

A family assessment is an essential part of a complete diagnostic workup of the child. The family assessment shifts the focus from the individual child to the family system. Each person is asked to identify what he or she sees as the problem in the family and what the family has done about it. An attempt is made to understand what the child's symptoms and current episode mean in terms of the family dynamics. Symptoms in other members or marital, sibling, or parent dyads are noted. An assessment is made of the potential for change within the system and the need for marital or family therapy. (See Chapter 33 for specifics.)

Nursing Diagnosis

Ideally, the diagnostic assessment of the child culminates in the formation of both nursing and medical diagnoses, which are summarized in a multidisciplinary staff conference. Examples of psychiatric nursing diagnoses and DSM-IIIR diagnoses related to children are discussed in the Nursing Care Plan later in this chapter. The DSM-IIIR Axis

IV rating is made more specific to children by using the Severity of Psychosocial Stressors Scale: Children and Adolescents in Table 12–3 in Chapter 12. The child's general social, psychologic, and academic functioning is described using the Global Assessment of Functioning Scale (GAF Scale) in Table 12–4 in Chapter 12.

Planning and Implementing Interventions

Although the medical and nursing diagnoses may suggest certain standard interventions, each child must be considered individually. Intervention with the emotionally disturbed child and family involves an interdisciplinary approach determined by the child's age, developmental level, symptoms, parents' commitment, economic resources, and accessibility of services. Nurses are involved in either primary or collaborative roles in the various treatment modalities, including:

- Psychotherapy, play therapy
- Social skills training
- Psychopharmacology
- Milieu (routines, rules, peer pressure)
- Group modalities (including milieu meeting, group therapy, psychodrama)
- Occupational therapy (including art therapy, recreation therapy, sensory-motor integration)
- Parent approaches (including counseling, psychoeducation, family therapy, parent education, support groups)
- Placement (in a regular classroom with teacher consultation, therapeutic classroom, therapeutic day school, partial hospitalization, in-patient care, or residential care)

If the child is in a therapeutic milieu, the Joint Commission on Accreditation of Hospitals (JACH) mandates weekly multidisciplinary staff conferences on every client. The plan is developed at the initial conference and revised as indicated. The components of the multidisciplinary treatment plan (MTP) include:

- Problems
- Goals (measurable, specific)
- Interventions (frequency)
- Responsible staff
- Target dates

Longitudinal follow-up of children with a severe emotional disorder is essential. Further episodes may be prevented with early detection of symptoms. In addition, children often regress following the return home from an in-patient hospitalization.

Nursing Goals

The following are some common nursing goals in working with children with severe psychiatric disorders:

- Meet the child's emotional/recognitional needs.
- Reduce the child's tension and need for defensive behavior.
- Help the child form a relationship with another person (a personal object relationship).
- Help the child develop a sense of self-identity.
- Offer the child an opportunity to regress and relive previous developmental stages that were unsuccessfully resolved.
- Help the child learn to communicate effectively.
- Prevent the child from hurting self or others.
- Help the child maintain physical health.
- Help the child form relationships with others.
- Promote appropriate reality testing by the child.

Play Therapy*

The treatment modality most widely used with children is **play therapy.** Play therapy lets children use their natural medium of expression to resolve conflicts (Figure 34–2). The play therapist adds the further resource of an accepting, understanding adult.

Functions of Play

Play has many functions. Children use play to:

- Master and assimilate past experiences over which they had no control
- Communicate with their unconscious constructs or needs
- Communicate with others
- Explore and experiment while learning how to relate to self, the world, and others
- Compromise between the demands of drives and the dictates of reality

Play therapy offers the child a safe place to explore all the uses of play, thus dealing with conflictual material, devel-

---

*This section was contributed to the second edition by Pamela Burton.

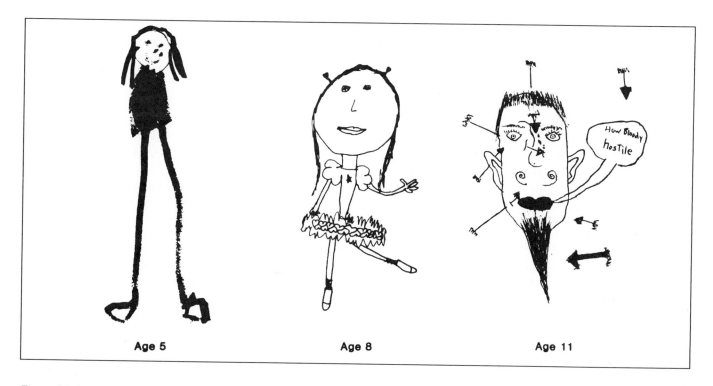

Age 5   Age 8   Age 11

Figure 34–2
Art therapy as a form of play therapy helps children communicate about their subjective
reality in these self-portraits.

oping a healthy self-image, and learning about self in relation to the therapist. In short, play therapy offers the
opportunity for growth under stable conditions.

Play is used in many different ways in child psychiatry:

- Recreation and socialization in day programs and in-
  patient milieus
- Rewards in therapeutic classrooms for children
  accomplishing their work (e.g., when you finish your
  math, you can play a board game with the staff)
- An activity during the child's one-to-one time with his
  or her primary nurse
- A method of evaluation or treatment of sensorimotor
  deficits

Role of the Play Therapist

The role of play therapist is not a passive one, but it is
essentially nondirective. The child sets the pace and does
the work. The therapist contributes personally as an
accepting and understanding adult whose goal is to foster
the child's development of self. The relationship between

the child and therapist is a new experience for the child,
one that does not translate effectively outside the play therapy situation. The therapist accepts these children fully as
they are, yet maintains the belief that they can change and
grow. As they begin to trust the relationship, children can
use it as a context for trying out new ways of behaving and
relating to themselves and others.

Dynamics of Play Therapy

The acceptance the therapist shows these children can help
them evolve a new self-image. Fearful and passive children
may be able to try out some assertive or aggressive behavior. Consistently aggressive children may explore new ways
to meet their needs. Children who perceive themselves as
worthless may eventually accept the therapist's message
that they are valuable, worthwhile people. In some cases,
it may be a matter of educating the child to the possibility
of different interactive patterns. It is difficult for young
children to think of theoretical alternatives. They may believe
that a dysfunctional family interactional pattern is the only
possible one. Given a new pattern, they can explore new
behavior. As their conflicts begin to be resolved and as

confidence and trust evolve from the therapeutic relationship, their tension decreases, and they can expand their new awareness outside the therapeutic relationship.

Setting for Play Therapy

Ideally, play therapy is done in a well-equipped playroom. Toys might include dollhouse and furniture, puppets, dolls, blocks, art materials (Play-Doh, clay, paper, crayons, paints, marking pens), toy animals, telephone, cars and trucks, play kitchen, musical instruments, toy soldiers and guns, checkers and other games, and clothes for make-believe. (This kind of equipment is not strictly necessary. The nurse who is helping the fearful child overcome a terror of injections by letting the child handle the injection paraphernalia is also doing play therapy.) The toys stay in the playroom, and children use them there.

In the initial session, the therapist tells the children the playroom is for them to use as they please during the time they are there, and sets the limits (usually the minimal ones of not hurting self or therapist or breaking equipment). Usually, therapists will try to find out children's perceptions of what's going on by asking them why they are there. Therapists will offer briefly their own understanding for the referral (i.e., you're having trouble in school). How things proceed from there is largely up to the child. Most children are eager to use the playroom situation and the presence of an accepting, consistent, and understanding adult to resolve conflicts and try out different ways of relating to self and others.

The following example illustrates a child's use of play.

A 12-year-old female had been sexually molested by her father. Her father was sent to prison for the sexual molestation of another preschooler. During the 12-year-old's therapy session, she asked the nurse therapist to go to the playroom. She built a fortress of large multicolor blocks. She put a chair inside the structure and sat down stating, "This is a dungeon. A rainbow dungeon." Her play demonstrated her ambivalent feelings toward her father (i.e., loss and resentment).

Group Therapy

Verbal group therapy with children tends to be most effective with adolescents or older prepubertal children. Verbal, insightful children are particularly good candidates. Children with a severe disruptive disorder may not be appropriate group candidates as they may disrupt the process

and require the sole attention of the therapist. Activity therapy may be more effective with the prepubertal age group. For example, a psychiatric nurse-psychodramatist in an in-patient unit developed a sociodrama play group where children are encouraged to improvise fairy tales, stories, or fantasies in a theater format followed by a discussion. (Psychodrama and sociodrama are discussed in Chapter 30.)

Psychopharmacology

Although the findings in psychopharmacology research with adults have been impressive (see Chapters 9 and 32), child psychopharmacology is less well developed. This can be explained by the typical lag between adult and child psychiatry, the unavailability of drug studies on children, and the concern for unknown developmental risks (e.g., Ritalin can cause growth retardation). Drugs have been used with children to decrease behavioral symptoms rather than to treat syndromes as with adults.

Medications Used With Children

Stimulants are the most commonly used medications with children and have been studied more often than other medications. Stimulants have been shown to increase ability to use cognitive skills, but not cognitive capacity, in hyperactive and normal children. These medications include amphetamine (Benzedrine), methylphenidate (Ritalin), and pemoline (Cylert).

Antidepressants are used to treat depression, school phobia, attention deficit disorder, and enuresis. Even though several studies have demonstrated the effectiveness of tricyclics in a limited number of cases of enuresis, the exact mechanism is not known. Children may become tolerant, have symptom breakthrough, or have only temporary responses (Greenhill 1985). A few clinicians and researchers have demonstrated the efficacy of antidepressants in prepubertal depression, although there is some disagreement about appropriate plasma levels (Weller 1983). The Food and Drug Administration limits the use of these medications with children because of cardiotoxicity. Imipramine (Tofranil) is the tricyclic antidepressant most commonly used with children as it is less cardiotoxic than other tricyclic medications. Nurses should administer these medications only under the orders of a physician with FDA exemption who uses strict procedure for monitoring cardiac effects and blood serum levels. MAO inhibitors are not used with children because of the severe side-effects and the difficulty in controlling children's diet.

Lithium (Lithonate) has been found to be the most effective drug for the treatment of mania. Since manic symptoms occur infrequently in children, this drug is not often used. Lithium is sometimes used to treat autistic, aggressive, and undersocialized conduct disordered children (Campbell 1985). This work is preliminary and there are few controlled studies.

Although frequently used in child psychiatry, neuroleptics do not have a specific target disorder in school-aged children. One study described the use of haloperidol (Haldol) in managing behavior such as fidgetiness, stereotypies, and hyperactivity in children with pervasive disorders (Campbell 1985). The most common use of neuroleptics in children is to sedate retarded children who are institutionalized, although this use is often inappropriate. Neuroleptics should be used sparingly with children because of side-effects and unknown effects.

Nurses play an important role in monitoring the child on medication and educating the child and parents about the medication. Side-effects of the pharmacologic agents most commonly used in children are listed in Table 34–1.

Side-effects should be monitored daily in in-patient settings and weekly in outpatient settings. Monitoring of side-effects is discussed in Chapter 32.

Educating the Child and Parents

Drug holidays are used to assess the difference between drugged and drug-free states and to prevent growth delays. The child and the parents should be prepared for an increase in symptoms when the medication is removed. The nurse records behavior of the child systematically and accurately to provide data by which the physician can make the decision about future medication. If the child is being treated in an outpatient setting, the nurse teaches the parents and teachers to record the behavior. It is also necessary to assess the concerns the child has about side-effects and social stigma with peers related to the medication or the child may fail to go to the school nurse to get the medication.

The nurse assesses parent's individual beliefs and fears about the medications. Parents are often concerned about the potential for the child to become dependent on medication, the side-effects, and stigma. The nurse gives parents an opportunity to discuss their worries and questions and become informed about the medication. This time can be used to guide the parents toward a realistic view of the uncertainty of the medication so they will not anticipate a magical cure. Client information sheets on particular medications are helpful.

Milieu Nursing in Child Psychiatry

The majority of generalists in child psychiatric nursing work in in-patient settings. These settings provide the most intense methods of diagnosis and treatment. In-patient admission is indicated for children in the following situations:

- The child has threatened his or her own life (suicide, eating disorder) or the life of others

- Extreme family pathology interferes with the child's achievement of developmental tasks
- Both physical and emotional disorders are present, and the contribution and interaction of each is unclear in terms of the child's difficulty
- Extended and round-the-clock assessment is indicated
- Initiation, monitoring, and maintenance of medication is indicated
- Outpatient treatment has not been effective
- The child's behavior is progressively deteriorating (regression, psychosis)

Common to milieu treatment of children is the notion that the milieu is a safe holding area for the child in which to accomplish the various therapeutic tasks of the treatment plan. Equally important is the child's need for a predictable environment. These needs are addressed in the structure and routines of a program, reinforced by behavioral management.

Child units have schedules that take up every time frame of the day. Some times, such as school, group therapy, and recreational therapy, are formally structured. Others are routines, such as early morning wakeup, meals, and bedtime, which tend to be more informal. Bedtime, for example, may have the structure of occurring at 9:30 after 9:00 P.M. relaxation, with lights out at 10:00 P.M. Routines include washing up, brushing teeth, putting dirty clothes in the laundry. The children get some personal time to prepare for sleep by putting the day behind them and looking ahead to the next day.

The behavioral focus of the program allows the nursing staff to give continuous feedback to the children about the appropriateness of their behavior within each time frame. The children receive cues such as verbal praise, a sticker, or points, depending on developmental level, for appropriate behavior. Often these cues go together. For example, children who have a problem hitting others all the time may receive a sticker and verbal praise for no hits on an hourly basis until they connect their behavior to the reward. At that time the need for feedback may decrease to a less frequent schedule and to the need for only verbal reminders of the desired behavior.

At the same time staff are trying to reward children for positive behavior, they also need to know that negative behavior will not be tolerated. Typically when children cannot tolerate an activity they are asked to take a "time-out" from the activity by sitting on a chair until able to pull themselves together. If that does not work, the time-out may be taken in a "quiet room" free of objects and stimulation. If isolation is also too difficult, staff may use a restraining hold to help children calm down. As children

	Table 34–1		
Common Side-Effects of Psychopharmacologic Agents in Children			
Category of Drug	**Side-Effect**	**Category of Drug**	**Side-Effect**
Neuroleptics	Blurred vision	Stimulants	Growth slowdown
	Constipation		Headaches
	Convulsions		Initial nausea and vomiting
	Decrease in cognitive functioning		Insomnia
	Difficulty in urination		Irritability
	Dizziness		Loss of appetite and weight
	Dry mouth		Mood changes
	Hypotension	Tricyclic antidepressants	Blurring of vision
	Increase in prolactin (unknown effect on development)		Constipation
			Difficulty in urination
	Jaundice		Dizziness
	Lethargy		Drowsiness
	Sedation		Dry mouth
	Sensitivity to extreme heat or cold or light		Hypertension
			Increased heart rate
	Tardive dyskinesia (long-term use)		Jaundice
			Rash
	Weight gain		Speech problems
Lithium	Constriction of veins		Weakness
	Decrease in cognitive functioning		
	Dizziness		
	Facial pallor		
	Increased blood pressure and pulse		
	Increased thirst		
	Increased urination		
	Nausea/stomach ache		

are able to calm down, staff help them to see how they get into time-outs and how they can avoid them. The goal is to have children learn what precedes episodes where they get out of control and learn ways to avoid the negative consequences of out-of-control behavior such as fights with other children.

Intensive Nursing Care

Staffing in child psychiatric units is based on a low staff-client ratio because of the intensive nature of children's care and meeting the needs of children at different development levels. Children with psychotic disorders present

---

Box 34–3
NURSING CARE OF THE PSYCHOTIC CHILD

1. Assess degree of thought disorder (content and behavior):

   a. Record observations.

   b. Inform physician of escalations.

   c. Note response to psychopharmacology.

2. Encourage reality testing:

   a. Do not reinforce experiences that are not real.

   b. Make simple statements about experiences the child describes that do not exist.

   c. Direct attention to real experiences.

   d. Limit number of thoughts nurse will listen to and number of people available to listen to pressured thoughts.

   e. Help child avoid experiences that increase delusions.

   f. Avoid the use of jokes and puns commonly used with children.

   g. Avoid the unnecessary use of stimuli (such as intercoms or whispering between staff in child's room).

3. Encourage socialization:

   a. Interrupt isolation.

   b. Maintain eye contact with child.

   c. Provide instructions and rewards for appropriate behaviors in social situations.

4. Orient child to routines:

   a. Provide child with frequent data for orientation (such as calendar, clock, references to time and place, the reason for hospitalization, and introducing the staff to the child).

   b. Set up a structured routine for child's day. A chart of the routine could be drawn with clocks and pictures representing the activities.

   c. Discuss child's typical daily routine with the parents.

   d. Explain each procedure clearly and simply.

   e. Keep communication direct, concrete, and simple.

   f. Perform procedures in a consistent manner.

   g. Provide a minimum of changes in nursing staff (provide a primary nurse for each shift).

5. Provide a safe environment for the child:

   a. Supervise child frequently.

   b. Remove dangerous materials from child's room.

---

some of the most difficult management problems. Box 34–3 discusses the nursing care for these children as an example of intensive nursing care in child psychiatry. Another example of the intensive nursing care in child psychiatry is the care of the suicidal child. Box 34–4 describes interventions for these children.

Countertransference in Child Psychiatric Nursing

Working with children, particularly children with emotional problems, may reactivate nurses' feelings about their family of origin or current family. Nurses may then react as if the client were part of that situation rather than responding to the current reality. Staff may also react to children or parents from their own stereotypes or beliefs rather than getting to know each child and parent as an individual. A third possibility is that the nurse can involve clients on the unit in their own conflicts or competition within the staff group. This phenomenon is known as countertransference and is also experienced by pediatric

nurses. The following vignette illustrates a common example of countertransference.

An 11-year-old girl had a history of living with extended family and several hospitalizations. The child's mother was ambivalent toward her, often openly rejecting her (i.e., limited visitations and missed family sessions). The child stimulated a lot of feeling among the staff about bad mothers and good mothers, and the staff was protective of the child and angry at the mother. The staff was encouraged to examine the mother's own deprivation by an abusive mother and the difficulties in raising this very troubled child.

Clinical supervisors and nursing managers can help staff reframe their view of the child and the family, identify personal experiences that limit their perception of the child, and identify unresolved staff issues. Through these explo-

---

Box 34–4
INTERVENTIONS FOR SUICIDAL BEHAVIOR IN CHILDREN AND ADOLESCENTS: A GUIDE FOR PROFESSIONALS, PARENTS, AND PEERS

Step 1: *Listen.* A person in a mental crisis needs someone who will listen to what the person is saying. Every effort should be made to understand the problems behind the statements.

Step 2: *Evaluate the seriousness* of the child's thoughts and feelings. If the child has made clear suicide plans, the problem is more acute than when the child's thinking is less definite.

Step 3: *Evaluate the intensity or severity of the emotional disturbance.* The child might be extremely upset but not suicidal. A change from depression to agitation and restless movement is a possible cause for alarm.

Step 4: *Take seriously every complaint and feeling the child expresses.* Do not dismiss or undervalue what the child is saying. In some instances the child might minimize the difficulty, but beneath an apparent calm profoundly distressed feelings may be present.

Step 5: *Do not be afraid to ask directly if the child has entertained thoughts of suicide.* Suicide might be suggested but not openly mentioned during the crisis period. Experience shows that harm is rarely done by inquiring directly about suicide at an appropriate time. As a matter of fact, the child is frequently glad to have the opportunity to open up and discuss it.

Step 6: *Do not be misled by the child's saying that the emotional crisis has passed.* A youth will often feel initial relief after talking about suicide, but the same thinking recurs later. Follow-up is crucial.

Step 7: *Be affirmative but supportive.* Strong, stable supports are essential in the life of a distressed child. Provide emotional strength by giving the impression that you know what you are doing and that everything possible will be done to help the child.

Step 8: *Evaluate available resources.* The child might have inner resources, including various mechanisms for rationalization and intellectualization, that can be strengthened and supported, and other resources, such as ministers, relatives, and friends, who can be contacted. If these resources are absent, the problem may be more serious.

Step 9: *Act specifically.* Do something tangible: that is, give the child something definite to hang on to such as arranging to see the child later or subsequently contacting another helpful person. Nothing is more frustrating to a child than to feel that nothing has been gained from the discussion.

Step 10: *Obtain appropriate assistance and consultation.* Do not try to handle the problem alone. Seek the advice of physicians, school specialists, mental health professionals, or other knowledgeable persons.

Source: Adapted from Frederick C: Trends in Mental Health: Self-Destructive Behavior Among Younger Age Groups. *US Department of Health, Education and Welfare DHEW Publication No. (ADM) 76-365. NIMH, 1976.*

---

rations staff can work more therapeutically with children and parents and increase their self-awareness.

Working With Families

Earlier milieu treatment tended to provide more of a custodial approach, while the current emphasis is on keeping the child involved with the family and helping the child return as quickly as possible to home and community. Inpatient care is generally becoming more family oriented. Each child participates in the routines and group activities of the unit while individual treatment and family activities are planned according to the special needs of the child.

Child disorders cannot be fully understood or managed without exploring the family context. Research studies have demonstrated that treating the family system produces more rapid and enduring changes.

Professionals often fail to recognize the overwhelming and confusing feelings parents may feel when confronted with the decision to provide psychiatric services for their child. Parents often describe feelings of guilt, depression, anxiety, denial, and embarrassment. In addition, one parent must often make this decision when the spouse is angry and nonsupportive of the plan. Grandparents frequently blame parents for the problem or push the parents not to follow through with treatment. The following example illustrates the anxiety and denial elicited in grandparents when confronted with serious emotional problems in a grandchild.

The maternal grandmother of a suicidal child who was scheduled for admission to an in-patient unit tried to block the admission. She told her daughter just to send the child to stay with her for a while. The child psychiatrist and the child psychiatric nurse spent time with the parents discussing the pressure they experienced from her mother. They reminded the parents of how psychiatric services are unfamiliar to the grandmother's generation. They also reviewed the basis for the recommendation of hospitalization. The parents were encouraged to make their own decision based on their experience with their child and their concerns for her safety. Possible explanations for the grandparents were suggested and the professionals offered to be available to discuss the grandparents' questions and concerns.

Nursing staff often need to help parents plan their visits with the child to avoid perpetuating dysfunctional parent-child interaction. The following example illustrates the type of family problems encountered.

The staff in an in-patient milieu found they needed to help the parents of a 12-year-old boy plan the weekend day passes. The child reported he barely saw his parents while home on pass, and he generally returned early. His mother went to work and his father had an outside activity. The child hung out at the local mall with his friends. This chain of events interfered with the goal of a transition of the child back into the family. The family therapist and primary nurse worked with the family unit to structure the passes to meet the goals of reentry and increase availability of the parents to the child.

Discharge Planning

Prior to discharge from in-patient hospitalization, the parents should meet with each member of the interdisciplinary team to discuss the treatment plan. Parents need to be given this information verbally and in writing. A model for discharge planning is provided in Table 34–2. Conferences are typically held between the interdisciplinary team, the parents, and representatives from the child's community school to develop an individualized educational plan.

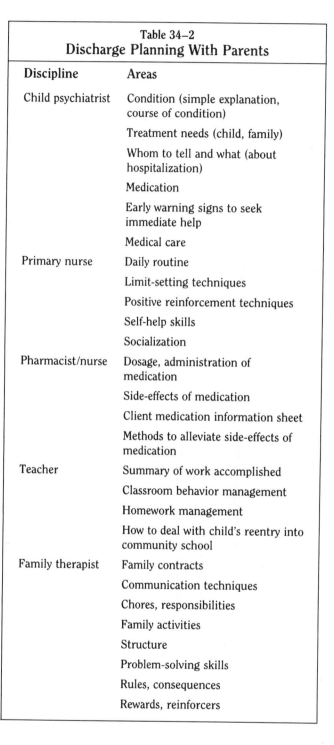

Table 34–2
Discharge Planning With Parents

Discipline	Areas
Child psychiatrist	Condition (simple explanation, course of condition)
	Treatment needs (child, family)
	Whom to tell and what (about hospitalization)
	Medication
	Early warning signs to seek immediate help
	Medical care
Primary nurse	Daily routine
	Limit-setting techniques
	Positive reinforcement techniques
	Self-help skills
	Socialization
Pharmacist/nurse	Dosage, administration of medication
	Side-effects of medication
	Client medication information sheet
	Methods to alleviate side-effects of medication
Teacher	Summary of work accomplished
	Classroom behavior management
	Homework management
	How to deal with child's reentry into community school
Family therapist	Family contracts
	Communication techniques
	Chores, responsibilities
	Family activities
	Structure
	Problem-solving skills
	Rules, consequences
	Rewards, reinforcers

Aftercare

Aftercare is a term used to refer to the plan and implementation for care and treatment after hospitalization of the child. Given the current limitations of third-party payment reimbursement for hospitalization, the priority in health care is abbreviated assessment and establishment of a plan of treatment within the context of limited or no outpatient benefits. Parents need to be involved in the decision-making process, and their wishes are the major determinant. All children who are hospitalized need some type of follow-up. The possible dispositions include:

- Discharge to home and return to the same school
- Foster care
- Day treatment program or special class
- Residential treatment

Family During the hospitalization, parents are encouraged to learn about their part in the child's difficulties. The parent's availability to the child and participation in the treatment is usually an indication of the degree of cooperation that can be anticipated in the outpatient treatment. Parents and children tend to get anxious and fearful at the time of discharge. The child may be concerned about failing and being sent away again. Parents are worried the child may become symptomatic again and they will not be able to manage. The child and parents may experience a honeymoon period following discharge. This is a period where the child shows little evidence of previous difficulties and seems to be making the transition well. During this period the parents may resist aftercare treatment. However, children often regress after a few months, and parents have difficulty maintaining the aftercare program developed in the hospital. The following is an example of the response of parents to the reemergence of their child's problems.

Following the discharge of an 11-year-old male with attention deficit disorder and mood disorder the parents reported everything was going well. School had begun, and the child started doing poorly on tests as he had prior to his admission. The parents were convinced he was going to be rehospitalized. They were frustrated with their own sense of incompetence and angry at the child for defeating himself. They generalized their worries to a longitudinal concern that the child would never accomplish anything worthwhile.

School Personnel

The child reentering school needs help with explaining the absence to peers, since peers tend to be very curious about absences. Often parents put pressure on the child to keep the hospitalization a secret. However, school personnel who do not know the nature of the child's hospitalization are handicapped in facilitating the child's reentry. School personnel may need to maintain an important monitoring role for recurrence of symptoms, particularly if limited outpatient service is feasible. Reentry may be facilitated by participation in a reentry group, encouragement to participate in at least one peer extracurricular activity, and identification of a particular support person for the child in school.

Evaluation

The use of evaluation as part of the nursing care plan for disturbed children has been established in the ANA Standards of Child and Adolescent Psychiatric and Mental Health Nursing Practice, standard VI. The standard states for process criteria that "The nurse (1) pursues validation, suggestions, and new information; (2) evaluates observations, insights, and data with colleagues; and (3) documents the results of evaluation of nursing care" (ANA 1985). The nurse looks to such routine data as vital signs, weights, sleep record, bowel and bladder charts, and other physical findings not only to confirm initial data base findings but also to note changes. Psychopharmacologic treatments are followed especially closely as children are known to reach toxicity quickly and to have many responses to medication not typical to the adult populations on which many drugs are initially tested. The more experienced nurse also develops an awareness of the physical findings that may be associated with emotional disturbance (such as encopresis and abdominal pains), as well as the physical problems that are accompanied by behavioral or psychiatric symptoms (such as Tourette syndrome and seizure disorders).

The behavioral record provides another constant source of information for the child psychiatric nurse. Most treatment units have some sort of provision for the periodic assessment of identified behaviors. To provide effective behavioral management the nurse must frequently evaluate for the client's progress toward identified goals and effectiveness of the reward system for the client. Such responsiveness to the individual needs of the client within a behavioral program enhances the effectiveness of such programs.

As the therapeutic milieu treatment of children involves a much more intense relationship between staff and clients and consistency of approach among staff interacting with the client, the exchange of information with colleagues is essential. The twenty-four-hour assessment of the child going through various daily routines and interactions with others contributes invaluable information to the formulation of care goals for the family as well as the client. Bringing together this information helps the nurse present to client and family a coherent plan, not just one based on a set of limited discrete observations by one person.

Text continues on p. 947.

CASE STUDY: A Child With a Disruptive Disorder and a Mood Disorder

Identifying Information

Rob is a 9-year-old white, Protestant male who is in the fourth grade. He is referred to the in-patient unit for diagnosis and treatment following an out-patient evaluation during which it was determined that his problems were too severe for out-patient management.

Client's Definition of Present Problem, Precipitatory Stresses, Coping Strategies, Goals for Care

Rob and his parents defined the problem as his behavior, primarily his self-destructiveness and aggression toward others. The precipitants for the current crisis include several losses and illnesses in the nuclear and extended family and the potential loss of the father's work. Rob is coping poorly with the losses, and long-term marital problems are accentuated. Rob's understanding of the hospitalization is poor, as he feels he's here because others "pick on me." The goals include:

1. Preventing injury to self or others
2. Providing an intensive twenty-four-hour evaluation
3. Determining appropriateness of psychopharmacologic treatment
4. Providing family support and intervention
5. Encouraging effective peer socialization

History of Present Problem

For the past two months, Rob has shown evidence of suicidal ideation (e.g., writing a note saying "I want to kill myself."). He draws morbid pictures and worries about family members dying. He also writes "I hate myself." Rob recently threatened to take his father's pills so he wouldn't have to go to school. Rob withdraws to his room and cries. Rob has been aggressive toward his peers (e.g., trying to choke a child) and has been destructive of school property. Rob's peers tease him and call him names. Rob exhibits school refusal on some days.

Rob was taking Ritalin for concentration problems but the medication was discontinued for the diagnostic evaluation. Rob appeared depressed and withdrawn while taking the Ritalin but became more volatile and aggressive once off the Ritalin. Rob's behavior problems have rapidly escalated following the illnesses and hospitalization of both parents and two grandparents and the death of one grandparent in the past seven months. Rob was placed on Ritalin seven months ago, and it was increased the month before the escalation of his symptoms. Rob previously did well academically, but this academic year his grades dropped. He enjoys bike riding, reading, and games. Peer relationships have been poor.

Psychiatric History

This is the first psychiatric hospitalization for this child. The only previous treatment was counseling in the school by a social worker in response to Rob's aggressiveness toward other children. Following the onset of the morbid and suicidal symptoms the school personnel referred the mother for out-patient treatment. There has been no previous psychiatric involvement with other family members. The Ritalin was prescribed by a neurologist.

Family History

The family has a routine for meal- and bedtimes. Rob's father is gone for long hours of working and often sleeps in the evening. Although Rob expressed no food dislikes, his mother states he is a "picky eater." He is small in stature but has not

continued

Case Study (continued)

lost weight. He has difficulty falling asleep and at times complains of nightmares. Rob's impulsivity sometimes keeps him from doing tasks well, but his self-care is appropriate for his age.

Social History

Rob lives in a suburban area with his parents who are in their twenties, and two siblings, 6 and 3 years old. Mrs. V is a housewife who has a history of depression, anxiety, and medical problems. Mr. V supports the family in a blue-collar job. The marital relationship is strained. The family lives in small quarters, and the siblings share a room. They live in the neighborhood where the father grew up, and the grandparents live close by. None of the family members has activities outside the home, and the family has few leisure activities in general. The family is isolated and extremely enmeshed with the extended family on both sides. Both parents were overprotected by their parents. Rob primarily plays with his siblings as there are no other children living in the area.

Family health has been poor recently. Four months prior to Rob's admission his mother had a medical admission to the hospital. One month later Rob's father suffered an industrial injury, which has necessitated a career change and financial uncertainty. Rob's paternal grandmother had an extreme weight gain following a move two years prior to his admission. Nine months prior to his admission, his maternal grandfather suffered a stroke. The maternal grandmother died two months prior to his admission after seven years with cancer.

A brother, age 6, is doing well in school and has friends, although he is impulsive and hyperactive and has mild developmental problems. A sister, age 3, is assertive and extroverted and is adjusting well in preschool and with her peers. The siblings are aggressive toward each other.

Significant Health History

Rob's physical health is good other than some difficulty in fine motor coordination and mild anorexia reported by his mother. This well-groomed child showed no physical problems except for some minor bruises on his arm, which were reportedly self-induced. Because of staring periods, Rob was referred to a neurologist in preschool to rule out epilepsy. Findings were negative. Immunizations were up to date.

Rob was the product of an unplanned pregnancy, which ran a difficult course including hospitalizations toward term for toxemia. He was delivered by forceps, a 9 pound, 2 ounce baby. Developmental milestones were within normal limits. Walking and talking were early, and though toilet training was difficult, he was trained by age 3.

Rob's long history of behavioral problems began with temper tantrums at 6 months. At 3 he cut up the family sofa. The parents removed Rob from preschool because they felt the school could not handle his behavior. He continued to be a behavioral problem with poor socialization resulting in aggressiveness toward himself and others. Rob's concentration was poor, and he appeared depressed.

Current Mental Status

Appearance: well-groomed, neat and clean
Mood: energetic, excited, enthusiastic
Thought process: changes topics quickly
Thought content: appropriate to age and circumstance
Speech: has lisp, talks a lot

continued

Case Study (continued)

Orientation: good to three spheres

Eye contact: fair

Attention: fair

Memory: good

Suicidal orientation: makes statements of intent to "punch myself because I'm no good"

Homicidal ideation: he would like "to get really strong and let them (school bullies) have it"

Other Subjective or Objective Clinical Data

A dexamethasone suppression test was done at admission and was in the borderline range. After four weeks of intensive observation, Rob was given a trial dose of lithium. This was ineffective in controlling his mood swings. He was then switched to desipramine and maintained at a dose of 50 mg.

Diagnostic Impression

Nursing Diagnoses (PND-I/NANDA)

01.04.01	Difficult transition to and from sleep* /Sleep pattern disturbance
02.03.03	Knowledge deficit* /Knowledge deficit
02.04	Altered learning processes associated with underachievement
02.04	Altered learning processes associated with learning disability
04.02.02	Anxiety* /Anxiety
04.02.07	Guilt
04.02.08	Sadness
05.02.01.02	Aggressive/violent behaviors toward others* /Violence, potential for: directed at others
05.02.01.03	Aggressive/violent behaviors toward self* /Violence, potential for: self-directed
05.03.03	Altered parenting role* /Parenting, alteration in: actual
05.03.05	Altered student role
05.97	Undeveloped interpersonal processes
06.01.01	Distractibility
06.03.04	Altered self-esteem* /Self-concept, disturbance in self-esteem
07.06.02.02	Altered systemic processes, less than body requirements* /Nutrition, alteration in: less than body requirements
07.99	Potential for altered physiologic processes associated with medication toxicity
08.01.01	Hopelessness* /Hopelessness
08.03.02	Inability to internalize values
08.99	Potential for altered valuation processes

DSM-IIIR Multiaxial Diagnosis

Axis I: Cyclothymic disorder
         Attention deficit disorder

Axis II: Speech disorder (articulation)

continued

Case Study (continued)

Axis III: Fine motor deficits
Axis IV: 4-Severe
Axis V: Current GAF: 50
          Highest GAF past year: 60

Nursing Care Plan

Nursing Diagnosis (PND-I/NANDA)	Client Care Goals	Nursing Planning/ Intervention	Evaluation
07.06.02.02 Altered systemic processes: less than body requirements* /Nutrition alteration in: less than body requirements	Rob will maintain or increase weight. Rob will enjoy meals.	Structure meals and snacks. Help Rob make appropriate choices.	Weigh Rob as ordered. Observe Rob during mealtime (intake and interaction).
07.99 Potential for altered physiologic processes associated with medication toxicity	Indications of toxicity will be noted early.	Monitor Rob's vital signs daily, including one standing and two sitting blood pressures. Report any abnormal vital signs or signs of illness (e.g., dehydration or an elevated temperature can influence metabolism of the medication). Monitor side-effects daily.	Compare daily and baseline physical assessment. Review laboratory results.
06.01.01 Distractibility	Rob will be able to attend to an activity long or well enough to complete tasks and progress in classwork.	Medicate as prescribed. Provide a low stimulus place to work in. Provide tasks that can be accomplished in pieces or in a short time to help Rob feel successful. Record success relative to intervention. Provide feedback about success to Rob.	Observe and document classroom behavior. Document Rob's report of ability to concentrate. Seek feedback from parents regarding progression of activity and concentration.
01.04.01 Difficult transition to and from sleep* /Sleep pattern disturbance	Rob will experience less anxiety at bedtime. Rob will feel safe in his bedroom.	Use relaxation exercise at bedtime. Do not allow Rob to nap during the day. Provide extra support at bedtime. Use extra time prior to bedtime to decrease physical activity.	Observe Rob at regular intervals during sleeping hours. Record sleep behavior. Evaluate Rob's level of restfulness and compare progression.

continued

Case Study (continued)

Nursing Diagnosis (PND-I/NANDA)	Client Care Goals	Nursing Planning/ Intervention	Evaluation
		Encourage Rob to talk about his fears.	
02.04 Altered learning processes associated with underachievement	Rob will achieve in school consistent with his ability.	Refer for comprehensive educational psychologic testing of Rob's abilities related to school activities. Implement recommendations.	Consult with unit teacher to compare academic functioning currently and at time of admission.
02.04 Altered learning processes associated with learning disability	Rob will compensate for his learning problem through awareness and development of new skills.	Provide learning materials that accent Rob's strengths in order to achieve academically. (The nurse acts in a supportive role and may work with Rob on individual academic tasks.)	Observe Rob in learning tasks for evidence of increased or decreased anxiety. Observe Rob for ability to learn new skills.
08.03.02 Inability to internalize values associated with refusing limits and running away	Rob will follow direction, including rules of conduct, without incident. Rob will use alternative means of managing stress and/or anxiety precipitating acting out behavior.	Medicate as prescribed, since some behavior may recede spontaneously with medication (especially if secondary to a depression or other condition responsive to pharmacology); e.g., school phobia has been treated successfully with imipramine. Monitor Rob's behavior prior to and following medication.	Measure incidence of problem behaviors. Evaluate effectiveness of stress management techniques.
08.03.01 Conflict with social order* /Social interaction (impaired)	Rob will develop positive relationship with adult authority figures.	Assist Rob in developing new responses if necessary. Broaden vocabulary relative to feelings. (Are you angry or hurt?) Teach Rob to identify what upsets him. Help Rob learn to remove himself from difficult situations and to tell adults he is having a difficult time. Encourage Rob to talk about feelings rather than act out.	Review record for evidence of decreased incidence of oppositional behavior.

continued

Case Study (continued)

Nursing Diagnosis (PND-I/NANDA)	Client Care Goals	Nursing Planning/Intervention	Evaluation
05.03.05 Altered student role	Rob will attend school and develop positive attitude toward school.	Provide constant and consistent feedback to Rob about how he is doing.	Review record to determine if Rob sets up situations to avoid school or leave the classroom.
			Assess for verbal evidence of positive statements regarding school.
05.02.01.02 Aggressive/violent behavior toward others* /Violence, potential for: directed at others	Rob will express feelings without harming another or losing control.	Develop a behavioral program to manage the aggressive impulses, using limit setting, time-outs, holding, and seclusion.	Review record for evidence of decreased incidence of problem behaviors.
			Evaluate effectiveness of medication on behavior.
		State clearly and repeatedly that aggression is not tolerated and that staff are present to provide a safe place for all the children.	
05.97 Undeveloped interpersonal processes	Rob will show improved social skills with peers, demonstrated by sharing, cooperation, healthy competition, and conflict resolution, as seen in a variety of milieu routines (meals, school, and play times).	Discuss with Rob basic expectations about social interactions with peers, stressing the basics of mutual respect and cooperation.	Make observations regarding number of nonconflictual interactions with peers.
		Plan a program of gradually increased expectations of social interactions for Rob.	
	Rob will enjoy and/or look forward to peer activities.	Begin with interactions with staff, doing tasks and games so staff can instruct and provide role models for the client.	
04.02.02 Anxiety* /Anxiety	Rob's anxiety level will decrease.	Provide ways for Rob to express feelings and worries.	Observe for evidence that Rob can verbalize feelings toward situations without feeling responsible for others.
04.02.07 Guilt	Rob will feel more secure.	Offer empathic comments about worries (e.g., "It must be hard to concentrate when you're worried about your Dad.")	
06.03.04 Altered self-esteem* /Self-concept, disturbance in self-esteem	Rob will begin to feel more positive about himself.	Help Rob label feelings.	Review verbal statements about self and staff interactions with Rob for evidence of insight.
	Rob will feel more hopeful about life.	Reflect Rob's feelings.	
04.02.08 Sadness		Acknowledge Rob's feelings.	
08.01.01 Hopelessness* /Hopelessness		Make connections with Rob's feelings and events.	
		Record verbal statements about self.	

continued

Case Study (continued)

Nursing Diagnosis (PND-I/NANDA)	Client Care Goals	Nursing Planning/ Intervention	Evaluation
05.02.01.03 Aggressive/ violent behaviors toward self* /Violence, potential for: self-directed	Rob will remain safe. Suicidal thought content will decrease. Rob will develop new outlets for aggression. Self-destructive behaviors will decrease.	Inquire about suicidal thoughts, wishes, or plans. Provide verbal reassurance to Rob that you will not allow him to hurt himself or others. Note and record observations of self-destructive behavior. Provide constant supervision of Rob. Place Rob on highest level of suicide precautions (Busteed and Johnstone 1983). Review suicide level daily. Do suicidal assessment during one-to-one with primary nurse (including physical assessment).	Assess interactions for a decrease in violent content. Observe for decreased incidence of self-destructive behaviors.
02.03.03 Knowledge deficit associated with condition and treatment* /Knowledge deficit	Rob will understand the medication at his developmental level. Rob will understand his condition at his developmental level. Rob will express negative and positive feelings associated with medication.	Inquire about Rob's understanding of medication and any changes associated with medication. Develop a teaching plan to teach Rob about his condition (e.g., depression). Provide opportunities for questions and discussion concerning condition, hospitalization, and treatment. Reinforce Rob's attempts to learn about his condition. Encourage Rob to express feelings related to medication. Provide support and education for Rob when he receives venipunctures to measure blood levels of antidepressant medication by preparing and educating Rob and his parents, comforting and reassuring Rob during the procedure,	Assess Rob's ability to describe to his primary nurse the reason for his hospitalization and his treatment. Evaluate for compliance to medication regimen and positive statements toward medications.

continued

Case Study (continued)

Nursing Diagnosis (PND-I/NANDA)	Client Care Goals	Nursing Planning/ Intervention	Evaluation
		and helping him master the trauma.	
05.03.03 Altered parenting role* /Parenting, alteration in: actual	Parents will understand Rob's normal and special needs. Rob's parents will understand the action and monitoring of the medication. Rob's parents will be prepared for handling the medication after discharge. Parents will begin to develop plan for suicide precautions at home. Rob will feel nurtured and supported by parents. Parents will deal with their losses so they do not provide additional stress for Rob. Parents will feel acknowledged and respected by the staff.	Meet with parents to understand treatment plan. Model support and nurturing of Rob. Attend the session between the physician and parents when medication is explained. Provide ongoing medication teaching for Rob and his parents, including the name of the medication, reason for taking it, description of what the child can expect, frequency and dosage, list of side-effects (including serious and annoying effects), and potential for overdose. Plan for discharge, for example, safety, storage, and administration of medication; danger of sudden withdrawal from medication; when and how to report problems and take vital signs. Explain that the plastic boxes are available in pharmacies with compartments for daily doses. Reinforce seriousness of Rob's suicidal threats to parents. Reinforce parents' concern for Rob's safety. Teach Rob and his parents about the unit philosophy and structure related to preventing suicide. Establish no-suicide contract with Rob and his parents. Develop a plan with parents	Parents increase participation in treatment plan. Parents are observed being supportive and nurturing. Parents will be able to describe use of medications, dosage, precautions, and side-effects. Parents show evidence of planning for suicide precautions including a safe home environment and signed no-suicide contract. Observe parent-child interaction in the milieu for evidence of appropriate parent-child boundaries, and parental nurturing of child. Observe parents for responses to staff.

continued

Case Study (continued)

Nursing Diagnosis (PND-I/NANDA)	Client Care Goals	Nursing Planning/ Intervention	Evaluation
		for supervision during passes.	
		Encourage frequent and regular visits and phone calls.	
		Involve parents in Rob's care.	
		Provide support to parents (e.g., difficulty dealing with separation).	
		Educate parents about depression in children (e.g., symptoms and approaches).	
08.99 Potential for altered valuation processes associated with medication	Rob and his parents will accept administration of medication.	Encourage Rob and parents to discuss their beliefs about the medication.	Evaluate compliance with medication on pass. Assess family's verbalization about medication.

PND-I diagnosis also in NANDA list.

Finally, evaluations of child treatment must be compared to appropriate developmental markers. The evaluation of frustration tolerance, for example, differs greatly between the 4-year-old and 14-year-old child. So evaluation of such behaviors must compare norms for age appropriateness. Individual and family norms also contribute to this problem. Often a child who exhibits what appear to be bad manners or poor boundaries with adults has been taught this behavior at home. While children need to learn socially useful behavior, they also need to fit in with their families.

Chapter Highlights

- Child psychiatric nursing concerns itself with the promotion of mental health in all children as well as the treatment of the emotionally disturbed child.

- The role of the nurse in child psychiatry is changing as a result of the increase in focus on biochemical disorders and dual diagnoses.

- Standards of practice for generalists and specialists in child psychiatric nursing have been published by the American Nurses' Association.

- The etiology of psychiatric disorders in children is multicausal and may include genetic and biophysical factors, social and cultural factors, family system factors, and acquired illness and injury.

- The manifestation of psychiatric disorders in children is influenced by the child's developmental level.

- Nursing assessment in child psychiatry is a multistep process that includes basic assessment of the child (psychosocial and physical), life space interview, and family assessment.

- Nursing diagnoses specific to child psychiatric clients have been developed and are being refined.

- The treatment of psychiatric disorders in children must be family oriented and multidisciplinary in nature.

- Child psychiatric nurses are involved in primary or collaborative roles in various treatment modalities including play therapy, psychopharmacology, milieu, group therapy, parent counseling, and psychoeducation.

- The use of psychopharmacologic agents in children has not been well tested. These agents must be used cautiously and closely monitored.

- Discharge planning and aftercare facilitate the child's reentry into the community and may help prevent problems with adjustment and rehospitalization.

References

Achenbach T: *Developmental Psychopathology,* ed 2. Wiley, 1982.

American Nurses' Association: *Standards of Child and Adolescent Psychiatric and Mental Health Nursing Practice,* ANA, 1985.

American Psychiatric Association: *Diagnostic and Statistical Manual of Mental Disorders* ed 3, revised. APA, 1987.

Babich K (ed): *A Workbook Assessing the Mental Health of Children.* Western Interstate Commission for Higher Education, 1982.

Burgess AW, et al: Child molestation: Assessing impact in multiple victims. *Arch Psychiatr Nurs* 1987;1(1):33–39.

Busteed E, Johnstone C: The development of suicide precautions for an inpatient psychiatric unit. *J Psych Soc Nurs Mental Health Serv* 1983;21(May):15–19.

Campbell M, Pali M: Measurement of tardive dyskinesia. *Psychopharm Bull* 1985;21:106–107.

Cantor S: *The Schizophrenic Child,* Eden Press, 1982.

Caplan G: *Prevention of Mental Disorders in Children.* Basic Books, 1961.

Cohen D, Leckman J Shaywitz B: The Tourette syndrome and other tics, in Shaffer D, Ehrhardt A, Greenhill L (eds): *The Clinical Guide to Child Psychiatry.* Free Press, 1985.

Endicott J, et al.: The global assessment scale: A procedure for measuring overall severity of psychiatric disturbance. *Arch Gen Psychiatry* 1976;33:766–771.

Eth S, Pynoos RS: *Post-Traumatic Stress Disorder in Children.* American Psychiatric Press, 1985.

Greenhill L: Pediatric pharmacology, in Shaffer D, Ehrhardt A, Greenhill L (eds): *The Clinical Guide to Child Psychiatry.* Free Press, 1985, chap 26.

Grossman J, et al.: *Alcoholism in Family Histories of Depressed Prepubertal Children,* unpublished manuscript. University of Illinois Medical Center, 1984.

Grossman J, Herrmann C: Nursing care of the child with a psychiatric or social disorder, in Mott S, Fazekas N, James J (eds): *Nursing Care of Children and Families.* Addison-Wesley, 1985, chap 15.

Herskowitz J, Rosman NP: *Pediatrics, Neurology, and Psychiatry—Common Ground: Behavioral, Cognitive, Affective and Physical Disorders in Childhood and Adolescence.* Macmillan, 1982.

Hoffman L: *The Evaluation and Care of Severely Disturbed Children and Their Families.* Spectrum Publications, 1982.

Looney JG: *Chronic Mental Illness in Children and Adolescents.* American Psychiatric Press, 1987.

Peck M, Farberrow N, Litman R: *Youth Suicide.* Springer Publishing, 1985.

Pothier P, Norbeck J, Laliberte M: Child psychiatric nursing: The gap between need and utilization. *J Psych Soc Nurs* 1985;23:18–23.

Poznanski E: The clinical phenomenology of childhood depression. *Am J Orthopsychiatry* 1982;52:308–313.

Poznanski E, et al.: *Cortisol Nonsuppression and Suicidal Ideation in Prepubertal Children,* unpublished manuscript. Rush-Presbyterian-St. Luke's Medical Center, 1987.

Puig-Antich J, Chambers W, Ryan W: *The Schedule for Affective Disorders and Schizophrenia for School-Age Children (K-SADS-P).* Western State Psychiatric Institute and Clinic, 1980.

Redl F: *When We Deal With Children.* Free Press, 1966.

Ross C: *Youth Suicide and What You Can Do About It.* Los Angeles: American Association of Suicidology, 1984.

Rothstein A: Hallucinatory phenomena in children: A critique of the literature. *J Am Acad Child Psychiatry* 1981;20:623–635.

Rutter M, Hensov L (eds): *Child and Adolescent Psychiatry: Modern Approaches.* Blackwell Scientific, 1985.

Shaffer D, et al: A children's global assessment scale. *Arch Gen Psychiatry* 1983;40:1228–1231.

Shaffer D, Erhardt A, Greenhill L (eds): *The Clinical Guide to Child Psychiatry.* Free Press, 1985.

Tanquay P, Cantor S: Schizophrenia in children: Introduction. *J Am Acad Child Psychiatry* 1986;25:591–594.

Trends in Mental Health: Self-Destructive Behavior Among Younger Age Groups. US Department of Health, Education, and Welfare Publication No. (ADM) 76-365, 1976.

Weiner J, Hendren R: Childhood depression. *J Dev Behav Pediatr* 1983;4:43–49.

Weissman M, et al.: Psychopathology in the children (ages 6–18) of depressed and normal parents. *J Am Acad Child Psychiatry* 1984;23:78–84.

Werry J: An overview of pediatric psychopharmacology. *J Am Acad Child Psychiatry* 1982;21:3–9.

Wilkinson T: *Child and Adolescent Psychiatric Nursing.* Blackwell Scientific, 1983.

Zimmerman ML: Art and group work: Interventions for multiple victims of child molestation. *Arch Psychiatr Nurs* 1987;1(1):40–46.

THIRTY-FIVE

Applying the Nursing Process with Adolescents

Carol Bradley

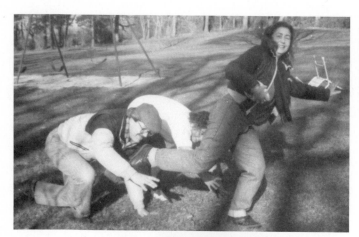

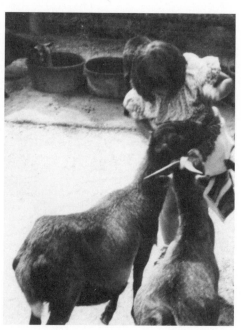

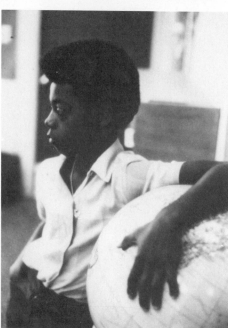

After reading this chapter, students should be able to

- Relate the importance of using a humanistic interactionist framework to a comprehensive assessment of adolescent problems

- Give a clinical example of difficulties within Erik Erikson's developmental stages of trust, autonomy, initiative, and industry

- Describe the roles and functions of the nurse in outpatient and in-patient treatment settings for adolescents

- Describe the roles and functions of the nurse working with families of adolescent clients

- List at least four functions of the staff nurse to maintain a therapeutic milieu

- Define the term *acting out*, giving an example of the adolescent's acting out a "life script"

- Discuss at least three theoretical explanations for anorexia nervosa

- Construct a client contract for use with the adolescent in treatment

- List seven steps for implementation by the nurse to prevent adolescent suicide

- Identify four risk factors for adolescent suicide

Other topics relevant to this content are: ANA Standards of Child and Adolescent Psychiatric Mental Health Nursing, Chapter 34 and Box 34–1; Depression, Chapter 18; Developmental stressors in parenting during adolescence, Table 6–12 in Chapter 6; Drug abuse, Chapter 16; Family therapy, Chapter 33; Normal adolescent growth and development, Chapter 6; Suicide, Chapter 29.

We are really all one in the form of many.

acting out	limit setting
anorexia nervosa	no self-harm contract
behavioral contract	obesity
bulimia nervosa	scapegoating
eating disorders	seduction of the nurse
life script	suicide cluster

What is adolescence? Some sources define it simply as the time of physical and psychosocial development between the ages of 12 and 20. Others have described it as a period of "normal psychosis." Still others see it as an attempt by a tyrannical subculture to overtake adult America. It is not necessary to accept these last two definitions verbatim to understand their implications. Most people recognize the immense stress that occurs during adolescence and the importance it holds for that person's future.

Trying to understand the adolescent is a challenge to anyone. For the nurse who chooses to work with adolescents, the challenge offers considerable rewards. Nurses who can recollect their own experiences and reactions during this tumultuous time will better appreciate the adolescent's dilemma.

THEORETICAL FOUNDATIONS

A sound theoretical knowledge base will help the nurse differentiate "normal" and "abnormal," usual and unusual, behaviors of the adolescent. In particular, the nurse can do a comprehensive assessment by focusing on the psychologic development of the individual and the evolution of the adolescent as a biopsychosocial being. The nurse can accomplish the first task with an understanding of developmental theory and the second with an appreciation of humanistic interactionist theory.

An understanding of developmental theory will help the nurse identify and intervene with deviations in the adolescent's growth and development processes. The theories of Sigmund Freud, Erik Erikson, and Harry Stack Sullivan provide considerable insight about the adolescent's struggle to attain adulthood. These theories as they relate to "normal" growth and development are discussed in Chapters 5 and 6. Erik Erikson's theory will be highlighted here to offer examples of pathologic beginnings along this developmental continuum.

The development of the adolescent's sense of identity entails a preoccupation with self-image. It also entails a connection between future role and past experiences. In the search for a new sense of sameness and continuity, many adolescents must repeat the crisis resolutions of earlier years to integrate these past elements and establish the lasting ideals of a final identity. According to Erikson, these crisis periods or stages are reviews of the adolescent's sense of trust, autonomy, initiative, and industry, in that order (Figure 35–1).

A Sense of Trust

In the first stage the adolescent must look for ideas and objects in which to believe or place trust. Simultaneously, however, the adolescent fears too strong a commitment and so expresses this need for faith in boisterous and doubtful mistrust.

Oral character is a term used to portray the individual with unresolved conflicts of this stage (Erikson 1968, p 102). Such persons may fear "being left empty" or simply "being left." They may display their insatiable needs simply, as with overeating. In more severe cases, they may make hostile or sarcastic remarks as an ineffectual way of getting what they need from others. They both need and fear trusting relationships, since they have not received satisfaction from them in the past.

Jimmy is an obese boy of 12 who was referred to the school nurse-counselor because of his boisterous classroom behavior. His parents were first separated when he was an infant, at the time when development of trust is so important. His mother was depressed during his early years and required several psychiatric hospitalizations. Since that time she has attempted to establish a good relationship with him but has received nothing but insults and sarcasm in return. Jimmy manifests all the unresolved feelings of this stage. These feelings are expressed in verbal pessimism, sarcasm, insatiable gratification of oral needs, and mistrust of others.

A Sense of Autonomy

In the second stage the adolescent must learn to perform or decide independently. This involves a venture into one of the available or necessary methods of service. Examples could be volunteer work at a hospital or participation in a church-related program. It must involve some free choice for the adolescent, however. Again, adolescents fear being forced to engage in activities that would result in ridicule or self-doubt. They prefer to perform possibly embarrassing activities voluntarily, and in the presence of adults, rather than under compulsion, and in the presence of peers.

Steven is a pert, independent boy of 13. His parents are divorced. In discussing them, Steven says, "Then my parents were divorced—thank goodness! My father has been much happier since she left. She was quite difficult to get along with." Although Steven boasts about his father and the attention he receives from him, the grade counselor views Steven as a neglected child whose father cares only about his achievements in school and elsewhere. Steven denies having any friends and says his greatest joy is in winning a chess game from his father. He tries hard to perform optimally at any task and is given to intellectualization in discussions with the nurse-counselor. He seems to have to prove himself continually to gain the sense of autonomy so important to his self-esteem.

A Sense of Initiative

The third stage originates in childhood when children are no longer concerned with *how* to walk but rather what they can do with that ability. They then experiment with what they *may* do rather than what they *can* do. The task in the third stage is to free the adolescent's initiative and sense of purpose for adult tasks that will fulfill the adolescent's range of capabilities. In this stage the individual seems unrestrained by any limitations of self-image. Ambition knows no bounds.

Before completing an intensive course of in-patient and outpatient psychotherapy, including two months' hospitalization on an adolescent psychiatric unit, 14-year-old Shirley had felt quite depressed and hopeless, taking a serious overdose of her mother's Valium. She is now hopeful about her future and is striving to attain a sense of initiative. At present Shirley is testing her imagination by mentally casting herself in various life roles. One day she avidly reads about a career in nursing. The next day she has plans to become a dancer and appear on Broadway. She shows much initiative in group work and in instituting activities that will contribute to her aspirations.

A Sense of Industry

In the fourth stage a sense of industry demands that the adolescent choose a career that not only promises financial success but also provides the satisfaction of performing well. The very reason that many young people postpone or even shun work is to avoid entering a field that would not yield these satisfactions. They may also wish to avoid being coerced into such work.

Matthew is a very interesting boy of 16 who is striving for a sense of industry. He is representative of other youths his age who must find themselves before they can begin seriously considering their life's work. He has moved from truancy to drugs to stealing and has now begun to reevaluate his life and what he hopes to gain from his experiences. He says that he now wants to "start over" and work toward a career as a police officer or probation officer.

Humanistic Interactionist Theory

In addition to having knowledge about developmental theories, the nurse will need to integrate humanistic interactionist principles into assessment and interventions to develop a trusting, caring interpersonal relationship with

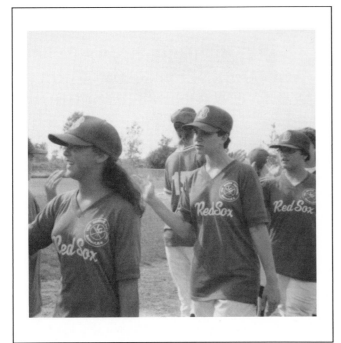

Figure 35–1
A sense of community in team work facilitates the development of a sense of trust, autonomy, initiative, and industry in adolescents.

the adolescent client. The adolescent developmental period is a time in the individual's life when identity, values, and goals are in a state of flux. The nurse should take into account not only the immediate situation but also the impact of the developmental stage, social and cultural factors, family influences, and psychodynamic conflicts on the adolescent's behavior.

To do this the nurse should explore the meaning of the identified problem or behavior including the answers to the following questions:

- What meaning does this behavior or problem hold for the adolescent?
- What is the adolescent saying with this behavior?
- What impact does this problem have on the client in this developmental stage? Is this a usual or unusual problem or behavior for the adolescent's peer group?
- How have resulting changes, if any, affected the adolescent and relationships with others?
- What goals does the adolescent have for the immediate and distant future?
- What personal strengths does the adolescent have to help deal with this problem?
- What considerations have we (the client and the nurse) given to other developmental, familial, biologic, or sociocultural factors involved?

To respond to the adolescent's needs and dilemmas based solely on behaviors without a more comprehensive evaluation of these other factors can yield ineffective treatment, a temporary surcease of the initial behaviors with an upheaval of symptoms in another area, and possibly a sterile treatment environment without any meaningful therapeutic alliance. Only by considering all aspects of the adolescent client as a biopsychosocial being can the nurse truly understand the meanings of such behaviors to the adolescent and intervene effectively in the situation.

HISTORICAL FOUNDATIONS

The evolution and significant changes in the role of the psychiatric nurse during the past century are well summarized in Chapter 2. The role of the nurse in the care and treatment of adolescents has dramatically changed during this time. Once regarded simply as a technician who monitored somatic therapies, the nurse is now acknowledged as a professional with numerous capabilities and skills that have a direct bearing on the favorable treatment outcome of adolescents.

The American Nurses' Association (ANA) now recognizes child and adolescent psychiatric and mental health nursing as a specialty area of psychiatric and mental health nursing practice. The ANA *Standards of Child and Adolescent Psychiatric and Mental Health Nursing Practice* (1985) are reproduced in Box 34–1 in Chapter 34.

Whether a generalist or clinical specialist, the nurse in today's health setting integrates these characteristics and role responsibilities to intervene with the adolescent within the significant social system toward optimal social, emotional, cognitive, and physical development. Using expertise in identifying relevant deviations in the developmental process, the nurse works closely with the systems (family, school, community, and institution) on which the adolescent is emotionally and economically dependent.

THE ROLE OF THE NURSE

In numerous roles within a variety of treatment modalities the nurse can help maintain the adolescent client's health and well-being and identify abnormal or problem-causing behavior during this difficult period of development.

In the Outpatient Setting

As a Community Health Nurse

In the school, clinic, or community health agency, the nurse has excellent opportunities to observe the adolescent engage in the normal activities of daily living. The nurse will have frequent occasions to counsel adolescents in the problems that confront them daily and to advise school or clinic staff members in their encounters with adolescents. The nurse who knows how to deal with normal adolescent problems will also be adept in identifying obstacles to effective resolution of emotional problems and suggesting further treatment.

School is the most influential experience in the adolescent's life outside of the home. The adolescent spends more waking time in school activities than in any other activity, and most of the adolescent's successes, problems, and conflicts are demonstrated within the school setting. Even adolescents who are supposedly "truant" from school can often be found on the school grounds, perhaps meeting their friends at lunchtime, playing cards in the library, or "hanging out" on the school steps. Such an "absent" student may suddenly appear at the school nurse's door because of "boredom" or a somatic complaint.

Unfortunately, the school nurse's role in the early rec-

ognition and treatment of predelinquent individuals has been minimized or has gone unrecognized. There are several reasons for this. First, school administrators and teachers tend to view the school nurse as a person who deals only with physical sickness and medical emergencies. They may not be aware that because of the intimate quality of a nurse-client relationship or the comprehensive and holistic nature of nursing assessments, the nurse may be helpful in exploring an area of conflict in the adolescent's life or intervening with a disruptive student. Such early intervention could prevent more serious problems in later years. Many studies have indicated a direct correlation between problems of early school life and the incidence of subsequent juvenile delinquency, depression, and suicidal behavior (Child et al. 1980, Glueck and Glueck 1972, Pfeffer 1984). Box 35–1 offers a list of possible problems demonstrated by the adolescent in the school setting that would benefit from early intervention.

Second, administrators tend to limit the nurse's activities to the school itself. They may see no need for the nurse to make home visits to meet with the sick student's family or view problems firsthand. Many school districts lack time and money to provide for counseling families or individuals in a formal setting. As the role of the independent nursing practitioner expands, and as legislation for third-party reimbursement for independent practice becomes a reality, nurses will be better able to assume more autonomy and responsibility and to meet the needs of the student in a more comprehensive and effective way.

Meanwhile, the nurse who is already employed in the school setting or community agency can seize every oppor-

---

Box 35–1

INITIAL PROBLEMS THAT WOULD BENEFIT FROM EARLY INTERVENTION IN THE SCHOOL SETTING

- Antisocial behavior (e.g., stealing, setting fires, bullying others)
- Avoidant social behavior
- Chronic illness
- Depression
- Disruptive classroom behavior
- Drug abuse
- Excessive daydreaming
- Hypochondriasis
- Learning difficulties
- Poor school performance or dramatic shift in school performance
- Temper tantrums
- Truancy

tunity to provide an active school health program and to educate school administrators and faculty to the importance of preventive care. For example, the nurse in a viable school health program can provide preventive counseling not only to troubled adolescents in school but also to their preschool siblings during routine home visits. Nurses can establish productive relationships with teachers, help other faculty members encourage parent-teacher conferences, take an active part in developing the curriculum, and help adolescents on probation or parole return to school.

As a Nurse Counselor/Therapist

Whether in the clinic, home, school, or community health setting, the psychiatric nurse has many opportunities to organize individual, group, or family counseling sessions. Nurses can function within a variety of treatment roles, depending on their experience and capabilities.

As an Individual Therapist

The nurse's qualifications and role in the clinic, school, or community setting may allow for counseling the adolescent on an individual basis. Sometimes the nurse can establish a trusting alliance and can facilitate communication with the client. On the other hand, the adolescent may be too threatened to talk openly with the nurse in this intimate setting. Some adolescents view the nurse as an authority figure and will resist all efforts to communicate. The nurse may make more headway with this mode of treatment when it is used in conjunction with group therapy. Unless certified to provide this service, the nurse should counsel the adolescent only for the purposes of identifying the problem area and referring the client to a qualified professional for individual psychotherapy.

As a Group Therapist

It is usually most effective to work with adolescents in a group. Because the values, acceptance, and recognition of peers are so important during adolescence, the group can provide the support the student needs to deal with problems and effect change. In addition, involving the adolescent's peers helps dilute the conflict with adults that may exist in one-to-one work. In the school setting, health education groups can provide an acceptable format for peer interaction and discussion of difficult topics. Otherwise, the nurse should practice as a group therapist only as a certified individual or with adequate supervision by a certified individual. Knowledge of group dynamics is crucial for the nurse to be an effective group leader.

As a Family Therapist

Being a parent of a "normal" adolescent is difficult at best. As the child grows into adulthood with all its perplexing questions and problems, parents normally worry about their

child's safety and well-being. They may feel rejected because they are no longer needed in the same way. Since many parents of relatively normal adolescents share this plight, they can usually find receptive listeners who will give them comfort and support.

The problems of the parents of emotionally disturbed adolescents are more complicated. Many such parents have a strong sense of failure because their children did not turn out "right." Their feelings of guilt, frustration, and helplessness are likely to increase if their child is institutionalized. They have probably felt confused and resentful when experts offered them smug and guilt-provoking advice. Unlike the parents of normal adolescents, they may have no one in whom to confide, either because they lack the support and understanding of others, or because their own self-incriminating feelings prevent them from seeking out confidants.

Meetings with family members may be indicated if the adolescent's role within the family seems to be compounded by the problems presented in the school or agency setting. The nurse should consider it an important part of the problem-solving process to organize initial interviews with parents and family members. The information gathered during these meetings can be used to determine whether the problems stem from difficulties posed by the larger system (the family), and, if so, whether family therapy is indicated.

The nurse should show compassion and understanding for the parents' dilemma without blaming them or their offspring. Parents will be more receptive to family therapy and to exploring their part in the adolescent's problems if they sense that the nurse will support them, too. Any tendency to feel self-righteous or superior to the disturbed adolescent's parents will become an obstacle to effective treatment. Such feelings are readily communicated to parents and can only validate their fear of blame and increase their reluctance to participate in therapy with their child. By the same token, the nurse should resist any temptation to overidentify with the parents, perpetuating the family system's problems further. The adolescent and the family need a "neutral" party who can play an objective, knowledgeable, and supportive role in helping them change. The adolescent's chances for resolving the underlying conflicts and maintaining a healthy life will be virtually nil if the family system remains unchanged.

Parents, school, and agency staff must understand the objectives and goals of treatment to appreciate the progress the client has made and avoid reinforcing the client's previously maladaptive behavior. The following incident illustrates the problems that arise when parents and school authorities, particularly those who must deal directly with behavior problems in the classroom, lack psychologic sophistication.

Jeremy, a 13-year-old boy, was referred to the school nurse because he was introverted and isolated. He made no contact with either his peers or teachers and rarely spoke unless addressed directly. After he had spent three months in group and individual therapy sessions with the nurse, Jeremy began to come to the grade counselor's office of his own accord to talk about his depression and the problems he had been having in his family. Both the grade counselor and the boy's family believed this to be an indication that his difficulties had worsened, and they began to complain to the nurse about his illness! Not only were Jeremy's parents and counselor ignorant of the goals of treatment and the behaviors expected to come with change, but apparently they were also uncomfortable with the changes in Jeremy's behavior and with the implications of these changes for their relationships with him.

The client's siblings may experience many different feelings. Sometimes they share in the parents' guilt and shame. On the other hand, they may be quite pleased and relieved that the "troublemaker" is out of the family and hospitalized. The nurse should extend the same degree of understanding to the siblings as to the parents and should help them see how each member of the family contributes to the problem. Often another member of the family, usually a sibling, will assume the role of the "bad" or "sick" person in the family, since the identified "bad" person is no longer at home. The nurse should be aware of this tendency. If the nurse is not skilled in assessing the need for family therapy or in providing this service, the family should be referred to a competent family therapist.

The nurse may identify a need for all of the above therapies in dealing with an individual's problem. In some cases, an informal discussion with the nurse is all that is warranted. In other cases, the nurse may identify problems that require considerable attention. Sometimes a period of unsuccessful treatment is necessary to determine that outpatient therapy is ineffective, and that hospitalization is indicated. In these circumstances, it is essential to establish a trusting relationship with the client and the parents in order to make such a recommendation.

In the In-Patient Setting

Admission into a hospital or other residential treatment facility may be indicated:

- If the adolescent lacks sufficient ego strength to control impulsivity

- If the degree of destructive or antisocial behavior escalates beyond normal limits
- If the adolescent cannot form meaningful, stable relationships within the everyday environment (e.g., due to family dysfunction)

The existence of any one of these criteria warrants counseling or professional treatment. A combination of two or more is likely to make treatment on an outpatient basis virtually ineffective and indicates the need for hospital or residential treatment.

There are many advantages of hospitalization for the disturbed adolescent:

- It provides additional structure within which to handle the physically and psychologically destructive elements of the adolescent's behavior.
- It removes the individual from the stresses of a disturbed family environment.
- It offers opportunities for supporting existing ego strengths and for promoting whatever ability the client has for forming relationships.

Adolescents are sometimes institutionalized because their ideas are strange or threatening to their families, or because the responsible authorities seek to punish the adolescent's unacceptable behavior. The results can be disastrous. Therefore, it is important that accurate assessments be made and that early treatment is implemented when indicated. The nurse has a valuable role in making such assessments, undertaking appropriate interventions, and educating parents, teachers, and school officials to recognize such needs.

As a Staff Nurse in a General Hospital Setting

Adolescents with an emotional problem may have symptoms of physical illness. This can result in admission to a general hospital setting for evaluation and treatment. Clients with anorexia nervosa in particular are often seen by their pediatricians or primary care clinicians, due to their dramatic weight loss, amenorrhea, or other physical symptoms, and then referred for in-patient treatment on general adolescent medical units.

As a Consultant in a General Hospital Setting

Staff nurses from a psychiatric in-patient unit within a general hospital may be consulted by other nursing staff regarding emotionally disturbed adolescents who have been admitted to their general medical or surgical units. Some general hospital settings are fortunate enough to have clinical nurse specialists in psychiatric liaison positions to consult with nursing staff.

As a Staff Nurse or Clinical Specialist in the Psychiatric Setting

In the in-patient psychiatric setting the staff nurse or clinical nurse specialist may assume any of the previously mentioned roles. Nurses in the in-patient setting will also have numerous opportunities to observe and assess the family dynamics among the adolescent's family members and possibly to intervene. Nurses who are involved in family therapy sessions can perceive maladaptive ways of relating more easily and take direct steps to work toward change. However, it is not necessary that the nurse works within the structured format of a therapy hour to have an impact on the family system. Table 35–1 delineates specific parent behaviors with helpful interventions for the nurse within the therapeutic milieu.

Since in-patient nursing entails around-the-clock care, the nurse has the responsibility to maintain the therapeutic milieu. The role of the in-patient staff nurse includes:

- Maintaining the physical and psychologic safety of the unit
- Setting verbal and physical limits on the clients' behavior
- Establishing meaningful one-to-one relationships with clients
- Identifying clients' strengths and promoting more adaptive coping skills

---

Table 35–1
Intervening With Specific Parent Behaviors

Parent Behavior	Nursing Interventions	Parent Behavior	Nursing Interventions

Initiates loud verbal arguments during visits with adolescent	1. Stop the immediate behavior, pointing out the disruptiveness to the unit.
	2. Refer adolescent and family to family therapists to resolve differences and learn more adaptive ways of relating in supportive atmosphere of family therapy.
	3. Suggest that family therapist contract with family for one or more of the following:
	  a. Staff will monitor visits.
	  b. Family will bring up potentially volatile topics only within the structure of family meetings and not on the unit during visits.
	  c. Staff will intervene if arguments ensue on unit.
	  d. Staff may limit visiting time on unit.
		Is unable to set limits with adolescent during unit visits (is adversely influenced by manipulative attempts, tolerates verbal abuse, etc.)	until progress is seen in family therapy.
			1. Intervene if demands or behavior could yield physical harm, unit rule breaking, or other negative results.
			2. Point out problem and refer adolescent and parents to family therapy.
			3. Role model appropriate and effective limit setting with adolescent if necessary.
			4. Offer to discuss situation with parents and adolescent if desirable in immediate situation.
			5. Offer emotional support to parent who needs to talk.

Has history of physical violence against adolescent	1. Upon admission, contract with adolescent and family for no acts of violence against people or property. 2. Monitor visits with adolescent on unit. 3. Limit or deny passes with parents until progress is demonstrated. 4. Depending on abilities with impulse control, refuse visiting privileges with adolescent	Has limited interaction with adolescent during unit visits	1. Initiate discussion among adolescent and family members related to visit and treatment goals. 2. Refer problem and give observations to family therapists. 3. Initiate discussion with parents to allow exploration of difficulty, if desired. 4. Suggest that family members and adolescent discuss the problem in family therapy. 5. Plan outings/special occasion celebrations to include families, if appropriate.

- Role modeling more socially acceptable behaviors
- Participating in group therapies and other structured activities

THE VALUE OF THE THERAPEUTIC MILIEU

Many authors have described the importance of the therapeutic milieu, indicating the strong influence of the treatment environment on the treatment outcome. Chapter 31 discusses the development of the milieu concept.

In considering adolescents' needs for peer acceptance, their overwhelming uncertainties and fears, and their ever-changing behaviors and attitudes about identity, it should be readily apparent that the adolescents' chances for success in in-patient treatment are increased by a peer group setting. Much has been written about the value of the therapeutic milieu in dealing with adolescent problems, including the problems of drug abuse and similar destructive activities (Amini and Salasnek 1975, Amini et al. 1976, Zilberg and Burke 1979). The peer group setting provides social interaction and living-learning situations without which psychotherapy of the adolescent may be sterile and ineffectual.

Box 35–2 lists the value of the therapeutic community for adolescents in treatment.

A Therapeutic Community

The Youth Service (Unit B) of the Langley Porter Psychiatric Institute (LPPI) in San Francisco is an example of a therapeutic community established on principles defined by Maxwell Jones and Harry Wilmer. In fact, Dr. Wilmer was the medical director during the unit's development. The Youth Service is a therapeutic community that provides twenty-four-hour care to a maximum of twenty-two clients. The program is offered to young men and women ranging in age from 13 to approximately 34 years of age. The average age is between 14 and 18 years.

The individual therapy focus for the Youth Service clients is primarily psychodynamic, but group therapies are an integral part of the treatment program. Treatment includes intensive participation in

- Community meeting
- Client government group
- Family therapy
- Small group therapy
- Psychodrama
- Art therapy
- School program
- Recreational therapy
- Vocational counseling
- Transitional group (to aid in transition from hospital to community)

Such a structured treatment focus helps the clients understand the meaning their behavior holds for them, develop controls and structure for their behavior, and identify the conflicts and behaviors that keep them from more useful and satisfying lives.

The clients present the gamut of psychiatric diagnoses, including schizophrenic disorders and acute behavioral disturbances. They are usually referred either through the court system after having committed such illegal acts as drug abuse or burglary, or by their families following antisocial behavior beyond their parents' control. The unit has a locked door policy, but clients are granted varying degrees of privilege depending on their status in the program.

The nursing staff, consisting of psychiatric nurses and technicians, have a vital role within the therapeutic com-

---

Box 35–2
VALUE OF THERAPEUTIC COMMUNITY FOR THE ADOLESCENT IN TREATMENT

1. Adolescent will more readily hear and accept limits from peers than from adults.
2. Adolescent will more readily respond to negative and positive feedback from peers.
3. Shared goals and objectives facilitate group process and development of cohesion among adolescent group members.
4. Group interaction allows for expression of appropriate feelings and identification with peers with similar feelings.
5. Group interaction provides learning opportunities in developing relationships with others.
6. Group structure allows for "testing" of new, more adaptive behaviors with peer group.
7. Adolescent receives feedback from peer group and has opportunity to give feedback in supportive environment.
8. Group format provides opportunity to work out specific issues of conflict with adult group leaders while receiving support and understanding of peers.

munity and in the clients' lives. Clinical nurse specialists also assume the role of primary therapist.

Several rules provide a nonthreatening atmosphere in which treatment objectives can be attained:

- There should be no acts or threats of physical violence to oneself, others, or the environment.
- There should be no sexual contact between clients or between clients and staff.
- While in treatment, clients should refrain from the use of all drugs, including alcohol.
- Clients should attend all meetings.

Enforcing these rules to the limit presents many problems. Given the nature of adolescents, particularly disturbed adolescents, there is a great deal of testing around rules. Indeed, strict adherence to rules is not the prime objective in successful treatment. Rather, it is the struggle around rules that provides nursing staff and clients with external evidence of the adolescent's internal struggle and forms a basis for the beginning of problem solving within the relationships. This process entails considerable acting out of past experience, as clients repeat earlier patterns of relating to others and attempt to use previously maladaptive measures to overcome obstacles to satisfaction. The concept of acting out is explained in the section Assessment.

A Residential Treatment Program

The Kansas Boys Industrial School is a good example of a residential treatment program that emphasizes the behavioral aspects of the clients' progress. Clients who are committed to the Boys School have been judged delinquent in juvenile court, tend to be impulsive and nonreflective, and usually resort to antisocial behavior when overwhelmed by their feelings.

The treatment program includes group and individual counseling, specially selected educational classes, and family therapy. The average length of stay is fourteen months, and the population ranges from 160 to 250. The institution maintains external control of the boys while it helps them learn to control their own behavior and impulses. Through the use of sports and other activities, the program teaches them to redirect some of their aggressive energy into more appropriate channels. Whenever a boy seems to be losing self-control, he is helped by reducing the number of his relationships and minimizing the demands placed on him.

Both the Kansas Boys Industrial School and the Youth Service of Langley Porter Psychiatric Institute illustrate the effectiveness of the group setting in dealing with the behavior problems of disturbed adolescents and helping them change their lives.

THE NURSING PROCESS AND ADOLESCENTS

Adolescents present behaviors and problems unique to their developmental stage. Without knowledge and understanding about potentially difficult areas, the nurse may respond with confusion, anger, and even hostility, which will cause feelings of frustration and failure for both the nurse and the adolescent. The following pages contain numerous examples of either typical behaviors expected of the "normal" adolescent or problem behaviors that may provide the impetus for referral to a treatment setting, or both. In many situations the nurse may simply need attention drawn to the difficult issues encountered in working with adolescents. That information is given in the Assessment section. Situations that represent an identified problem necessitating treatment are categorized under Planning and Implementing Interventions.

Assessment

Accurate and comprehensive assessments can be obtained only by viewing the adolescent as a biopsychosocial being. By integrating knowledge from the biologic and psychologic sciences and humanistic interactionist theory, the nurse will be able to understand what a particular behavior means to the adolescent. Nurses who can recollect their own adolescent experiences—the conflicts and uncertainty as well as the elation and the triumphs—can better appreciate the adolescent's turmoil. On the other hand, it is equally important that the nurse discover who the individual adolescent is. Meanings of behavior, values, and actions can vary from client to client and may not reflect similar meanings or values held by the nurse. For example, an invitation from the adolescent's peers to play a game of Trivial Pursuit may not receive an appreciative response, particularly if the client has trouble with competitive feelings. In addition, since adolescents are between childhood and adulthood, they frequently have the feelings and choices of adulthood without an adult's abilities in verbal discourse and impulse control. As a result, feelings and decisions may get "acted out" nonverbally, in a childlike way. This is particularly true of the emotionally disturbed adolescent.

Acting Out

The concept of **acting out** is complex. The term has been used to describe a variety of behaviors, ranging from antisocial, destructive acts to unconscious impulses expressed in action rather than in symbolic words or symptoms. Acting out may, and often does, include destructive actions and seemingly undefinable behaviors. The term describes a recreation of the client's life experiences, relationships with significant others, and resulting unresolved conflicts.

These are all components of what is commonly called the client's **life script**, which unfolds as the client relates, reacts, and behaves in accustomed ways. Through observation of and interaction with the client, the nurse can uncover the meanings that various behaviors and actions hold for the individual. For example, the child who has assumed the "black sheep" role in the family will seek to recreate that familiar role in relation to others outside the home, particularly in the in-patient setting. The following clinical example illustrates one girl's relationship with her parents as replayed with the nursing staff on an in-patient unit.

Liza is 14 years old. She has been on the unit for six days. She is an attractive, engaging young person who has been friendly with both staff and clients. Liza has been on the periphery of several rule-breaking incidents but has not been directly involved. She has begun to establish close ties with Jim, a nurse, and engages in frequent lengthy discussions with him about her innermost feelings and fears. One evening she candidly talks to him about the callous way in which she was treated by one of the other nurses, a woman, in regard to a gynecologic problem. Liza says with undisguised fear and embarrassment that she is afraid the situation will repeat itself. She expresses great respect for Jim's knowledge and style and asks him to attend to any subsequent problems himself rather than report her dissatisfaction with Jane, the other nurse.

The implications for treatment are many. The most important factors for Jim to consider are what meaning Liza's behavior has for her and what would be the most therapeutically effective way to deal with the situation. The client's presenting problems and the expectation that the client will act out previous conflicts and life scripts have provided Jim adequate information on which to base an appropriate intervention. The client's attempt to seduce the nurse, and the need for nurses to examine their own behavior and motivations, are discussed in detail later in this chapter.

Jim recognizes the "pull" from Liza to feel that only he can adequately handle the situation. He remembers that Liza's home situation is chaotic. Liza's mother and father frequently fight over who is the better parent. Jim surmises that Liza also plays a part in these fights. The present situation seems to indicate that he is about to be played off against Jane, just as Liza perhaps plays one parent against the other. Jim responds by reiterating his concern for her dilemma and suggesting that Liza speak with Jane about the situation.

In this situation it is clear that the client is attempting to recreate her home situation, using two of the nurses to reenact the roles of her parents. Had Jim been seduced into playing the father's role in the script, he would have recreated the family's conflict on the ward. The ideal solution is for staff to interrupt this pathologic process by substituting a healthier way of resolving the problem. Thus Jim does not react with compliance or with anger to Liza's attempts. Instead he recognizes the significance of her behavior and deals with the situation in a concerned yet healthy way, suggesting a resolution to the immediate problem that demonstrates respect for both Liza's and Jane's abilities to resolve the conflict.

Such situations are commonplace on an adolescent service. They require nursing staff to evaluate the client's psychodynamics and psychopathology as well as their own inner feelings and behavior. But these situations are not limited to the in-patient setting. This fact alone obliges nurses to be alert in observing and assessing verbal and nonverbal communication and to understand their own feelings and behavior in order to make accurate assessments and appropriate interventions.

Communication

Communication with adolescents is an art in itself. To become proficient in this area it is necessary to accept and understand that:

- Feelings and conflicts tend to get acted out rather than verbalized
- Adolescents have an unconventional language of their own
- Profanity may be in frequent use, especially by the disturbed adolescent
- Many clues can be obtained simply by observing the adolescent's behavior, dress, or environment

The nurse who learns the skills of interviewing and the use of nonverbal cues and messages can use them comfortably and naturally in communicating with the adolescent.

Adolescents give many nonverbal cues to the specific emotional struggles, underlying confusion, or simply transitory moods that they are experiencing (Figure 35–2). A glance around their rooms or a brief study of their dress can tell the nurse more than several direct questions would elicit. Sometimes adolescents give obvious cues. A client who wears a coat around the unit may be planning to run away. Other less obvious behaviors, which are often outside the client's conscious awareness or control, can also yield vital information. A sudden escalation of horseplay among the boys around bedtime is an example. The nurse would probably be correct in identifying this behavior as an expression of anxiety related to sexual identity and fears of homosexual feelings. Interactionist theory holds that the adolescent boy's newfound sexual feelings and changing body image provide unfamiliar ways of relating to members of his own sex. As a result, he regresses to preadolescent behavior, which served him well in handling close feelings up to now, but which now proves inappropriate. In this instance, firm limit setting is in order. The nurse should avoid interpreting the behavior or paying undue attention to the specifics. Testing and limit setting are discussed later in this chapter.

Adolescents seek to create a language all their own. This takes some understanding and acceptance. In seeking their identity, adolescents establish a form of communication unique to the group. To gain acceptance into the adolescent world, the adult must accept this need to employ ambiguous (to the adult) yet specific (to the adolescent) terms to express themselves. In many cases, the nurse must communicate with adolescents by using their own jargon.

This jargon often includes obscene and profane words. This is particularly true of disturbed adolescents, who have an especially difficult time expressing anger and fear appropriately. The words employed often reveal the nature of the emotional conflict. For example, a young male adolescent grappling with his sexual identity and aggressive feelings may resort to sexually graphic words when he feels anxious or afraid. The nurse may sometimes find it productive to use similar words to give explanations or to clarify communication. Understandably, some nurses have difficulty tolerating profane or sexually graphic language. However, nurses need to evaluate their clients' underlying reasons for using such language to help clients understand their feelings. Only then can they encourage clients to use more appropriate means of expression. Needless to say, if clients sense that the reason the nurse wants them to speak more appropriately is only to make the nurse more comfortable, the end result will not be satisfactory.

Anger and Hostility

How effectively we deal with expressions of anger and hostility will depend on how effectively we handle our own angry or hostile feelings. Nurses compromise their own

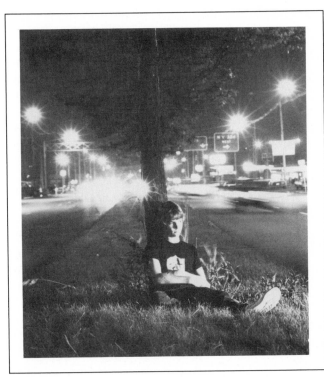

Figure 35–2
This adolescent's nonverbal behavior gives some clues to his sense of aloneness and isolation. His moodiness reflects this stormy period in his life when conflicting ideas and feelings intensify on all fronts.

effectiveness if they are uncomfortable with expressions of anger or hostility or view them as negative or to be avoided at all costs.

Nurse's Self-Assessment

This brings up a subject that is rarely considered—anger felt and expressed by the nurse toward the client. The general focus on the client's need for understanding and good care seem to make it unacceptable for the nurse to display negative feelings toward the client. In the nursing care of adolescents, however, a constant all-giving and all-accepting attitude by the nurse, particularly during times of testing, would be not only nontherapeutic but also illogical and dishonest. Testing behavior is at an all-time high, and adolescents need honest feedback. The adolescent will sometimes escalate the provocative behavior to evoke an angry reaction from the nurse. For nurses to pretend that they are not angry in such a situation is as undesirable for treatment as it would be for them to pretend that they were fond of the client. Honesty with one's feelings is a prime prerequisite in establishing and maintaining meaningful and productive relationships with adolescent clients. This does not mean that nurses should give vent to all their thoughts or impulses. They should be aware of their own reactions and use good judgment in handling them.

Chapters 27 and 28 offer help to nurses evaluating the integration of personal and professional role identifications and give suggestions for taking care of themselves. In addition, the following questions could be of help in assessing the nurse's own ways of dealing with anger:

- What kinds of things make me angry?
- How do I deal with my anger? Do I tend to ignore or hide it, or do I show that I am angry?
- Do I sometimes use profanity or act out my feelings in a physical way? How do I feel about others who do this?
- What do I think about how I handle anger?
- How do I feel about how I handle anger?
- How do I react to others when they are angry?

The discussion of anger and hostility expressed by the adolescent found in the section on Planning and Implementing Interventions can help the nurse decide what actions to take, if any.

Anxiety and Resistance

Normal adolescents frequently feel anxious as they experience change and inner turmoil in adapting to a new identity. The anxiety evidenced by the disturbed adolescent in treatment can indicate many other things. The changes required of the disturbed adolescent are much more threatening than those required of the normal adolescent. If treatment is to be successful, clients must look at the meaning of their behavior and must change many of their earlier interactional patterns. This can be frightening. For example, it is more comfortable to play the role of the "bad seed" or "bad kid," with its known pitfalls and expectations, than to attempt a change that entails many uncertainties and unknowns.

Clients feel threatened and anxious when the nurse does not act according to the familiar life script because they must then find other ways of handling the situation. They must also deal with the anxiety. Frequently this anxiety will be channeled into a game of "cops and robbers" as the client once again assumes a familiar role and maintains the negative or unhealthy image. The anxiety caused by unfamiliar roles will be dissipated by further testing and

acting out. The nurse should not take this as an indication that therapy is not working. It may simply indicate that the client needs to move ahead more slowly with insightful discoveries and needs the nurse's support in doing so.

The nurse should keep in mind that to such adolescents, "opening up" in a trusting way does not hold the same positive promise as it does for the nurse. From a humanistic interactionist perspective, the adolescent who has been rejected or experienced loss following close relationships in the past will feel wary of the nurse's expressions of interest or concern and will be cautious about repeating such experiences. These adolescents may respond to the nurse with testing behaviors, anger and mistrust, or outright rejection. Adolescents who expect rejection assume some control over the relationship if they reject others before being rejected themselves.

Sometimes nurses find it difficult to allow adolescents to grapple with their anxieties and fears. At other times, the nurse may not recognize the client's behavior as a symptom of anxiety or depression. The following clinical example demonstrates the value of a comprehensive assessment, of exploring all possible reasons for a client's resistance to the nurse's efforts before implementing action.

Kathy was the quietest and most aloof client on the ward. She had isolated herself from the other clients during the week that followed admission and avoided conversing with staff members outside meetings. One evening she seemed especially receptive to the new nurse, Ellie, who was able to interest her in a sewing project. Ellie, who was a new graduate, felt pleased that Kathy had responded warmly to her during their time together. The next day Kathy did not speak to Ellie and seemed to avoid her at all costs. Later Ellie noticed that the dress Kathy had been sewing was torn into shreds and stuffed into the wastepaper basket. Ellie interpreted this quite personally. She felt deeply hurt and rejected. In her discussion with her supervisor, Ellie showed her disappointment and anger. Her supervisor observed that, although the good time and feelings that Ellie and Kathy had shared the evening before were genuine, Kathy had not experienced many such times before with her parents or other adults. She suggested that Kathy was probably angry with Ellie for pointing up what she, Kathy, had missed. The supervisor suggested that Ellie be patient with Kathy. Perhaps later Ellie could reestablish the bond, and they would be able to talk about what had happened.

Fortunately, Ellie did not act on her angry feelings. Had she done so, she might have impulsively assessed Kathy's behavior as "hopeless," relating Kathy's anxiety and resistance to an inability to trust, or she may have begun to relate to the client in a vindictive way, withdrawing from

Kathy in turn. Instead, she sought advice. Ellie's supervisor recognized that Ellie wanted badly to do well and needed positive feedback. She also realized that Ellie did not understand the nature of giving to emotionally disturbed adolescents. Had Ellie not sought advice, she might have acted on her angry feelings, further alienating Kathy and causing herself more anger and frustration. Without an understanding of Kathy's actions, Ellie would have continued to expect kindness in return for kindness and would have been keenly disappointed.

Seduction of the Nurse

In working with adolescents there is always a risk of **seduction of the nurse**, or being manipulated into relating in a nontherapeutic way, due to:

- The intimate nature of the nurse's involvement with the adolescent

- The narcissism inherent in this age group
- The nurse's all-accepting attitude in working with the adolescent

Narcissism in this age group is caused by the child's withdrawal from the parents and their value system. This withdrawal leads to a general self-centeredness, overevaluation of the self, heightened self-perception, decreased ability for reality testing, and extreme self-absorption. The result is that the people to whom adolescents turn become all-important and perfect in their eyes. Nurses may be strongly tempted to respond accordingly.

The dangers inherent in this situation are not simply the two possible extremes—total submission to temptation and participation in a sexual relationship with the client,

RESEARCH NOTE

Citation

Thomas SP, Groer MW: Relationship of demographic, life-style, and stress variables to blood pressure in adolescents. Nurs Res 1986;35(3):169–172.

Study Problem/Purpose

To examine the relationship of selected anthropometric, life-style, demographic, and stress factors to blood pressure of freshman high school students.

Methods

The subjects were 323 students in rural, suburban, and urban high schools in eastern Tennessee. Information was obtained from the Adolescent Life Change Event Scale, a questionnaire involving standard health hazard appraisal items (age, sex, and race; diet, smoking, and aerobic exercise; family history of heart disease, diabetes, hypertension, and stroke), questions regarding stress management techniques, and body mass index (calculated from measurements of blood pressure, height, and weight).

Findings

There was a notable difference observed in life stress scores for subjects with good health habits (lower stress scores) compared to individuals with poor health habits. The three most frequently reported stressors for participants were arguments with parents, arguments with siblings, and making new friends. Dietary practices of females were generally better than males although females were more likely to smoke and had more family members with heart disease, diabetes, hypertension, and stroke. Females

exercised less than male subjects. Females were more likely to report being stressed by appearance changes, size problems, and relationship issues; males reported lower stress scores, feeling more stressed by poor academic achievement and adjusting to a new job. Systolic pressures were higher in urban subjects. Males had higher mean systolic pressures than females for each geographic area.

Implications

Further research is needed to establish relationship between poor health and high stress factors for the adolescent: Do health habits deteriorate as life stressors increase or is neglect of health a contributing factor to high stress levels? In either instance there are important implications for the nurse who works with adolescents, regardless of the setting. In the educational setting, health education classes within the peer group setting, which provide opportunities for frank and candid discussion and validation of fears, myths, and problems, may help improve health habits of the adolescent population and identify or possibly deter related stress factors. In the acute care, community, or clinic setting, questions regarding life-style and recent stressors may yield valuable clues. Information regarding stress management techniques, more adaptive coping skills, and validation of the adolescent's concerns as not uncommon may offer amelioration of physical difficulty. In the psychiatric setting adolescents may do well to attend more to health habits and life-style choices as contributors to the accumulation of life stress. This seems particularly true for males since the results raise the question: Do adolescent males encounter fewer stress factors or have they been socialized to ignore or not to acknowledge their stressors?

or strong denial of temptation by maintaining a rigid, unapproachable stance that makes it impossible to establish a meaningful, trusting relationship. Neither of these extremes is unknown, but the greatest danger is actually intrinsic to the role of the helping professional. It is tempting to respond to the adolescent's idealized view, to be the "savior" who succeeded with this difficult person where everyone else has failed, to feel superior to the imperfect parents, the harassed school teacher, the skeptical juvenile judge, or the other staff on the unit. However, the nurse should not give in to such temptations. Complications will most certainly develop that at best will temporarily compromise the nurse's effectiveness and at worst will render the treatment program completely ineffective. Liza's example of acting out demonstrates this. Jim, the evening nurse, could have been seduced by Liza to collude with her against the day nurse, Jane, had he not been keenly aware of the possibility.

Nurses who work intensively with adolescents often face situations in which their own unresolved feelings are aroused. They must choose whether to act on these impulses or to explore their origin. Of course, one is not always conscious of these unresolved feelings. It would be absurd to expect nurses to be totally aware of the meaning of their behavior at any given moment. On the other hand, the skilled clinician is usually acquainted with the issues or conflicts that have caused problems in the past. In doubtful cases the knowledgeable nurse will seek consultation from such a clinician. The clinician can help the nurse assess the situation and understand what part the nurse may have played in initiating it. Nurses who wish to explore their personal conflicts further may then seek counseling or therapy. The nurse can use the following questions to assess the nature of such interactions with the client:

- Is this client's friendliness compromising the professional role boundaries between us to "personalize" our relationship?

- Do I feel compelled to respond in a personal rather than a therapeutic way, possibly revealing information about my own life and life-style?

- Do I feel uncomfortable with the client's flattering comments or probing questions?

- Do I tend to forget that this person is a client?

- Is the client encouraging me to keep secrets from other staff or to "side" with the client against other staff?

In addition to the above, nursing staff would benefit from establishing one or more of the following to provide a consistent format for assessing and evaluating ongoing situations with adolescent clients:

- Each nurse's own ongoing supervision with preceptor or nurse supervisor

- A regularly scheduled meeting (perhaps monthly) for all nursing staff to discuss difficult situations and conflicting feelings

- A staff meeting (perhaps weekly) in which all disciplines identify interpersonal obstacles and plan interventions toward more optimal treatment

Given the nature of their work, the staff—particularly the nursing staff—undergo considerable stress as accepted ideas and values are constantly challenged by the adolescents. However, in a research study evaluating the levels of stress in an in-patient psychiatric adolescent unit, the nursing staff reported only low to moderate stress in what seemed to be high-stress situations (Campbell 1977). This raises the question of the extent to which staff members use denial in dealing with stressful issues and suggests how much denial may indeed be necessary in working with disturbed adolescents on a daily basis.

Sexual Behavior of the Adolescent

Jersild (1978, p 109) says, "Sexual development is a meeting ground of the biological, psychological, and moral influences that shape an adolescent's life." The nurse should not underestimate the importance of the adolescent's experimentation and attitude in sexual matters. Likewise, nurses should evaluate their own attitudes and feelings about sexual issues as they relate to their own past experiences and current activities. Conflicts in such matters or residual resentments left over from the past will certainly affect their decisions or interaction with the client regarding sexual matters. Again, while it is not necessary that the nurse resolve all these issues, it is highly desirable to be aware of areas of conflict that might make it difficult to view a situation objectively or set rational limits. Nurses may find the following questions helpful in increasing their self-awareness about sexual attitudes and feelings:

- How would I describe my adolescence as it related to my developing sexuality?

- What do I remember about the development and changes in my body?

- How did I feel about these changes?

- How would I describe my adolescent relationships with members of my sex?

- How would I describe my adolescent relationships with members of the opposite sex?

- What event stands out in my mind when I recall my sexual experiences during adolescence?

- How have these past relationships, events, and feelings influenced me today?

Until adolescents master their anxieties and fears about their sexual identity and gain control over sexual urges, they will exhibit a variety of behaviors and attitudes that may confuse or trouble the nurse. The following sections focus specifically on three related issues: heterosexual behavior, homosexual behavior, and pregnancy.

Heterosexual Behavior

Heterosexual activity is normal and desirable during adolescence. However, the nurse who works with either normal or disturbed adolescents will sometimes see them engage in sexual activities that do not seem healthy or growth producing. For example, the adolescent girl who seeks punishment rather than true pleasure in her sexual exploits will display them in an overt, exhibitionistic way in a place where a particularly moralistic person will discover her and give her the reprimands she desires. She may be testing her mother's values in an attempt to resolve her own inner conflicts about this. Adolescents in an in-patient treatment setting where sexual intercourse is forbidden may engage in sexual intercourse where a staff member will be sure to discover them. The experience may reinforce their image of sexual behavior as "bad" behavior. Or it may simply provide a means of acting out their defiance of the rules, thereby earning the familiar "bad kid" label. The incident involving the nurse Barbara and the clients Laurie and Bill in the Planning and Implementing Interventions section is an excellent example of this.

Homosexual Behavior

During preadolescence, people normally choose a member of the same sex with whom to experience intimate or loving feelings. This does not necessarily mean that a sexual relationship will ensue, although it often does. Homosexual activity may continue into the adolescent years.

Generally, however, adolescents begin to view homosexual feelings as a threat to the development of their identity. As a result, they may ward off such feelings by engaging in frantic sexual activity with a member of the opposite sex. This is particularly true for boys. It is normal for the adolescent boy to be afraid of his own passive wishes and to label them homosexual. He has probably been brought up to relate to physical displays of strength or aggressive displays of power. Thus, an incident in which he feels threatened or powerless would produce feelings of sexual impotence, a fear of castration, a feeling of dependency or weakness, and a greater fear of homosexuality. The adolescent boy in treatment may act out these feelings, or he may attempt to reaffirm his masculinity with inappropriate displays of aggression or destructive behavior. See the Planning and Implementing Interventions section for nursing actions.

At the other extreme are adolescents who engage in predominantly homosexual activities. Many of these individuals find relationships with the opposite sex threatening and continue to seek intimacy and solace with people like themselves. Some feel more comfortable with companions of the same sex and are satisfied with these relationships. Others use their homosexual affiliation to express and act out hostility directed against their parents and their parents' values.

Since nurses who work with adolescents may encounter any or all of these situations, they must attempt to understand the meaning of clients' homosexual activities or life-style. The clients may need to explore their feelings and anxieties openly. Open discussion with an understanding yet knowledgeable professional may resolve many of the conflicts inherent in the choice between homosexual and heterosexual life-styles. Many professionals believe that homosexual behavior in any age group is abnormal, and that particularly during adolescence feelings about sexual identity may be acted out before the identity conflict is resolved. This group advocates psychotherapy as the only way to help such people deal with their feelings and resolve the conflicts.

Clients who use homosexuality to express hostility toward their parents will undoubtedly act out with the staff as well. The nurse would be wise to remain objective and relatively nonjudgmental with these clients, allowing them to deal with the feelings of anger or depression that may result from addressing the conflict.

Although adolescence is a very young age at which to make lifelong decisions regarding homosexual relationships, some may decide on homosexuality as a satisfactory alternative. These people will not experience conflicts about such relationships or need to flaunt them or act out with the staff in an angry or hostile way. In such cases, however, nurses may have to deal with their own negative feelings about homosexuality. It is important that nurses consider what their relationships mean to clients and respect their right to make life-style choices for themselves.

Pregnancy

The etiology of adolescent pregnancy includes social and family expectations and unconscious motivations. Some teenage girls are quite pleased with the state of motherhood and suffer no emotional consequences from the decision to become a mother. Generally speaking, however, a conscious, deliberate decision for pregnancy at this age is manipulative. The goal may be to escape a difficult family situation, to express hostility toward parents, or to act out a life script in which the daughter is seen as "bad." In cases where the adolescent failed to receive adequate nurturing as a child, she could be acting out dependency needs in an attempt to give the baby the love and caring she herself did not receive. In so doing, she feels loved and cared for in turn.

The nurse should be sensitive to motivational factors in dealing with emotionally deprived adolescents. It is important to use existing educational tools and interpersonal relationships to help adolescent girls understand their needs and motivations in becoming pregnant. It is also important to provide teenagers of both sexes with knowledge about sex and birth control. Many high schools are now recognizing this need and providing such information in birth control clinics or through health education classes. Too often parents and professionals alike deny the adolescent's sexual activity until an unwanted pregnancy occurs and it is too late to discuss the meaning or possible consequences of sexual behavior.

Dietary Problems

Food Fads and Diets

The eating habits and food preferences of disturbed adolescents can reveal a lot about the nature of their inner turmoil. A comparison between the client's diet and that of a normal adolescent may show little difference in variety but probably a great difference in quantity. Adolescents who have been deprived of early nurturing tend to eat more than normal adolescents and will probably place a higher value on mealtimes and on their "share" of the food. The nurse may notice that adolescents consume more milk than usual during periods of stress or anxiety. Generally speaking, girls will want to follow food fads or unreasonable dietary regimens in order to become slim and attractive. This usually gives the nurse an opportunity to engage in health teaching about food and exercise and to express a cooperative interest in their developing feminine identity.

Obesity

In the American culture, slimness is admired, and many adolescent girls will go to great lengths to fit into that size five dress. By the same token, the obese adolescent often feels unattractive and unpopular. In both "normal" and disturbed adolescents the need to overeat may have deep-rooted psychologic implications. Adolescents may eat compulsively in an attempt to compensate for the love and nurturing that they did not receive as children. They may also turn to obesity as a defense against intimacy with the opposite sex. While they keep this emotional distance, they frequently use excuses such as, "I would be popular if I weren't so fat," or "When I lose weight, I'm going to learn to dance." The nurse should recognize these defenses for what they are but generally should not challenge them

until the obese adolescent has progressed far enough to look at their meaning.

On the other hand, the compulsion to overeat may be borne out of sociocultural factors. Some feminists have suggested that overeating may reflect a need to fill oneself "up and out" to attain the stereotypic all-giving, nurturant role that women have been encouraged to assume. Others hold the opposite viewpoint that the obese individual is simply rejecting the stereotypical "thin is in" ideal. Moreover, research has shown strong familial implications for obesity, either biologic or psychosocial in origin, such as learning family eating habits. Etiology may also entail hypothalamus dysfunction.

While assessing the nature of the client's problem with overeating, the nurse will also want to assess the nature of the client's relationships with peers. Other adolescents may tease and ostracize their obese peer. When this happens, the nurse can support the client while asking, in as nonthreatening a way as possible, what the obesity does for him or her.

Whether the underlying cause relates to psychologic, sociocultural, or familial issues, the nurse should constantly encourage the client to understand the implications of obesity and try to further a healthier sexual identity for the client. The nurse should not let this persistence take on the same character as teasing from the adolescent's peers. Nor should the nurse assume any one of the above reasons for the client's obesity. The nurse will do well to keep in mind the tenets of interactionist theory while discovering what meaning obesity has for the client and establishing mutually desirable goals warranting intervention.

Eating disorders, on the other hand, are conditions that will most likely warrant treatment. They are discussed in the next two sections as well as in the Planning and Implementing Interventions section.

Eating Disorders

Anorexia Nervosa

There has been an increasing prevalence of **anorexia nervosa** during the past decade. The clinical picture is of a person, usually a young woman, who is obsessed with the idea of being thin. Although the client does not lose appetite, she consistently restricts food intake to the extreme of dangerous emaciation. At other times, she may indulge in enormous eating binges, alternating them with periods of fasting. The following are commonly seen with these clients:

- The client has an intense fear of becoming obese that does not diminish with weight loss.

- The client's body image is disturbed; for example, the client claims to "feel fat" even when emaciated.

- The client refuses to maintain body weight over the minimum norm set for age and height (weighs 15% below expected weight).

- There is no known physical illness (such as cancer, tuberculosis, hyperthyroidism, pyloric obstruction) that would account for the weight loss.

- Weight loss is usually accomplished by reduction in total food intake with a disproportionate decrease in high carbohydrate and fat-containing foods, self-induced vomiting, use of laxatives and/or diuretics, and extensive exercise.

- Amenorrhea often appears before noticeable weight loss has occurred: i.e., absence of at least three consecutive menstrual cycles.

- Significant weight loss is usually the primary reason the individual comes to medical attention.

- Numerous physical signs accompany profound weight loss: hypotension, hypothermia, dependent edema, bradycardia, lanugo (neonatal-like hair), and a variety of metabolic changes.

- The client most commonly undergoes a single episode with full recovery; however, the course may be episodic or even unremitting until death by starvation.

- The severe weight loss often necessitates hospitalization to prevent death by starvation.

- In some cases the onset of illness is associated with a stressful life situation.

- The disorder is more common among sisters and mothers of individuals with the disorder than in the general population.

There have been many theoretical explanations for anorexia nervosa:

- From a developmental perspective, its incidence among adolescent females has been linked to a fear of growing up, concerns with sexual identity, and rejection of the feminine form.

- A family systems perspective would focus on the increased incidence among sisters and mothers of individuals with the disorder as well as the family triad constellation of a controlling, domineering mother and an emotionally distant, perhaps physically absent, father.

- Biologic research studies point to metabolic changes, such as electrolyte imbalances, or evidence of structural changes, such as enlarged ventricles in the brain.

- Some feminists assess the condition as a reaction against development of the stereotypic all-giving, maternal figure.

- A number of authors have linked the sociocultural pressures for thinness to the apparent increase of this disorder.

Hilde Bruch (1978) called this increase a "sociocultural epidemic," suggesting that vulnerable adolescents may come to believe that weight control is equivalent to self-control, leading to success and beauty as depicted by fashion's ideal. During the last decade there seems to have been

a shift in the idealized female form from a voluptuous hourglass shape to the lean, angular look popularized in magazines today. As evidence of this, one study examined data from Playboy centerfolds and Miss America Pageant contestants between 1960 and 1980 (Garner et al. 1980). Results showed that in the Playboy centerfolds bust measurements decreased, waists became larger, and hips became smaller, evolving toward a more "tubular" body form and away from the characteristic "hourglass" shape previously idealized. In the past decade both centerfolds and pageant winners have been thinner than their historical counterparts. The authors of this same study report that over the same period there was a significant increase in diet articles in six popular women's magazines, providing additional evidence for a growing emphasis on weight reduction in pursuit of this idealized thinner image.

See the Planning and Implementing Interventions section for discussion of nursing actions and the use of client contracts.

Bulimia Nervosa

A disorder characterized by binge eating, **bulimia nervosa** is commonly encountered in adolescent and young adult women. Recent statistics show it escalating among older women and younger men as well. Individuals with bulimia rapidly consume large quantities of high-calorie food, such as ice cream, cake, or bread, over a limited time, such as a couple of hours. There must be a minimum average of two binge-eating episodes per week for at least three months to warrant this DSM-IIIR diagnosis. Although the binges may be pleasurable, they are commonly followed by disparaging self-criticism and depression. Self-induced vomiting is commonly associated with this disorder since it decreases the physical pain of abdominal distention and may reduce postbinge anguish. However, severe dieting, fasting, cathartics, diuretics, and laxatives may provide alternative or additional methods of self-control. Bulimic episodes may occur as part of anorexia nervosa, but not all individuals with bulimia have the disturbances of body image characteristic of anorexia nervosa, and, although weight may fluctuate, clients with bulimia rarely become as emaciated as clients with anorexia nervosa.

B, a 17-year-old student, came to the mental health center because of binge eating. She complained that although she was very concerned with her weight and very invested in her physical image, she regularly went on gluttonous eating binges for one to two days. These would leave her nauseated, exhausted, and disgusted with herself. Her inability to control the behavior voluntarily was making her depressed.

In the course of her therapy, it became apparent that although B consciously wanted certain improvements to occur in academic and social life, and in her appearance, she had subtle ways of sabotaging any movement in that direction. Binge eating destroyed any attempts she made to control her weight and thus feel positive about her body image.

Movement in a self-interested direction had become attached in B's mind to repudiation of her depressed mother, with whom she felt very close. Individual successes, she felt, were antagonistic toward her mother, since they might lead to her own greater independence. Although she wished such independence for herself, she also feared losing her mother's support, which she needed. Thus she developed ways of undermining her own efforts.

Psychotherapeutic work with B involved discovering these meanings, bringing her concerns to the surface for discussion, and attempting to resolve issues of fear of separation and dependency needs. When this material was directly discussed, B had less need for indirect expression of conflict, and the binge-eating behavior subsided.

Client contracts can be particularly helpful with the adolescent with eating disorders. Contracts are discussed in the Planning and Implementing Interventions section.

Depression and Suicide

The incidence of suicide among adolescents has risen dramatically during this decade. About 6000 teenagers committed suicide nationwide in 1983, and for every successful suicide, some researchers say there are 100 attempts. The National Center for Health Statistics ranks suicide as the second leading cause of death for youth between 15 and 24 years of age in the United States. Moreover, there is real concern about a contagion of suicides, known as **suicide clusters,** in which one suicide appears to set off another. Such clusters were reported in several communities in 1984: In Plano, Texas, seven adolescents died within a year; in Westchester County, New York, five teens killed themselves within one month.

Why has there been such an increase—a 173 percent increase since 1950—in adolescent suicides? Many say it has been linked to decreased family stability, a more pressured childhood, or greater competition for grades in the schools and for jobs in the workplace. Some speculate that the complexity and dangers in the world (nuclear threats, terrorism, etc.) contribute to a sense of depression or futility about the adolescent's future.

Some maintain that the very nature of adolescence greatly contributes to the problem: that adolescent grandiosity and narcissism make the potentially suicidal adolescent believe, "I cannot die. Someone will find me before this overdose kills me." Others put responsibility for the increase in adolescent suicides on the media reporting of suicides. They insist that the reporting has a sensational and romantic quality that actually precipitates suicides, particularly the suicide clusters described earlier, which these critics allege would never have happened in the absence of publicity.

Numerous studies and varied agencies are working on these issues but few, if any, definitive answers have been found. However, we do know there are stressors and risk factors that can help the nurse identify a potentially suicidal adolescent.

Most suicides or suicide attempts are preceded by verbal or action threats, a statement of intent or a suicidal gesture. However, this is less true of adolescents, unless they have a history of long-standing problems and behavior change. Often adolescent suicides occur without warning. Frequently, they are triggered by a seemingly trivial incident—a fight with a boyfriend or a quarrel with parents. The suicide is a sudden, impulsive reaction to a stressful situation.

What may be extremely stressful to one adolescent, however, may be a minor matter to another. The nature and severity of the precipitating stress can reveal a lot about the adolescent's coping abilities. However, there are events and situations that have special significance as potential stressors for the adolescent. Table 35–2 lists some stressors with the possible meanings they may have for the adolescent. Rather than assume a meaning, however, the nurse with an appreciation for interactionist theory will explore a stressor with the client to identify the significance of the event and work toward mutually satisfactory goals and behaviors.

Which adolescents are most likely to commit suicide? It is known from retrospective studies of suicides, from interviews with attempted suicide victims, and from reports of effective interventions with potentially suicidal individuals that there are risk factors that can help the professional identify the potentially suicidal adolescent. For example, it is possible to recognize individuals who are suffering from depression before it interferes with their ability to function in everyday life and before the depression becomes so oppressive that the adolescent considers suicide. Box 35–3 lists risk factors that can give a warning signal to the nurse to explore and assess further.

The most common precursor of adolescent suicide is certainly depression. Since adolescence is such a volatile time, with rapid mood swings and great intensity of feelings as the norm, adults may have trouble recognizing depression in adolescents. Moreover, adults tend to idealize adolescence and may refuse to accept the idea of adolescent

Table 35–2
Stressors That Have Special Significance for the Adolescent

Stressor	Possible Meaning
Anniversary date of death of loved one (particularly if death was suicide)	Can rekindle feelings of loss and mourning; may evoke feelings of guilt or anger, if unresolved; may prompt ideas of "rejoining" the loved one
Developmental milestone (e.g., menarche, leaving grammar school and entering high school)	Can represent loss of childhood and decreasing dependency on parental figures; can evoke performance anxiety and fear of failure or embarrassment
Holidays	Can represent unfulfillment and disappointment; can trigger or intensify unmet needs and longings; can be a source of increased family tension and fighting
Loss, real or imagined	Can intensify feelings of low self-esteem and unworthiness; can cause feelings of acute loss and loneliness, resulting in depression and despair
Performance failure (e.g., failed exam, embarrassing school situation)	Can devastate the adolescent, particularly the overachieving adolescent with uncompromising parents; at the other extreme, can provide the "last straw" for an adolescent with many failures

depression. Mental health professionals have suggested that adolescent depression is underreported, with one researcher estimating that as many as 20 percent of youth of all ages may be depressed (Yahraes 1978). Moreover, one study showed that among youth referred for psychiatric emergency care due to suicidal behavior, 40 percent had symptoms of depression for at least one month before being seen (Child et al. 1980).

How can the nurse effectively assess depression in individuals who characteristically act out their feelings rather than express them verbally? In fact, largely because of this acting out behavior, the nurse in a setting frequented by adolescents has numerous opportunities to make such assessments. Not only will adolescents who are depressed exhibit certain behavioral cues but also comparisons of their behavior can be made with their peers who are not depressed. Assessments and interventions by the school or community nurse can be critical in this respect. Table 35–3 lists possible behavioral cues indicative of adolescent depression.

The section on Planning and Implementing Interventions contains specific actions for the nurse. See Chapter 29 for other information.

Drug Use and Abuse

Experimentation with drugs among the adolescent population is widespread. Surveys have reported that 50 to 95 percent of the adolescent subjects have used drugs, including alcohol, at least once.

Adolescents give many reasons for using drugs: to experiment, to get high, to "get inside my head," to have fun, to understand more about life. Although the general public may disagree about whether drugs are harmful, the fact remains that using drugs is acceptable to most adolescents—at least on an experimental level.

Box 35–3
FACTORS PUTTING ADOLESCENTS AT RISK FOR SUICIDE

1. Depression, particularly related to the loss of someone or something of great value to the adolescent (e.g., the death of a parent, sibling, or pet, separation following divorce, or a lengthy hospitalization).

2. Low self-esteem and lack of basic trust in self and others.

3. Family unit factors:

   - Psychiatric illness within the family unit, particularly in one or both parents.

   - Chronic depression within the family unit, particularly in one or both parents.

   - Marital discord and unhealthy interactions between parents or among parents and adolescent. Parents may use the adolescent as a scapegoat, displacing their feelings of dissatisfaction and disappointment and leading the adolescent to accept blame.

   - Suicide of a relative or someone else significant to the adolescent.

   - Situations characterized by long-term neglect, abuse, or an unstable home and family life.

   - Rigid parents with strict, uncompromising standards yielding helpless and hopeless feelings as a result of the adolescent's not "measuring up."

4. Handicap making the adolescent "different" and unworthy (e.g., a learning problem, a chronic illness, or a physical deformity); it is not this handicap per se that yields an unworthy reaction but the negative messages the adolescent may receive if the family is unable to provide frequent and consistent positive and accepting emotional experiences.

Table 35–3
Behavioral Cues Indicative of Adolescent Depression

1. Changed mood	Reflects a persistent and pervasive unhappy mood rather than the transient and situation-specific mood typical of adolescence; may project a global anger that interferes with interpersonal relationships.
2. Low self-esteem	Results in feelings of unworthiness, guilt, and rejection; leads to behaviors that "set up" failure and rejection.
3. Decreased energy	Marked by extreme fatigue that is incapacitating at times; adolescent may "wake up tired"; leads to concern about possible underlying illness.
4. Problems with school involvement	Includes both academic performance and social activity; low grades or decrease in academic performance can provide marker of emotional difficulty; changes in interpersonal relationships, particularly social withdrawal and isolation, are cues for the nurse.
5. Somatic complaints	Will most likely be reason to see nurse in school or community clinic; symptoms usually fall into three major categories: physical complaints with fatigue, alterations in sleep patterns, and changes in appetite and body weight.

How can the nurse determine when drug *use* becomes drug *abuse*? Generally, the adolescent who abuses drugs, including alcohol, exhibits at least one of the following characteristics:

- The adolescent's performance at school or work increasingly deteriorates.

- The adolescent is frequently caught high or in the act of getting high by parents or other authority figures.

- The adolescent increasingly resorts to drugs in times of stress or boredom.

- The adolescent has seriously deficient interpersonal relationships and can relate only when under the influence of drugs.

- The adolescent may lose interest in interpersonal relationships altogether, preferring to be high alone rather than to be with others.

Nurses are most effective when they can discern what the particular drug or high does for the client. A boy with a poor self-image and low self-esteem may say that it makes him "feel like a man." A particularly shy or introverted girl may say that it makes her "outgoing and friendly." The nurse may discover that being high helps rid disturbed adolescents of angry or depressed feelings. Indeed, in the treatment setting the client will frequently resort to smoking marijuana or "popping" uppers or downers in an attempt to escape uncomfortable feelings. Specific nursing actions related to drug abuse are included in the Planning and Implementing Interventions section of this chapter.

Nursing Diagnosis

The use of nursing diagnoses with adolescent clients can lend meaning and substance to the clients' behavior that might be overlooked with a DSM-IIIR diagnosis alone. For example, a DSM-IIIR diagnosis of "Disruptive behavior disorder, conduct disorder, solitary aggressive type" identifies the nature of the adolescent's difficulty. With various subsystems provided by nursing diagnoses (e.g., 05.02.01.01 Altered conduct/impulse processes, and 05.02.01.03, Aggressive/violent behaviors toward environment and self, respectively), however, the nurse can establish a more comprehensive picture of the client's difficulty and immediately become more goal-oriented in assessing and planning care. Moreover, in many treatment settings with adolescents mental health professionals are reluctant to give a DSM-IIIR diagnosis to the client during these early formative years lest the adolescent be psychiatrically labeled (possibly erroneously), which may result in inadequate treatment, self-fulfilling prophesy, or both in subsequent mental health contacts. Table 35–4 offers suggestions to help the nurse make correlations among NANDA diagnoses, PND-I diagnoses, and DSM-IIIR diagnoses. Nursing diagnoses are also identified with specific adolescent behaviors in the Planning and Implementing Interventions section of this chapter.

Planning and Implementing Interventions

Client Contract with the Adolescent

Contracts can be particularly useful with adolescents since they can feel powerless in a treatment setting, especially when "referred" by parents or the legal system. Moreover,

Table 35–4
Comparison of DSM-IIIR and Psychiatric Nursing Diagnoses

DSM-IIIR	PND-I	NANDA
Conduct disorder 312.00 Solitary aggressive type 312.20 Group type	05.02.01.01 Aggressive/violent behaviors toward environment 05.02.01.02 Aggressive/violent behaviors toward others	Violence, potential for Coping, ineffective individual
312.90 Undifferentiated type		
Eating disorder 307.10 Anorexia nervosa	07.06.02.02 Altered nutrition processes, less than body requirements	Nutrition, altered: less than body requirements
307.51 Bulimia nervosa	07.06.02.01 Altered nutrition processes, more than body requirements	Nutrition, altered: more than body requirements
	06.03.01 Altered body image	Self-concept, disturbance in body image
305.90 Psychoactive substance use disorder, NOS	05.02.01.03 Aggressive/violent behaviors toward self	Coping, ineffective individual Violence, potential for: self-directed
300.40 Dysthymia	08.01.01 Hopelessness	Hopelessness
	08.01.03 Loneliness	
	04.02.08 Sadness	
	05.05.02 Social isolation/withdrawal	Social isolation
	05.03.02 Altered leisure role	Social interaction, impaired
	05.03.04 Altered play role	Self concept, disturbance in: self-esteem
	06.03.04 Altered self-esteem	

with this increased sense of control over their own behavior adolescents become allies with the nurse in their treatment rather than the object of the nurse's treatment.

In most situations with adolescents, it seems most desirable to have the concrete form of a written contract because:

- The goals and expectations are written in black and white.

- They are less easily forgotten.

- The process seems more formal and "serious" to the adolescent.

- There is less room for misinterpretation and manipulation.

Contracts seem especially helpful in situations of substance abuse, eating disorders, suicidal behavior, and impulsive or manipulative behaviors (as with some personality disorders; see Chapter 21).

Whether verbal or written, the contract can be simply stated to promote clarity, consistency, and cooperation. For example:

I will not take drugs or bring drugs into the unit.

I will not call or accept calls from my drug friends while in the treatment program.

I will go directly to my outpatient therapy appointment and return immediately to the unit.

I will not harm myself or others. If I feel like hurting myself, others, or property, I will tell the staff.

If written, the contract is signed by the client, dated, and cosigned by the nurse. The contract is renegotiated at regular intervals, hourly, daily, or weekly, depending on the goals, the severity of the symptoms, and the degree of compliance with the agreement. In implementing a client contract, the form of the contract is less important than how the nurse and the adolescent jointly set the goals and expectations, carry out the contract, set limits and renegotiate changes, and evaluate the final outcome as demonstrated by the nursing care plan. Chapter 27 discusses contracting with clients in general.

Anger and Hostility

Expressions of anger and hostility are common on an adolescent ward. Verbal expressions usually take the form of profanity. Depending on the degree to which the client is experiencing and expressing these feelings, the nurse may choose any of a variety of interventions. These range from doing nothing other than observing the client's behavior to physically restraining someone who is attempting destructive action. In some situations a disturbed adolescent's ability to express anger directly to another person can be a sign of success in treatment. The choice of interventions also depends on the nurse's own experiences with such feelings, the nurse's knowledge and understanding of this client's life experiences with anger, and the external limits imposed by the agency. See the Anger and Hostility discussion in the Assessment section of this chapter.

In choosing an appropriate nursing intervention the nurse can question what meaning the adolescent's anger and hostility has for him or her by asking the following questions:

- How has the adolescent handled his or her anger in the past?
- Does the client have a history of aggression toward objects or persons?
- If so, what have been the consequences of this behavior?
- How does the adolescent feel following such a reaction?
- What kinds of things make the adolescent angry? Which of these would be most likely on the unit or in our setting?

Steve had expressed great interest in building a model airplane. He had saved up his money and had taken a long time to choose "just the right one" at the hobby shop. After spending most of the afternoon constructing and painting it, he was interrupted by a phone call from his mother. She told him that she would not be able to attend the family meeting that week, giving a number of specious-sounding reasons. This was the third consecutive week that she had missed. Each time she gave questionable reasons for being unable to attend. Steve was disappointed and angry. He slammed down the receiver, yelling obscenities in response to the nurse's questions, and ran into his room. There he began to destroy the plane by throwing it repeatedly on the floor.

In the preceding example, Steve was not hurting himself or another. Although he did destroy property, the plane belonged to him, and he was free to do with it as he chose. The nurse resisted any impulse to stop Steve from damaging his plane. Since it was of significant value to him, he later regretted having taken out his aggressions on it. However, the situation provided Steve with an opportunity to explore his actions, and he later asked the nurse why he would destroy something that he valued so much after his mother had disappointed and angered him. The parallel between this situation and hurting himself with drugs right after he had argued with his mother was only too apparent.

Incidents in which the nurse bears the brunt of a client's anger or hostility do not offer such obvious solutions. Disturbed adolescents may not think twice about addressing a female nurse as "bitch" and coupling such a greeting with a request for a favor. Adolescents direct insults and hostile remarks at nurses for many reasons, most of which have little to do with the nurses as people but a lot to do with them as adults or authority figures.

There are as many suggestions for intervention as there are people who will be involved in such exchanges. In choosing interventions, nurses should consider the meaning behind the client's behavior, their own relationship with this client, their own immediate feelings, and the end result desired. For example, if the client calls the nurse "bitch" the first time they meet, the nurse may interpret this as a form of testing. She may choose to respond immediately with a bewildered look at this unwarranted display of hostility. Later, the nurse may approach the client, expressing a naive curiosity as to the origin of the hostile feelings: "Hey, I don't understand what happened between us a few minutes ago. We just met, and you're calling me a bitch. What's that all about?" This simple question conveys two messages. First, it indicates to the client that the nurse is not accustomed to this kind of salutation. Second, it indicates that the nurse is more interested in the motivation for the remark than she is in curtailing its use.

On the other hand, if the client resorts to name calling only when angry or under stress, the nurse may decide to ignore the words and deal only with the feelings involved. For example, if a client has angrily left an ongoing family meeting, and then calls the nurse who attempts to talk with him a bitch, the nurse can probably assume that the anger is displaced. It is probably a result of overwhelming feelings experienced during the meeting. The nurse may elect simply to say, "I know you're not angry at me right now. It seems like the meeting is pretty heavy, though. Do you want to talk about why you don't want to be in there now?" In neither situation is the name calling intended as a personal affront. However, the way the nurse handles it will determine both the outcome of the immediate situation and the nurse's chances of furthering the relationship with the client.

The adolescent's reaction to the nurse's intervention will largely determine its effectiveness. For example, in the situation with Steve and the destruction of his plane, the nurse's goal was to help Steve understand the impulsive reaction that destroyed something he loved and to encourage a more appropriate and direct expression of anger at his mother. He was able to do this as well as draw a parallel between anger at his mother and his drug abuse, which hurt himself. If the nurse's goal had been simply to stop the destruction of his property, Steve could have felt even greater anger and frustration, and he might have turned his aggression toward himself, the nurse, or the environment. Certainly if the client had not stopped with destruction to his own property and had escalated his destructive behavior, turning his aggression toward himself or others, then direct **limit setting**, including physical restraints, would have been indicated.

In first-time encounters with any client new to the setting, the nurse should not be surprised or dismayed about less-than-optimal success with intervention. It may take some time and trial and error to assess the client's behaviors and choose the most effective interventions. See the beginning of this section for a discussion of client contracts. A nursing care plan for clients who act out aggression against themselves, others, and/or property is on the next page.

Testing and Limit Setting

As young adolescents attempt to adjust to the upheaval in their emotional lives and begin to emancipate themselves from parental figures, a good deal of testing is to be expected. This is normal. However, the meaning that testing holds for the disturbed adolescent is a more complicated matter.

As the clients in the Youth Service demonstrate, adolescents who lack early nurturing have difficulty with interpersonal relations. In most cases, the parents were emotionally unable to provide parenting. In a few cases, they chose not to impose their values on their children. In either case, the children never developed the internalized values that reduce conflict and avert crisis in adolescence. This causes identity diffusions, which in turn result in emptiness, a lack of basic trust, and difficulties with intimacy on any level.

In the treatment setting, testing for these clients seems to consist of making limitless and absolute demands. Although the limits the staff impose on these clients' behavior are frequently met with cries of injustice, the clients often really seem to be asking for limits as an indication of caring.

Julie had been on the unit only two days. During that time she had seen several of the older clients run away from the unit, commonly known as going AWOL, and had witnessed the staff members' attempts to encourage those remaining on the ward to deal with whatever feelings they were experiencing. Toward the end of her second evening, Julie abruptly jumped up from a conversation with a nurse and ran toward the open door. The surprised nurse immediately followed, running down the stairs after her. A smiling Julie was waiting at the bottom step when the nurse arrived, quite breathless and thoroughly confused, and began her barrage of questions. Julie quickly answered, "I just wanted to see if you cared enough to come after me."

In this situation no further action was necessary.

Sometimes the client may use annoying or destructive behavior to test the nurse. At these times, firm limit setting without further interpretation or exploration may be indicated. In other instances, the client may not be testing the nurse but be reacting to some real threat or uncomfortable situation.

Joanne was quietly playing pool by herself when she noticed her therapist talking to a new female client. Her volatile nature gave way to jealousy and rage, and she immediately began to hit the billiard balls off the table, making a lot of noise and startling everyone around her. The nurse who had been observing her witnessed the change in her behavior and understood the reaction. Without questioning Joanne's apparent anger, she stepped up to the table and challenged her to a game, which Joanne immediately accepted. Since Joanne prided herself on her pool-playing ability, she quickly channeled her energy and competitive feelings into the game and won. She then sought out her therapist and happily announced her victory.

Had the nurse not understood what had triggered Joanne's outburst, she might have become angry with her for making noise. She might have seen this as a form of testing and might even have begun to set limits on Joanne's privilege of playing pool. This would certainly have produced a helpless and even angrier Joanne, who would probably have escalated her behavior. Since the nurse was perceptive and adept in handling such situations, the results were

Nursing Care Plan: An Adolescent Client with a Disruptive Behavior Disorder

Nursing Diagnosis (PND-I/NANDA)	Client Care Goals	Nursing Planning/ Intervention	Evaluation
05.02.01.01 Aggressive/ violent behaviors toward environment (associated with destruction of property) 05.02.01.02 Aggressive/ violent behaviors toward others* /Violence, potential for: directed at others	Client will show increased impulse control. Client will verbally express difficult feelings prior to acting out feelings and impulses. Client will manifest more appropriate use of physical activities to cope with anxieties about potentially explosive situations.	Provide for physical safety of unit, ensuring that all sharp objects are confiscated. Anticipate angry or potentially explosive situations, allowing time to talk about it, or at least acknowledge existence of present situation, e.g., "I think you're trying to get me angry now by throwing those things around the room. I would rather talk about what's happening between us." Set firm limits on behavior while client can still hear them, before behavior escalates out of control. Expect that client will control actions. Ask client to come to talk to nurse in quiet area away from peers. If client does not stop behavior, direct to room for "time-out" until calm. If client continues to be violent against objects or with threats of violence against others, tell client you are going to help with controls. Implement procedure for use of physical restraints or seclusion room. Reinforce good behavior and give feedback at times when out of control, e.g., "I liked the way you handled John's provocative behavior today. You were cool when you told him that you were angry without storming around." Spend time with client when not acting out. Do not wait for negative behavior to give attention.	Client is able to gain attention in positive, more adaptive ways. Client asks directly for one-on-one time with assigned nurse and will set a later time if nurse not readily available. Client asks for time to talk in groups (at least one per day) about thoughts, feelings, and treatment plans. Client talks with staff if feels like hurting self, others, or property rather than acting out impulses. Nurse documents interventions, client response, and client's progress with impulse control and in potentially volatile situations. With increasing anxieties and inability to deal with feelings, nurse assesses need for increasing levels of limits and structure, evaluating and documenting client's response with each level. Nurse evaluates and revises behavioral contract in collaboration with client.

*PND-1 diagnoses also in NANDA list.

continued

Nursing Care Plan: An Adolescent Client with a Disruptive Behavior Disorder (*Continued*)

Nursing Diagnosis (PND-I/NANDA)	Client Care Goals	Nursing Planning/ Intervention	Evaluation
05.02.01.03 Aggressive/ violent behaviors toward self /Violence, potential for: self-directed	Client will show increased impulse control to curb self-directed violence.	Directly address the underlying feelings of sadness, loneliness, confusion, etc., when appropriate.	Client responds to staff prompts toward increased impulse control to curb violent acts.
		Ask other clients to give feedback in group meetings, particularly community meeting and small group therapy.	Client follows through with a no self-harm contract, outlining all the above.
		Encourage more appropriate coping skills, e.g., use of physical activities.	
		Promote involvement with peers in activities and comment on socially acceptable behaviors.	
		Update and renegotiate no self-harm contract as necessary—at least daily as an initial plan. (See Box 35–5.)	
		Encourage client to accept responsibility for behavior rather than blaming other people or circumstances for problems or using anger to avoid dealing with painful feelings.	

Source: Carrie McRae, RN, BSN, Langley Porter Psychiatric Institute, Unit B, San Francisco, California.

more satisfying to both parties. Because of the nurse's action, Joanne was able to save face by winning at pool and was not forced to feel more helpless.

Scapegoating

Scapegoating is common in many groups, but particularly in adolescent groups. It occurs in three stages.

1. Frustration generates aggression.
2. Aggression becomes displaced on relatively defenseless others.
3. Through a process of blaming, projecting, and stereotyping, this displaced aggression is rationalized and

finally justified, since the identified scapegoat is "different" in some real way.

The members of a group tend to attack the scapegoated individual because they are afraid to attack the person on whom their feelings are actually focused.

Adolescents readily identify peers who are "different" and project on them their own fears and insecurities about their changing images. Moreover, MacLennan and Felsenfeld (1968) discovered that adolescents use scapegoating to test operations. In the group they studied, adolescents attempted to "feel out" the leader, to test his style, his objectives, and his patience. They essentially scapegoated the leader and combined with each other in what the therapists called "collaborative resistance." In so doing, they developed a group identity and cohesiveness that would otherwise have been difficult to achieve.

Scapegoating, then, can be therapeutic or nontherapeutic. At any rate, scapegoating does occur within the group, and the nurse will need to know what to expect and how to deal with it. The client identified as the scapegoat will be the object of much teasing and many hostile remarks. The nurse should refrain from attempting merely to rescue the scapegoat, since this may augment the other clients' anger and frustration and encourage an escalation of the hostility. The nurse would do better to set limits on the behavior and then ask the group to focus on what is going on, to acknowledge the anxiety or other uncomfortable feeling that preceded the scapegoating incident. If possible, the nurse should anticipate the occurrence of scapegoating in times of stress and attempt to circumvent the process before it gets out of control.

The nurse should also be aware that identified scapegoats share some responsibility for their predicament by presenting themselves to the other clients in a different or provocative stance. In some instances the scapegoat of choice has an inner need to be punished and meets the group's urgent need to punish as well. The nurse can be valuable to these clients by helping them to explore whatever function this role serves for them.

Examples of effective results in dealing with the scapegoating phenomenon are outlined in the nursing care plan below. As described earlier, the best results will be obtained if the nurse recognizes that the problem and need for change

Nursing Care Plan: A Client Who Is a Scapegoat

Nursing Diagnosis (PND-I/NANDA)	Client Care Goals	Nursing Planning/ Intervention	Evaluation
05.02.02 Social isolation/ withdrawal /Social isolation /Social interaction, impaired	Client will increase peer group participation. Client will show decreased evidence of being "different" from peers. Client will have more appropriate verbal expression of fears related to rejection or hostility from others.	Encourage participation in group activities and offer opportunities for one-to-one exchanges with other clients. Discourage monopolizing of staff members' time, pointing out how this isolates client from peers. Give feedback on how client's behavior affects others. Encourage peers to say how they feel when client rejects them, e.g., when client refuses to play pool with them. Intervene when peers are being sadistic toward client, pointing out the process rather than simply rescuing client. Encourage role modeling of healthy figures of client's sex on ward. Encourage direct expression of feelings when client begins to act out anger or rejection passively. Help client check out motivations for staff members' or peers' behavior when client suspects rejection or hostile intentions.	Client participates in group activities and will lessen need to be scapegoat for group. Client accepts offers to engage in activities with peers and will initiate offers. Client recognizes pattern of being "different" and feeling outcast, e.g., "I want them to like me, but I never want to do the things they want to do." Client spends less time with staff and feels more comfortable with peers. Client is able to express anger and negative feelings in more direct ways. Client is able to check out beliefs about others, identifying their motives for seeking contact with client and dealing more directly with own suspicious ideas. Nurse evaluates client's progress with peer relationships each day and evening shift. Nurse documents course of assessments, interventions, and evaluations in progress notes.

lies with the identified scapegoat as well as with the rest of the group members.

Sexual Behaviors

With a self-awareness and understanding of feelings and attitudes about sexual issues, the nurse can more readily plan interventions with sexual behaviors of the adolescent client. Masturbation, heterosexual behavior, and homosexual behavior are addressed in this section.

Masturbation

Masturbation is a normal sexual activity for people of all ages, from the beginning of sexual awareness to senescence. If the nurse has a relatively healthy attitude toward masturbation, it is not likely to cause problems unless the client masturbates in inappropriate places or uses masturbation to express hostility. There may be times when the nurse will be confronted with an adolescent boy who fondles his genitals when he is anxious or feels threatened. Understanding his behavior as an indication of anxiety, the nurse may elect to ignore the gesture and explore the nature of his anxiety with him. At other times, the boy may make a masturbatory gesture to convey contempt or hostility to the nurse. In this case it would be ludicrous to feign indifference in response.

The nurse's reaction will depend on all the previously mentioned factors, such as his or her relationship with the client and the behavior that preceded the gesture. Generally, however, it would be wise to comment on the client's gesture, for example, by mentioning it as an attempt to "make me uncomfortable," and then to allow the client the opportunity to express verbally what he is feeling. It is unlikely that this intervention will produce a tumultuous outpouring of feeling resulting in immediate resolution. However, it does allow the nurse to acknowledge both the client's and the nurse's own feelings, perhaps paving the way for a more appropriate exchange in the future.

Heterosexual Behavior

The adolescent often uses sexual behavior as a means of acting out other conflicts and as a testing ground for the nursing staff's feelings and attitudes.

This was the third time Barbara, a nurse, had gone into Laurie's room to check on two clients, Laurie and Bill, who were an identified couple on the ward. Although there was a rule against clients having sexual intercourse with each other, Laurie and Bill had been discovered in the act each evening Barbara was on duty. Barbara found these discoveries disconcerting. She began to wonder whether she was the only staff member who checked on clients, since no one else had reported any sexual activity. She decided to bring the subject up in the next nursing care plan meeting to find a more effective way of dealing with the situation.

Imagine Barbara's surprise when the group agreed that Barbara was actually partly responsible for Laurie and Bill's acting out! While they supported Barbara, they evaluated the problem and gave Barbara feedback regarding her nonverbal messages. It seemed that her frequent checking on clients conveyed her expectation that they were up to something. Barbara acknowledged that she expected that sort of behavior from them and was quite afraid of discovering them in the act of intercourse. The group helped Barbara see that her own expectations were being met. Laurie and Bill were doing exactly what she expected them to do— maybe even wanted them to do. Laurie and Bill were following their scripts of being "bad" and expressing their hostility to Barbara. When Barbara heard how other staff members spent time with the couple to encourage them in indirect ways to join the larger group activities and compared her own behavior to that of her peers, it became apparent to her how obvious her anxiety and unconscious messages actually were! She then began to question her own attitudes about sexual matters and to explore why she feared discovering the couple engaged in sexual intercourse.

In the previous clinical example, the client couple used sexual behaviors to act out their own underlying feelings. Had Barbara's assessment been limited to the immediate situation, she would have focused only on their unacceptable behavior and would not have been open to the implications for her. By seeking out information and feedback from her peers she made a discovery about herself and realized more effective ways of anticipating and possibly circumventing such client behaviors rather than having to intervene after the fact. Had Barbara not asked for feedback, the problem would have continued with an increase in the sexual behaviors and in Barbara's frustration. The situation would have then demanded intervention by an astute supervisor or an empathetic colleague.

Homosexual Behavior

See the Assessment section of this chapter for information pertaining to homosexual behavior as a developmental step, a life-style choice, an expression of weakness, or an expression of defiance against authority figures. In situations where such behaviors indicate an expected developmental step or a life-style choice without expressions of anger or hostility toward parents or staff, little or no intervention from the nurse may be indicated. On the other hand, when homosexual behavior is used to act out feelings of impotence, or aggressive behavior is used to counteract feelings of intimacy, limits must be imposed.

The nurse would do well to anticipate such behavior and provide other ways for the adolescent to demonstrate his masculinity, perhaps by organizing a game of football or tennis, if he is fairly proficient at these skills, or engaging him in some other activity in which he excels. The point is to reestablish the adolescent's feeling of competency and control. Without such intervention his feelings of impotence will escalate to the point where he will most certainly act them out in a negative way.

The client who uses homosexuality to express defiance against authority figures will most assuredly flaunt homosexual activities and consistently incur the anger, embarrassment, or both of staff and clients alike. The nursing care plan on page 980 contains some helpful suggestions for relating to the client who uses homosexuality in a hostile way.

Eating Disorders

See the discussion of anorexia nervosa and bulimia nervosa in the Assessment section of this chapter. Client contracts can be particularly helpful with eating disorders. Contracts are discussed earlier in this section.

Anorexia Nervosa

The client with anorexia nervosa can be found in any setting, school and clinic, outpatient and in-patient. But while the clinical picture among the diverse settings will be a consistent one, the client's needs and expectations for treatment may vary. For example, to make effective recommendations for treatment nurses in the school or community setting should:

- Realize that the client who seeks help from the medical setting will have certain expectations for care: e.g., may anticipate physiologic tests and medical treatment but may resist psychiatric intervention
- Know that family may be ambivalent but must not sabotage treatment plan if outpatient care is to be effective
- Be alert to recognize the problem

Furthermore, the nurse may readily see that in-patient treatment is indicated if the following exist:

- Dramatic weight loss or deteriorated physical condition necessitating hospitalization for hydration and nutrition

- Indication of marital discord yielding greater likelihood of unhealthy coalition between one of parents and client
- A client's opinion regarding the better site; when client says she needs to be in the hospital, she is usually correct (Anyan and Schowalter 1983)

In-patient treatment within the therapeutic milieu in conjunction with behavior therapy generally yields positive results. The nurse plays an important part in planning and implementing dietary and behavioral regimens during the client's hospitalization. The nursing care plan on pages 981–983 outlines interventions for the hospitalized adolescent.

It can be helpful to incorporate interventions into a client behavioral contract for weight gain for the client with anorexia nervosa. Figure 35–3 provides an example of such a contract.

Whether in the acute care setting or in the in-patient psychiatric setting, the adolescent client with anorexia nervosa offers a unique challenge. In general, the nurse in the in-patient setting will need to keep the following in mind:

- Invariably the client will have extensive knowledge regarding nutritional and caloric value of foods.
- The client may have lack of knowledge or awareness of the complications of illness.
- In many cases the client will deny the severity of the illness.
- The client will represent middle to upper socioeconomic classes.
- Degrees of family cooperation and involvement in care may vary from overwhelming attempts at control to ambivalence and even sabotage of the treatment plan.

Moreover, in monitoring the staff reaction to this client, nurses:

- Know that it can be exhausting dealing with structured demands of an anorectic's care plan, even when the task seems minimal
- Should recognize and deal with the manipulations and demands that evoke a variety of responses in the nurse, ranging from identification with or overprotectiveness of the client to feelings of annoyance, anger, and sadism toward the client
- Need to have a staff outlet to vent anger and frustration (e.g., nurses' meeting)
- Need to be alert to attempts at "staff splitting" and must keep lines of staff communication open

The nurse in the acute care setting may be challenged by client needs along a wide continuum of care: The client may have extreme needs for physiologic and nutritional care or may need little physical care, in contrast to others on the unit.

Text continues on p. 983.

Client's Name: _____   Weight: _____

Date of Birth: _____   Age: _____   Height: _____

Goal Weight Range: _____

You will be weighed daily in the morning after voiding, wearing only a johnny coat and no jewelry. Nothing is to be consumed prior to being weighed.

No exercising, jogging, etc. is to be done.

Ensure or Ensure Plus is given as a medication. It must be taken within 15 minutes while sitting at the nurses' station. No conversation, reading, knitting, other activity while drinking Ensure.

Must drink _____ cans of Ensure per day if weight gain is 1/4 pound or more over your last highest weight.
Ensure will be dispensed at: _____   _____   _____   _____   _____   _____

Must drink _____ cans of Ensure per day if weight gain is less than 1/4 pound over your last highest weight.
Ensure will be dispensed at: _____   _____   _____   _____   _____   _____

Weights to be attained for status change/privileges:

    Independent Status: _____ pounds
    Monitor Status: _____ pounds for _____ consecutive days
    Buddy Status: _____ pounds
    Passes: _____ pounds for _____ consecutive days

Ensure can be made optional, at the discretion of your primary clinician, once you reach Buddy Status weight.

To use Buddy Status or take passes, a weight gain of 1/4 pound above your last highest weight must be attained on that day.

Participation in dance therapy and walks: at Monitor Status weight and/or with staff permission.

Participation in gym: at Buddy Status weight and/or with staff permission.

Additional comments/issues:

Signature of Client _____
Signature of Primary Clinician _____

Date: _____

Figure 35–3
Client contract for weight gain.
Courtesy Patricia Worthy, Head Nurse, and the nursing staff of the Adolescent and Young Adult Treatment Unit, Yale-New Haven Hospital, New Haven, Connecticut.

Nursing Care Plan: Homosexuality as an Expression of Hostility in an Adolescent

Nursing Diagnosis (PND-I/NANDA)	Client Care Goals	Nursing Planning/ Intervention	Evaluation
04.02.01 Anger 05.05.01 Social intrusiveness 08.03.01 Conflict with social order	Client will manifest more appropriate expression of hostility toward parents and other authority figures. Client has increased ability to verbalize feelings and impulses rather than act them out. Client will increase peer relationships in more socially appropriate activities. Client will show increased trust in staff.	Seek client out and attempt to engage in appropriate activities, using areas of strength or activities that interest client (e.g., candle making). Initiate contact around this and help client obtain materials. Attempt to establish close, trusting relationship, recognizing client's value as an individual and not focusing on the struggle between client and others. Attempt to include client's partner in appropriate activities with group, recognizing partner's importance to the client and demonstrating acceptance of partner's positive traits. Set the same limits on passionate displays as with heterosexual relationships, expressing how you feel during them, e.g., "Your behavior makes me uncomfortable, and I don't want to take you out if you and Felice are going to continue fighting with me about this." Encourage peers to express how they feel about client, both when client behaves acceptably and when client behaves unacceptably with partner. Point out the struggle client sets up with off-unit passes. Refuse inappropriate passes, encourage appropriate visits, and give clear messages that you are concerned about client and what the relationship means. Encourage client to participate in individual and family therapy sessions to deal more directly with the underlying conflicts.	Client gains insight into need for relationship, decreasing the need to express hostility indirectly. Client ceases to use homosexual activities in blatantly hostile manner. Client establishes relationships with others. Client is able to express hostility and anger at parents and staff directly. Client is able to plan acceptable passes from unit with partner and use relationship in a constructive way, if possible. Nurse documents effectiveness of plan and interventions each day and evening shift. Nurse evaluates and documents client's ability to correlate hostile behaviors with anger at staff and parents.

Nursing Care Plan: A Client with Anorexia Nervosa

Nursing Diagnosis (PND-I/NANDA)	Client Care Goals	Nursing Planning/ Intervention	Evaluation
07.06.02.02 Altered nutrition processes: less than body requirements*/Nutrition, altered: less than body requirements	Client will show adequate nutritional intake. Client will return to normal weight for height and age.	Client is first in line for meals and has thirty minutes to eat. Give one-to-one supervision during meals and observe closely for any indication of hiding food. Client sits with staff member who is supervising at a table separate from other clients. Do not encourage client to eat during the thirty minutes. Keep other clients away from the table. Staff member will pick up tray from dietary personnel, checking diet slip to make certain all items are there, including milk and dessert. No omissions or substitutions. After thirty-minute mealtime, pick up tray without speaking. Check the tray for uneaten food, looking under plates and napkin. Any food remaining on tray after thirty minutes will be blended and tube fed. Limit fluids to 500 cc. at one time. Client is to be in dayroom for thirty minutes with one-to-one supervision after meals; no bathroom privilege at this time. Client is to be supervised by staff in bathroom. Set limits on physical activities. Client is not to take part in activities that involve exercise not prescribed in doctors' orders.	Client has adequate dietary intake for weight gain. Client behaviors associated with food ambivalence cease. Client eats a standard nutritional diet. Client eats all the meal to avoid negative reinforcement for not eating. Client follows behavioral contract outlining the above. Nurse documents in progress notes on Monday, Wednesday, and Friday client's compliance with plan. Nurse evaluates client's progress as evidenced by weight gain and ability to focus on difficulties other than food and eating habits. Nurse documents each shift the amount of liquids consumed.

*PND-I diagnosis also in NANDA list.

continued

Nursing Care Plan: A Client with Anorexia Nervosa (*Continued*)

Nursing Diagnosis (PND-I/NANDA)	Client Care Goals	Nursing Planning/ Intervention	Evaluation
		Chart activity level on the ward (pacing, standing, isometrics).	
		Client is to be weighed at 7 a.m. on Tuesday, Thursday, and Saturday in hospital gown and pajamas.	
		Note frequency and consistency of bowel movements to avoid constipation.	
		One staff member will work with physician to establish regimen and weight goals before these are presented to client.	
		One staff member will be present while the regimen is presented to client.	
		Regimen will be presented clearly and in full detail.	
		The nurse will answer client's questions at the time of the initial presentation.	
		No staff member will answer questions or respond directly to comments about the regimen once the physician and nurse have explained it. They will direct the client to the doctor for any discussion of regimen. They will not converse with client about food or weight.	
		Staff will acknowledge client's anger when it is verbalized but will not deal with issues of weight or food.	
		In all aspects of regimen, staff will be extremely consistent.	
		Staff member's questions about the regimen will be referred to team or client's nurse.	

continued

Nursing Care Plan: A Client with Anorexia Nervosa (*Continued*)

Nursing Diagnosis (PND-I/NANDA)	Client Care Goals	Nursing Planning/ Intervention	Evaluation
07.08.01 Altered skin integrity* /Skin integrity, impairment of	Client will show improved skin integrity. Client will manifest improved hydration.	Daily bathing will be discouraged. Lanolin cream will be provided after bathing and twice a day. The nurse will massage skin over bony prominences twice a day and teach client to do likewise frequently throughout the day. The nurse will carefully monitor vital signs and blood pressure.	Client is adequately hydrated; skin integrity is maintained; vital signs are clearly monitored as an aid in evaluating health status. Client follows behavioral contract for adequate amounts of liquids consumed each shift.

*PND-I diagnosis also in NANDA list.
Source: Nursing staff of the Inpatient Treatment and Research Service (ITRS) at Langley Porter Psychiatric Institute, San Francisco, California.

Nurses in the in-patient psychiatric setting need to:

- Realize that often clients will present the picture of the "model client" in contrast to the seemingly "more disturbed" other psychiatric clients. It may be difficult for the novice nurse to appreciate the degree of pathology in contrast to the hallucinating or belligerent adolescent.

- Know that occasions for "splitting" are more numerous in the in-patient setting, especially in the therapeutic milieu where participation with others in treatment is crucial to successful outcome. Since clients are ambulatory and involved with others in treatment, it is more difficult to monitor self-defeating behaviors (e.g., vomiting after meals); as a result, clients may need to be closely monitored by staff at first.

- Be alert to recreation of family dynamics, particularly the tendency to reenact the power struggle from home around mealtimes, weights, etc.

- *Remember that consistency is the key.* Ideally, one caregiver is in charge of the treatment plan, with all client complaints, requests for changes, etc., referred to and handled by that person.

Bulimia Nervosa

As part of developing the treatment approach for the bulimic client, the nurse may find it useful to include a client contract. The contract is developed by the client and the nurse and renegotiated at periodic intervals, for example, hourly, daily, or weekly, depending on the client's goals, severity of symptoms, and compliance with the contract. Such a contract might include agreements related to undesirable symptoms of the illness, such as binging, vomiting, or hoarding food. The contract might include the following:

I will sit at the nurses' station for one-half hour following my meal.

I will not attempt to vomit after my meal.

I will not hoard food.

I will not take laxatives or diuretics.

I will not bring any such substances onto the unit.

I will tell the nursing staff if I feel like binging.

I will avoid the kitchen if I feel like binging.

Signed _____

Date _____

Nurse _____

Depression and Suicide

Prevention and treatment of adolescent suicide can be facilitated by the following seven steps:

1. Recognize and accept the warning signals as appeals for help from the client. Warning signals might include *verbal statements* such as, "They'll be better off with-

out me," or "Everyone would be happier if I were no longer around" or statements closer to suicidal threats such as, "You won't have to worry about me anymore," or "I'm going to sleep and never wake up." Treat such statements, no matter how casually made, as serious. Such a statement, even an offhand remark, is meant to get the nurse's attention. If the nurse discusses it lightly or regards it contemptuously, the adolescent may feel that all hope of support is gone and proceed with suicidal action.

Behavioral signals might be any of the following:

- Changes in academic performance
- Depression
- An elated mood following a chronic depression
- Excessive use of drugs or alcohol
- Giving away treasured possessions
- Failure to communicate with family and school personnel
- Changes in social behavior
- Isolation and withdrawn behavior
- Morose behavior
- Insomnia
- Apparent "accidents," especially if more than one

An adolescent who is not contemplating suicide might also make these statements or show these behaviors, but they should be treated as warning signals and not ignored. The nurse cannot give the adolescent the idea of committing suicide. It is much better to err on the side of caution and concern than to overlook the behavior for fear of annoyance or embarrassment.

2. Talk to the adolescent. Confront the adolescent with the changes you have observed. Depending on the behaviors, the nurse may begin with an exploratory statement such as, "I've noticed that you seem 'down' lately. Is something bothering you?" If the adolescent is depressed but not suicidal, simply listening closely with a nonjudgmental attitude and possibly helping with coping abilities, lending some ego strength, and helping with problem solving may be the only necessary step. Repeat the adolescent's statements, using your own words. If you have not interpreted the information accurately, the adolescent will correct you.

3. If you do not already have a careful history at this point, get one now. Ask some well-directed questions to uncover possible risk factors (outlined in the Assessment section)

> Have you had any recent losses or disappointments?
>
> What about separations from people you care about?
>
> Have there been recent deaths in your family?

You say you have been sad for some time. Is there someone else in your family who gets sad a lot?

Adolescents who give evidence of depression should be questioned about the extent of their depressed symptoms and about thoughts or wishes about death. Such questions could focus on possible stressors and behavioral cues outlined in Tables 35–2 and 35–3. For example:

> Have there been any changes in relationships with your friends?
>
> Have you experienced any embarrassing situation in school or any disappointment in social activities or with achievements?
>
> Who's your best friend? (Such questions also help to identify use of supports.)
>
> How have you been sleeping lately? Is that a change from usual?
>
> What kinds of dreams have you had recently? Are they troublesome?
>
> Have you ever felt so bad that you wished you were dead?
>
> Have you ever felt so bad that you wanted to kill yourself?
>
> Have you ever thought about suicide?
>
> (If yes to the above) Do you feel like hurting or killing yourself now?
>
> (And to detect a plan) How would you go about it?
>
> Have you ever tried to hurt yourself or commit suicide?
>
> Have you ever known someone who tried to hurt himself or tried to kill himself?
>
> Have other members of your family committed suicide?

4. Assess the nature of the stressor that precipitated the behavior. This indicates the adolescent's tolerance for stress: the milder the stress, the weaker the defenses and coping mechanisms and the greater the chance for recurrence. Since this may warrant a judgment call, the nurse should explore with the adolescent the meaning and value of the stressor without devaluing it based solely on the nurse's feelings.

5. Evaluate the nature and depth of the inner conflict and the degree of disharmony that exists in the family living situation or equivalent environment. Include an evaluation of the resources available to the client and the willingness of these resources to help. If in a school setting, talk to the adolescent's teachers to get a sense of the family situation and the adolescent's resources.

6. Talk to the parents. If the adolescent says he or she confided only in you about suicidal thoughts and wants you to keep it a secret, you can explain that you do care what happens and you would not be a friend if you kept it quiet. The nurse can offer to be with the

adolescent to talk to the parents. Sometimes the nurse can facilitate this process and encourage trust in the beginning when met with the initial plea, "I want to tell you something but you have to promise not to tell anyone." The nurse can respond with, "I can do that as long as it doesn't mean harm to you or to someone else."

This one step may be all that is needed to open the door between the adolescent and the parents. For others there may be no one at home to help. The nurse may be the person then to alert the school psychologist, social worker, family and children's services, whatever means is appropriate to the setting when a useless or dangerous situation exists at home.

7. If indicated, take steps to remove the client from the source of anxiety or danger and refer for appropriate treatment. It is desirable to obtain therapy, when indicated, on an outpatient basis for the nonhospitalized adolescent whenever possible since hospitalization may exacerbate feelings of isolation, helplessness, and inadequacy. However, perhaps the adolescent needs to be removed from a lethal situation at home (e.g., physical or sexual abuse) to obtain treatment as well as a sense of safety and well-being. Placement in a residential treatment setting may be indicated to provide safety as well as supportive controls.

With knowledge and observational skills the nurse, especially in the school and community setting, can play a key role in preventing adolescent suicide (see The school nurse's dilemma 1984).

In the treatment setting the nurse will be faced with the challenge of establishing a trusting relationship with the adolescent client while helping the client deal with suicidal impulses. The use of a **no self-harm contract** can be instrumental in meeting both objectives. (See Box 35–4.) Disturbed adolescents frequently act out their aggression against themselves in self-mutilating ways, against other people, and/or against objects in the environment (Bradley 1980). (See the nursing care plan in the case study for the client who does all of these.)

Drug Abuse

The nurse will benefit from self-awareness and appreciation for the feelings that working with drug abusers can evoke. For example, the nurse who feels angry and punitive with the client who abuses drugs or overidentifies with the client and finds adventure in the client's drug stories cannot establish a therapeutic relationship with the client. Feelings of disdain or envy for the drug user can compromise nursing care and, indeed, may make the client's treatment ineffective. Only by viewing drug abuse as a symptom of a broader illness can the nurse be effective in dealing with adolescents. Following the case study is an example of a nursing care plan for working with the drug abuser. Nurses who have contact with adolescents, especially in

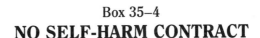

Box 35–4
NO SELF-HARM CONTRACT

A no self-harm contract can be effective without being lengthy. See the discussion of client contracts earlier in this section. To prevent self-mutilating or suicidal behaviors, the nurse can obtain a mutually satisfactory contract by writing out or having the adolescent write out any or all of the following sentences:

- I will not hurt myself or others.

- If I feel like hurting myself, others, or property, I will tell the staff.

- I will not bring scissors or other sharp objects onto the unit.

- I will not ask visitors to bring me harmful objects or substances, including medications or other drugs.

- I will ask for a one-to-one talk with staff on day and evening shifts to talk about my treatment goals and how I am feeling.

---

school or community settings, would be well advised to familiarize themselves with the general effects of various drugs and the first aid treatment for each.

In 1982 researchers completed the National Survey on Drug Abuse and High School Senior Survey. Results indicate a decline for high school seniors in the daily use of marijuana, cigarette smoking, and the hallucinogenic drug PCP. However, sources report no changes in the use of alcohol, cocaine, heroin, and sedatives and a marked increase in the use of stimulants (US Public Health Reports 1983). Following this report, national objectives were established to provide a measure of progress with quantifiable goals designed to improve health, reduce risk factors, increase awareness, and improve protection and surveillance. These objectives were developed by the Alcohol, Drug Abuse, and Mental Health Administration of the Public Health Service and are identified as priority objectives for the year 1990. Of the nineteen alcohol and drug prevention or treatment goals, those pertaining to adolescents are listed in Box 35–5.

To achieve these objectives, the Department of Health and Human Services plans to:

- Develop and disseminate factual literature on alcohol and drugs

- Support mass media campaigns on alcohol and drug abuse

Box 35–5
1990 PRIORITY DRUG USE AND ABUSE GOALS FOR ADOLESCENTS

By 1990 per capita consumption of alcohol should not exceed current levels. (In 1978 for individuals 14 years of age and older about 2.82 gallons of absolute alcohol were consumed per year per person.)

By 1990 the proportion of adolescents 12 to 17 years old who abstain from using alcohol or other drugs should not fall below 1977 levels. (The proportion of abstainers in 1977 was 46.5 percent for alcohol; for other drugs it ranged from 83.9 percent for marijuana to 99.9 percent for heroin.)

By 1990 the proportion of adolescents 14 to 17 years of age who report acute drinking-related problems during the past year should be reduced to below 17 percent. (It was estimated to be 19 percent in 1978 based on 1974 survey data.)

By 1990 the proportion of adolescents 12 to 17 years old reporting frequent use of other drugs should not exceed 1977 levels. (In 1977 it was 8.7 percent and 1 percent for drugs other than marijuana.)

By 1990 80 percent of high school seniors should state that they perceive great risk associated with frequent regular cigarette smoking, marijuana use, barbiturate use, or alcohol intoxication. (In 1979 high school seniors perceived "great risk" as follows: 63 percent with one or two packs of cigarettes daily; 42 percent with regular marijuana use; 72 percent with regular barbiturate use; and 35 percent with five or more drinks per occasion once or twice each weekend.)

- Provide technical assistance to states, business and industry, and schools developing prevention, intervention, and treatment programs
- Support drug and alcohol abuse prevention demonstration projects
- Support research on the social, psychologic, and biochemical factors underlying drug and alcohol dependence
- Support activities to monitor drug and alcohol use patterns

Whether in school, community, in-patient, or outpatient settings, nurses will have key roles in the design, implementation, and research of these plans.

Evaluating nursing interventions with the adolescent client can be tricky for numerous reasons:

- The adolescent client may need to test the limit one more time following a nursing intervention to avoid appearing "too compliant" or to "save face" with his or her peer group.
- While it is important to set limits with the adolescent, it is equally important to be flexible. To set a limit and immediately "draw the line" with the next infraction is to invite the adolescent to step over that line to test its seriousness.
- Quick judgments should not be made if immediate results are not obtained. Persistence and consistency are the keys to success.
- The behaviors that brought the adolescent to psychiatric treatment will continue long after treatment and nursing interventions are begun. Despite a well-designed nursing care plan and client contract, the adolescent will resort to previous maladaptive ways, immature and impulsive acts, or destructive behaviors in the face of change, particularly if this change represents improvement or growth (e.g., an increase in privileges or an impending discharge). The nurse who thinks the nursing interventions are not effective as a result may feel hopeless about progress and convey that hopelessness to the client and the rest of the treatment team.
- Use of a behavioral contract without understanding the underlying reasons or contributing factors to the adolescent's problems will result in a superficial approach with an equally superficial evaluation.

If the adolescent had the desire or the impulse control simply to "act right" after being given the rules and consequences, then the client would be doing so already and psychiatric treatment would not have been necessary. The adolescent needs the structure and consistency of a nursing care plan and client contract without the rigidity that can be imposed by a "now or never" behavioral plan with absolute consequences.

The nurse can make a more adequate evaluation if aware of the social context and meaning of the behavior to the adolescent. For example, the nurse may be wrong in determining that an indicator of increased self-esteem for a female client would be to stop dyeing her hair purple. Perhaps dyeing one's hair an unusual color may have been an indication of low self-esteem during the nurse's adolescent years, but for the client in question, that may or may not be the case. For that adolescent client and her peer group, purple hair may be a well-defined status symbol.

Evaluation is determined to be effective or ineffective by the use of various subjective and objective behavioral criteria reflecting the client care goals. See the nursing

Text continues on p. 993.

CASE STUDY: A Suicidal Adolescent Client

Identifying Information

Cindy is a 15-year-old, single, white, female, nonpracticing Protestant, who is referred to the in-patient psychiatric unit by a social worker who is a friend of Cindy's mother. Cindy is a sophomore in high school. Third party insurance will cover full cost of hospitalization.

Client's Definition of Present Problem, Precipitatory Stresses, Coping Strategies, Goals for Care

Cindy is voluntarily admitted to the unit because "my mother says I'm impossible." She describes a three-year history of drug abuse, including marijuana, Valium, Seconal, and LSD. The precipitating stressor for this hospitalization was Cindy's slashing her wrist with a razor blade following an argument with her mother. Cindy says this is the first time she has "attempted suicide." Cindy reports that she frequently resorts to smoking marijuana or "sneaking" her mother's Valium when under stress, particularly following arguments with her mother. Her goals for treatment are "to gain control of my impulses and to learn more about myself." She says that she would like to get along better with her mother but says that is "unrealistic."

History of Present Problem

It is difficult to determine the exact date on which Cindy's problem first appeared (see Psychiatric History and Social History). It seems evident that her depression and related difficulties worsened around puberty at the age of 12, compounded by the abuse of drugs and the increased competitiveness among Cindy's siblings. Her parents state that she is now beyond control and they are at their "wit's end," having endured three years of "fighting, manipulation, and unhappiness."

Cindy describes herself as a "loner," who has few friends and keeps to herself at home and at school. She lives with her parents and two sisters. Cindy leaves the house each morning for school before the others are awake "to avoid the hassles with my mother and sisters." She has average to poor school grades. She reports frequent physical complaints, admitting that she frequently feigns illness to the school nurse to avoid certain classes. Cindy describes one female classmate to whom she feels close but states that their time together is brief and usually involves smoking marijuana in the morning just before school.

Psychiatric History

Cindy's parents have complained of difficulties with her "hyperactive, impulsive" behavior since she was 2 years old. According to her mother, Cindy was diagnosed at an early age as hyperkinetic following numerous visits to clinics and doctors' offices in quests for help for her uncontrollable behavior. Cindy's mother reports that Cindy could never be satisfied, cried all the time, and was never "still" once she was able to crawl.

During the past three years Cindy's difficulties have increased as she began to abuse drugs. Two months prior to this admission she underwent a four-week residential drug treatment program. The precipitant for this treatment was Cindy's suspension from school as a result of the school principal's discovery of Cindy and her friend smoking marijuana outside the cafeteria. The treatment modality was primarily a behavioral one, using a strict behavioral protocol of "time-outs" in a room alone or lost pass privileges for failure to attend or being late for meetings. The purpose of the program was educational. Meetings structured around films

continued

Case Study (Continued)

and discussions detailing the physical and legal risks of drug abuse consumed most of their waking hours. No attempts were made to explore the meaning of Cindy's drug-taking behaviors, her relationship to her parents, or the life events leading up to this difficult time. Cindy considers the program "helpful since I didn't take any drugs while I was there," but she acknowledges that she feels like a failure because she continues to use drugs.

Family History

Cindy lives with her parents, John and Kate, and two sisters (Katherine, 16 years old, and Janice, 14 years old). John is a chemist for a local pharmaceutical firm. Kate is a housewife. All three children are students at the same high school. On admission Cindy's parents explained that competition among the girls has been the primary problem at home, adding that Cindy's behavior makes it impossible to handle the problems. Since an early age Cindy has been identified as the "black sheep" of the family, according to Cindy. She has consistently been told she is "impossible" because she behaves badly and does poor to average school work, whereas her sisters have both been honor students and model children, according to her parents. Cindy's mother, Kate, frequently made favorable comparisons between herself and Katherine, her oldest daughter. She made disparaging comparisons between Cindy and Kate's younger sister, who Kate felt had "stolen the show and my father away from me when I was 4 years old."

Social History

Although Cindy's pediatrician reports normal developmental milestones, Cindy's mother states she has always been "slow at everything." Her school record validates the report of poor to average grades, except for the third grade when Cindy achieved As and Bs. Cindy's teacher wrote in her report that Cindy's performance can improve with encouragement and personal attention. All accounts of Cindy's social development consistently support the idea of an isolated individual with few friends. Her leisure time has characteristically involved watching TV and occasionally spending time with her younger sister. According to Cindy, her three-year history of drug abuse has involved regular marijuana use one to two times a week, occasional use of Valium (5 mg tablet prescription for Cindy's mother), Seconal ("street reds") on two occasions, and LSD on two occasions. Cindy's mother insisted that Cindy was a heavy drug abuser "who takes anything and everything," but she acknowledged that the only times she was aware of Cindy's taking drugs had been those identified by Cindy on admission.

Significant Health History

Cindy's health history is unremarkable. She reports no allergies or hospitalizations. Her wrist slashing consisted of a superficial laceration of the left wrist, requiring no sutures in the emergency room.

Current Mental Status

Cindy is an alert, articulate bright female who is slightly overweight and appears older than her stated age. During the psychiatric examination she was cooperative and spontaneous, answering questions readily, although often giving vague responses necessitating more detailed inquiry. She was oriented to time, place, and person and denied having any hallucinations or delusions. Cindy performed adequately with most of the examination. She did rather poorly on serial sevens, however,

continued

Case Study (Continued)

making four mistakes in the four-minute period it took her to complete this exercise. Her explanations of proverbs were quite concrete. Cindy tended to minimize her depression, wanting to project a happy and healthy image to the interviewer. She revealed that her happiness is a front so that others would not know what is going on in her head. Cindy seems to have little insight into her current situation. Her primary defenses include denial, rationalization, and introjection.

Other Subjective or Objective Clinical Data

Cindy is on no prescription medications at this time. She denies any suicidal feelings but agrees to the terms of the client contract that she will tell staff if she feels like hurting herself.

Diagnostic Impression

A long-standing depression and extreme feelings of worthlessness stem from the treatment Cindy received from her parents as an abnormal, hyperactive child. The onset of puberty combined with increasing competitiveness among the females in the family provided additional stress, leading to drug abuse and a suicidal gesture.

DSM-IIIR Multiaxial Diagnosis

Axis I: 300.40 Dysthymia, primary type, early onset
          305.20 Cannabis abuse

Axis II: 799.90 Deferred. (There is insufficient information to make any diagnostic judgment about an Axis II diagnosis or condition.)

Axis III: None

Axis IV: Psychosocial stressors:
1. Onset of puberty with resulting physical and psychologic changes
2. Increased competitiveness among siblings and mother with resulting arguments
3. Suspension from school
4. Suicidal gesture
5. Four weeks out-of-home drug treatment with unsuccessful results

Axis V: Severity: 3-Moderate (predominantly acute events)
       Current GAF: 43
       Highest GAF past year: 55

Nursing Diagnoses (PND-I/NANDA)

05.02.01.03 Aggressive/violent behaviors toward self (associated with substance abuse and suicidal gestures)*
           /Violence, potential for: self-directed

05.05.02   Social isolation/withdrawal*
           /Social isolation

05.03.04   Altered play role

05.03.05   Altered student role*
           /Social interaction, impaired

08.01.01   Hopelessness

04.02.08   Sadness

06.03.04   Altered self-esteem*
           /Self-concept, disturbance in: self-esteem

continued

Case Study (Continued)

Nursing Care Plan

Nursing Diagnosis (PND-I/NANDA)	Client Care Goals	Nursing Planning/ Intervention	Evaluation
05.02.01.03 Aggressive/ violent behavior toward self (associated with substance abuse and suicidal gestures)* /Violence, potential for: self-directed	Client will abstain from use of drugs or harmful substances. Client will talk with staff if she feels like hurting herself. Client will ask for one-to-one time with nurse on day and evening shifts. Client will ask for time to talk in groups (at least once daily) about her thoughts, feelings, and treatment plans.	Provide for physical safety of unit, ensuring that all sharp objects are confiscated. Search clients' and visitors' packages to ensure no drugs or harmful substances are brought onto unit. Implement behavioral contract regarding one-to-one contacts, group therapy participation, and increased freedoms. Spend time with her when she is not acting out. Do not wait for negative behaviors to give her attention. Reinforce positive behaviors.	Document each day and evening shift one-to-one conferences with nurse. Document content and progress of discussions both individually and in groups. If client demonstrates a worsening of suicidal thoughts and diminished impulse control, assess need for limitations on privileges and freedoms (e.g., reverse status level; consider one-to-one observation, suicide precautions, visitor limitations). Document on day and evening shifts compliance and progress with plan.
05.05.02 Social isolation/ withdrawal /Social isolation	Client will initiate social contact with peers at least once daily. Client will not isolate self in room except for "earned" time. Client will ask for one-to-one time with nurse on day and evening shifts to discuss feelings. Client will participate in all planned social activities of unit. Client will attend family meetings.	Establish mutually acceptable goals and objectives for socialization: e.g., "Who would you like to get to know here? How do you think you could approach her/him?" Implement behavioral contract including reinforcement for positive behaviors (e.g., "earned" time in room alone for 15- to 30-minute periods). Encourage to participate in social activities. Evaluate progress with client regarding social interaction attempts, successes, and difficulties. Encourage to explore feelings regarding interpersonal relationships with peers, parents, and other authority figures. Encourage and support participation in group therapies.	Document nursing interventions and client results each shift in progress notes. With each attempt to initiate contact with peers, offer encouragement and constructive criticism, evaluating results with client.

continued

Case Study (Continued)

Nursing Diagnosis (PND-I/NANDA)	Client Care Goals	Nursing Planning/ Intervention	Evaluation
05.03.04 Altered play role* /Social interaction, impaired 05.03.05 Altered student role 08.01.01 Hopelessness 04.02.08 Sadness 06.03.04 Altered self-esteem* /Self-concept, disturbance in: self-esteem	Client will attend unit school program. Client will complete assignments. Client will ask for help when needed rather than passively fail to do work. Client will recognize and accept sad, lonely feelings as long-standing problem. Client will identify at least three strengths and discuss them in one-to-one and group therapy contacts. Client will talk about negative feelings rather than acting out.	Implement behavioral contract, including school attendance and completion of assignments as criteria for rewards (e.g., "earned" time in room). Help identify her strengths and areas of interest. Encourage school participation and completion of work. Give praise for assignments well done. Help identify her strengths. Explore helpless, hopeless, sad, or lonely feelings. Attempt to correlate feelings with precipitating event (e.g., fight with sister). Promote activities that use her strengths. Give praise for successes.	Document daily difficulties and successes with school attendance and assignments in progress notes. Document content and progress of one-to-one and group discussions. Evaluate ability to correlate feelings with behavior. If the client demonstrates worsening of feelings and social interaction, set limits and provide structure of one-to-ones. Document interventions and results.

*PND-I diagnosis also in NANDA list

Nursing Care Plan: An Adolescent with Psychoactive Substance Use Disorder

Nursing Diagnosis (PND-I/NANDA)	Client Care Goals	Nursing Planning/ Intervention	Evaluation
05.02.01.03 Aggressive/ violent behaviors toward self* (associated with substance use) /Violence, potential for: self-directed	Client will live in drug-free environment. Client will show increased impulse control. Client will verbally express feelings rather than act out feelings and impulses. Client will show increased sense of responsibility for self and behaviors.	Be clear in defining acceptable versus unacceptable behavior. Design client contract to stop drug use. Search client's and visitors' packages. Set limits on visits and interactions with others. Closely monitor client when off unit on outings, since client may attempt to obtain drugs or have contact with outside friends. Immediately confront client	Client attends admission orientation meeting with peers and nursing staff to discuss unit rules related to substance use. Client is able to recognize and admit to drug use and makes verbal commitment to remain drug free in compliance with unit rules and client contract. Client abstains from use of drugs or other harmful psychoactive substances (e.g., sniffing aerosol cans).

*PND-I diagnosis also in NANDA list.

continued

Nursing Care Plan: An Adolescent with Psychoactive Substance Use Disorder *(Continued)*

Nursing Diagnosis (PND-I/NANDA)	Client Care Goals	Nursing Planning/ Intervention	Evaluation
		in direct, nonjudgmental manner if any drug-related activity is suspected.	Client is able to understand and verbalize the meaning of his or her drug use, identifying precipitants and factors that contribute to the drug habit (e.g., will be able to relate it to feelings of anger or loneliness).
		Set firm and consistent limits. Point out manipulative or acting out behaviors in matter-of-fact manner.	
		Keep the focus on the client's responsibility for self.	Client learns to use supports and more adaptive measures for dealing with difficult feelings and situations; e.g., seeks out nursing staff and peers when urges to get "high" come up.
		Avoid intellectualizations about family problems or staff faults. Do not support client's efforts at denial; support realistic thoughts and concerns: e.g., client attempts to minimize degree of drug use, giving current abstinence on unit as evidence.	
		Suggest that client use a "mood journal"; encourage client to write daily in a notebook, the content of which will be shared with primary nurse. Nurse may choose to give structured questions for reflection/ response.	
		Recognize and discuss with client that life-style without drugs is a major change and loss. Help client identify and use strengths, interests, and capabilities toward more adaptive and healthier life.	Nurse documents in admission note assessments, interventions and evaluation of orientation meeting with peers and staff.
		Identify sources of community support for client and family: e.g., Alcoholics Anonymous, Al-Anon, etc.	Nurse assesses and documents client's impulse control ability and correlates difficult behaviors with feelings.
		Design a highly structured plan for discharge while still in hospital: e.g., emphasize importance of attendance at all client group activities, including recreational activities.	Nurse evaluates and documents content and frequency of contacts initiated by client with nursing staff and peers.
			Nurse evaluates and revises client contract on daily basis, in collaboration with client.

continued

Nursing Care Plan: An Adolescent with Psychoactive Substance Use Disorder (*Continued*)

Nursing Diagnosis (PND-I/NANDA)	Client Care Goals	Nursing Planning/ Intervention	Evaluation
		Address all behavior, positive and negative, in staff-client groups, particularly community meetings.	
		Use individual supervision and group staff meetings to identify and deal with staff issues of countertransference, such as anger, resentment, and frustration in dealing with the drug abuser.	

Source: Carrie McRae RN, BSN, Unit B, Langley Porter Psychiatric Institute, San Francisco, California.

care plans in the Planning and Implementing Interventions section for specific problems and their criteria for evaluation.

Chapter Highlights

- Adolescence is a stormy time of conflicting ideas and feelings when identity, values, and goals are in a state of flux. The individual is no longer a child with investment in play or parental approval but is not yet an adult with abilities in verbal discourse or impulse control.

- A more comprehensive assessment of this developmental period and the adolescent's problems is possible with the use of humanistic interactionist principles and information related to the developmental stage, social and cultural factors, familial influences, and psychodynamic conflicts.

- Roles and functions for both the generalist and the clinical specialist are clearly delineated in the ANA's Standards of Child and Adolescent Psychiatric and Mental Health Nursing Practice.

- Nurses work with adolescents in the outpatient setting as a community health nurse in the school, home, or clinic and nurse counselor-therapists (including individual, group, or family therapist roles). In the in-patient setting (hospital or residential treatment) nurses work with adolescents as staff nurses, consultants, or clinical specialists in either a general hospital setting or a psychiatric setting.

- In the home, school, or clinic environment, the general hospital setting, or the in-patient psychiatric setting, the nurse can perform a central role in counseling parents and families of adolescent clients.

- The nurse can maintain a therapeutic milieu by providing a physically and psychologically safe environment, setting verbal and physical limits on the client's behavior, establishing meaningful relationships with the adolescent, identifying clients' strengths, promoting more adaptive coping skills, role modeling more socially acceptable behaviors, and participating in therapy groups and structured activities.

- The peer group setting provides social interaction and living-learning situations without which psychotherapy of the adolescent may be sterile and ineffectual.

- Adolescents can present "normal" behaviors and problems unique to this developmental stage that could give the nurse difficulty. To be effective with nursing interventions, the nurse needs to understand typical adolescent behaviors as well as extremes in behavior.

- Specific issues and problems frequently related to psychiatric nursing care of adolescents include attempts to manipulate the nurse into relating in a nontherapeutic way, use of unconventional language and profanity, testing and limit setting, anxiety and resistance, anger and hostility, scapegoating, adolescent sexual behavior, dietary problems such as obesity, eating disorders such as anorexia nervosa and bulimia nervosa, drug use and abuse, and suicidal behavior.

- *Acting out* is often misused to describe antisocial destructive acts. It may include destructive actions, but it is much more than that. The term describes a recreation of the client's life experiences, the relationships with significant others, and the resulting unresolved conflicts.

- Nurse interventions with adolescents may be most effective if designed within the format of a client contract.

- Scapegoating is common to adolescent groups. The nurse will be most effective if he or she identifies the need that the scapegoat has to be "different," as well as setting limits on the scapegoating behaviors.

- Nurses can perform a key role in preventing adolescent suicides by recognizing risk factors, identifying behavioral cues, and acknowledging stressors.

- Experimentation with drugs among the adolescent population is widespread, but the nurse can recognize certain characteristics that distinguish the adolescent drug abuser from the user.

- Nurses should be aware of the social contexts and meaning of the behavior to the adolescent in order to evaluate it adequately.

References

American Nurses Association: *Standards of Child and Adolescent Psychiatric and Mental Health Nursing Practice.* American Nurses' Association, 1985.

Amini F, Salasnek S: Adolescent drug abuse: Search for a treatment model. *Compr Psych* 1975;16:379–389.

Amini F, Salasnek S, Burke EL: Adolescent drug abuse: Etiological and treatment considerations. *Adolescence* 1976;11:281–299.

Anyan WR, Schowalter JE: A comprehensive approach to anorexia nervosa. 1983;22(March):122–127.

Bradley C: Personality disorders, in Kalkman ME, Davis AJ (eds): *New Dimensions in Mental Health-Psychiatric Nursing,* ed 5. McGraw-Hill, 1980.

Bruch H: *The Golden Cage: The Enigma of Anorexia Nervosa.* Harvard University Press, 1978.

Burke E: Patient values on an adolescent drug unit. *Am J Psychother* 1970;24:400–410.

Busteed EL, Johnston C: The development of suicide precautions for an inpatient psychiatric unit. *J Psychosoc Nurs* 1983;21:15–19.

Campbell C: Perception of stress by staff members in an adolescent milieu. Unpublished research, 1977.

Child AA, Murphy CM, Rhyne MC: Depression in children: Reasons and risks. *Pediatr Nurs* 1980;6(July/August):9–13.

Ciseaux A: Anorexia nervosa: A view from the mirror. *Am J Nurs* 1980;80:1468–1470.

Deering C: Developing a therapeutic alliance with the anorexia nervosa client. *J Psychosoc Nurs* 1987;25(3):11–17.

DeMaio D, DeMaio-Esteves M, Shuzman E: Technological society: Its impact on youth. *Top Clin Nurs* 1983;5(April):55–65.

Edmands MS: Overcoming eating disorders: A group experience. *J Psychosoc Nurs* 1986;24:19–25.

Erikson E: *Identity, Youth and Crisis.* W.W. Norton, 1968.

Fagin CM (ed): *Child and Adolescent Psychiatric Nursing.* C.V. Mosby, 1974.

Garner DM, et al.: Cultural expectations of thinness in women. *Psych Rep* 1980;47:483–491.

Glaser K: Suicide in children and adolescents, in Abt LE, Weissman SL (eds): *Acting Out: Theoretical and Clinical Aspects.* Jason Aronson, 1976.

Glueck S, Glueck E (eds): *Identification of Predelinquents.* Intercontinental Medical Book, 1972.

Jersild AT: *The Psychology of Adolescence,* ed 3. Macmillan, 1978.

Jones M: *Beyond the Therapeutic Community: Social Learning and Social Psychiatry.* Yale University Press, 1968.

Keidel GC: Adolescent suicide. *Nurs Clin N Am* 1983;18(2):323–332.

Kelter NL: Bulimia: Controlling compulsive eating. *J Psychosoc Nurs* 1984;22:24–29.

Keicott-Glaser J, Dixon K: Postadolescent onset: Male anorexia. *J Psychosoc Nurs* 1984;22(1):11–20.

Kneisl CR, Ames SA: *Adult Health Nursing: A Biopsychosocial Approach.* Addison-Wesley, 1986.

MacLennan BW, Felsenfeld N: *Group Counseling and Psychotherapy With Adolescents.* Columbia University Press, 1968.

Mahon NE: Developmental changes and loneliness during adolescence. *Top Clin Nurs* 1983;5(April):66–76.

Marks R: Anorexia and bulimia: Eating habits that can kill. *RN,* January 1984, pp 44–47.

Pallikkathayil L, McBride AB: Suicide attempts: The search for meaning. *J Psychosoc Nurs* 1986;24(August):13–18.

Pfeffer CR: Clinical aspects of childhood suicidal behavior. *Ped Annals* 1984;13(January):56–61.

Potts NL: Eating disorders: The secret pattern of binge/purge. *Am J Nurs* January 1984, pp 32–35.

Sanger E, Cassino T: Eating disorders: Avoiding the power struggle. *Am J Nurs* January 1984, pp 31–33.

Swift W, et al.: A follow-up study of 30 hospitalized bulimics. *Psychosom Med* 1987;49(1):45–55.

The school nurse's dilemma, interview. *J Psychosoc Nurs* 1984;22(August):31–34.

Trygstad LN: Stress and coping in psychiatric nursing. *J Psychosoc Nurs* 1986;24(August):23–27.

U.S. Public Health Reports: Promoting health/preventing disease: Public Health Service implementation plans for attaining objectives for the nation. *US Pub H Svc,* September/October 1983(Suppl), pp 116–132.

Valente S: The suicidal teenager. *Nursing 85,* December 1985, pp 47–49.

Vandereycken W, et al.: Body-oriented therapy for anorexia nervosa patients. *Am J Psychother* 1987;41(2):252–259.

White JH: Bulimia: Utilizing individual and family therapy. *J Psychosoc Nurs* 1984;22(4):22–28.

Wilmer HA: *Social Psychiatry in Action: A Therapeutic Community.* Charles C Thomas, 1958.

Wilson P (ed): *Fear of Being Fat.* Jason Aronson, 1983.

Yahraes H: *Causes, Detection and Treatment of Childhood Depression.* US Department of Health, Education, and Welfare publication (ADM) 79-612. Government Printing Office, 1978.

Zilberg NG, Burke EL: Inpatient versus outpatient treatment of delinquent drug-abusers: An outcome study. Presented at the 87th Annual Convention of the American Psychological Association, New York, September 1979.

THIRTY-SIX

Applying the Nursing Process with the Elderly

Colleen Love

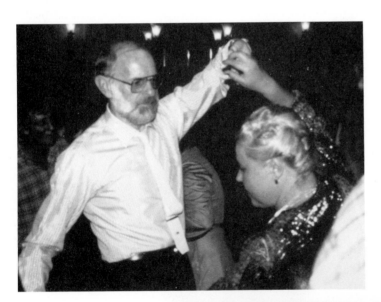

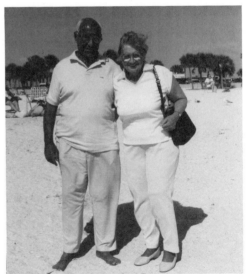

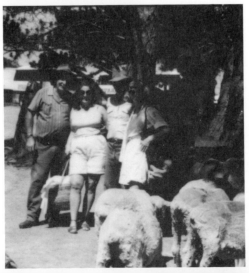

Learning Objectives

After reading this chapter, students should be able to

- Discuss three significant age-related demographic projections and their implications for future health services for the elderly

- Describe the normal physical and psychosocial changes accompanying the aging process

- List the major theories of aging and three main points of each

- Apply the nursing process to care of elderly clients

- List the important components of a multifactorial assessment of an elderly client

- Complete a psychosocial assessment of an elderly client

- Explain the importance of distinguishing between depression, dementia, and delirium

- Contrast attitudes of older persons experiencing ego integrity with those of elders experiencing despair

- Identify the most common DSM-IIIR mental disorders and associated nursing diagnoses among elderly psychiatric clients

- Comprehend interventions that will foster ego integrity late in life

Cross References

Other topics relevant to this content are: Elder abuse, Chapter 25 (Part II); Human growth and development, Chapter 6; Organic mental disorders, Chapter 15; Psychobiology, Chapter 9; Psychotropic medications, Chapter 31; Social support, Chapter 8; Substance abuse, Chapter 16.

Some say that we're moving toward our own destruction whether by nuclear war or by pollution of the environment. It just may happen unless we do something to stop it.

Key Terms

agism
delirium
delusions
dementia
elder abuse
excess disability
family burden
frail elderly

gerontophobia
lethality index
mental mediators
polypharmacy
psychogerontology
reactive drinker
somatization

Nurses have enormous potential to influence the health of the elderly. Of all the health professions, nurses have the most contact with elderly persons (Institute of Medicine 1983). Nursing's emphasis on interaction, humanism, and promotion of health, self-care, and autonomy are particularly important for meeting the unique psychosocial needs of the elderly. The aim of this chapter is to provide a comprehensive discussion of health promotion, advocacy, and application of the nursing process to mental health care for the elderly. It provides a broad overview of important age-related, biopsychosocial nursing considerations for advocacy and health promotion in later life; discusses the DSM-IIIR (1987) mental disorders commonly seen in later life; and presents guidelines for applying the nursing process to the mental health care of the aged.

ADVOCACY AND HEALTH PROMOTION FOR THE ELDERLY

Roadblocks to Mental Health Services for the Elderly

It is important to note that the elderly are the most underserved population in need of supportive and tertiary mental health services (Figure 36–1). This discussion highlights four roadblocks (agism, myths, stigma, and access) to mental health services and examines the demographic realities that compel us to break down these disabling roadblocks through health promotion and client advocacy.

Agism

A primary roadblock to mental health services for older persons is agism, which refers to negative, hostile attitudes toward the elderly (Butler 1980). In contemporary social environments, aging is often viewed with disdain and contempt. The elderly are criticized for being unattractive,

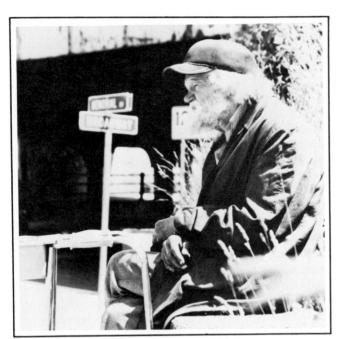

Figure 36–1
Percy Joe confronts us with our own aging. With elders like him we can reflect on the past; gain the beginnings of wisdom; and develop awareness of adaptability, courage, and humanity.

uable support, insight, and feedback to colleagues who are working with the elderly. We now know the elderly are as responsive to mental health services as any other age group. By modeling positive attitudes toward aging and by advocating quality of life and health care for the aged in all settings and at all levels of function, nurses can help dispel agist and gerontophobic influences on health care of the elderly.

Myths

Health professionals, and elders themselves, often equate growing old with growing sad, disengaged, and depressed. The myths that depression, disengagement, and senility are part of growing old all too often inhibit the elderly from seeking treatment for feelings and behaviors they think are a "normal" part of aging. Misled by these myths, professionals are less inclined to refer elderly clients for mental health services. We now know that advancing age does not condemn an individual to senility, isolation, loneliness, and depression. The majority of elderly persons live independently and contentedly well into late life.

Nurses can serve as advocates to the elderly by educating the public, health professionals, and the elderly themselves to differentiate between normal and pathologic states in later life. Dispelling the myths surrounding the aging process will help promote the notion that aging itself is not a "problem," so that when problems do arise, they will be identified and treated.

incompetent, socially irrelevant, and unhealthy. For many years, the elderly were considered inappropriate candidates for mental health interventions. Freud's contention that the elderly lacked the needed mental elasticity for analysis was a major factor in forming an agist bias among mental health professionals. This bias has until recently delayed advances in the study of mental health in late life. Agism also stems from the belief that the elderly present a financial and emotional drain to the family and society. **Gerontophobia**, a phenomenon related to agism, refers to fear of interacting with the elderly (Chaisson-Stewart 1985). Agist attitudes can be internalized by elderly persons, causing decreased self-worth and self-esteem (Ebersole and Hess 1985).

Researchers have recently identified six attitudes or countertransference responses elicited in therapeutic work with the elderly (Poggi and Berland 1985). These countertransference responses (see Box 36–1) reflect agist and gerontophobic influences that may deter a professional from engaging in mental health work with the elderly. These responses may also affect the quality of work of clinicians who do interact with the elderly.

Nurses caring for the elderly must be aware of their feelings and make a conscious effort not to let countertransference responses influence clinical assessment and interventions with the elderly. Nurses can provide inval-

---

Box 36–1
COUNTERTRANSFERENCE RESPONSES FROM WORKING WITH THE ELDERLY

1. The work stirs feelings in the clinician about his or her own age and issues surrounding death.

2. Working with the elderly touches on the clinician's conflicts about relationships with parents and parental figures.

3. The clinician believes the elderly are too rigid and set in their ways and cannot change.

4. The clinician feels his or her skills are wasted because clients are old and want to die anyway.

5. The clinician feels his or her interventions are in vain because elderly clients may die during treatment rather than improve.

6. The clinician's colleagues do not support his or her work with the elderly for any of all of the above reasons.

Source: Adapted from Poggi RG, Berland DI: The therapist's reactions to the elderly. The Gerontologist *1985;25(5):508–513.*

Stigma

Despite recent advances in mental health care, the stigma associated with mental illness remains very real to elderly people who were socialized when psychiatric treatment was less sophisticated than it is today. The elderly rarely seek psychiatric or mental health services and often deny or hide their psychic pain for fear of being labeled "crazy."

Nurses have tremendous access to persons at all levels of the health care and social systems. By educating the public about mental disorders and state-of-the-art mental health care, nurses can decrease the stigma associated with mental illness and psychiatric treatment and thus help allay the fears of the elderly who require mental health services.

Access

Perceived financial barriers, physical disability, and transportation problems limit the older adult's access to mental health services. While certain kinds of mental health treatment are time-consuming, expensive, and often not reimbursable (e.g., psychoanalysis), other interventions, such as support and therapy groups, time-limited cognitive and behavioral therapy, exercise programs, and group meals, are often reimbursable, free, or priced on a sliding scale for the elderly.

Nurses can play an important role in upgrading the quality and availability of mental health services for independent as well as homebound and institutionalized elderly. In-home services and handicapped transportation are becoming more available. Nurses have been gaining access to grant funding and research programs geared toward documenting the need for, and increasing the availability of, services for the elderly. Nurses must remain politically active to promote community-funded programs to meet the special needs of the aged.

Demographic Realities

The elderly population is growing faster than that of the nation as a whole. In 1980 the US Bureau of Census reported that by the year 2000 there will be almost thirty-five million people aged 65 and over. Forty-two million persons will be 60 and over. Figure 36–2 illustrates the demographic trend toward a greater percentage of older persons in the population. The over-75 population, which includes the "middle-aged old" (71–80), the "old-old" (81–90), and the "very old-old" (91–100), is estimated to reach 17.4 million by the year 2000.

It is important to examine the age distribution of the over-65 population carefully. Grouping the elderly arbitrarily into an aggregate of all persons over the age of 65 tends to blur important distinctions between elderly age groups. The "old-old" group of elders tends to have the greatest incidences of depression, organic mental disor-

ders, and chronic disabling illnesses. This group averages four to five times as many days in acute care hospitals as the national average, and 70 percent more than individuals aged 65 to 75 (Blazer 1980). Thus, the stereotypic **frail elderly**, who need many health care and maintenance services, constitute only 5 percent of the over-65 population. This differentiation by age group indicates that there is a large proportion of well elderly, particularly older women living alone (who outnumber single elderly men by 2.5 to 1), who will benefit from supportive psychosocial services.

The implications of a growing population of aging individuals is important for projecting needs and planning for social programs and fund allocation. The figures point to the need for greater numbers of health care professionals versed in the multiple needs of the elderly. Nursing's role in geriatrics and **psychogerontology** is expanding as the needs and real numbers of elderly increase (Ebersole 1985).

Theories of Aging

Defining mental health in late life is a difficult task. Many variables affect mental health as persons age, including:

- Health status
- Cultural factors
- Heredity
- The environment
- The family network
- Meaningful relationships
- Life losses
- Personality composition
- Economic and social support
- Spirituality

Late-life research efforts and theory development have focused on biologic aging, development, and social and interactional factors to explain "normal aging." Yet the many variables to consider and the complex interface of physical and emotional factors necessarily impose limitations on any single theory of aging. The most frequently cited theories of aging, and the major points of each, are presented in Table 36–1.

All the theories on aging must be viewed tentatively at this time because the research remains inconclusive. For example, the disengagement theory, which views withdrawal from social activities as a normal aspect of later life, is considered by some to be particularly controversial and potentially damaging to the elderly. When working with elderly individuals, it is crucial to consider the individual needs and unique characteristics of each aging person rather than attempting to fit an individual into a theoretical mold.

Philosophic Perspectives

The Value of Interaction

Each elder is unique. The philosophic tenets of interactionism provide us with a dynamic view of mental health in later life that focuses on the personal meaning each individual assigns to situations, behavior, life events, and relationships in his or her life. Essentially, interactionist theory tells us there is no one "right" way to age. Aging is processed and interpreted by each individual in his or her own way. The following case studies illustrate the individuality of elders as they find personal meaning in their unique life situations.

The nurses respected 92-year-old Mrs. Fee's need to refer to her diapers as "envelopes," and her desire to be "dressed for work," wear makeup, and carry a purse every day. Her many years as an executive secretary brought her much satisfaction and a sense of identity and self-esteem, which she maintains in her present situation by integrating aspects of her past.

Mr. Floyd had never been socially active or considered a "joiner." He looked forward to the day when he would be able to retire and spend long idle hours relaxing, just "doing nothing."

Mrs. Baptista became depressed for a time after her enforced retirement at age 65. She found herself bored and down in the dumps with the excess free time and decreased social contact. She came across a senior's organization and soon replaced her busy work schedule with active participation in elderly social activities and volunteer programs for handicapped children.

Mr. Stanwyck became despondent when he was forced to move into a nursing home, interpreting it as a prelude to his death. His roommate, Mr. Cliff viewed nursing home residency as a welcome haven, providing him with needed care, companionship, and three square meals a day.

Mental health for each elder is defined differently and expressed in unique ways. Through client interactions nurses can help elderly persons reflect on and integrate the past and find new meaning and purpose in the present.

Individuality versus Obsolescence

A rich history of life experiences adds to the complexity and individuality of each elder. In the past elderly people were revered for their knowledge and wisdom. In our present culture, information and technology are advancing so rapidly that the elderly are often viewed as obsolete and out of touch. Interactions influenced by agist attitudes convey a sense of worthlessness and obsolescence, which is internalized by elderly persons and predisposes them to mental illness.

A long life is evidence of strength and wisdom. Certainly living to a ripe old age is indicative of adaptive strength and coping ability. The elderly have much to share with younger people. Contemporary elders have lived through more dramatic changes in culture and technology than any former generation. The elderly must be respected for their individual strengths and the life-wisdom they have accumulated.

Ego Integrity versus Self-Despair

Erickson (1963) noted that the developmental task of late life is to achieve a sense of ego integrity versus self-despair. People who look back on their lives with satisfaction and a sense of wholeness, accomplishment, and a life well lived have achieved ego integrity. They convey a sense of serenity and wisdom and a desire to change little of their past. Despair results when an elder experiences a sense of loss and meaninglessness, a feeling that life's goals have not been achieved. Respect and worth must be conveyed to the elderly by their caregivers and significant others to foster trust and ego integrity. Nurses caring for elderly people in all settings can promote ego integrity in each unique elderly individual through interactions focusing on personal strengths. Teaching family members and caregivers to emphasize these personal strengths will enhance the ego-strengthening, interactive processes available to the elderly.

Physiologic Perspectives

The rate of physical aging, which begins at birth, varies tremendously among individuals. Different tissues and body systems vary widely in the rate at which they age. Some persons appear old at age 50, whereas others appear vibrant and energetic into their eighties and nineties (Busse and Blazer 1980). Factors believed to influence the aging process include heredity, cultural influence, the amount and regularity of exercise, past illnesses, the presence of chronic illness, and the stresses experienced throughout life.

Changes in physical functioning can dramatically affect a person's ability to cope with daily stress and perform the activities of daily living. Age-related metabolic, circulatory, nutritional, and neurochemical disturbances have been

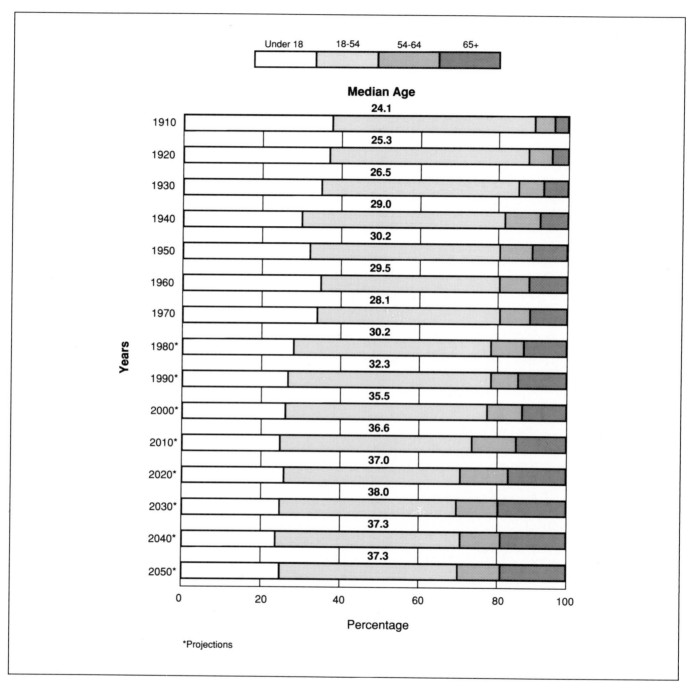

Figure 36–2
Percentage distribution of the total population by age group, 1910–2010.
Source: From Allan C, Brotman H: Chartbook on Aging in America.
White House Conference on Aging, 1981.

identified as physiologic antecedents in certain mental disorders. Hallmarks of aging and the psychosocial implications of each are listed in Table 36–2.

While normal age-related changes cannot be prevented, nurses can assess the extent of these changes and help elderly clients adapt by encouraging ventilation of feelings about the aging process, suggesting environmental alterations, and increasing social support.

Table 36–1
Theories of Aging

Theory	Key Ideas	Theory	Key Ideas
Biologic theories		Activity theory	Controversial theory widely debated
Deliberate biologic programming	Cellular level theory of aging		Contrasts with disengagement theory
	Diminished capacity for spontaneous change		Activity is desired by the elderly
	Each cell holds a finite capacity for reproduction and a preprogrammed termination		Older adults remain active and involved
	Aging is the result of intrinsic destiny		Lost roles and pastimes are replaced with meaningful substitutes
	Decline of biologic, cognitive, and motor function is inevitable		Assumes homogeneity or individual uniqueness
Wear-and-tear theory	Over time the human organism wears out	Symbolic interactionist theory	The individual's experience is constructed socially through an ongoing process of interpretation
	Structural and functional changes may be accelerated by abuse and stress accumulation		The social context is crucial to understanding aging, since all values and meanings are dynamic and evolving
	The rate of organ system degradation varies from individual to individual		Satisfaction in life is influenced by the symbolic significance of things and social interactions encountered
	Decremental model of aging		
Stress-adaptation	Emphasizes the effects of positive and negative stress on aging		Expansive theory, useful for studying many aspects of the aging process
	Perception influences stress response		Social values and views of aging influence each individual's experience
	Stress may deplete reserves, predisposing to illness	Life review/ reminiscence	Reminiscence is normal and universal
	Stress may lead to more effective adaptation and growth		Past experiences return to the conscious level
	Stress generally presumed to accelerate aging		Reintegration of unresolved conflicts desirable
Interactional theories			Successful integration of the past provides ego integrity and existential meaning
Disengagement	Characterized by mutually satisfying withdrawal between older adults and society		May result in anxiety, fear, and depression related to unresolved issues
	Disengagement is seen as a gradual, intrinsic, inevitable process		
	Cohorts prefer company of same age groups		
	Little recognition of the heterogeneity of the elderly		

continued

		Table 36–1 (*Continued*) Theories of Aging	
Theory	Key Ideas	Theory	Key Ideas
Personality theories			Acknowledges individual differences and uniqueness
Erikson's eight stages of man	Developmental sequence of eight psychosocial stages		Aging patterns differ from individual to individual
	Each stage characterized by specific developmental tasks	Developmental theories	Elders desire control over living situation
	Predetermined structural order to maturation		Continuity of intimacy (including sexual activity)
	Assumes inborn coordination to average expectable environment		Strive to maintain optimum level of health
	Eighth stage: ego integrity versus despair		Desired contact with family and extended family
	Ego integrity requires integration of the past		Pursue former and new activities
Continuity theory	Personality is stable over time		Find meaning after retirement
	Habits, preferences, associations, commitments are relatively unchanged with age		Refinement of personal philosophy
	"You are like you always were, only more so"		Adjustment occurs to losses of significant others

Source: Love CC, Buckwalter KC: Reactive depression, in Nursing Diagnosis and Interventions for the Institutionalized Elderly. *Addison-Wesley, in press.*

Psychologic Perspectives

Just as age-related physical changes vary from person to person, so do the psychologic changes that occur as one ages. The goal of research into the psychologic aspects of aging is to describe, understand, and predict the changes that come with age and differentiate normal age-related changes from abnormal, illness-related changes. While studying intelligence, memory, problem solving, learning ability, motor performance, personality, coping, and adaptation in later life, researchers have identified methodologic difficulties that are relevant to clinical practice. For example, cultural factors have been shown to influence test results. The time of day and length of testing also influences performance of elders because of fatigue and boredom. The elderly are often intolerant of gadgetry such as stopclocks and computerized test formats. Different age groups often include a variety of backgrounds and life experiences, which must be considered when designing and interpreting test results, thus making comparison across different groups difficult.

Intelligence

The idea that intelligence declines with age is widely debated among researchers. Disagreement centers around the timing and extent of age decrements, the causes of the decrements that do appear in the elderly, and the validity and reliability of IQ tests in measuring intelligence in older subjects (Belsky 1984). It now appears that the most important factors affecting intelligence have to do with the individual's lifelong patterns and abilities. Older persons who have been intellectually active in their lifetime and continue to be challenged intellectually and socially active and to relate well to others have been found to show a minimum decrease, and in some cases an increase, in IQ scores with advancing age (Braudis 1986).

Learning and Memory

Learning and memory are closely related. It is commonly believed that as people age their memory starts "slipping,"

Table 36–2
Age-Related Changes

Hallmarks of Physical Aging	Psychosocial Implications
Graying and loss of hair Wrinkling of skin Subcutaneous body fat redistribution	Loss of self-esteem related to social ideals, physical appearance, less emphasis upon grooming and self-presentation
Sensory losses: hearing (presbycusis), sight (presbyopia, cataracts), taste, smell, touch	Decreased pleasure from foods, communication problems, potential dehydration and inadequate food intake, safety risk factors, decreased sensitivity to pressure, temperature, and pain
Decreased muscle mass and strength Osteoporitic joint and bone changes	Decreased ability to perform certain routine tasks (e.g., ADL, hobbies), changes in dexterity
	Increased potential for bone fracture, immobility, fear of falling; possible chronic pain from arthritis; decreased agility
Organ shrinkage with decreased efficiency, metabolic and endocrine changes, adult-onset diabetes	Necessary diet changes, decreased activity tolerance, increased potential for drug toxicity and alcohol intoxication, increased susceptibility to illness, sleep pattern disturbance, depression
Arterial changes: athlerosclerosis with decreased tissue perfusion	Potential cognitive impairment, heart disease, decreased activity tolerance
Renal excretory changes: bladder hypertrophy	Decreased ability to excrete medications, urinary frequency, urgency and increased nocturia, incontinence
Reproductive changes	Menopause, hormonal changes, alterations in sexual functioning, grief reaction to loss of child-bearing capacity and perceived loss of femininity/masculinity

and they are not as quick to learn as they used to be. Elders often cite these changes themselves. According to the information-processing model, memory is an active process that passes through three stages: (1) encoding or receipt of the information, (2) storage of the information, and (3) retrieval of the information. One factor that has been noted to affect the storage and retrieval of information in older persons has to do with the use of **mental mediators**. Mediators are cues used to enhance memory and learning (Belsky 1984, p 132). Nursing students often use the phrase, "On old Olympus' towering top a Finn and German viewed all hops," to remember the twelve cranial nerves. This is an example of a mediator. Elderly subjects were found not to use mediators spontaneously to help them remember. When mediators were suggested to these subjects, however, their performance on tests improved. This information is useful for clinicians when helping the elderly to remember things.

Mr. O'Brien began to forget his apartment keys when he left the house to go to the senior center for lunch every day. He never forgot his pipe and tobacco, however. The nurse at the center suggested Mr. O'Brien mentally connect his tobacco pouch with his keys. When he places his tobacco pouch in his pocket she suggested he get into the habit of putting his keys in his pocket at the same time. This solved Mr. O'Brien's problem of forgetting his keys.

As persons age they tend to think and move more slowly than younger people. Part of this slower pacing is related to adaptation to sensory deficits and part to a more cautious approach to life. Older people perform better if information is meaningful to them. As illustrated in the research box, when the elderly are permitted to pace themselves, rather than being rushed, their performance improves significantly. When trying to teach elderly clients a new skill such as progressive relaxation or assertion, the following guidelines will be useful:

- Present the information so that its utility to the clients' life-style is clear.
- Allow clients to pace themselves.
- Provide time for repetition of material.
- Suggest mediators when appropriate.
- Be sincere and focus on small positive steps.

Overall memory, learning, intelligence, coping and adaptation, and personality remain relatively stable as individuals age. The elderly *can* be taught new ways of coping and handling the stressors of aging. Subtle, minimal changes are normal as people adapt to age-related changes in functioning and life experiences. Any marked variation in cognitive functioning or affective status of older people, whether sudden or progressive, should not be regarded as a normal part of aging. Gross alteration in mental status, personality, and cognition suggest the presence of a mental or physical disorder or both. The following section provides an overview of the most common mental disorders in later life.

MENTAL DISORDERS IN LATER LIFE

Epidemiology

The agist attitudes in our culture are responsible for many misperceptions about mental disorders in the elderly. Older people are believed to be more prone to mental disorders

than the young. It is difficult to obtain exact incidence and prevalence rates of mental disorders in later life for several reasons. Often the elderly are difficult to reach with community-wide surveys. Researchers have noted that the elderly are reluctant to respond to research questions dealing with emotions. As mentioned earlier, the elderly often do not seek treatment, so elderly subjects are underrepresented in clinical samples. Different researchers diagnose mental problems differently, making comparisons between community-wide surveys difficult. Symptoms of mental illness

RESEARCH NOTE

Citation

Kim KK: Response time and health care learning of elderly patients. Res Nurs Health *1986;9:233–239.*

Study Problem/Purpose

The purpose of this study was to determine if elderly clients perform better in health care learning when they are provided with slower or self-paced response conditions. The hypothesis tested was: Elderly clients will differ in learning performances, with the slow-paced group superior to the fast-paced group and the self-paced group superior to both the slow- and fast-paced groups.

Methods

This study was conducted at a midwestern hospital serving adult clients with chronic diseases. After screening 122 eligible clients with a mental status questionnaire, 105 subjects (70 men and 35 women) were randomly assigned to one of three experimental groups: (1) a fast-paced response group, (2) a slower-paced response group, and (3) a self-paced response group. All participants were given nutrition instruction on ten calcium-rich foods. Approximately twenty-four hours after receiving the nutrition instruction, the subjects were given a posttest via videotape. In the fast-paced group, respondents were required to answer each question within three seconds. In the slower-paced group the respondents were given six seconds to respond, and in the self-paced group, respondents could take as long as they needed to respond.

Findings

The group means on the nutrition knowledge posttest for the fast-, slow-, and self-paced groups were 12.37, 12.74, and 14.11 respectively. To strengthen the statistical power of the analysis, covariant analysis was performed to take into consideration pretest nutrition knowledge, mental status questionnaire scores, race, and posttest scores of the respondents. Although the slow-paced group performed

better on the nutrition knowledge posttest, the difference failed to reach statistical significance, thus failing to support the first hypothesis. The second hypothesis was supported, however, showing significantly higher scores in the self-paced group over the slow- and fast-paced groups. The author concluded that the self-paced response condition was superior.

Implications

This study supports the importance of self-paced learning situations for the institutionalized elderly. The findings suggest that stress and anxiety related to the timed-response requirement adversely affect elderly clients' performance. The statistical analysis indicated that prior nutrition knowledge and mental status questionnaire scores also affected the subjects' performance on the posttest. These findings illustrate the need for assessing the client's baseline knowledge and cognitive functioning and tailoring teaching interventions individually. In questioning elderly clients, the nurse should provide the client as much time as needed to respond. If elderly clients are not given enough time to respond to a question, their performance may be poor, even if they know the information. Although the present study focused on response time of elderly subjects in health care learning, the findings have implications for other aspects of nurse-client interactions. For example, in health assessment and data collection in clinical practice, if response slowness is not taken into consideration, client data may be incorrect or incomplete. Clients in mental health settings usually have medical and emotional problems that affect their ability to learn and respond to questions. Response slowness is difficult to provide for in busy clinical environments. In situations where nurses are assessing and caring for the elderly, data such as those presented in this study may provide clout for clinicians seeking to "buck the system" and gain the necessary staffing to allow for the slower pace so essential for comprehensive, effective nursing care of elderly individuals.

in the elderly often differ from those of other age groups. While the DSM-IIIR (APA 1987) has greatly enhanced our ability to make reliable and valid diagnoses of mental disorders, there are few age-specific categories for mental disorders in later life. Thus, in spite of the DSM-IIIR's extensive detailed description of each problem category, clinicians and researchers continue to have difficulty applying the written descriptions to symptoms in later life (Belsky 1984, Zung 1980).

The epidemiologic studies to date tell us that the elderly suffer no more than other groups from disorders, such as adjustment disorders, personality disorders, and grief reactions. The elderly do have a disproportionately high incidence of depression and are somewhat more likely to become paranoid. Organic brain syndromes are much more prevalent in the elderly, particularly the chronic organic dementias. The elderly also frequently complain of sleep disturbances. A recent area of exploration, for which there is very little epidemiologic data at present, is the area of substance abuse in later life.

Mood Disorders

Mood disorders are primarily characterized by a disturbed affect or emotional experience. Mood disturbances in the elderly, as in other age groups, may present as:

- Sustained elation and hyperactivity, as seen in a manic episode
- Changes from elation to depression, as seen in a bipolar disorder
- Pervasive depressed mood not accompanied by mania, as seen in a major depression

Depression is the most prevalent and most treatable mental disorder in later life.

Depression in the Elderly

Depression robs the elderly of late life satisfaction, inhibits ego integrity, and may substantially decrease the life expectancy of a depressed elder, since symptoms may precipitate or aggravate physical deterioration. Suicide rates among the elderly are more than three times the rates seen in the general population (Osgood 1985).

While the signs and symptoms of depression are relatively consistent throughout the life span (see Chapter 18), there are certain characteristics of depression particular to the elderly. It is crucial for clinicians to note that depres-

sion in the elderly, which responds well to treatment, may present with cognitive changes similar to other organically based, irreversible disorders. Tyler and Tyler (1984) suggest that nearly half the elderly clients thought to be demented actually have a depressive disorder with misleading cognitive symptoms such as disorientation, agitation, and memory loss.

In addition to cognitive changes, another flag for depression in elderly persons is excessive preoccupation with physical symptoms, which is known as **somatization**. Expressing discomfort through the body may be more familiar to older persons than bringing forth symptoms of psychic pain. Chronic complaints of constipation, headaches, musculoskeletal pain, chest tightness and dyspnea with no physical basis, and chronic gastrointestinal upset may be the result of a depressed elder's unconscious shifting of attention away from distressing emotions to what they may feel are more acceptable, familiar, and less stigmatized physical complaints. Clinicians have noted that due to the stigma associated with mental illness, depressed elderly clients sometimes "cover up" a dysphoric mood by maintaining meticulous grooming and feigning a cheerful affect (Love and Buckwalter, in press). Nurses must be persistent and perceptive in foraging for signs of depression. Depressed apathetic elders may believe they are supposed to feel blue and "down in the dumps" as they age. It should be explained to depressed elders and their families that depression is a pathologic condition often caused by biochemical imbalances. Interventions should be instituted to correct depressive states in the elderly as aggressively and comprehensively as with any other age group.

Suicide

The depressed elderly are more prone to commit suicide than any other age group in the United States (Stenback 1980). The **lethality index** (ratio of suicide attempts to successful suicides) is also higher in the elderly, and these data do not even begin to tap the passive, indirect suicides accomplished by starvation and "accidental" overmedication. The dramatically high rates clearly indicate that suicide is a significant problem in later life.

Elders who present a greater suicide risk include:

- Elderly males
- The unmarried
- Caucasians
- Lower socioeconomic classes
- Elders with chronic pain and terminal illness
- The lonely and isolated in urban settings
- The elderly who use alcohol and medication to cope (Osgood 1985)

The suicidal elderly have been known to seek help (often for a vague or nonspecific physical problem) from physicians, clergy, and nurses prior to their self-destructive act.

Thus accurate assessment of suicide potential in the elderly is crucial and requires perception, active listening, and direct questioning. The suicidal elderly individual may present with:

- Verbal cues (e.g., "I'm going to end it all; life is not worth living; I won't be around much longer")
- Behavioral cues (e.g., completing a will, making funeral plans, "acting out," withdrawing, somatic complaints)
- Situational cues (e.g., recent move, loss of a loved one, diagnosis of a terminal illness) (Osgood 1985)

For more information on suicide and assessment of suicide potential including a lethality index, see Chapter 18. Osgood (1985) has provided a comprehensive volume covering the topic of suicide in the elderly.

Organic Mental Syndromes and Disorders

The diagnostic group termed *organic mental syndromes* (OMS) refers to a temporary or permanent dysfunction of the brain, which is either caused by an illness unrelated to a mental illness listed on the DSM-IIIR Axis I or has no known etiology. Organic mental disorders (OMD) are progressive pathophysiologic brain processes of known etiology. Both OMS and OMD cause a variety of psychologic, cognitive, and behavioral abnormalities. The elderly present with both OMS and OMD more than any other age group. The challenge for clinicians is to identify and treat reversible organic mental syndromes, whether they exist alone or with an irreversible condition.

Delirium

Delirium refers to an acute confusional state that usually appears within hours or days. Delirium is characterized primarily by confusion and an obvious decrease in attention span and level of consciousness that may fluctuate over the course of the day. Other symptoms may include perceptual disturbances, psychomotor retardation or agitation, incoherent speech, and disorders of the sleep-wake cycle. When an elderly client becomes acutely confused, thorough and prompt assessment will often uncover a specific organic factor or combination of factors such as infection; congestive heart failure; trauma; hepatic, pulmonary, and renal insufficiency; and drug toxicity.

The treatment of delirium, which is usually reversible, must be directed toward correcting the underlying disorder. Symptomatic treatment may be necessary, particularly if agitation, anxiety, perceptual disturbances, delusions, or other behavioral features are endangering the client's safety or interfering with the evaluation and treatment of the underlying disorder. Nursing interventions for a client with delirium include:

- Calm, consistent low level of stimuli (avoid sensory deprivation and overstimulation)
- Reassurance from trusted caregivers and significant others
- Physically secure, carefully monitored environment
- Night lights to aid orientation
- Judicial use of low-dose psychotropic medication

Dementia

Dementia, or loss of cognitive function, once thought to be an inevitable part of growing old, is now known to be a pathologic condition afflicting only 5 to 7 percent of the over-65 population (Mortimer et al. 1981). There are reversible conditions that mimic dementia that improve markedly with treatment. While the dementias are irreversible, some have a progressively downward course ending in death. The causes of dementia vary and, as in the case of Alzheimer's disease, are not well understood. Multiinfarct dementia, caused by a series of small strokes, results in a variety of stepwise, focal, neurologic signs and symptoms. The reversible dementia-like symptoms are listed in Table 36–3.

Alzheimer's disease and multiinfarct dementia are the most prevalent dementias. Senile dementia–Alzheimer's type (SDAT), the fourth leading cause of death in the elderly, has received a great deal of publicity recently, heightening the public's awareness of the tragedy of dementia and its impact on family and caregivers. It has been noted by Zarit et al. (1985) that since Alzheimer's disease has received a large amount of publicity, increasing numbers of people have been incorrectly diagnosed with SDAT when in fact they have had a reversible dementia-like condition. The definitive diagnosis of SDAT can be made only on autopsy.

Family Burden

Perhaps no other illness is as devastating to family members and caregivers as an irreversible dementia. The anguish of family members seeing loved ones becoming progressively more dependent is profound. The stress of looking after demented individuals, who often become delusional, suspicious, angry, and sometimes unmanageable, is being studied in a growing area of research called **family burden.** Coping abilities will vary markedly, depending on the family's emotional, financial, and environmental resources. To prevent burnout and elder abuse, family members caring for a demented elder need emotional support and information about specific interventions aimed at problem solving and stress reduction. Nurses are in key positions to

	Table 36–3 Reversible Causes of Dementia Symptoms and Delirium		
	Dementia	Delirium	Either or Both
Therapeutic drug intoxication			Yes
Depression	Yes		
Metabolic			
a. Azotemia or renal failure (dehydration, diuretics, obstruction, hypokalemia)			Yes
b. Hyponatremia (diuretics, excess antidiuretic hormone, salt wasting, intravenous fluids)			Yes
c. Hypernatremia (dehydration, intravenous saline)		Yes	
d. Volume depletion (diuretics, bleeding, inadequate fluids)			Yes
e. Acid-base disturbance		Yes	
f. Hypoglycemia (insulin, oral hypoglycemics, starvation)			Yes
g. Hyperglycemia (diabetic ketoacidosis or hyperosmolar coma)		Yes	
h. Hepatic failure			Yes
i. Hypothyroidism			Yes
j. Hyperthyroidism (especially apathetic)			Yes
k. Hypercalcemia			Yes
l. Cushing's syndrome	Yes		
m. Hypopituitarism			Yes
Infection, fever, or both			
a. Viral			Yes
b. Bacterial			
Pneumonia		Yes	
Pyelonephritis		Yes	
Cholecystitis		Yes	
Diverticulitis		Yes	
Tuberculosis			Yes
Endocarditis			Yes
Cardiovascular			
a. Acute myocardial infarct		Yes	
b. Congestive heart failure			Yes
c. Arrhythmia			Yes
d. Vascular occlusion			Yes
e. Pulmonary embolus		Yes	
Brain disorders			
a. Vascular insufficiency			
Transient ischemia		Yes	
Stroke			Yes
b. Trauma			
Subdural hematoma			Yes

continued

	Dementia	Delirium	Either or Both
Table 36–3 (*Continued*) **Reversible Causes of Dementia Symptoms and Delirium**			
Concussion/confusion		Yes	
Intracerebral hemorrhage		Yes	
Epidural hematoma		Yes	
c. Infection			
Acute meningitis (pyogenic, viral)		Yes	
Chronic meningitis (tuberculosis, fungal)			Yes
Neurosyphilis			Yes
Subdural empyema			Yes
Brain abscess			Yes
d. Tumors			
Metastatic to brain			Yes
Primary in brain			Yes
e. Normal pressure hydrocephalus	Yes		
Pain			
a. Fecal impaction			Yes
b. Urinary retention		Yes	
c. Fracture		Yes	
d. Surgical abdomen		Yes	
Sensory deprivation states such as blindness or deafness			Yes
Hospitalization			
a. Anesthesia or surgery			Yes
b. Environmental change and isolation			Yes
Alcohol toxic reactions			
a. Lifelong alcoholism	Yes		
b. Alcoholism new in old age			Yes
c. Decreased tolerance with age producing increasing intoxication			Yes
d. Acute hallucinosis		Yes	
e. Delirium tremens		Yes	
Anemia			Yes
Tumor—systemic effects of nonmetastatic malignant neoplasm			Yes
Chronic lung disease with hypoxia or hypercapnia			Yes
Deficiencies of nutrients such as vitamin B_{12}, folic acid, or niacin	Yes		
Accidental hypothermia		Yes	
Chemical intoxications			
a. Heavy metals such as arsenic, lead, or mercury			Yes
b. Consciousness-altering agents			Yes
c. Carbon monoxide			Yes

Source: NIA Task Force: Senility reconsidered. Journal of the American Medical Association, *October 1980. Copyright 1980, American Medical Association.*

provide psychoeducative programs for the caregivers of demented individuals. Community support programs and publications are now available to provide emotional support, strategies, and practical information for persons choosing to care for a demented individual at home, including *The 36 Hour Day* (Mace and Rabins 1981) and *Alzheimer's Disease: A Guide for Families* (Powell and Courtice 1983). For further discussion of dementia and delirium, see Chapter 15.

It is crucial to perform a comprehensive physical and neurologic assessment whenever an elderly client presents with cognitive impairment. Nurses must become skilled at differentiating treatable disorders such as delirium and depression from irreversible dementia. It is also important to note that depression can exist with dementia or delirium, and the cognitive impairment may be worsened by the depressive overlay. Depression superimposed on dementia may cause increased cognitive problems, a situation described as **excess disability**. In these cases treatment with antidepressant medication may improve the cognitive status worsened by the depression. Table 36–4 provides guidelines for distinguishing depression from dementia.

Anxiety Disorders

Anxiety is a universal sensation experienced subjectively as worry, fear, restlessness, and terror stemming from fear of a real danger or the anticipation of danger or a threat. Anxiety is accompanied by physiologic "fight or flight" somatic responses such as shortness of breath, palpitations, and chest tightness. When anxiety recurs to the point that it interferes with an individual's ability to function, it is considered an anxiety disorder. Anxiety disorders, causes, and treatment in the elderly are outlined in Table 36–5.

Clients with anxiety disorders require interventions geared primarily toward symptom relief, followed by insight-oriented therapy. Until clients are less anxious, they are not likely to benefit from psychotherapy. Judiciously administered, medication in small doses often provides symptomatic relief of an acute anxiety state.

Delusional Disorders

Delusions are defined as an important personal belief that is almost certainly not true and resists modification (Wilson and Kneisl 1984, p 75). The elderly are more prone than any other age group to persecutory and somatic delu-sions. Persecutory delusions involve the belief that the elder is under investigation, being harassed, or at the mercy of some powerful force. With somatic delusions the predominant theme is an imagined physical disorder or abnormality of appearance. Somatic delusions in older persons are frequently characterized by extremely morbid content.

Delusional processes in the elderly are often associated with delirium, depression, dementia, or anxiety disorders. Persecutory delusions may be a response in the elderly to a diminishing sense of self-mastery. Among the various symptoms exhibited by elderly people with psychiatric problems, delusions involving suspiciousness and persecutory ideation are among the most disturbing and unsettling for their families and caregivers. As older adults gradually give up important areas of function, such as financial management, cooking, and shopping, they may begin to develop delusions that people are robbing them or poisoning their food. They respond to these delusional processes by "dismissing" or rejecting their caregivers in an effort to regain control over these areas of life. Delusions may also result from internalized agist attitudes, sensory losses—particularly hearing impairment—and social isolation.

Caregivers must work to establish trust and consistency with delusional elders. It is important to assess the situation to validate that the persecutory and somatic content is not reality based. Clients need consistent social interaction, with caring, consistent reality orientation. Relieving social isolation and correcting sensory losses may solve the problem. Delusional processes associated with delirium often abate when the cause of the delirium is treated. Medication in small doses, geared toward relieving an underlying anxiety or depressive disorder, may be helpful, although compliance is often a problem due to suspicion.

Substance Use Disorders

The extent of alcoholism and drug- and alcohol-related problems in the elderly is unknown. Typical signs of alcoholism, such as absence from work, difficulties in the family, and driving while intoxicated are often not apparent in older people, because they often are retired, live alone, and do not drive. It is known that the elderly use a disproportionately high amount of prescribed hypnotics and over-the-counter sleep medications. Elderly persons also often take a variety of medications for one or more chronic medical conditions. **Polypharmacy**, or mixing medications, with or without alcohol use, is potentially dangerous and adds to the chance of untoward drug interactions in the elderly (Colling 1983).

There seem to be two categories of older drinkers. The first category includes those who have a long history of alcohol abuse. The second category, the late-onset, **reactive drinker**, includes those who drink in response to one or more age-related stressors, such as social isolation, loss of

Table 36–4
Guide to Differentiating Dementia from Depression

Dementia	Depression	Dementia	Depression

Affect

Observe the client's overall mood and self-presentation throughout the interview. Enlist interpretations from family and caregivers. "How has your mood been lately?"

Dementia	Depression
Labile, fluctuating from tears to laughter, not consistent or sustained; may show apathy, depression, irritability, euphoria or inappropriate affect. Normal control impaired, suggestible to content of interview.	Depressed, feelings of despair that are pervasive, persistent. May be anxious or hypomanic. Not influenced by suggestions. May be flat, withdrawn, sad, tearful.

Memory

Ask specific questions geared toward assessing recent and remote memory. Ask client to recall recent events, details from a classic, personal, or well-known story. Ask client to repeat a series of three or four words at five-, ten-, and fifteen-minute intervals.

Dementia	Depression
Decreased attention. Decreased for recent events. Confabulation, covers up memory loss. Shows irritability when memory tested. Perseveration, dwells on certain topics inappropriately.	Difficulty in concentration. Impaired learning of new knowledge. Decreased attention with secondary decrease in recent memory. May not respond when tested or will admit can't remember.

Intellect

Assess the client's cognitive functioning, taking into account cultural and educational factors, which will influence results. Ask the client to perform simple math equations and solve simple problems.

Dementia	Depression
Impaired, decreased as tested by serial 7s, similarities, recent events. Decreased capacity for abstract thinking.	Impaired but can perform serial 7s and usually remember recent events.

Orientation

Elicit level of orientation regarding person, time, place date, etc. May vary with different times of the day.

Dementia	Depression
Fluctuating with varying levels of awareness. Disoriented for time, place.	May have some confusion, not as profound as in dementia.

Judgment

Ask the client to solve hypothetical problems (e.g., What would you do if you saw a fire across the street?)

Dementia	Depression
Poor judgment with inappropriate behavior, dress. Deterioration of grooming, personal habits, and hygiene. Loss of bowel and bladder control.	May be poor, especially if suicidal. May be careless with medication, and may risk personal safety.

Somatic Complaints

Ask the client specific questions regarding physical status. (How is your health?)

Dementia	Depression
Fatigue, failing health complaints with vague complaints of pain in head, neck, back.	Typical complaints as: decreases in sleep, appetite, weight, libido, energy, and constipation.

Psychotic Symptoms

Enlist interpretations from family and caregivers. Often (but not always) psychotic material will become evident during interview. (Are you being plotted against? Do you ever see/hear/smell things others do not?)

Dementia	Depression
Mainly visual, hallucinations, delusions.	May occur in psychotic depressions, mainly auditory hallucinations and delusions of a morbid quality.

Source: Adapted from Zung WWK: Affective Disorders, in Busse EW, Blazer DG (eds): Handbook of Geriatric Psychiatry. *Van Nostrand Reinhold, 1980, p 357.*

Table 36–5
Anxiety Disorders Seen in Later Life

Anxiety	Etiology	Treatment
Acute traumatic anxiety	Adjustment reaction to a real life loss	Social support
		Psychotherapy
		Medication
Chronic neurotic anxiety	Lifelong pattern, usually ego-dystonic	Medication
		Psychotherapy
		Relaxation training
Helplessness anxiety	Anticipated loss	Social support
	Powerlessness	Ventilation of feelings
	Loss of control and mastery	Environmental alterations to restore security
Depression anxiety	Despair	Medication
	Fear of impending death	Psychotherapy
	Grief reaction	Relaxation training
Phobic disorders	Projection and externalization to relieve anxiety	Medication
		Behavior modification
		Relaxation training
		Systematic desensitization
Obsessive-compulsive disorders	Often seen in depression	Behavior modification
	May be lifelong personality disorder	Medication (if depressed)
Anxiety associated with psychosis	Psychosis: delusional phobias, persecutory anxiety, paranoia paraphrenia, schizophrenia	Medication
		Psychotherapy

Source: Adapted from Verwoerdt A: Anxiety, dissociative and personality disorders in the elderly, in Busse EW, Blazer DG (eds): Handbook of Geriatric Psychiatry. *Van Nostrand Reinhold, 1980.*

---

a loved one, and loss of social status (Blazer and Penny-backer 1984).

When older drinkers seek medical help for alcohol-related problems (e.g., malnutrition, injuries from falling, sleep problems), the alcoholism is rarely the presenting problem. Often a drinking problem is not diagnosed in an elderly client; the presenting symptoms are treated and other symptoms are attributed to "normal" age-related changes. Glassock (1982) has suggested that a "conspiracy of silence" exists between the client, the client's family, and the health care provider to keep the client's drinking problem hidden and avoid the stigma associated with alcoholism.

Assessment for drug and alcohol abuse in elderly clients, especially socially isolated elders who have suffered recent life losses, should be approached with a high index of sus-picion. Elderly alcoholics usually drink daily but in lower quantities than other age groups. Special problems may arise in older drinkers because of the:

- Decreased metabolic efficiency in older people
- Interaction of alcohol with medication
- Presence of chronic illness
- Sensory losses that occur with aging

All elderly clients must be educated about the danger of mixing and altering medications. Nurses must approach elderly clients nonjudgmentally to educate them and their families about the risks of mixing medications and alcohol. Preventing reactive drinking may be accomplished by providing social support and preventive mental health services for elderly people who, by suffering one or more life losses, are at risk for social isolation and depression.

Disorders of Arousal and Sleep

The quantity and quality of sleep changes with aging. In a comprehensive review of research on sleep and aging, the elderly demonstrated more frequent awakening during the night than younger adults, increased total time awake, and longer time spent in bed before finally falling asleep (Miles and Dement 1980). Changes in sleep patterns are believed to be related to changes in internal body rhythm (circadian asynchrony), emotional stress, physical illness, and drugs (Colling 1983). Over one-third of people over 60 complain of sleep disturbances (Woodruff 1985). The elderly have been found to nap more during the day and to use a disproportionately high amount of over-the-counter and prescription sleeping aids.

Problems With Use of Sleep Medication

The chronic use of sedatives and hypnotics by elderly people has *not* been shown to improve the quality of sleep and can lead to many undesirable and dangerous side-effects. The elderly excrete these drugs slower than the young and thus are prone to develop toxic effects, including delirium, daytime drowsiness, and loss of equilibrium. Respiration can be significantly disturbed with the use of sleeping medication, which may lead to a physiologically adaptive response of frequent arousal to stimulate respiration (Wynne et al. 1978).

Guides to Improve Sleep

The following guidelines can be used to improve sleep in the elderly (Busse and Blazer 1980):

- Increased physical activity, particularly in the late afternoon and early evening hours, has beneficial effects.

- A cool room is usually more conducive to sleep than an overly warm room.

- A light bedtime snack containing calcium combined with sugar may help induce sleep.

- Stress reduction and progressive relaxation can be taught to older persons to help them relax.

- Elderly people should be encouraged to arise at the same time every day rather than try to catch up on lost sleep by "sleeping in" late in the morning.

- Elderly people should avoid napping during the day.

- The sleep "milieu" is very important in promoting sleep. Bed linen should be clean and made up each day.

- The elderly should spend as little time as possible in the bedroom during the day, thus associating the bedroom with sleep.

THE NURSING PROCESS AND THE ELDERLY

The Nursing Assessment Interview

The variety of theories on aging and the complex interface between physical, emotional, and environmental factors point to the importance of an individualized, multifactorial approach to assessment. The assessment information must be comprehensive and multidimensional. If available, a multidisciplinary team approach is usually most effective in securing comprehensiveness and providing validation of assessment impressions, leading to accurate diagnoses and effective intervention strategies.

The interview is the initial step in the assessment process and the most important procedure in differentiating between psychiatric disorders in the elderly. Interviewing requires skill and heightened sensitivity and typically takes more time with the elderly than with other age groups. The interviewer should attempt to make the interview pleasant for the elderly client, conveying a sense of respect and caring. The interviewer should be close to the client, use touch when appropriate to relieve anxiety, and be clear in stating the purpose of the interview and length of time it will take. A skilled diagnostician attends to verbal, nonverbal, and environmental cues, as well as the cognitive and behavioral aspects of the client. During the course of the interview, it may become necessary to repeat the purpose and time frame of the interview, since the elderly may tend to wander and reminisce.

Sensory loss, confusion, communication disorders, cultural influences, shame, and fear of stigmatization may inhibit expression of feelings by elderly persons. Older people may be unaware of changes in their behavior or expect negative changes as a "normal" part of aging. It is important to enlist interpretations from family and staff members to help fill in aspects of the clinical picture and validate the information the client has provided. Box 36–2 provides a framework for a multidimensional nursing assessment of an elderly client. The following discussion highlights salient features of the nursing assessment guide, focusing on the psychosocial dimensions. Sample questions are provided to guide the novice interviewer.

Physiologic Status

Whenever a mental disorder is suspected in an elderly client, a complete physical and neurologic exam must be performed. While still remaining independent and highly functional, most persons over age 65 have at least one chronic illness. Physical factors often affect the mental health of the elderly, and a definitive psychiatric diagnosis must not be made until all possible physiologic causes, including drug-induced (iatrogenic) disorders, have been ruled out. Nutritional status, as well as medication and alcohol intake (past and present use), affects the mental status of an elder and therefore should be assessed.

Cognitive Status

When interviewing the elderly, the *presence* and *extent* of cognitive impairment should be included in the assessment. The interviewer should include the family and caregivers to gain a description of the course of the mental changes. Did the changes happen gradually (e.g., SDAT, drug toxicity, metabolic imbalances), suddenly (e.g., depression, CVA, drug toxicity), or in a graduated, stepwise fashion (e.g., multiinfarct dementia)? A thorough mental status examination is essential. Pfeiffer's (1975) Short Portable Mental Status Questionnaire (SPMSQ) is a simple, reliable, and valid ten-item cognitive performance evaluation tool (Figure 36–3). It was designed for use with the elderly and can be used by most nurses to assess and monitor cognitive changes in an elderly client. The SPMSQ is not capable of distinguishing delirium from dementia, however.

It is important to remember that the elderly are sensitive to fatigue, boredom, medication, and environmental influences, which can affect their performance. Any tool used to assess an elderly client must have been determined reliable and valid for use with older persons. Tools designed for use with other age groups are not likely to be accurate or complete for use with older persons.

Psychologic Status

Strengths and Coping Strategies

Aging is a continuous process, punctuated by positive and negative stress-producing life events. The elderly are individuals who have learned to cope with stress. Information regarding an elder's coping strategies and strengths is as important as their psychologic symptomatology. Bringing up the subject of adaptive strengths, you might begin by asking, "You have certainly lived a long, full life. Would

---

Box 36–2
MULTIDIMENSIONAL NURSING ASSESSMENT GUIDE

- **Physiologic status:** Assess general appearance, sensory losses. Health history should include past illnesses, surgeries, past medication use and efficacy of medication, family health and psychiatric history, eating habits, activity patterns, sleep-wake cycle; must include a thorough medical and neurologic exam.

- **Cognitive status:** Perform thorough mental status examination, level of orientation, memory (short- and long-term), decision making and judgment, abstract thinking, reality testing, self-care abilities and limitations. Describe the nature of changes in cognition over time (e.g., gradual, stepwise, or sudden); consider educational level and cultural influences on assessment.

- **Psychologic status:** Include adaptive strengths, past coping skills, emotional resources, psychiatric symptomatology, suicidal ideation, history of suicide attempts, self-harm and homicidal tendencies, religious and spiritual expression, sexuality, past and present family functioning, and the client's perception of the problem, expectations, and primary concerns.

- **Social and financial status:** Assess quality and quantity of social support, marital status, financial status, home situation, abuse potential, environmental factors, use of leisure time, transportation, cultural norms and expectations, and previous and current use of health care resources.

---

you be willing to share some of your survival secrets with me?" Sample questions to gather information regarding the psychologic strengths of the elderly client are listed in Box 36–3.

Having gained an understanding of an elderly client's strengths and coping strategies (e.g., spiritual expression, listening to music, reading, reaching out to others), the nurse can foster these strengths and adaptive strategies by including them in the care plan and encouraging significant others and the client to mobilize them to deal with the situation at hand.

Sexuality

Sexuality in later life is an important assessment area often overlooked by health care professionals. Sexual activity can and does continue into later life. It should be remembered that sexuality does not refer only to sexual activity (intercourse or masturbation); it includes a broad multidimensional component of personhood and identity. Sexual expression includes body image, affection and love, flirtation, and social roles and interaction. Older people may abstain from sexual activity because they are denied the

Instructions: Ask questions 1–10 in this list and record all answers. Ask question 4A only if patient does not have a telephone. Record total number of errors based on ten questions.

+   -

____   1.   What is the date today?_____ (month/day/year)

____   2.   What day of the week is it?_____

____   3.   What is the name of this place?_____

____   4.   What is your telephone number?_____

____4A.   What is your street address?_____

____   5.   How old are you?_____

____   6.   When were you born?_____

____   7.   Who is the president of the U.S. now?_____

____   8.   Who was the president before him?_____

____   9.   What was your mother's maiden name?_____

____ 10.   Subtract 3 from 20 and keep subtracting 3 from each new number, all the way down.

____   Total Errors

To be completed by interviewer

Patient Name:_____

Sex: 1. Male   2. Female   Race: 1. White   2. Black   3. Other

Years of Education:_____

1. Grade School   2. High School   3. Beyond High School

Interviewer's Name:_____

The total number of errors constitutes the score in the SPMSQ. The test is sensitive to educational attainment. For persons with 9–12 years of education, the following scoring applies:

0-2 Errors: Intact intellectual functioning

3-4 Errors: Mild intellectual impairment

5-7 Errors: Moderate intellectual impairment

8-10 Errors: Severe intellectual impairment

For persons with 8 or fewer years of education, one additional error is allowed for each scoring category. Persons with more than 12 years of education, one less error is allowed for each category.

Figure 36–3

Short Portable Mental Status Questionnaire (SPMSQ).

Source: From Pfeiffer E: The psychosocial evaluation of the elderly client, in Busse EW, Blazer DG (eds): Handbook of Geriatric Psychiatry. Von Nostrand Reinhold, 1980. Copyright © E. Pfeiffer, 1974.

- Delusions
- Hallucinations
- Suicidal ideation/gestures
- Anxiety states
- Psychomotor and speech changes
- Personality and mood changes
- Impaired judgment
- Substance abuse
- Obsessive-compulsive behavior
- Irrational guilt
- Aggressive behavior
- Impairment in concentration and abstract thinking

Symptomatology provides important clues for identifying a mental disorder.

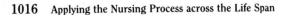

Box 36–3

PSYCHOLOGIC STRENGTHS ASSESSMENT

What are some things you like about yourself?

What are some of the upsetting (stressful, difficult) times you can remember?

What did you do to comfort yourself when your (husband/wife) died?

How did you make it through the death of your son?

What kinds of things do you do to cheer yourself up?

What things make you happy? Content?

What do you do to nurture yourself?

What do you do to relax? To have fun?

What things do you think you can do to get you through these rough times?

How have the passing years affected your sexuality?

Do you enjoy sex as much as you used to?

Are you happily married?

What are you most concerned about right now?

How can I (we) help you through this difficult time?

Social and Financial Status

The quality and quantity of social support (past and present) available to the elderly person must be assessed (Figure 36–4). Quantity does not guarantee quality. Social support has important implications for recovery from psychologic disturbances. The more social support available, the better equipped an elderly person will be to overcome a stressful life event (Chaisson-Stewart 1985). Maintenance of an abundant, meaningful social network suggests strong interpersonal skills that can be mobilized to help negotiate late life stresses and losses. Formation of a new social network, when others have dissolved, will be easier for an elderly person with the social skills and personal resources (e.g., assertiveness, friendliness, and warmth) to form new social bonds and friendships. Elderly people who have been unsuccessful or disinclined to develop strong ties and friendships may benefit from exploring the interpersonal factors that prevented them from reaching out to others in the past.

The elderly, who often survive on a low, fixed income, may be plagued by financial problems that affect their mental and physical health. Some communities have services that help the elderly manage finances and learn about financial aid and assistance programs. Removal of financial strain may dramatically improve the health of an elder pressured by inadequate funds and inexperience with financial management. Sample questions to gain information about the social and financial status of the client are listed in Box 36–4.

opportunity or they perceive negative social pressure and social norms regarding sexuality among persons their age. Broaching the subject of sexuality with an older person may be just the thing they need to give them permission to explore an untapped source of pleasure they may have long since forgotten. Approaching the topic in a tactful, caring, nonjudgmental manner is important. If the elderly client does not wish to discuss sexual issues, he or she most likely will make that clear, by stating it directly, not answering the question, or changing the subject. An older person who was socialized in a different, more conservative time, may not feel comfortable discussing his or her sexual life. However, bringing up the subject of sexuality may give an elderly client the opportunity to explore that part of themselves privately or with a significant other.

Symptomatology

Psychologic symptomatology should be recorded, as well as the client's perception of his or her status and priorities. Symptoms to look for include:

- Somatization
- Changes in eating behavior

Elder Abuse

It has been suggested that **elder abuse** is at least as serious, in terms of incidence, as child abuse (Hirst and Miller 1986). Elder abuse can take many forms, including active physical, emotional, or sexual maltreatment, as well as passive emotional neglect and omission on the part of the responsible person to provide for the normal physical and

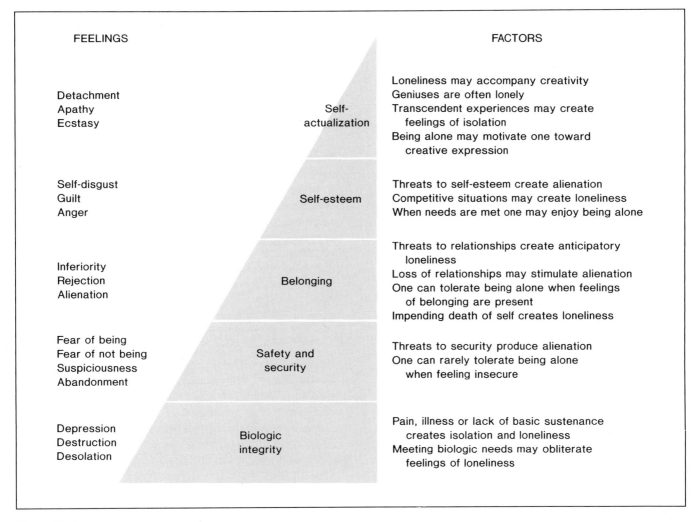

Figure 36–4
Loneliness and isolation.
Source: Adapted from Ebersole P, Hess P: Toward Healthy Aging:
Human Needs and Nursing Response. *Mosby, 1981.*

financial needs of the elder in their care. Hirst and Miller (1986) note that the elder at highest risk for abuse is often:

- Female
- Caucasian
- Physically and/or cognitively impaired
- Dependent
- Presenting behavior problems

The person at risk for abusing an elderly person is often:

- A family member (usually a daughter)
- Ill-equipped or reluctant to provide care

- Disorganized with marital problems
- An alcohol and/or drug abuser
- Lacking communication skills
- Lacking effective coping patterns
- Unrealistic in expectations of the older adult

The abused elderly may exhibit wariness of contact with adults, extreme withdrawal or aggressiveness in certain situations, infantile behavior, poor social interaction with peers, and ambivalent feelings toward family (Hirst and Miller 1986, p 30). Assessment of the elderly, particularly those seeking treatment in emergency rooms, must include observation for signs of abuse, including:

Box 36–4
SOCIAL AND FINANCIAL ASSESSMENT GUIDELINES

How many phone calls do you get in a week?

How frequently do you receive visitors?

How frequently do you go visiting?

Are you happily married?

How would you describe your relationship with your (family, daughter, husband, wife, etc.)?

Who do you know well enough to go visiting at their home (room, if in nursing home)?

Do you have someone you can trust and confide in?

Do you find yourself feeling lonely?

Do you have someone who can drive you to the doctor or the hospital if you need it?

How is your financial situation? Do you worry about money?

- Overmedication or deprivation of life-sustaining medications
- Falls and injuries, particularly bruises on face, arms, legs, and buttocks
- Malnutrition
- Extended periods of neglect or restraint evidenced by contracture pressure sores and long, curved fingernails and toenails
- Agitation when certain persons appear (family, friends, or caretakers)

The elderly rarely report abuse themselves out of fear of disbelief, reprisal, or institutionalization. The elderly often feel loyal to their abusers and may believe they deserve the maltreatment. Several tools have been developed to help with this essential portion of the assessment of the older adult (Ferguson and Beck 1983, Ross et al. 1985). Most states have mandatory reporting laws to protect the elderly from abuse. Nurses must be alert for signs of elder abuse and report any suspected cases in accordance with the legislation in their states. Through detection, education, clinical intervention, and research, nurses can reduce this serious threat to the health and quality of life of the elderly.

Psychiatric Nursing Diagnosis

Table 36–6 provides the most commonly seen psychiatric nursing diagnoses associated with the mental disorders discussed in the assessment section.

Nursing Interventions

There is a notable lack of studies comparing different nursing interventions used to treat mental disorders in later life. The few studies available concur that the elderly are more amenable to therapy than was previously believed. Several studies have demonstrated that a combination of psychotherapy and medication has been more efficacious in relieving depression in the elderly than either intervention alone. The studies available also support the use of reminiscence and life review, cognitive-behavioral approaches, group work, and somatic therapies. The choice of treatment is determined by the specific needs of the client and the nature of mental and physical disorders presented (Dye 1986).

Reminiscence and Life Review

Reminiscing normally occurs to some degree throughout the life span, but the activity acquires special significance for elderly individuals (Ebersole 1976, 1978). Robert Butler coined the term *reminiscence* and has noted that it is a universal activity in the elderly, reinforced by personal and environmental factors (e.g., personality, isolation, retirement, and relocation) and precipitated by the imminence of death (Butler 1963). Reminiscence provides a chance for working through issues from the past. Reminiscing is necessary for ego integrity, providing a means by which the elderly maintain a sense of identity and self-esteem. Life review, which is a part of the reminiscing process, may involve a more structured goal-oriented examination of the past.

Unfulfilled expectations, lifelong maladaptive patterns of interacting and coping, the unresolved death of a significant other, lack of accomplishment, "sins," ineffectiveness, rigidity, and failures are examples of issues that may need to be reckoned with as death approaches (Figure 36–5) (Butler 1963).

When an elder expresses despair over the past, comments like, "Oh, just don't think about it," or "Why don't you focus on the happy times," while said with good intentions, may abruptly halt the resolution process necessary for reintegration of a distressing past. Nurses are socialized to supply answers, provide comfort, and relieve suffering. Encouraging an elderly person to work through painful and distressing memories may seem antithetical to the nurse's ethics of care and nurturance. It may be necessary for an elderly client to experience psychic pain during the

Table 36–6
Comparison of Common DSM-IIIR Diagnoses and Psychiatric Nursing Diagnoses for Elderly Clients

DSM-IIIR	PND-I Diagnoses	NANDA Diagnoses
296.2x Major depression, single episode	04.02.05 Grief	Grieving, dysfunctional
	01.03 Altered self-care*	Self-care deficits: feeding, dressing/grooming
296.3x Major depression, recurrent	01.03.01 Altered eating	
	01.03.02 Altered grooming	
	01.03.03 Altered health maintenance	
	01.03.04 Altered hygiene	
	01.03.05 Altered participation in health care	
	06.03 Altered self-concept*	Self-concept: disturbance in self-esteem
	05.04 Altered sexuality processes	Sexual dysfunction
	05.05 Altered social interaction*	Social interaction, impaired
	05.05.02 Social isolation/withdrawal*	Social isolation
	08.01.01 Hopelessness*	Hopelessness
	04.02.02 Anxiety*	Anxiety
203.00 Delirium	04.02 Altered feeling patterns	Sensory/perceptual alterations
	04.02.06 Fear*	Fear
		Injury, potential for
	01.04 Altered sleep/arousal patterns	Sleep pattern disturbance
	01.04.04 Nightmares	
	02.07 Altered thought content	Thought processes, altered
	02.07.01 Delusions	
	02.06.02 Delirium	
	05.02 Altered conduct/impulse processes	
	05.02.01.02 Aggressive/violent behaviors toward others	Violence, potential for: self-directed or directed at others
	05.02.01.03 Aggressive/violent behaviors toward self	
	05.02.02 Dysfunctional behaviors	
	05.02.02.02 Bizarre behaviors	
	05.02.02.05 Unpredictable behaviors	
	07.05 Altered neurosensory processes	
	07.05.01 Altered levels of consciousness	

PND-I diagnosis also in NANDA list

continued

Table 36–6 (*Continued*)
Comparison of Common DSM-IIIR Diagnoses and Psychiatric Nursing Diagnoses for Elderly Clients

DSM-IIIR	PND-I Diagnoses	NANDA Diagnoses
290.00 Multiinfarct dementia	05.01.02 Altered verbal communication*	Communication, impaired: verbal
		Coping, ineffective family
		Home maintenance management, impaired
	08.01.01 Hopelessness*	Hopelessness
	08.01.04 Powerlessness*	Powerlessness
	07.02.01 Altered bowel elimination	
	07.02.01.03 Incontinence*	Incontinence, total
	07.02.02 Altered urinary elimination	
	07.02.02.03 Incontinence	Mobility, impaired physical
	05.03 Altered role performance*	Role performance, altered
	05.03.01 Altered family role	
	01.03 Altered self-care*	Self-care deficits: dressing/grooming
	05.05.02 Social isolation/ withdrawal*	Social isolation
		Sexual dysfunction
300.00 Generalized anxiety disorder	04.02.02 Anxiety*	Anxiety
		Coping, ineffective individual
	01.03 Altered self-care	
	01.03.01 Altered eating	Nutrition, altered: less than body requirements
	01.01 Altered motor behavior	
	01.01.04 Hyperactivity	
	01.04 Altered sleep/arousal patterns	Sleep pattern disturbance
	01.04.01 Difficult transition to and from sleep	
	01.98 Altered activity processes NOS	
	02.01 Altered decision making	
	02.02 Altered judgment	
	02.02 Altered physiologic processes NOS	
293.81 Organic delusional disorder		Health maintenance, altered
		Home management, impaired
		Noncompliance (with eating, taking medication)
		Nutrition, altered: less than body requirements
	02.07 Altered thought content	Thought processes, altered
	02.07.01 Delusions	
	02.07.02 Ideas of reference	
	04.02 Altered feeling patterns	

continued

Table 36–6 (*Continued*)
Comparison of Common DSM-IIIR Diagnoses and Psychiatric Nursing Diagnoses for Elderly Clients

DSM-IIIR	PND-I Diagnoses	NANDA Diagnoses
	04.02.01 Anger	
	04.02.01 Anxiety*	Anxiety
	06.03 Altered self-concept	
	06.03.03 Altered personal identity	
307.45 Sleep-wake schedule disorder	01.04 Altered sleep/arousal patterns	Sleep pattern disturbance
	01.04.01 Difficult transition to and from sleep	
	01.04.03 Insomnia	

PND-I diagnosis also in NANDA list.

PROBLEMS	SYMPTOMS	NEEDS	INTERVENTIONS
Social clocks Self-fulfilling prophesies Routinized life	Apathy Rigidity Boredom Ennui	**Self-actualization** Self-expression New situations Self-transcendence Stimulation	Creative pursuits Meditation Reflection Fantasy Teaching/learning Relaxation
Social devaluation Lack of role Meaninglessness Little autonomy	Delusions Paranoia Depression Anger Indecisiveness	**Self-esteem** Control Success To be needed	Reminiscing Control of money Activate latent interests Allowed to help others Identify legacy
Displacement Losses	Depression Hallucinations Alienation Loneliness	**Belonging** Territory Friends Family Group affiliation Philosophy Confidante	Significant objects Pets, plants Soap opera families Touch group participation Listening Fictive kin
Sensory losses Limited mobility Translocation	Illusions Hallucinations Confusion Compulsions Obsessions Fear/anxiety	**Safety and security** Safe environment Sensory accoutrements Mobility	Familiar routines Spaced stimulation Explanations Environmental cues
Homeostatic resilience Poor nutrition Medications Income Subclinical disease (Birren) Pain	Confusion Depression Fear Anxiety Disorientation	**Biologic integrity** Food Shelter Sex Rest Body integrity Comfort	Adequate resources Knowledge of medications Conservation of energy Napping Small, frequent meals Choice of food

Figure 36–5
The nursing process and Maslow's hierarchy of needs among the aged.
Source: Adapted from Ebersole P, Hess P: Toward Healthy Aging: Human Needs and Nursing Response. *Mosby, 1981.*

integration process (Ebersole 1978). Skilled, sensitive nursing interactions can facilitate the reintegration process for an elder by establishing a trusting, caring relationship in which active listening (even to repetitive material) and nonjudgmental validation prevail. The nurse's interactive role is to help the client establish his or her own answers while moving through the life review process (Love and Buckwalter, in press).

Reminiscing can and should be stimulated for elders, individually and in groups. Creative uses of food, music, pets, and special events can facilitate the process and make it fun. Materials such as photo albums, journals, and tape and video recorders provide a means for elders so inclined to establish a permanent record of their life review, creating a legacy for those who follow.

Social Support and Group Interventions

Loss of affiliation with significant groups (family, professional and work group, bridge club, etc.) and social support can lead to identity dissolution, isolation, loneliness, and despair in the elderly. Yalom (1975) identified "curative factors" in group psychotherapy, five of which are particularly beneficial to elderly persons. See Table 36–7.

Group therapy is considered by many to be the treatment of choice for the elderly. It is efficient, because eight to ten persons can benefit at one time. Long-term care facilities are ideally suited for group work because the members are easily accessible and transportation is not a problem.

Special Focuses of Group Work With Elders

A geriatric group may be designed for a variety of purposes. Severely depressed and cognitively impaired elders will benefit from remotivation, resocialization, and reality orientation. Table 36–8 provides a summary of the differences between groups with these different focuses. "Mixing affects" may be beneficial in stimulating withdrawn clients and calming anxious members. A cohort or specific age group focusing on reminiscing and life review may facilitate these processes for members reluctant to engage in reminiscing on a one-to-one basis. Movement, music, art, and role playing may bring forth creativity and expression of feelings (catharsis). The curative factors of "universality" and "instillation of hope" will be beneficial for members of a "grievers" or widows group, in which the members can share their loss experiences.

Group work, when applied with sensitivity, caring, planning, organization, skill, and self-investment, can be fun and rewarding. Anecdotal evidence and an increasing body of research supports the effectiveness of this inter-

---

Table 36–7
Curative Factors in Group Interventions With the Elderly

Socialization	Provides replacement of meaningful relationships and stimulation of social skills. Allows for celebration of holidays and social events, reality orientation and reminiscing among cohorts. Provides opportunities to resume former roles (e.g., chairman, secretary, president).
Group cohesiveness	Refers to the "stick togetherness" characterized by group membership. Provides a sense of belonging (e.g., an old-old cohort group may begin to view themselves as the "biological elite" within a facility). Reaffirms ability to be liked and make friends. Provides for expression of affection and physical contact, esteem, and validation.
Universality	Provides a sense of, "We're all in this together." Enables members to see themselves in others and to share experiences, successes, and losses.
Instillation of hope	Compliments universality. Enables members to see others have suffered and survived similar situations. Members can share adaptive strengths and coping skills.
Altruism	Very important. Members are provided opportunities to feel needed and help others. Reinforces self-esteem. Often the support and advice received from peers is integrated more readily than "professional advice."

Source: Love CC, Buckwalter KC: Reactive depression, in Nursing Diagnosis and Interventions for the Institutionalized Elderly. Addison-Wesley, in press.

---

vention with the elderly. Nurses are in key positions to explore this cost-effective, therapeutic intervention through ongoing research efforts.

Milieu Therapy

Behavioral principles and group process theory form the major theoretical foundation for constructing a therapeutic milieu. No other psychotherapeutic intervention has such strong implications for nursing in acute and long-term care facilities as the scientific structuring of the environment to promote health, foster individual strengths, and effect personal growth in clients and staff. Milieu therapy has preventive as well as therapeutic value and must be a major consideration in all settings providing services to elderly populations.

Table 36–8
Differences Between Remotivation, Resocialization, and Reality Orientation

Reality Orientation	Resocialization	Remotivation
1. Correct position or relation with the existing situation in a community. Maximum use of assets	1. Continuation of reality living situation in a community	1. Orientation to reality for community living; present oriented
2. Called reality orientation and classroom reality orientation program	2. Called discussion group or resocialization to differentiate between a social function and a therapeutic need	2. Called remotivation
3. Structured	3. Unstructured	3. Definite structure
4. Refreshments and/or food may be served for identification	4. Refreshments served	4. Refreshments not served
5. Appreciation of the work of the world. Constant reminders of who and where clients are, why they are present, and what is expected of them	5. Appreciation of the work of the world. Reliving happy experiences. Encourages participation in home activities relating to subject	5. Appreciation of the work of the group stimulates the desire to return to function in society
6. Class range from 3 to 5, depending on degree/level of confusion or disorientation from any cause	6. Group range from 5 to 17, depending on mental and physical capabilities	6. Group size: 5 to 12
7. Meeting ½ hour daily at same time in same place	7. Meetings three times weekly for ½ to 1 hour	7. Meeting once or twice weekly for 1 hour
8. Planned procedure: reality-centered objects	8. No planned topic; group-centered feelings	8. Preselected and reality-centered objects
9. Response of resident is responsibility of teacher	9. Clarification and interpretation is responsibility of leader	9. No exploration of feelings
10. Periodic reality orientation test pertaining to residents' level of confusion or disorientation	10. Periodic progress notes pertaining to residents' enjoyment and improvements	10. Progress ratings
11. Emphasis on time, place, person orientation	11. Any topic freely discussed	11. Topic: no discussion of religion, politics, or death
12. Use of portion of mind function still intact	12. Vast stockpile of memories and experiences	12. Untouched area of the mind
13. Resident greeted by name, thanked for coming, and extended handshake and/or physical contact according to attitude approach in group	13. Resident greeted on arrival, thanked, and extended a handshake on leaving	13. No physical contact permitted. Acceptance and acknowledgment of everyone's contribution
14. Conducted by trained aides and activity assistants	14. Conducted by RN, LPN/LVN, aides, and program assistants	14. Conducted by trained psychiatric aides

Source: Adapted by permission of The Gerontologist/The Journal of Gerontology, *from Barns E, Sack A, Shore H:* The Gerontologist 1973;13:513.

Table 36–9 Interventions Within a Therapeutic Milieu			
Structure	**Containment**	**Support**	**Validation**
Regular meal times	Physical aspects of the facility include the interior design, safety features, atmosphere, space, privacy, lighting location, temperature, noise, odors, colors, infection control, restraints, confinement, isolation, "homey" atmosphere of client rooms, roommates, access to public transportation, "knock before entering" policy	Nourishment	Reality orientation
Scheduled activities		Medication	Feedback and acceptance
Predictability and routine		Social support	Interaction and contact with the world
Consistency		Reassurance	
Bowl/bladder program		Visitors	Music, touch, warmth, and creative expression
Shift change		P.T. and O.T.	Sensory stimulation
Medication time		Spiritual expression	Focus on positive aspects of behavior
Vital signs		Consistent positive staff attitudes	
Regular MD visits			"Downplay" of negative
Bedtime		Handrails	Newspaper and TV
Primary nursing		Mutual goal setting	1 to 1 relationships
Care planning		Exercise	Client autonomy and decision making
Evaluation			Excursions outside

Source: Adapted by Patricia Schroeder, Menninger Clinic from Gunderson JG: Principles and Practice of Milieu Therapy. *Aronson Jason, Inc. 1983.*

A geriatric milieu must be dynamic and evolving to meet the needs of each unique elder within a diverse and changeable patient-staff community. Staff-related factors (e.g., nurse-patient ratio, interpersonal variables, attitudes and interactions, staffing patterns and composition, and level of skill) have a profound influence on the prevailing atmosphere and therefore must be included in the milieu assessment and structuring. Table 36–9 provides a useful framework for organizing the complex concept of milieu into a workable format with some examples illustrating how to categorize interventions in the environment. Once categorized, the "milieu committee" (composed of staff and residents if at all possible) can determine which interventions should be manipulated or altered to promote health, foster growth, and prevent deterioration. The concepts of structure, containment, support, and validation may also be applied to home-based elders to ensure that their environment contains essential health promotion and preventive features.

Cognitive-Behavioral Therapy

Vague, abstract, and "mysterious" approaches to therapy are not tolerated well by elderly persons. The elderly seek a therapeutic relationship that provides some reciprocity.

Nurses caring for the elderly must invest themselves through active involvement and judicious self-disclosure to foster trust and a warm, caring relationship.

A combination of cognitive and behavioral approaches has been found to work best with the elderly. These approaches are "practical" and very specific, providing concrete goals (i.e., behavior change or correcting negative thought patterns) and ongoing evaluation of progress through self-monitoring of goal accomplishment.

Cognitive-behavioral therapy is based on the notion that the way we think about something influences the way we behave and feel. Negative patterns of thinking tend to be automatic and pervasive, coloring individuals' perceptions of the world around them and affecting their mood and self-esteem. Cognitive-behavioral therapy, used often and successfully with depressed older people, suggests that the depressed elder's unrealistic negative thought processes are central to his or her becoming and staying depressed (Belsky 1984). Box 36–5 lists common cognitive distortions and provides examples of alternatives the nurse might present to challenge the distorted thought processes of elderly clients.

Because cognitive-behavioral therapy focuses on symptoms and thought processes (rather than a hypothetical unconscious cause) and fosters a sense of self-responsibility and self-control, the elderly are often receptive and

Box 36–5

COGNITIVE DISTORTIONS

Over-generalization: Thinking in absolute terms, exaggerating or drawing broad conclusions from limited evidence or a single incident. Statements beginning with "I'll never . . . , He always . . . , No one wants . . ." are probably irrational generalizations.

Situation: A new widow bounced a check.
Distortion: "I'll never make it on my own."
Alternative thought: "I'm taking new risks and learning new things."

Polarizing: Insisting on extremes (other people and things are either good or bad, helpful or harmful, safe or dangerous) without any middle ground.

Situation: A physician made a diagnostic error.
Distortion: "All physicians are incompetent and should not be trusted."
Alternative thought: "Everyone makes mistakes occasionally."

Using shoulds: Following a list of inflexible rules about how people should act. Any deviation from the rule is perceived as bad.

Situation: A wife is depressed about placing her husband in a nursing home.
Distortion: "All wives should care for their aging husbands."
Alternative thought: "I haven't failed since he's getting the best care. Now I can help by visiting."

Mind reading: Making snap judgments based on hunches, feelings, and perhaps a few experiences.

Situation: An elderly woman walks by a group of teens who are laughing.
Distortion: "They were all laughing at me because I am old."
Alternative thought: "I have no proof that they were laughing at me. They could be laughing at any number of things."

Expecting fairness: Thinking that each person's actions deserve a specific reaction from others.

Situation: An elderly woman is no longer able to care for herself.

Distortion: "I took care of my children, now they should take care of me."
Alternative thought: "Everyone has the right to make choices in life. I made my choices and my children have the right to make theirs."

Catastrophizing: Thinking the worst in any situation.

Situation: An elderly man lost his house keys for the first time.
Distortion: "I must be getting senile."
Alternative thought: "I've misplaced things on occasion all my life, and my mind is still as sharp as ever."

Externalizing: Blaming external events and persons for problems, thereby shifting the responsibility to other persons and things.

Situation: An elderly man spends long hours in front of the television.
Distortion: His wife blames her loneliness on her husband's inattention.
Alternative thought: "I am responsible for my own feelings, my husband does not control me. I made the decision to stay home, likewise, I can choose to go out and find alternatives to staying home and watching television."

Internalizing: Blaming oneself for all problems, illustrated by the comment, "I am responsible for everyone's happiness, well-being, safety, etc."

Situation: An elderly diabetic woman refuses to adhere to her diabetic diet, resulting in repeated hospitalizations.
Distortion: Husband expresses irrational guilt, "If I would only eat the foods my wife is supposed to eat, she wouldn't have this problem."
Alternative thought: "I cannot control my wife's behavior. I can support her, but it is ultimately her responsibility to remain on her diet."

Source: Adapted from McKay M, Davis M, Fanning P: Are you listening to yourself? Increase your self awareness for more control over your life. Nursing Life, January/February, 1983. Intermed Communications, Inc.

willing to try it. Furthermore, in cognitive-behavioral therapy, the elderly are not required to reveal their private thoughts to the clinician. Instead they focus on their problems and symptoms and receive advice from the clinician on how to make improvements. The advice gives the elderly a sense that they are getting something for their personal and financial investment. The self-monitoring of progress (often with a journal and/or homework assignments) provides inspiration for the elderly to proceed. For further information on cognitive-behavioral therapy see Yost et al. (1986).

Somatic Therapies

Medications

Used judiciously, medication can be an effective *adjunct* to psychotherapy for mental disorders in later life. The high

Text continues on p. 1030

CASE STUDY: A Client With Major Depression, Single Episode

Identifying Information

Mr. Rozello is an 85-year-old Italian immigrant who is currently residing on the health-related floor in a long-term care facility. He is married to Mrs. Rozello, age 80, who resides in the same facility on the skilled nursing floor. They are both devout Catholics.

    The long-term care facility contacted a geropsychiatric nurse clinician to come to the facility to assess Mr. Rozello, who had become increasingly unmanageable.

History of Present Problem

The Rozellos lived independently up until about a year ago, when Mrs. Rozello suffered a massive stroke, leaving her comatose. She is described as having been a doting wife and a meticulous housekeeper. Despite living in this country since they were both 18, she spoke little English, relying on her husband for all interactions outside the immediate household. Since his admission Mr. Rozello has refused to visit his wife and has demonstrated a variety of behavior changes, becoming progressively agitated and unmanageable. He has lost 15 pounds since admission. Mr. Rozello's attending physician ordered Valium 5 mg p.o. t.i.d. to control his anxious and combative tendency and Restoril p.r.n. for sleep. The medication seemed to decrease his agitation, although he became more withdrawn during the day, refusing to participate in any activities. His disturbed sleep pattern remains unchanged; he wakes between 2 and 4 A.M. every morning and anxiously paces the hall, talking to himself.

Psychiatric History

Negative

Family History

Mr. Rozello's parents were both laborers in Italy. He has lost contact with his only sibling, an older brother who resided in Italy. No other family information was available.

Social History

Mr. Rozello immigrated to America with his wife when he was 18. Mr. Rozello completed the equivalent of eighth grade in Italy before immigrating to the United States. He was employed as a mason for forty-seven years. He was affiliated with a fraternal organization for twenty-five years. Mr. Rozello was active in several church-related activities up until several years before his admission to the facility. Mr. Rozello is visited weekly by the parish priest, and several parishioners visit him occasionally. He has no surviving relatives and no close friends. Mr. Rozello smoked cigars occasionally and drank one or two glasses of wine daily with dinner prior to admission. He has had no tobacco and no alcohol since admission.

    Mr. Rozello enjoyed gardening, tending his own grapevines and making wine annually, until his admission. He also mentioned that he enjoyed caring for the family dog, who died shortly before his wife became ill.

Significant Health History

Medical records revealed Mr. Rozello had been essentially healthy during his adult years. Family health history was not available. He was on no medication at home. He has no allergies. His appetite has been poor since admission, and he had lost

Adapted from Love CC, Buckwalter KC: Reactive depression, in Mass MM, Buckwalter KC: Nursing Diagnosis and Interventions for the Institutionalized Elderly. Addison-Wesley, in press.

continued

Case Study (Continued)

15 pounds in the past eight months. He was treated for frequent fecal impactions for which he received Colace b.i.d. He had no physical limitations and had been physically active, gardening and taking daily walks with the family dog, prior to admission.

Current Affective and Mental Status	Mr. Rozello appeared gaunt, disheveled, and tired, with uncombed hair and several days worth of stubble on his face. He emitted a pervasive feeling of despair with an undercurrent of anger and despondency. His mood was severely depressed. Mr. Rozello was oriented in all spheres, with judgment and remote and recent memory intact. He scored 1 on the SPMSQ, which indicates intact intellectual functioning. His thoughts flowed logically, although he was easily distracted with some loosening of associations. Reality testing was intact, with no delusional thought content, nor signs of psychosis. He did not demonstrate any perceptual difficulty. His gait was obviously steady though slow. He spoke hesitantly of the many losses he had encountered in his life both long past and recently.

He noted that he and his wife had been sexually active occasionally until her illness. Currently he admits to decreased energy and libido.

When asked what things he did to get through difficult times in the past he looked puzzled and then explained he never considered his needs, since his wife's were more important. He indicated that his wife grieved quite openly and demonstratively, and he often felt the need to console her rather than himself. He noted their marriage was a good one and he loved his wife. When the subject of his wife's condition was mentioned, it became apparent that he felt irrationally guilty, blaming himself for not having insisted she see a physician when she had complained of dizziness. He abruptly blocked any further conversation about his wife's condition. Well into the assessment interview the following conversation between the nurse and Mr. Rozello took place:

Nurse: Mr. Rozello, do you ever think about killing yourself?	Assessment of suicidal ideation
Client: (Withdrawing, angrily) You think I'm crazy don't you?	Fear of stigmatization
Nurse: (Touching his arm, emphasizing her response with direct eye contact) Mr. Rozello, You are *not* crazy. Everything you have said makes perfect sense to me. You are thinking very clearly and logically. (Pause) The staff and I are concerned about you because you seem blue and down in the dumps most of the time. You aren't eating or sleeping well. You've lost weight, and these things suggest to me that you are feeling depressed. I can understand fully why you are feeling blue. It seems very *normal* to me that you feel sad. (Pause) I would like to help you to feel better and maybe even be happy again. (Pause, nurse takes his hand) Sometimes when people have suffered great losses in their life, they are able to feel better if they can share their feelings with another person. You have	Validation, support, emphasis on strengths

Provides concrete evidence of disorder

Validation

Expression of caring

Touch, contact, instillation of hope
Validation
Education |

continued

Case Study (Continued)

been holding your sadness inside for a long time, and now it's affecting your health. (Pause) I would like to help you. You don't have to suffer alone. I think together we can work this out. Would you be willing to share your feelings with me? (Long silence) Only you can tell us how you feel.

Empathy

Reassurance

Seeking client input, reinforcing client's control

Client: (Withdraws his hand and wipes away a tear) If I could sleep better I'd feel better.

Shifting focus from feelings to somatic symptoms

Nurse: That's probably very true. Maybe a goal we could work on would be to help you sleep longer at night. (Pause) Do you think if you shared your upsetting feelings with me during the day you might feel more restful at night? (Long silence, no answer)

Validation, mutual goal setting
Redirecting

Reluctance, use of silence

Nurse: I imagine it feels uncomfortable for you to think about sharing your sadness with me. You don't know me very well. (Pause) Maybe we could start by talking about some of the good times you've had in your life? Would that feel more comfortable to you?

Validation, empathy, establishing trust by refocusing temporarily on less painful issues, being direct, using feeling words

Client: (Pause) Will you come every day?

Client's seeking clarification suggests acceptance

After much encouragement Mr. Rozello agreed to see the nurse regularly. She continued the interaction and determined he was not suicidal.

Client Strengths/Signs of Growth

In excellent physical condition, chronic illness absent, completely mobile, agile, and fully ambulatory; nonsuicidal; resides on the Health-Related Unit, among many other highly functional peers; financially secure (SSI, private health insurance, and pension); has been assisting his roommate to the dining room recently; bilingual, had enjoyed translating magazines and newspapers to his wife; knowledgeable about gardening; possesses adaptive strengths, has endured significant losses in his life; had a solid marriage, good relationships with his neighbors in the community, and belonged to a fraternal organization much of his life indicating the ability to maintain meaningful relationships; has strong religious beliefs; is physically attractive; has a rich life history, having immigrated from Italy; used to make his own wine; agreed to meet with the geropsychiatric clinician.

Diagnostic Impressions

Nursing Diagnosis (PND-I/NANDA)

04.02.06   Grief*
/Grieving, dysfunctional

07.06.02.02 Altered nutrition: less than body requirements*
/Nutrition, altered: less than body requirements

*PND-I diagnosis also in NANDA list.

continued

Case Study (Continued)

04.02.02	Anxiety*/Anxiety	
05.05.02	Social isolation/withdrawal*/Social isolation	

DSM-IIIR Multiaxial Diagnosis

Axis I: 296.34 Major depression, first episode
Axis II: V71.09 No diagnosis on Axis II
Axis III: None
Axis IV: Psychosocial stressors: 5, Extreme (death of wife, loss of independence)
Axis V: Current GAF: 35
          Highest GAF in the past year: 60

Nursing Care Plan

Nursing Diagnosis (PND-I/NANDA)	Client Care Goals	Nursing Planning/ Interventions	Evaluation
04.02.06 Grief*/Grieving, dysfunctional	Client will begin expressing feelings. Client will explore guilt associated with wife's illness with staff. Client will visit his wife. Client will attend "griever's group."	Offer "feelings list" daily to help in feeling expression and identification. Arrange for client to meet with geropsychiatric nurse twice a week. Assist in recognition of grieving behavior during 1 to 1 interactions. Encourage "griever's group" membership. Staff will meet with client's parish priest to establish consistent approach and spiritual component.	Client will engage in normal grief work: work through grief process, recognize reality of loss. Client will visit wife, assist in her basic care, read to her. Client will express feelings in preparation for wife's impending death.
07.06.02.02 Altered nutrition: less than body requirements*/Nutrition, altered: less than body requirements	Client will begin eating small amounts. Client will gain 2 lb/week. Client will have regular BM.	Offer small frequent feedings. Meet with dietitian twice a week for menu planning. Provide liquid supplement as tolerated. Offer small frequent feedings. Give wine before dinner. Encourage fiber and physical activity.	Client will regain 15 lbs. Client will be free from impactions.
04.02.02 Anxiety*/Anxiety	Client will reduce pacing and combative behavior.	All staff will provide active listening.	Client will accurately appraise stress level.

*PND-I diagnosis also in NANDA list.

continued

Case Study (Continued)

Nursing Diagnosis (PND-I/NANDA)	Client Care Goals	Nursing Planning/ Interventions	Evaluation
	Client will sleep past 5 A.M.	Encourage diversional activities through mutually developed plan with OT.	Client will establish adequate coping resources.
		Provide calm milieu; firm, calm staff.	
		Reduce guilt through cognitive restructuring in 1 to 1 sessions.	
05.05.02 Social isolation withdrawal* /Social isolation	Client will explore ways needs can be met through interpersonal contact.	Respect client's need for time alone.	Client will demonstrate precrisis communication skills.
		Recognize efforts to participate with positive feedback.	Client will express one positive statement about self per day.
		Use touch appropriately.	
		Encourage budding interaction with roommate.	Client will express satisfaction with interactions.

*PND-I diagnosis also in NANDA list.

incidence of adverse drug reactions in the elderly under-scores the need for careful monitoring and conservative dosages.

The elderly almost always require only a third to half as much medication as other age groups. Dosages of medication should be divided over the course of the day. The action of drugs in elderly clients is affected by the following factors:

- Biochemical and biologic changes
- Stress
- Nutritional status
- Drug and alcohol use
- Genetics
- Changes in metabolism, absorption, distribution, and excretion

The elderly are more susceptible to the side-effects of psychotropic medications, such as:

- Constipation
- Extrapyramidal symptoms (dystonias, akasthesia, peri-oral tremor, pseudo-Parkinsonism)
- Anticholinergic effects (urinary retention, blurred vision, dry mouth, sexual dysfunction, anticholinergic psychosis)
- Cardiovascular effects (postural hypotension, arrhythmias)
- Drug interactions (delirium, confusion, disorientation)

Yanchick (1986) suggests that a realistic therapeutic goal be established before starting pharmacotherapy, noting that few medications will be successful at relieving *all* symptoms. Usually the desired effects have to be weighed against bothersome side-effects in determining the course of treatment.

It is generally recommended that the elderly client be started on dosages 30 to 50 percent of the recommended starting dosage for younger clients of similar size. The medication should be titrated until the desired therapeutic effect is established.

Ideally psychotropic drug therapy should be supervised by a geropsychiatrist. General medical practitioners unfamiliar with psychopharmacokinetics in the elderly often unknowingly overmedicate older clients. Medication should never take the place of psychotherapeutic modalities. Psychotherapy should always be continued along with medications. For more information on psychopharmacologic interventions, see Dye (1986), Carnevali and Patrick (1986), and Chapter 32 of this text.

Electroconvulsant Therapy

The two- to three-week lag time between onset of antidepressant drug therapy and symptom relief is significant for severely depressed elders whose health is in danger. When suicide or starvation is a real threat, or when antidepressants are ineffective or contraindicated, electroconvulsant therapy (ECT) should be considered. The main criteria for selecting ECT as the treatment of choice in the elderly are severity of depression and need for immediate results (Zung 1980).

ECT is rapidly effective and safe with judicious screening and advances in the use of muscle relaxants and anesthesia. The unilateral method has been shown to decrease the confusion and recent memory loss associated with ECT. Essentially, ECT may serve as a lifesaving measure in the elderly. Ignorance and negative emotions associated with early, less sophisticated use of ECT should not enter into decisions regarding the appropriateness of this intervention with the severely depressed elderly.

Evaluation

The evaluation of nursing interventions is an essential step in the nursing process. Evaluations are based on the quantifiable goals and desired outcomes outlined in the nursing care plan, and may include objective and subjective data. Whenever possible the client should be involved in the evaluation process. Many tools used for client assessment (e.g., SPMSQ) can also be used for evaluation to document changes in client status.

Chapter Highlights

- The aging population is increasing at a faster rate than the general population.
- Most elderly people remain relatively healthy, active, and vital well into later life.
- The elderly are the most underserved population in need of mental health services due to agist biases, stigmatization, myths regarding normal aging, and inaccessibility of care.
- Mental health in later life is linked closely to intrapersonal, environmental, and interpersonal interactive processes.
- Depression is the most prevalent, most treatable mental disorder in later life.
- Somatization, or excessive preoccupation with bodily functions, may be a sign of depression in an older adult.

- The suicide rate for elderly persons is nearly three times the rate of the general population.
- Electroconvulsant therapy may be a lifesaving intervention for severely depressed, suicidal older adults.
- Comprehensive, accurate, ongoing assessment is essential for differentiating treatable mental disorders from irreversible states.
- The elderly metabolize and excrete medication less efficiently, and are at risk for drug toxicity, which can mimic different mental disorders.
- Medication is not a substitute for psychotherapy. Medication should be prescribed primarily to enhance the effectiveness of psychotherapeutic interventions by reducing disabling symptomatology.
- When the elderly are given psychotropic medication, they require only one-half to one-third the amount prescribed for younger adults of comparable weight, in doses divided over the course of the day.
- Family members caring for a dependent older adult need much emotional support and psychoeducative interventions.
- The elderly respond best to therapy that is goal oriented and practical and has built-in short-term goals that enable them to monitor their accomplishments and progress over time.
- For the older adult, social support and group affiliation is an important means for maintaining orientation, self-esteem, and a sense of identity and belonging.
- Reminiscing can be a significant therapeutic tool for enhancing self-esteem and maintaining a sense of identity in the older adult.

References

American Psychiatric Association: *Diagnostic and Statistical Manual of Mental Disorders,* ed 3, revised. APA, 1987.

Belsky JK: *The Psychology of Aging: Theory, Research and Practice.* Brooks/Cole, 1984.

Blazer DG: The epidemiology of mental illness in late life, in Busse EW, Blazer DG (eds): *Handbook of Geriatric Psychiatry.* Van Nostrand Reinhold, 1980.

Blazer DG, Pennybacker MR: Epidemiology of alcoholism in the elderly, in Hartford JT, Samorajski T (eds): *Alcoholism in the Elderly.* Raven Press, 1984.

Braudis EM: Later adulthood, in Edelman C, Mandle CL (eds): *Health Promotion Throughout the Life Span.* Mosby, 1986.

Busse EW, Blazer DG: Disorders related to biological functioning, in Busse EW, Blazer DG (eds): *Handbook of Geriatric Psychiatry.* Van Nostrand Reinhold, 1980.

Butler RN: The life review: An interpretation of reminiscence in the aged. *Psychiatry* 1963;26:65–76.

Butler RN: Meeting the challenges of health care for the elderly. *J Gerontol Nurs* 1980;8(February):87–96.

Carnevali D, Patrick M: *Nursing Management for the Elderly,* ed 2. Lippincott, 1986.

Chaisson-Stewart MG: *Depression in the Elderly: An Interdisciplinary Approach.* Wiley, 1985.

Cole M, Dastoor D: A new hierarchic approach to the measurement of dementia. *PSO* 1987;28(6):298–304.

Colling J: Sleep disturbances in aging: A theoretic and empiric analysis. *Adv Nurs Science,* October 1983, pp 36–44.

Dye CA: *Assessment and Intervention in Geropsychiatric Nursing.* Grune and Stratton, 1986.

Ebersole PE: The therapeutic value of reminiscing with the aged. *Am J Nurs* 1976;76(August):601–602.

Ebersole PE: Establishing reminiscing groups, in Burnside IM (ed): *Working With the Elderly: Group Process and Techniques.* Duxbury, 1978.

Ebersole PE: Gerontological nurse practitioners: Past, present and future. *Geriatr Nurs* 1985;6:219–221.

Ebersole PE, Hess PA: *Toward Healthy Aging: Human Needs and Nursing Response,* ed 2. Mosby, 1985.

Erickson E: *Childhood and Society,* ed 2. W.W. Norton, 1963.

Ferguson D, Beck D: H.A.L.F.: A tool to assess elder abuse within the family. *Gerontol Nurs* 1983;4(5):301–304.

Glassock JA: Older alcoholics: An underserved population. *Generations* 1982;192(Spring):23–24, 64.

Gunderson JG: *Principles and Practice of Milieu Therapy 1983.* Aronson, 1983.

Hirst SP, Miller J: The abused elderly. *J Psychosocial Nurs* 1986;24(October):28–34.

Institute of Medicine: *Nursing and Nursing Education: Public Policies and Private Actions.* National Academy Press, 1983.

Love CC, Buckwalter KC: Reactive depression, in Mass M, Buckwalter KC (eds): *Nursing Diagnosis and Interventions for the Institutionalized Elderly.* Addison-Wesley, in press.

Mace NL, Rabins PV: *The 36 Hour Day.* Johns Hopkins University Press, 1981.

McKay M, Davis M, Fanning P: Are you listening to yourself? Increase your self awareness for more control over your life. *Nurs Life,* Jan/Feb 1983, pp 57–63.

Miller F et al.: Formed visual hallucinations in an elderly patient. *Hosp Community Psychiatry* 1987;38(5):527–529.

Miles LE, Dement WC: Sleep and aging. *Sleep* 1980;3:119–220.

Mortimer JA, Schuman LM, French LR: Epidemiology of dementing illness, in Mortimer JA, Schuman LM (eds): *The Epidemiology of Dementia.* Oxford University Press, 1981.

Osgood NJ: *Suicide in the Elderly.* Aspen Publications, 1985.

Pavkov J: Suicide in the elderly. *Ohio's Health* 1982;34(1):21–28.

Pfeiffer E: A Short Portable Mental Status Questionnaire for the assessment of organic brain deficit in elderly patients. *J Am Geriatr Soc* 1975;23:443–441.

Pfeiffer E: The psychosocial evaluation of the elderly patient, in Busse EW, Blazer D (eds): *Handbook of Geriatric Psychiatry.* Van Nostrand Reinhold, 1980.

Poggi RG, Berland DI: The therapist's reactions to the elderly. *The Gerontologist* 1985;25(5):508–513.

Powell LS, Courtice K: *Alzheimer's Disease: A Guide for Families.* Addison-Wesley, 1983.

Roca R: Bedside cognitive examination: Usefulness in detecting delirium and dementia. *PSO* 1987;28(2):71–76.

Ross M, Ross P, Ross-Carson M: Abuse of the elderly. *Can Nurs* 1985;81(2):36–39.

Stenback A: Depression and suicidal behavior in old age, in Birren JE, Sloane RB (eds): *Handbook of Mental Health and Aging.* Prentice-Hall, 1980.

Tyler KT, Tyler HR: Differentiating organic dementia. *Geriatrics* 1984;39(3):38–50.

Verwoerdt A: Anxiety, dissociative and personality disorders in the elderly, in Busse EW, Blazer DG (eds): *Handbook of Geriatric Psychiatry.* Van Nostrand Reinhold, 1980.

Wilson HS, Kneisl CR: *Handbook of Psychosocial Nursing Care.* Addison-Wesley, 1984.

Winger J et al.: Aggressive behavior in long-term care. 1987;25:4:28–33.

Woodruff DS: Arousal, sleep and aging, in Birren JE, Schaie KW (eds): *Handbook of the Psychology of Aging.* Van Nostrand Reinhold, 1985.

Wynne J, Block AJ, Hunt LA: Disordered breathing and oxygen desaturation during day time naps. *Johns Hopkins Med J* 1978;143:3–7.

Yalom ID: *The Theory and Practice of Group Psychotherapy,* ed 2. Basic Books, 1975.

Yanchick VA: Drug therapy, in Dye CA (ed): *Assessment and Intervention in Geropsychiatric Nursing.* Grune and Stratton, 1986.

Yost EB, Beutler LE, Corbishley MA, Allender JR: *Group Cognitive Therapy: A Treatment Approach for Depressed Older Adults.* Pergamon Press, 1986.

Zarit SH, Orr NK, Zarit JM: *The Hidden Victims of Alzheimer's Disease.* New York University Press, 1985.

Zung WWK: Affective disorders, in Busse EW, Blazer DG (eds): *Handbook of Geriatric Psychiatry.* Van Nostrand Reinhold, 1980.

THIRTY-SEVEN

Applying the Nursing Process with Dying Clients and Their Families

Hannah Dean

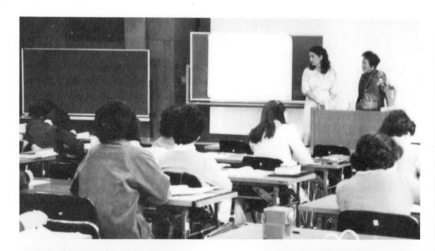

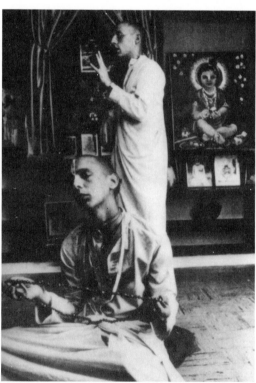

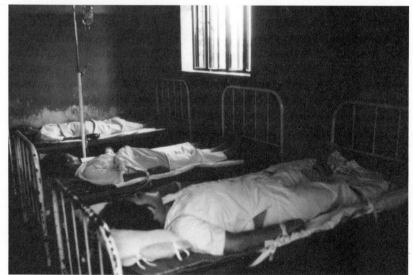

Learning Objectives

After reading this chapter, students should be able to

- Describe how a humanistic interactionist nursing philosophy influences the care of the dying

- Identify factors that have an impact on the effect of a loss for clients and families

- List four phases of dying and the expected features characteristic of each

- Enumerate the tasks of dying and the role of the nurse in helping clients achieve them

- Raise ethical questions about the care of the dying client

- Identify the barriers to effective communication with dying clients

- Apply the nursing process in providing humanistic interactionist care to dying clients

- Assess the psychosocial needs of the dying client

- Describe the nursing diagnoses the nurse will expect to see manifested in dying clients

- List factors that necessarily influence planning the care of dying clients

- Identify nursing interventions most frequently described by families as helpful in the care of clients dying at home

Cross References

Other topics relevant to this content are: Communication skills, Chapter 11; Dying clients in general hospital settings, Chapter 24; Ethics, Chapter 10; Human growth and development, Chapter 6.

Only by facing that nuclear war is a possibility can we avert it.

Key Terms

appropriate death
death anxiety
decline and deterioration
existential plight

mitigation and
  accommodation
preterminality and
  terminality

The issues inherent in loss, dying, and death afford the nurse an opportunity to practice psychiatric nursing according to the conceptual framework presented in this text. The theoretical bases, the practice processes, and the intervention modes of the entire book, in addition to those in this chapter, provide nurses with knowledge and skills appropriate for application to the human responses encountered with dying clients and their families.

This chapter concludes the section on applications across the life span. The perspective presented for working with dying clients and their families should be considered in the context of the entire text. Principles from the chapters in Part III and from the other chapters in Part V apply to dying clients and their families. In addition to impending death, dying clients and their families are subject to stressors such as those addressed in other parts of this book. Effective nurses attend to the range of distress, disorder, and developmental issues applicable to clients and their families. Nurses should assess clients thoroughly to determine the factors affecting the clients' responses to actual or impending losses.

THEORETICAL BASES

Humanistic Perspective

The humanistic interactionist philosophy of this text provides all nurses, including generalists and specialists, basic premises on which to operate. Nurses who approach clients with caring and compassion, affirming the joys, beauties, and values of human life, express a commitment to the interests of clients whatever their status. Dying clients and their families require such qualities in their professional caregivers.

In Chapter 1 the basic philosophical premises of the interactionist model are identified:

- Human beings act toward things on the basis of the meaning that things have for them.

- The meaning of things in life is derived from the social interactions a person has with others.

- People handle and modify the meanings of the things they encounter through an interpretive process.

These basic philosophic premises imply that nurses need to develop skill in determining the meaning of client behavior through observing, interpreting, and validating with clients to arrive at negotiated meanings. Accurate interpretations of client behaviors require examination of the social context in which they occur. Meanings can be modified by interactions between nurses and clients. These implications applied assiduously to the care of dying clients and their families place nurses in a position to improve the quality of life. In the effort to find a common ground of negotiated meanings, nurses must know themselves well, must examine their feelings about death, and must be open to exploring the meaning of dying and death to dying clients and their families.

Fear of Death and Death Anxiety

Lepp (1968) distinguishes between fear of death and **death anxiety**. Fear of death is essential to life in that it protects us from premature death. Death anxiety, on the other hand, serves death to the extent that it paralyzes us from action, deprives us of the desire to live. Diagnosis of a terminal illness may carry a set of meanings for clients and families that may or may not accurately predict their actual experiences. Terminally ill clients may express the desire to die rather than suffer pain or perceived indignity. Dying clients express concern about the dying process, abandonment, and pain above all other anxieties. Nurses can attend to these anxieties by providing excellent physical care and helping clients and families achieve a realistic view of and plan for the future.

Loss

Loss is the central theme in dying. Marris (1975) describes loss in terms of its effects on meaning, a perspective appropriate to the premises of a humanistic interactionist philosophy and the implications for psychiatric nursing practice. Marris states, "loss disrupts our ability to find meaning in experience, and grief represents the struggle to retrieve this sense of meaning when circumstances have bewildered or betrayed it."

The impact of loss on clients and families depends on the meaning of relationships, the timing of the loss in relationship to other stressors, the social context in which the loss occurs, and the perceptions of the persons involved.

The nurse must explore each of these aspects with clients and families in order to provide acceptable and effective care. The careful reader will notice the compatibility of the humanistic interactionist premises with the factors that affect the impact of a loss.

Rando (1984) identifies two kinds of loss: physical and symbolic. Both types of loss result in grief. Physical or tangible loss refers to the loss of the being or object; symbolic or psychosocial loss includes loss of role or status. The death of a loved one involves both types of loss, thus compounding the grief experienced.

Dying persons face the loss of themselves, loved ones, possessions, roles, and status. The dying person experiences anticipatory grief, which is influenced by the meaning of the various losses, the interaction the dying person has with others in the environment, and the dying person's interpretation of the meaning of the death.

The recognition of loss as the central theme in dying enhances our ability to identify with clients. Most of us have experienced both physical and symbolic losses through divorce, moving (or our friends' moving), changing jobs, or finishing phases of schooling. Graduation involves loss of student status, friends, a familiar environment, and teachers. Moving may mean loss of treasured possessions, friends, and a job. For each loss, we experience anticipatory grief, the loss (dying) process, and grief. The intensity of the experience varies from person to person and from loss to loss depending on the meaning of the lost object, relationship, or role; past experiences with loss; the social context in which the loss occurs; and our interpretation of the meaning of our loss.

Phases of Dying

Weisman (1980) identifies four psychologic phases of dying more or less tied to the physical process:

- Existential plight
- Mitigation and accommodation
- Decline and deterioration
- Preterminality and terminality

The first phase, **existential plight**, encompasses the numbness and shock experienced at the realization that one's life is coming to a foreseeable end. Although we have a concept of death, the reality of our own death is difficult to imagine. Few of us live our lives with the thought that they will end soon. We exist and conduct ourselves as if we have unending time in which to accomplish our dreams and work. The realization that we are personally and imminently vulnerable to death constitutes Weisman's first phase.

Mitigation and accommodation represent clients' and families' attempts to maintain function, balance, and control in the face of the reality of foreshortened life expectancy. This second phase may include efforts to achieve a remission or a cure. Some clients will make attempts to resume or continue normal activities such as work roles. Denial may be evident and may be adaptive or maladaptive depending on its effect on clients' abilities to achieve appropriate death. *Appropriate death* is defined in the next subsection.

As clients' conditions worsen, the third phase, **decline and deterioration**, becomes evident. Clients and families become increasingly aware of the symptoms and the progression of the disease. Although the struggle to maintain function, balance, and control continues, the effort becomes more difficult, roles begin to alter, activities are influenced by physical limitations, and positive attitudes become more and more difficult to maintain.

The final phase, **preterminality and terminality**, occurs when the imminence of death is apparent. Dying persons continue to need care; in this phase, however, they begin to withdraw, to focus their energies inward, to detach.

Kübler-Ross (1969) identified five stages of dying in her popular work *On Death and Dying*:

- Denial
- Anger
- Bargaining
- Depression
- Acceptance

Although she admonishes the reader against applying her framework to all dying persons in a stepwise fashion, many clinicians expect clients to pass through each stage from denial to anger, bargaining, depression and, finally, acceptance. Such an approach oversimplifies and overgeneralizes the process and misleads caregivers who are surprised by the reappearance of denial at later phases or by continuous expressions of anger throughout the dying process.

Weisman's phases provide a clearer, less equivocal framework than Kübler-Ross's stages. An additional aspect of Weisman's work that facilitates understanding of the process is the recognition that dying persons alternate between denial and acceptance; that denial is necessary and adaptive at times; and that the dying person will choose to whom to express denial or acceptance. One family member may hear only expressions of denial; another may hear only expressions of acceptance; and others may hear expressions of both depending on the dying person's mood or the circumstances of the interaction.

Appropriate Death

In his classic work, *On Dying and Denying,* Weisman (1972) proposes the concept of **appropriate death**. This concept offers guidance to caregivers as a goal toward which to strive in caring for dying persons. Weisman distinguishes appropriate death as a way:

- Of living to the end of life
- Of maintaining function at as high a level as possible

- Of being pain free to the extent possible
- Of being able to make choices, resolve conflicts, and fulfill wishes

Weisman encourages us to believe that such a goal is possible and that as caregivers we play a significant role in its realization.

In the context of the humanistic interactionist model of this text, appropriate death must be defined individually. What is appropriate for one client may differ from what is appropriate for another client. Client A may choose to face the end of life by selling a business, updating a will, planning the funeral, settling debts, and saying good-bye to each family member. Client B may choose to continue involvement in religious activities through healing services, prayer, and other efforts to forestall death of the earthly body. The second client might be seen by some as denying the reality of impending death and avoiding preparing for the end of life. However, in the context of Client B's value system, this approach may constitute an appropriate death and should be respected and supported by professional caregivers.

Tasks of Dying

Awareness of and sensitivity to the tasks facing dying clients help nurses provide comprehensive care. Rando (1984) identifies seven tasks of dying, thus offering another framework from which to view caring for dying persons. The tasks are:

- Controlling pain and other symptoms
- Managing stress related to treatment
- Developing and maintaining relationships with professional caregivers
- Preserving emotional balance
- Preserving self-image
- Managing relationships with family and friends
- Preparing for the future

Controlling Pain and Other Symptoms

Death anxiety is often caused by anticipation of pain and other troublesome symptoms. Dying clients and their families focus considerable attention on this aspect of the dying process. Concern about maintaining control to the end of life raises questions about the effect of narcotics on clients' abilities to remain fully conscious; the potential for loss of bowel and/or bladder control; or the ability to perform the activities of daily living. Professionals skilled in the care of the terminally ill use a wide array of techniques to assist clients and families with this task. Discussion of such techniques goes beyond the scope of this chapter; however, readers are encouraged to become familiar with the extensive professional literature that addresses this concern.

Managing Stress Related to Treatment

Even when clients, families, and physicians have recognized that curative measures are ineffective, clients may be treated to control pain and other symptoms. Such treatments might include nasogastric suction (to prevent vomiting), radiation or chemotherapy (to reduce the size of a tumor thereby relieving painful pressure), or immobilization of a body part (to control pain or prevent fractures). Hospice programs have influenced care of the terminally ill by encouraging clients and caregivers to choose treatments and settings that provide the most comfort in the least restrictive setting in order to reduce the stresses of both the treatment and the treatment setting.

Developing and Maintaining Relationships with Professional Caregivers

Dying clients must clarify the expectations they have for the caregivers and the expectations the caregivers have for them. Dying clients may encounter professionals unwilling or unable to follow their lead or involve them fully in decision making. If the choice of caregivers is limited, clients may be compelled to continue in a less-than-desirable relationship to have access to needed medical or nursing care. Nurses practicing within a humanistic interactionist framework make every effort to facilitate this task.

Preserving Emotional Balance

The physiologic changes occurring in the body, the medications used to control pain and other symptoms, anticipatory grief, and signs of decline influence clients' emotional states. Emotional reactions commonly noted in dying clients include anger, sadness, anxiety, depression, and a sense of satisfaction or disappointment with life.

Preserving Self-Image

Dying clients often must reevaluate the standards against which they measure themselves. Competency may take the form of successfully telling someone else how to bake sticky buns rather than doing it oneself, for example. Goals set

should be achievable within the limitations of the effects of the terminal illness so that dying clients can feel a sense of accomplishment.

Managing Relationships with Family and Friends

Relationships with family and friends may change over the course of the terminal illness. Roles may change, conflicts may be resolved, relationships may end, other relationships may become more intimate. The stresses of the terminal illness may strain some relationships and strengthen others. Sarton (1981) portrays this task exceedingly well in her novel, *A Reckoning,* chronicling the final months of a woman's life. The protagonist seeks to resolve her difficult relationship with her elderly mother, reconsiders her relationship with each of her children, develops a new relationship with a hired caregiver, and evaluates the most important relationships in her life including the one with her late husband. Sarton's sensitive approach to this difficult subject offers an excellent literary review of the importance and complications of this task.

Preparing for the Future

Preparation for the future encompasses planning for care needs until the end of life, completing unfinished business, and planning the funeral. The cofounder of the Older Women's League (OWL) named her successor to the presidency, established an endowment fund to ensure the stability of the organization, and, within a week of her death, made a videotape presentation to be shown to the membership at the convention to be held a year later. She knew she was dying and participated in planning the future of the organization and the memorial for her at the convention.

PROCESSES FOR PRACTICE

Ethical Reflections

The ethical issues encountered in caring for dying clients are somewhat different from those pertaining to the care of psychiatric clients, although they have similar general areas of concern: individual freedom, client rights, confidentiality, and the politics of treatment in an era of perceived limited resources. The framework for analyzing an ethical issue and the principles of bioethics described in Chapter 10 provide crucial information for nurses caring for terminally ill clients as well as for psychiatric or mental health clients. The principles provide a set of criteria against which to measure one's choices in an ethical dilemma. Nurses caring for dying clients should review the analysis framework and principles frequently to ensure familiarity with them.

Individual Freedom

The questions of suicide and euthanasia often arise in the care of dying clients. These questions are addressed in Chapter 10 with reference to both physically and mentally ill clients. Professional caregivers are in a position to affect the quality of life of dying clients to a certain extent. If a client expresses a wish to die based on the experience of uncontrolled pain, for example, the professional caregivers are obliged to treat the pain to the extent that it is possible to control it. But if the professional is confident that the pain is manageable and the client refuses to allow the treatment, what then?

What about the issue of intravenous or gastric feedings? What if the client refuses such treatments? Can the professional caregiver reasonably comply with a client's refusal, which will likely result in the client's starvation?

The question of individual freedom for the dying person is complicated by the family. What happens if the client refuses treatment and the family demands it? The professional caregiver is faced with a client who will die and a family who will continue and may decide to pursue legal action against the caregiver. A disagreement between the client and family puts the caregiver in a serious ethical dilemma, which is complicated by the implied threat of legal consequences.

Client Rights

Dying persons have the same rights as all other clients. They have a right to humane treatment, to integrity of the body, to control of treatment, and to accurate information. The question of truth telling in the case of terminal illness continues to be debated in the professional literature and in the back stairwells of hospitals. The trend in the professional literature supports clients' rights to know and understand the truth about their terminal illnesses. In practice some caregivers question whether the truth may rob the client of the will to live and actually do more harm than good.

The importance of trust in the caregiver-client relationship must influence the decision about truth telling. Clients must be able to trust the veracity and good will of their caregivers. Lack of trust may lead clients to refuse treatment that would benefit their quality of life. When one considers death anxiety and its potential for paralyzing clients from action or depriving them of the ability to think clearly about their futures, the imperativeness of trust in the caregiver-client relationship is clear.

Confidentiality

Ordinarily the family is integral to the care of dying clients. In most hospice programs the client and family are viewed as the unit of care. However, there are clients who prefer not to discuss their condition with family members for a

variety of reasons. Some people do not want to make their family members sad; some do not want their families to worry; and some want to project a positive image at all costs. The client may expect the caregiver to maintain confidentiality about the reality of the condition. The professional caregiver faces an ethical dilemma, especially if forewarning of the impending death has particular importance in the health and well-being of the family member. The timing and circumstances of a death and the significance of the relationship influence the grieving process; lack of preparation might cause dysfunctional grief in the surviving family member. The professional caregiver must wrestle with the choice of maintaining or breaking confidentiality.

Occasionally the nurse is in the opposite position; that is, the family member may know the truth and forbid the nurse from discussing it with the client. If the client asks questions requiring answers that would reveal the truth, the professional is in a difficult position.

The importance of trust in the caregiver-client relationship also guides decision making in this area. The nurse may approach the situation by attempting to convince the client or the family member of the value of truth telling. A trusting relationship with the family is as vital as trust between the caregiver and client. However, nurses will find that some clients and families remain adamant in their viewpoints.

Politics of Treatment

Care of dying clients is influenced by so-called limited resources. The debate about whether resources are actually limited goes beyond the scope of this chapter. However, the perception of limited resources perpetuates policies that influence the care available to all clients including those who are dying. Occasionally one hears the argument that expensive treatments ought not to be wasted on certain individuals because of their age, their mental capacity, or their terminal illness. Such reasoning has been used to argue in favor of hospice programs on the assumption that acceptance of the terminality of the illness decreases the use of expensive technology. In fact, radiation therapy can be beneficial in pain management; surgery may be employed to debulk a tumor and make the client more comfortable; continuous intravenous morphine therapy may be necessary to relieve pain; physical therapy might help a client remain mobile for a time; and occupational therapy may help teach the client methods of self-care as disabilities worsen. When the goal is quality of life and helping the client remain in control to the end of life, use of resources may be extensive.

The attempt to curtail such services to the terminally ill is evident in the rules and regulations of third party payers. Some insurance policies exclude physical therapy for clients with terminal illnesses, for example. Nurses involved in the care of the terminally ill should be aware of treatment decisions based on financial resources.

The rules and regulations governing the Medicare hospice benefit also raise ethical problems for professional caregivers in that they require the client to sign a statement acknowledging that the illness is terminal, and they strongly favor home care and home death. To maintain financial stability, hospice programs may be forced to screen referrals carefully to ensure that potential clients will not survive beyond the number of days for which reimbursement can be received or that they are good candidates for being maintained at home for the greatest percentage of time prior to death. Dying clients who have no one to care for them at home or whose life expectancy is less predictable are unlikely to be acceptable referrals.

Communication

The humanistic interactionist model demands attention to communication. The basic premises require that nurses be skilled at arriving at negotiated meanings with clients and families. Chapter 11 presents a thorough discussion of communication, including theory, criteria for effective communication, and techniques. Communication with dying clients uses the techniques and meets the criteria for effective communication. The underlying principle must prevail; that is, communication occurs in a relationship in a social context with multiple factors affecting it. Techniques applied according to a formula are likely to miss the mark. Nurses skilled in communicating with clients and families will adjust their communications to fit situations and interactions with clients.

Communicating with dying clients concerns caregivers due to the perceived delicacy of the subject. General discussion of dying and death is no longer taboo; however, specific discussion of dying and death with terminally ill persons or their families continues to be difficult. Gonda and Ruark (1984) describe the barriers to effective communication with dying clients, including:

- The authority of the caregiver
- Disclosure of information
- Withholding information
- Strong emotions
- Mixed messages

Although Gonda and Ruark's intended audience is physicians, their discussion is also instructive to nurses.

Authority of the Caregiver

Caregivers who assume an air of authority run the risk of creating a barrier between themselves and their clients. Nurses who approach the care of their clients from an authoritarian stance are less effective in the care they deliver. Engaging the client and family in the process of care communicates respect.

Mr. A cared for his dying wife at home for six months, attending to her needs with tenderness and sensitivity. When her pain became difficult to control she was admitted to the hospital for intravenous morphine therapy. Mr. A tried to teach the nursing staff how to move Mrs. A without hurting her, but the nurses told him to leave the room so they could care for her without his interference. Mrs. A winced in pain as the nurses moved her in the bed. Mr. A was furious that he was ignored and that his wife was being handled in a way that caused her discomfort. The nurses wrote "belligerent husband" on the care plan. Mr. A sought assistance from a clinical specialist nurse who suggested to the staff that they create an alliance with Mr. A, recognizing his skill in caring for Mrs. A and allowing him to direct them in areas of her care in which he had considerable experience. When the nurses dropped their air of authority and established a partnership with Mr. A, he became cooperative and complimentary about her care.

Disclosure of Information

Professional caregivers have knowledge and information that is not available to clients except through the caregivers' abilities to communicate. The criteria for successful communication (see Chapter 11) apply in this instance particularly. Information must be shared in language that is understood, in amounts that can be managed, and in settings designed to facilitate communication. Disclosing information about terminal illness is likely to be complicated by the client's reactions, so caregivers must be flexible enough to adjust the approach to the client's needs. It may be necessary to have a series of interactions clarifying information and the import of the information to the client.

Mrs. C was diagnosed with an inoperable brain tumor. The physician told her the diagnosis and referred her to the hospice program. The hospice nurse counseled with Mrs. C over several days to clarify the diagnosis and the prognosis. Mrs. C understood what she heard but required continuing clarification as questions occurred to her between interactions. The impact of the information was such that she needed time to absorb it and consider its meaning. The hospice nurse answered questions, provided information, clarified the medical terminology, and checked Mrs. C's understanding.

Staff nurses commonly express concern about what clients have been told and how much they should reveal. An effective strategy is to ask clients what the physician said, what they understand is wrong with them based on what the physician said, and what they think it means for their future. This allows interactions to proceed with the direction dictated by the client rather than the nurse.

Withholding Information

Gonda and Ruark (1984) maintain that withholding information is likely to do more harm than good. Openness to sharing information and feelings in the face of terminal illness facilitates interactions and adjustment.

Mrs. D approached a clinical specialist nurse to request assistance in communicating with her husband. Mr. D had been treated for cancer for many months but continued to deteriorate. Mr. D never discussed his illness with anyone and had refused a hospice referral. Mrs. D was sure that Mr. D was dying, but she was afraid to talk about it openly because he was so adamant that he was going to "beat this thing." The clinical specialist nurse suggested that Mrs. D talk about her feelings to Mr. D without expecting Mr. D to agree that he was dying. Mrs. D told Mr. D that she loved him very much and that she was sad because she was afraid he was dying. She said that she wanted to be sure that he knew how much she cared about him. Mr. D said that he loved her also and asked her to call his lawyer to come to the hospital. Mr. D revised his will, which had been written prior to his marriage to Mrs. D. Mr. and Mrs. D spent the afternoon talking about their good memories of their life together. Mr. D died that evening never having acknowledged that he was dying.

Strong Emotions

The expression of strong emotion is considered inappropriate in some cultures. Professional caregivers are often taught that they must maintain a cool demeanor in their relationships with clients and families. Men are often taught restraint in the expression of strong emotions. Some ethnic groups, such as Scandinavians, are also taught to restrain the expression of strong emotion. Stoicism may block effective communication.

Mr. E told the home health nurse that he felt fine and needed nothing for pain management. The nurse noticed that Mr. E was sitting in a contorted position. She touched

him on the shoulder and he shouted in pain. In Mr. E's culture it was unacceptable for him to express "weakness." He felt compelled to manage his own affairs and to tolerate pain. The nurse was constantly challenged to negotiate shared meanings with Mr. E and to offer assistance in ways he could define as acceptable.

Mixed Messages

Professional caregivers may inadvertently give mixed messages that confuse clients and families. When the information being conveyed is emotionally laden, the possibility for confusion is even greater. Consider this example.

Mr. L underwent an exploratory thoracotomy and was discovered to have inoperable lung cancer. The surgeon reported the results to the family in the gravest terms. Mr. L was admitted to the Intensive Care Unit (ICU) for several days after surgery. During his stay in the ICU Mr. L suffered from disorientation caused by the constant activity and lack of uninterrupted rest afforded clients in that setting. His family was very concerned. They questioned the medical director of the ICU who told them Mr. L was recovering beautifully and was coping as expected. Mr. L's family physician approached the family during the height of Mr. L's confusion to tell them that he was concerned about Mr. L's condition. He wanted to move him out of the ICU as soon as possible to begin a program of rehabilitation so Mr. L could go home.

Mr. L's eldest daughter sought consultation with a clinical specialist nurse. The family believed they were receiving conflicting messages from the three physicians. They heard that he would die very soon, that he was recovering beautifully, and that he would be going home! With the help of the clinical specialist nurse, it became clear that Mr. L was terminally ill; that he was reacting to the ICU in an expectable manner; that he was recovering from the surgical procedure very well; that although he had incurable cancer, it would take some time before it took his life; and that he could expect to live for some time at home before the period of decline and deterioration began.

The messages from the physicians reflected their varying perspectives and their varying responsibilities for Mr. L. The intervention of the clinical specialist nurse allowed the family to come to an understanding about Mr. L's condition and what to expect in the future.

Research

In 1983 Benoliel thoroughly reviewed the nursing research on death, dying, and terminal illness. The earliest nursing studies cited focus on psychosocial and emotional support. Benoliel categorized the research into three areas: responses of nurses to death and terminal illness, adaptations of clients and families, and environmental and social processes influencing adaptation. She indicated that the nursing research in these realms of concern is sparse. Most of our knowledge comes from related disciplines such as psychology and sociology. The nursing research is largely descriptive and devoid of conceptual frameworks that would allow a systematic building of nursing knowledge. Few studies attempt to explain or predict client behavior or the effectiveness of nursing interventions. Such efforts are necessary to improve the quality of services nurses offer. Clinical anecdotes are useful but limited in giving valid and reliable information about dying, death, and effective nursing interventions. (See Chapter 14 for an in-depth discussion of research in psychiatric nursing.)

THE NURSING PROCESS AND DYING CLIENTS AND THEIR FAMILIES

The nursing process is a powerful tool to guide professional nursing practice. Careful attention to each step—assessing, diagnosing, planning, implementing, and evaluating—ensures a systematic approach to caregiving; facilitates communication among nurses and with other professionals; provides a basis for quality assurance; and creates a base from which clinical nursing researchers can build the science of nursing.

Assessment

The assessment format presented in Chapter 12 provides a common framework with which to assess all clients. Dying clients may or may not have accompanying psychiatric symptoms; however, the psychosocial assessment of dying persons is essential. Some clients will be managed effectively by generalists, others may be better served by clinical specialists.

Nurses counseling dying clients should perform complete assessments to ensure that physical needs are being managed effectively. Clients preoccupied with pain and other troublesome symptoms are less able to engage in meaningful interactions.

The assessment of dying clients should specifically address a number of issues (Box 37–1). The approaches for gaining information may need to be adjusted to build and maintain successful communication among nurses, clients, and families.

What is the meaning of the terminal illness to the client and family? Some people see terminal illness as a punishment either for the client or the family. Others see terminal illness as a challenge to their religious beliefs or as an assault on their expectations for their lives. Some may see it as an injustice, some as an overwhelming burden. The meaning may change from time to time, or several meanings may exist side by side. The meaning to the client might be quite different from the meaning to the family.

What do the client and family expect to happen during the course of the illness? Often peoples' expectations are worse than the reality; on the other hand, sometimes the expectations are unrealistically positive. Nurses need to know clients' and families' expectations to begin developing mutually understood meanings. In the case of Mr. L the family believed that he would stay in the hospital until he died; they did not expect a period of time when he would be home. Much of the work of counseling dying clients and their families involves clarifying and helping them anticipate the future realistically.

What social influences may have an impact on clients' and families' perceptions of the dying process? Many persons have known other people who died and may compare their own to the other person's experience.

Mrs. Q had a friend who died from breast cancer many years ago under exceedingly painful and difficult circumstances. Mrs. Q expects her experience to be similar in spite of advances in cancer treatment and care of the terminally ill that have improved the quality of life for dying persons.

Another source of social influence might be from the client's religious affiliation.

Mrs. R was inclined to accept and prepare for the finality of her terminal illness, but members of her religious sect encouraged her to pray for release from her illness as a sign of her faith. They told her that if she had enough faith she would be healed. Mrs. R was in a bind because her primary reference group would not accept the prognosis.

Are the client and family receptive to the modification of meanings through interaction with the nurse? The third premise of the interactionist model described earlier is cru-

Box 37–1
ASSESSMENT QUESTIONS

- What is the meaning of the terminal illness to the client and family?

- What do the client and family expect to happen during the course of the illness?

- What social influences may have an impact on clients' and families' perceptions of the dying process?

- Are the client and family receptive to the modification of meanings through interaction with the nurse?

- Which losses are of greatest concern to the client?

- What other stressors influence the effect of the impending death?

- What are the roles of the various players? Of what significance are the players to the dying client?

- What promises have been made among the persons involved, and of what significance are they in the context of the dying process?

- What is the prognosis, and what is the expected cause of death?

- To whom does the client express what? How can the nurse facilitate negotiated meanings among the persons involved?

- What constitutes "appropriate death" for this client?

cial to the complete picture. Clients or families may reject any modification of the views they hold about the illness or the death.

Mr. S asked to see the hospice nurse after the physician told him the extent of his illness. While Mr. S was talking to the nurse, Mrs. S entered the room. Mrs. S interrupted the interaction, adamantly ordering the nurse to cease any discussion about dying or death. Before Mrs. S could dismiss the nurse, the nurse suggested to Mrs. S that hospice could help her manage Mr. S's physical needs when he went home. Mrs. S softened her tone immediately and began to ask questions about Mr. S's care. Mrs. S was unwilling to negotiate a shared meaning about Mr. S's illness and prognosis but she was willing to negotiate a different relationship with the hospice nurse.

Which losses are of greatest concern to the client? The client faces multiple losses, some physical and some symbolic. The effective nurse will identify those of greatest importance to the client.

Mr. P was estranged from his family, including his three children. His two oldest children were married and lived in another town. His son lived with Mr. P's wife from whom he was legally separated and whom Mr. P believed was developing Alzheimer's disease. He maintained a close relationship with a woman who considered herself to be his significant other. Mr. P had been a successful businessman with the same company for 25 years; he maintained excellent relationships with his customers and his long-time secretary.

As he began to deteriorate, Mr. P began the process of terminating his relationships. He arranged for his accounts to be taken over by another firm; he worked with his secretary to notify all his customers about the

RESEARCH NOTE

Citation

McGinnis S: How can nurses improve the quality of life of the hospice client and family?: An exploratory study. Hospice J 1986;2:23–36.

Study Problem/Purpose

This study aims to determine which supportive nursing behaviors are needed by the family or primary caregiver for a person dying at home to maintain quality of life.

Methods

A convenience sample of twenty bereaved primary caregivers (family or friends) completed a Q-sort of sixty nursing behaviors modified from a previously designed and tested instrument. The nursing behaviors were in categories related to the client's physical needs, the client's psychosocial needs, and the caregiver's psychosocial needs.

Findings

Of the ten behaviors ranked most helpful, eight were related to psychosocial care of the client or the caregiver. The findings of this study compare to previous studies identifying three behaviors among the top ten most helpful: Answer my questions honestly, openly, and willingly; let me know about changes in the client's condition; and talk to the client to reduce his or her fears.

Implications

The findings imply that the nurse's skills in psychosocial care of clients and families are significant.

disposition of their accounts and to sell his office furniture; he found another position for his secretary; he contacted his married children and reestablished a relationship with one of them; he redrafted his will to protect his estate for his son and wife; he worked with the hospice team to ensure that his woman friend would be supported at the time of his death and funeral; and he arranged for a gift for his son's 16th birthday. Mr. P identified his significant losses and involved the hospice nurse in helping him terminate his relationships in a way that satisfied him that he was meeting his obligations.

What other stressors influence the effect of the impending death? Mr. P's circumstances illustrate this point as well as the previous one. His estrangement from his family and his relationship with his woman friend caused him considerable distress. He felt strongly that his funeral should be a family affair and he worked hard to ensure that it would be. At the same time he did not want his woman friend to be without support. He was further bothered that his woman friend devoted much of her time to him and served as his primary caregiver but would receive no compensation through his estate. She assured him that she freely chose to be with him through the dying process. The stress of his impending death for his woman friend was complicated by the fact that she was a widow whose husband had died from cancer very suddenly.

What are the roles of the various players? Of what significance are the players to the dying client? Sarton (1981) portrays the roles of multiple players in the death of an old woman. The physician, the hired caregiver, and a maiden aunt play significant roles in the immediate life of the protagonist. Each of them is involved in her physical care and in helping her maintain a routine of living. Family members come and go, helping her sort out the meaning of her life and her relationships but having only very limited involvement in her activities of daily living.

Mr. J, dying from metastatic lung cancer, had no interest in seeing his children. His wife's adult daughter lived in Florida but maintained close contact with Mr. and Mrs. J. When Mrs. J challenged the physician about various treatments, it was because her daughter had called and was upset over the course of Mr. J's illness. She was not even his daughter, and she lived more than a thousand miles away, but her influence was strongly felt by Mr. and Mrs. J and the professional caregivers.

What promises have been made among the persons involved, and of what significance are they in the context of the dying process?

Mrs. A had been faithful to her husband through some very difficult times during which he drank heavily. When Mrs. A was diagnosed with a terminal illness, Mr. A promised her that he would care for her at home until she died. He provided superb care for many months during which Mrs. A was bedridden. She never developed a pressure ulcer and she spent every day in the center of activity. He moved her from the bedroom to the living room daily and built his activities around caring for her. He seldom left their small apartment for more than thirty minutes at a time. After six months Mr. A was becoming exhausted and experiencing pain in his legs but he would not seek help from their adult children or see a physician about his legs. His promise to Mrs. A was more important to him than his own health.

What is the prognosis, and what is the expected cause of death?

Mrs. B had a gastric tumor that threatened to erode the aorta. She wanted to die at home, and her son and his family were willing to be her caregivers. The physician was reluctant to discharge Mrs. B because he expected her to bleed to death when the tumor destroyed the wall of the aorta. The nurse counseled Mrs. B, her family, and the home health nurse, helping them understand the physician's concerns. Mrs. B was discharged when she and her family assured the physician that they understood the risks and were prepared to deal with them with the home health nurse's help.

To whom does the client express what? How can the nurse facilitate negotiated meanings among the persons involved?

Mr. T had several adult children who visited regularly. His interactions with each varied to the extent that one thought he had given up hope, another thought he was unrealistically optimistic, another thought he was preparing for his death with equanimity, and another thought he vacillated in his reactions to his illness. Mr. T was honest with each of his children, but expressed his different moods to each child according to his relationship with each of them.

What constitutes "appropriate death" for this client? Assessment of this aspect of the dying process for individual clients helps nurses establish the outcome measures for the evaluation of nursing care. Weisman's definition gives guidance but the specific characteristics will vary from client to client as the result of arriving at negotiated meanings with the family and the professional caregivers.

Nursing Diagnosis

Counseling dying clients may be complicated by the simultaneous occurrence of physical or mental disorders other than the terminal illness. Generalist nurses should refer complex clients to a clinical specialist nurse. The care of such clients requires sophistication beyond the skills of

generalists. The physical effects of a terminal illness and accompanying medical treatments may also cause a variety of problems that must be diagnosed and treated by nurses. This chapter focuses on diagnoses that may result from the dying process. Nurses expecting to work with dying clients are urged to become acquainted with the literature addressing all aspects of caring for terminally ill clients.

Nursing diagnoses offer a rich array of possibilities in the care of dying clients.

Box 37–2 lists the nursing diagnoses from PND-I that have the most potential for use with dying clients. The diagnoses included in the biologic human response pat-

---

Box 37–2
COMMON PND-I DIAGNOSES FOR DYING CLIENTS

01. Human Response Patterns in Activity Processes

01.03   Altered self-care
   01.03.01   Altered eating
   01.03.02   Altered grooming
   01.03.03   Altered health maintenance
   01.03.04   Altered hygiene
   01.03.05   Altered participation in health care
   01.03.06   Altered toileting

02. Human Response Patterns in Cognition Processes

02.02   Altered judgment
   02.03.03   Knowledge deficit
02.08   Altered thought processes
   02.08.02   Altered concentration
   02.08.03   Altered problem solving

04. Human Response Patterns in Emotional Processes

04.02   Altered feeling patterns
   04.02.01   Anger
   04.02.02   Anxiety
   04.02.05   Fear
   04.02.06   Grief
   04.02.07   Guilt
   04.02.08   Sadness

05. Human Response Patterns in Interpersonal Processes

05.03   Altered role performance
   05.03.01   Altered family role
   05.03.02   Altered leisure role
   05.03.03   Altered parenting role
   05.03.04   Altered play role
   05.03.05   Altered student role
   05.03.06   Altered work role
05.05   Altered social interaction
   05.05.02   Social isolation/withdrawal

06. Human Response Patterns in Perception Processes

06.02   Altered comfort patterns
   06.02.01   Discomfort
   06.02.02   Distress
   06.02.03   Pain
06.03   Altered self-concept
   06.03.01   Altered body image
   06.03.05   Altered social identity

08. Human Response Patterns in Valuation Processes

08.01   Altered meaningfulness
   08.01.01   Hopelessness
   08.01.02   Helplessness
   08.01.03   Loneliness
   08.01.04   Powerlessness
08.02   Altered spirituality
   08.02.01   Spiritual distress
   08.02.02   Spiritual despair

Box 37–3
PLANNING GUIDELINES

- Manage physical symptoms
- Include all persons involved
- Anticipate the likely cause of death
- Identify least restrictive, most supportive setting possible
- Clarify relationships and expectations
- Reassess frequently

---

terns are not specified because their applicability will vary depending on clients' terminal illnesses. The activity, cognition, emotional, interpersonal, perception, and valuation processes of the human response patterns offer a complete range of specific nursing diagnoses likely to be encountered in dying clients. For example, depressive behavior includes defining characteristics that may or may not be applicable in every instance.

Planning Interventions

Planning care for dying clients encompasses physical care and psychosocial care. Physical problems, such as alterations in respiratory function, may be physiologically based but aggravated by anxiety. Effective care plans address the full range of problems experienced by clients, using an array of physical and interpersonal approaches to alleviate distress (Box 37–3).

Predesigned Plans

Predesigned nursing care plans provide general guidelines for nurses caring for dying clients and their families. Ulrich et al. (1986) include care plans for terminal care specific to anxiety, alteration in respiratory function, fluid volume deficit, alteration in comfort: pain, alteration in comfort: nausea and vomiting, alteration in comfort: pruritus, alteration in comfort: gas pain and abdominal distention, alteration in comfort: hiccoughs, impairment in skin integrity: irritation or breakdown, alteration in oral mucous membrane: dryness, impaired physical mobility, self-care deficit, alteration in pattern of urinary elimination: incontinence, alteration in bowel elimination: constipation, alteration

in bowel elimination: diarrhea, alteration in bowel elimination: incontinence, alteration in thought processes, sleep pattern disturbance, injury: physiologic, grieving, and ineffective family coping.

This listing illustrates the potential range of nursing diagnoses for which nurses might need to plan care for terminally ill clients. Only three (anxiety, grieving, and ineffective coping) are specific to psychosocial issues; however, the interaction of these diagnoses with the physiologic diagnoses complicates the picture and demands a holistic approach to planning.

The Oncology Nursing Society (ONS) Clinical Practice Subcommittee on Guidelines published a comprehensive set of guidelines organized according to the standards of oncology nursing practice and NANDA nursing diagnoses (McNally et al. 1985). The ONS guidelines identify the populations at risk, expected outcomes, and nursing management including assessment and client teaching. Many of the guidelines address nursing diagnoses commonly seen in dying clients as identified in Box 37–2.

Words to the Wise

Care planning should reflect the humanistic interactionist premises and the goal of "appropriate death." Nurses planning care for dying clients should keep several factors in mind, including the following:

1. Manage physical symptoms with the utmost care. Meticulous attention to the physical care of the client is essential; wrinkle-free beds, clean skin, bowel and bladder care with accompanying pericare, careful grooming, and any other aspect of care with which the client needs assistance must be the concern of the nurse. Failure to ensure that clients are as comfortable as possible will complicate and undermine any other efforts nurses may make.

2. Include all the persons involved (client, family members, significant others, other health care providers) in planning. The impact of the social context on meanings dictates that negotiated meanings include those persons who might have an influence on the client or on the plans being made.

3. Anticipate the likely cause of death and build a plan that takes it into account. Nurses help clients and families prepare, thereby relieving anxiety.

4. Work with the persons involved to identify the least restrictive, most supportive setting possible. Home death became an acceptable choice with the advent of hospice care; however, some clients do not have willing or able caregivers and hospice services are not available in every community.

5. Clarify relationships and expectations. Plan for emergencies. Determine whether resuscitation is expected or desired. If the client wants to die at home, plan with the family whom they should call for assistance. An

ambulance crew is likely to institute life-saving measures; they should be called only if that is what the client and family want.

6. Reassess frequently. Perceptions and physical conditions change frequently in dying persons. An effective plan is flexible enough to reflect the changes as they occur.

Implementing Interventions

The key to successful interventions lie in the philosophy of care, communication skills, assessment, and planning. Nurses who intervene according to the philosophic premises and practice processes presented in this chapter and throughout this text provide quality care acceptable to clients and families.

An intervention that can be particularly useful is silent presence. Although dying persons do not want to be abandoned, neither do they want continuous interaction. Sometimes the most effective thing nurses can do is sit quietly with clients, assuring them of their presence and not expecting them to interact.

Evaluation

Nursing care that facilitates individually defined appropriate death can be considered quality care. The specific interpretation of appropriate death depends on the client, the social context, and the meanings negotiated among the persons involved. The character of the dying process and death varies from client to client; what is appropriate for one may not be appropriate for another.

It may be necessary in the course of caring for dying clients to set priorities with clients and families with respect to their perception of appropriate death.

Mrs. A wanted to die at home, but Mr. A became too exhausted and her pain became very difficult to manage. Mrs. A died in the hospital with Mr. A and her children at her side. The nurse helped Mr. A accept hospitalization with managed pain and rested family members in round-the-clock attendance as preferable to dying at home with an exhausted caregiver unable to manage her pain.

Working with dying clients and their families offers nurses the opportunity to practice humanistic care using the interactionist model. The quality of the relationships that develop between nurses and dying clients reinforces the significance of nursing and of the humanistic approach to caring for clients.

Chapter Highlights

- Nursing care of dying clients affords the nurse an opportunity to practice nursing humanistically.

- Fear of death protects us from premature death; death anxiety deprives us of the desire to live.

- Loss is the central theme in dying. The impact depends on the meaning of the relationship, the timing of the loss, the social context in which the loss occurs, and the perceptions of the principals.

- Death involves physical and symbolic loss.

- The dying process includes four phases: existential plight, mitigation and accommodation, decline and deterioration, and preterminality and terminality.

- Dying clients alternate between denial and acceptance.

- Appropriate death is a way of living to the end of life and is realizable.

- The tasks of dying include controlling pain and other symptoms; managing the stress associated with treatment; developing and maintaining relationships with professional caregivers; preserving emotional balance; preserving self-image; maintaining or resolving relationships with family and friends; and preparing for the future.

- The tasks of dying provide a framework that helps nurses focus the nursing process.

- Caring for dying clients and their families raises ethical questions related to individual freedom, client rights, confidentiality, and the politics of treatment.

- Barriers to communication between professional caregivers and dying clients include the professional's air of authority, disclosure of information, withholding information, difficulty in expressing strong emotions, and mixed messages.

- Nursing research in the area of death and dying is sparse and poorly developed.

- A humanistic interactionist philosophy, communication skills, assessment, and planning are the keys to successful interventions with dying clients and their families.

References

Ahana DN, Kunishi MM: *Cancer Care Protocols: For Hospital and Home Care Use.* Springer, 1981.

Ahmed P: *Living and Dying with Cancer.* Elsevier, 1981.

Amenta MO, Bohnet NL: *Nursing Care of the Terminally Ill.* Little, Brown, 1986.

Benoliel JQ: Nursing research on death, dying, and terminal illness: Development, present state, and prospects, in Werley HH, Fitzpatrick JJ (eds): *Annual Review of Nursing Research,* vol 1. Springer, 1983.

Cassileth BR, Cassileth PA: *Clinical Care of the Terminal Cancer Patient.* Lea and Febiger, 1982.

Collison C, Miller S: Using images of the future in grief work. *Int J Nurs Studies* 1987;19(1):9–11.

Gonda TA, Ruark JE: *Dying Dignified: The Health Professional's Guide to Care.* Addison-Wesley, 1984.

Kirschling JM: Support utilized by caregivers of terminally ill family members: Clinical implications for hospice team members. *Am J Hospice Care* 1985;2:27–31.

Kübler-Ross E: *On Death and Dying.* Macmillan, 1969.

Lepp I: *Death and Its Mysteries,* Murchland B (trans). Macmillan, 1968.

Marris P: *Loss and Change.* Anchor Books, 1975.

McFarland GK, Wasli EK: *Nursing Diagnoses and Process in Psychiatric Mental Health Nursing.* Lippincott, 1986.

McGinnis SS: How can nurses improve the quality of life of the hospice client and family?: An exploratory study. *Hospice J* 1986;2:23–36.

McGoldrick M, et al.: Mourning rituals: How culture shapes the experience of loss. *Fam Ther Networker.* 1986; Nov–Dec:28–36.

McNally JC, Stair JC, Somerville ET (eds): *Guidelines for Cancer Nursing Practice.* Grune and Stratton, 1985.

Meinhart NT, McCaffery M: *Pain: A Nursing Approach to Assessment and Analysis.* Appleton-Century-Crofts, 1983.

Rando TA: Bereaved parents: Particular difficulties, unique factors, and treatment issues. *Social Work* 1985;30(1):19–23.

Rando TA: *Grief, Dying and Death: Clinical Interventions for Caregivers.* Research Press, 1984.

Rigdon I, Clayton B, Dimond M: Toward a theory of helpfulness for the elderly bereaved: An invitation to a new life. *Adv Nurs Science* 1987;9(2):32–43.

Sarton M: *A Reckoning.* WW Norton, 1981.

Saunders C (ed): *The Management of Terminal Malignant Disease,* ed 2. Edward Arnold, 1984.

Ulrich SP, Canale SW, Wendell SA: *Nursing Care Planning Guides: A Nursing Diagnosis Approach.* WB Saunders, 1986.

Weisman AD: *On Dying and Denying: A Psychiatric Study of Terminality.* Behavioral Publications, 1972.

Weisman AD: Thanatology, in Kaplan HI, Sadock BJ (eds): *Comprehensive Textbook of Psychiatry,* ed 4. Williams and Wilkins, 1985, pp 1277–1286.

Worden JW: *Grief Counseling and Grief Therapy: A Handbook for the Mental Health Practitioner.* Springer, 1982.

Zimmerman JM: *Hospice: Complete Care for the Terminally Ill.* Urban & Schwarzenberg, 1981.

PART SEVEN

Social, Political, Cultural, and Economic Environments for Care

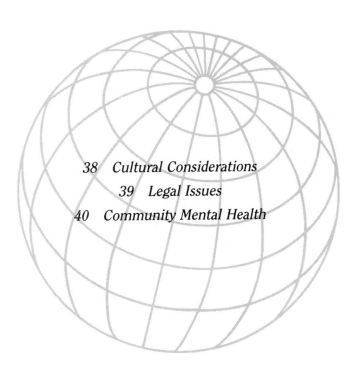

THIRTY-EIGHT

Cultural Considerations

Carol Ren Kneisl
Sally A. Hutchinson

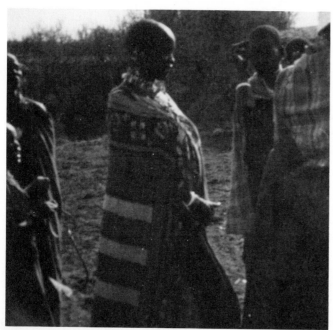

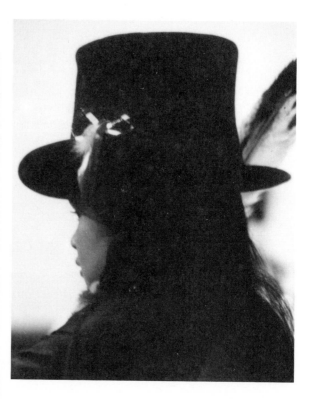

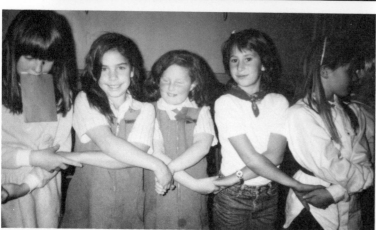

After reading this chapter, students should be able to

- State the relevance of cultural factors in psychiatric nursing practice

- Discuss cultural forces that influence mental health

- Explain the concepts of culture, holism, world view, ethnocentrism, and cultural relativism and their value for nursing practice

- Describe the process of obtaining a cultural profile

- Compare the three domains of health care

- Identify the inherent dangers in cultural stereotyping

- Analyze their own cultural heritage and its effect on the nurse-client relationship

- Discuss some of the folk beliefs and healing practices of four minority groups

- Develop culturally aware strategies for implementing the nursing process

Cross References

Other topics relevant to this content are: Assessment, Chapter 12; Communication skills, Chapter 11; Ethics, Chapter 10; Nurse's values, Chapter 3; Psychiatric theories, Chapter 5; Social support systems, Chapter 8.

To be loyal to this country does not compel us to be disloyal to the human species.

Key Terms

barrio	ethnocentrism
cao gio (coining)	faith healers
cultural relativism	folk health care systems
cultural stereotyping	mal de ojo
culture	root doctor (Voodoo man or
culture-bound syndromes	woman)
culture broker	Santeria
culture shock	shaman (medicine man)
Curanderismo	susto
curandero	world view
Espiritismo	yin and yang
espiritisto	

In a remote Eskimo village, a 34-year-old woman sits quietly, seemingly preoccupied with her own thoughts, in a trancelike state. Suddenly she leaps to her feet, throwing objects at the wall and heaping verbal abuse on her husband. His attempts to calm her do not work, and when he attempts to restrain her physically, she wrests herself from his grasp, tears off her clothing, and runs screaming out into the snow. Hearing her shrieks most of the adults of the village run after her across the snowfields. Although she initially outdistances them, she begins to tire, and the villagers finally catch up with her as she drops exhausted into the snow. They carry her back to her home where she falls into a deep sleep. When she awakens she recalls nothing of the episode. The people of the village are not surprised by her behavior. *Pibloqtok* can happen to anyone. No treatment is necessary; on awakening the next day the person behaves as usual.

On a busy downtown street walks a shy, introverted young Southeast Asian refugee, who has just been fired from his job as a restaurant dishwasher. The job was hard to come by in the first place, and now he and his family are faced with the discouraging prospect of trying to feed six people on the few dollars that remain from his last paycheck. At a crowded intersection the young man suddenly pulls a knife and begins to slash wildly at the startled people around him. He appears to be in a murderous rage and struggles with great strength, despite his small frame, against several people who are attempting to restrain and disarm him. A passing police cruiser picks him up and takes him to the police station. However, by this time he seems to be in a deep depression and fails to respond to their questions. The police take him to the community mental health center, where he is admitted to the in-patient unit and treated for depression. In Southeast Asia he would have been known as a victim of *amok,* the condition on which the phrase "run amok" is based.

RELEVANCE OF CULTURE TO PSYCHIATRIC NURSING PRACTICE

The behavior of the Eskimo woman and the Southeast Asian refugee has deep meaning for them and for others interacting with them.

In the Eskimo village, the hysterics of *pibloqtok* are a culturally sanctioned release in a society that stresses conformity and repression. In Western society, we might label the Eskimo woman as hysterical, sexually repressed, or acting out. In American psychiatric terminology she might be said to be suffering from a dissociative disorder.

In the sixteenth century in Southeast Asia, *amok* referred to the behavior of brave fighters who chose to die in battle rather than lose. Those who ran amok fighting colonial oppression were honored and treated with respect. Although no longer socially acceptable, the cultural tradition remains, and maladjusted persons who have been humiliated still occasionally run amok, although episodes of amok are becoming less frequent. Outdated diagnostic practices in psychiatry might have led to a diagnosis of paranoid schizophrenia, or manic-depressive psychosis in the pre–DSM-IIIR days.

Culture plays a major role in shaping how people think, behave, and feel. Culture determines how and by whom children are raised; how they are cuddled and fed; how they acquire rules of behavior; how they are punished; and how they learn about sex, gender roles, and marriage. Culture may affect personal psychology and shape character. Culture provides standards and values according to which we evaluate ourselves, our groups, and outsiders. Culture provides guidelines and rules for recognizing or diagnosing mental disorder and for its management and, sometimes, treatment (Foulkes 1980).

In both of the examples above, the culture has an idea of what insanity *should* be and of the meaning of the behavior of its members. Culture shapes the very way we conceive of illness. Culture determines not only who is labeled mentally ill and under what circumstances, but also the nature of the treatment and the identity of the helper. Therefore, a humanistic position in psychiatric nursing care must take account of culture and its influence on both client and nurse.

This chapter pinpoints the relevance of culture to psychiatric nursing practice, discusses cultural complexity and diversity, biosocial factors and sociopolitical forces influencing mental health, folk beliefs and healing practices,

the importance of cultural self-analysis for caregivers, and culturally aware strategies for nursing intervention blending insights from nursing, anthropology, sociology, and social psychology. It also explores the ways in which culture influences the perception, classification, process of labeling, explanation, symptoms, and treatment of what is called mental illness.

HISTORICAL FOUNDATIONS

Psychiatric nursing has not traditionally focused on culture and its influence on psychiatric nursing practice. Various psychologic and psychoanalytic interpretations of client experience and behavior have predominated. The biochemical and physiologic aspects of mental illness have received increasing attention since the 1950s. But only within the last few years has culture been recognized as a relevant variable in nursing care. Note the following significant historical events.

- 1900–1909: Public health nurses wrote of their experiences with, and observations of, immigrants such as Italians, Russians, and Portuguese.

- 1904: Emil Kraepelin studied the relationship between culture and mental disorder. He focused on the mental disorders prevalent in Java and Germany and determined that the different frequencies in mental disorder were due to hereditary rather than cultural factors.

- 1913: In *Totem and Taboo,* Sigmund Freud proposed that the Oedipus complex and incest taboo were universal.

- 1927: Bernard Malinowski, an anthropologist doing fieldwork in the Trobriand Islands, disproved the universality of the Oedipus complex. He noted that in the Trobriands, the taboo has to do with a boy's mother's brother (not the boy's father) because of the matrilineal descent pattern in which the boy inherits his name and position from this uncle (his mother's brother), and not from his biologic father.

- 1930–1939: The culture and personality school in anthropology was founded with psychoanalytic psychology as the theoretical underpinning. *Cultural determinism,* the belief that culture determines personality much more than biology, became dominant. Anthropologic researchers such as Margaret Mead, Ruth Benedict, Ralph Linton, Clyde Kluckhohn, and Gregory Bateson initiated psychiatric research in foreign cultures in an attempt to define how culture affects personality. In *Coming of Age in Samoa,* Mead described the seemingly nonstressful behavior of adolescent Samoan girls, which contrasted distinctly from that of adolescent American girls. Based on this difference, she concluded that culture, not biology, was responsible for the nature of this developmental stage. In *Patterns of Culture,* Benedict also emphasized the importance of taking cultural context into account when describing normal and abnormal behavior.

- 1930–1969: As anthropologists studied all over the world, they published the results of their findings on "culture-bound syndromes." For example, amok was studied in Southeast Asia. Esther Lucille Brown, an anthropologist, studied nursing and wrote of the need to include the social sciences in the nursing curriculum (see Chapter 2). In 1937 the National League for Nursing (NLN) officially supported this view by recommending that nursing students complete ten semester hours in the social sciences.

- 1940–1949: Experiences during and after World War II brought the reality of cultural differences home to military nurses. These nurses, hired by schools of nursing, brought cultural content to the curriculum.

- 1950–1959: Anthropologic and sociologic studies about nurses and nursing proliferated. Cornell University School of Nursing invited anthropologists and sociologists to lecture. Margaret Mead wrote an article for *Nursing Outlook* entitled "Understanding Cultural Patterns."

- 1960–1969: Nursing theorists focused on understanding how culture influences mental illness. Interest in indigenous (native) mental health workers (spurred on by the community mental health movement; see Chapter 40) and health care beliefs increased. This interest continues today, along with the desire to work toward giving culturally relevant care to different ethnic groups within our pluralistic society. Madeleine Leininger, a nurse anthropologist, developed and popularized the field of *transcultural nursing,* the study of different cultures, their health care belief systems, and their caring and curative practices. These understandings are used to provide culturally specific nursing care. During the sixties several nurses obtained doctoral degrees in anthropology. In 1969, the Council of Nursing and Anthropology was established within the American Anthropological Association in an effort to bring together people with interests in both fields to study cultural practices relevant to nursing.

- 1970–1979: The Transcultural Nursing Society was established in 1974 and began presenting national transcultural nursing conferences in 1976. In 1977 the NLN required cultural content in all nursing curricula. In 1978 the President's Commission on Mental Health expressed its belief in the value of traditional cultural health belief systems and indigenous healing practices. During that same year the American Psychiatric Association created a Task Force on Cultural and Ethnic Issues in Psychiatry. The chief aims of the task force were to suggest culturally differentiated diagnostic and treatment techniques for various ethnic groups and to include cultural psychiatry in residency training programs for psychiatrists. In 1979 the NLN published a Position Statement on Nursing's Responsibilities to Minorities and Disadvantaged

Groups. In this document the NLN advocated that nursing curricula include information on culture, that disadvantaged or minority group nursing students receive tutoring and assistance if needed, that hospitals hire nurses from different ethnic groups, and that research on nursing care of different ethnic groups be initiated.

- 1980: The American Nurses' Association established the Council on Intercultural Nursing to focus on minority issues in health care.

THEORETICAL FOUNDATIONS

To appreciate the relevance of culture to psychiatric nursing, it is vital to understand several key concepts derived from anthropologic theory. These concepts offer a theoretical framework to guide nursing practice. Although they may appear simplistic and almost self-evident, in practice they are complex. They are much more clearly "felt" and understood when one works with or cares for a person from a different cultural group.

Holism

A distinguishing feature of anthropology and nursing, *holism* is the idea that every part of culture/behavior must be seen within the larger context. Only then can it make sense. From an anthropologic perspective a holistic view encompasses environment, material culture, world view, social structure, and symbolic systems and the interchanges among them. To isolate one component or subsystem is to ignore cultural complexity. One must transcend the individual parts in an effort to see the whole. In practice, nurses are considered to have a holistic approach if they view the client as participating in a specific environment, with its own material culture, ways of communicating, and beliefs about the world. Such nurses recognize that biopsychosociocultural variables influence health and therefore need to be assessed both separately and as part of the entire system.

Culture

Culture consists of the abstract values, beliefs, and perceptions of the world that lie behind people's behavior and are reflected by that behavior. Culture is shared by the members of a society, and when acted on it produces behavior considered acceptable within that society. Cultures are learned, through the medium of language, rather than inherited biologically, and the parts of a culture function as an integrated whole (Haviland 1983). Margaret Mead (1955, pp 12–13) defines culture as:

> an abstraction from the body of learned behavior which a group of people who share the same tradition transmit entire to their children, and, in part, to adult immigrants who become members of the society. It covers not only the arts and sciences, religions and philosophies, to which the word culture has historically applied, but also the system of technology, the political practices, the small intimate habits of daily life, such as the way of preparing or eating food, or of hushing a child to sleep, as well as the methods of selecting a prime minister or changing the constitution.

The following incident illustrates the abstract concept of culture. The headline reads "A Tragedy in Santa Monica" (Reese 1985, p 10):

> On a cold, windy afternoon last January, Fumiko Kimura walked slowly across the beach in Santa Monica, clutched her two young children to her and then, facing her native Japan, waded into the sea. Rescuers spotted the submerged bodies too late to save Kazutaka, four, and Yuri, six months, who gave a tiny gasp for breath and then died. But Kimura survived, consumed with anguish and resentment at herself and those who saved her. "They must have been Caucasians," she thought. "Otherwise they would have let me die."

This scenario, tragic from an American perspective, dramatically reveals how culture influences human beings. In America we view suicide as a negative nihilistic act, a coward's way out. To take one's children is clearly murder and is against the law. In Japan, parent-child suicide is illegal, yet suicide is traditionally viewed as an honorable act. A mother who commits suicide with her children is more honorable than a mother who commits suicide alone, leaving her children to survive without her. The latter woman is viewed as "demonlike." Interestingly, Kimura's grief- and guilt-stricken husband also expressed envy of the bond his wife felt with their children. This story illustrates Margaret Mead's famous statement: "The worlds in which different societies (and individuals) live are distinct worlds, not merely the same worlds with different labels attached." Caring for culturally different clients requires nurses to be aware of this fact.

Culture refers more to the values and beliefs that underlie behavior than to the behavior itself. Culture is always in process, never static. According to Haviland (1983, p 33) subcultural variation is "a distinctive set of standards

and behavior patterns by which a group within a larger society operates."

Value Orientations

Brink (1984) describes value orientations as a part of culture. She examines value orientations as a theoretical construct and as a tool to assess cultural diversity. Brink used the tool with the Annang of Nigeria and suggests its usefulness in trying to understand the cultural perspectives of individual cultures and individual clients. Table 38–1 presents the four different value orientations that Brink adapted from Papajohn and Speigel (1975, p 268).

Subculture

There is some controversy about what exactly is a culture and a *subculture,* or culture within a culture. Recently researchers have referred to the "culture" of the hospital, the operating room, or the nursing school and the "subculture" of the mentally ill, the physically handicapped, or the elderly. Tripp-Reimer (1984) points out that just because people share some common characteristics does not make them members of a culture or subculture. There must be considerable data to indicate more homogeneity for a group to be considered a culture or a subculture. For example, the Choctaw Indians living on a reservation in Philadelphia, Mississippi, are a subculture because they share a language, values and beliefs, and behavioral patterns. They are part of the larger American Indian culture. In contrast, the physically handicapped are not a subculture because they have various disabilities, come from different socioeconomic levels, and may only rarely come into contact with other physically handicapped people.

A case can be made for viewing a hospital or part of it as a culture or subculture. Within the hospital there is a shared language, learned acceptable behavior, and a similar world view. This can be seen even more clearly in specialty units such as intensive care or psychiatric units. People can be viewed as working within a hospital culture while living within the American culture. Using the term *culture* or *subculture* in situations like this may help in understanding a hospital, an emergency room, a school, or a church. Leininger (1970) and Spector (1979) view nursing as a subculture (the health care providers subculture) and document how it has a definite set of beliefs, practices, habits, rituals, and values, often stemming from dominant American cultural values.

World View

The concept of **world view** refers to how a group of people (culture or subculture) see their social world, symbolic system, and physical environment and their own place in

---

Table 38–1
Value Orientations and Preferences: An Interpretative Key

Modalities	Value Orientation Preferences		
Activity	Doing: Emphasis is on activity measurable by standards conceived as external to the acting individual, i.e., achievement (American core culture).	Being: Emphasis is on activity expressing what is conceived as given in the human personality, i.e., the spontaneous expression of impulses and desires (Mexican rural society).	Being-in-becoming: Emphasis is on the kind of activity that has as its goal the development of all aspects of the self as an integrated whole (classical Greek society, yoga, gestalt psychology).
Relational	Individualism: Individual goals are preferred to group goals. Relations are based on individual autonomy; reciprocal roles are based on recognition of the independence of interrelating members (American core culture).	Collaterality: Individual goals are subordinated to group goals; relations are based on goals of the laterally extended group; reciprocal roles are based on a horizontal, egalitarian dimension (Italian extended family).	Lineality: Group goals are preferred to individual goals; relations on a vertical dimension are hierarchically ordered, reciprocal roles are based on a dominance-submission mode of interrelation (British upper class).
Time	Future: The temporal focus is based on the future; emphasis is on planning for change at points in time extending away from present to future (American core culture).	Present: The temporal focus is based on the present; the past gets little attention; the future is seen as unpredictable (Italian and Latin American societies).	Past: The temporal focus is based on the past; tradition is of central importance (traditional Chinese society).
Man-Nature	Mastery-over-nature: Man is expected to overcome the natural forces and harness them for a purpose (American emphasis on technology to solve all problems).	Subjugation-to-nature: Humans can do little to counteract the forces of nature to which they are subjugated (Spanish rural society).	Harmony-with-nature: A sense of wholeness is based on a continual communion with nature and with the supernatural (Japanese and Navaho Indian societies).

Source: Brink P: "Value orientations as an assessment tool in cultural diversity," from Nursing Research, *Vol. 33, No. 4, page 199. Copyright © The American Journal of Nursing Company. Adapted from Papajohn J, Speigel J:* Transactions in Families. *Jossey-Bass, 1975.*

---

each. World view is revealed in people's religion, art, language, values, and health care beliefs and practices. A people's world view provides a sense of identity as an American Indian, a Puerto Rican, or a Masai tribesman. It encourages a group's survival and gives members a generally useful picture of the universe.

A naturalist world view, which is held by hunters and gatherers, reveals a respect for animals and nature. Animals are killed only for food, and even then they are valued and respected. Farmers, pastoralists, and modern humankind share an exploitative world view in which the land and its products exist to be used or exploited. These two different belief systems, to live with nature or to control and improve it, clearly influence a group's approach to the world.

Snow (1974) proposes that Southern rural blacks essentially view the world as a hostile place with inaccessible resources. Consequently, they rely on supernatural solutions to health problems. Roberson (1985) disagrees with Snow, believing that the spiritual beliefs of Southern rural blacks indicate a positive world view—that God is beneficent and loving and, in spite of the difficulties in day-to-day life, God is always there. Roberson points out the interrelationship of religion and health and how religion helps people with the process of living.

Ethnocentrism

Ethnocentrism is the belief that one's own culture is more important and better than any other culture. It is frequently revealed in the form of negative value judgments or selective reporting that criticizes or emphasizes negative aspects of other cultures (Beals 1979).

Health care providers need to be confronted with their own ethnocentric, medicocentric, psychocentric views (see

Kleinman et al 1978). The following are examples of medicocentric beliefs:

- The doctor or nurse knows best.

- Clients must be compliant if they want to get better.

- If clients aren't compliant they don't want to get better and therefore are not worthy of our time.

- Psychiatric clients can be classified according to the DSM-IIIR.

- Because of the nature of their illness psychiatric clients are often noncompliant.

- The description of feelings and thoughts is very important in mental health.

These views are responsible for such professional beliefs as, "Why bother explaining her medication to her; she is ignorant," or "Hispanics have those crazy beliefs in their own witchdoctors. They never do what we say." Such ethnocentric beliefs, spoken or unspoken, inevitably create antagonism among clients and health care personnel. In the present litigious environment, antagonism can easily escalate to legal problems. To avoid this, nurses need to be aware of their own beliefs and values and recognize how these may be different from, not better than, those of the clients they care for. Taking a holistic view reduces the likelihood of ethnocentrism.

Cultural Relativism

Cultural relativism is the fundamental anthropologic concept that all cultures are equally valued. It argues against passing judgments about practices that are unfamiliar, strange, or even shocking to us, suggesting instead that all cultures can be evaluated only on their own values in context.

Combating ethnocentrism is not easy. It takes energy and work and constant assessment of oneself and society. Client problems need to be seen from a cultural relativist's perspective; that is, what does the problem seem like to the client? Only by understanding the client's view can nurses provide effective care. How to do this will become clearer in the next section.

CULTURALLY AWARE STRATEGIES FOR IMPLEMENTING THE NURSING PROCESS

Quality nursing care is culturally sensitive; that is, the nurse is aware of cultural issues that are important to the

client and may affect the client's response to treatment. In planning nursing interventions the nurse does not follow a predetermined plan but plans care that is culturally congruent for each person. For example, if a Hispanic teenage girl is obese and wants to lose weight, the nurse would not hand her a printed 500-calorie diet but would work with her and a nutritionist to create a diet based on the foods she prefers. The nurse would also discuss the care plan with the girl's father and would expect many family members at visiting time. If an Asian client who is a Buddhist wants time each day to meditate, the nurse would build that time into the care plan rather than imposing our frenetic Western pace in which every hour is filled with "constructive," "growth-producing" activity.

Taking a client's culture into consideration when planning care is not an easy task. It is time-consuming and requires patience, insight, and creativity on the part of the nurse.

Transcultural Nursing Premises

Cultural and social class differences between client and nurse may impede a nurse's best intentions. Some fundamental transcultural nursing premises (Henderson and Primeaux 1981) that will help nurses avoid ethnocentric problems are:

- Nurses cannot solve clients' problems, but they may be able to help clients solve their own problems.

- The easiest, least-creative response to transcultural conflict is to pretend that it does not exist.

- Every client behaves according to unwritten ethnic customs and traditions.

- Every successful effort by nurses to teach clients the elements of scientific medicine alienates clients from relatives and friends who do not have this knowledge.

- Previous transcultural experience is a valuable asset when used as a general guide. However, such experience can be a liability if the nurse believes it provides the answer to every transcultural problem.

- Nurses will make mistakes in transcultural interactions, but they should learn from those mistakes and not repeat them.

Understanding One's Own Sociocultural Heritage

Gaining awareness of sociocultural differences requires that nurses first come to understand their own backgrounds and the influence of that background on their practice. Chapter 3 explored some dimensions of self-knowledge through an examination of the concept of professional and personal integration. This chapter urges nurses to

---

Box 38–1
QUESTIONS THAT ACKNOWLEDGE SOCIOCULTURAL HERITAGE

- What ethnic group, socioeconomic class, religions, age group, and community do you belong to?
- What experiences have you had with people from ethnic groups, socioeconomic classes, religions, age groups, or communities different from your own?
- What were those experiences like? How did you feel about them?
- When you were growing up what did your parents and significant others say about people who were different from your family?
- What about your ethnic group, socioeconomic class, religion, age, or community do you find embarrassing or wish you could change? Why?
- What sociocultural factors in your background might contribute to being rejected by members of other cultures?
- What personal qualities do you have that will help you establish interpersonal relationships with persons from other cultural groups? What personal qualities may be detrimental?
- What assumptions do you hold about the people who populate our world?

Box 38–2
EXPLORING SPECIFIC SOCIOCULTURAL ATTITUDES

- I accept opinions different from my own.
- I respond with compassion to poverty-stricken people.
- I think interracial marriage is a good thing.
- I feel uncomfortable in a group in which I am the ethnic minority.
- I consider failure a bad thing.
- I invite people I don't like to my home.
- I believe that the Ku Klux Klan has its good points.
- I set realistic life goals.
- I would enjoy serving as a juror in a rape case.
- I am concerned about the treatment of minorities in employment and health care.
- I feel uncomfortable in low-income neighborhoods.
- I prefer to conform rather than disagree in public.
- I value friendship more than money.
- I maintain high ethical standards as a professional.
- I would not object to premarital sex for my children.
- I spend a lot of time worrying about social injustices without doing much about them.
- I believe that almost anyone who really wants to can get a good job.
- I have a close friend of another race.
- I would rather attend a concert than an athletic contest.

---

acknowledge and explore their own sociocultural heritage. Nurses are better able to meet the sociocultural needs of a client when they acknowledge that a culture and a society influence their beliefs, values, attitudes, and behavior. The questions in Box 38–1 are designed to facilitate acknowledgment of the nurse's own sociocultural heritage. Answering these questions honestly and completely is the important first step in self-awareness. The second step involves exploring beliefs and attitudes that may be different from or the same as those held by the client. Nurses might ponder the statements in Box 38–2 (Henderson and Primeaux 1981, p 55).

Nursing Assessment: Obtaining a Cultural Profile

Fong's (1985) CONFHER model (Table 38–2) is an excellent model for obtaining the client's *cultural profile.* Each variable in Fong's model is elaborated below, primarily in questions designed to elicit the relevant information. Some of this information can be gleaned from observation or from information on the chart. Some is more relevant to nurses caring for clients with biologic illnesses. Depending on the situation some questions may be more useful than others. They should function as a comprehensive guide for gathering and assessing information and for planning care.

Fong suggested that before completing a client's cultural profile, the nurse should complete her or his own cultural profile so that differences and similarities between the client and nurse will be clear, and similarities can be emphasized to help in forming a close therapeutic relationship. Differences may serve as topics for discussion. An open, ongoing dialog is beneficial for both parties. With such a dialog each person will surely learn to understand the other culture better.

Communication Style

Does the client speak English fluently? If not, how limited is the client's ability to communicate in English?

Does the client understand common health terms like *pain, fever,* and *nausea?*

Orientation

Does the client identify with a particular racial (e.g., Asian, African, or American Indian) or ethnic group (e.g., Chinese, Japanese, or Korean)?

Where was the client born?

Where has the client lived and for how long?

How long has the client or the client's ancestors been in America?

How closely does the client adhere to traditional habits and values of his or her cultural system?

The nurse should identify the client's beliefs about:

1. Human nature (basically evil, both good and evil, or basically good)

2. The relationship between humans and nature (people in subjugation to nature, in harmony with nature, or having mastery over nature)

3. Time orientation (past, present, or future)

4. The main purpose of life (being, being in becoming, or doing)

5. People's relationships to one another (lineal, collateral, or individualistic)

Table 38–2 A Cultural Profile: Fong's CONFHER Model	
Cultural Component	**Variable**
Communication style	Language and dialect preference
	Nonverbal behaviors
	Social customs
Orientation	Ethnic identity
	Acculturation
	Value orientation
Nutrition	Symbolism of food
	Preference and taboos
Family relationships	Family structure and roles
	Family dynamics and decision-making style
	Life-style and living arrangements
Health beliefs	Alternative health care
	Health, crisis, and illness beliefs
	Response to pain and hospitalization
	Disease predisposition and resistance
Education	Learning style
	Informal and formal education
	Occupation and socioeconomic level
Religion	Preference
	Beliefs, rituals, and taboos

Source: Fong C: Ethnicity and nursing practice. Top Clin Nurs 1985;7(October):4. Aspen Systems Corp., Rockville, MD. Reprinted by permission.

Would the client like an interpreter or to have the question rephrased in simple English?

Can the client read and write in English?

Are there ethnic behaviors or styles of nonverbal communication to which the client adheres (e.g., the bowing of the head to show respect in the traditional Japanese culture, or frequent smiling and speaking softly in the Southeast Asian culture)?

Does the client mean what he or she says or, does the client give a pleasant, agreeable answer when a literal, factual answer might be unpleasant and embarrassing?

How much physical touching is appropriate in the client's culture?

Nutrition

Are there ethnic foods that the client prefers?

Are there foods the client is encouraged to eat when sick?

Are there foods to be avoided because of ethnic origin, health status, or illness?

Family Relationships

Who is in the family?

Is the client's definition of family nuclear, extended, or tribal?

Who is the head of the household?

Is the family matriarchal or patriarchal?

What is the role and position of women, the aged, male children, and female children within the household?

Who controls the rearing and socialization of children?

How are decisions made in the family?

Who manages financial matters?

How important is it to have the family nearby when the client is sick?

What are important social customs or taboos (e.g., table manners, forms of greetings, and customs between men and women or adults and children)?

What are family priorities and goals (e.g., family solidarity, more children, more money, more material possessions, better housing, higher social status, and optimal health)?

Where does the family live: inner city or suburbs; ethnic enclave; or white or black middle-class neighborhood?

Are art, music, and recreational amenities available?

Health Beliefs

Does the client rely on any self-care or traditional folk medicine practices?

Is the client currently being treated by a cultural healer (e.g., medicine man, Voodoo doctor, Chinese herbalist, or curandero)?

How does the client explain illness (e.g., germ theory, imbalance of yin and yang, or evil spirits)?

How does the client generally respond to pain (e.g., with stoic endurance, with loud cries, or with quiet withdrawal)?

How does the client respond to hospitalization?

Are there any illnesses that are more prevalent in the client's ethnic group (e.g., sickle cell anemia and hypertension among blacks, lactose intolerance among Asians and blacks, myopia among Chinese, or Tay-Sachs among Jews)?

Are there any diseases that the client would have increased resistance to because of ethnic background (e.g., cervical cancer among Jews or skin cancer among blacks)?

Education

Does the client prefer printed literature or audiovisual learning tools?

Does the client learn by trial and error or didactic methods?

What is the client's informal and formal education level?

What is the client's life experience?

Who in the family works?

What is the annual income of the family?

Does the family have health and dental insurance?

Religion

Does the client believe in God or gods?

Does the client have a religious preference?

What religious beliefs, sacred rites, and religious sanctions or restrictions does the client adhere to (e.g.,

beliefs of Christian Scientist, Seventh-Day Adventist, Buddhist, Native American Church, or West African Voodoo)?

What religious persons will be involved in the client's health care (e.g., Catholic priest, Buddhist monk, Islamic imam, or black minister)?

Nursing Assessment: Eliciting the Client's Explanatory Model of Illness

Often health professionals are unaware of or insensitive to the reality that each client has his or her own explanatory model of illness. The medicocentric view envisions a patient as suffering from disease. Kleinman et al. (1978, p 251) define *disease* as abnormalities in structure and function of body organs and systems. In contrast *illness* is the experience of being sick. Whereas disease can be viewed and observed objectively, illness is culturally constructed. It depends on the meanings clients assign to it, which are determined by culture. Frank (1964, p viii) emphasizes the importance of illness:

> Illness always implies certain meanings. Never merely bodily pathology, it has implications for the patient's view of himself and society's view of him . . . Illness may create noxious emotions, cause moral issues, disturb the patient's image of himself, and estrange him from his compatriots. Barred from the front door, these intangibles sneak in at the back, and unless the physician takes them into account, he will often fail.

In this view the physician focuses on the disease while the client focuses on the illness. Given the different perspectives of the health care provider and the client it is easy to see how communication difficulties may arise, clients may not "comply," and anger may build.

The nurse might use the following simulation as a guide to eliciting the client's explanatory model of illness.

I know that nurses and the other staff here sometimes have different ideas about diseases and what causes them. It's important to get clear how both you and I think about it. That's why I'd like to know more about your ideas about (whatever symptom or disorder is relevant to the situation). That way, I can know what your concerns are, and we can work together to help you get better.

Illness Beliefs and Practices

The following questions will help the nurse reveal the client's illness beliefs and practices (Randall-David 1985):

What do you think caused your problem?

Why do you think it started when it did?

What do you think your sickness does to your body? How does it work?

How severe is your sickness? How long do you think it will last?

What are the main problems your sickness has caused for you?

Do you know anyone else who had this problem? What did they do to treat it?

Did you discuss your problem with any of your relatives or friends? What did they say?

What kinds of home remedies, medicines, or other treatments have you tried for your sickness? (Quantity, dosage, frequency, how prepared) Did it help? Are you still using it/them?

What type of treatment do you think you should receive?

What are the most important results you hope to receive from this treatment?

Do you think there is any way to prevent this problem in the future? How?

Is there any other information that would be helpful for designing a workable treatment plan?

It is far more useful to spend time getting answers to these questions and planning culturally relevant interventions than to waste time planning care that will be irrelevant to the client and thus ignored. Besides resulting in ineffective treatment plans, blocked communications will make both clients and professionals resort to their original stereotypes of each other.

Medications and Compliance

One of the biggest problems identified by mental health professionals concerns psychiatric clients' noncompliance with medication orders. The frustrated professional cannot make the client understand that taking medicine "is necessary for the rest of your life" and "is what is keeping you out of the hospital." Amarasingham (1980) recognizes that clients have explanatory models not only about their illness but also about medications. She identifies some common beliefs about medication in our culture:

- Medicine is only necessary as long as you feel sick.
- Diseases can be cured by diet manipulation or exercise.
- Medicine is a contaminating substance.
- Drugs are a "crutch"; it is virtuous not to take drugs.
- You may become immune to drugs if you take them often.

These beliefs directly influence whether a client complies with medication orders. The terms *complies* and *orders* reveal the medicocentric view that the client should do what doctors and nurses think is necessary. Since this method is ineffective, new strategies are required. The concepts of explanatory models, cultural assessment, and negotiation are as useful with the problem of medications as with the more general problem of mental disorder. When medications are prescribed for psychiatric clients, the nurse should attempt to understand the client's beliefs and assumptions about the medication. Then the negotiation process described later in this chapter can begin.

Two problems in the nurse-psychiatric client interaction make the negotiation more difficult:

1. Psychiatric clients generally appear confused about the fact that taking medications helps keep them out of the hospital. Being out of the hospital generally implies wellness, and taking medication implies sickness. This apparent contradiction will need to be clarified over time.

2. Clients with psychiatric illnesses that require medication (depression, bipolar affective disorder, and schizophrenia) often are confused and disorganized and have memory impairment. Consequently, repeated negotiation and explanations are necessary.

The timing and environment for such interactions need to be taken into consideration. The environment should be peaceful and private and the client fairly lucid and relaxed, or the interaction will be unrewarding and ineffective.

Negotiating Health Care Practices

Negotiating among professionals and the client and family about health care practices is aimed at increasing the effectiveness of treatment. A cultural assessment reveals the client's explanatory model of illness. The professional answers similar questions to clarify his or her own explanatory model for the client's "disease." Through discussions and negotiations the client and professional should come to an agreement about treatment. Ideally the treatment will be congruent with both models, and if not actually congruent it will not be counterproductive or harmful. For example, if a Hispanic client wants to eat certain foods to restore the balance and harmony that has gone out of his or her body due to illness, and is also willing to take antidepressant medications, no harm is done and both client and professional are doing what they believe is correct. In contrast, if a hospitalized Buddhist refugee wants to meditate and remain isolated all day and night, additional negotiations will be needed. Perhaps a closely monitored outpatient treatment plan could be devised in which the client agrees to spend a certain number of hours a day with family or friends doing certain activities. The negotiation phase of the process requires excellent interviewing skills, creative listening, and ingenuity in adapting health care practices. However, the labor-intensive work of negotiating shared care plans will pay off in "compliance," and a close therapeutic relationship that is egalitarian rather than hierarchical.

Circumventing the Language Barrier

An interpreter may be necessary if language is a barrier. If the client attempts to speak English, his or her thoughts may appear distorted when language is the real problem. There have been a number of documented instances in which persons have been diagnosed as mentally disordered and confined to a mental hospital because mental health professionals erroneously diagnosed a language problem or value difference as disordered thinking or psychosis. Nonverbal behavior may also be misinterpreted. Boxes 38–3, 38–4, and 38–5 provide specific guidelines for circumventing the language barrier.

Avoiding Cultural Stereotyping

One person cannot be aware of all the cultural factors that should be taken into consideration in planning and implementing a particular psychiatric nursing intervention. A frequent solution to this dilemma is to go to the literature or the resource person likely to know the most about the culture in which we are interested. In doing so, however, we must put the data in the proper perspective. There is a danger of cultural stereotyping, that is, assuming that all members of one ethnic heritage are alike without taking steps to verify the assumption. The following example from Chapman and Chapman (1983) dramatizes a health care team's experience of overenthusiasm for group data about Indian culture.

Maria was brought to the medical center because she seemed to "not be learning right." As a result of an evaluation elsewhere—with which the parents were not happy—they became aware of her epilepsy and that her neurological difficulty was caused by a disease that would be fatal in several years, no matter what was done. The staff at our center immediately developed in their consideration of the family a high sensitivity to their being "special," since they were urban Navajo and had a child soon to die. The staff

> **Box 38–3**
> # GENERAL COMMUNICATION GUIDELINES FOR MONOLINGUAL PROVIDERS IN A CROSS-CULTURAL ENVIRONMENT
>
> 1. Unless you are thoroughly effective and fluent in the target language, always use an interpreter.
>
> 2. Avoid using family members as interpreters.
>
> 3. Learn basic words and sentences in the target language. Asking interpreters about words or comments that have not been translated prompts attention to detail.
>
> 4. Use dictionaries of languages used by your client population. Beware of brief "definitions" that serve only as labels.
>
> 5. Become familiar with special terminology. Specific beliefs, practices, and traditions are often referenced by indirect language or special terms. Local beliefs and moral tenets may lead to overemphasis or underreporting of certain symptoms, issues, and events.
>
> 6. Check the quality of translated health-related materials by having them back-translated.
>
> 7. Meet with your interpreters on a regular basis. They will provide both a window and a mirror when you deal with another language and another culture.
>
> 8. Personal information is often closely guarded and difficult to obtain. Clients often request a specific interpreter or even bring their own.
>
> 9. Evaluate the interpreter's style and approach to clients. For special situations and problem cases, try to match the interpreter to the task.
>
> 10. Be patient. Careful interpretation often requires the interpreter to use long explanatory phrases.
>
> *Source: Adapted from Putsch R: Crosscultural communication. JAMA 1985;254:3347–3348.*

did not know much about the Navajo people and assumed that perhaps the other evaluation center had not fully appreciated that particular culture.

The staff became enthusiastic about formal review of the literature on the Navajo culture and a large workshop conference was held on religious medicine of the Indian culture in general and the practices of the Navajo in particular. Indian participants conferred with us, as did several staff members who had worked on an Arizona Navajo

Box 38–4
GUIDELINES FOR NURSE-INTERPRETER-CLIENT INTERACTIONS

1. Address clients directly. Avoid directing all of your commentary to and through the interpreter.

2. Be certain the interpreter is thoroughly involved with the client during an interview.

3. Develop alternatives to gathering information by direct questions. People who are strangers to direct, Western-style inquiry may respond better to conversational modes.

4. Invite correction and induce the discussion of alternatives: "Correct me if I'm wrong, I understand it this way . . . Do you see it some other way?"

5. Pursue seemingly unconnected issues raised by the client. These issues may lead to crucial information or uncover difficulties with the interpretation.

6. Come back to an issue if you suspect a problem and get a negative response. Be certain the interpreter knows what you want. Use related questions, change the wording, and come at the issue indirectly.

7. Provide instructions in list format. Ask clients to outline their understanding of the plans.

8. If alternatives exist, spell each one out.

9. Emphasize by repetition.

10. Clarify your limitations. The willingness to talk about an issue may be viewed as evidence of "understanding" it or the ability to "fix" it.

11. Rumors, jealousy, privacy, and reputation are crucial issues in closely knit communities. Acknowledge the problem and assure the client of confidentiality.

12. Unless the correct circumstances are devised, it may be impossible to address certain male/female problems by way of discussion or physical examination.

Source: Adapted from Putsch R: Crosscultural communication. JAMA 1985;254:3347–3348.

reservation. The in-service experience was excellent, and we *factually* learned much about the Navajo people.

It was a double-edged experience, however. Many assumptions we had made about this family went by the wayside, since we now "knew" about Navajos; yet it became clear as we talked enthusiastically about applying our new-found knowledge that we were making new assumptions that tended to lump them into a group like "all Navajos." We knew that we had not fallen into the trap of lumping them into Anglo culture. Neither did we feel that we were failing to be "culture conscious." But something was wrong.

Only after we reflected on what *they* had come to us for and began to struggle with what kinds of helping action *they* wanted did we realize that we did not have much detail about *these particular* parents' notion of help—regardless of culture. We retracked with them. Our first surprise was that although they originally came "from the reservation" they knew less about Navajo culture factually than we and experientially less than they both had wanted. They both had been separated from their parents at 5 years of age and spent most of their life in government schools. They related in an embarrassed fashion that they believed that they knew nothing that could be learned from either the Anglo or Navajo cultures. They were lost between two cultures.

They said that they knew that Maria was not going to live a long time. Their anxiety was long and deep and they had to live with that fact in their own way, but *right now* they could not live *with* her happily. She was an overactive, resistive, hard-to-manage child and would allow them to go nowhere without her. She was described as "ruling the roost." Yes, they wanted her to live and learn, but in the here and now they felt helpless and at a loss as to "how to raise her" or any other child whom they might have.

Our other surprise was that they trusted us more than we had assumed that they possibly could. We knew that they periodically used their medicine man when they went back home. We had assumed that they trusted him more and perhaps would not hear us. However, when asked, they stated that they would not have come to us if they did not think that we could help and that they could have gone back to the reservation for help anytime and chose not to with their immediate concerns.

In looking back on this, I sometimes wonder if we would not have saved a lot of time and been more effective if right at the beginning we had simply said to them: "We don't know anything about *you*: we are different; let us spend some time in finding out about each other."

Acting as a Culture Broker

When nurses work with clients from different cultural groups, they can work toward assuming the role of culture broker or helping another person in that role. A **culture broker** essentially functions as a mediator between the people or groups from two cultures. Culture brokers are effective if they have knowledge of the two systems. There are two types of mediators: a hierarchical mediator, who works within the health care system, and a representative mediator, who is from the same ethnic community as the client (LaFargue 1985). The culture broker understands both the health care belief systems and the perspectives of client, family, and professional in the particular situation. Given this understanding the culture broker essentially moves back and forth between groups to ensure client care that is effective, efficient, and viewed as helpful by the client. The culture broker can prevent problems merely by explaining to the professional a client's wish to have numerous visitors or worship in his or her own way with special candles and chanting. Or the culture broker may explain to the client and family that the chanting is fine but that there are hospital rules against candles because of the fire hazard. The aim is to have both sides understand and accept each other and to negotiate the issues either group believes to be important.

Mobilizing Support Systems

The concept of social support has been discussed in general in Chapter 8. Nurses will want to assess a client's support systems and mobilize them when necessary. Support systems are vital to a client's well-being and can be most useful in keeping them out of the hospital. Their functions can be incorporated into the nursing care plan.

Using the knowledge she derived from her anthropologic research with mentally ill Hispanics, Garrison (1978) offers some practical suggestions:

- Mental health services should be localized in small neighborhood units, staffed by persons who are or can become thoroughly acquainted with the concrete social systems of that specific neighborhood.

- Acquaintance with the concrete social systems of the neighborhood can be brought about through interviews with clients in all degrees of disturbance. Influential, potentially helpful members of the community can be identified through reports from clients of their daily lives.

- Severely disturbed persons might be located alone or in pairs in community apartments as long as there are supportive others outside the household.

- Mapping the distribution of clients' residences within the area would show clusters of clients who might be organized into neighborhood-based groups or supportive networks.

- Supportive psychotherapy groups might be based in homes rather than the clinic, particularly in the homes of severely disturbed persons who require assistance to maintain the household.

- Neighbors, "good friends," Pentecostal people, spiritualist mediums, and bodega (a general store or apothecary in a Hispanic community) proprietors are particularly likely candidates to participate in recreated support systems, to provide or recommend foster home placement, or to alert mental health professionals to problems.

- "Living network therapy," or the maintenance of a network of natural associates in the neighborhood context, could probably be accomplished with no greater

---

Box 38–5
GUIDELINES FOR LANGUAGE USE IN INTERPRETER-DEPENDENT INTERVIEWS

1. Use short questions and comments. Technical terminology and professional jargon, like "psychotropic medication," should be reduced to plain English.

2. When lengthy explanations are necessary, break them up and have them interpreted piece by piece in straightforward, concrete terms.

3. Use language and explanations the interpreter can handle.

4. Make allowances for terms that do not exist in the target language.

5. Try to avoid ambiguous statements and questions.

6. Avoid abstractions, idiomatic expressions, similes, and metaphors. It is useful to learn about these usages in the target language.

7. Plan what you want to say ahead of time. Avoid confusing the interpreter by backing up, inserting a proviso, rephrasing, or hesitating.

8. Avoid indefinite phrases using *would, could, if,* and *maybe.* These can be mistaken for actual agreements or firm approval of a course of action.

9. Ask the interpreter to comment on the client's word content and emotions.

Source: Adapted from Putsch R: Crosscultural communication. JAMA 1985;254:3347–3348.

---

expenditure of money or professional time than is now spent on the same group of clients in medication maintenance.

- Quasi-groups and action sets can be mobilized in the support of clients, or can be cued to mobilize themselves in times of crisis for a client discharged into the community.

- Mental health services would probably be used more readily, and dropouts would be fewer, if time and attendance were structured less rigorously than is conventional in most mental health clinics. Walk-in services without fixed appointments and group activities without fixed membership are two examples of patterns congenial with those found in the natural community.

- Mental health services integrated with general medical clinics would be more acceptable to this population and probably better used than freestanding facilities.

Incorporating Research Findings

Lawson (1986) reviewed research that concerns itself with racial and ethnic factors in pharmacotherapy and biologic psychiatry. The findings of these many research projects are as follows:

- Black and Hispanic clients with bipolar affective disorder may hallucinate more than white clients. This may contribute to misdiagnoses of schizophrenia.

- Black schizophrenics may show more paranoia, hallucinations, and delusions than whites.

- Black clients with mood disorders may have more hallucinations, delusions, hostility, and somatization. Whites may have a greater degree of mania, depression, or guilt.

- Because depression is often unrecognized in racial and ethnic minorities, biologic assessment tools may be useful for diagnosis.

- Asians require lower dosages than whites for numerous psychotropic medications, such as lithium, antidepressants, and neuroleptics.

- Asians experience side-effects at lower doses of psychotropic medications than blacks or whites.

- Asians show higher plasma levels of diazepam at a given oral dose than whites.

- Asians tolerate better the sedating effects of diphenhydramine.

- Hispanics require less antidepressant medication and report more side-effects at dosages half the Anglo therapeutic dose.

- Black schizophrenics and depressed clients improve more than whites with phenothiazines and tricyclic antidepressants.

- Blacks have greater anxiety reduction with antianxiety and antidepressant agents.

- Blacks show more improvement with a tricyclic antidepressant in one week.

- Blacks who overdosed on amitriptyline had higher levels of antidepressants than whites who overdosed.

- Blacks show a significantly longer plasma lithium half-life and a higher ratio of red blood cell lithium to plasma lithium than whites or Asians.

Racial and ethnic differences have been found in serum creatinine phosphokinase (CPK), platelet serotonin, and HLA-A2. Consequently, when researchers aim to evaluate these biologic markers they must control for race. Lawson advocates more research on safe and effective doses of medications for different racial and ethnic groups. Not to do so and not to have different dose ranges for different ethnic groups can have dangerous consequences for clients.

Racial and ethnic factors also play a role in perceptual and diagnostic research. For example:

- An in-patient staff in one study perceived blacks as more violent than whites, although objective findings revealed blacks to be less violent.

- Other studies show blacks receive more p.r.n. medication and may spend more time in seclusion than whites.

- Blacks are more often diagnosed as schizophrenic when they really suffer from mood disorders (Jones and Gray 1986).

Jones and Gray believe such misdiagnoses result from cultural differences in language and mannerisms, difficulties in relating between black clients and white therapists, and the myth that blacks rarely suffer from affective disorders. They point out that in physical illness, physicians search for the causative agent and examine it in the context of symptoms. In psychiatry, by contrast, professionals can determine no causative agent, so they diagnose based on signs, symptoms, and behaviors. Different illnesses may involve the same symptoms, and particular symptoms and behaviors are culturally determined in part, making diagnosis difficult. Misdiagnosis may occur because white therapists don't understand black clients' use of language and therefore may believe it is indicative of a thought disorder; they may view a black client's style of relating as a disturbance of affect and his or her mannerisms as bizarre.

The essence of all this research is that racial and ethnic factors are clearly linked to people's biologic makeup. Much more knowledge in this area is needed so safe treatment can be given to clients. The research also shows that racial bias can have serious consequences in terms of diagnosis and treatment.

FOLK BELIEFS AND HEALING PRACTICES

Folk beliefs and healing practices are culture-specific ways of handling physical problems and emotional conflicts. For example, members of some cultural groups, such as Chicanos and Appalachian whites, believe that illnesses caused by witches' spells may not respond to drugs. This may account for a client's seeming noncompliance with a treatment plan. In some other ethnic groups—such as the Indians of North, Central, and South America; Chinese Americans; and Japanese Americans—herbal products are used to treat both physical and mental disorders. The culturally unaware mental health team member may not know that such herbs are being used or that they may produce both positive or negative interactions with medications.

Folk beliefs and healing practices reflect the world view of the particular culture. In most Western societies disease is viewed as the result of such natural phenomena as microbes, viruses, chromosomal abnormality, or chemicals. Many Third World people, however, believe that supernatural forces cause illness, and that cures can be effected by appealing to the supernatural force through witches or sorcerers or by controlling the force with magic.

Despite the fact that many people from different cultures become "westernized" in appearance and overt behavior when they move to the United States, they often retain their folk beliefs. One study of 450 college students in the United States and Ireland revealed that about 70 percent of the students relied on such magic as carrying good luck charms to an exam, crossing their fingers, having a lucky number, or knocking on wood. Reliance on magic can be seen even in technologically advanced groups. People often use magic to control things they feel they cannot control.

Being aware of **folk health care systems** will help the nurse provide better health care to particular groups of people. Culturally aware nurses will be able to devise more meaningful nursing care plans and perhaps discover ways in which the middle-class Western system of health care can be humanized by incorporating folk beliefs and practices. The clinical example below demonstrates how an understanding of folk health care systems can be used to facilitate mental health treatment.

Henri, a 21-year-old Haitian refugee, was brought by his family to the emergency room of a large general hospital in Miami. Family members believed Henri to be possessed by an evil spirit. They told the emergency room staff that they had been unable to control him for two days. He had been breaking dishes and glasses in the family's small apartment, shouting obscene curses in Creole at his mother, and attacking his brother on a number of occasions, screaming, "I am God the Son." Psychiatrists summoned by the ER staff prescribed massive doses of tranquilizers, and arranged for his transfer to the in-patient psychiatric unit, where Henri remained for three more days with no decrease in his violent behavior. A surgical staff nurse who had been raised in Cuba and was familiar with Santeria (Cuba's folk blend of Catholicism and mysticism) heard of Henri's strange behavior. She suggested to one of her colleagues on the psychiatric unit that a Voodoo practitioner might be helpful. After the psychiatric nurse confirmed that the family did believe in Voodoo, she brought the suggestion to a team conference. After much heated discussion the team decided to try an exorcism by a Voodoo priest if the family agreed. The exorcism was carried out at the offices of a community mental health outreach center in Miami's Little Haiti. The in-patient psychiatric staff who observed the exorcism ceremony found that their client became very quiet after it. Henri returned to their unit where professional treatment was continued and he improved rapidly.

The unique aspect of this situation is that the psychiatric team was able to allow for a folk health care system that stood in opposition to the system of health care they espoused. There is a strong contradiction between professional and folk health systems in terms of the relationship between practitioners and clients. In folk systems, both practitioner and client define the nature of illness and health, while in professional systems practitioners are likely to have a monopoly on defining the nature of illness and health. The process of treatment is another basis for comparison. In folk systems, the process of treatment is a social act, while in professional systems it is a technologic act. The folk systems of some specific groups—Black Americans, Hispanic Americans, Asian Americans, and American Indians—are discussed more thoroughly in the following sections.

Professional, Folk, and Popular Domains of Health Care

The *professional domain of health care* refers to psychiatrists, social workers, and nurses—institutionally sanctioned health care workers. These people generally focus on the disease process through a process of scientific assessment and diagnosis. As the professionals become enlightened to the possibly conflicting explanatory models of disease and illness, it is hoped they will learn to treat illness along with disease. Interestingly, 90 percent of clients who come to health care providers have already attempted to treat their illness with folk or popular methods.

Folk healers, the *folk domain of health care,* are healers such as root doctors, high priests from the cult of Santeria, or faith healers. Although these healers are considered nonprofessional, they are experts within their system. Some of the practices of these healers may sound bizarre, primitive, and unscientific, but the people who believe in them can document their healing abilities.

A young Hispanic girl had been admitted to the adolescent psychiatric unit for agitated behavior and apparent hallucinations and delusions. An interview revealed that she was being treated by a Santeria priestess (described later in the chapter). She chanted periodically, fondled a cluster of charms around her neck, and later told the nurse that she had been cured before by the priestess and she felt that with time the priestess would cure her again.

The effectiveness and power of folk healers should not be underestimated. A more useful approach is to find out everything possible about the healing practice to determine how it fits in with professional treatment. It is generally recognized that folk practitioners work on treating the illness and not the disease. Often if they view a problem as being out of their realm of expertise they will refer the client to a medical professional.

The *popular domain of health care* refers to family and friends who function in the role of healer by offering health information, emotional support, prayers, and advice.

Peg was a real "health nut" and believed that one's mental outlook was directly related to food intake and exercise. When her friends or family became depressed she lectured them on exercising to increase endorphins and told them what kinds of foods encouraged or prohibited sleep. According to Peg, almost any type of mental or physical problem could be treated by disciplined eating and exercise habits.

A client's explanatory model of illness does not simply derive from one or two domains of health care. It represents a blend of information from past and present experiences and education. Aiming for clarity in understanding the client's model encourages a therapeutic relationship based on mutual respect.

Black Americans

Black Americans, the largest racial minority group in America, are a large and diverse group of people who have one thing in common: African ancestors. Black Americans are young, old, poor, rich, rural, urban, tall, short, light, dark, religious, atheist, educated, and uneducated (Capers 1985). Ever since the slaves arrived in 1619, blacks have lived parallel to white American society. Capers (1985) points out that although they move in and out of white society, blacks are generally socialized among blacks and still suffer from racial prejudice and discrimination.

It is not easy to categorize the folk systems and healing practices of black Americans for a number of reasons. The system is a unique blend of African folklore, fundamentalist Christianity, the Voodoo religion of the West Indies, and some tenets of both classic and modern medicine. Folk medicine is more likely to be important to black Americans who live in the southern United States or rural areas or who are recent immigrants, because they are less likely to

have been thoroughly assimilated into the larger culture. However, folk practices may also be important to black Americans living in the urban Northeast and the West.

Health Care Beliefs and Practices

Blacks have historically been responsible for their own health care because the white American health care system did not accept them. Thus indigenous healing beliefs and practices are a core part of black culture. These health beliefs and practices did not originate in isolation but are integrally linked to the people's world view. Some of these beliefs are (Roberson 1985):

- Physical and mental illness and spiritual problems are all interrelated (see the Research Note).
- Some illnesses are natural and can be treated by natural agents (herbs), while others are supernatural, that is, caused by witchcraft and evil people.
- Conflict in one's life can cause illness.
- Magic and witchcraft can counteract evil spells.
- People determine the cause of their illness and then go to the practitioner of their choice.
- People can be treated simultaneously by representatives of three domains of health care: a professional health care provider (professional domain); a faith healer or a root doctor (folk domain); and a grandmother or head of the family (popular domain).
- God is the ultimate healer.
- The bible has much useful information about health care.
- Prayer and belief in God are helpful healing strategies.
- Sin, stress, the devil, and a negative attitude may cause sickness.

Rootwork or Voodoo

If a person believes he or she has been hexed by another person a **root doctor (Voodoo man or woman)** is necessary to remove the hex or put a hex on someone else. The hex can cause illness, which frequently mimics mental disorder, by infusing the person with evil spirits. People believe they are hexed by ingesting food with something in it or by walking over the offending object. Plants, herbs, ground glass, and other substances can be used in putting on or neutralizing the hex ("fix," "mojo").

Voodoo is a West African word that means god or spirit. According to Voodoo, a religion, the spirits of the dead can visit the world of the living to bless or curse people. In Haiti, a blend of Voodoo and Catholicism called *Vodun* is of prime importance in the religious life of Haitian peasants. Voodoo priests (*Houngan*) or priestesses (*Mambo*) may exorcise evil spirits or may cause injury to an enemy by sticking pins into a wax image of the enemy. Voodoo and other forms of spiritualism are integral to the folk medicine of black Americans.

Faith Healing

Spiritual or **faith healers** deal with illness ascribed to spiritual or supernatural causes. The client may have somatic symptoms but will seek out a faith healer in one of two places:

1. In the community, faith healers function autonomously and are not part of organized religion.
2. Within a church, usually the Church of God, faith healers have revivals, during which people make testimonials or present themselves to be healed.

Nursing Practice Issues

In order to give good nursing care to black clients it is vital for nurses to understand their historical background and cultural values and beliefs. Racism is an additional issue. The long history of racism has resulted in an often unarticulated and even unrealized lack of trust, with prejudice and often discrimination on both sides. Racism is rooted in our culture and cannot be denied. Griffith, a black psychiatrist, believes that the central problem throughout American life is that "black and white perceptions of reality, of what is important, are discordant" (1986, p 5). Therefore, white nurses must be sensitive to racial issues when working with black clients. Racism in psychiatric-mental health care will increase clients' feelings of inadequacy, powerlessness, and frustration, and can deprive them of a sense of control and hope (Brantley 1983). Such issues directly affect transference and countertransference and therefore should be confronted openly. For example, "How do you feel about having a white nurse?" Some black clients may desire a black nurse and, if possible, their request should be granted. If not, part of the therapeutic process can focus on dealing with the black-white problems. Black professionals working with black clients need to be careful not to overidentify with the client's aggression. Instead, they need to help the client view racism as a reality and to learn useful coping strategies (Brantley 1983). Psychiatric nurses in in-patient units have often discussed how black nurses and attendants are often much more effective than white staff with black male patients. Such realities should be considered when client assignments and interventions are initiated as the example below demonstrates.

John G, a 35-year-old black male, was brought into the locked unit screaming, kicking, and hallucinating. He was extremely paranoid and cowered in the corner for five days, withdrawing from the staff. He appeared frightened and became hostile and violent when approached. Bill, a black male attendant, was the only staff member who could talk with him. Bill began to check on John hourly and slowly began to increase the time he spent talking quietly and calmly to John. The bond between John and Bill was considered central to John's progress.

Nurses also need to recognize that cultural variables are directly related to client behavior. For example,

Georgia, a 50-year-old black woman, was admitted to the psychiatric unit for the third time for depression. An

---

RESEARCH NOTE

Citation

Allen L, Graves P, Woodward E: *Perceptions of problematic behavior by southern female black fundamentalists and mental health professionals.* Health Care Women Int 1985;6:87–104.

Study Problem/Purpose

The purpose of the study was to compare the perceptions of problematic behavior by mental health professionals with those of a sample of black female fundamentalists.

Methods

The sample was composed of twenty black female fundamentalists and twenty mental health professionals. In personal interviews, ten vignettes, each describing problematic behaviors, were used to elicit responses that were dichotomized as "mental illness/no mental illness," and "treatment/no treatment." Data were analyzed by chi-square test.

Findings

Mental health professionals were more likely to classify the behavior as indicative of mental illness than the fundamentalist minority group. Among the fundamentalists, most "no mental illness" responses were related to religious beliefs. Other responses labeled behaviors as immoral, criminal, or psychic. Types of management recommended by black subjects often included prayer and religious counseling.

Implications

Transcultural nursing studies should pay attention to those religious beliefs that may underlie what is perceived as "normal" or "abnormal."

examination of her progress notes indicated she had been treated with a variety of antidepressants. An interview revealed she had severe financial problems that influenced her housing situation, she was in the middle of a crisis with one of her children, and her husband had recently died.

In this situation, which is common with poor blacks and poor people generally, antidepressants were not enough. Nurses need to assess the realities of a client's life and their relationship to the presenting illness. Instead of viewing Georgia as the disease category *depressed,* the nurse needs to plan intervention strategies that take into account the sociocultural variables. Helping her decide how to manage her finances and find an acceptable place to live are good beginning goals. When these basic needs are taken care of, the nurse can focus on Georgia's concerns about her child's crisis and her grief about her husband's death.

Asian Americans

People whose ethnic heritage is identified with China, Japan, Korea, Southeast Asia, and such Pacific islands as Samoa, Guam, and the Philippines are identified as Asian American. According to Chang (1981), American nurses are more likely than ever before to have contact with clients from Asian backgrounds because of the recent influx of new immigrants from these countries. No one set of characteristics describes or categorizes Asian Americans, since there are similarities as well as differences among these various groups of people. Most of the specific examples in this section relate to Chinese Americans and Japanese Americans because together they constitute the largest Asian American population in the United States.

A strong Chinese influence pervades the folk systems of all Asian people. Traditional Chinese medicine is a well-organized system of medical theory with a strong philosophical character. It uses herbs, other flora, acupuncture, acupressure, massage, and nutrition principles, which also figure prominently in the holistic health movement. A resurgence of interest in traditional Chinese medicine in the People's Republic of China is resulting in the integration of these traditional forms of healing with Western biomedical science. "Barefoot doctors" in China are agricultural workers in rural communes who receive special training as part-time medical workers to provide integrated health care (Weisberg and Graham 1977). Unlike much of Western medicine, this form of health care focuses on preventing illness.

Health Care Beliefs and Practices

Some of the health beliefs and practices of Asian Americans are:

- Health is present when natural forces are balanced; illness prevails if these forces are out of balance.
- There is no difference between physical and emotional illnesses.
- Mental disorder is stigmatized.
- The popular culture (family and friends) is used for mental health problems, which are reported as somatic complaints; hospitalization is suggested only for psychotic clients.
- As authorities, physicians and nurses are to be respected and obeyed. They tell the client what to do.
- Emotional control of feelings (fear, pain, anger) is good; self-assertion and expressions of individuality are not good.
- Treatments include herbs prescribed for specific ailments, nutritional therapy, moxibustion, cupping, acupuncture, and skin scraping.

Chinese folk medicine evolved from a systems view of the universe. Each organism in the universe interacts with and is affected by all others in the universe. The system derives its energy from the **yin and yang,** two opposing forces that must be perfectly balanced to maintain physical and mental health and social harmony (Campbell and Chang 1981). The yang is a positive force that produces light, warmth, and fullness, while the yin is a negative force that produces darkness, cold, and emptiness. In Asian American folk systems some parts of the body are yang and others are yin. Yin and yang are also symbols for hot and cold with yin being a cold energy force and yang a hot energy source. Hot foods are used to treat yin illnesses and cold to treat yang illnesses. See Table 38–3 for a general guide to hot and cold diseases or conditions and their treatment. Many Hispanic Americans also share these beliefs.

Certain foods can restore balance, and herbs are also used to correct an energy imbalance. Louie (1985a) also describes other treatments.

Skin scraping: Corn is dropped in water and rubbed over the skin—for heat stroke, headaches, indigestion, and colic.

Cupping: A cup filled with heat is put on the skin and adheres due to the heat—for arthritis, stomachaches, bruises, and paralysis.

Moxibustion: A plant is burned in a small wooden box and then the box is placed on the skin—for mumps, convulsions, nosebleeds, and backaches.

Acupuncture: Needles are inserted into certain areas of the body—for many illnesses and for surgery.

Tai-Chi exercises, which are graceful and appear to be almost a slow motion ballet, are performed regularly by many Chinese people.

Cao gio (coining), a treatment that is similar to skin scraping, is practiced by Cambodians and Vietnamese for fever or headache. The caregiver uses great pressure and rubs a coin up and down the person's body until red marks appear. In numerous instances children with such marks have been considered child abuse victims when they entered our Western health care system.

The Japanese code of behavior, Wabi-Sabi (Box 38–6), has some similarities to the Chinese belief system. However, the professional should never assume that all Asians are alike. Differences among these varied cultural groups will be revealed in a cultural assessment and in the negotiation for treatment.

Nursing Practice Issues

Social harmony is of vital importance to Asian Americans. In an effort to maintain this harmony many avoid conflict and confrontation. This means they may smile and agree when they really disagree, and their conversation may appear vague and unfocused.

In assessing all Asian clients it is important to attempt to understand how they adjust to American society. Sue (1981) describes three possibilities:

1. The *traditionalists* retain their traditional values and reject Western beliefs and practices. Generally the older generation, traditionalists feel much conflict with the later generation, i.e., their children and grandchildren, who often give up some traditions.

2. The *marginal people* essentially "go native" and completely embrace Western values. Marginal people may have an identity crisis that is discovered during psychiatric treatment. Young refugees are often in this category. In an effort to cope they put down traditional values and those who represent them because they appear so out of place in Western society.

3. *Asian Americans* are able over time to develop a new integrated identity while both retaining traditional beliefs and acquiring Western beliefs and practices.

Table 38–3
Hot and Cold Diseases or Conditions and Their Treatment

Hot Diseases or Conditions	Cold Diseases or Conditions	Hot Foods	Cold Foods	Hot Medicines and Herbs	Cold Medicines and Herbs
Constipation	Cancer	Aromatic beverages	Barley water	Anise	Bicarbonate of soda
Diarrhea	Common cold	Cereal grains	Bottled milk	Aspirin	Linden
Hypertension	Earache	Cheese	Cod	Castor oil	Milk of magnesia
Infections	Headache	Chili peppers	Fresh vegetables	Cinnamon	Orange flower water
Kidney diseases	Joint pain	Chocolate	Honey	Cod liver oil	Sage
Liver complaints	Malaria	Coffee	Low-prestige meats (goat, fish, chicken)	Garlic	
Rashes and other skin eruptions	Menstrual period	Eggs	Raisins	Ginger root	
Sore throat	Paralysis	Goat milk	Tropical fruits	Iron preparations	
Ulcers	Pneumonia	Hard liquor		Mint	
Upset stomach	Postpartum	High-prestige meats (beef, water fowl, mutton)		Penicillin	
Venereal disease	Pregnancy	Oils		Tobacco	
Warts	Rheumatism	Onions		Vitamins	
	Stomach cramps	Peas			
	Teething	Temperate-zone fruits			
	Tuberculosis				

Box 38–6

WABI-SABI: THE TRADITIONAL JAPANESE CODE OF BEHAVIOR

- The tendency is to act in groups and to respect others.

- The aim is to achieve harmonious accord between men and man and to avoid discord and dissent.

- The Japanese physician is as much a minister as a medical attendant.

- The Japanese prefer not to be told the "truth" about illness so they can maintain faith and hope. They believe the truth isolates clients.

- A characteristic proverb is, "The nail that protrudes will surely be hammered down." This is also expressed in the statement, "If it makes one person happy to wear black, we want everyone to be happy wearing black."

Source: Adapted from Schor J: Wabi-sabi: The traditional Japanese code of behavior. JAMA 1984;252:3173.

The type of adjustment has implications for client care. For example, a marginal person may prefer individual therapy while a traditionalist may accept only medication.

Since the extended family unit is so important to Asians, and because the individual is subjugated to the group, individual psychotherapy may not be a useful treatment modality. Family therapy may be more useful. Because Asians are private and do not generally discuss personal or family issues with strangers, an extended time period may be necessary for therapy. The nurse should be cautious in raising issues that appear conflictual or that evoke strong feelings (Louie 1985a). Because Asians will express their symptoms physically, many will want medication for relief.

Traditional Asians are suspicious of negotiation with a professional. They expect the professional to know best and prefer to be told what to do. Consequently, structure and education are useful.

Hospitalization poses a severe threat to Asians. Because they deplete all the family resources before they come to the hospital, the fear of separation from the family and the fear of death are present in the entire family system. Permitting the family to bring food and be involved in therapy is useful. Food is very symbolic to Asians. Certain foods even have medicinal purposes. In hospitals in China families cook the food for their family members as often as possible. In China people don't say "How are you?" but "Have you eaten?" Drinking tea, an omnipresent ritual in the East, may help the client feel more welcome. Drinking tea together is an act of sharing, friendship, and social will.

Asians feel that touching between strangers, boys and girls, or parents and children (after the age of 8) is inappropriate. Touching the head of a person may be construed as an attempt to rob the spirit. While Americans communicate with a wide range of facial expressions, Asians communicate primarily with their eyes.

Hiring Asian nurses and psychiatrists is a logical answer for Asian clients. However, Asian psychiatrists suggest that traditionalist clients may "lose face" by expressing their private thoughts and familial difficulties to an Asian therapist; a Western therapist would be more nonthreatening. As with blacks, the issue of countertransference (overidentification with or rejection of the client) is also significant (The Asian Pacific American 1978).

Two additional points are useful for nurses to know:

1. Asians give gifts as appreciation rituals. They are offended if the gift is rejected.

2. Our focus on time—the therapy "hour"—is offensive to Asians. They spend hours getting to know people and see predetermined abrupt endings as rude. More flexible time schedules are useful in enhancing a trusting relationship.

American Indians

The category *American Indians* refers to numerous groups of people in the United States who have different cultures but share the fact that they have been oppressed by the American majority. Some were sheepherders, others farmed or fished, and still others raised livestock. Most lost their land and consequently suffered from social and cultural disintegration. Today the various groups are in different stages of economic development. Generally, however, Indians are poor, are discriminated against, and have a high incidence of alcoholism. Violence, suicide, and family breakdown are additional problems. Probably because of rapid culture change, some Indian tribes have been described as "self-destructing."

Health Care Beliefs and Practices

Some general characteristics of American Indian health care beliefs and practices are:

- Medicine and religion are inextricably linked.

- Illness occurs because a person is out of balance with nature and the universe.

- The Native American Church (the peyote religion) is essentially a healing ritual.

- The shaman (medicine man) heals with herbs and plants.

- Chanting, incantations, charms (to ward off evil), and fetishes are used in healing rituals, along with dance and the shaking of a rattle.

- Native American languages do not have clear-cut terms for mental disorders, which are seen as a lack of harmony.
- Private thoughts are kept to oneself.

In American Indian culture, the word *medicine* can be equated with *mysterious*. It is linked to the supernatural religious experience central to the existence of the American Indian. According to Henderson and Primeaux (1981, p 244), it is impossible to separate Indian medicine and religion or to make distinctions between physical and mental illness.

The shaman is the central healing figure. Because the Native American theory of disease includes physical, social, psychologic, and environmental aspects, closely intertwined with spiritual and religious aspects, the germ theory is rejected. The shaman conducts a tribal healing ceremony, a highly ritualized and religious way of coping with illness and death. The shaman may also involve family members in the healing ritual, because family members (including a large extended family of cousins, aunts, uncles, etc.) are important sources of support during periods of crisis. It may be important to the family and to the client to have the healing ceremony carried out at the bedside of a hospitalized person. A medicine bundle containing charms or fetishes to ward off evil; a bag of herbs, plants, or roots to provide the curative aspect; a drum or rattle; and a special costume for the shaman may all be integral parts of the healing ceremony. The rattle may be shaken, or the drum beaten, while the healer chants the remedies revealed to him by the spirits.

Foods have symbolic meaning as well as nutritional value to Native Americans. For example, before visitors enter a home, the occupants sprinkle cornmeal on their shoulders in order to prevent them from bringing illness inside. Cornmeal may also be sprinkled around the bed of a hospitalized person or directly on the client (Henderson and Primeaux 1981, p 245).

A few authors have written about the concepts of disorder indigenous to certain Indian tribes. These authors point out the bias that exists because the descriptions of these disorders, also called **culture-bound syndromes**, are not analyzed within the cultural context. Studies that attempt to understand how these illnesses fit in with the life-style and world view of the people would be a useful contribution. Briefly, these disorders and their symptoms are (Trimble et al. 1984):

- *Windigo psychosis.* In this disorder, the person has symptoms of melancholia and a craving for human flesh and believes that he or she has been transformed into a windigo, who has a heart of ice. There is disagreement over whether cannibalism really occurs.
- *Pibloqtok,* or active hysteria. In this convulsive hysterical seizure, the person at first is withdrawn and then becomes wildly excited, experiences convulsive seizures, and collapses. After sleep the individual appears

perfectly normal and does not remember the experience. (See the first clinical example at the beginning of this chapter.)

- *Soul loss.* This disorder is characterized by sudden and repeated fainting, withdrawal, self-deprecation, and preoccupation with death and dead relatives.
- *Spirit intrusion.* A variety of symptoms are associated with spirit intrusion, including anorexia, insomnia, and apathy alternating with restlessness, crying spells, nostalgic dependency, dyspnea, pericardial sensations, and vague spastic pains. This disorder appears similar to what is known as agitated depression and is believed to be caused by evil spirits or ghosts.
- *Taboo breaking.* This disorder is brought on by broken taboos, usually involving sexual behavior. Symptoms can include mild weight loss, sleeplessness, fatigue, edema, headaches, heavy or irregular menstruation among women, mood swings, paranoia, and epileptic-like seizures.
- *Ghost sickness.* Believed due to evil power, ghost sickness can cause weakness; nightmares; feelings of danger, futility, and suffocation; confusion; loss of appetite; fainting; dizziness; and fear.

Dietary deficiencies are also suggested as possible causes for windigo psychosis and pibloqtok.

Nursing Practice Issues

In caring for American Indians the nurse needs always to be aware of the meaning given to nature and the environment. See Box 38–7 for an Indian prayer that conveys this sense of harmony with nature. Keeping this in mind, the nurse can thoughtfully develop a nursing care plan that takes these needs into consideration. Perhaps a home health nurse can care for Indian clients in their own environment. Nurses can also permit many family members to visit in the hospital since the family is so important. Permitting the shaman or an Indian healer to come into the hospital for curing rituals may also aid the Indian client's recovery. See Box 38–8 for a contemporary update on what it's like to be an Indian.

Hispanic Americans

By the year 2000 Hispanics will comprise 40 percent of the United States population. The Hispanic population is generally a young population that has difficulties with education, housing, and employment, all of which affect their mental health needs (Hispanic Americans 1978). The Hispanic American population includes a number of diverse ethnic groups from Spanish-speaking countries in Central and South America and some Caribbean islands. It would be an error to assume that all Spanish-speaking groups share the same beliefs. Some of the subcultural differences between Mexican Americans, Puerto Ricans, and Cubans, for example, are discussed below.

It is important to recognize that many Chicanos (Mexican Americans) are not immigrants but were born in the United States. Many live in the Southwest. Puerto Ricans are United States citizens and enter and leave the country as they desire. They tend to live in New York and other areas of the Northeast. Many Cubans left their homes for political reasons and now reside in southern Florida. The group differences are directly related to their varied histories. Even the most apparent commonality, language, is not always shared, since several Spanish dialects are spoken in the United States.

Health Care Beliefs and Practices

The list below summarizes many of the health care beliefs and practices of Hispanic Americans.

- The family is central to Hispanic culture. If a problem exists, the family is the first source of support.
- Older family members (especially males) must be consulted before treatment or hospitalization is accepted.
- Families keep very sick family members at home for a long time. (This can be a problem with certain physical illnesses, schizophrenia, or bipolar affective disorder.)
- If a person is hospitalized, the family wants to care for and eat and spend the night with the person. They want to share in the suffering.
- Males are responsible for elders, women, and children, so they require authority over the system and family members.
- Three concepts are basic to a Hispanic's way of life: *respeto* (intrinsic worth of the individual and subsequent pride in oneself), *carino* (giving and receiving love at the same time), and *dignidad* (strong belief in the dignity of individuals and their value as human beings (Hispanic Americans 1978).
- Independence and interdependence are positively valued.
- There is no differentiation between physical and emotional illnesses because the mind and the body are inseparable.
- Mental illness (hospitalization or a medical diagnosis) implies stigma and loss of respect.

Box 38–7
AN INDIAN PRAYER

O GREAT SPIRIT,
Whose voice I hear in the winds,
and whose breath gives life to all the world,
hear me! I am small and weak, I need your
strength and wisdom.
Let me walk in beauty, and make my eyes
ever behold the red and purple sunset.
Make my hands respect the things you have
made and my ears sharp to hear your voice.
Make me wise so that I may understand the
things you have taught my people.
Let me learn the lessons you have hidden
in every leaf and rock.
I seek strength, not to be greater than my
brother, but to fight my greatest
enemy—myself.
Make me always ready to come to you with
clean hands and straight eyes.
So when life fades, as the fading sunset,
my spirit may come to you
without shame.

- The popular system (family and friends) is the first system people turn to for help, the second is a folk healer, and the third is a medical professional.
- People are innocent victims of malevolent external or internal forces.
- **Susto** (fright sickness) has a natural cause.
- Many folk beliefs have a religious basis; accidents and illnesses are caused by the wrath of God or a saint, by the evil eye (*mal de ojo*), or susto.
- A hot-cold (*caliente-frio*) imbalance of body humors is responsible for disease.

Mal de Ojo

Mal de ojo is thought to be the result of a witch purposefully casting a spell or a person involuntarily injuring a child by looking admiringly at it. Magical amulets of coral and jet, scapulars of the saints, and tiny bags of salt or garlic around the neck or wrist are used to help protect one from the evil eye. The fear of severe injury or death from the evil eye is so great that it may contribute to what Engel (1971) calls a *lethal life situation,* an otherwise sudden and unexplained rapid death under conditions of psychologic stress.

Espiritismo and Santeria

Among Mexican Americans, Cubans, and Puerto Ricans the **espiritisto,** spiritualist, or medium, is believed to be capa-

Box 38–8
BEING INDIAN IS . . .

Being Indian is—having a Christian missionary tell you it is wrong to believe in more than one Divine Being, then listening to him tell you about God, Jesus Christ, the Holy Ghost, The Virgin Mary, St. Joseph, St. Patrick, St. Christopher, St. Francis, etc., etc.

Being Indian is—paying 15 to 20 bucks apiece for eagle tail feathers.

Being Indian is—knowing the so-called peyote cult is probably a better way of worshipping the Great Spirit than any other Christian way or denomination.

Being Indian is—trading your surplus commodities to a local farmer (who used them for hog feed) in exchange for fresh eggs, butter, milk, etc.

Being Indian is—respecting your elders who have earned it.

Being Indian is—masking your emotions in times of stress.

Being Indian is—never giving up the struggle for survival.

Being Indian is—having your liberal white friends continually urging you to do as your black brothers have done.

Being Indian is—meeting at least two dozen anthropologists before you are 21.

Being Indian is—having the option of joining at least three dozen Indian unity organizations.

Being Indian is—calling your kinsmen "Apples" for selling out their Indianness for the white man's values. Red on the outside; white on the inside.

Being Indian is—not rioting in the streets, but occupying godforsaken places like Alcatraz, Mount Rushmore, the New York-Canadian bridge, etc.

Being Indian is—cutting off your cast after two weeks because it is in the way and isn't needed anyway.

Being Indian is—having your friends and relatives accuse you of being a traitor if you earn more than $6000 a year, wear a tie and white shirts, drive a car less than three years old, and have a three bedroom home.

Being Indian is—having heard grandparents, parents, and yourself say "When we get our land claims payment" then suddenly realizing you are hearing your children use the phrase also.

Being Indian is—sad.

Being Indian is—tough.

Being Indian is—hard.

Being Indian is—to cry.

Being Indian is—great.

Being Indian is—to laugh.

Being Indian is—beautiful.

Being Indian is—forever!

Source unknown.

ble of putting a person in touch with the dead. **Espiritismo**, a religious cult of European origin, is a way to counteract or prevent mal de ojo and is also concerned with moral behavior. In contrast to the espiritisto, the Cuban *santero,* who is a practitioner of **Santeria** (the unique blend of Catholicism and mysticism referred to in the earlier case study involving Henri), is not concerned with the client's moral behavior. Both espiritistos and santeros prescribe folk remedies, such as teas, herbs, salves, and lotions, which may be purchased in a *botanica,* a store that sells these items along with religious articles such as statues and scapulars.

Santeria is a healing practice that essentially is a combination of African (Yoruba) religion, Catholicism, and Espiritismo. The many cults of Santeria are different, but all worship the Oricha-Santo, a divinity that evolved from the blending of the Yoruba god (Oucha) and a Catholic saint. People who "make saints" are initiated into the cult of Santeria for a cost of up to several thousand dollars. These people may or may not become practicing priests. Initiation is a lengthy ritualistic process. Noninitiated believers may pay for an espiritisto to heal them. Meetings occur in the espiritisto's home in a room that may have an altar, pictures of saints, and candles. Many complex rituals are performed, depending on the nature of the presenting symptoms. Occasionally several mediums are present and all help in the communication between the material and the spirit world.

The fundamental belief of Espiritismo is that all who have ever lived reside in the spiritual world and continue to influence the living. Facilitating communication between the two worlds can help minimize conflict and solve problems. Animal sacrifices may be used to give thanks or to appease the supernatural beings. In Miami, Florida, police are being educated about the cult of Santeria, including the belief of animal sacrifice, so they can be more effective when they are called to a "disturbance" (which often is a group of people practicing Santeria).

According to Sandoval (1983), Santeria offers a type of magic to people who can use it to control the supernatural forces that threaten their lives. Santeria is a source of power and strength, a form of support for the believers.

Curanderismo

Curanderismo is a folk healing system derived from Aztec Indian and Spanish cultures. The curandero, or folk healer, functions in the role of advisor to the Mexican-American family (especially the father) and the client. The **curandero** is chosen by God to help people with folk illnesses such as susto, mal de ojo, or empacho (indigestion, a ball in the stomach). Unlike Espiritismo, Curanderismo has no relationship to evil spirits; the curandero functions more like a health care provider in that good will and the aim of holistic care is there.

The major philosophic premises of Curanderismo are (Maduro 1983, p 868):

- Disease or illness may follow strong emotional states (such as rage, fear, envy, or mourning of painful loss).

- Disease or illness may result from being out of balance or harmony with one's environment.

- A person is often the innocent victim of malevolent forces.

- The soul may become separated from the body (loss of soul).

- Cure requires the participation of the entire family.

- The natural world is not always distinguishable from the supernatural.

- Sickness often serves the social function, through increased attention and rallying of the family around a person, of reestablishing a sense of belonging (resocialization).

- Latinos respond better to an open interaction with their healer.

Hot-Cold Theory of Disease

The hot-cold theory of disease espoused by many Hispanic Americans stems from the classic theory spelled out by Hippocrates, the father of medicine. In the Hippocratian theory, it is necessary to balance blood, phlegm, black bile, and yellow bile (the four body humors) to achieve or maintain health. In her discussion of the health care needs of Spanish-speaking clients, Murillo-Rohde (1981) identifies the characteristics of each of these body humors in relation to both temperature and moisture: Blood is hot and wet, phlegm is cold and wet, black bile is cold and dry, and yellow bile is hot and dry. When the four humors are balanced and the body is warm and somewhat wet, the body is healthy. When the humors are not balanced and the body is very hot, cold, dry, wet, or any combination of these, the body may become diseased.

Treatment by using the proper "hot" (*caliente*) or "cold" (*frio*) foods, herbs, or medicines is thought to restore the body to its normal balance. Hot diseases are treated by cold foods, herbs, or medicines, and vice versa. Although hot and cold foods, illnesses, and treatments vary from ethnic group to ethnic group, Table 38–3 can be used as a general guide in considering both the Hispanic American population discussed here and the Asian American population discussed earlier in the chapter.

"Bad air" is another explanation for illness that seems to be related to the hot-cold theory of disease. "Bad air" is often night air, particularly cold air or a cold draft, thought to cause illnesses such as earache, rheumatism, facial paralysis, and tuberculosis. There is no simple explanation of "bad air," however, since it also seems to be connected to some extent with the belief that "aire" is an evil spirit, the result of witchcraft, or a dangerous emanation from a corpse or from the moon (moonlight).

Nursing Practice Issues

Hispanic Americans, unlike Asian Americans or American Indians, are an effusive people who want health care professionals both to show respect (respeto) and to be friendly (personalismo). Shaking hands and smiling is expected. The nurse who admires a child should also touch that child; not to do so may inspire fear of the evil eye.

In assessing a client who believes in spirits, witches, or Santeria, it is important for the nurse to determine if the client's beliefs are acceptable to Santeria or to his or her subculture. If the belief system is out of the ordinary for the client's family or friends the possibility of a mental disorder is greater. Symptoms attached to witchcraft or the supernatural often mimic mental disorder.

Initial interviews should include the entire family, and the nurse needs to assume an authoritative role at first. Hispanics want advice and suggestions and rely on the authority of the professional. Although Americans openly discuss sex with caregivers, Hispanics view sex as a private topic. The nurse needs to ascertain what topics the individual or family are comfortable discussing. More sensitive areas may be saved until later. Remember also that Hispanics frequently have somatic symptoms that may indicate anxiety or depression.

After assessing whether the client is experiencing a culture conflict, the nurse determines how the conflict affects the client's mental state. Hispanics (and others from other cultural groups) often feel pressures to remain Hispanic, but must become Americanized to survive. They feel familial demands not to leave the culture yet may date Anglos. All this causes discomfort and possible identity problems.

Hispanics who are still tied to their culture and believe in Santeria or go to a curandero may feel too embarrassed or guilty to tell the nurse. The nurse should convey acceptance of this and ask directly if they are seeking help from other sources. Then perhaps all the healers can work together for the benefit of the client, or at least the nurse can make sure that one treatment or medication is not counteracting another.

Some researchers have suggested having health clinics in the **barrio** (Hispanic neighborhood) because Hispanics prefer not to go to a mental health clinic that is distant. Research has shown that they, more than whites or blacks, take advantage of neighborhood mental health services.

Recognition that the Hispanic culture is heterogeneous should help prevent cultural stereotyping. Efforts to understand and accept the client's world view and values will help ensure a positive therapeutic encounter.

Immigrants and Refugees

In the last decade the United States has become home for increasing numbers of immigrants and refugees. *Immigrants* often leave their country by choice with varying degrees of distress; *refugees* are actually fleeing their homes, usually because of social or political upheaval. Recent immigrants generally are from China, the Middle East, and South America; refugees have flooded the United States from Cambodia and Haiti.

Both immigrants and refugees arrive in the United States in an extremely vulnerable condition. However, refugees, who have witnessed a devastating war in which friends and loved ones have been killed or injured, are by far the most vulnerable. Increased rates of mental illness are the result of such physical and psychic trauma and of sociocultural disintegration. Refugees and immigrants who appear disturbed are often taken to a psychiatric hospital. An appreciation for the stresses they have undergone and are experiencing is necessary for nurses to plan culturally relevant care.

According to Lipson and Meleis (1985), immigrants and refugees initially experience a personal and social disorganization that may culminate in a cultural exhaustion syndrome. Being in a new and totally different world where people speak and act strangely and where they (immigrants and refugees) are usually not understood is extremely stressful. **Culture shock** is another term used to describe the feelings of depression and frustration that result from immersion in a totally different environment. The nurse may also experience culture shock when working in a different country or caring for many clients from another culture, as in a refugee center. The more different the host culture, the more potential there is for problems (Lipson and Meleis 1985).

Refugees must first meet their basic needs for survival—food, work, a home; this requires considerable energy but keeps them occupied. After these needs are met, more generalized anxiety and depression may occur. Physical illness and somatic problems are common. Ideally, a nurse coming in contact with an immigrant would obtain a cultural profile. However, if there was not enough time (for example, if a client were admitted for a psychiatric evaluation in the emergency room), a few key questions would be useful (Lipson and Meleis 1985, p 50):

How long has the client been in the states and where was he or she raised?

What language does the client speak? How well does the client know English?

What is the client's nonverbal communication style?

What are the client's religious practices?

What is the client's ethnic affection and ethnic identity?

Who makes decisions in the family?

What systems of social support exist for the client?

On the basis of this interview and a brief mental health assessment, the nurse can begin to assess if and how cultural exhaustion or the stress of immigration contributes to the total picture. Interviews often have to be conducted with the help of an interpreter (see Boxes 38–3, 38–4, and 38–5 earlier in this chapter). Care that is relevant and focuses on the problem as perceived by the client will have a greater possibility of being effective. As nurses increase their understanding of what refugees and immigrants experience, they can better plan for their clients' needs.

Chapter Highlights

- Culture (learned behavior) shapes the way we conceive of illness. Culture determines not only who is labeled mentally ill and under what circumstances but also the nature of the treatment and the identity of the helper.

- Recently culture has been recognized as a relevant variable in nursing care.

- Understanding the following key concepts from anthropology is vital in appreciating the relevance of culture to psychiatric nursing: holism, culture, world view, ethnocentrism, cultural relativism.

- Culturally relevant and sensitive nursing care requires that the nurse take a client's culture into consideration when planning care.

- Obtaining a cultural profile and eliciting the client's explanatory model of illness are vital steps in the nursing process.

- Nurses need to be careful not to stereotype clients from different cultural groups.

- Nurses are in a good position to function as culture brokers and to mediate between people or groups from two cultures.

- Being aware of clients' folk health care systems will help the nurse provide better health care to particular groups of people.

- Understanding the three domains of health care—professional, folk, popular—and the client's use of them is helpful to the nursing process.

- Natural support systems are vital to a client's well-being.

- Racial and ethnic factors are linked to people's biologic

makeup, which directly affects their responses to medication.

- Cultural heritage also affects what health care professionals believe about clients and how they care for clients.

References

Ailinger R: Beliefs about treatment of hypertension among Hispanic older persons. *TCN* 1985;7:26–31.

Allen L, Graves P, Woodward E: Perception of problematic behavior by southern female black fundamentalists and mental health professionals. *Health Care Women Int'l* 1985;6:87–104.

Amarasingham L: Social and cultural perspectives on medication refusal. *Am J Psychiatry* 1980;137:353–58.

The Asian Pacific American. *Cultural Issues in Contemporary Psychiatry* (tape). Smith, Kline and French, 1978.

Aylesworth L, Ossorio P, Osaki L: Stress and mental health among Vietnamese in the United States, in Endo R, Sue S, Wagner N (eds): *Asian-Americans: Social and Psychological Perspectives.* Basic Books, 1978.

Beals A: *Culture in Process.* Holt, Reinhart and Winston, 1979.

Brantley T: Racism and its impact on psychotherapy. *Am J Psychiatry* 1983;140:1605–1608.

Brink P: Value orientations as an assessment tool in cultural diversity. *Nurs Res* 1984;33:198–203.

Campbell T, Chang B: Health care of the Chinese in America, in Henderson G, Primeaux M (eds): *Transcultural Health Care.* Addison-Wesley, 1981.

Capers C: Nursing and the Afro-American client. *TCN* 1985;7:11–17.

Chang B: Asian-American patient care, in Henderson G, Primeaux M (eds): *Transcultural Health Care.* Addison-Wesley, 1981.

Chapman J, Chapman H: *Psychology of Health Care: A Humanistic Perspective.* Wadsworth Health Sciences, 1983.

Chaves D, LaRochelle D: The universality of nursing: A comprehensive framework for practice. *Int Nurs Rev* 1985;32:10–13.

Dougherty MC, Tripp-Reimer T: The interface of nursing and anthropology. *Am Rev Anthropology* 1985;14:219–241.

Egan M: A family assessment challenge: Refugee youth and foster family adaptation. *TCN* 1985;7:64–69.

Eisenthal S, et al.: Adherence and the negotiated approach to patienthood. *Arch Gen Psychiatry* 1979;36:393–398.

Engel G: Sudden and rapid death during psychological stress: Folklore or folk wisdom? *Ann Int Med* 1971;74:771–782.

Flaskerud J: Perceptions of problematic behavior by Appalachians, mental health professionals, and lay non-Appalachians. *Nurs Res* 1980;29:140–149.

Fong C: Ethnicity and nursing practice. *TCN* 1985;7:1–10.

Foreman J: Susto and the health needs of the Cuban refugee population. *TCN* 1985;7:40–47.

Foulkes E: The concept of culture in psychiatric residency education. *Am J Psychiatry* 1980;137:811–816.

Frank J: Foreword, in Kiev A (ed): *Magic, Faith and Healing.* Free Press, 1964.

Garrison V: Support systems of schizophrenic and non-schizophrenic Puerto Rican migrant women in New York City. *Schizophrenic Bull* 1978;4:561–596.

Griffith E: Blacks and American psychiatry. *Hosp Community Psychiatry* 1986;35:5.

Harwood A: *Ethnicity and Medical Care.* Harvard University Press, 1981.

Haviland W: *Cultural Anthropology.* Holt, Reinhart and Winston, 1983.

Henderson G, Primeaux M (eds): *Transcultural Health Care.* Addison-Wesley, 1981.

Hispanic Americans. *Cultural Issues in Contemporary Psychiatry* (tape). Smith, Kline and French, 1978.

Hutchinson SA, Wilson HS: American nurses on safari: An illustration of coping with cultural complexity. *Pub Health Nurs* 1985;2(3):153–158.

Jones B, Gray B: Problems in diagnosing schizophrenia and affective disorders among blacks. *Hosp Community Psychiatry* 1986;37:61–65.

Kleinman A, Eisenberg L, Good B: Culture, illness and care: Clinical lessons from anthropologic and cross-cultural research. *Ann Int Med* 1978;88:251–258.

LaFargue J: Mediating between two views of illness. *TCN* 1985;7:70–77.

Lawson W: Racial and ethnic factors in psychiatric research. *Hosp Community Psychiatry* 1986;37:50–53.

Leighton A: Culture and psychiatry. *Can J Psychiatry* 1981;26:522–529.

Leininger M: *Nursing and Anthropology: Two Worlds to Blend.* John Wiley and Sons, 1970.

Lin T: Psychiatry and Chinese culture. *West J Med* 1983;139:862–874.

Lipson J, Meleis A: Culturally appropriate care: The case of immigrants. *TCN* 1985;7:48–56.

Louie K: Providing health care to Chinese clients. *TCN* 1985a;7:18–25.

Louie K: Transcending cultural bias: The literature speaks. *TCN* 1985b;7:78–84.

MacDonald A: Folk health practices among north coastal Peruvians: Implications for nursing. *Image* 1981;13:51–55.

Maduro R: Curanderismo and Latino views of disease and curing. *West J Med* 1983;139:868–884.

Manson S, et al.: Psychiatric assessment and treatment of American Indians and Alaska natives. *Hosp Community Psychiatry* 1987;38(2):165–173.

McGoldrick M, Rohrbaugh M: Researching ethnic family stereotypes. *Family Process* 1987;26(1):89–99.

Mead M (ed): *Cultural Patterns and Technical Change, UNESCO.* New American Library, 1955.

Murillo-Rohde I: Hispanic American patient care, in Henderson G, Primeaux M (eds): *Transcultural Health Care.* Addison-Wesley, 1981.

Nichter M: Idioms of distress: Alternatives in the expression of psychosocial distress: A case study from south India. *Culture Med Psychiatry* 1981;5:379–408.

Orque M, Bloch B, Monrroy L: *Ethnic Nursing Care.* Mosby, 1983.

Papajohn J, Spiegel J: *Transactions in Families.* Jossey Bass, 1975.

Putsch R: Cross-cultural communications. *JAMA* 1985; 254:3344–3348.

Randall-David E: *Mama Always Said: The Transmission of Health Care Beliefs among Three Generations of Rural Black Women*, dissertation. University of Florida, Gainesville, Florida, 1985.

Reese M: A tragedy in Santa Monica. *Newsweek* May 6, 1985, p 10.

Reeves K: Hispanic utilization of an ethnic mental health clinic. *J Psychosoc Nurse* 1986;24(2):23–26.

Roberson M: The influence of religious beliefs on health choices of Afro-Americans. *TCN* 1985;7:57–63.

Rozendal N: Understanding Italian American cultural norms. *J Psychosoc Nurs* 1987;25(2):29–33.

Ruiz M: Open-closed mindedness, intolerance of ambiguity and nursing faculty attitudes toward culturally different patients. *Nurs Res* 1981;30:177–181.

Sandoval M: Santeria. *J Fla MA* 1983;70:620–628.

Schor J: Wabi-sabi. *JAMA* 1984;252:3173.

Schwartz D: Caribbean folk beliefs and Western psychiatry. *J Psychosoc Nurs* 1985;23(11):26–30.

Snow L: Folk medical beliefs and their implications for care of patients. *Ann Int Med* 1974;81:82–96.

Sobralske M: Perceptions of health: Navajo Indians. *TCN* 1985;7:32–39.

Spector R: *Cultural Diversity in Health and Illness.* Appleton-Century-Crofts, 1979.

Stern P: Solving problems of cross-cultural health teaching: The Filipino childbearing family. *Image* 1981;13:47–50.

Sue D (ed): *Counseling the Culturally Different: Theory and Practice.* Wiley, 1981.

Trimble J, et al.: American Indian concepts of mental health, in Pederson P, Santorious N, Marsella A (eds): *Mental Health Services and the Cross-Cultural Context.* Sage, 1984.

Tripp-Reimer T: Barriers to health care: Variations in interpretation of Appalachian client behavior by Appalachian and non-Appalachian health care professionals. *West J Nurs Res* 1982;4:179–191.

Tripp-Reimer T: Reconceptualizing the construct of health: Integrating emic and etic perspectives. *Res Nurs* 1984; 7:101–109.

Tripp-Reimer T, Brink P, Saunders J: Cultural assessment: Content and process. *Nurs Outlook* 1984;32:78–82.

Tripp-Reimer T, Dougherty M: Cross-cultural nursing research. *Am Rev Nurs Res* 1985;3:77–104.

Weisberg M, Graham J: *A Barefoot Doctor's Manual.* Cloudburst Press of America, 1977.

Westermeyer J: Clinical considerations in cross-cultural diagnosis. *Hosp Community Psychiatry* 1987;38(2):160–165.

Wilson HS, Hutchinson SA: Contemporary mental health care in the People's Republic of China. *Am J Nurs* 1983;83(3):393–395.

Zhi-Zhang L: Traditional Chinese concepts of mental health. *JAMA* 1984;252:3169.

THIRTY-NINE

Legal Issues

Joanne Keglovits

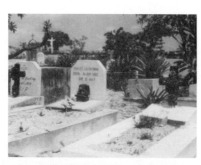

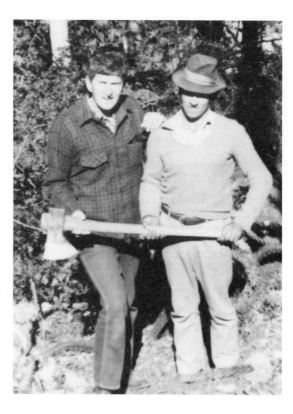

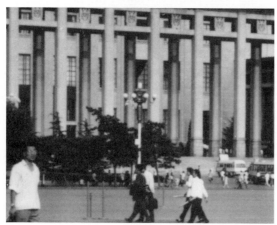

After reading this chapter, students should be able to

- Describe the historical roots of current mental health law
- Relate mental health legislation to humanistic psychiatric nursing practice
- Describe the relationship between the legal and civil rights of mental health clients and humanistic psychiatric nursing practice
- Identify and discuss advocacy interventions in psychiatric nursing
- Identify the major components of mental health legislation
- Analyze key court decisions about mental health laws
- Identify liability issues and safeguards
- Compare the four major rules or tests that are used in an insanity defense

Cross References

Other topics relevant to this content are: Clients rights regarding electroconvulsive therapy, medication, and other biologic therapies, Chapter 32; Deinstitutionalization, Chapter 40; Ethical dilemmas, Chapter 10; History of moral treatment, Chapter 2; Milieu aspects, Chapter 31; Monitoring treatment compliance among the chronically mentally ill, Chapter 22.

The truth is on our side. All that must be done is to allow that truth to be told boldly, fearlessly, and persistently.

Key Terms

American Law Institute (ALI) Model Penal Code	malpractice
	M'Naughten rule
commitment	parens patriae
elopement	privileged communication
involuntary commitment	tort
irresistible impulse	voluntary commitment
least restrictive alternative	writ of habeas corpus

Judicial, legislative, political, and economic decisions profoundly influence mental health practice. Many factors provoke changes in the understanding and practice of mental health intervention. These changes challenge the psychiatric nurse to examine central issues such as the definition of *mental health*, decision-making, clients' and society's rights, liability, and accountability. This examination requires a surrender of past ideas and generally improves care, but it often confuses the boundaries of mental health practice and the law. This confusion entraps mental health professionals, lawyers, families, clients, and the public in a muddle of conflicting policies and procedures reflecting ignorance and ambivalence about mental health that often shifts with newspaper headlines, political elections, and general public opinion.

The philosophy of humanism has at its core the individual's ability freely to choose among alternatives. Each person is believed to have the potential to solve life's problems. Humanistic psychiatric nursing is interacting with a person (couple, family, community) in such a way that the person moves toward his or her definition of happiness and growth while contributing to the community.

The individual rights of minority groups, including the mentally disordered, have taken on new meaning over the past fifteen years. Many of the values that follow from a humanistic perspective are now mandated by law. These values, however, blur the boundaries between public and individual good, voluntary and involuntary treatment, and informed and uninformed consent, which makes the development and implementation of policies difficult. In addition, a client's right to privacy, to receive and refuse treatment, and to define happiness and growth pivot on society's values.

The humanistic perspective seeks not perfection but growth in the delivery of mental health services. Negotiation demonstrates respect for the client, society's values, and the law and offers hope of growth.

This chapter will attempt to bring some clarity to the ever-changing relationship between the law and mental health services so that nurses can not only practice with confidence but also exercise their power as citizens and professionals to influence the direction of mental health care in this country.

HISTORICAL AND THEORETICAL FOUNDATIONS

Before reviewing contemporary legal practice, this chapter takes a brief historical look at the relationship between the law and the state of mind known by many names, including madness, lunacy, and mental illness.

Laws develop in a social context, ideally in response to the problems and needs of the governed. Traditionally, mental disability was considered a private matter, except where either public safety or legal issues (usually regarding property) were at stake. Only in the last few hundred years has society been seeking out its mentally disturbed members to do something for them.

Greek and Roman Law

Greek and Roman law took account of "mad" people chiefly in relation to protection of the community and protection of the mad person's property. From Plato's *Laws* we learn that the insane were generally not held responsible for criminal actions. Slaves defective in mind or body could not be sold, and a fine was levied against both slaveholders and families who let their mad members loose in the city.

English Law

In early England the feudal lord assumed guardianship of a mentally disordered person and control of the person's property. After consolidation of the crown in the thirteenth century, this function was assumed by the king, who, as parens patriae (father of his country), was considered the protector of the personal and property interests of his subjects. The parens patriae doctrine is one rationale for present day commitment statutes.

Law in Colonial America

The American colonists brought to the New World not only their worldly possessions but also much of the culture and tradition of their mother countries.

In 1677 Massachusetts passed a statute directing the selectmen of towns having any dangerously distracted persons to "take care of them so that they do not damify others." This Massachusetts statute provided the legal basis for the forcible restraint of the violent and served as model legislation for other New England colonies.

Mental disorder was generally not recognized as a major medical problem or a pressing social concern in the United States in the seventeenth and eighteenth centuries. American society was still largely rural, and in most cases the insane could be dealt with in an informal manner.

In the second quarter of the nineteenth century a number of factors combined to make traditional and informal mechanisms ineffectual. It was a time of immigration of ethnic minorities, of rapid population growth, and of periodic economic depressions and unemployment. The emphasis was on the establishment of institutions to take care of those who could not take care of themselves. This could take the form of the poorhouse, almshouse, jail, or asylum. Mental hospitals were built in response to the philosophy of the Enlightenment and the success of moral treatment by Philippe Pinel in France and William Tuke in England. Massachusetts and New York established state hospitals in which to segregate and treat the insane. Recovery rates were reported as high as 91 percent for acutely ill persons with moral treatment.

The movement for state mental hospitals was also accelerated throughout the country by the crusade of Dorothea Dix. Dix's determination about this single issue gained her a broad base of support, and she was eventually responsible for founding or enlarging over thirty mental hospitals. It is suggested by J. Sanborn Bockoven (1956), an authority on moral treatment, that Dix's reform movement, with its emphasis on bringing people into asylums without any planning for effective treatment, was responsible at least in part for the downfall of moral treatment in the United States.

Early Commitment Laws

Even though mental hospitals increased in size and number, **commitment** procedures continued to be easy and informal, without much concern for the individual's right to liberty. During the 1840s two lawsuits in particular captured the legal profession's, and to a certain extent the public's, attention regarding the problem of personal liberty and wrongful civil commitment. In 1845, Josiah Oakes, using the common law right of habeas corpus (a writ requiring the agency holding a person in custody to show that it is doing so legally and properly), successfully petitioned the Massachusetts Supreme Court for his release from McLean Asylum in Massachusetts on the grounds that he had been illegally committed by his family. In its decision, *Matter of Oakes,* 8 Law Rptr 123 (Mass Sup Ct 1845), the court acknowledged that no person should be deprived of life or liberty without due process of law and that both dangerousness and need for treatment were commitment criteria.

This decision is said to have set a new precedent for the detention of the alleged insane. The old standard of "detention of the violent" was not applicable in this case. Oakes had been detained for "therapeutic reasons," because he was thought to suffer from hallucinations and was conducting his business affairs in an unsound manner. The charge grew out of the fact that Oakes, an elderly and generally judicious man, had become engaged to a woman of questionable character shortly after his wife's death.

The second case that drew attention, particularly from physicians and hospital employees who were regularly involved in commitment proceedings, was that of Hinchman (Brakel et al. 1985). Hinchman, a patient at the Friends' Asylum in Philadelphia, instituted a civil suit for wrongful detention. The suit was filed against his family, the physician, and the hospital employees involved in his commitment. In addition to regaining his freedom, he succeeded in obtaining damages.

Commitment legislation was seen as necessary not only to safeguard the prospective client but also for the protection of hospital employees. With recovery rates declining and reports that a large number of insane persons were still in almshouses despite the increase in the number and cost of asylums, mental hospitals came under attack. The publication of exposés by former mental clients including those of Mrs. E.P.W. Packard added fuel to the fires of public mistrust of these hospitals.

Much of the lunacy legislation enacted in the United States during the 1870s was a reaction to public distrust of mental hospitals. The emphasis in the legislation was on preventing the commitment of sane individuals. Once the question of sanity was settled, protective legislation usually ended. The model for lunacy legislation was the criminal law system, with its procedural safeguards of sworn complaints, open hearings, and jury trials. Unlike criminal sentences, however, commitments were for an indefinite period of time. Civil rights were automatically taken away during confinement.

In 1890 New York passed the State Care Act, making the state primarily responsible for the cost of hospitalizing its indigent clients. Other states followed suit, and the state system continued to predominate until the middle of the twentieth century.

Mid-Twentieth-Century Mental Hygiene Laws

Despite many advances in psychiatric theory and treatment, nineteenth-century legal practices remained on the statute books of most states well into the twentieth century. Over the years, however, commitment procedures lost many of their protective elements. After World War II, prominent psychiatrists and psychiatric organizations began attacking these commitment laws on the ground that they were hindering the delivery of good psychiatric care to the mentally ill. Words such as *escapee* and *parole* were believed to stigmatize the mentally disordered, and jury trials were said to be traumatizing rather than helpful. This reform movement in the late 1940s and early 1950s reasoned that "railroading" or wrongful commitment was a myth.

One of the results of this movement was the model

legislation published in 1952 by the National Institute of Mental Health, which advocated:

- Increased use of admission on a voluntary basis
- Admission on medical certification
- Nonjudicial proceedings for involuntary hospitalization
- Opportunities for clients to protest after admission

Many states followed the recommendations and updated their mental health statutes. New York State added a new statewide agency, the Mental Health Review or Information Service, to make sure the procedural rights of involuntary clients were followed.

In the last fifteen years the courts have had an impact on the direction of mental health legislation and state statutes. As a review of history tells us, the courts have traditionally been concerned with the possibility of wrongful commitment. Little attention was paid to the restrictions placed on the legal and civil rights of an individual once hospitalized. In recent years, however, the courts have become more concerned with the substantive rights of a hospitalized individual, including the right to treatment, the right not to perform institutional labor, and retention of civil rights such as the rights to communication, visitation, religious activities, and medical self-determination. This is reflected in many state statutes, along with an emphasis on procedural safeguards centering on involuntary commitment.

HUMANISTIC INTERACTIONIST FOUNDATIONS

Implementation of Clients' Rights

This chapter reviews important aspects of mental health legislation and key court decisions as they relate to practice issues and clients' rights. However, the rights clients have in theory and those in actual practice are often quite different. Richard Price and Bruce Denner (1973, p 7) aptly comment on this phenomenon: "Although Pinel was able to remove the chains from the inmates of the Bicêtre by declaring that they were mentally ill, today many people lose a substantial portion of their human and civil rights when the same declaration is made about them." This discrepancy between rights in theory and practice is often cited but has received little systematic attention.

This discrepancy exists for two basic reasons: (1) the struggle between client and provider rights and authority and (2) the "medical model" approach. For example, Szasz and others contend that within the medical model an individual is labeled "mentally ill" because of certain behavior or "symptoms." The label implies that sickness will prevent the client from knowing what is good in the way of treatment.

Two studies that have been done on this gap between clients' rights in theory and practice point to a knowledge deficit on the part of treatment providers (Tancredi and Clark 1972, Laves and Cohen, 1972). Treatment providers were not against the idea of clients' rights, but they often did not know what those rights were. This presents a real problem as clients in many circumstances depend on treatment providers for this information. (See the Research Note on the following page for the client's knowledge of in-hospital rights.)

Another study (Freddolino 1980) found that support for clients' rights among state hospital personnel (psychiatrists, psychologists, social workers, nurses, and therapy aides) was affected most strongly by:

1. The person's power or level of responsibility
2. Professional prestige
3. Socioeconomic factors, such as sex, race, and education, which are linked to power in our society
4. Extent of direct client contact

Direct care providers, of which nurses were a large number, were found to be least supportive of extending clients' rights. It was hypothesized that extension of clients' rights is perceived as threatening to staff responsible for both maintaining order and dealing directly with clients who often are angry over their involuntary confinement. A recommendation was made for administrators, legislators, and judges to provide some outside mechanism of enforcement when extensions of clients' rights are considered and not simply to rely on institutions to implement a pro-rights philosophy.

While the client advocacy clause of the Mental Health Systems Act was not funded, there has been some recent judicial and legislative movement for the establishment of mandatory clients' rights advocacy programs, independent of the mental health system. Legislation is pending in Congress that would either encourage or require states accepting federal block grants for mental health to have advocacy programs. These programs would have the authority to investigate the abuse of the mentally ill in public or private hospitals, residential facilities, and nursing homes. Almost every major mental health organization has testified in favor of the pending legislation. While an external advocacy program may become a reality, the need for advocacy interventions by the nurse will undoubtedly remain.

Although laws can protect certain aspects of human rights, there is a far greater area that laws cannot protect. Laws rarely have a direct effect on a person's beliefs, values, and attitudes, which to a great extent determine whether the letter or the spirit of the law will be carried out. Psychiatric nurses practicing from a humanistic perspective are often in a position to advocate both the letter and the spirit of clients' rights.

Clients are particularly vulnerable to both physical and psychologic abuse and often do not have the ability or power to defend themselves. There is little actual data on how much client abuse exists within treatment settings. One advocate group ranked client abuse to be the most frequent rights violation complaint. Another ranked it third. The types of abuse reported to occur with some frequency are listed in Box 39–1. Psychiatric nursing intervention would be directed at some of the identifying causes that may lead to client abuse, including:

- Unsuitability of certain staff who do not have the patience or understanding to work with clients having trouble with control
- A buildup of stresses that have reduced both the staff's patience and ability to problem solve (burnout)
- An actual lack of knowledge of other means of interacting with clients in a high-stress situation

Other areas of advocacy include:

- Educating clients and their families about their legal rights

---

Box 39–1
TYPES OF CLIENT ABUSE FOUND BY ADVOCACY GROUPS

- Supplying clients with drugs or alcohol in return for favors
- Making privileges contingent on favors from clients
- Slapping and kicking clients when staff felt frustrated
- Using restraints when other less intrusive alternatives were available
- Verbal harassment including threats, sarcasm, and other "put-downs"
- General threats of harm if clients do not behave "appropriately" or as they are told
- Inhumane physical facilities

- Monitoring treatment planning and delivery of service for abuse of clients' rights

- Evaluating policies and procedures regarding clients' rights infringement

- Making sure clients have the necessary information to make an informed decision or give an informed consent

- Questioning other health professionals when their care is based more on stereotypic ideas than an assessment of the client's needs

- Speaking out for safe practice conditions when threatened by budget cutbacks

OVERVIEW OF MENTAL HEALTH LAWS AND JUDICIAL DECISIONS

Christoffel (1982) lists the two functions of law as social control and conflict settlement, advises that law is best understood as a political mechanism, and suggests that it be approached with common sense. The four primary sources of law in this country, at both the state and federal level are: (1) constitutional law, (2) statutory law, (3) administrative law, and (4) common law.

Constitutional law legitimizes statutory, administrative, and common law. *Statutes* are the written laws passed by the legislatures in response to the perceived need for social regulation. Each state has a mental health statute. Individuals or groups can influence the process not only by voting for specific candidates but also by testifying before committees and submitting written proposals or briefs for public hearings on proposed changes in mental health legislation. Nursing practice acts are another example of statutory law. Each state has statutes spelling out procedures for mental hospital admission and discharge. Some states also have statutes on the medical and legal rights of individuals once they are in the hospital.

Administrative law comes from the rules and regulations promulgated by administrative departments and offices as they operationalize the broadly worded statutes into standards. For example, each state mental health statute also has an accompanying book of regulations spelling out the implementation process.

The fourth source of law is *common,* or court-made, law. Common law develops as the courts decide specific cases. A ruling by a court establishes precedent for all lower courts within its jurisdiction. Interpreting the statutes and their compliance with basic constitutional rights is the primary function of the United States Supreme Court. A Supreme Court ruling sets precedent for all courts in the United States. The Supreme Court accepts only a small percentage of the cases referred to it and will accept only those cases involving a right guaranteed by the constitution. The Supreme Court usually chooses and rules on narrow issues. However, the decision sets precedent for further litigation.

Admission

The two major categories of hospitalization are **voluntary** and **involuntary commitment.** Admission and release procedures differ between them.

Voluntary

All states now have some provision for voluntary admission. Basically voluntary admission comes about by written application for admission by prospective clients, or someone acting in their behalf, such as a parent or guardian. As the word *voluntary* implies, the client has a right to

RESEARCH NOTE

Citation

Mills MJ, Gutheil TG, Igneri MA, Grinspoon L: Mental patients' knowledge of in-hospital rights. Am J Psychiatry 1983;140:225–228.

Study Problem/Purpose

The purpose of the study was to identify any discrepancy between the actual information clients had about their rights and the chart entry "rights brochure given."

Methods

Fifty-two recently admitted clients were questioned about formally receiving information regarding clients' rights and their knowledge of that information. Charts were checked for notation of "rights brochure given" and clients' receptivity to material on rights.

Findings

Almost all day-hospital clients but only half of the inpatients recalled receiving written information on clients' rights. Two-thirds were receptive at the time of admission to clients' rights information; one-third was not. No difference in actual knowledge was found between those who remembered receiving the information and those who did not.

Implications

Not all clients are going to be receptive to discussion of their rights at time of admission and may need to be approached on several occasions. Written material, along with posting of the information, can supplement discussions.

demand and obtain release. However, all states but California have what is called a "grace period" in which the client agrees to give notice, usually in writing, of intention to leave. Depending on the statute, this grace period can last from twenty-four hours (in Arizona) to fifteen days (in Oklahoma). It is justified on the ground that the hospital staff needs time to examine the client to determine whether a change to involuntary status is indicated. The extra time also gives family and staff the opportunity to persuade the client to remain voluntarily. This "conditional provision" is seen by some as a covert form of involuntary hospitalization.

There are now statutory assurances in over half the states, compared with just nine a decade ago, that voluntary clients must be adequately informed of their rights and status.

Informal voluntary admission, an alternative to the structure and personal concessions required in voluntary admission, is an option in at least ten states, including New York, Pennsylvania, Connecticut, and Illinois. This procedure is akin to that required in a medical admission. The prospective inpatient verbally requests admission and is free to leave the institution at any time. Informal voluntary admission procedures are more likely to be an option in general and private facilities than in state institutions, and they account for a small percentage (less than 1 percent to 9 percent) of all admissions in states that have this provision.

Involuntary

The state's ability to hospitalize or commit an individual involuntarily is sanctioned by one of two state powers:

1. Police power enables the state to hospitalize people who are considered dangerous to others because of their illness.
2. Parens patriae power enables the state to take on the role of protector and assume responsibility for people considered dangerous to themselves or unable to care for themselves in a potentially dangerous situation because of a mental disability.

Most states provide for more than one involuntary hospitalization procedure. Involuntary hospitalization can come about if the designated body, such as a court, an administrative tribunal, or the required number of physicians, find that the prospective client's mental state meets the statutory criteria for involuntary admission. The criteria vary from state to state according to the type of involuntary hospitalization. However, all state involuntary admission statutes can be expected to include one or more of the following criteria:

- Dangerous to self or others
- Unable to provide for basic needs
- Mentally ill

In an increasing number of states (now 25) involuntary admission is justified only if the individual is dangerous to self or others as a result of a mental disorder. The remaining states augment this by stating that the client's need for care and treatment may also justify commitment. See Brakel et al. (1985) for specific state laws governing civil commitment.

Lessard v Schmidt, 349 F Supp 1078, 1092 (ED Wis 1972), a class action suit decided by a federal district court, provided the precedent for overthrowing several outmoded commitment statutes. Before October 17, 1972, an individual in Wisconsin could be committed if the court was satisfied that the person had a mental disorder to such an extent that care and treatment was required for his or her own welfare or that of the community.

After the decision in *Lessard,* commitment could be made only if there was an extreme likelihood that the person would do immediate harm to self or others unless confined. Not only were the commitment criteria more stringent but the mechanism of commitment also became tighter. The court ruled that, under the due process provisions of the Constitution, individuals facing involuntary commitment were entitled to the same procedural safeguards present in criminal proceedings. The safeguards were to include:

- A hearing within forty-eight hours after detention
- Court-appointed counsel if the individual was unable to afford a private attorney
- The right of the individual to be present and heard
- Notification to the person's family about the proceedings
- Proof beyond a reasonable doubt that the person was dangerous and imminently harmful to self or others
- The right of the person to remain silent to avoid self-incrimination
- Consideration of a less restrictive alternative

While the *Lessard* decision was applauded by civil libertarians, it appalled others and evoked articles citing cases of individuals who were felt to have "died with their rights on" as a result of the court's ruling. Although the *Lessard* decision was vacated twice by the Supreme Court, the decision eventually was reinstated by the federal district court and continues to influence other courts and commitment legislation.

Involuntary hospitalization can be divided into three categories: (1) emergency, (2) temporary or observational, and (3) extended or indeterminate.

Emergency involuntary hospitalization is available in all but Alabama, Arkansas, and Mississippi. It is a temporary measure with limited, short-range goals, and it deals largely with the prevention of behavior likely to create a "clear and present" danger to the client or others. Under common law any official or private person has the right to detain a dangerous mentally disordered person.

Some formal application is required to initiate emergency detention. In some states any citizen may make the application. In others it is limited to police officers, health officers, and physicians. Because this type of involuntary admission is an emergency measure and is warranted only until the appropriate legal steps can be taken, the statutes limit the amount of time an individual can be detained. The limits range from twenty-four hours in states such as Arizona, Georgia, and Michigan to twenty days in New Jersey. The usual practice is to allow detention for three to five days.

Temporary or Observational

Provisions for temporary or observational involuntary hospitalization started appearing in the statute books in the late 1940s. This detention can be described as the involuntary commitment of an allegedly mentally deranged individual for a specified period of time to allow for adequate observation so that a diagnosis can be made and treatment instituted. The actual time period varies. It can be as short as forty-eight hours (in Alaska) and as long as six months (in West Virginia).

Application for the temporary hospitalization of a person in need of aid can be made by any citizen in some states. Others require a family member or guardian, a health or welfare officer, or a physician to apply. Temporary hospitalization may be brought about by the medical certification of one or two physicians or may require further approval by a judge, justice, or district attorney in some jurisdictions.

At the end of the observation period, several options are available. The treating physician may (1) discharge the client, (2) have the client stay voluntarily, or (3) file an application for extended hospitalization. In at least nine states, observational hospitalization is mandatory before a court ruling in favor of extended hospitalization.

Extended or Indeterminate

Indeterminate or extended involuntary hospitalization can come about through either judicial or nonjudicial procedures. Judicial hospitalization procedures require that a judge or jury determine whether the person is mentally ill to a degree that requires extended hospitalization. If so, the court orders the client hospitalized for an extended period (60 to 180 days) or an indeterminate time.

Although at least forty-eight states have judicial hospitalization procedures, they vary widely from state to state. They range from those that require a full judicial hearing and determination to those that eliminate the courts from the initial decision but permit court review of it.

Proceedings are usually initiated by an application for hospitalization of an allegedly mentally ill person. About half the states permit any responsible person or citizen to make or swear to the application. Others allow only one or more of the following groups: relatives, public officers, physicians, and hospital superintendents. Supporting medical evidence may or may not be required at the time of application.

Most states having judicial hospitalization procedures make some provision for a prehearing medical examination in addition to the medical certification required to support the application. In all forty-eight jurisdictions having judicial hospitalization procedures, it is mandatory to notify the person proposed to be hospitalized of the proposed hearing. The large majority of states also require notice to the client's attorney, family, or guardian.

A hearing is mandatory in most states, although a few states leave it to the client to request it. While the client's presence is required at the hearing in a few states, most states merely permit attendance if it is not thought to be harmful to the client's condition or if the client in fact demands it. Few states require the hearing to be held in a courtroom. Most say the place is entirely discretionary.

Jury trials are no longer mandatory in any state, but fifteen states still have provisions for the use of a jury to decide the question of hospitalization.

Nonjudicial procedures for extended or indeterminate involuntary hospitalization include both administrative and medical certification, but such procedures are much less prominent on the statute books than they were a decade ago. Three states (Nebraska, South Dakota, and West Virginia) have provisions for administrative hospitalization procedures. Extended hospitalization is brought about by an administrative board, which basically follows the same procedure used in judicial hospitalization.

Involuntary hospitalization by medical certification, an alternative to the more traditional judicial commitment, is possible in eight states and the District of Columbia. It is usually advocated for clients who are incapable of consenting to voluntary treatment, although they do not protest hospitalization. These individuals are generally called "nonprotesting" clients. The need for hospitalization is usually determined by an examination by one or more physicians and documented by a medical certificate. All states having medical certification provide either for judicial proceedings if the client contests the hospitalization at any time after certification or for expanded habeas corpus proceedings.

	Voluntary Admission		Involuntary Admission		
	Informal	Voluntary	Emergency	Temporary	Extended
Release	Anytime	Usually conditional	Average after 3 to 5 days	48 hours to 6 months	After from 60 to 180 days or an indeterminate time
Use	Limited	Increasing	Increasing	Increasing	Decreasing
Criteria for admission	Client request	Client request	Usually client dangerousness	Client dangerousness or need of care and treatment	Client dangerousness or need of care and treatment

Table 39–1
Voluntary and Involuntary Hospitalization Compared

A comparison of voluntary and involuntary admissions is presented in Table 9–1.

Dilemmas Associated with Involuntary Commitment

Involuntary hospitalization is an exercise of power and like all power can be abused. Because of this potential for abuse, commitment criteria are important. In this country, a person's loss of liberty can be justified only under certain circumstances. Loss of individual freedom through incarceration is generally accepted as justified if one is charged with a crime. In the past individuals were quarantined if they had a contagious disease such as tuberculosis. Today debates continue regarding the restriction of activities of individuals with AIDS and the public's right to safety.

As the review of mental health statutes shows, a degree of "dangerousness" is the favored justification for loss of liberty by involuntary hospitalization. The "dangerousness" criterion is not without its inherent problems. Some of these are considered to be:

- Definitions of "dangerousness" vary from state to state.
- It is impossible to predict dangerous behavior reliably.
- In the absence of other criteria, "dangerousness" will be overused to justify admission.
- The stigma of *dangerous* will be added to that of *mentally ill.*
- The stereotype of *mentally disabled* will be reinforced and thus will work against the development of community programs.
- The media will be encouraged to continue selective reporting of instances in which mental illness and criminal behavior appear to be linked.

- Clinical practice shows "dangerous" individuals are often not treatable, while the most treatable individuals are not dangerous.

Discharge or Separation from a Mental Institution

A client can separate from a mental institution in one of four ways: death, escape, transfer, and discharge.

Death

In 1969 the death rate accounted for roughly 7 percent of the separations from mental institutions. Estimates for 1981 put the death rate in public and county mental institutions at 2 percent compared with a 1 percent death rate in the general population. Alarmingly, however, Slovenko (1981) reports that 13 percent of the clients discharged from New York's state mental hospitals to community facilities were dead within two months.

Escape

A client may take the initiative and decide to terminate his or her relationship with the institution by informally leaving the hospital grounds. This is commonly referred to as escape, **elopement**, or being **AWOL** (absent without leave). Voluntary clients cannot generally be returned to the hospital against their will. However, involuntarily committed clients may be brought back to the hospital against their will with the assistance of the police, if necessary.

Transfer

Transfers account for approximately 3 percent of the separations from a mental facility. Most are transfers within the state and county mental health system. A smaller number are transfers from state to federal facilities or from one state to another.

Discharge

Like admission, discharge from a mental hospital can have various layers of complexity. Discharges occur in one of two ways—conditionally or absolutely.

Conditional

As implied by the word *conditional*, complete discharge in this situation depends on whether the person fulfills certain conditions over a specified period of time, usually six months to a year. Compliance with out-patient care, demonstrated ability and willingness to take medications, and ability to meet the needs of daily living are a few of the many possible prerequisites.

An individual who is unable to meet the specified conditions can be reinstitutionalized without going through any legal admission procedure. An individual committed for an extended or indeterminate time is more likely to be a candidate for conditional than absolute discharge.

Absolute

The legal relationship between the institution and the client is terminated by an absolute discharge. If the client should require readmission to the hospital at any time, even a few hours after discharge, a new hospitalization proceeding would be required.

An absolute discharge can be brought about in three ways:

1. An administrative discharge is issued by the hospital officials.
2. A judicial discharge is ordered by the courts.
3. A writ of habeas corpus is ordered by the courts on the client's application.

As a rule, the authority for discharging involuntary clients rests in the hands of the hospital superintendent, and these clients are given administrative discharges. However, a few statutes extend this power to the central agency responsible for supervising mental institutions in the state, such as the Department of Mental Hygiene. The client has no formal method of initiating an administrative discharge.

Twenty-seven states have provisions for judicial discharge, which is initiated by an application to the court by the client, the client's family, or any citizen who is in disagreement with hospital authorities over the client's

need to be hospitalized. A few states require the application to be accompanied by a medical certificate supporting the idea that the client is ready for discharge. In many states, judicial discharge does not depend on complete recovery. A degree of improvement may be sufficient. Twenty-one states guard against frequent applications for discharge by the same clients by imposing a three-month to one-year waiting period between requests.

All but a few states recognize the right of clients, or persons acting in their behalf, to question their detention in a mental hospital by means of a **writ of habeas corpus**. This writ, dating back to English common law, is available not only to mental clients but also to any person deprived of liberty through illegal detention. In thirty-five states the writ is used only to test the legality of the original detention. The question of the need for continued confinement of the client is not addressed by habeas corpus. In the last few years, some courts have expanded the writ to include an examination of the client's mental status at the time of the proceedings. In these cases the basic criterion for further detention or release is the client's present mental status. This expanded use of the writ is reflected in the statutes of at least sixteen states.

Rights of Clients

The current concern for clients' rights has not developed overnight. It actually has been evolving since the 1960s when there was an increased interest in the underrepresented minority groups including blacks, the poor, women, and the mentally disabled.

In 1980 the United States Congress passed the Mental Health Systems Act, which included a model mental health client's bill of rights. This model bill of rights is summarized in Box 39–2. The review of admission and discharge procedures underscores the fact that there is a great deal of variability from state to state. This is also true for the rights of people receiving mental health treatment. The Omnibus Budget Reconciliation Act of 1981 provoked the repeal of parts of the Mental Health Systems Act but did retain the bill of rights. Unfortunately, the provisions for protection and advocacy were repealed and not funded.

Right to Treatment

The first argument for a right to treatment for involuntarily committed individuals came from Morton Birnbaum, a lawyer and a physician, in an article published in 1960. However, the ground-breaking cases did not come from the familiar circles of civil commitment but from individuals who had been sidetracked from the prison system into hospitals.

Rouse v Cameron

The first case to address the right to treatment issue directly and gain national attention was *Rouse v Cameron*, 373 F2d 451 (DC Cir 1966). In 1962, Charles Rouse had been brought to trial for carrying a dangerous weapon, which is a misdemeanor in the District of Columbia and carries a maximum sentence of one year. Instead of being convicted and sent to trial, Rouse pleaded "not guilty by reason of insanity," and was sent to the maximum security pavilion at Saint Elizabeth's Hospital for treatment.

Four years later, Rouse questioned his detention by means of a writ of habeas corpus on the ground that he had not received any psychiatric treatment. His lawyer argued that this was the quid pro quo to which he was entitled— that is, treatment in exchange for loss of liberty. Under District of Columbia law the plea of insanity takes away criminal responsibility and subjects the defendant to an automatic involuntary commitment. State laws vary tremendously on how the committed person obtains release. Some state statutes require the person to remain committed until pardoned by the governor. Others require the person to meet the same criteria for discharge as any other civilly committed individual.

Judge David Bazelon, speaking for the United States Court of Appeals for the District of Columbia, stated that involuntary commitment is imposed because it is assumed that the criminal offender needs treatment for a mental condition. If treatment is not given, as in Rouse's case, the court held, the offender is deprived of basic rights. Although Judge Bazelon said Rouse was entitled to treatment on the basis of the present District of Columbia statute, he indicated that there might be a constitutional basis for the right as well. Whenever possible, however, courts will base their decisions on statutory rather than constitutional grounds.

Nason v Bridgewater

Another important decision was the Supreme Judicial Court of Massachusetts ruling in *Nason v Bridgewater*, 233 NE2d 908 (Mass 1968). John Nason, a man indicted for murder, had been sent to Bridgewater State Hospital because he was found incompetent to stand trial. After spending five years at Bridgewater, the Massachusetts facility for the dangerously insane, he filed a writ of habeas corpus for his release on the ground that he was not receiving adequate treatment, and he requested transfer to another facility. Through expert testimony, Nason's attorneys were able to show that staffing at Bridgewater was so grossly inadequate

---

BOX 39–2
MENTAL HEALTH SYSTEMS ACT BILL OF RIGHTS

1. Right to appropriate treatment in the least restrictive setting.

2. Right to individualized treatment plan, subject to review and reassessment. To include assessment of mental health services needed after discharge.

3. Right to active participation in treatment, with the risk, side-effects, and benefits of all medication and treatment to be discussed, as well as treatment alternatives.

4. Right to give or withhold consent. May be treated without personal consent only in emergencies or with the consent of a guardian after incompetency has been determined by a court.

5. Right to be free of experimentation unless it follows the recommendations of the National Commission on Protection of Human Subjects.

6. Right to be free of restraints except in an emergency and unless restraints are specifically part of the treatment plan, always subject to the participation and consent requirements. Applies also to behavior modification techniques involving restraints and seclusion.

7. Right to a humane environment.

8. Right to confidentiality of mental health information.

9. Right of access to personal treatment records unless two mental health professionals believe it to be detrimental.

10. Right to as much freedom as possible to exercise constitutional rights of association and expression. Restriction of specific visitors is allowed only if freely documented and part of the treatment plan.

11. Right to information about these rights in both written and oral form, presented in an understandable manner at the outset of treatment and periodically thereafter.

12. Right to assert grievances through a grievance mechanism that includes the power to go to court.

13. Right to obtain advocacy assistance.

14. Right to criticize or complain about conditions or services without fear of retaliatory punishment or other reprisals.

15. Right to referral to complement the discharge plan.

---

that Nason was simply receiving custodial care. The court acknowledged the existence of a constitutional right to treatment, at least for incompetent people awaiting trial, and even went on to suggest what a proper treatment plan for Nason would be.

While *Rouse* and *Nason* may have had little impact on the actual delivery of care in most institutions around the country, they did articulate the right to treatment and provided a statutory and tentative constitutional rationale for that right.

Wyatt v Stickney (Wyatt v Aderholt)

The next step in the move to establish a right to treatment through the court system was taken in Alabama in 1970, with the filing of *Wyatt v Stickney*, 344 F Supp 373 (MD Ala 1972). It was the first class suit successfully brought against a state's entire mental health system. The issue was detention without treatment of individuals committed civilly and involuntarily. The court established that involuntary clients have a constitutional right to individualized treatment that will give each of them a realistic chance to be cured or at least improve. The court found that the treatment program in Alabama state institutions was deficient in three fundamental areas. It did not provide:

1. A humane psychologic and physical environment
2. Qualified staff to administer adequate treatment
3. Individualized treatment plans

To remedy these defects, the court promulgated a lengthy and detailed set of standards, including:

- Provisions against institutional peonage (against institutional use of clients for work)
- A number of protections to ensure a humane psychologic and safe physical environment
- Minimum staffing requirements
- Establishment of a human rights committee at each institution
- A requirement that every client have a right to the least restrictive setting necessary for treatment

If the standards could not be met and clients were denied adequate treatment, the court stated, they had to be released from custody. In the words of Judge Johnson, "to deprive any citizen of his or her liberty upon the altruistic theory that confinement is for humane therapeutic reasons and then fail to provide adequate treatment violates the very fundamentals of due process" (*Wyatt v Stickney*, 325 F Supp 781, 785 [MD Ala 1971]).

For a time there was some question whether the *Wyatt* ruling, recognizing the constitutional basis for the right to treatment, would be upheld in subsequent decisions. In 1972 a neighboring federal district court in Georgia held that there was no constitutionally guaranteed right to treatment (*Burnham v Georgia,* 349 F Supp 1335 [MD Ga 1972]). But since then, the *Wyatt* decision has been affirmed by the federal court of appeals (503 F2d 1305 [5th Cir 1974]).

Donaldson v O'Connor

Another important development in the constitutional right to treatment controversy was *Donaldson v O'Connor*, 493 F2d 507 (5th Cir 1974). Kenneth Donaldson, an involun-

tary patient in a Florida mental hospital for over fourteen years, brought suit against the hospital superintendent, alleging that the superintendent had maliciously deprived him of his constitutional right to liberty. At trial, the jury found that (1) Donaldson had received not merely inadequate treatment but no treatment at all, (2) he was not dangerous, (3) acceptable community alternatives were in fact available for Donaldson, and (4) the doctor, knowing all this, had "maliciously" refused to release him.

On appeal, the federal court of appeals held that there is a constitutional right to treatment, and it awarded $38,000 in compensatory and punitive damages to Donaldson. However, the United States Supreme Court declined to affirm the court of appeals finding of constitutional right to treatment. The court said that the case raised a single question concerning every person's constitutional right to liberty—that is: Does one have the right to be discharged from custodial care if not dangerous to self or others, the right not to receive treatment if one can survive safely in freedom? The unanimous answer was yes (*O'Connor v Donaldson*, 43 USLW 4929 [1975]).

This precedent-setting decision in June 1975 did not decide the damage issue in the case, however. The Supreme Court remanded that issue for reconsideration by the lower court in light of the decision in another case dealing with the liability of a civil service employee. In February 1977, at the age of sixty-seven, Kenneth Donaldson was awarded $20,000 from two defendant psychiatrists. Donaldson's lawsuit had been undertaken in the public interest by the American Civil Liberties Union and the Mental Health Law Project, and a ruling in early May 1977 entitled Donaldson to recover reasonable attorneys' fees. Donaldson has written a book about his confinement, *Insanity Inside Out* (1976), and is reported to spend much of his time now lecturing and writing.

The right to treatment comes from the philosophical point of view that the deprivation of liberty, whether voluntarily or involuntarily, must have an overriding purpose. Review of court cases indicates the right to treatment came about because there was no overriding purpose: Due to overcrowded conditions, inadequate staffing, financial and programmatic deficiencies, there were not enough resources to deliver the bare minimum of treatment. "Right to treatment" ensures that clients are not in a treatment setting for custodial purposes only. Box 39–3 lists some of the necessary elements in a treatment-oriented program.

The following clinical example illustrates a lack of treatment from the client's perspective.

Mary, a 22-year-old woman with an eating disorder, was admitted to the psychiatric unit of a general hos-

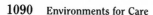

Box 39–3
NECESSARY ELEMENTS IN A TREATMENT-ORIENTED PROGRAM

1. Physical examination and social and psychologic assessment on admission and then as indicated
2. Treatment plans with clear objectives and interventions
3. Evidence of client participation in treatment planning and consent for all treatment methods
4. Up-to-date medical records
5. Treatment in as normal an environment as possible
6. Staff in adequate numbers and with sufficient training to provide quality care
7. Availability of treatment that meets the needs of the client identified in the treatment plan
8. Necessary support services such as dental, speech, physical, and rehabilitation therapy
9. Ongoing treatment plan evaluations
10. Programs to help clients develop skills needed for independent versus institutional living
11. Adequate discharge planning matching client's needs to a less restrictive setting.

---

pital. She signed out against medical advice on the eleventh day saying to her out-patient therapist she didn't know what she was doing there. She had kept track of the time she spent talking with the staff about herself and her difficulties. It totaled one and a half hours, so she signed out! Did Mary fail to notice the "milieu therapy" or was the programming so deficient that no treatment was given?

Some of the unresolved problems or questions regarding the "right to treatment" issue are the cost in tax dollars and the difficulty in providing effective treatment for all conditions. If effective treatment does not exist, is custodial care enough?

Right to Refuse Treatment

The courts articulated a committed client's right to treatment over a decade ago. More recently the courts have been asked to rule on whether the client in a mental institution has the right to refuse treatment.

One of the first cases is that of *Price v Sheppard*, 239 NW 2d 905 (Minn 1976), in which electroconvulsive therapy was felt to be an "intrusive" treatment and not allowed to be given against a competent client's wishes. The two most recent and well-known cases are *Rennie v Klein* and *Rogers v Okin*.

Rennie v Klein

Rennie v Klein was initiated in December 1977 by John Rennie, an involuntarily committed client at a New Jersey state hospital who claimed that the hospital and the New Jersey Department of Human Services were violating his constitutional rights by forcibly administering medication. Mr. Rennie had objected to the side-effects produced by Thorazine and lithium carbonate.

Judge Stanley Brotman ruled that involuntarily committed clients have a qualified right to refuse psychotropic medication. Involuntary clients were addressed because New Jersey statutes already stated that voluntary clients have an absolute right to reject medication. His decision was based on the constitutional right to protect their mental processes from governmental interference. Judge Brotman, impressed by the side-effects of psychotropic medication, stated, "Individual autonomy demands that the person subjected to the harsh side-effects of psychotropic drugs have control over their administration" (*Rennie v Klein* 462 F Supp at 1145).

Judge Brotman did qualify the right to refuse, listing four factors to be considered in overriding a client's objection:

- *Safety.* Is the client a physical threat to other clients or staff?
- *Competency.* Is the client competent to make treatment decisions?
- *Less restrictive means.* Do less restrictive means of treatment exist, and are they available?
- *Risk versus benefit.* What are the risks of permanent side-effects from the proposed treatment?

In 1979 Mr. Rennie's complaint was amended to include class action allegations, and the court went on to add more specific steps to be followed in implementing an involuntarily committed client's qualified right to refuse treatment. These included:

- Notify clients that they have a right to refuse medication.
- Provide clients with information regarding potential side-effects from the medication.
- Obtain written consent prior to initiation of medication.

If written consent is withheld by a client already declared "legally incompetent" by the court, or certified "functionally incompetent" by a treating psychiatrist, the decision to medicate forcibly would be referred to a "client advocate." It would be in the client advocate's discretion to request a hearing before an independent psychiatrist, who would base a decision on the four factors mentioned above. In the case of a competent though involuntarily hospitalized person, a hearing before an independent psychiatrist would be required at which the client would have the right to legal counsel. The commissioner of the Department of Human Services would be the person responsible for appointing client advocates and independent psychiatrists.

Rogers v Okin

Another important case in the establishment of a client's right to refuse medication is *Rogers v Okin*, 478 F Supp (D Mass 1979). In 1975 a class action suit was initiated by clients at Boston State Hospital who contended that their constitutional rights were being violated by the hospital's practice of using forced seclusion and medication in nonemergency situations. Judge Joseph Tauro issued a temporary restraining order against the use of seclusion and medication without the client's informed consent. In the case of a person declared incompetent by the court, informed consent would need to be elicited from the client's guardian. This restraining order applied to both voluntary and involuntary clients. In 1979, after a lengthy trial, the court made the temporary restraining order permanent.

Judge Tauro based his decision on the constitutional right to privacy (right to be left alone) and the first amendment right to freedom of thought. While Judge Tauro recognized that safety considerations might necessitate forcible administration of medication, he allowed much less discretion on the part of the hospital staff than did Judge Brotman in *Rennie*. Only in emergencies that create a substantial likelihood of physical harm to the client or others could medication be forcibly administered. Judge Tauro did not include a set of procedures to be followed in the case of client refusal, as had been done in *Rennie*. Instead, hospital staff were directed to apply to the court for a competency hearing and subsequent appointment of a guardian for clients they believed were incompetent to make treatment decisions. The decision in *Rogers* is considered to be more far-reaching than that in *Rennie*, since it grants competent clients and guardians of incompetent clients an absolute right to refuse medication in nonemergency situations. The United States Supreme Court remanded both cases to lower courts for reconsideration. No right-to-refuse-treatment cases have yet been decided by the court.

Other recent court decisions support a qualified right to refuse psychotropic medication, unless a legitimate emergency exists. It is vital to remember that overriding a client's right to refuse treatment is legally complicated and related to safeguards in place to manage such situations. These safeguards protect the rights of all people.

Dilemmas Associated with Right to Refuse Treatment

There are a number of areas of judicial disagreement in the right to refuse treatment that will create dilemmas for the mental health professional. For example, there is no common definition for the term *psychiatric emergency*.

The traditional definition of *emergency* refers to an overt and immediate threat to a person's life. The contemporary definition centers on the immediate, impending, and significant deterioration of the client's condition.

Another area of controversy is: At what point can the state override an involuntarily committed client's right to refuse psychotropic medication in a nonemergency? Is it only when a person has been judged incompetent, or does danger to self or others provide a legitimate reason under the state's police power to administer treatment?

In the case of an incompetent individual, there is disagreement over who should decide for the person and what standard should be used. Is it to be a guardian, the hospital staff, or the judiciary? Is the standard to be what the best interests of the client seem to be as judged by an informed outsider, or is it what the client would want if competent to make the choice?

Henebery (1982) gives some criteria (listed in Table 39–2) that a court is likely to use in ruling on a right-to-refuse-treatment case. Despite the difficulties and issues raised by the client's right to refuse treatment some very real positive outcomes are:

- Clients must be involved in treatment choices, process, and outcome.
- Clients must be informed of choices and offered alternatives.
- Staff must acquire a second opinion on potentially harmful procedures.

Least Restrictive Alternative

The idea of least restrictive alternative has become an important component of both the deinstitutionalization and clients' rights movements (see Chapters 22 and 40). The term **least restrictive alternative (LRA)** generally refers to the placement of clients in the therapeutic setting that will provide care while allowing maximum freedom. The concept of LRA evolved from the legal term "least drastic alternative" as mentioned in a series of court cases.

The first of these was *Lake v Cameron*, 364 F2d 657(DC Cir 1966). Mrs. Lake, a 61-year-old woman, had difficulty caring for herself because of periods of confusion secondary to arteriosclerotic brain disease. While not considered a danger to others, she did wander when confused and was subsequently admitted to St. Elizabeth's Hospital. The court ruled that Mrs. Lake did not need twenty-four-hour psychiatric supervision and a less restrictive form of treatment should be found. Ironically, even though Mrs. Lake won her case, she ended up dying at St. Elizabeth's as no other facility was available.

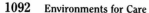

ical issues implicit in the term." To help nurses begin to judge the restrictiveness of an intervention, Garritson suggests consideration of the following dimensions:

- Treatment setting
- Institutional policy
- Enforcement
- Treatment
- Client characteristics

Treatment Setting

Treatment setting is evaluated on such criteria as the limitations it places on physical freedom (locked or unlocked), choice of activities, and the presence of "adult status" as shown by locked bedrooms and unsupervised use of private bathroom facilities. In this scheme, total institutions would be considered the most restrictive, half-way houses less so, and family or independent living the least. It is doubtful the client in the following example would have needed LRA defined.

It was Sarah's first day of her mental health nursing rotation. She met Mrs. M, a short, unkempt, overweight, middle-aged woman dressed in typical hospital attire, in the hall shuffling from one foot to the next muttering something in an excited manner. With some effort, Sarah realized she was saying repeatedly "I just spoke to my group home worker . . . I'm welcomed back . . . I don't have to go to the state hospital. . . ."

Institutional Policy

Institutional policy is the degree of restriction that comes from the rules and regulations necessary to run the institution. Criteria to evaluate a setting would include such items as the amount of supervision in daily living tasks, the amount of client involvement in treatment planning, and the priority of activities that increase the client's autonomy.

Enforcement

The enforcement dimension includes the methods sanctioned to enforce the institution's rules. Is coercion or threat of punishment used? Is the standard for socially acceptable behavior higher in the institution than it would be in the client's own environment? For example, a nurse says to a client, "We don't use that foul language here . . . I don't think you're ready for that pass." How readily and to what extent is the client's autonomy compromised to meet organizational needs? The following clinical example illustrates this point.

Table 39–2
Right-to-Refuse-Treatment Litigation: Factors a Court May Consider in Its Ruling

Factor	Significance
Client competency	If the client is competent, informed consent is possible.
Intrusiveness of treatment	As intrusiveness increases, so does court's scrutiny. Also look at what other treatment has been tried.
Permanence of treatment effect	If side-effects are adverse and permanent, a court is less likely to override refusal.
Experimental nature of treatment	The treatment must have scientific merit, and the client must give informed consent.
Risk-benefit ratio	The benefits of the treatment must outweigh the risk.
Motivation for treatment	The treatment cannot be used to punish or "quiet" the client for the staff's benefit; it must be an acceptable course of treatment or an emergency.
Motivation for refusal	Religious objections are usually upheld.

Wyatt v Stickney (previously cited under right to treatment) extended the idea of LRA to life within the institution. In *Dixon v Weinberger* 405 F Supp 974(DDC 1975), a class action in the District of Columbia, a judge ruled that "suitable care and treatment under the 'least restrictive' condition is required for all patients in Washington, DC." The court required the government to develop less restrictive alternatives if they were not readily available.

The right to LRA is listed in the bill of rights in the Mental Health Systems Act. The ANA's Standards for Psychiatric and Mental Health Nursing Practice expect that the nurse will "set limits in a humane and least restrictive manner to assure the safety of client and others."

While in principle the right to LRA is relatively straightforward, its implementation is often not so clear-cut. Work is being done on defining the concept (see Killebrew et al. 1982, Ransohoff et al. 1984) so that the restrictiveness of a given setting can be measured more accurately.

In looking at the degrees of restrictiveness in psychosocial nursing Garritson (1983) views the LRA concept as "more than just a set of techniques . . . involving the adoption and incorporation of underlying social and philosoph-

Eight out of the thirty clients on a VA's in-patient unit were Vietnam veterans, and today as a group they had been quite vocal in their complaints to the hospital director and local congressional representatives about the lack of programs specific to their perceived needs. An administrative decision was made to cancel their evening passes to attend a Vietnam veteran rally downtown with the rationale of needing to defuse an explosive situation.

Treatment

The treatment dimension has to do with the intrusiveness of the treatment used. Pychosurgery and electroconvulsive therapy would be considered more intrusive than medication. Long-acting medication such as fluphenazine decanoate would be considered more intrusive than oral medication. The clarity of treatment goals is also a consideration. Nebulous or nonexistent goals increase restrictiveness.

Client Characteristics

The client's characteristics or illness is seen by some as restricting behavior to a much greater degree than any locked door. Some believe it is simplistic to think that moving a client from an institutional setting to the community will automatically result in less restriction. Without effective community-based treatment, including safe housing, the chronically ill clients frequently end up in "psychiatric ghettos." As one headline in a newspaper exposé entitled "After the Institution," put it, "the cost of freedom is heavy for many mental patients."

Communication and Visitation

All but three states (Alabama, Mississippi, West Virginia) have some statutory provisions on client correspondence. The basis for laws granting communication rights is that such communication can expose cases of wrongful hospitalization. Generally, communication is unrestricted or guaranteed to named public officials or the central hospital agency for the state. Twenty-seven states extend this guarantee to include correspondence with attorneys. Most states require that any correspondence limitation be part of the client's clinical record. Approximately half the states require the client to have reasonable access to writing materials and postage.

All but five states (Alabama, Mississippi, Pennsylvania, Virginia, and West Virginia) have some statutory provisions concerning visitation. However, hospital authorities are generally given broad discretionary powers to curtail this right. Before implementing any restriction in communication or visitation the nurse should ask: Is it fair and reasonable? Could I defend it to a noninvolved professional?

Restraints and Seclusion

Though improvements in treatment have decreased the use of mechanical or physical restraints, such restraints still play a role in some treatment programs. Most states have attempted to regulate their use by statute. Twenty-six states specify that restraints can be used when the client presents a risk of harm to self or others. Eight states also permit the use of restraints for therapeutic purposes. Some states specifically say restraints are not to be used for punishment or staff convenience. In those states not having statutory provisions regarding restraints the procedures to be followed usually are found in the administrative regulations.

Half the states have laws relating to seclusion. Prevention of harm to self or others is the most common criterion, followed by treatment or therapeutic reasons. Colorado specifically prohibits the use of seclusion but does allow a time-out period. The use of either restraints or seclusion must be documented in the client's medical record in most states.

Electroconvulsive Therapy and Psychosurgery

In almost all states, electroconvulsive therapy (ECT) is closely regulated by statute. Most state statutes specify that ECT can only be administered if informed consent is obtained from the client. In the case of an incompetent client, consent must be obtained from the guardian or next of kin. The client's right to refuse ECT is specifically mentioned in many state statutes.

Psychosurgery, referred to in various state statutes as "brain surgery," "lobotomy," or "experimental" or "hazardous" procedures, is also closely regulated by state statute. Most state statutes specify that psychosurgery can be performed only if informed consent is obtained from the client. In a number of states, psychosurgery can only be done upon a court order if the client is incompetent. The client's right to refuse psychosurgery is also specifically mentioned in many state statutes.

Periodic Review

Thirty-one states and the District of Columbia have some provision for periodic review of involuntary clients. Periodic review provides some protection for the individual against spending more time than necessary in the hospital. Review is required every thirty days in some states, every year in others. A few states require review "as frequently as necessary," or "from time to time." The actual scope of the review is usually not governed by statute. The trend in recent years has been away from hospitalization for indeterminate periods of time. In New York and California, short-term commitment is the rule, and court review is necessary to extend commitment for another short period.

Participation in Legal Matters

Contracts

Clients committed to a mental hospital generally maintain their right to make a valid contract, unless they have also been judged incompetent. In most states commitment proceedings are separate from those for competence. Therefore, an individual who is "legally incompetent" is not necessarily subject to commitment, and an individual committed to an institution is not automatically legally incompetent. Even though the issue of contracts may seem clear-cut, in reality, a client's right to contract may be restricted by the administrative regulations of hospitals and state mental health agencies. A contested contract would most likely be a matter for the court to decide.

Wills

To make a valid will, an individual must:

- Be aware of making a will
- Be familiar with the property being disposed of
- Know the names, identities, and relationship of the people named in the will

An individual with a psychiatric diagnosis, whether in or out of the hospital, can make a valid will as long as these requirements are met. Psychosis with accompanying delusions does not by itself negate a valid will. The delusions have to produce a significant distortion of the person's perception of the property, family, or personal relationships to invalidate the will.

Marriage and Divorce

According to statute and common law, a valid marriage contract hinges on the individual's possession of sufficient mental capacity to give consent. Sufficient mental capacity implies that the person:

- Understands the nature of the marriage relationship
- Knows the duties and obligations involved

The statutes of a small number of states prohibit marriage by mentally disordered persons because they are believed to be incapable of making a contract. More states, however, prohibit marriage by the mentally disordered on the grounds that they are "insane" or "of unsound mind," without specifically defining these terms. Despite these prohibiting statutes, few states even try to enforce the prohibition outside mental institutions.

Most states have provisions for annulment or divorce on the ground of prenuptial mental disability. Within the last twenty years, divorce on the grounds of postnuptial mental disability has been incorporated in the statutes of most states.

Voting

The majority of states do not actually prohibit hospitalized persons from voting. In fact, some specifically preserve this right by legislation. The institutionalized are eligible to register to vote in twelve states. In eighteen others the ability to vote depends on a hospitalized client's legal competence. Only in Maryland and Missouri are individuals confined to an institution ineligible to vote. All states except Louisiana allow absentee voting by disabled persons. The hospitalized client's right to vote is probably more restricted by caretaker and community apathy than it is by statute.

Right to Drive

Statutes on driving privileges are difficult to interpret. Most states will not issue a driver's license to mentally disturbed persons. In some states this restriction also applies to epileptics, drug addicts, and alcoholics. Several states suspend a driver's license as soon as the individual enters a mental institution. Other jurisdictions limit the restriction to individuals admitted involuntarily, while still others base suspension on legal competence.

Right to Practice a Profession

The ability of a hospitalized client to practice a profession is usually impaired simply by the physical confinement. However, the majority of states have some statutes prohibiting the practice of a profession by a mentally disturbed person. The vagueness of the statutes often makes it difficult to know when they are applicable. As a rule, it is up to the professional licensing board to suspend or revoke the license of a member who is believed to be too mentally incapacitated to practice a profession safely, even though not hospitalized.

Rights of Children

The rights of children, along with those of other groups frequently considered politically powerless, have been the subject of judicial and legislative action over the last fifteen years. Up until this time children or minors had few rights of their own. Under early common law children were the parent's "property" and owed them strict obedience.

In most states an individual is considered a minor or juvenile if younger than 18 years of age. As a minor the person is considered legally incompetent. Legal consent for medical treatment must come from parents or guardian. There are, however, a number of exceptions to this general rule of presumed legal incompetence in some state statutes, these include the rights to:

- Seek treatment for drug abuse
- Consent to contraception
- Seek psychiatric treatment

Other factors such as military service, marriage, emancipation, pregnancy, and parenthood may also affect the age at which a minor may be considered competent.

The most controversial issue of a minor's role in the mental health system involves involuntary commitment. Like adults, minors can be committed to a mental hospital against their will. But, unlike adult admissions, the admission of a minor who objects is considered "voluntary" if the parents have authorized it. Because of the realization that parents may not always be acting in the best interests of the child, a number of lawsuits challenging this practice were filed in the 1970s. It was argued that "voluntary" admission of minors without procedural safeguards was unconstitutional, and that a court hearing should always be held to determine if commitment is warranted. The Supreme Court had already ruled in 1967 *In re Gault*(387 US 1) that juveniles in the criminal justice system were entitled to some of the same procedural safeguards accorded adult defendants. Many states did change their commitment statutes to include procedural safeguards. However, in the 1979 case of *Parham v J.R.* (442 US 584), the United States Supreme Court upheld the rights of parents to admit their children to psychiatric facilities as long as a "neutral factfinder" (physician) believes medical standards for admission have been met.

The trend for inclusion of procedural safeguards, though slowed by the ruling in *Parham v J.R.*, continues as an increasing number of states have modified their "voluntary" parental commitment statute by one or more of the following factors:

- Lowering the age of required consent: In four states (Alaska, Idaho, Vermont, and Pennsylvania) the age is 15 or older, the majority of states specify 16 to 18, with New Jersey alone remaining at 21 years of age.
- Requiring consent of the child.
- Providing for a court hearing if the child protests.
- Providing for self-initiated institutionalization for minors: In New Mexico a child 12 years or older qualifies for self-initiated hospitalization, six other states cite age 14 years, and the rest are divided between 16 and 18 years of age.

Therapist-Client-Public Relations

Confidentiality

Almost all states have a specific statute regarding confidentiality of client information, and the specific steps to be taken for release of that information. The confidential nature of the client information is also cited in the American Nurses' Association Code of Ethics, as it is in most professional codes.

The goal of confidentiality is to ensure the client's privacy. There is a significant amount of stigma attached to being the recipient of psychiatric treatment. Though professionals may argue that this is unfair, it is a fact. Because of this, it is important that clients be the ones to give out this information about themselves. Instructors, students, supervisors, or team members who receive information about a client in the course of supervision or in providing treatment for the client are also obligated to treat this material as confidential.

For disclosure of information to occur, a client will need to sign a release form. To be a valid release, the information to be released should be as specific as possible. The client should know the following prior to signing:

- What information is going to be released?
- Who needs it?
- Why do they need it?
- When will they need it?
- How will it be used?

Emergency situations may arise. For example, a client may be in a car accident or take an overdose while out on pass and end up being treated in another hospital's emergency room. In these situations, release of information can occur without the client's approval. It is important to document such a breach of confidentiality.

Confidentiality of information is not easy to maintain. Medical records are generally kept, not in locked files, but at an easy access point in the nurses' station. Medical files usually travel all over the hospital with the client and are often available for the perusal of others not directly involved in the client's treatment. The increased use of computers for communication and data storage, along with the information requested by the government, third party payers, and employers, often poses a threat to a client's privacy. More mundane incidences of breaches of confidentiality occur when staff talk about clients in the halls, elevator, and cafeteria.

Privileged Communication

Privileged communication is a narrower concept than confidentiality. It is established by state statute to protect possibly incriminating disclosures made by the client to specified professionals. Privileged communication has traditionally existed between husband and wife, attorney and client, clergy and church member, and physician and client. In some states, communications between psychologist and client are also accorded privileged status. Arkansas, New York, Oregon, Vermont, and Wisconsin recognize privileged communication between nurse and client. The privilege is the client's and can only be claimed if a therapeutic relationship exists. The professional can reveal the information at the client's request.

Each state that grants a privilege also specifies exceptions to that privilege. The most common exceptions include:

- When the therapist suspects child abuse
- When the therapist is seeking civil commitment
- When the court ordered the exam
- When the client introduced into litigation proceedings a defense of mental illness (likely to happen in child custody disputes, malpractice suits against therapists, personal injury suits, workers' compensation cases, and will contests)
- When the client poses a danger to others (establishes the therapist's duty to warn)

Therapist's Duty to Warn: Disclosure to Safeguard Others

An exception to confidentiality and privilege that has developed from a recent California Supreme Court decision illustrates the competition between two responsibilities of the mental health professional:

1. Confidentiality to the client
2. Protection of the public from the "violent" client

The court's ruling underlines the therapist's responsibility to balance the two.

In *Tarasoff v Regents of the University of California*, 13 CAL3d 177, 529 P2d 553, 118 Cal Rptr 129 (1974), the parents of Tatiana Tarasoff successfully sued the University of California, claiming that a psychotherapist on the staff of the university's student counseling center had a responsibility to warn their daughter that his client, Prosenjit Poddar, had threatened to kill her when she returned from a trip abroad. At the time, the psychologist did notify campus security officers that he believed his client was dangerous and should be involuntarily committed for observation and treatment. However, Poddar appeared rational to the police and promised them he would stay away from Ms Tarasoff. Poddar terminated treatment, and two months later killed Tatiana Tarasoff.

The suit was brought on two accounts: (1) failure to warn Tarasoff, and (2) failure to detain Poddar for treatment. Although the suit was dismissed by the lower courts, on appeal the California Supreme Court reversed the dismissal, saying that, despite the unsuccessful attempt to confine Poddar, the therapist knew that Poddar was at large and dangerous and had a duty to warn Tarasoff of the danger. The court recognized the client's right to confidentiality but said this must be weighed against the public's need for safety against violent assault, especially when an individual in danger can be identified. The *Tarasoff* concept or at least some version of it has continued to be reaffirmed in a number of state and federal jurisdictions. In two cases, therapists were held liable for not taking some action to protect potential unidentified victims.

Appelbaum (1985) suggests a change from the idea of "a duty to warn" to that of a "duty to protect." With that in mind he suggests a model, presented in Table 39–3 to help mental health caregivers decide on a course of action.

Table 39–3 The Appelbaum Model for Implementing the Duty to Warn or Protect	
Do	**How**
Assess dangerousness.	1. Compare data to factors believed to correlate with dangerous behavior, such as previous threats and subsequent violence. 2. Ask: Can victim be identified? Are the threats repeated?
Select a course of action to protect victim.	1. Suggest either voluntary or involuntary hospitalization. 2. If the client is already hospitalized, is a more secure ward needed? 3. If the client is an outpatient, is medication needed? Is more intensive out-patient care needed, such as day programs? 4. Is intensive, systems-oriented therapy indicated to include intended victim? 5. If containment or control is not possible, contact identified victim.
Implement decision.	Continue to monitor: If initial course of action fails, take other measures.

Situations in which reporting by physicians to authorities is required by law include child and elder abuse, knife or gunshot wounds, certain contagious diseases, and the driving of a car by a person with unstable epilepsy. Kjervik (1981) notes that in court cases so far a client's voicing of suicidal ideation does *not* create a duty to warn. The duty to warn or protect applies only when there is danger to others.

The "duty to warn" has stirred up controversy in the mental health community. There is concern about the fact that clients with aggression problems will drop out of therapy, not use it effectively, or be less likely to seek treatment for fear of being betrayed. Remember also that no mental health professional can reliably predict the future violence of a mentally disordered person.

Liability and the Psychiatric Nurse

As the practice of nursing is moving toward greater independence and accountability, nurses are more likely to be named as defendants in lawsuits. Taub (1983) gives the following reasons for increases in claims against mental health professionals:

- The emphasis on clients' rights in recent court decisions
- The public's more open attitude and greater expectations of treatment
- The new legal duties identified in the therapist-client relationship, such as the "duty to warn"
- The publicity given the sizable sums awarded in some psychiatric malpractice cases

According to the American Psychiatric Association, the most frequent sources of claims (listed in order of decreasing frequency) for psychiatrists are:

- Client suicide
- Improper treatment
- Ineffective or improper medication
- Breach of confidentiality
- Wrongful commitment
- Injuries from electroconvulsive therapy
- Sexual misconduct
- Failure to obtain consent

Box 39–4 clarifies pertinent legal terminology regarding malpractice.

The basic elements of every nursing malpractice suit are:

- The client claims that a special duty of care is owed; that is, a nurse-client relationship existed.

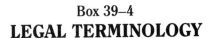

Box 39–4
LEGAL TERMINOLOGY

Criminal and civil are the two main classes of law. *Criminal law* pertains to behavior considered to be a threat to the order of society as a whole, such as murder, assault, and robbery. *Civil law* is concerned with the legal rights and duties of private parties.

An important division of civil law is known as *tort law.* The term **tort** comes from the Latin word meaning twisted. A tort is a wrongful act resulting in injury for which the injured party files a civil suit requesting legal redress, usually in the form of monetary damages. Torts may be intentional, as in assault, battery, defamation of character, invasion of privacy, false imprisonment, fraud, and misrepresentation, or unintentional, as in negligence.

Medical **malpractice** refers to the negligent acts of health care professionals when they fail to act in a responsible and prudent manner in carrying out their professional duties.

- Because of this the nurse is required to meet a specific standard of care.
- The nurse's failure to meet that standard resulted in injury or harm.
- The client claims compensatory damages.

The most important legal element in a nursing malpractice case is whether the nurse met the required standard of care. A court may determine the expected standard of care by the profession's standards of practice and testimony of expert witnesses.

The case of *Abille v U.S.* (482 F Supp 703 Calif) illustrates a breach of the American Nurses' Association's Standards of Psychiatric and Mental Health Nursing Practice and emphasizes the importance of written communication between nurse and physician.

Aramul Abille was admitted to a U.S. Air Force base hospital after becoming increasingly depressed and suicidal secondary to the reserpine used to treat his hypertension. As a new client he was not allowed to leave the unit. Four days later the nursing staff assumed without a verifying written medical order (later a verbal order would be claimed) that Mr. Abille was allowed to leave the unit with permission of the nurse on duty. Mr. Abille left the unit unescorted to attend Mass and returned without incident. The following morning he was allowed to go to breakfast unescorted. This time he committed suicide by jumping out a seventh floor window. The court ruled that the nurse involved with Mr. Abille's care breached the standard of care due under Alaska law. The nurse failed to exercise reasonable care to protect a suicidal client against foreseeable harm to himself.

Another case shows the importance of nursing observation and documentation, even though in this case it did not prevent a tragedy.

Distraught with problems and a pending divorce, Matthew Wassner was voluntarily admitted to a psychiatric hospital. During his admission he expressed thoughts of suicide and also thoughts of killing his wife and her mother. Three weeks after his discharge he was readmitted again voluntarily after a suicide attempt. Nurses' notes revealed close observation of Mr. Wassner and his repeated homicidal threats. Three weeks after his second admission, he was given a pass. He subsequently secured a gun and shot and killed his wife and her friend. He was tried and convicted on two counts of murder. The children brought a wrongful death action against the hospital, seeking damages for the murder of their mother by their father. The court granted substantial damages to the children. No liability was attributed to the nurses involved, but the physician was judged negligent.

In another case the court found that a nurse who forcibly administered medication to a competent adult client had committed an intentional tort.

The client was involuntarily committed to a mental hospital. She was a practicing Christian Scientist and refused medication. The court held that medication could be given over the client's religious objections only if she were harmful to herself or others. The court allowed her damages for assault and battery.

It is important to remember the nature and purpose of hospital records and to follow prudent, appropriate, and ethical procedures in record maintenance. Records that have been changed for whatever reason need to include the date, the reason for the change, and the signature of the person making the change. If the change was dishonest it could result in the charge of fraud or misrepresentation as in *Pisel v Stamford Hospital et al.* 430 A2d (Conn 1980).

A 23-year-old woman was admitted with a diagnosis of schizophrenia. She spent three days in a furniture-less quiet room for safety reasons. On the fourth day the bed was returned to the room but no rationale was noted in the chart. A few days later, an order on the client's chart for an antipsychotic medication was not noted, and the client was without medication for three days. The client was later found in a semicomatose condition with her head lodged between the side rails and mattress. Subsequently, the nursing director ordered the nursing staff to "rewrite" the nursing notes. The substituted record clearly conflicted with other records and staff testimony. A $3.6 million verdict against the hospital has been upheld.

Many factors contribute to the initiation of a malpractice suit by a client. As long as a nurse is involved in practice, lawsuits are a possibility. The nurse may be sued without necessarily being singled out. A number of ways to protect against a successful lawsuit are to:

- Be aware of provisions in the state nurse practice act.
- Follow standards of care.
- Know the relevant law.
- Review hospital procedures and policies with both the standards of care and relevant law in mind, clarify any conflict with legal counsel if necessary, and then follow procedures.
- Document the nursing process.
- Have malpractice insurance.

INTERSECTION OF PSYCHIATRY AND CRIMINAL LAW

Review of mental health statutes and court decisions has shown the impact of the legal system on the practice of psychiatry. Psychiatry also affects the resolution of such legal questions as the credibility of witnesses, competency to make a will or contract or to stand trial, compensation of injured persons, custody of children, and, most controversial, criminal responsibility.

Competency to Stand Trial

Competency to stand trial is based on our common law tradition that defendants must have the mental capacity to defend themselves in a court of law. The process of determining competency to stand trial is the issue most frequently leading to the hospitalization of individuals in the criminal justice system. Until 1972, pretrial commitment was widely used as the final disposition. The defendant failed to become "competent" and remained in the institution indefinitely. Such was the case in *Jackson v Indiana*. The defendant was a 27-year-old retarded, hearing impaired, mute individual who was accused of stealing property valued at nine dollars and confined to a maximum security unit awaiting trial. Because of his disabilities it was doubted that he would ever become competent to stand trial. In its ruling the United States Supreme Court set out some general limitations on the length of pretrial commitments, saying a person cannot be held more than a "reasonable period of time." If the person is unlikely to become competent to stand trial, the civil commitment standards must be met, or the person must be released.

A psychiatric nurse clinician is qualified in some states to perform competency evaluations by interviewing the defendant to determine his or her:

- Understanding of the nature of the legal process
- Recognition of the consequences of the accusation
- Ability to assist counsel in his or her defense

A competency evaluation no longer requires an inpatient stay and may be done in a prison outpatient setting. While not many nurses may actually do competency evaluations, nurses employed in state systems may work with clients transferred from the prison system for treatment to regain their competency. The following are a few clinical examples.

Mrs. L has been transferred from the county prison to the state hospital for a pretrial competency determination. She is a 31-year-old married woman, who three weeks ago was charged with murder in the death of her 9-day-old son. Mrs. L recalls little except what people have told her. The baby was found suffocated in a plastic bag on top of a Salvation Army drop-off box.

Ms. S has been transferred from the county prison to the state hospital for a competency evaluation. She is charged with the murder of two people and the wounding of eight in a shooting spree at a local shopping mall. She is withdrawn and talking incoherently about a "black box."

Insanity Defense

All civilized cultures have had some form of insanity defense. It has been recognized in English courts for over 700 years. Insanity tests or rules that are influential or currently in

use include wild beast, M'Naghten, irresistible impulse, Durham or "product," and model penal code.

Wild Beast Test

The wild beast test, articulated in 1723, essentially said a man must be so totally deprived of his understanding and memory that he knows no more of what he is doing than an infant or wild beast. Legislation submitted by the Reagan administration in the aftermath of the Hinckley verdict is characterized by some as going back to the wild beast test.

The wild beast test remained the standard for judging responsibility until a case involving the assassination attempt of a head of state in 1800. The defense successfully argued that if the person's mental condition either produced or caused the criminal act, the person should not be held legally responsible for it. This was considered a landmark decision as it broke with the ideas that a person must be totally deprived of reason, and did not link insanity with the inability to tell right from wrong. Subsequent cases did not follow this precedent but reverted back to the wild beast test. However, this reasoning is found in the Durham test or "product rule" in 1954.

M'Naghten Rule

From the trial of *The Queen v Daniel M'Naghten* in 1843 came a set of rules that for many years has provided the basis for the majority of American federal and state courts' decisions on the insanity plea.

Daniel M'Naghten was a Scottish woodcutter who felt persecuted by the Tories, who were in power. He believed they were following him, preventing him from sleeping, accusing him of crimes, and planning to murder him. He decided to take action and shoot the prime minister, but he mistakenly shot the prime minister's secretary. Nine physicians testified for the defense, relying heavily on the ideas of Isaac Ray in *A Treastise on the Medical Jurisprudence of Insanity* published in 1838. The jury found M'Naghten not guilty by reason of insanity. Even though M'Naghten was committed to an asylum and spent the rest of his life there, his acquittal was met with anger and outrage, much like the recent outcry in the Hinckley acquittal. M'Naghten's attack had been the fifth attempt on a political figure in forty years, and the government and press believed the court's action would not help to stem this tide. The fifteen judges of the common law court were called to task for their ruling and asked to clarify and tighten the concept of criminal responsibility. Their clarification has come to be known as the **M'Naghten rule**, which states that for an insanity plea to be valid, the defendant at the time of committing the offense must have been functioning under such a defect of the mind, or reasoning power, as not to know the nature and quality of the act or that it was wrong.

The M'Naghten rule was adopted in the federal and most state courts in the United States by 1851. Until recently only New Hampshire had judged insanity pleas by a rule not in line with the M'Naghten formula.

Irresistible Impulse Test

The claim that the M'Naghten rule focused exclusively on cognition led to the development of the **irresistible impulse** doctrine as a supplement to the M'Naghten rules in some states. The irresistible impulse test refers to the inability of a person to control his or her behavior as a result of a mental disorder even though he or she may know it is wrong. A popular question asked in making the determination is: "Would the person have yielded to that impulse had a policeman been at his (her) elbow?"

Durham Test or "Product Rule"

In 1954 the Supreme Court of Appeals for the District of Columbia handed down its decision in *Durham v US,* discarding the M'Naghten rule and introducing another basis for determining criminal responsibility. Known as the "product rule" this had actually been articulated by the New Hampshire Supreme Court in 1870. The rule stated that a person is not criminally responsible if his or her behavior at the time of the crime was a "product" of mental illness. The Durham rule did not gain wide acceptance and was generally discarded in 1972.

American Law Institute's Model Penal Code

In 1955 the **American Law Institute (ALI)** drafted the **Model Penal Code** test, which states that a person is not responsible if because of a mental disease he or she lacks the capacity either to appreciate the criminality (wrongfulness) of an act or to conform his or her conduct to the requirements of the law. The ALI formulation includes both cognitive (knowledge) and volitional (control) criteria. It is used in all federal circuit courts and was used in the Hinckley case. More than half the states also use these criteria. Approximately one-third of the states use some variation of the M'Naghten rule and irresistible impulse test. New Hampshire is the only state still using the product rule. See Table 39–4 for a listing of the insanity defense and allocation of burden of proof in individual states.

Despite its infrequent use, the insanity defense is the subject of much debate since the 1982 "not guilty by reason of insanity" verdict in the trial of John Hinckley, Jr., would-be assassin of President Ronald Reagan. The verdict drew a mixed reaction from the American public. Some believed Hinckley to be insane. Others felt frustrated that punishment had not been administered. To some people the success of the insanity plea seemed linked to the ability to afford an expensive legal defense.

Prior to the Hinckley verdict the insanity defense had been raised in a number of other sensational cases. The media focus on the "Twinkie defense"—so called because of the argument that junk food affected Dan White's mental functioning and diminished his responsibility in the murder of a San Francisco mayor and councilman—did not exactly portray psychiatry in a positive light. David Berkowitz, a bizarre multiple murderer known as "Son of Sam," was initially found incompetent to stand trial. Once competent, he surprisingly pleaded guilty to second-degree murder, and the insanity issue was never presented at trial.

Prior to more effective treatment of mental disorders a verdict of not guilty by reason of insanity (NGRI) saved a person from the death penalty, but not from lifelong incarceration. With modern treatment, however, individuals who were found NGRI are often released or discharged quite early. Movie and television portrayals of ex-mental clients as "mad killers" and "homicidal maniacs" have primed the public to fear the worst.

Since the Hinckley verdict there have been various proposals to limit drastically or abolish the insanity defense. Montana and Idaho have already done so. The National Commission on the Insanity Defense was an independent commission established by the National Mental Health Association to broaden the public debate on the insanity defense and make recommendations of its own. Based on its investigations, public hearings, and analysis the commission concluded that much of the outcry for change in the insanity defense is based more on myths and displaced frustration over the multiple problems of the criminal justice system than on facts. The myths and realities of the insanity defense are summarized in Box 39–5.

Policy statements regarding the insanity defense have been issued by the American Bar Association (ABA), American Psychiatric Association (APA), National Commission on the Insanity Defense (NCID), and the American Medical Association (AMA). The policies of these four influential groups can be summarized as follows:

- All favor retention except the AMA.
- The ABA and APA support a narrowing of the defense to delete the volitional component.
- The ABA believes the burden of proof regarding the defendant's sanity should be on the state.
- The NCID believes the burden of proof of insanity should be on the defendant.

	Table 39–4		
	Current Tests for Insanity and Allocation of Burden of Proof*		
State	**Test**	**Burden**	**Proof**
Alabama	ALI	Defendant	Reasonable satisfaction of jury
Alaska	ALI modified	State	Beyond reasonable doubt
Arizona	M'Naghten	State	Beyond reasonable doubt
Arkansas	ALI	Defendant	Preponderance of evidence
California	ALI(§1)	Defendant	Preponderance of evidence
Colorado	M'Naghten/irresistible impulse	State	Beyond reasonable doubt
Connecticut	ALI	State	Beyond reasonable doubt
Delaware	ALI/irresistible impulse	Defendant	Preponderance of evidence
Dist. Columbia	ALI	Defendant	Preponderance of evidence
Florida	M'Naghten modified	State	Beyond reasonable doubt
Georgia	M'Naghten	Defendant	Preponderance of evidence
Hawaii	ALI modified	State	Beyond reasonable doubt
Idaho*	—	—	—
Illinois	ALI	State	Beyond reasonable doubt
Indiana	ALI	Defendant	Preponderance of evidence
Iowa	M'Naghten	State	Beyond reasonable doubt
Kansas	M'Naghten	State	Beyond reasonable doubt
Kentucky	ALI	Defendant	Preponderance of evidence
Louisiana	M'Naghten modified	Defendant	Preponderance of evidence
Maine	ALI modified	Defendant	Preponderance of evidence
Maryland	ALI modified	State	Beyond reasonable doubt
Massachusetts	ALI(§1)	State	Beyond reasonable doubt
Michigan	ALI modified	State	Beyond reasonable doubt
Minnesota	M'Naghten	Defendant	Preponderance of evidence
Mississippi	M'Naghten	State	Beyond reasonable doubt
Missouri	ALI modified	Defendant	Preponderance or greater weight of evidence
Montana	Unique	Defendant	Preponderance of evidence
Nebraska	M'Naghten	State	Beyond reasonable doubt
Nevada	M'Naghten	Defendant	Preponderance of evidence
New Hampshire	Unique	Defendant	Preponderance of evidence
New Jersey	M'Naghten	Defendant	Preponderance of evidence
New Mexico	M'Naghten/irresistible impulse	Defendant	Preponderance of evidence
New York	M'Naghten modified	State	Beyond reasonable doubt
North Carolina	M'Naghten	Defendant	Satisfaction of jury
North Dakota	Unique	State	Beyond reasonable doubt
Ohio	ALI(§1)	Defendant	Preponderance of evidence

(continued)

	Table 39–4 *(Continued)*		
Current Tests for Insanity and Allocation of Burden of Proof*			
State	**Test**	**Burden**	**Proof**
Oklahoma	M'Naghten	State	Beyond reasonable doubt
Oregon	ALI	Defendant	Preponderance of evidence
Pennsylvania	M'Naghten	Defendant	Preponderance of evidence
Rhode Island	ALI modified	Defendant	Preponderance of evidence
South Carolina	M'Naghten modified	Defendant	Preponderance of evidence
South Dakota	M'Naghten modified	State	Beyond reasonable doubt
Tennessee	ALI	State	Beyond reasonable doubt
Texas	ALI	Defendant	Preponderance of evidence
Utah	ALI	State	Beyond reasonable doubt
Vermont	ALI modified	State	Beyond reasonable doubt
Virginia	M'Naghten/irresistible impulse	State	Beyond reasonable doubt
Washington	M'Naghten	Defendant	Preponderance of evidence
West Virginia	ALI	State	Beyond reasonable doubt
Wisconsin	ALI	Defendant	Reasonable certainty by greater weight of credible evidence
Wyoming	ALI	State	Beyond reasonable doubt

*All federal circuits use the ALI-Model Penal Code test and, pursuant to Davis v United States, *160 US 469 (1895)*, the burden of proof is on the prosecution on a beyond a reasonable doubt standard.
Source: Myths and Realities: Report of the National Commission on the Insanity Defense. National Mental Health Association, 1983, p. 42a.

- The ABA, APA, and NCID all reject the "guilty but mentally ill" (GBMI) verdict enacted by a few states. The GBMI verdict gives a jury another alternative when they find a defendant does not meet criteria for a successful insanity plea.

- The ABA, APA, and NCID all support the creation of "special" dispositional commitment statutes for all persons acquitted of a violent crime on the basis of insanity. All reject using the ordinary civil commitment statute.

No definitive answers are available on the fate of the insanity defense, which reflects society's ambivalence and discontent with this issue. However, it is a moral and ethical dilemma worthy of the attention of psychiatric nurses.

Chapter Highlights

- Law develops in a social context—ideally in response to the problems and needs of the governed.

- Factors influencing the development of laws about the rights of mentally disturbed persons include the state of medical knowledge, the community's acceptance of some responsibility, and the legal profession's sensitivity to the social and civil liabilities that befall the mentally disturbed.

- Knowledge of existing mental health legislation is essential for nurses to become politically active and protect the legal rights of individuals using mental health services.

- Early commitment procedures were easy and informal without much concern for the rights of the individual.

- Not until communities started to offer treatment that necessitated confinement did laws become concerned with the mentally disordered person's loss of freedom and basic civil rights.

- Mental health legislation varies considerably from state to state. In every state, mental hygiene laws identify procedures for admission to and discharge from mental hospitals, but only some states deal with the medical and legal rights of hospitalized persons.

Box 39–5
MYTHS AND REALITIES OF THE INSANITY DEFENSE

Myth: Many criminal defendants plead insanity and most are acquitted.

Reality: The insanity plea is rarely used; acquittals are extremely rare.

Myth: The insanity defense causes major problems for the criminal justice system.

Reality: The insanity defense has a minor practical role in the criminal justice system but a very important moral role.

Myth: Mentally ill people are dangerous and are capable of violent behavior at any time.

Reality: The overwhelming majority of the 35 million mentally ill people in this country are neither dangerous nor unpredictable; they are victims of stigma.

Myth: Most insanity defendants are murderers who commit random acts of violence.

Reality: Most of the crimes committed by insanity defendants are nonviolent crimes. Only 14 percent of insanity defendants are charged with homicide or other violent crimes, most of which are directed not at strangers but at family members and authority figures.

Myth: The insanity defense allows defendants to fool juries and escape punishment.

Reality: The overwhelming majority of acquittees suffer from the most serious forms of mental illness.

Myth: The insanity defense is a rich man's defense.

Reality: Most insanity defendants are likely to be as poor as most other criminal defendants.

Myth: Insanity trials are a "circus" of conflicting expert testimony that confuses the jury.

Reality: Most insanity cases reflect agreement among the experts, the defense, and the prosecution; few go to trial, and even fewer go to a jury. The celebrated cases are the exception not the rule.

Myth: Most insanity acquittees go free immediately or within a short time after trial.

Reality: The majority of acquittees are confined for significant periods of time.

Myth: Insanity acquittees repeat the same crime when they are released.

Reality: Crimes committed by insanity acquittees upon release tend to be less violent in nature. Recidivism rates are no higher than for convicted felons.

Myth: The "guilty but mentally ill" verdict means that the defendant will receive mental health treatment.

Reality: A "guilty but mentally ill" verdict does not guarantee treatment beyond what a convicted felon would receive.

- The Mental Health Systems Act of 1980 provides some direction for states to review and revise their mental health laws to ensure that clients receive the protection and services they require.

- Members of the health professions are being held increasingly accountable for their behavior. They need to become familiar with the state laws that govern their responsibilities and actions.

- Contemporary issues concerning rights of hospitalized clients include access to communication, use of restraints and seclusion, use of psychosurgery and electroconvulsive therapy, and provision for periodic review of involuntary clients.

- Contemporary legal issues important in humanistic psychiatric nursing practice include involuntary admission criteria, the right to treatment, civil rights of hospitalized persons, client-therapist relations, the controversial right to refuse treatment, and treatment in the least restrictive alternative.

- Theory about rights of mental clients often is not reflected in practice.

- Effective implementation of client's rights frequently depends on awareness, support, and advocacy by the psychiatric nurse.

- Mental health statutes and court decisions impact on the practice of psychiatry. Psychiatry also affects the resolution of such legal questions as the credibility of witnesses; competency to make a will, contract, or to stand trial; custody of children, and, most controversial, criminal responsibility.

References

Alexis A: Body searches and the right to privacy. *J Psychosoc Nurs* 1986;24(11):5–20.

Annas GJ, Glantz LH, Katz BF: *The Rights of Doctors, Nurses and Allied Health Professionals.* Avon, 1981.

Appelbaum P: Refusing treatment: The uncertainty continues. *Hosp Community Psychiatry* 1983;38:11–12.

Appelbaum P: *Tarasoff* and the clinician: Problems in fulfilling the duty to protect. *Am J Psychiatry* 1985; 142:425–429.

Bachrach L: Is the least restrictive environment always the best? Sociological and semantic implications. *Hosp Community Psychiatry* 1980;31:97–103.

Banes J: An ex-patient's perspective of psychiatric treatment. *J Psychosoc Nurs* 1983;21:11–20.

Birnbaum M: The right to treatment. *ABAJ* 1960;46:499–505.

Bockoven JS: Moral treatment in American psychiatry. *J Nerv Ment Dis* 1956;125:167–194, 292–321.

Brakel SJ, Parry J, Weiner BA: *The Mentally Disabled and the Law.* American Bar Foundation, 1985.

Burgdorf MP: Legal rights of children—Implications for nurses. *Nurs Clin N Am* 1979;14:405–415.

Bursten B: Posthospital mandatory outpatient treatment. *Am J Psychiatry* 1986;143(10):1255–1258.

Christoffel T: *Health and the Law—A Handbook for Health Professionals.* Free Press, 1982.

Code For Nurses With Interpretive Statements. American Nurses' Association, 1976.

Davis PK: What nurses should do when a patient says "No! I don't want treatment." *Nurs Life* 1984;4:41–45.

Donaldson K: *Insanity Inside Out.* Crown, 1976.

Fenner KM: *Ethics and Law in Nursing.* Van-Nostrand Reinhold, 1980.

Freddolino P: Factors affecting the patients' rights ideology of mental health personnel, in Lippsett P, Sales B (eds): *New Directions in Psycholegal Research.* Von-Nostrand Reinhold, 1980.

Garritson SH: Degrees of restrictiveness in psychosocial nursing. *J Psychosoc Nurs* 1983;21:9–16.

Gutheil TG, Bursztajn H: Clinicians' guidelines for assessing and presenting subtle forms of patient incompetence in legal settings. *Am J Psychiatry* 1986;143:1020–1023.

Geller, JL: Rights, wrongs, and the dilemma of coerced community treatment. *Am J Psychiatry* 1986;143(10): 1259–1263.

Hannah GT, et al.: *Preservation of Client Rights.* Free Press, 1981.

Henebery JK: The right of the psychiatric patient to refuse treatment. *Leg Med Annu* 1982;137–159.

Killebrew JA, Harris C, Kruckeberg K: A conceptual model for determining the least restrictive treatment–training modality. *Hosp Community Psychiatry* 1982;33:367–370.

Kjervik DK: The psychiatric nurse's duty to warn potential victims of homicidal psychotherapy outpatients. *Law Med Health Care* 1981;9:11–16.

Laben JK, Maclean CP: *Legal Issues and Guidelines for Nurses Who Care for the Mentally Ill.* Slack, 1984.

Laves R, Cohen A: A preliminary investigation into the knowledge of and attitudes toward the legal rights of mental patients. *J Psychiatry Law* 1972;June:49–78.

Mental Health Systems Act: Summary and Analysis. *Ment Disability Law Rep* 1980;4:383–390.

Myths and realities: *A Report of the National Commission on the Insanity Defense.* National Mental Health Association, March 1983.

Oriol M, Oriol D: Involuntary commitment and the right to refuse medication. *J Psychosoc Nurs* 1986;24(11):5–20.

Pavlo A, et al.: Weighing religious beliefs in determining competence. *Hosp Community Psychiatry* 1987;38(4): 350–352.

Price R, Denner B: *The Making of a Mental Patient.* Holt, Rinehart and Winston, 1973.

Ramik-Finneran M, Schell-King M: The role of forensic psychiatry and the insanity defense. *Perspect Psychiatr Care* 1982;20:55–64.

Randall JP: Avoiding legal liability, in Bullough B (ed): *The Law and the Expanding Nursing Role.* Appleton-Century-Crofts, 1980.

Ransohoff P, et al.: Restrictiveness of care among the severely mentally disabled. *Hosp Community Psychiatry* 1984;35: 706–709.

Sanders JB, DuPlessis D: An historical view of right to treatment. *J Psychosoc Nurs* 1985;23(9):12–17.

Slovenko R: The past and present of the right to treatment: A slogan gone astray. *J Psychiatry Law* 1981; Fall:263–282.

Standards of Psychiatric-Mental Health Nursing Practice. American Nurses' Association, 1982.

Steiner J: Ethical issues in the institutionalization of patients, in Rosenbaum M (ed): *Ethics and Values in Psychotherapy—A Guidebook.* Free Press, 1982.

Stone A: The right to refuse treatment. *Arch Gen Psych* 1981;38:358–362.

Szasz T: *Law, Liberty and Psychiatry.* Macmillan, 1963.

Tancredi L, Clark D: Psychiatry and the legal rights of patients. *Am J Psychiatry* 1972;129:328–330.

Taub S: Psychiatric malpractice in the 1980s: A look at some areas of concern. *Law Med Health Care* 1983; 11:97–103, 135.

Wexler D: An offense-victim approach to insanity defense reform. *Ment Phys Disabil Law Rep* 1984;8:146–149.

Ziegenfuss JT: *Patients' Rights and Professional Practice.* Van-Nostrand Reinhold, 1983.

FORTY

Community Mental Health

Holly Skodol Wilson
Carol Ren Kneisl

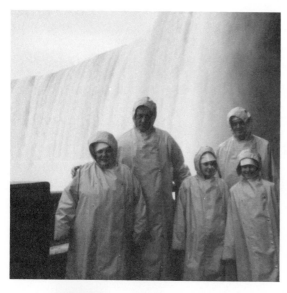
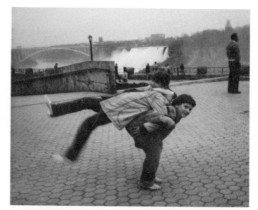
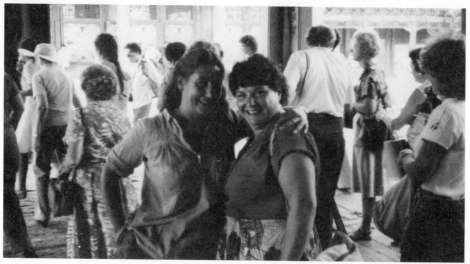

Learning Objectives

After reading this chapter, students should be able to

- Identify the social conditions that led to the development of the community mental health movement

- Discuss the impact of legislation on community mental health

- Explain six concepts basic to community mental health philosophy

- Relate the ANA Psychiatric-Mental Health Nursing Standards of practice and professional performance to community mental health nursing

- Identify community mental health nursing roles appropriate to the educational preparation, skills, and experience of the individual nurse

- Describe community mental health nursing roles and functions in terms of primary, secondary, and tertiary levels of prevention

- Evaluate the problems of the community mental health and deinstitutionalization movements

- Discuss the NSGAE and the psychoeducational approach as two examples of innovations in community care of the severely and chronically mentally disordered

Cross References

Other topics relevant to this content are: Assessment, Chapter 4; Chronically mentally ill, Chapter 22; Families, Chapter 33; Family burden in schizophrenia, Chapter 17; History, Chapter 2; Legal issues, Chapter 39; Social Support, Chapter 8.

Human life is like a tapestry—rich woven magic—a lasting vision of ever-changing views.

Key Terms

block grant
broker for community resources
caseworker model
catchment areas
community mental health centers
Community Mental Health Systems Act
deinstitutionalization
diagnostically related groups (DRGs)
diagnostic creep
dumping

Nursing Adaptation Evaluation (NSGAE)
paraprofessional extender model
primary prevention
prospective payment (PP)
psychoeducation
revolving door syndrome
secondary prevention
skimming
team model
tertiary prevention
transinstitutionalization
true chronics

In the cavernous interior of a large railroad terminal, a 39-year-old woman actually makes her home on an old wooden bench, surrounded by three large plastic bags that hold all her earthly possessions. She is one of an estimated 18,000 homeless men and women in New York City thought by various observers to be former residents of state psychiatric hospitals. In another city a 24-year-old community college student attends classes during the day and lives, along with six other young adults, in a well-kept house on a quiet residential street staffed by mental health counselors and community volunteers. In yet another metropolitan area, a 62-year-old man walks to a storefront clinic in his neighborhood where he tells the receptionist in his native Italian that his pill bottle is empty and he needs another prescription.

What these three people have in common are their experiences with a system for delivery of mental health services called **community mental health**. This chapter explores the dimensions of their experience in which the locus of care has shifted in two decades from large, often isolated, state institutions to the community itself.

TURNING POINTS IN PSYCHIATRIC CARE

Psychiatric professionals are fond of calling the turning points that have occurred in psychiatric care "revolutions." The community mental health movement is often referred to as the third revolution in psychiatry (the first was the provision of treatment for, rather than incarceration of, the mentally ill; the second was the emphasis on intra-psychic causes, an outgrowth of psychoanalysis). However, a number of other turning points have been responsible for creating the social conditions that led to the development of the community mental health movement:

- In the late 1700s Philippe Pinel of Paris cast off the chains and irons that bound the mentally disordered and ushered in the era of moral management and mental institutions (the first revolution).

- At the turn of this century Sigmund Freud of Vienna developed a method of investigation, therapeutic technique, and body of scientific concepts and propositions called psychoanalysis (the second revolution).

- During World War II almost 2,000,000 late adolescent and young adult men were found unfit for military service because of psychiatric and neurologic findings, and large numbers of military personnel and veterans required psychiatric treatment and hospitalization.

- The National Institute for Mental Health was created in 1946, heralding the beginning of a new federalism in the provision of mental health services.

- Drug treatment for mental illness began in the early 1950s.

- In 1955 the National Mental Health Study Act established the Joint Commission on Mental Illness.

- In his 1963 message to Congress, President John F. Kennedy called for a "bold, new approach" to the problems of mental illness and mental retardation.

The first five turning points have been discussed in other chapters. This chapter is concerned with the events that began in 1955 and shaped the social movement that we know as community mental health. It also suggests future directions.

EMERGENCE OF THE COMMUNITY MENTAL HEALTH MOVEMENT

- In the ten years following the end of World War II, the in-patient population of state psychiatric institutions grew from 450,000 to 550,000. New institutions were built and old ones became more crowded. This had a profound impact on the economic health of many states and drew the attention and concern of politicians at local, state, and national levels. They were the moving force responsible in 1955 for legislating the National Mental Health Study Act that established the Joint Commission on Mental Illness and Health. This group

was charged with the responsibility of studying the mental health needs of the nation and making recommendations for a national mental health program.

- Psychotropic drugs, especially tranquilizers, were being used more and more. They helped staff members manage large numbers of clients in crowded conditions. Research into chemotherapy and the etiology of mental illness seemed to promise that an answer or cure could be discovered any time.

- Group therapy and short-term (five to six sessions) individual psychotherapy instituted to treat large numbers of military personnel began to be used for other segments of the population. Mental health professionals began to consider options other than costly long-term individual psychotherapy or long-term hospitalization.

- Milieu therapy, sometimes called sociotherapy, began to develop based on the efforts of Maxwell Jones, who established therapeutic communities in English hospital settings (1953), and Alfred Stanton and Morris Schwartz (1949) and Milton Greenblatt, Richard H. York, and Esther Lucille Brown (1955), who studied milieus in the United States.

The 1960s: A Bold New Approach

By 1961, the Joint Commission on Mental Illness and Health had presented its report, *Action for Mental Health,* to Congress. The report concluded that psychiatric services in this country were woefully inadequate. The landmark recommendations of the group called for:

- A shift from institutional to community-based care
- A more equitable distribution of mental health services
- Preventive services
- Consumer participation in both the planning and delivery of mental health services
- The hiring and training of citizens in the community as nonprofessional mental health workers
- The education of increased numbers of mental health professionals
- Public support for research
- Shared federal, state, and local funding for the construction and operation of a system of community mental health centers

President John Kennedy appointed a cabinet-level committee to study the Joint Commission's recommendations, and on February 5, 1963, he delivered the first presidential message concerned with the mental health of the nation. In it Kennedy called for "a bold new approach" in which mental health services would be integrated with community life. Congress responded by passing legislation to implement the president's proposal in the form of the Mental Retardation Facilities and Community Mental Health Centers Construction Act (PL88–164; frequently called the Community Mental Health Centers Act) before the end of the year. This legislation authorized 150 million dollars in federal funds to be matched by state funds over three years for the construction of comprehensive community mental health centers. In order to qualify for federal funding, the five essential services outlined in Table 40–1 had to be offered.

A center could continue to receive federal support in decreasing proportions for an eight-year period. It was expected that after this time centers would be able to operate on state and local funds and fees received from services. In 1965 legislation extended federal funding for community mental health services through 1968, and the program was extended once again in 1970. At this time funding for services to children and adolescents was specifically provided in response to the 1969 report of the Joint Commission on the Mental Health of Children, which cited inadequate programs for young people. This amendment also provided for services to drug and alcohol abusers, and for mental health consultation.

The 1970s: Realistic Problems

Unfortunately the Community Mental Health Centers Act program often did not work as planned. Some states and local municipalities did not have funds to match those available at the federal level. Some centers, especially those in poverty areas or predominantly rural areas, were unable to generate sufficient revenue through fees. Services that generated little or no income, such as public education and mental health consultation, began to suffer.

Table 40–1
Essential Community Mental Health Services

1963	1975	1981
In-patient care: 24-hour hospitalization for any person in the community requiring around-the-clock care	Five essential services mandated in 1963 plus:	Outpatient care
Outpatient care: Psychiatric treatment for clients living at home	Follow-up care: Ongoing programs for community residents after discharge from a mental health facility	Partial hospitalization
Partial hospitalization: Treatment programs for clients not requiring around-the-clock care; day treatment programs allowing clients to return home at night; night treatment programs allowing clients to maintain jobs during the day and return to the hospital at night	Transitional services: Living arrangements for persons unable to live on their own but not requiring hospitalization, or newly discharged from a mental health facility and requiring assistance in adjusting to living on their own	24-hour hospitalization and emergency care
Emergency care: 24-hour emergency services	Services for children and adolescents: Mental health diagnostic treatment, liaison, and follow-up services for children and adolescents	Consultation and education
Consultation and education: To professionals or community groups in schools, health clinics, churches, courts, law enforcement agencies, etc.	Services for elderly: Mental health diagnostic, treatment, liaison, and follow-up services for the elderly	Screening services
	Screening services: Assistance to courts and other agencies to screen persons referred to mental health agencies	
	Alcohol abuse services: Programs geared toward prevention, treatment, and follow-up in alcohol abuse	
	Drug abuse services: Programs geared toward prevention, treatment, and follow-up in drug abuse	

The 1975 amendments to the 1963 law (Community Mental Health Center Amendment PL94–63) not only reemphasized the goals of the 1963 legislation, but also required that each center provide the seven additional mental health services outlined in Table 40–1. This requirement meant that in order to receive funds, a community mental health center might have to provide services not necessarily needed by the population it served.

The next major assessment of the mental health needs of the nation began in 1977 when President Jimmy Carter established a twenty-member President's Commission on Mental Health. Unlike the Joint Commission of 1955, which was dominated by physicians, this group included a nurse, Martha Mitchell, the chairperson of the ANA Division on Psychiatric and Mental Health Nursing Practice. Three other professional nurses served on adjunct committees. *Report to the President of the President's Commission on Mental Health* (1978) focused on the following major areas:

- Providing community-based services as the keystone of the mental health system

- Improving community support systems and networks among families, neighbors, community organizations, and existing service components

- Establishing national health insurance that would include coverage for mental health care

- Encouraging mental health coverage (including outpatient) in all health insurance plans

- Continuing the phaseout of large public mental hospitals and improving services in the remainder

- Providing funding to increase the number of mental health professionals, especially those working with minorities, children, and the aged

- Establishing a center with a strong emphasis on primary prevention within the National Institute for Mental Health

- Protecting the human rights of persons in need of mental health care

- Improving the delivery of services to underserved populations and high-risk populations, such as minorities and the chronically ill, through a new federal program

- Developing an advocacy program for the chronically mentally ill

- Increasing support for research related to mental health and illness

- Providing health education to the public and increasing the public understanding of mental health problems

- Centralizing the evaluation efforts of governmental agencies concerned with mental health

The commission's report had special significance for psychiatric nurses. It was hailed as the first official high-level document to give visibility to the professional competence of nurses in mental health care (Hadley 1978). The document specifically mentioned nurses in sections concerned with staff shortages, training and education for primary care practitioners, and mental health care providers whose services should be reimbursed by insurance companies.

The 1980s: Dismal Prospects

The Community Mental Health Systems Act of 1980 was a major achievement of the outgoing Carter administration. It was designed to implement the recommendations made by the president's commission authorizing the funding of community mental health centers, services to high-risk populations, ambulatory mental health care centers, a prevention unit and associate director for minority concerns at NIMH, rape research and services, and recommending a model mental health patient's bill of rights. Its basic task was to coordinate the two-tiered system of mental health care that had evolved since President Kennedy's 1963 efforts. The severely mentally disordered continued to inhabit state institutions, and those with less acute problems used the services of federally funded community mental health centers. Unfortunately, there was little coordination between these two systems. Clients discharged from state institutions often failed to receive follow-up services, and certain populations—the chronically mentally ill, the elderly, and youth—fell between the two systems. This act was intended to coordinate federal and state efforts.

Before the programs authorized by this legislation to start in 1982 could get off the ground, the political climate changed and significantly altered the role of the federal government in the nation's mental health. The 1980 Community Mental Health Systems Act was essentially repealed in 1981 when the 97th Congress passed the new Reagan administration's Omnibus Budget Reconciliation Act (PL97–35). The new budget placed the mental health services programs formerly administered by NIMH into an alcohol, drug abuse, and mental health services block grant, shifting the decision-making about allocation of funds to the states and decreasing the federal role in coordination.

The decrease in the federal budget has had and will continue to have far-ranging effects on the community mental health movement. It cuts funding for community mental health centers and other mental health care delivery programs. Community mental health centers were no longer funded after 1984, and funding reductions were felt as early as 1983. Mandated services have been reduced from twelve to five (see Table 40–1), and their continuing existence and quality depends on state support, private funding, and earned revenue. Legislative impact on the community mental health movement is outlined in Table 40–2.

Table 40–2
Legislative Impact on the Community Mental Health Movement

1955	National Mental Health Study Act (PL840–182) establishes the Joint Commission on Mental Illness and Health.		National Institute for Drug Abuse and National Institute for Alcoholism and Alcohol Abuse established.
1961	Joint Commission on Mental Illness and Health presents its report *Action for Mental Health* to Congress.	1975	Community Mental Health Centers Amendments, Title III (PL94–63) extends services of CMHC to include specific underserved groups, etc., and increases mandated essential services to twelve.
1963	President John F. Kennedy's special message to Congress on mental illness and mental retardation advocates federal participation in mental health programs.	1977	President Jimmy Carter establishes President's Commission on Mental Health to identify the mental health needs of the nation.
	Mental Retardation Facilities and Community Mental Health Centers Construction Act (PL88–164) provides matching funds of $150 million for construction of community mental health centers and mandates five essential mental health services.	1978	*Report to the President from the President's Commission on Mental Health* published in April.
		1980	Mental Health Systems Act to coordinate services between state institutions and community mental health centers passed.
1965	Funding for community mental health centers extended through 1968.	1981	Omnibus Budget Reconciliation Act (PL97–35) of new Reagan administration and 97th Congress requires drastic federal funding cuts. Alcohol, drug abuse, and mental health services put under block grant under state control. Essential services reduced to five.
1969	Joint Commission on the Mental Health of Children report, *Crisis in Child Mental Health: Challenge for the 1970s* addresses the problems of inadequate mental health services for children and adolescents.		
1970	Amendment to 1963 Community Mental Health Centers (CMHC) Act extends program funding and increases service provision to include children, drug and alcohol abusers, and consultation.	1982–1983	States begin to apportion funding for mental health services under block grant.
		1984	Termination of funding for community mental health under terms of 1981 Budget Act.

Budget reductions have already decreased the staff at NIMH, which has lost a number of key people.

The 1990s: DRGs Spell Change

On October 1, 1983, the single largest payer for health care services (Medicare) started paying hospitals according to a system called **prospective payment (PP)**. With that development, hospitals of this nation embarked on a new and uncharted course. Nurses throughout the country have been engaged in discussions about the impact of this new direction and about how to shape and influence it in ways consistent with nursing's values and philosophy.

Cost-based, retrospective reimbursement is a complicated term for the way hospital care had been paid for prior to October 1983. It was a system that current policy makers

argue rewarded hospitals for spending more. "Retrospective payment for services put most of the financial risk on the payer and provided hospitals with incentives to maximize use" (Davis 1984). The United States reportedly spent $322 billion dollars for health care, reflecting a 12.5 percent increase in national health expenditures over 1982 and an increase of three times the general rate of inflation during the same time period. Medicare in 1982 was spending *each month* what it had spent *each year* 15 years before. Congress and the Reagan administration chose prospective payment as an effort to rescue Medicare and to contain health costs. The concept of prospective payment is presumably intended to provide incentives for efficient hospital management. If a hospital is paid a fixed amount for each client admitted for a hysterectomy, for example, it has an incentive not to exceed that specified payment for each type of client. The assumption is of course that **diagnostically related groups (DRGs)** (groups of diagnoses for which a set payment is made) correlate well with use of hospital resources. Experts have reported, however, that conventional DRGs (all 467 of them) have accounted for only 26 percent of the variance in nursing workload, while nursing diagnoses, as primitive as they are, accounted for 52 percent. Clearly DRGs are based on clients' medical needs and are inadequate predictors of clients' nursing needs. They are overly focused on technical and physical providers with little inclusion of psychosocial intervention, client teaching, and social support. At the time of this text's publication, psychiatric care is exempt from DRGs, but some believe that DRGs, occasionally called "dumb regulatory garbage," lurk in psychiatric nursing's near future with the potential to:

- Immerse us in overregulation of clinical decisions by fiscal concerns (resulting in **diagnostic creep**—the alteration of diagnoses to attain maximum benefits)
- Deny access to care for vulnerable groups like the poor and elderly (through patient **dumping** or **skimming**)
- Force nursing to shoulder the burden of hospital cost cutting and justify squeezes on employment of well-educated nurses
- Stagnate the American health care industry with particularly devastating consequences for underserved groups

On the other hand, prospective payment systems may provide unique opportunities to:

- Document the impact of psychiatric nursing's contribution to mental health care
- Justify the value of sophisticated nurse clinicians and researchers with the advanced education to devise innovative approaches and scientifically evaluate their outcomes
- Transform psychiatric nursing into its own revenue-generating system

Whether the 1990s prospective payments systems such as DRGs will have favorable or unfavorable effects on psychiatric care is up to the social inventiveness, strategic vision, and industry nurses bring to shaping state-of-the-art practice. Some view self-help as the bold new approach needed, and nurses are crucial to the implementation of such strategies. Self-help, self-care, and **psychoeducation** are consistent with trends toward realignment of power, control, and responsibility with givers and receivers of health care. Self-help has the potential to meet the increasing demands being placed on formal and institutional mental health services in the next decade.

The psychiatric community has learned some important lessons from its experience with **deinstitutionalization** and the community mental health movement over the last decades. Caregivers have learned to think about the needs of the chronically mentally ill (CMI) in new ways. We have learned about:

- The importance of social support
- The necessity of involving natural or family caregivers
- The importance of planning creative, residential alternatives
- The need to direct treatment approaches to both the disorder itself and the associated disability through social skills training
- The possibility that nursing could provide a cadre of specialists in psychoeducation and chronic care management to transform these lessons into renewed opportunities for mental health care

Many psychiatric services are still exempted from prospective payment, but caregivers must address the issues of cost shifting, quality of care, and evaluating severity of disorders and related resource use that have resulted from this major American health policy change (Widem et al., 1984). Prospective payment is expected to become the predominant method of reimbursement despite efforts to continue psychiatry's current exemption (Beigel 1986).

ORIGINAL CONCEPTS

The original basic philosophy of the community mental health movement was that health care is a right and, therefore, mental health services should be available to all people. The six concepts basic to community mental health are discussed below.

Systems Perspective

The systems perspective provides a holistic view of people and their environment and has already been described in other chapters. Basic to community mental health is the notion that people constantly interact with the environment. A systems perspective requires broadening the scope of mental health care beyond the individual to the system (community) as a whole with holistic awareness of the biologic, psychologic, and sociocultural forces that influence interacting systems.

Levels of Prevention

Since its origin, the community mental health movement has emphasized prevention. Initially, Gerald Caplan (1964) adapted the concepts of preventive medicine for application to psychiatry in general and to community mental health in particular. The levels of prevention in mental health care—primary, secondary, and tertiary—are the foundation for the nursing role in community mental health, and are described later in this chapter.

Interdisciplinary Collaboration

The essential services of community mental health cannot be totally provided by the members of any one discipline or paraprofessional group. Blurring of roles between and among mental health professionals is even more apparent in community mental health programs. It can be traced to the 1961 report of the Joint Commission on Mental Illness and Health that recommended that nurses provide brief, short-term psychotherapy to psychiatric clients. While some nurses in some sections of the country were already doing so, it further legitimated their psychotherapy role. The 1963 legislation funded graduate level clinical specialist programs to prepare nurses at the psychotherapist level. The lines between psychiatric nursing and the other mental health professions became even more indistinct and

even psychiatric nurses have experienced difficulty in defining what is unique to nursing. Fortunately, increased nursing research and the development of nursing theories have helped define this area for psychiatric nurses.

Interdisciplinary collaboration is also influenced by the setting in which the community mental health nurse practices. The following settings (Leininger 1969) also influence practice today:

- *Undifferentiated.* In these settings the roles of mental health professionals are flexible. They are based on the individual's abilities, experience, and interests. It is difficult to distinguish the professional disciplines to which members belong. These settings are most common in multiservice agencies and community mental health centers.

- *Traditional.* Traditionally based roles are determined primarily by the profession to which each individual member belongs. Each profession makes its own con-

---

RESEARCH NOTE

Citation

Wilson HS: Deinstitutionalized Residential Care for the Mentally Disordered: The Soteria House Approach. *Grune & Stratton, 1982.*

Study Problem/Purpose

In the absence of conventional, elaborate, psychiatric control structures (such as formalized authority lines, hierarchical division of labor, formal organizational goals, schedules, therapies, and locked doors), how are problems of social control solved?

Methods

Data were collected using field research strategies. These strategies included 200 hours of field observation, eleven in-depth interviews with eight staff members, analysis of all available documents related to the facility (i.e., grant proposals, journal articles, correspondence, and records), attendance at four formal presentations about the setting, review of a documentary film, and self-examination of the investigator's own experiences.

Findings

Conventional, formal techniques for social control are negated and avoided at Soteria House. Instead of restrictive, controlling approaches to manage others' behaviors, an infracontrol process emerges. Infracontrol consists of three implementing processes: presencing, fairing, and

limiting intrusion. *Presencing* refers to ways in which the physical presence of other people influence and shape resident behavior. Presencing consists of mere physical presence, purposeful monitoring, and active intervention. *Fairing* refers to the management and distribution of work according to implicit understanding of fairness. *Limiting intrusion* refers to the process of restricting involvement and control by external agencies in the activities of Soteria House.

Implications

The deinstitutionalization movement aimed to provide vigorous early treatment to mentally disordered individuals close to their home and aimed to avoid the debilitating impact of prolonged hospitalization with its loss of social and interpersonal skills. Yet community mental health treatment has become governed by rigid standards, policies, procedures, and regulations. Clients are screened, labeled, medicated, and discharged with the same lack of attention to their self-control and self-determination as occurred in institutional treatment. Soteria House operationalized the deinstitutionalization philosophy and showed that successful experience provides direction to nurses wishing to intervene in a less rigid, controlling, and routinized fashion. The Soteria approach has the capacity to humanize care of the increasing numbers of chronically mentally disordered. Additionally, humane treatment philosophies and techniques are applicable in all health care settings.

tributions. The setting is often a traditional hospital-based program.

- *Ambivalent.* These are settings characterized by confusion and uncertainty over who should do what. In actual practice vacillation occurs between undifferentiated and traditional roles.

The challenge in mental health team work is to balance flexible role boundaries with areas of unique expertise to deliver more effective and higher quality mental health care.

Consumer Participation and Control

Consumer participation and control is another outgrowth of the 1960s era. Although the 1961 Joint Commission report recommended community involvement and was supported by the subsequent legislation, the practical aspects were not clear.

In many instances, citizen participation continued as it had in the past; socially prominent citizens, wealthy contributors, and health care providers continued to serve on the governing bodies of mental health agencies. The 1975 amendments provided clarifying guidelines for citizen participation by requiring governing bodies of new community mental health centers to be composed of people living in the area served by the community mental health center, at least half of whom should not be health care providers. In addition, it required that centers in operation before 1975 appoint community members in an advisory capacity to their governing boards. This legislation aimed to ensure that the services provided by community mental health centers would respond to the needs of the citizens. This demonstrated both the philosophic and policy commitment to a decision-making role for the citizens of a given community.

Members of the community also participate in other ways. Large numbers of indigenous nonprofessionals have been employed by community mental health programs as human service workers. Because they understand the problems of the community and the language and customs of ethnic groups specific to that community, they have been quite successful in delivering personalized mental health services.

Comprehensive Services

The community mental health philosophy is committed to providing a full range of comprehensive services to all the members of a community. These services are described throughout this chapter and are outlined in Table 40–1.

The community as client is defined in terms of **catchment areas,** geographically circumscribed areas comprising a city, or several rural communities, with from 75,000 to 200,000 residents. This effectively divides a population into segments whose mental health needs can be met by a specifically designed system of services. Optimally, the segments are small enough to promote collaborative relationships within the system of services.

Continuity of Care

Continuity of care means that, while providing comprehensive services to clients, caregivers also assume the responsibility of monitoring or assisting clients in their move from one program to another. In traditional mental health care systems, separate programs rarely interface, and clients may feel that they have been shuttled from one mental health agency to another. In some instances, clients become discouraged or embarrassed about obtaining needed services. Others are unable to be persistent or seek help in the first place. The continuity of care concept in community mental health was intended to correct these problems. Unfortunately, the community mental health movement has not fulfilled its promise in relation to the concept.

NURSING ROLES IN COMMUNITY MENTAL HEALTH

Community mental health nursing roles consist of a wide scope of activities from the maintenance of mental health and prevention of illness to treatment and rehabilitation. In the broadest sense of the words, the community is the client. Since people are constantly interacting with the environment, when community mental health nurses provide direct services to individual clients, they also direct attention toward the client's community.

Applying the ANA Standards

One of the ANA Psychiatric Nursing Professional Performance Standards (see Chapter 3 for the complete list of the recently revised standards) provides an umbrella for community mental health nursing practice at the clinical specialist level:

> **Standard 10: Utilization of Community Health Systems** The nurse participates with other members of the community in assessing, planning, implementing, and evaluating mental health services and community systems that include the promotion of the broad continuum of primary, secondary, and tertiary prevention of mental illness.

While demonstrating competence in meeting Standard 10 has been determined by the ANA to be in the province of the specialist, the community mental health nurse generalist uses all the other standards as guidelines for practice.

Levels of Community Mental Health Nursing

There is no one set of skills, educational preparation, or nursing experience that determines who is and who is not a community mental health nurse. Both generalists and specialists practice in community settings. They are identified by their commitment to the philosophy and concepts presented earlier in this chapter. However, their roles vary according to the educational preparation, skills, and experience they possess. Table 40–3 identifies three different levels of community mental health nursing in regard to education and experience, professional responsibilities, licensure and certification, and employment settings.

Table 40–3
Levels of Community Mental Health Nursing

Practitioner	Community Mental Health Nurse I	Community Mental Health Nurse II	Clinical Nurse Specialist in Community Mental Health
Education and experience	Nursing diploma or associate degree with minimum one year of psychiatric nursing experience Baccalaureate degree graduate	Baccalaureate degree plus two years of clinical experience	Master's degree in psychiatric/mental health nursing
Professional responsibilities	Interviewing techniques, interpersonal relationship skills, basic knowledge of prevention, assessing client's level of functioning, observations/data collection, facilitation and use of community resources	Mental health education, supportive therapy, behavioral management of psychiatric disorders, therapeutic one-to-one relationship, crisis intervention technique, assessment of client's functioning, knowledge of family theory, group dynamics, personality development, sociopsychologic principles, theories, methods of mental health treatment	Insight-oriented psychotherapy, family therapy, group therapy, psychoanalytic theory, psychopathology, diagnostic evaluation, community organization, mental health consultation, supervision, eclectic approach to mental health and treatment
Licensure and certification	Professional licensure by state	Professional licensure by state, American Nurses' Association Certification as Psychiatric and Mental Health Nurse	Professional licensure by state, after two years of clinical experience: eligible for American Nurses' Association Certification in Psychiatric and Mental Health Nursing; clinical specialist in psychiatric and mental health nursing—adult or children and adolescent
Employment settings	Community mental health centers, community nurse for psychiatric inpatient setting, preventive programs	Community mental health centers, crisis intervention teams, high-risk populations—child abuse, rape, drug abuse, preventive programs	Community mental health centers, crisis intervention multiservice center, mental health consultant and/or supervisor, private mental health facilities, individual private practice, administration, teaching, research

Source: Berns JS, Hamilton MS: Nursing role in community mental health, in Jarvis LL: Community Health Nursing: Keeping the Public Healthy. FA Davis, 1981, p 328.

sible alternatives to hospitalization and to promote the goal of deinstitutionalization for clients.

Primary, Secondary, and Tertiary Prevention

Community mental health nurses hold the principles of primary, secondary, and tertiary prevention as central to their clinical work.

- In **primary prevention**, the nurse is concerned with preventing new cases of mental disorder by counteracting harmful stressors. Nursing activities are directed toward fostering mental well-being and identifying potential stressors and segments of the population that may be at high risk.

- In **secondary prevention**, the nurse attempts to shorten the duration of a mental disorder through early case-finding and treatment and to reduce its prevalence in a given segment of the population.

- In **tertiary prevention**, the nurse implements treatments and rehabilitative services for clients who have been diagnosed as mentally disordered.

Table 40–4 gives specific examples of community mental health nursing roles and functions in all three levels of prevention.

CRITIQUE OF COMMUNITY MENTAL HEALTH AND THE DEINSTITUTIONALIZATION MOVEMENT*

Lest the following critique be used to justify a retreat from the principles of community psychiatry, we have tried to make the apparent criticisms understandable in light of the circumstances. Leaving aside these contextual considerations makes it easier to find community mental health's deficiencies sufficient to conclude the whole thing was a mistake. This conclusion is particularly tempting at a time when we are witnessing a swing of the pendulum of opinion away from a social conception of the cause and treatment of mental disorders to a much more biologic one. Our point is not that the old state hospital system is preferable to community health systems. It is that a system originally set up as a competitive alternative to the state hospital has done so little to define the breadth and limitations of pos-

---

*Adapted by permission from Wilson HS: *Deinstitutionalized Residential Care for the Mentally Disordered: The Soteria House Approach.* Grune & Stratton, 1982.

Lack of True Innovation

The community mental health movement represents the essence of the new hospital psychiatry. Its purposes are to:

- Deemphasize long-term hospitalization
- Institute the notion of brief hospitalization for the stabilization of acute crises
- Develop community resources to treat and support the mentally ill person without resorting to institutionalization

Some professionals believe these changes have brought significant economic and legal forces into the context of contemporary psychiatric treatment. Government planners and managers now set health policy and establish priorities. The demands made by these new systems of monitoring and control have substantially altered the practice of psychiatric care and led to the development of complicated mechanisms for processing clients through treatment. These new processes are designed to negotiate a complex maze of nonclinical considerations peripheral to the actual treatment programs themselves.

In short, conventional treatment in the community mental health system has become a highly prescriptive, elaborately formal structure of policy, regulations, and standards. Complying with these procedures demands increasing attention from mental health professionals. *The old state hospital warehouse has been replaced by a similarly bureaucratized clearinghouse* where care and treatment consist primarily of an institutionalizing process that denies self-care, self-determination, and self-control to clients. Instead, in what Wilson (1982) calls "a dispatching process," they are held, screened, patched together, stamped with a diagnostic label, sorted into a legal category, and returned to an unwelcoming community placement.

Inpatient hospital units under the community mental health system must fill the social control gap left by the closing of traditional state hospitals. Mental health clinicians in such settings must become agents of the community. Regardless how much the community desires successful treatment and rehabilitation of the mentally disordered, it demands safe custody of those individuals it rejects. Viewed in this light, the community mental health inpatient psychiatric facility must respond to multiple and contradictory messages. It stands at the intersection of community care and traditional institutionalism with its emphasis on isolation and custodialism. It must protect the community but at the same time guarantee the client's rights. It must provide for custodial needs of individuals whom society rejects and yet facilitate return as quickly as possible to the rejecting community.

Table 40–4
Community Mental Health Nursing Roles and Functions

Primary Prevention	Secondary Prevention	Tertiary Prevention
Identifying potentially stressful conditions in the community and high-risk populations	Providing brief psychotherapy to individuals, groups, and families	Helping plan for a client's discharge from the hospital
Holding effective parenting classes for adolescent parents, at day-care centers, in schools	Suicide prevention hot line counseling and staffing crisis intervention programs	Coordinating and monitoring follow-up care in home, half-way house, foster care home, or other transitional service
Holding divorce therapy groups for couples, families, and individuals	Providing counseling to victims of violence and their significant others	Teaching clients self-care activities before discharge from the hospital
Providing mental health consultation to health care providers	Holding stress reduction groups for health care providers	Serving as a client advocate
Providing mental health education to members of the community	Case-finding and referring clients in need of treatment	Providing individual, group, and family psychotherapy
Consulting with self-help groups	Providing emergency mental health services	Referring clients to self-help groups or aftercare services
Being politically active in relation to mental health issues	Intake, screening, and assessment of clients	Staffing partial hospitalization programs

Conceptual Confusion

Between 1955 and 1975 the new term *deinstitutionalization* was introduced into the writing and practice of American psychiatric professionals. Under the banner of deinstitutionalization the census of resident clients in American state mental hospitals decreased from 559,000 to 193,900, approximately 60 percent. The quantitative goal set for the deinstitutionalization movement was a 50-percent reduction in the client population of state hospitals for the mentally ill within two decades (Minkoff 1978).

One might expect that a concept with the apparent power and impact of deinstitutionalization would have considerable consensus of meaning for its advocates and users. On the contrary, deinstitutionalization is surrounded with definitional disorder. According to Bachrach (1978), deinstitutionalization is simultaneously a fact, a philosophy, and a process. The well-known fact is that the resident population of state hospitals has decreased from about half a million to about 190,000 or about 62 percent. The philosophy represents an expression of civil libertarian emphasis on rights of individuals and modification of environments as the primary avenue of social change. The process refers to the avoidance of traditional hospital settings for treatment of the mentally ill and the concurrent expansion of community-based facilities.

Bassuk and Gerson (1978) equate deinstitutionalization with a massive reform movement in the delivery of mental health services parading under the banner of community mental health. But they raise questions about whether deinstitutionalization represents an enlightened revolution or an abdication of responsibility. Due to shortcomings in legislation, lack of funding, and the unanticipated impact of discharged clients on communities, the dual promise of an extensive support system of comprehensive, coordinated community care and prevention programs has never been fulfilled. Instead, according to these critics, hospitalized clients have been released haphazardly to a nonsystem of aftercare that has meant real hardship and even tragedy. Roughly half of the homeless are former residents of state psychiatric hospitals. Critics of the deinstitutionalization movement cite inadequate discharge planning, weak follow-up efforts, scarce supportive housing, rampant inflation, rising rents, fixed subsistence income, and a shrinking supply of low-income dwellings as reasons for the swelling ranks of the homeless. Most of the discharged clients whose releases from hospitals were to "unknown" living arrangements had unknown destinations because they had no place to go. Critics argue that basic human needs for shelter and food must be satisfied before more sophisticated therapeutic measures can have any chance of success. Others challenge that the aims of social reform and effective treatment have become entangled and that while social justice may be a necessary condition for successful treatment, it is not a sufficient one.

Klerman (1979) views deinstitutionalization as primarily a shift from a state-owned and operated monopoly to a pluralistic and diversified system of services that resulted from a short-lived consensus between lawyers interested in civil rights, budget advisors pressured by economic forces to shift mental health financing from state to national levels, and theorists and researchers in social psychiatry. In this view, deinstitutionalization is first and foremost a shift in location and funding arrangements.

Talbott (1979) calls deinstitutionalization a misnomer and substitutes his own terminology, including **transinstitutionalization**, a circumstance in which chronically mentally ill clients have been shifted from a single lousy institution to multiple wretched ones, a shuffle to despair and a national tragedy. He characterizes the outcomes of the deinstitutionalization movement as:

- The dramatic appearance of large numbers of dirty, hallucinating, strange faces on city streets, in low-cost ghettos, and deteriorating neighborhoods, in his terms "naked men dancing on Broadway and bag ladies on Park Avenue"

- Transfer of thousands more clients to nursing homes

- Mental health service patterns of use characterized by falling between the cracks, a total lack of follow-up, and the revolving door of continued readmissions

- Demoralization, demedicalization, and deterioration within remaining state hospitals

An analysis of data collected at NIMH made three conclusions about deinstitutionalization (Goldman et al. 1983):

1. Outpatient care has not replaced in-patient care.
2. Public institutions have not been replaced by community-based facilities.
3. Private resources have not replaced public ones as the bearer of cost for the mentally ill.

DEINSTITUTIONALIZED ALTERNATIVES

Deinstitutionalization is one of the most important developments in the history of psychiatry, yet the well-intentioned reform movement has from its beginning been plagued by a variety of problems. In addition to the **revolving door syndrome** (i.e., short stay with rapid turnover and eventual repeated readmissions to the hospital), large numbers of discharged former clients who are still disturbed endure bleak lives in board and care homes, in nursing homes, and on skid row. The problem rests with the erroneous notion that institutionalization is merely a matter of the location and funding arrangements of psychiatric care and the widespread devaluation of any form of long-term residential care for anyone. However, if we view institutionalization as the process by which an individual is denied self-care and self-determination to the point of exchanging personal independence for institutional control and decision-making, the shortest possible hospitalization need not be the crucial goal. Instead, mental health professionals can begin to define and study the full range of possible innovative alternatives to institutionalizing modes of care—alternatives specifically directed toward relinquishing institutional dependency and control and fostering self-care and self-control. Our disenchantment with deinstitutionalization should be used to rethink the concept from its origins. The following list of proposals offers a starting point:

- We must continue to pursue the goals of deinstitutionalization, confused as they might be. We must remember that deinstitutionalization is both a process and an effect.

- The most significant problem in the contemporary American mental health care system is dealing effectively with psychiatric chronicity.

- We need sustained, and not merely transitional, life support settings for many chronic clients: alternative living situations that balance the restriction of clients' freedom with protection for the client and the community.

- Key processes in such settings include training in self-care and community living skills, improvement of employability, incentives for taking increasing responsibility, development of social skills, and provision of leisure time activities.

- A successful program for deinstitutionalization would be enhanced by the contributions of a cadré of specialists for chronic clients who could teach self-care and adaptive functioning and provide psychoeducational programs for family caregivers.

Nurses have always had the primary responsibility for creating an environment for client care. Therefore, nurses are a likely source of the cadré of specialists in residential alternatives where chronic clients can be taught and supported in developing skills of self-care and self-determination.

Community Support Programs

Community support programs are becoming the cornerstone of current national mental health policy for long-term mentally disordered clients (Reinke and Greenley 1986). Some follow a **caseworker model**, which emphasizes basic living skills and day-to-day problem solving. Others use the **paraprofessional extender model**, in which natural helpers in a rural area are paid to assist clients in the community, or the **team model**, in which staff members share responsibilities for all clients (Figures 40–1, 40–2, 40–3). Of the three models tested, the caseworker model serves the widest range of clients at the least cost (Reinke and Greenley 1986).

Self-Care Nursing Centers for True Chronic Clients

Clinical observations, the psychiatric literature, and most recently the diagnostic categories of the DSM-IIIR raise the possibility that there are some chronic clients for whom community living is unrealistic. These people are described as the **true chronics** by Goldman (1981). True chronics are clients who suffer severe and persistent mental or emotional disorders that interfere and substantially limit primary aspects of daily life, such as personal self-care, interpersonal relationships, work, or schooling. Such prolonged functional disability caused or aggravated by severe mental disorders has now become the chief distinguishing characteristic of this population of chronic clients. These are the people who have required institutional care for an extended time and have become institutionalized.

Despite our recognition that such clients exist, it is not as easy to identify them as Goldman's reference might suggest. The general definition of chronic disease established by the Commission on Chronic Illness is:

All impairments or deviations from normal which have one or more of the following characteristics: Are perma-

nent; Leave residual disability; Are caused by nonreversible pathological alterations; Require special training of the patient for rehabilitation; May be expected to require a long period of supervision, observation, or care.

The American Psychiatric Association Conference on the chronic mental client used the following general definition by Bachrach (1979): "Those individuals who are, have been, or might have been but for the deinstitutionalization movement on the rolls of the long-term mental institutions, especially state hospitals." Bachrach has attempted to define chronic clients by location. She identified five subgroups of the population that at one time would have been the residents of state hospitals. In the community are clients released from the hospital and clients who have never been hospitalized. In hospitals are old long-term clients, recent short-term clients, and new long-term clients who probably will not be discharged. Minkoff (1978) refined Bachrach's general definition by distinguishing three separate but overlapping chronic populations:

1. The chronic mentally ill—people who are continuously ill for two years according to DSM-IIIR

2. The chronic mentally disabled—subgroup of the chronic mentally ill characterized by partial or total impairment of instrumental role performance

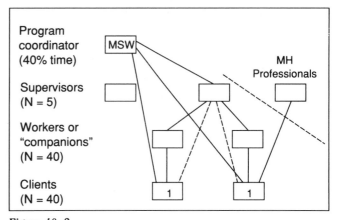

Figure 40–2
Organizational structure of a community support program based on the paraprofessional extender model. Note that the full organizational chart would show five supervisors and forty workers, each of the latter with responsibility for one client. Supervisors and workers are indigenous neighborhood people, mostly with a high school education. Each client is also connected with a mental health professional outside the community support program.
Source: Reinke B, Greenley JR: Organizational analysis of three community support program models. Hospital and Community Psychiatry, *37(6), 624–629. Copyright 1986, The American Psychiatric Association. Reprinted by permission.*

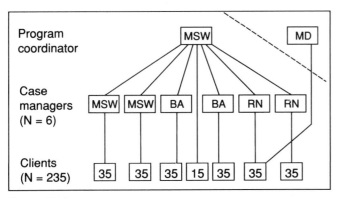

Figure 40–1
Organizational structure of a community support program based on the caseworker model. Note that physicians (MD) routinely perform medication checks but are not administratively part of the community support program.
Source: Reinke B, Greenley JR: Organizational analysis of three community support program models. Hospital and Community Psychiatry, *37(6), 624–629. Copyright 1986, The American Psychiatric Association. Reprinted by permission.*

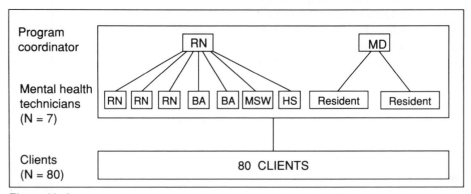

Figure 40–3

Organizational structure of a community support program based on the team model. The nurse (RN) is a program coordinator and supervises mental health technicians. The physician (MD), who is one-third time, functions as a coequal to the program coordinator and supervises two psychiatric residents on six-month rotations.

Source: Reinke B, Greenley JR: Organizational analysis of three community support program models. Hospital Community Psychiatry, *37(6), 624–629. Copyright 1986, The American Psychiatric Association. Reprinted by permission.*

3. Chronic mental clients—people who have continuously or for a long time been hospitalized or received mental health services

However we define chronic clients, they have certain identified needs or services. These needs include material resources such as food, clothing, decent housing, medical and psychiatric care, transportation, and money; vocational rehabilitation resulting in marketable skills and job opportunities; and less tangible needs such as resocialization, day-to-day coping skills, reduction of bizarre behavior, motivation to remain involved with life and a source of nurturing, affirming, and helpful interpersonal alliances. The self-care approach describes psychiatric nursing's strategies for meeting these needs of chronic psychiatric clients (Underwood 1978).

Self-Care Model of Nursing*

Nursing education for psychiatric nurses has for the past few decades emphasized psychotherapeutic and psychologic models rather than nursing models, thus raising questions about the potential for any unique nursing contribution to the mental health team. Psychiatric nurses need a model of nursing in order to make a unique and valued contribution to the mental health services team beyond services in areas where roles are blurred. The self-care model offers a clearer picture of the nature of nursing and nurs-

ing's valuable part in the community mental health movement. It draws heavily from existing knowledge and skills in nursing and organizes them to guide the client care offered by psychiatric nurses. Nursing evolves from a tradition and present day pattern that emphasizes a twenty-four-hour-a-day, seven-day-a-week commitment to client care, a holistic view of mind-body relations, an emphasis on care rather than cure, and a focus on client strengths. Nursing also includes knowledge about mental disorder, chronicity, institutionalizing processes, and effective approaches to clients in residential settings. The processes or skills nurses use include problem solving, decision making, health teaching and interpersonal communication.

In brief, the self-care model originated by Orem (1980) and adapted to psychiatric clients by Underwood (Morrison et al. 1985) guides nurses in using nursing processes to help clients establish, maintain, or increase self-care and self-determination in day-to-day living. Using this approach, the psychiatric nurse can minimize the institutionalizing effects of psychiatric care and psychiatric disabilities and thus help the client avoid a life-style of institutionalized psychiatric chronicity and dependency.

Nursing actions according to Orem (1980) include:

- Acting or doing for clients when they are critically ill, unconscious, or unable to participate in decision making

- Guiding clients when they require direction or supervision to make choices or take action

- Supporting clients (by a look, a touch, or simple physical presence, as well as verbal exchange) by acting as an advocate in their attempts to obtain resources essential to life, health, and well-being

---

*This section is based on clinical and research work of Patricia R. Underwood. Summarized with permission.

Assessment: The NSGAE Scale

Using a proposed extension of Axis V of DSM-IIIR, psychiatric nurses in the San Francisco Bay Area have devised and begun pilot testing the **Nursing Adaptation Evaluation** or **NSGAE scale** (Morrison et al 1985). The NSGAE uses a six-digit code to record the current overall level of adaptive self-care functioning and additional assessments of functioning or self-care level in five basic areas for which nurses assume responsibility, particularly in residential treatment (Box 40–1 and Figure 40–4): (1) nutrition, (2) solitude and social interaction, (3) grooming and hygiene, (4) activity and rest, and (5) elimination. They are based on Underwood's (1978) adaptation of Orem's original 1971 self-care concepts. The goal of treatment plans based on NSGAE level assessments is to help clients maintain, regain, or attain self-care and self-determination in day-to-day living.

Periodic evaluation using this approach can provide a clear indication of progress during care or treatment and document the effectiveness of nursing intervention expressly directed to client teaching in basic areas of routine living. The NSGAE scale can also provide a basis for estimating costs of psychiatric nursing care (Box 40–2). Clearly, higher levels of client self-care require lower levels of nursing resources, thus decreasing costs. Behavioral criteria for each of the four levels in all NSGAE categories are being developed by nurses in the San Francisco Bay Area, particularly those working at Langley Porter Psychiatric Institute with Underwood's Self-Care Approach (Box 40–3).

Planning and Implementing Interventions: Applying the NSGAE

Nursing interventions are directed toward goals of supporting optimum self-care functioning, preventing and controlling disability, and compensating for lack of independence. The nursing care plan later in this chapter is only one example of those used by psychiatric nurses at Langley Porter Psychiatric Institute in San Francisco who work with the Self-Care Approach.

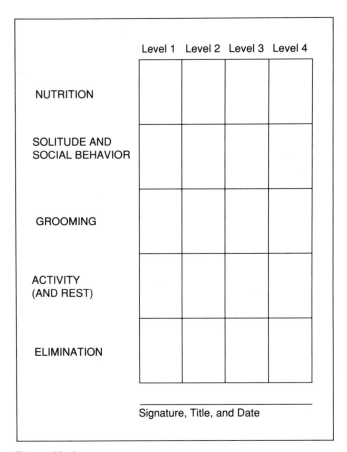

Figure 40–4
NSGAE adaptation categories and assessment levels.

Evaluation: Outcome Criteria for the NSGAE

Empirical research is needed to establish the validity and reliability of the NSGAE as an assessment and care-planning approach directed toward increasing the level of self-care functioning of individual clients; the notion of "self-care residential centers" for chronically disordered and disabled clients; the economic value of nursing interventions that emphasize teaching self-care to clients; and the use of the NSGAE to predict psychiatric nursing costs. Implementation of the NSGAE may:

- Create a milieu that supports acquisition of community living skills rather than hospital adjustment for clients
- Encourage program clarity, clear communication, and systematic treatment plans for staff
- Offer a realistic basis for a *prototype* client classifica-

---

Box 40–1
SAMPLE CODE USING NSGAE

Axis	6.323232	Very poor/limited
V	Overall functioning in past year	6
V	Overall current adaptive functioning	3
V	Nutrition	2
V	Solitude and social interaction	3
V	Grooming	2
V	Activity/rest	3
V	Elimination	2

Box 40–2
OPERATIONAL DEFINITIONS OF NSGAE LEVELS

Level 1: The client demonstrates self-care abilities in meeting all the basic biologic needs and consistently uses appropriate resources when difficulties become manifest.

Level 2: The client demonstrates the ability to accomplish specific self-care activities independently, but limited ability to use available resources.

Level 3: The client has limited ability to accomplish self-care activities and requires verbal direction or consistent verbal reminders to ensure needs are met.

Level 4: The client has severely limited ability to accomplish self-care and requires either physical assistance or consistent verbal direction to ensure needs are met.

Source: Adapted from Underwood, P. Nursing Care as a Determinant in the Development of Self-Care Behavior by Hospitalized Adult Schizophrenics. *DSN dissertation, University of California, San Francisco, 1978.*

---

tion system for costing out psychiatric nursing care for administrators and executives

Certainly the NSGAE represents one pragmatic example of true innovation in the era of deinstitutionalization and prospective payment.

Psychoeducational Approaches for Family Caregivers

Theoretical and scientific interest in the relationships between support and outcomes for disabled and dependent disordered clients have resulted in an innovation known as the psychoeducational approach (Anderson et al. 1981; 1986). Reports from successful treatment programs for the chronically ill underscore the importance of mobilizing interpersonal and environmental supports to maintain biologic, psychologic, and social functions and community tenure (Test and Stenn 1978). Erosion of social supports leaves the disabled vulnerable to extreme isolation and to the recidivism, treatment inadequacy or instability, and social disaffiliation that this isolation frequently implies.

Box 40–3
NSGAE BEHAVIORAL CRITERIA

Nutrition Level

1. Is able to maintain nutrition and hydration independently.
2. Needs assistance with culturally accepted table manners. Is able to understand teaching about medications.
3. Needs assistance selecting food or staying with meal.
4. Inadequate/excessive intake due to fear of food, inability to be with others, medications, or physical handicap.

Solitude and Social Interaction Level

1. Is able to use nonhospital support system constructively to meet basic needs.
2. Is able to use nurse-client relationship to problem solve and validate feelings and perceptions of self and others.
3. Is preoccupied with internal stimuli but responds when approached. Is verbally provocative with peers or staff.
4. Is withdrawn or mute. Is unable to control excitement, intrusiveness, or abusiveness.

Grooming and Personal Hygiene Level

1. Is able to dress and groom self at own initiative according to environmental demands and cultural norms.
2. Is able to use hospital structure to care for own clothes, personal space, and grooming.
3. Needs assistance to prepare and complete hygiene tasks. Has no belongings and needs interventions to obtain basic articles of clothing or grooming tools.
4. Cannot dress self according to environmental demands or cultural norms. Cannot perform basic hygiene tasks.

Activity and Rest Level

1. Is able to select and participate in activities. Is able to sleep restfully.
2. May still have sleeping difficulties but is able to verbalize and problem solve solutions.
3. Is overactive or underactive, but has some control over behavior and responds to direction.
4. Cannot sleep for restful periods or sleeps continuously. Is unable to control harmful activity without locked seclusion, restraints, and medications.

Elimination Level

1. Is able to regulate elimination pattern independently.
2. Is able to ask for help to maintain elimination pattern.
3. Cannot maintain elimination without medication or other active treatment.
4. Cannot report bowel/bladder function. Antisocially urinates, defecates, or smears feces.

Source: Adapted from Underwood PR: Facilitating self-care, in Pothier P: Psychiatric Nursing. *Little, Brown, 1980.*

Nursing Care Plan Using NSGAE for Hospitalized Client

Asset/Problem	Goal	Nursing Interventions
1. *Nutrition* No problem.	Client will continue to eat 3 meals a day independently.	Observe and document client's independent functioning.
2. *Solitude and social interaction* Client cannot express his need for interaction verbally. He giggles inappropriately and becomes intrusive when anxious.	Client will be able to tolerate limited interaction with staff (at least 5 minutes 3 times per shift).	Introduce self each shift. Attempt to meet needs despite his inability to verbalize them. Set up three times per shift to be together. Spend the time in structured ways, i.e., do grooming tasks, go for a walk. Client does not tolerate intense verbal interaction and becomes more inappropriate with direct questions. Allow him time to be alone if he starts to giggle. Assist him to join activities as tolerated. Verbally redirect client from situations with too much stimuli. Give encouragement and positive feedback when appropriate.
3. *Solitude and social interaction*	On discharge, client will be able to tolerate limited interaction with others in a structured environment as evidenced by his ability to follow his schedule (see problem 4).	Role model social interaction and use group activities to increase social skills. Use nurse-client relationship to help him learn new social skills.
4. *Grooming* Client is unable to care for hygiene and clothing due to the disorganization of psychosis.	Client will do the following: • be up, dressed, and shaved by 9 A.M. • make bed and clean area by 9:30 A.M. • do laundry Monday and Thursday P.M. • shower Monday, Wednesday, and Friday P.M.	Arrange schedule with client for hygiene. Review schedule early in the shift and give reminders as necessary of tasks to be done. Monitor and give further assistance if needed. Give positive feedback for all tasks accomplished. Allow him to do as much as possible for himself.
	At discharge, client will do the above tasks independently.	Be alert for progress and allow the client as much independence as he tolerates. Give positive feedback.
5. *Activity and rest* Client has impulsive behavior, inability to concentrate, and an	Client will develop a schedule with nurse and follow through on ward expectations.	Assist client to develop a schedule that will include grooming tasks, free time, and therapeutic activities.

continued

Nursing Care Plan Using NSGAE for Hospitalized Client (continued)

Asset/Problem	Goal	Nursing Interventions
increased activity level with decreased sleep due to response to internal stimuli.		Assist client to identify and participate in free time activities.
		Be familiar with schedule and redirect questions regarding what to do back to the schedule.
		Give reminders to follow schedule if necessary.
		Validate the client's ability to problem-solve and regulate own rest and activity schedule.
		Give positive feedback for successes in this area.
	Before discharge client will develop a schedule to follow at the board and care home.	Assist him to develop a schedule consistent with expectations at the home and other discharge plans.
		Give positive feedback for this and encourage own decision making without overwhelming him.
	Client will sleep 6–8 hours a night.	Set up (with client) nightly routine for sleep and include this on his schedule.
		Remind him to follow this routine.
		Document if this routine helps him get to sleep.
6. *Elimination* No problem.	Client will continue to have BM daily according to prehospital routine.	Observe and document client's independent functioning

Source: Adapted from model used by clinical nurses at Langley Porter Psychiatric Institute. Original by Geoffry McEnany, RN, MS.

Goals

The psychoeducational approach to family treatment combines two basic goals:

1. Decreased client vulnerability to environmental stimulation through a program of educated maintenance chemotherapy and other treatment regimens
2. Increased predictability and stability of the family environment achieved by decreasing the anxiety of family members about the client, increasing their knowledge about chronic mental disorders, and increasing their repertoire of strategies to deal with the problems that need confident management

When rehospitalization rates are used to reflect outcomes, the rate is significantly less in families who have undergone psychoeducation than in control groups whose family members were treated exclusively with drug or surgical therapy (Anderson et al. 1981).

Phases in the Psychoeducation Approach

The two goals of psychoeducation can be achieved through interventions that fall into four somewhat overlapping categories:

1. Connecting
2. Survival skills training
3. Individualization
4. Continuation or disengagement

Psychoeducation with families of chronically disordered and dependent clients is based on the central premise that families can be a pivotal resource for the care and long-term management of their relatives if they are given emotional and practical support and information. The approach begins as early in contacts with the family system as possible with sessions devoted to connecting, or building an alliance, with the family. Such sessions typically include discussion of the pain, frustration, embarrassment, and anger associated with the burdens of caring for a chronically disordered, disabled, and dependent relative. The intent of these sessions is to obtain a good grasp of the type and degree of difficulties being experienced by the family. The nurse in this role should realize that most families have met at least one health professional who has implied that they directly or indirectly caused their relative's illness and should strive to be viewed as the family's ombudsman. Moreover, the nurse should realize that feelings of helplessness and hopelessness prevail even among caring and concerned families and should emphasize the family's strengths and power to influence the course of things positively. The family's performance of care tasks can have a positive effect on the client and become important to keeping him or her alive, out of the hospital, or at a higher level of self-care adaptive functioning. The final task of this initial phase in the psychoeducational approach is to establish a mutual agreement about the goals, content, length, rules, and methods of family counseling. The point here is to establish a treatment contract.

Survival Skills Training

Often survival skills training takes the form of multiple family workshops that provide information about the symptoms, onset, course, and outcome of the client's disability and disorder and about different families' experiences living with it. It is important to try to distinguish between factual data and opinions about these topics. Information about medications should include the mechanisms of action, main effects, and possible side-effects. The nurse should stress the evidence that medication compliance is associated with control and even survival but encourage each family to weigh the costs and benefits of all and any medications. Information about management should include how to set reasonable limits, decrease overstimulation, avoid blow-ups, create helpful structures such as labels for those with Alzheimer's disease, and reevaluate and modify expectations for the client and his or her behaviors. The nurse should support family members' needs to normalize their own lives as much as possible and to establish networks for social and psychologic support as well as practical help.

Individualization

The individualization category of family meetings customarily includes both client and caregiving family. The overall goals of these meetings involve applying strategies to the individual situation, and the sessions usually address family boundaries and client responsibilities.

The goals with respect to family boundaries are to increase the structure within the family (e.g., the boundaries between the client and his or her family) and decrease the boundaries between the family and sources of social support. The goal with respect to client responsibilities is to increase the client's assumption of self-care tasks and enhance his or her competencies in these areas. Problems that emerge often revolve around the client's lack of energy and motivation to decrease dependency and increase self-care levels and the family's guilt about providing for their own needs rather than concentrating on the client's needs. Often the psychiatric nurse can provide invaluable help by becoming a broker for community resources, directing and coordinating family members toward respite care, support groups, and the like. (See Appendix C.)

Continuation or Disengagement

Usually when maximally effective family functioning has been attained, the family either moves into more conventional family therapy or elects "maintenance sessions," which become less frequent and ultimately terminate. The intent of these sessions is to maintain initial gains and to abort potential new problems by anticipating stress and reinforcing knowledge about the client's illness—be it schizophrenia, substance abuse, or Alzheimer's disease—its characteristics, and family burdens.

FUTURE DIRECTIONS: TOWARD TRUE INNOVATION

The self-care nursing model and the NSGAE are approaches emphasizing a practical orientation and the teaching of community survival skills to chronic clients. The psychoeducational approach is directed toward enhancing social support for family caregivers. In a future characterized by cutbacks in resources, increased needs for self-determination, family caregivers, and power based on knowledge and information, psychiatric nurses have a unique opportunity for designing true innovations.

Chapter Highlights

- The community mental health movement (known as "the third revolution" in psychiatry) is a social movement as well as a system for the delivery of community-based mental health services.

- Landmark recommendations made in 1961 by the Joint Commission on Mental Illness and Health drew the attention and concern of politicians and mental health professionals toward the woefully inadequate psychiatric services in the country.

- Millions of dollars of federal funding were provided for the construction of comprehensive community mental health centers, mental health research, and training programs for mental health care providers.

- Other major studies, such as the 1978 report of the President's Commission on Mental Health, gave visibility to the professional competence of nurses in mental health care and made significant recommendations toward coordinating the two-tiered system of mental health care that had evolved.

- In the two-tiered system of mental health care the severely mentally ill continued to inhabit state institutions, and those with less acute problems used the services of community mental health centers. Certain populations (recently discharged clients, the chronically mentally ill, the elderly, youth, and minority groups, for example) fell between the two categories and were not served.

- The 1980 Community Mental Health Systems Act (which was intended to coordinate the two-tiered system) could not be implemented without a change in the political and economic climate. In addition, decreases in the federal budget caused increasing concern over the possible demise of community mental health programs.

- Introduction of prospective payment systems in the form of DRGs may lead to changes in psychiatry's future.

- The basic philosophy of the community mental health movement is that health care is a right, and, therefore, mental health services should be available to all people.

- Six concepts central to community mental health are (1) a systems perspective; (2) an emphasis on prevention; (3) interdisciplinary collaboration, balancing flexible role boundaries with unique areas of expertise; (4) consumer participation and control; (5) the provision of comprehensive services to the community as client as defined by geographic catchment areas; and (6) continuity of care for clients in their movement from one program to another.

- Community mental health nursing roles include such diverse activities as effective parenting classes; divorce therapy groups; suicide prevention counseling; case finding; planning for a client's discharge; teaching self-care activities; staffing partial hospitalization programs; and providing individual, group, and family psychotherapy.

- The ANA Standards provide guidelines for both nursing generalists and specialists who practice in community settings.

- Conventional treatment under the community mental health system has become a highly prescriptive, elaborately formal structure of policy, regulations, and standards in which the old state hospital warehouse has been replaced by a similarly bureaucratic clearinghouse.

- Part of the community mental health system's dilemma is that it must protect the community and, at the same time, guarantee the client's rights.

- Deinstitutionalization is simultaneously the *fact* that the resident population of state hospitals has decreased about 62 percent, and a *philosophy* of civil-libertarian emphasis on clients' rights and expanded-care services based in the clients' communities.

- Shifting the location and funding arrangements for the chronically and severely mentally disordered has not solved their problems.

- Genuine innovation is needed to devise alternative-care approaches, particularly for the severely and chronically mentally disordered.

- The NSGAE self-care nursing model and the psychoeducational approach for family caregivers create new roles for psychiatric nurses of the future.

References

Anderson CM, Hogarty GE, Reiss DJ: The psychoeducational family treatment of schizophrenia, in Goldstein M: *New Directions for Mental Health Services*. Jossey Bass, 1981.

Anderson CM, Reiss DJ, and Hogarty GE: Schizophrenia and the Family, the Guilford Press, 1986.

Bachrach LL: A conceptual approach to deinstitutionalization. *Hosp Community Psychiatry* 1978;29:573–578.

Bachrach LL: Planning mental health services for the chronic patient. *Hosp Community Psychiatry* 1979;30:387–392.

Bassuk EL, Gerson S: Deinstitutionalization and mental health services. *Sci Am* 1978;238:46–53.

Beigel A: Planning psychiatry's future. *Hosp Community Psychiatry* 1986;37(6):551–554.

Berns JS, Hamilton MS: Nursing role in community mental health, in Jarvis LL (ed): *Community Health Nursing: Keeping the Public Healthy* FA Davis, 1981, pp 319–353.

Caplan G: *Principles of Preventive Psychiatry*. Basic Books, 1964.

Davis CK: The status of reimbursement policy and future projections, in Williams C (ed): *Nursing Research and Policy Formation: The Case of Prospective Payment*. American Academy of Nursing, 1984.

Dumas RG: The psychiatric-mental health clinical nurse specialist: A future view. Keynote address at the Third Southeastern Regional Conference of Clinical Specialists in Psychiatric Nursing, Virginia Beach, VA, September 24, 1981.

Goldman HH: Defining and counting the chronically mentally ill. *Hosp Community Psychiatry* 1981;32:21–27.

Greenblatt M, York RH, Brown EL: *From Custodial to Therapeutic Patient Care in Mental Hospitals.* Russell Sage Foundation, 1955.

Hadley R: President's commission sets national mental health goals. *Am Nurse* 1978;10:1.

Joint Commission on Mental Health of Children: *Crisis in Child Mental Health: Challenge for the 1970s.* Harper & Row, 1969.

Jones M: *The Therapeutic Community.* Basic Books, 1953.

Kennedy JF: Mental illness and mental retardation. Presented at the 88th Congress, 1st Session. House of Representatives Document 58, 1963.

Klerman GL: National trends in hospitalization. *Hosp Community Psychiatry* 1979;30:110–113.

Leininger M: Community psychiatric nursing: Trends, issues, and problems. *Perspect Psychiatr Care* 1969;7:11.

Minkoff K: A map of chronic mental patients, in Talbot J (ed): *The Chronic Mental Patient.* APA 1978, pp 11–73.

Morrison E, et al.: The NSGAE: A proposed axis for DSM-III. *J Psychosoc Nurs* 1985;23(8):10–13.

Orem D: *Nursing Concepts of Practice,* ed 2. McGraw-Hill, 1980.

Reinke B, Greenley JR: Organizational analysis of three community support program models. *Hosp Community Psychiatry* 1986;37(6):624–629.

Report to the President of the President's Commission on Mental Health. Vol. I. US Government Printing Office, 1978.

Stanton A, Schwartz M: The management of a type of institutional participation in mental illness. *Psychiatry* 1949;12:13–26.

Talbott JA: Deinstitutionalization: Avoiding the disasters of the past. *Hosp Community Psychiatry* 1979;30:621–624.

Test MA, Stern LI: Community treatment of the chronic patient: Research overview. *Schizophrenia Bull* 1978;14:350–364.

Underwood PR: *Nursing Care as a Determinant in the Development of Self-Care Behavior by Hospitalized Adult Schizophrenics,* DSN dissertation. University of California, San Francisco, 1978.

Underwood PR: Facilitating self-care, in Pothier P: *Psychiatric Nursing,* Little, Brown, 1980.

Washington Report on Medicine and Health, The Changing Mission of ADAMHA, January 11, 1982.

Widem P, et al: Prospective payment for psychiatric hospitalization. *Hosp Community Psychiatry* 1984;35(5):447–451.

Wilson HS: *Deinstitutionalized Residential Alternatives for the Severely Mentally Disordered: The Soteria House Approach.* Grune & Stratton, 1982.

APPENDIX A

Comprehensive Mental Health Assessment

Erie County Department of Mental Health

Completion of the forms on pages 1138–1145 follows the "Initial Contact" and provides more detailed demographic and client information. It may take anywhere from one to several contacts with the client in order to complete all the relevant items on these forms.

RATING SCALES

The rating scales are designed to provide a more objective picture of an individual's level of function or dysfunction by rating the person in ten Life Areas and six areas called Signals of Distress on a 5-point scale with standard definitions attached to each scale. Crises or mental health problems arise from broken life attachments in one of the ten life areas. Such broken attachments are also often manifested by signals of distress. The assessment rating scales enable workers to describe and evaluate individuals in a sufficiently comprehensive way so that specific service goals can be identified.

Source: Hoff, LA, *People in Crisis,* ed 2. Addison-Wesley, 1984, pp 95–104. Reproduced by permission of the Erie County Department of Mental Health; Mental Health Services, Erie County, Corporation IV, South East Corporation V, and Lakeshore Corporation VI. For samples of forms not included here and for complete specifications for use of these forms, the reader is referred to Erie County Department of Mental Health, 95 Franklin Street, Buffalo, New York 14202.

Since assessment is an *ongoing process* over time, these forms should assist the worker in recording changes in a client's level of functioning, which then has implications for revising the service contract.

Initial Assessment Phases

During the Initial Assessment Phase, the worker records a composite of several viewpoints or perspectives (Worker [W], Client [C], and Significant Other [O]) in relation to each life function or signal of distress. During or after the clinical interview(s), the worker should decide on a rating for the sixteen items. This decision is based on his/her observation and interviewing skills. Assessment can be further expanded by asking the client and/or significant others to rate the client's level of functioning. All the areas may not be assessed at any one time, but should be completed prior to completion of the service contract.

Working Phase

Reassessment may be done at any time during the service interval if the worker finds significant life changes or progress made on goals to *warrant* an interim assessment.

Termination Phase

At the completion of the service contract, when the client and counselor have worked toward termination, a final assessment is done to (a) suggest whether the level of functioning desired has been achieved, and (b) make a comparison between the initial and termination functional levels.

Follow-Up

After termination of service, the person should be contacted periodically to ascertain whether any further service is needed or desired. The follow-up contact should be negotiated as part of the service contract and carried out unless the person states that he or she does not wish to be contacted after termination of service. Follow-up contacts are particularly important for the person who finds it very difficult to ask for and use help during the early stages of a problem before a serious crisis develops.

ASSESSMENT RATING SCALE DESCRIPTIONS AND DEFINITIONS

Rating scale descriptions and definitions are intended to provide the worker with a more comprehensive understanding of the meaning of each assessment area. The examples cited in the definitions of each scale are just that, examples. The worker should recognize that there will be numerous other examples of real-life situations that will be analogous to those provided. Also, while no rating of a person can be *completely* objective, the scale definitions provide a framework for eliminating subjective assessment as much as possible.

A. LIFE FUNCTIONS

1. Physical Health

Description

This scale is intended to focus on a person's physical health needs as well as ability to identify, regulate, anticipate, and seek treatment for those needs. Physical illness refers to symptoms, whether real or imagined. Ratings should be made considering severity of illness and need for an immediate medical response. Considerations include: sleeping, eating, drinking, alcohol and drug use/abuse, weight, posture, motor mannerisms, physical complaints, general nutrition, personal hygiene, dental hygiene, activity level, medication, physical impairments/disabilities.

Ratings

1. *High:* Person is involved in pursuit of physical health as a part of living. Is aware of and follows through on physical health problems when they occur. Enjoys good physical health with no present need for medical services.

2. *Moderate High:* Person has health problems and can identify, regulate, and anticipate them.

3. *Moderate:* Person has physical problems and can identify them; however, is inconsistent in seeking medical attention; e.g., sees physician for prescription, but self-medicates.

4. *Low/Moderate:* Person has physical symptoms that indicate medical attention is needed. Has knowledge that a problem exists but is not making an effort to seek assistance. Person requires regulation by others and reminders that physical needs are important.

5. *Low Functioning:* Person has physical symptoms that require immediate medical attention and are potentially life threatening (malnutrition, heart pain, dehydration, excessive obesity). The person is not concerned about the problem and is not making any efforts to seek medical treatment.

2. Self-acceptance/Self-esteem

Description

This scale is intended to assess an individual's feelings toward the self as a person—the degree to which he or she feels capable, adequate, and valuable as a person.

Ratings

1. *High Functioning:* Individuals are enthusiastic about life and confident of their resources and capacities for personal adjustment. They employ a realistic standard of self-appraisal based upon awareness of both positive and negative traits. While not viewing themselves as perfect, they see themselves as capable and adequate. Their goals are realistically based upon their capacity for achievement and they choose appropriate means for goal solutions. They are capable of feeling guilt and anxiety when they have violated their own internalized standard of personal conduct. Their aspirations are consistent with their capacities and are organized within a systematic life-style that permeates the past, present, and future. Failure can be accepted without damaging their basic sense of personal adequacy. They adjust relatively easily to frustrations of daily life and can change their goals consistent with personal and/or situational changes. Since they feel basically adequate, they are capable of total personality development and can creatively actualize the full range of their inner potential. Basic self-acceptance translates into basic acceptance of others and allows them to freely enjoy social interactions. It is important to distinguish those individuals with a genuine positive self-regard from those who practice denial of negative self-regard.

2. *High/Moderate:* Individuals are usually productively involved in many areas of life. Their expectations are realistic and they usually set goals consistent with their ability. Since they realistically accept having some negative traits, they are relatively free from anxiety, guilt, and blame. They are committed to the development of their potential and usually view themselves as being in relative control of their life situation. They accept frustration as a fact of life and adjust their goals accordingly. Under extreme stress they may question their ability and self-worth and many experience a minor and temporary decline in functioning. They rarely have feelings of depression and they advance beyond personal responsibility to being able to assume responsibility in relationships with others.

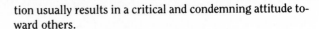

3. *Moderate Functioning:* These individuals characterize the majority of the population. Their sense of adequacy and competence is sufficiently strong to allow self-management and responsibility to others within the context of their daily lives. While there is awareness of both negative and positive traits, there may be some distortion of either. They may have some difficulty in accepting failure and may rely upon support from others in dealing with frustration. At times, they protect themselves through falsification of their own ability or the circumstances relating to failure of goal achievement. With sufficient stress they may temporarily underaspire or overaspire to goals and may engage in self-depreciation and/ or blaming of others. Guilt and anxiety are determined by an appropriate internalized standard of personal conduct, but at times they may accept responsibility for events over which they lack control. Some negative traits may be denied and some positive traits exaggerated. While being reasonably self-confident, they may become defensive when their behavior or accomplishments are challenged. Their means-goals relationships are appropriate and usually consistent with their capacity, although they usually do not develop their full potential. At times they may experience mild depression and have fleeting fantasies of suicide that are not acted out in actual behavior. They usually have a few close friendships and are capable of interpersonal relationships based upon the acceptance of others.

4. *Low/Moderate:* Individuals are inconsistent in their self-evaluations. While usually feeling inadequate in managing their problems, they have sporadic periods of renewed confidence in their coping ability. They basically feel inadequate, guilty, and self-condemning with frequent fantasies of suicide and possible attempts. While they are cognitively aware of some positive traits, they generally feel negatively toward themselves and act accordingly. Periods of positive mood are reactions to situational determinants rather than to positive self-regard, which may also represent attempts to overcome unwanted depression. They experience their daily life as stressful and feel unable to manage ordinary problems.

5. *Low Functioning:* Individuals are preoccupied with a sense of personal failure and guilt. They generally feel inadequate and incompetent and characteristically focus upon their negative traits and are unaware of and deny having positive traits. The tendency to condemn themselves is overt and prominent to the extent of self-punishment, including frequent suicide ideation or actual attempts. There is obvious defenselessness and open admission of worthlessness. Frustration tolerance is weak with a lack of capacity for coping with stress resulting from personal and situational changes. There is a pronounced inability to plan objectives realistically. Individuals may underaspire or overaspire to goal achievements, which leads to actual failure due to their unrealistic standard of self-expectation. There is a sense of hopelessness, pessimism, self-doubt, and acute depression. Unfavorable comparison with others often leads to social withdrawal. These people cannot accept responsibility for themselves or for others. Basic self-rejec-

tion usually results in a critical and condemning attitude toward others.

3. Vocational/Occupational

Description

This area focuses on the person's present employment/vocational role in terms of:

- Extent to which it meets his or her financial needs.
- Individual's degree of satisfaction with present employment or role, e.g., Are you working to your level of capacity—or above it? If unemployed, do you have any job skills or education that could be developed? If unemployed, ascertain the degree of activity around job search, e.g., What have you done to find a job? Are you working two jobs that interfere with family life?

Occupation refers to student, homemaker, retired, as well as usual occupations.

Ratings

1. *High:* Person is employed and working at full capacity. Person expresses satisfaction with job or retirement.

2. *Moderate/High:* Person is employed. Satisfied with job, not actively seeking for better paid work, but says, "I wish I could make more." Or, person is retired and quite satisfied with self-support.

3. *Moderate:* Person is employed but expresses dissatisfaction with present job in terms of (a) pay, (b) advancement, (c) hours, and/or (d) nature of work. Has fairly stable job history and can get and keep jobs. Is aware of skills, but does not show much activity around changing jobs for self-betterment. Person is only moderately happy with retirement role and lacks options for use of time.

4. *Low/Moderate:* Person is unemployed at present, has worked in past, but work history is sporadic. Takes jobs when he or she can get them, but leaves, gets fired, or laid off. Has some skills but is not aware of them. Is retired and has few options for satisfying use of time.

5. *Low:* Person is unemployed. Has no vocational goals. Cannot assess self in terms of future employment. No skills. Is retired and has no satisfying outlets.

4. Immediate Family

Description

This scale is intended to assess the ability of family members to provide support and problem-solving assistance during crisis as well as on a day-to-day basis.

Ratings

1. *High:* Person is able to rely on the family as a unit during times of emotional crisis as well as on a day-to-day basis. Family is usually able to meet the person's needs and can

offer both positive and negative feedback in a constructive way.

2. *Moderate/High:* Person relies on family members in times of crisis; however, family members are not always able to respond completely or in a consistently constructive way.

3. *Moderate:* Person relies on at least two family members and can depend on them in times of need. Person has no real sense that these people would help for extensive periods of time.

4. *Low/Moderate:* Person has one family member that he or she talks to; however, does not rely on them except in extreme cases. Feels family doesn't care about him or her.

5. *Low:* Person feels like family is never around when needed—acts as if he or she were not a member of the family. Person depends on nonfamily members when in trouble. Person is isolated and does not have a regular support system.

5. Intimate Relationships

Description

Intimate relationship is defined as "a close, familiar, and usually affectionate or loving relationship" which is usually limited to one or a few people. This rating measures the extent to which a person can have such a relationship in which there is mutual sharing of positive/negative feelings. Such relationships are often characterized by a sense of openness, honesty, and feelings of support. Although sexual intimacy may also be an important part of this relationship, the scale is intended to emphasize social or psychological intimacy even when a sexual relationship may not exist, e.g., a close brother-sister relationship.

Ratings

1. *High:* Person has intimate contact with a few others and the intimacy is acknowledged by all. There is a strong sense of permanency and future interactions are seen as important to maintain. Relationships are relaxed, open, and mutual understanding exists through honest interaction. Time is spent together by choice and significant moments are treasured.

2. *Moderate/High:* Person has intimate contact with (at least) a few others and the feeling of closeness is shared by both. The relationship has permanent qualities and though it may be closed in some areas, time is spent together by choice and for extended periods.

3. *Moderate:* Person can identify a close relationship in which there is intimacy and an honest sharing of feelings. A sense of permanence has existed or does exist, at least potentially, and some time is spent together.

4. *Low/Moderate:* Person has or had some marginal intimate relationships that were seen as somewhat supportive. These relationships may be strained, but feelings about the other can be discussed and there is a possibility for developing a relationship.

5. *Low:* Person has no intimate contacts with others, real or fancied. Is closed, defensive, and resistant to talking about feelings for others at present or in the past.

6. Residential Situation

Description

This area refers to a person's basic shelter needs, how he or she meets those needs, and the degree of satisfaction the person expresses about his or her residence; e.g., How do you judge your housing situation?

Is the person concerned about poor housing or is there little awareness that housing is substandard: e.g., If living situation is poor, what are you doing to improve your living situation? Does your living situation contribute to other problems, or (if the situation is good), does it improve your functioning? Is there overcrowding, rent too high, safety hazards, adequate heat and plumbing, lead paint, etc.?

Ratings

1. *High:* Living conditions are more than adequate. Owns home or lives in excellent surroundings. Person expresses satisfaction with present living situation and privacy is available at any time. Living situation is stable.

2. *Moderate/High:* Living conditions are adequate in terms of size and state of repair, with some degree of privacy, but not entirely satisfactory to the person. Is actively searching for better housing that is affordable. May include a transitional living situation that is adequate but temporary.

3. *Moderate:* Living conditions are adequate, but premises need repair or lack the degree of privacy that would be considered appropriate. Person expresses dissatisfaction, but is not actively looking for alternatives or is complaining about the state of disrepair of an unsafe neighborhood; does not do anything to correct the situation.

4. *Low/Moderate:* Living conditions are below standard, with no activity around improvement; or person is being evicted, not actively searching for other placement. Eviction due to nonpayment of rent or other problems is viewed as the landlord's fault. Feels there is not much that can be done about living conditions.

5. *Low:* Currently has no place to live, is living in temporary housing, or is living in conditions that require a change due to health problems. There is a definite need to provide alternative housing immediately. Living conditions are unstable.

7. Financial

Description

This area includes:

- Extent to which a person's financial needs are met; e.g., Do you make enough money to comfortably support yourself?

- Source of income. If unemployed or retired: Are you on welfare? Social Security? Veteran's benefits?

- Ability of the person to budget the money which he or she does have.

Ratings

1. *High:* Person has a sufficient source of income and moderate to extensive savings. Anyone would be willing to lend him or her $500 without concern. Has excellent credit rating. Has some potential for finding other sources of income if current job were terminated. Budgets income well and is capable of making good investments.

2. *Moderate/High:* Person has a good source of income and perhaps some savings or investments to fall back on if income were suddenly discontinued. Has some friends/family or a good credit rating that could be drawn upon if necessary.

3. *Moderate:* Person has a fixed source of income or a job that permits basic needs to be met, but requires some careful budgeting in order to purchase desired "extras." Has limited borrowing power from a few friends or other resources. Is generally able to budget funds but would be hard pressed if income were suddenly terminated.

4. *Low/Moderate:* Person has income either through public assistance or from a job, but it meets only the most basic needs. Person may or may not be able to meet the stringent budgeting required for living on a fixed income.

5. *Low:* Person has no source of income at present. May also owe money on some/several debts. There is no money to cover the coming week's expenses. His or her credit rating is nil and he or she has no one whom he or she could borrow from. Must have immediate assistance in order to cover basic living costs.

8. Decision-Making Ability

Description

The purpose of this scale is to assess the strategy, process, and effectiveness of the person's decision-making and problem-solving performance relative to goals and actual outcomes. Emphasis should be focused upon the person's cognitive functioning with less attention paid to emotional factors that are involved in the decision-making process.

Ratings

1. *High:* Individual is very task oriented and sets realistic goals consistent with ability. He or she thinks before acting and shows evidence of logical thought process in goals-means-ends relationships. Individual feels basically secure and self-confident as decision maker. He or she approaches problem-oriented situations with necessary emotional detachment— appropriately scanning the field; collecting relevant information, while holding extraneous factors constant; reviewing alternative solutions to the problem; and considering consequences of each alternative before implementing actions. If the choice is incorrect, the person shifts to a more appro- priate alternative rather than clinging compulsively to the original one, and he or she accepts responsibility for the decisions.

2. *High/Moderate:* The individual enjoys a full emotional life but is quite capable of task orientation when making decisions. There is usually no apparent emotional interference with the continuity and logic of thought processes, except when numerous problems occur simultaneously or when individual problems have severe consequences. The belief in oneself as a decision maker is stable, and the person more often than not accepts the consequences of his or her decisions, even during those infrequent times of acting impulsively. The individual sometimes chooses a particular course prematurely; considers consequences of alternative solutions before acting, sometimes acting impulsively; usually shifts to a more appropriate alternative if actual experience shows original alternative to be incorrect; and usually accepts responsibility for decisions, although sometimes he or she will blame the situation or other people for mistakes. At times, feelings may confuse thought processes, and the person may either temporarily withdraw or rely upon others for help in problem situations.

3. *Moderate:* Individual shows a blending of task- and self-orientation. At times, goal priorities may be in mutual conflict or goals-means relationships may be inconsistent. Nevertheless, the person is reasonably capable of making effective decisions most of the time. He or she collects relevant information, sometimes scanning either too narrowly or broadly; reviews alternative solutions, sometimes choosing a particular one prematurely; and considers consequences of alternative actions before acting, sometimes acting impulsively. The person usually shifts to a more appropriate alternative if actual experience shows the original alternative to be incorrect; and usually accepts responsibility for his or her decisions, although sometimes either blaming the situation or other people for personal mistakes. At times feelings may confuse thought processes, and the person may either temporarily withdraw or rely upon others for help in problem situations.

4. *Low/Moderate:* Individual is mainly self-preoccupied and is unable to concentrate for the necessary period of time to arrive at a problem solution. Thought processes are scattered and shifting; and impulsively arrived at solutions are implemented without considering alternatives. There is a noticeable degree of compulsive clinging to alternatives in spite of their ineffectiveness in actual experience. The person will quite desperately accept advice from others and will doubt his or her own capacity for decision making. Beliefs are often without foundation in reality and the person frequently thinks in a fatalistic way that he or she is incapable of altering surrounding situations.

5. *Low:* Individual is quite disorganized and reveals an obvious emotional interference with thought processes. He or she is self-preoccupied, impulsive, inconsistent, and distracted. When faced with a problem situation, the person becomes frightened and withdrawn and may either seek support and advice from others or avoid social contact altogether. Solutions to problems are impulsive and later regretted and disowned. Goals are inconsistent and unrealistic and means-goals relationships are inappropriate. Thought processes are scattered with considerable distractedness and shifting. Beliefs may take the form of compulsions and delusions and, at

times, hallucinations may be present. Events taking place in the person's life appear to have no order or purpose and seem to be outside the individual's control.

9. Life Philosophy

Description

This area examines the extent to which a person has life goals and a system of values. One's values guide a person in determining the "rightness" or "wrongness" of an idea or action. It is essential to assess whether there exists a system of values upon which goals and actions follow; not whether a person's value system is consistent with and/or acceptable to society's view of life. Certain life styles have special ritual/taboos or "laws"/guidelines/norms, which are consciously followed or ignored. A client's ability to "judge" a certain situation or to have a sense of a "good" or "bad" conscience are indicators of the existence of a value system. The person's value system forms the basis for various life goals and aspirations.

Children and persons with certain mental handicaps (e.g., mental retardation or psychosis) will tend to utilize their parents' or significant other's value system to guide their behaviors and attitudes.

Ratings

1. *High:* A system of values exists that reflects the origins of "right" and "wrong" judgments. This system can be described by the person and is used as a guide for goals and behaviors in ambiguous or ill-defined situations of varying kinds. The person's behavior reflects actions that are consistent with this value system. The person has set meaningful goals and has achieved them to his or her satisfaction.

2. *Moderate/High:* Person is in the process of defining his or her own value system and goals, and recognizes the need for same. Is usually satisfied with knowing "right" from "wrong." Experiences occasional confusion or ambivalence when facing complex situations involving "ethical" issues or decisions that are neither "black" nor "white" but in "gray" areas. May also be confused occasionally about what he or she wants out of life.

3. *Moderate:* A hierarchy or degrees of "rightness"/"wrongness" exists with some things being considered "forbidden." Behaviors are not entirely consistent with these judgments. Person can acknowledge the existence of a value system but it is "imposed" or "inherited" from others rather than truly integrated and acknowledged as one's own. Goals very often are those set for the sake of others or in response to pressure rather than for self. The value systems of most children would fall into this category.

4. *Low/Moderate:* Person has a value system that allows individual actions to be labeled as "right" or "wrong." There is no underlying scheme, so behaviors may not always be consistent. Similar situations can produce unexpected or different reactions. Person has poorly defined life goals and is generally frustrated in his or her attempts to achieve goals.

5. *Low:* Has no value scheme that expresses itself in a consistent pattern of behavior. Actions and decisions appear inconsistent and haphazard. Person appears at times to have "no conscience at all" and is generally directionless.

10. Leisure Time Use/Community Involvement

Description

This area refers to how a person uses leisure time and the degree of satisfaction that he or she obtains from it. Leisure time can be monitored by the extent the person uses available community resources appropriately and the extent to which these resources are sought out. Community involvement is determined by the extent the person participates in the community outside of his or her home. Leisure time is any time when the person is not at place of employment or not occupied with childrearing and/or other housekeeping activities. It would include going to the movies, the pool hall, playgrounds, etc. Is a person's leisure time so limited that there is no time for self, significant other, or family relationships to develop (as in the case of the person who works two jobs)? Does a person have too much leisure time (as in the case of being unemployed or retired)? For example, Do you have ample leisure time that helps you function in other life areas? Is leisure time a burden? A lonely period? A real bore?

Ratings

1. *High:* Feels comfortable with amount of leisure time. Realizes the necessity for leisure and uses this time for constructive projects, meetings, and recreational activities. Does not become over-involved. Regulates leisure time use very well. Is quite aware of community resources and actively involves self in several community activities. Has some sense of responsibility to his or her community.

2. *Moderate/High:* Has definite ideas about how to use leisure time and is aware of the need for it. Expresses satisfaction, but sees room for improvement and actively pursues it. Has knowledge of his or her community and becomes involved in the community on occasion.

3. *Moderate:* Recognizes the need for leisure time and has some available. Tends to become over-involved on occasion, but does not recognize this as a pattern. Has difficulty in regulating use of leisure time. Only occasionally will the person seek community activities or involvement due to some limited social skill or lack of transportation to community resources/activities.

4. *Low/Moderate:* Uses leisure time inappropriately. Is interested in some activities, but is inconsistent in pursuing them. Wants to do something, but doesn't know what. Has a talent or interest but cannot bring self to pursue it. Participates in community activities if encouraged, but would not initiate such activities for him/herself. Depends almost totally on others for knowledge of community resources.

5. *Low:* Never has any time to relax. Never knows what to do with leisure time. Sits and ruminates, feels like nobody cares. Not interested in anything outside of home. May engage largely in passive activities, e.g., watching television. Has never developed or engaged in outside interests, or did so only in the distant past. Person is almost totally unaware of potential community resources.

11. Feeling Management

Description

The intent of this rating is to measure the person's awareness of feelings and ability to appropriately use and manage feelings in various situations. This rating concerns the way in which a person's defense mechanisms protect him or her against problems in living; the person's ability to regulate impulsive behavior; the person's ability to control or work through painful feelings, e.g., How would you judge your ability to handle your feelings, or your ability to accept and value positive feelings?

Ratings

1. *High:* Person is aware of feelings, can express them at will, and can take appropriate action to discharge or regulate them. Person can effectively acknowledge and appreciate the value of both negative and positive feelings, which can lead to the "actualizing" state of living.

2. *Moderate/High:* Person can generally express and regulate feelings in all but a few situations. Can discriminate between positive and negative feelings most of the time.

3. *Moderate:* Person has an awareness of feelings that can be expressed and behavior is usually appropriate to the feelings, but mechanisms for working out feelings are not generally available.

4. *Low/Moderate:* Self-corrective and control capacities are limited to survival activities on a physical level. Person is a "victim" of feeling states. Cannot regulate actions in accordance with appropriateness of acts, but responds to feelings in a reactive way. Tends to be able to identify only strong negative feelings, for example, anger.

5. *Low:* Has no self-corrective or control capacity and requires structure and control to be imposed upon him or her from others. Has no awareness of feelings that can be expressed. Feelings tend to "erupt" and tend to be quite destructive to the individual or to others. Behavior tends to be incongruent with feelings after inappropriate over- under-reactions.

B. SIGNALS OF DISTRESS

12. Lethality Toward Self

Description

This scale is intended as a guide to assess the suicide potential of a particular individual at the time of assessment. Specific signs (based on the study of completed suicides) are applied to the individual in an effort to predict as accurately as possible whether or not a person is likely to commit suicide. The person should be assessed as to:

- *Suicide Plan:* a person with a well-thought-out plan including specific time, place, circumstances (e.g., excluding possible rescue) with a readily available high lethal method (gun, jumping, carbon monoxide poisoning, barbiturates, hanging, car crash) is a high risk for suicide; e.g., How are you planning to kill yourself? Do you have a gun? Do you have pills? What kind? How many?

- *History of Suicide Attempts:* a person who has made previous high lethal attempts or changes plan from low lethal to high lethal is a higher risk than a person with history of low lethal or no attempts.

- *Resources and Communication with Significant Other:* any person with poor coping ability and loss of interpersonal support system or inability to maintain communication with existing resources is a high risk; e.g., Is there anyone you feel you can turn to when you're really down? Does _____ know that you're feeling like killing yourself? What is _____'s response to your threat, plan, etc.? This last question is included because significant others may, in fact, encourage would-be attempters by not caring or, in fact, telling them to go ahead.

- *Age, Sex, Race:* suicide risk increases with age for white males. More white males than females commit suicide. Among racial minority persons, there are more suicides under the age of 40 than among older persons.

- *Marital Status:* more divorced, separated, and single persons commit suicide than married persons.

- *Physical Illness:* presence of physical illness increases suicide risk.

- *Drinking and Drug Abuse:* drinking or other drug abuse, accompanying impulsiveness, and loss of control increase suicide risk, especially in the presence of available high lethal methods. In addition, use of either legal or illegal drugs such as barbiturates, sleeping medications, or LSD may also raise impulsiveness and cause loss of control.

- *Recent Loss:* personal loss or threat of loss such as of a spouse, parent, status, money, or job increases suicide risk. In some situations a job promotion may actually be perceived as a loss because the individual feels he or she no longer has the capabilities to handle the situation, or the supports to carry through.

- *Unexplained Change in Behavior:* e.g., sudden reckless driving and drinking by a previously careful, sober driver can be an indicator of suicide danger. Another unexplained behavioral change to look for is the giving away of valued possessions suddenly, making a will, or purchasing a large life insurance policy.

- *Isolation:* a person who is isolated both emotionally and physically is at greater risk than a nonisolated person. This may sometimes be a sudden and unexplained withdrawal or self-imposed isolation.

- *Depression:* signs include sleeplessness, early wakening, weight loss, anorexia, amenorrhea, sexual dysfunction, crying, agitation, hopelessness: e.g. How is your appetite? Do you sleep well? Have you lost weight lately? Depression is not *universally* present in all high lethal persons.

- *Critical Life Event:* a person experiencing the stress of a life crisis situation who lacks internal/external resources for satisfactory resolution of the crisis is a greater risk for suicide than others.

Explicit, direct questions must be asked of the person regarding all these signs if the information is not already available through other assessment data.

Ratings

1. *High Functioning:* No predictable risk of suicide now. No suicidal ideation or history of attempts, has satisfactory social support system, and is in close contact with significant others.

2. *High/Moderate:* Low risk of suicide now. Person has suicidal ideation with low lethal method, no history of attempts, or recent serious loss. Has satisfactory social support system.

3. *Moderate Function:* Moderate risk of suicide now. Has suicidal ideation with high lethal method but no plan, or threats. Has plan with low lethal method, history of low lethal attempts: e.g., employed female, age 35, divorced, with tumultuous family history.

4. *Low/Moderate:* High risk of suicide now. Has current high lethal plan, obtainable means, history of previous attempts, is unable to communicate with a significant other; e.g., female, age 50, living alone, with drinking history; or black male, age 29, unemployed, and has lost his lover.

5. *Low Functioning:* Very high risk of suicide now. Has current lethal plan with available means, history of suicide attempts, is cut off from resources; e.g., white male, over 40, physically ill and depressed, wife threatening divorce, is unemployed.

13. Lethality Toward Others

Description

This scale is intended as a guide to assess the homicide potential or danger of assault by a particular individual at the time of assessment. The following signs are applied to the potentially homicidal individual:

- *Homicide plan:* the person with a high lethal specific plan and available means for homicide is a high risk; e.g., Do you ever get so angry that you feel like killing? How do you plan to do it? Do you have a gun?

- *History of homicide, impulsive acting out, or homicide attempts:* for example, Have you ever felt like hurting anyone before? Did you carry out your urge to kill someone? If so, what happened? Did someone stop you? Were you able to stop yourself? Do you ever feel like you are losing control of yourself? What do you usually do when you feel you are losing control?

- *Resources and communication with significant other(s):* most homicides occur within family units between/among individuals previously acquainted; e.g., How do you usually express your anger toward someone close to you? Is there someone you feel you want to get even with? Are you open to exploring other more constructive ways of expressing your anger?

- *Drinking/drug use/abuse:* a person who drinks frequently and also has a history of impulsive acting out behavior is a higher risk for homicide or assault than a nondrinker. Drinking and accompanying impulsivity and loss of control through substance use and abuse may also raise homicidal lethality, especially in the presence of available high lethal methods.

- *Other criteria:* the person who is suicidal as well as homicidal is an even higher risk because the consequential effects of homicide are not a possible deterrent. In the event that homicidal threats or references are made, however trivial these may seem, such references should be thoroughly checked out.

Ratings

1. *High Functioning:* No predictable risk of assault or homicide now; e.g., no homicidal ideation, urges, or history of same; basically satisfactory support system, social drinker only.

2. *High/Moderate:* Low risk of homicide now; e.g., has occasional assault or homicidal ideation with some urges to kill, no history of impulsive acting out or homicidal attempts, occasional drinking bouts, basically satisfactory social support system.

3. *Moderate Functioning:* Moderate risk of homicide now; e.g., has frequent homicidal ideation and urges to kill, no specific plan; history of impulsive acting out, but no homicide attempts; episodic drinking bouts; stormy relationships with significant other with periodic high tension arguments.

4. *Low/Moderate:* High risk of homicide now; e.g., has homicidal plan; obtainable means; drinking history; history of impulsive acting out, but no homicide attempts; stormy relationships and much verbal plus occasional physical fighting with significant others.

5. *Low Functioning:* Very high risk of homicide now; e.g., has current high lethal plan; available means; history of homicide attempts or impulsive acting out and feels a strong urge to "get even" with a significant other; history of drinking with possibly also high lethal suicide risk.

14. Substance Use

Description

This area refers to use and abuse of prescription or nonprescription drugs of all kinds (e.g., heroin, methadone, hallucinogens, amphetamines, barbiturates, tranquilizers, antidepressants, LSD) and alcohol.

The emphasis is on the person's ability to control consumption of drugs (social drinking and prescription diet pills can be examples of controlled consumption). When the controls break down, use changes to abuse. Abuse can be measured by how and to what degree it is self-destructive, the potential lethality (e.g., alcohol and barbiturates—high lethal combination), the degree to which use interferes with usual everyday functioning, or actually prevents the person from functioning.

This area also considers the person's awareness of drug use as a potential problem, current abuse as a problem, and the person's level of activity around alleviating or changing the self-destructive behavior.

Also, a clear picture should be obtained of what charges are pending against the person, and the severity of those charges, i.e., violations, misdemeanors, or felonies.

Divorce action generally does not include a legal problem.

Ratings

1. *High:* Never a problem. All substance use is constructive and controlled.

2. *High/Moderate:* Rarely a problem. Usually drinks or takes drugs within socially acceptable limits or on prescription, but feels a need every now and then to get drunk or high. However, this generally does not interfere with his or her social and family network or normal functioning.

3. *Moderate:* Some problems. An occasional "drunk," or periodic consistent drug intake. Drug use sporadic and can be traced to a precipitating event, e.g., "I got depressed because. . . ." Person realizes danger of becoming potential substance abuser and shows some activity around preventing this.

4. *Low/Moderate:* Frequent problems. Usually drinks or takes drugs "to get/keep going." Frequently the pattern gets out of control; person goes on binges or has "weekend highs." Constantly promising to improve. Social and family network weak, but intact. Tends to be cyclical. Potential danger not perceived because person is always "starting over."

5. *Low:* Constant problems. Currently abusing drugs/alcohol to the extent that it has caused a breakdown in social and family network; actual or threatened loss of employment due to absences; financial problems. Person denies problem with abuse, little activity around changing or alleviating situation, even though situation is perceived as stressful. There is an expression of "no hope."

15. Legal Problems

Description

This area focuses on the *degree* to which the person's current legal involvement is a problem that interferes with everyday functioning and the *nature* of the legal involvement.

On the "degree of involvement" continuum, how do his or her legal problems interfere with:

- Job possibilities
- Mental health
- Physical health

Under "kind of involvement," assaultive behavior toward others is included, as well as differentiation between crimes against persons vs. crimes against property, or both.

If the arrests and charges concern driving while intoxicated, or include other drug involvement, the degree of substance use needs to be better assessed.

The person's concern or lack of concern about the consequences of his or her actions should be taken into consideration and should be related to a homicide/suicide lethality assessment.

Ratings

1. *High:* Has never been arrested, convicted, or charged with any misdemeanor or felony, or has never been to family court. Is about to retain an attorney if he or she needs one, or knows how to obtain one through Legal Aid or the Public Defender's Office.

2. *High/Moderate:* Has been arrested or fined or charged with a family (civil) and/or criminal offense once, but has had no subsequent arrests or problems with the law. The person has or knows of an attorney to handle legal problems.

3. *Moderate:* Person has been arrested or fined or charged with a family offense or a criminal offense but did not serve time. May be on probation, but accepts responsibility of probation.

4. *Low/Moderate:* Person has a history of offenses, has served time, and when on probation/parole goes to probation/parole officer only when he or she feels like it.

5. *Low:* Has presently pending charges and is awaiting court hearing or trial. Is currently on probation, parole, or both, and may have to serve time if convicted of present charge.

16. Agency Use

Description

This area refers to the person's ability to negotiate with helping systems in the community in order to obtain his or her goals for service. Assessment should consider:

- Individual's degree of knowledge about existing services; e.g., Do you know where to get the help you need?
- Ability to contact agency.
- Ability to follow through with contacts.
- Ability to ensure that he or she gets the service from the agency or goes to a more appropriate agency; e.g., When you don't get help you need, what do you usually do?

Agencies are defined as service clusters that exist in the community or within reachable distance; e.g., lawyers, doctors, and welfare system.

Ratings

1. *High:* Always successful. Has knowledge of agencies and is able to contact the appropriate agency to fill need. Follows through on contacts. Is able to find out about new agencies and use them appropriately. Expresses satisfaction with agencies. Can relate to the agency as a whole.

2. *High/Moderate:* Usually successful. Has good knowledge of agencies. Is able to contact agencies and follow through. Usually contacts agencies appropriate to needs. Has had favorable experience with some agencies, but not with others.

Does not understand that requests for services may be inappropriate to a particular agency. Feels it depends on the person you contact whether or not you get services.

3. *Moderate:* Sometimes successful. Has fair knowledge of resources and contacts agencies for help. Follows through only if agency follows up or contacts person after "dropping out." Feels like he or she doesn't "want to bother anyone" with problems.

4. *Low/Moderate:* Seldom successful. Has limited knowledge of resources. Has understanding of needs, but cannot select appropriate agency. Contacts agencies but does not follow through: "agency shops." Feels "nobody really understands" his or her problem.

5. *Low:* Never successful. Has no knowledge of existing services. Does not understand own needs or how an agency can meet them. Feels no one can help, no one can do anything about his or her problems.

COMPREHENSIVE MENTAL HEALTH ASSESSMENT

ID # _____

Name _____

First   Middle   Last

Assessment Date _____ Time _____ AM / PM   Place of Assessment _____

Rating Scale

1	2	3	4	5
High Functioning	High/Moderate Functioning	Moderate Functioning	Low/Moderate Functioning	Low Functioning

A. Life Functions

1. *Physical Health*
   Medical information (include relevant items: e.g., illnesses, surgery, physical impairment, allergies, pregnancy, birth defects)

   Current medical care   Yes ___ No ___
   Family Physical or Medical Clinic(s) Name _____
   Address _____ Last time seen _____
   Phone _____

	Medication Use	Name	Dosage	Duration	Physician/Clinic
1.					
2.					
3.					
4.					
5.					

   Comments:

   W   C   O*

   __ __ __

2. *Self-Acceptance/Self-Esteem*
   Comments:

   W   C   O

   __ __ __

3. *Vocational/Occupational*
   Employed ___   Homemaker ___   Student ___   Other ___
   Employer/School:
   Name _____ Job Title (Functional) _____
   Address _____ How long? _____
   Phone # _____ Unemployed _____ How long? _____
   (Optional) Education/Training _____
   Comments:

   W   C   O

   __ __ __

   *W = worker; C = client; O = other

4. *Immediate Family*
Parental status:
Children? Yes ___ No ___ How many? _____
Comments:

W   C   O

___ ___ ___

(Refer to Child Screening Checklist if appropriate)

5. *Intimate Relationships*
Marital status
Never married ___   Married ___   Widowed ___   Divorced ___   Separated ___   Living together ___   How long? ___
Comments:

W   C   O

___ ___ ___

6. *Residential*
Living situation
Lives alone ___ Lives with family ___ Other ___ (specify) _____
Comments:

W   C   O

___ ___ ___

Significant Other Information

Name	Nature of Relationship	Within Household	Age	Grade*	Outside Household	
					Address	Phone

Special Class Placement

continued

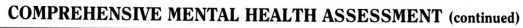

COMPREHENSIVE MENTAL HEALTH ASSESSMENT (continued)

7. *Financial*   Source of income _____
   Comments:

                                                                    W C O

                                                                    __ __ __

8. *Decision Making/Cognitive Functions*
   Comments:

                                                                    W C O

                                                                    __ __ __

9. *Life Philosophy/Goals*
   What are your life goals?
   1. _____
   2. _____
   3. _____
   Comments:

                                                                    W C O

                                                                    __ __ __

10. *Leisure Time/Community Involvement*
    Comments:

                                                                    W C O

                                                                    __ __ __

11. *Feeling Management*
    Comments:

                                                                    W C O

                                                                    __ __ __

B. Signals of Distress

12. *Lethality—Self*
    History of self-injury
    Method _____

    _____ within last month
    _____ within last 6 months   _____ High lethal
    _____ within last year   _____ Low lethal
    _____ over 1 year ago
    Total number of suicide attempts _____ Date of last attempt _____

    Comments (include ideation and threats):

    Outcome
    _____ Medical treatment only
    _____ Hosp. intensive care
    _____ Hosp. psychiatric
    _____ Out-pt. follow-up
    _____ No treatment

                                                                    W C O

                                                                    __ __ __

continued

COMPREHENSIVE MENTAL HEALTH ASSESSMENT (continued)

13. *Lethality—Other*

History of injury to other

Method _____

_____ within last month

_____ within last 6 months   _____ High lethal

_____ within last year   _____ Low lethal

_____ over 1 year

Total number of assaults _____ Date of last assault _____

Comments (include ideation and threats):

Client	Outcome	Victim
_____	Medical treatment only	_____
_____	Hosp. intensive care	_____
_____	Hosp. psychiatric	_____
_____	Out-pt. follow-up	_____
_____	No treatment	_____
_____	Other (_____)	_____

W   C   O

___ ___ ___

14. *Substance Use* (Drug and/or Alcohol)

Other drug use (include alcohol use)

	Type	Present Use	Past Use	Duration
1.	_____	_____	_____	_____
2.	_____	_____	_____	_____
3.	_____	_____	_____	_____
4.	_____	_____	_____	_____
5.	_____	_____	_____	_____
6.	_____	_____	_____	_____

Comments:

W   C   O

___ ___ ___

15. *Legal*

a. Pending court action   Yes _____ No _____   Where _____

b. On probation   Yes _____ No _____   When _____

c. On parole   Yes _____ No _____   Probation officer _____

d. Conditional discharge   Yes _____ No _____   Parole officer _____

Comments: Judge _____

W   C   O

___ ___ ___

16. *Agency Use*

Previous Mental Health Service Contacts

Outcare: Name of agency _____ Phone # _____

Contact person _____ Date of last contact _____

Address _____

Incare: Name of agency _____ Phone # _____

Contact person _____

Address _____

Date of last hosp. _____

Reason for admission _____

How often _____ How long _____ Avg. length of stay _____

Comments:

W   C   O

___ ___ ___

continued

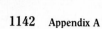

COMPREHENSIVE MENTAL HEALTH ASSESSMENT (continued)

Optional Information

Religious concerns _____Yes _____No _____What _____

Ethnic cultural background problems Yes _____No _____What _____

Narrative Summary of Assessment

Assessed by _____ Date _____

continued

COMPREHENSIVE MENTAL HEALTH ASSESSMENT (continued)

Client Self-Assessment Worksheet

Date _____   Name _____

Circle one for each question

1. *Physical Health*
   How is your health?
   Comments: _____
   _____
   _____
   _____

   Excellent
   Good
   Fair
   Poor
   Very poor

2. *Self-Acceptance/Self-Esteem*
   How do you feel about yourself as a person?
   Comments: _____
   _____
   _____
   _____

   Excellent
   Good
   Fair
   Poor
   Very poor

3. *Vocational/Occupational* (includes student and homemaker)
   How would you judge your work/school situation?
   Comments: _____
   _____
   _____
   _____

   Excellent
   Good
   Fair
   Poor
   Very poor

4. *Immediate Family*
   How are your relationships with your family and/or spouse?
   Comments: _____
   _____
   _____
   _____

   Excellent
   Good
   Fair
   Poor
   Very poor

5. *Intimate Relationship(s)*
   Is there anyone you feel really close to and can rely on?
   Comments: _____
   _____
   _____
   _____

   Always
   Usually
   Sometimes
   Rarely
   Never

6. *Residential*
   How do you judge your housing situation?
   Comments: _____
   _____
   _____
   _____

   Excellent
   Good
   Fair
   Poor
   Very poor

continued

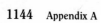

COMPREHENSIVE MENTAL HEALTH ASSESSMENT (continued)

7. *Financial*
How would you describe your financial situation?
Comments: _____

Excellent
_____ Good
_____ Fair
_____ Poor
_____ Very poor

8. *Decision-Making Ability*
How satisfied are you with your ability to make life decisions?
Comments: _____

_____ Always very satisfied
_____ Almost always satisfied
_____ Occasionally dissatisfied
_____ Almost always dissatisfied
_____ Always very dissatisfied

9. *Life Philosophy*
How satisfied are you with how your life goals are working for you?
Comments: _____

_____ Always very satisfied
_____ Almost always satisfied
_____ Occasionally dissatisfied
_____ Almost always dissatisfied
_____ Always very dissatisfied

10. *Leisure Time/Community Involvement*
How satisfied are you with your use of free time?
Comments: _____

_____ Always very satisfied
_____ Almost always satisfied
_____ Occasionally dissatisfied
_____ Almost always dissatisfied
_____ Always very dissatisfied

11. *Feeling Management*
How comfortable are you with your feelings?
Comments: _____

_____ Always very comfortable
_____ Almost always comfortable
_____ Occasionally uncomfortable
_____ Almost always uncomfortable
_____ Always very uncomfortable

12. *Lethality (Self)*
Is there any current risk of suicide for you?
Comments: _____

_____ No predictable risk of suicide now
_____ Low risk of suicide now
_____ Moderate risk of suicide now
_____ High risk of suicide now
_____ Very high risk of suicide now

continued

COMPREHENSIVE MENTAL HEALTH ASSESSMENT (continued)

13. *Lethality (Other)*
Is there any risk that you might physically harm someone?
Comments: _____
_____
_____
_____

No predictable risk of assault now
Low risk of assault now
Moderate risk of assault now
High risk of assault now
Very high risk of assault now

14. *Substance Use (Drug and/or Alcohol)*
Does use of drugs/alcohol interfere with performing your responsibilities?
Comments: _____
_____
_____
_____

Never interferes
Rarely interferes
Sometimes interferes
Frequently interferes
Constantly interferes

15. *Legal*
What is your tendency to get in trouble with the law?
Comments: _____
_____
_____
_____

No tendency
Slight tendency
Moderate tendency
Great tendency
Very great tendency

16. *Agency Use*
How successful are you at getting help from agencies (or doctors) when you need it?
Comments: _____
_____
_____
_____

Always successful
Usually successful
Moderately successful
Seldom successful
Never successful

Any additional comments?

APPENDIX B

DSM-IIIR Classification: Multiaxial Categories and Codes

All official DSM-IIIR codes are included in ICD-9-CM. Codes followed by a * are used for more than one DSM-IIIR diagnosis or subtype in order to maintain compatibility with ICD-9-CM. A long dash following a diagnostic term indicates the need for a fifth digit subtype or other qualifying term. The term *specify* following the name of some diagnostic categories indicates qualifying terms that clinicians may wish to add in parentheses after the name of the disorder. The abbreviation NOS = Not Otherwise Specified.

The current severity of a disorder may be specified after the diagnosis as:

Mild
Moderate } currently meets diagnostic criteria
Severe

In partial remission (or residual state)

In complete remission

DISORDERS USUALLY FIRST EVIDENT IN INFANCY, CHILDHOOD, OR ADOLESCENCE

Developmental Disorders

Note: These are coded on Axis II.

Mental Retardation

317.00	Mild mental retardation
318.00	Moderate mental retardation
318.10	Severe mental retardation
318.20	Profound mental retardation
319.00	Unspecified mental retardation

Pervasive Developmental Disorders

299.00	Autistic disorder. *Specify* if childhood onset
299.80	Pervasive developmental disorder NOS

Specific Developmental Disorders

Academic skills disorders

315.10	Developmental arithmetic disorder
315.80	Developmental expressive writing disorder
315.00	Developmental reading disorder

Language and speech disorders

315.39	Developmental articulation disorder
315.31*	Developmental expressive language disorder
315.31*	Developmental receptive language disorder

Motor skills disorder

315.40	Developmental coordination disorder
315.90*	Specific developmental disorder NOS

Other Developmental Disorders

315.90*	Developmental disorder NOS

Disruptive Behavior Disorders

314.01	Attention-deficit hyperactivity disorder

Source: American Psychiatric Association: *Diagnostic and Statistical Manual of Mental Disorders,* ed 3, revised. APA, 1987.

Conduct disorder

312.20 Group type

312.00 Solitary aggressive type

312.90 Undifferentiated type

313.81 Oppositional defiant disorder

Anxiety Disorders of Childhood or Adolescence

309.21 Separation anxiety disorder

313.21 Avoidant disorder of childhood or adolescence

313.00 Overanxious disorder

Eating Disorders

307.10 Anorexia nervosa

307.51 Bulimia nervosa

307.52 Pica

307.53 Rumination disorder of infancy

307.50 Eating disorder NOS

Gender Identity Disorders

302.60 Gender identity disorder of childhood

302.50 Transsexualism. *Specify* sexual history: asexual, homosexual, heterosexual, unspecified

302.85* Gender identity disorder of adolescence or adulthood, nontranssexual type. *Specify* sexual history: asexual, homosexual, heterosexual, unspecified

302.85* Gender identity disorder NOS

Tic Disorders

307.23 Tourette's disorder

307.22 Chronic motor or vocal tic disorder

307.21 Transient tic disorder. *Specify:* single episode or recurrent

307.20 Tic disorder NOS

Elimination Disorders

307.70 Functional encopresis. *Specify:* primary or secondary type

307.60 Functional enuris. *Specify:* primary or secondary type. *Specify:* nocturnal only, diurnal only, nocturnal and diurnal

Speech Disorders Not Elsewhere Classified

307.00* Cluttering

307.00* Stuttering

Other Disorders of Infancy, Childhood, or Adolescence

313.23 Elective mutism

313.82 Identity disorder

313.89 Reactive attachment disorder of infancy or early childhood

307.30 Stereotypy/habit disorder

314.00 Undifferentiated attention-deficit disorder

ORGANIC MENTAL DISORDERS

Dementias Arising in the Senium and Presenium

Primary degenerative dementia of the Alzheimer type, senile onset

290.30 With delirium

290.20 With delusions

290.21 With depression

290.00* Uncomplicated (Note: code 331.00 Alzheimer's disease on Axis III)

Code in fifth digit: 1 = with delirium, 2 = with delusions, 3 = with depression, 0* = uncomplicated

290.1x Primary degenerative dementia of the Alzheimer type, presenile onset, _____ (Note: code 331.00 Alzheimer's disease on Axis III)

290.4x Multi-infarct dementia, _____

290.00* Senile dementia NOS. *Specify:* etiology on Axis III if known

290.10* Presenile dementia NOS. *Specify:* etiology on Axis III if known (e.g., Pick's disease, Jakob-Creutzfeldt disease)

Psychoactive Substance-Induced Organic Mental Disorders

Alcohol

303.00 Intoxication

291.40 Idiosyncratic intoxication

291.80 Uncomplicated alcohol withdrawal

291.00 Withdrawal delirium

291.30 Hallucinosis

291.10 Amnestic disorder

291.20 Dementia associated with alcoholism

Amphetamine or similarly acting sympathomimetic

305.70* Intoxication

292.00* Withdrawal

292.81* Delirium

292.11* Delusional disorder

Caffeine

305.90* Intoxication

Cannabis

305.20* Intoxication

292.11* Delusional disorder

Cocaine

305.60* Intoxication

292.00* Withdrawal

292.81* Delirium

292.11* Delusional disorder

Hallucinogen

305.30* Hallucinosis

292.11* Delusional disorder

292.84* Mood disorder

292.89* Posthallucinogen perception disorder

Inhalant

305.90* Intoxication

Nicotine

292.00* Withdrawal

Opioid

305.50* Intoxication

292.00* Withdrawal

Phencyclidine (PCP) or similarly acting arylcyclohexylamine

305.90* Intoxication

292.81* Delirium

292.11* Delusional disorder

292.84* Mood disorder

292.90* Organic mental disorder NOS

Sedative, hypnotic, or anxiolytic

305.40* Intoxication

292.00* Uncomplicated sedative, hypnotic, or anxiolytic withdrawal

292.00* Withdrawal delirium

292.83* Amnestic disorder

Other or unspecified psychoactive substance

305.90* Intoxication

292.00* Withdrawal

292.81* Delirium

292.82* Dementia

292.83* Amnestic disorder

292.11   Delusional disorder

292.12   Hallucinosis

292.84* Mood disorder

292.89* Anxiety disorder

292.89* Personality disorder

292.90* Organic mental disorder NOS

Organic Mental Disorders Associated with Axis III Physical Disorders or Conditions, or Whose Etiology Is Unknown

293.00   Delirium

294.10   Dementia

294.00   Amnestic disorder

293.81   Organic delusional disorder

293.82   Organic hallucinosis

293.83   Organic mood disorder. *Specify:* manic, depressed, mixed

294.80* Organic anxiety disorder

310.10   Organic personality disorder. *Specify* if explosive type

294.80* Organic mental disorder NOS

PSYCHOACTIVE SUBSTANCE USE DISORDERS

Alcohol

303.90   Dependence

305.00   Abuse

Amphetamine or similarly acting sympathomimetic

304.40   Dependence

305.70* Abuse

Cannabis

    304.30   Dependence
    305.20* Abuse

Cocaine

    304.20   Dependence
    305.60* Abuse

Hallucinogen

    304.50* Dependence
    305.30* Abuse

Inhalant

    304.60   Dependence
    305.90* Abuse

Nicotine

    305.10   Dependence

Opioid

    304.00   Dependence
    305.50* Abuse

Phencyclidine (PCP) or similarly acting arylcyclohexylamine

    304.50* Dependence
    305.90* Abuse

Sedative, hypnotic, or anxiolytic

    304.10   Dependence
    305.40* Abuse
    304.90* Polysubstance dependence
    304.90* Psychoactive substance dependence NOS
    305.90* Psychoactive substance abuse NOS

SCHIZOPHRENIA

Code in fifth digit: 1 = subchronic, 2 = chronic, 3 = subchronic with acute exacerbation, 4 = chronic with acute exacerbation, 5 = in remission, 0 = unspecified.

Schizophrenia

    295.2x   Catatonic, _____
    295.1x   Disorganized, _____

    295.3x   Paranoid, _____ . *Specify* if stable type
    295.9x   Undifferentiated, _____
    295.6x   Residual, _____ . *Specify* if late onset

DELUSIONAL (PARANOID) DISORDER

    297.10   Delusional disorder. *Specify* type: erotomanic, grandiose, jealous, persecutory, somatic, unspecified

PSYCHOTIC DISORDERS NOT ELSEWHERE CLASSIFIED

    298.80   Brief reactive psychosis
    295.40   Schizophreniform disorder. *Specify:* without good prognostic features or with good prognostic features
    295.70   Schizoaffective disorder. *Specify:* bipolar type or depressive type
    297.30   Induced psychotic disorder
    298.90   Psychotic disorder NOS (atypical psychosis)

MOOD DISORDERS

Code current state of Major Depression and Bipolar Disorder in fifth digit: 1 = mild, 2 = moderate, 2 = severe, without psychotic features, 4 = with psychotic features (*specify* mood-congruent or mood-incongruent), 5 = in partial remission, 6 = in full remission, 0 = unspecified.

For major depressive episodes, *specify* if chronic and *specify* if melancholic type.

For Bipolar Disorder, Bipolar Disorder NOS, Recurrent Major Depression, and Depressive Disorder NOS, *specify* if seasonal pattern.

Bipolar Disorders

Bipolar disorder

    296.6x   Mixed, _____
    296.4x   Manic, _____
    296.5x   Depressed, _____
    301.13   Cyclothymia
    296.70   Bipolar disorder NOS

Depressive Disorders

Major depression

296.2x   Single episode, _____

296.3x   Recurrent, _____

300.40   Dysthymia (or depressive neurosis). *Specify:* primary or secondary type. *Specify:* early or late onset

311.00   Depressive disorder NOS

ANXIETY DISORDERS
(or Anxiety and Phobic Neuroses)

Panic disorder

300.21   With agoraphobia. *Specify* current severity of agoraphobic avoidance. *Specify* current severity of panic attacks

300.01   Without agoraphobia. *Specify* current severity of panic attacks

300.22   Agoraphobia without history of panic disorder. *Specify* with or without limited symptom attacks

300.23   Social phobia. *Specify* if generalized type

300.29   Simple phobia

300.30   Obsessive compulsive disorder (or obsessive compulsive neurosis)

309.89   Post-traumatic stress disorder. *Specify* if delayed onset

300.02   Generalized anxiety disorder

300.00   Anxiety disorder NOS

SOMATOFORM DISORDERS

300.70*   Body dysmorphic disorder

300.11   Conversion disorder (or hysterical neurosis, conversion type). *Specify:* single episode or recurrent

300.70*   Hypochondriasis (or hypochondriacal neurosis)

300.81   Somatization disorder

307.80   Somatoform plain disorder

300.70*   Undifferentiated somatoform disorder

300.70*   Somatoform disorder NOS

DISSOCIATIVE DISORDERS
(or Hysterical Neuroses, Dissociative Type)

300.14   Multiple personality disorder

300.13   Psychogenic fugue

300.12   Psychogenic amnesia

300.60   Depersonalization disorder (or depersonalization neurosis)

300.15   Dissociative disorder NOS

SEXUAL DISORDERS

Paraphilias

302.40   Exhibitionism

302.81   Fetishism

302.89   Frotteurism

302.20   Pedophilia. *Specify:* same sex, opposite sex, same and opposite sex. *Specify* if limited to incest. *Specify:* exclusive type or nonexclusive type

302.83   Sexual masochism

302.84   Sexual sadism

302.30   Transvestic fetishism

302.82   Voyeurism

302.90*   Paraphilia NOS

Sexual Dysfunctions

Specify: psychogenic only, or psychogenic and biogenic. (Note: If biogenic only, code on Axis III.) *Specify:* lifelong or acquired. *Specify:* generalized or situational.

Sexual desire disorders

302.71   Hypoactive sexual desire disorder

302.79   Sexual aversion disorder

Sexual arousal disorders

302.72*   Female sexual arousal disorder

302.72*   Male erectile disorder

Orgasm disorders

302.73   Inhibited female orgasm

302.74   Inhibited male orgasm

302.75   Premature ejaculation

Sexual pain disorders

302.76   Dyspareunia

306.51   Vaginismus

302.70   Sexual dysfunction NOS

Other Sexual Disorders

302.90*   Sexual disorder NOS

SLEEP DISORDERS

Dyssomnias

Insomnia disorder

307.42* Related to another mental disorder (nonorganic)
780.50* Related to known organic factor
307.42* Primary insomnia

Hypersomnia disorder

307.44   Related to another mental disorder (nonorganic)
780.50* Related to a known organic factor
780.54   Primary hypersomnia
307.45   Sleep-wake schedule disorder. *Specify:* advanced or delayed phase type, disorganized type, frequently changing type

Other dyssomnias

307.40* Dyssomnia NOS

Parasomnias

307.47   Dream anxiety disorder (nightmare disorder)
307.46* Sleep terror disorder
307.46* Sleepwalking disorder
307.40* Parasomnia NOS

FACTITIOUS DISORDERS

Factitious disorder

301.51   With physical symptoms
300.16   With psychological symptoms
300.19   Factitious disorder NOS

IMPULSE CONTROL DISORDERS NOT ELSEWHERE CLASSIFIED

312.34   Intermittent explosive disorder
312.32   Kleptomania
312.31   Pathological gambling
312.33   Pyromania
312.39* Trichotillomania
312.39* Impulse control disorder NOS

ADJUSTMENT DISORDER

Adjustment disorder

309.24   With anxious mood
309.00   With depressed mood
309.30   With disturbance of conduct
309.40   With mixed disturbance of emotions and conduct
309.28   With mixed emotional features
309.82   With physical complaints
309.83   With withdrawal
309.23   With work (or academic) inhibition
309.90   Adjustment disorder NOS

PSYCHOLOGICAL FACTORS AFFECTING PHYSICAL CONDITION

316.00   Psychological factors affecting physical condition. *Specify* physical condition on Axis III

PERSONALITY DISORDERS

Note: These are coded on Axis II.

Cluster A

301.00   Paranoid
301.20   Schizoid
301.22   Schizotypal

Cluster B

301.70   Antisocial
301.83   Borderline
301.50   Histrionic
301.81   Narcissistic

Cluster C

301.82   Avoidant
301.60   Dependent
301.40   Obsessive compulsive
301.84   Passive aggressive
301.90   Personality disorder NOS

V CODES FOR CONDITIONS NOT ATTRIBUTABLE TO A MENTAL DISORDER THAT ARE A FOCUS OF ATTENTION OR TREATMENT

V62.30   Academic problem

V71.01   Adult antisocial behavior

V40.00   Borderline intellectual functioning. (*Note: This is coded on Axis II*)

V71.02   Childhood or adolescent antisocial behavior

V65.20   Malingering

V61.10   Marital problem

V15.81   Noncompliance with medical treatment

V62.20   Occupational problem

V61.20   Parent-child problem

V62.81   Other interpersonal problem

V61.80   Other specified family circumstances

V62.89   Phase of life problem or other life circumstance problem

V62.82   Uncomplicated bereavement

ADDITIONAL CODES

300.90   Unspecified mental disorder (nonpsychotic)

V71.09*   No diagnosis or condition on Axis I

799.90*   Diagnosis or condition deferred on Axis I

MULTIAXIAL SYSTEM

Axis I   Clinical syndromes
           V codes

Axis II   Developmental disorders
           Personality disorders

Axis III   Physical disorders and conditions

Axis IV   Severity of psychosocial stressors

Axis V   Global assessment of functioning

SEVERITY OF PSYCHOSOCIAL STRESSORS SCALE: ADULTS

Code	Term	Acute events	Enduring circumstances
1	None	No acute events that may be relevant to the disorder	No enduring circumstances that may be relevant to the disorder
2	Mild	Broke up with boyfriend or girlfriend; started or graduated from school; child left home	Family arguments; job dissatisfaction; residence in high-crime neighborhood
3	Moderate	Marriage; marital separation; loss of job; retirement; miscarriage	Marital discord; serious financial problems; trouble with boss; being a single parent
4	Severe	Divorce; birth of first child	Unemployment; poverty
5	Extreme	Death of spouse; serious physical illness diagnosed; victim of rape	Serious chronic illness in self or child; ongoing physical or sexual abuse
6	Catastrophic	Death of child; suicide of spouse; devastating natural disaster	Captivity as hostage; concentration camp experience
0	Inadequate information, or no change in condition		

SEVERITY OF PSYCHOSOCIAL SCALE: CHILDREN AND ADOLESCENTS

Code	Term	Acute events	Enduring circumstances
1	None	No acute events that may be relevant to the disorder	No enduring circumstances that may be relevant to the disorder
2	Mild	Broke up with boyfriend or girlfriend; change of school	Overcrowded living quarters; family arguments
3	Moderate	Expelled from school; birth of sibling	Chronic disabling illness in parent; chronic parental discord
4	Severe	Divorce of parents; unwanted pregnancy; arrest	Harsh or rejecting parents; chronic life-threatening illness in parent; multiple foster home placements
5	Extreme	Sexual or physical abuse; death of a parent	Recurrent sexual or physical abuse
6	Catastrophic	Death of both parents	Chronic life-threatening illness
0	Inadequate information, or no change in condition		

GLOBAL ASSESSMENT OF FUNCTIONING SCALE (GAF SCALE)

Consider psychological, social, and occupational functioning on a hypothetical continuum of mental health-illness. Do not include impairment in functioning due to physical (or environmental) limitations.

Note: Use intermediate codes when appropriate, e.g., 45, 68, 72.

Code	
90 | 81	Absent or minimal symptoms (e.g., mild anxiety before an exam), good functioning in all areas, interested and involved in a wide range of activities, socially effective, generally satisfied with life, no more than everyday problems or concerns (e.g., an occasional argument with family members).
80 | 71	If symptoms are present, they are transient and expectable reactions to psychosocial stressors (e.g., difficulty concentrating after family argument); no more than slight impairment in social, occupational, or school functioning (e.g., temporarily falling behind in schoolwork).
70 | 61	Some mild symptoms (e.g., depressed mood and mild insomnia) *or* some difficulty in social, occupational, or school functioning (e.g., occasional truancy, or theft within the household), but generally functioning pretty well, has some meaningful interpersonal relationships.
60 | 51	Moderate symptoms (e.g., flat affect and circumstantial speech, occasional panic attacks) *or* moderate difficulty in social, occupational, or school functioning (e.g., few friends, conflicts with co-workers).
50 | 41	Serious symptoms (e.g., suicidal ideation, severe obsessional rituals, frequent shoplifting) *or* any serious impairment in social, occupational, or school functioning (e.g., no friends, unable to keep a job).
40 | 31	Some impairment in reality testing or communication (e.g., speech is at times illogical, obscure, or irrelevant) *or* major impairment in several areas, such as work or school, family relations, judgment, thinking, or mood (e.g., depressed man avoids friends, neglects family, and is unable to work; child frequently beats up younger children, is defiant at home, and is failing at school).
30 | 21	Behavior is considerably influenced by delusions or hallucinations *or* serious impairment in communication or judgment (e.g., sometimes incoherent, acts grossly inappropriately, suicidal preoccupation) *or* inability to function in almost all areas (e.g., stays in bed all day; no job, home, or friends).
20 | 11	Some danger of hurting self or others (e.g., suicide attempts without clear expectation of death, frequently violent, manic excitement) *or* occasionally fails to maintain minimal personal hygiene (e.g., smears feces) *or* gross impairment in communication (e.g., largely incoherent or mute).
10 | 1	Persistent danger of severely hurting self or others (e.g., recurrent violence) *or* persistent inability to maintain minimal personal hygiene *or* serious suicidal act with clear expectation of death.

APPENDIX C

Resources

AIDS Project Los Angeles, Inc
7362 Santa Monica Boulevard
West Hollywood, CA 90046
Phone: (213) 876-8951

An organization that provides support groups, information, and referral services for persons with AIDS. Publishes Living with AIDS: A Self Care Manual.

Al-Anon Family Group Headquarters
PO Box 862
Midtown Station
New York, NY 10018-0862
Phone: (212) 302-7240

For relatives and friends of alcoholics. Includes Alateen for children of alcoholics. Functions separately from Alcoholics Anonymous.

Alcoholics Anonymous World Services, Inc
PO Box 459
Grand Central Station
New York, NY 10163
Phone: (212) 686-1100

A self-help organization of people who share experiences with alcoholism and provide support for each other in overcoming alcoholism.

Alzheimer's Disease and Related Disorders Association (ADRDA)
70 E Lake Street
Chicago, IL 60601
Phone: (800) 621-0379; in Illinois (800) 572-6037 or (312) 853-3060

Provides information to the public and to health professionals, advocates and aids research, provides emotional support to family and friends, and makes referrals to other appropriate services.

American Alliance for Health, Physical Education, Recreation, and Dance
1900 Association Drive
Reston, VA 22091
Phone: (703) 476-3400

Provides information about recreation and fitness opportunities for the handicapped.

American Anorexia/Bulimia Association, Inc
133 Cedar Lane
Teaneck, NJ 07666

Phone: (201) 836-1800

A self-help group that provides information and help as well as referrals to physicians and therapists. On Wednesdays from 10 AM to 2 PM, a recovered person takes calls.

American Association of Retired Persons
1909 K Street, NW
Washington, DC 20049
Phone: (202) 872-4700

An association that provides informational material related to retirement and aging, a monthly newsletter, educational seminars, discounts on purchases and health insurance, etc.

American Association of Sex Educators, Counselors, and Therapists
11 Dupont Circle, NW, Suite 220
Washington, DC 20036
Phone: (202) 462-1171

Certifies sex educators, sex counselors, and sex therapists and provides other services associated with sex education and sex therapy.

American Humanist Association
7 Harwood Drive, PO Box 146
Amherst, NY 14226-0146
Phone: (716) 839-5080

A philosophical association that provides information on various social and health issues as well as referrals to local and national groups. See also the listing for Division of Humanist Counseling.

American Nurses' Association
Council on Psychiatric and Mental Health Nursing
2420 Pershing Road
Kansas City, MO 64108

A specialty division of the American Nurses' Association that provides information on the specialty and certification at both generalist and specialist levels.

Anorexia Nervosa and Associated Disorders (ANAD)
Box 7
Highland Park, IL 60035
Phone: (312) 831-3438

A self-help organization for people with eating disorders.

Anorexia Nervosa and Related Eating Disorders, Inc (ANRED)
PO Box 5102

Eugene, OR 97401
Phone: (503) 344-1144

Provides information and referrals for people with eating disorders.

Association for Voluntary Surgical Contraception
122 E 42d Street
New York, NY 10168
Phone: (212) 351-2500; for information call (212) 351-2555

Refers clients considering tubal ligation or vasectomy to specialists and treatment centers for consultation. Offers information and sponsors educational programs.

Autism Society of America
1234 Massachusetts Avenue, NW
Suite 1017
Washington, DC 20005
Phone: (202) 783-0125

A self-help organization for professionals, caregivers, and educators as well as for parents of children and adults with autism.

Biofeedback Society of America
10200 W 44th Avenue, Suite 304
Wheat Ridge, CO 80033
Phone: (303) 422-8436

Provides referrals and information on biofeedback.

Children of Alcoholics Foundation
540 Madison Avenue
New York, NY 10022

Provides information and free materials.

Committee on Pain Therapy
American Society of Anesthesiologists
515 Busse Highway
Park Ridge, IL 60068
Phone: (312) 825-5586

Distributes literature and provides information on chronic pain and its treatment.

Concern for Dying
250 W 57th Street, Room 831
New York, NY 10107
Phone: (212) 246-6962

Distributes literature, promotes research on death and dying, and works for the right of dying individuals to refuse extraordinary life-prolonging measures. Formerly called the Euthanasia Educational Council.

Division of Humanist Counseling
Arthur M. Jackson
3032 Warm Springs Drive
San Jose, CA 95127
Phone: (408) 251-3030

Provides referrals to humanist counselors and other professionals to meet individual needs.

Drugs Anonymous
PO Box 473, Ansonia Station

New York, NY 10023
Phone: (212) 874-0700

Modeled after Alcoholics Anonymous, has the goal of helping people live a drug-free life. Most members have or have had dependence problems with tranquilizers, sedatives, or analgesics.

Family Service Association of America, Inc
254 W 31st Street
New York, NY 10001
Phone: (800) 424-6268; in New York (212) 967-2740

Provides mental health services to families under stress and information and research on family living.

Fear Clinic
Crossroads Counseling Center
670 Washington Street
Braintree, MA 02184
Phone: (800) 426-2546; in Massachusetts (617) 843-7550

Provides individual and family counseling and publishes a monthly newsletter.

Gay Men's Health Crisis
Box 274
132 W. 24th Street
New York, NY 10011
Phone: (212) 807-6655

Provides information, support groups, and health care services to persons with AIDS.

Gerontological Society of America
1411 K Street NW, Suite 300
Washington, DC 20005
Phone: (202) 393-1411

Provides information on aging and advocacy for the elderly.

Hazelden Foundation
PO Box 176
Center City, MN 55012
Phone: (800) 257-7800; in Minnesota (612) 257-4010. For educational materials call (800) 328-9000; in Minnesota (800) 257-0070.

Provides dependency treatment programs at sites in Minnesota and Florida. Treatment is followed by a stay in a halfway house or participation in an outpatient program. Publishes literature related to chemical dependency and recovery.

The Hemlock Society
PO Box 66218
Los Angeles, CA 90066
Phone: (213) 391-1871

Promotes tolerance of the right of terminally ill persons to end their lives in a planned manner. Publishes the "Hemlock Quarterly" newsletter, various legal declarations and documents such as a "living will" and a durable power of attorney for health care, and the only guide to self-deliverance ("Let Me Die Before I Wake") for the dying in the United States.

Huntington's Disease Society of America, Inc
140 W 22d Street, 6th floor
New York, NY 10011
Phone: (800) 345-HDSA [345-4372]; in New York (212) 242-1968

Sponsors educational programs, raises funds for research, and maintains a comprehensive listing of specialists.

Impotence Information Center
PO Box 9
Minneapolis, MN 55440
Phone: (800) 843-4315; in Minnesota (612) 933-4666

Sponsored by American Medical Systems. Provides information on causes and treatment of impotence. Several booklets and pamphlets are available.

Impotents Anonymous
119 S Ruth Street
Maryville, TN 37801
Phone: (615) 983-6064

Offers information about the causes of impotence, treatments available, and emotional support. Meetings are held once a month at chapters throughout the United States. An associated organization, I-Anon (modeled after Al-Anon), gives impotent men's partners the chance to share their concerns and to benefit from the experience of others. Both organizations guarantee anonymity.

J2CP Information Service
PO Box 184
San Juan Capistrano, CA 92693
Phone: (714) 496-J2CP [496-5227]; recording only

Clients who are considering a sex change operation or who have questions about transsexualism can obtain information from this facility. Requests for information must be accompanied by a minimum contribution ($25.00 in 1987) to cover costs of materials, handling, and postage.

Lamaze Childbirth Education, Inc.
PO Box 88, Waverly Branch
Belmont, MA 02179
Phone: (617) 489-4030 [9 AM to 2 PM EST]

All the childbirth educators are registered nurses. Provides preparation for childbirth through a psychoeducational approach; offers guidance, knowledge, and support to groups, couples, and individuals during pregnancy and the postpartum period.

Masters and Johnson Institute
24 S Kingshighway
St. Louis, MO 63108
Phone: (314) 361-2377

Provides research, therapy, and education on matters related to sex.

Medic-Alert Foundation International
Turlock, CA 95381-1009
Phone: (800) ID-ALERT [432-5378] for entire US, including California; or (209) 632-2371

For a single lifetime membership fee ($20 as of 1987), this organization provides a bracelet or necklace with a medallion stating the wearer's medical problem; a wallet-sized card with personal information about allergies and medicines being taken; a computer information file containing the wearer's complete medical history; and a 24-hour answering service with operators available to relay the medical history to emergency personnel (the phone number is engraved on the medallion). The computer file can be updated for a minimal fee. This organization has over 700,000 members in the United States and Canada; the emblem is registered in over 40 other countries.

Mothers Against Drunk Driving (MADD)
5330 Primrose, Suite 146

Fair Oaks, CA 95628
Phone: (916) 537-9045

Acts as a voice for victims of drunk-driving accidents and their families, supports highway patrol programs, and lobbies for state and federal legislation for reform of drunk-driving laws. MADD also provides counseling services for victims and families and publishes brochures and a newsletter aimed at widespread public education.

Nar-Anon Family Group
PO Box 2562
Palos Verdes Peninsula, CA 90274
Phone: (213) 547-5800

An organization for the partners and families of persons who abuse narcotics. There are groups in both the United States and Canada (check local telephone book).

Narcotics Anonymous
PO Box 622
Sun Valley, CA 91352
Phone: (818) 997-3822

Recovered narcotics addicts meet regularly to help one another stay off drugs, based on the Alcoholics Anonymous philosophy. Local chapters publish the Narcotics Anonymous Newsletter.

National Alliance for the Mentally Ill (NAMI)
1901 Fort Myer Drive, Suite 500
Arlington, VA 22209
Phone: (703) 524-7600

A self-help advocacy organization for families of persons with schizophrenia and major depressive disorders, and those who have the disorders themselves. The philosophic approach of this organization is that serious mental disorders are biologically caused brain diseases without cure or prevention at this time, and that they are not caused by family interaction. There are affiliates in all fifty states, Canada, Guam, Puerto Rico, and the Virgin Islands. In addition to advocacy, NAMI also provides family self-help/support, public education, and research.

National Association to Aid Fat Americans, Inc (NAAFA)
PO Box 43
Bellerose, NY 11426
Phone: (516) 352-3120 [9 AM to 3:30 PM EST]

Fights prejudice and discrimination against obese people and promotes self-acceptance and societal acceptance.

National Association of Anorexia Nervosa and Associated Disorders
Box 7
Highland Park, IL 60035
Phone: (312) 831-3438

Provides information and referrals as well as advice on joining or forming a self-help group.

National Clearinghouse on Alcohol and Drug Information
PO Box 2345
Rockville, MD 20852

or:

1776 E Jefferson Street
Suite 400 South
Rockville, MD 20852
Phone: (301) 468-2600

This branch of the National Institute on Alcohol Abuse and Alcoholism and the National Institute on Drug Abuse makes available current information on alcohol and drug use and abuse, conducts computerized searches for specific materials, provides bibliographies and referrals to local alcohol and drug abuse programs, and gives notification of newly published research results. Several pamphlets and books are available.

National Committee for Prevention of Child Abuse
332 S Michigan Avenue
Suite 950
Chicago, IL 60604
Phone: (312) 663-3520

An organization concerned with physically and emotionally abused and neglected children.

National Committee on the Treatment of Intractable Pain
9300 River Road
Potomac, MD 20854
Phone: (202) 944-8140

Promotes education and research on more effective management of intractable pain. Information on the latest methods of pain management and current research can be obtained by contacting their Pain Control Information Clearinghouse. Referrals to other agencies for pain control information or treatment are available upon request.

National Council on the Aging, Inc
600 Maryland Avenue, SW
West Wing 100
Washington, DC 20024
Phone: (202) 479-1200

Provides information on aging to the public and to health professionals.

National Council on Alcoholism, Inc
12 W 21st Street, 7th floor
New York, NY 10010
Phone: (800) NCA-CALL [622-2255]; in New York (212) 206-6770

Consists of state and local affiliates. Supports and cooperates with self-help groups. The NCA Publications Office invites questions by telephone or letter.

National Crisis Prevention Institute
3315K N 124th Street
Brookfield, WI 53005
Phone: (800) 558-8976; or (414) 783-5787

Offers programs on nonviolent physical crisis intervention in facilities for health, education, social welfare, security, and corrections. Staff is trained in the prevention and management of disruptive, assaultive, or out-of-control behavior.

National Health Information Center
PO Box 1133
Washington, DC 20013-1133
Phone: (800) 336-4797; in Washington, DC area (202) 429-9091

A service of the Office of Disease Prevention and Health Promotion (ODPHP), US Department of Health and Human Services. Provides health and medical information, lists of other toll-free numbers, and referrals to appropriate organizations and researches answers to health questions. Also provides government-produced pamphlets such as "Healthstyle: A Self Test."

National Hospice Organization
1901 N Fort Myer Drive, Suite 307
Arlington, VA 22209
Phone: (703) 243-5900

An organization of hospices and individuals that encourages public and professional education on caring for the terminally ill, monitors legislation affecting the hospice movement, and publishes a quarterly newsletter.

National Institute of Mental Health
Public Inquiries Branch
Room 15C05
5600 Fishers Lane
Rockville, MD 20857
Phone: (301) 443-4517

This division of the federal government provides information on mental health, mental disorders, and programs and resources throughout the country.

National Mental Health Association
1021 Prince Street
Alexandria, VA 22314-2971
Phone: (703) 684-7722

A voluntary agency concerned with mental health.

National Nurses Society on Addictions (NNSA)
2506 Grosse Pointe Road
Evanston, IL 60201
Phone: (312) 475-7300

Publishes a newsletter four times a year for nurses working in the addiction field. Provides information on treatment and research in addiction, certification for nurses working in the field, and a network for nurses working with chemically dependent clients.

National Self-Help Clearinghouse
Graduate School University Center
City University of New York
33 W 42d Street
New York, NY 10036
[Letters only, please]

Monitors hundreds of self-help organizations throughout the United States and Canada.

Nightingale
77 Warren Street
Brighton, MA 02135
Phone: (617) 783-3522

A back-to-practice 18-bed in-patient recovery program for the licensed health care professional having trouble with alcohol and other chemical dependencies.

Nursing Transitions, Inc
PO Box 797
Williamsville, NY 14221
Phone: (716) 631-9706

This nurse-owned and -operated continuing nursing education company provides national psychiatric-mental health nursing conferences as well as conferences on AIDS nursing and topics of interest to nurses in other fields. Carol Ren Kneisl is president and educational director.

Overeaters Anonymous (OA)
PO Box 92870
Los Angeles, CA 90009
Phone: (213) 542-8363

Patterned after the philosophy of Alcoholics Anonymous, this self-help organization views compulsive eating as a disease that can be arrested but not cured. Literature available on request.

The Parent Connection
290 Massachusetts Avenue
Arlington, MA 02174
Phone: (617) 641-2229

A parents' resource group. Publishes an informative newspaper and sponsors support groups.

Parents Anonymous
7120 Franklin Avenue
Los Angeles, CA 90046
Phone: (800) 421-0353; in California (800) 352-0386

Provides confidential assistance about possible child abuse cases. Offers referrals to local chapters for help or information.

Parents without Partners, Inc
8807 Colesville Road
Silver Spring, MD 20910
Phone: (301) 588-9354

A self-help organization concerned with single, widowed, or divorced parents and their children. Provides referrals to local chapters throughout the United States.

Parkinson's Disease Foundation
Columbia University Medical Center
640–650 W 168th Street
New York, NY 10032
Phone: (212) 923-4700

Provides information and referral for people with Parkinson's disease and other diseases of the basal ganglia. Serves as a clearinghouse for clients, families, and health professionals.

Phobia Society of America
133 Rollins Avenue, Suite 4B
Rockville, MD 20852-4004
Phone: (301) 231-9350

Provides information on phobias and referrals to therapists and support groups.

Recovery, Inc: The Association of Nervous and Former Mental Patients
802 Dearborn Street
Chicago, IL 60610
Phone: (312) 337-5661

A self-help organization for people with mental problems and former mental patients.

Resolve, Inc
5 Water Street
Arlington, MA 02174
Phone: (617) 643-2424

Assists people who face problems of infertility. Offers counseling, information, and support concerning issues such as treatment and options for becoming parents (e.g., adoption). Branch offices available in many areas.

Salvation Army
132 W 14th Street
New York, NY 10011
Phone: (212) 807-4200

Sponsors both alcohol and drug rehabilitation programs, half-way houses, drop-in centers, and family service bureaus.

Salvation Army
National Information Service
799 Bloomfield Avenue
Verona, NJ 07044
Phone: (201) 239-0606

San Francisco AIDS Foundation
333 Valencia Street, 4th floor
San Francisco, CA 94103
Phone: (415) 864-4376

Provides AIDS education information for people with AIDS/ARC, people at risk, health care personnel, ethnic communities, and the general public. Their free catalog of educational materials is called AIDS Educator.

Sex Information and Education Council of the United States (SIECUS)
New York University
32 Washington Place, Room 52
New York, NY 10003
Phone: (212) 673-3850

Maintains an information clearinghouse on all aspects of human sexuality and will help clients locate information.

Stepfamily Foundation, Inc
333 West End Avenue
New York, NY 10023
Phone: (212) 877-3244

Offers a newsletter, awareness workshops, telephone counseling, and private and group counseling for stepparents and complex households with children of both spouses.

Therapeutic Communities of America, International
54 W 40th Street
New York, NY 10018
Phone: (212) 354-6000

Monitors the activities of drug-free therapeutic communities throughout the United States and makes referrals to those that meet its standards. Referral resources do not include methadone maintenance programs.

Toughlove
PO Box 1069
Doylestown, PA 18901
Phone: (215) 348-7090

A parent support group for parents whose children are in trouble.

Wellness Associates
PO Box 5433
Mill Valley, CA 94942
Phone: (415) 383-3806

Publishes the Wellness Inventory, a broad-based paper-and-pencil questionnaire that individuals can use to determine stress levels and promote wellness. It does not require laboratory testing or computer analysis, as other more detailed health risk appraisals do, and its results are more general.

Women for Sobriety, Inc
PO Box 618
Quakertown, PA 18951
Phone: (215) 536-8026

A network of over 200 self-help groups for women alcoholics only.

Youth Suicide National Center
1811 Trousdale Dr.
Burlingame, CA 94010
Phone: (415) 877-5604

Provides resource material on youth suicide.

In Canada

Alcoholics Anonymous, Intergroup Office
272 Eglington Avenue, West
Toronto, Ontario M4R 1B2
[Letters only]

Alcoholism and Drug Addiction Research Foundation
33 Russell Street
Toronto, Ontario M5S 2S1
Phone: (416) 595-6000

Canadian Association for Community Living
4700 Keele Street
Kinsmen Building
Downsview, Ontario M3J 1P3
Phone: (416) 661-9611

Supports and encourages community living for people with mental handicaps. Divisions are also located in Winnipeg, Manitoba; Fredericton, New Brunswick; St. John's, Newfoundland; Dartmouth, Nova Scotia; and Charlottetown, Prince Edward Island.

Canadian Association on Gerontology
Suite 1080
167 Lombard Avenue
Winnipeg, Manitoba R3B OV3
Phone: (204) 944-9158

Canadian Centre for Toxicology
645 Gordon Street
Guelph, Ontario N1G 1Y3
Phone: (519) 837-3320

Canadian Psychological Association
Vincent Road
Old Chelsea, Quebec J0X 2N0
Phone: (819) 827-3927

Canadian Rehabilitation Council for the Disabled (CRCD)
One Yonge Street, Suite 2110
Toronto, Ontario M5E 1E5
Phone: (416) 862-0340
(A chapter is also located in Fredericton, New Brunswick.)

Dying With Dignity
175 St. Clair Avenue, West
Toronto, Ontario M4V 1P7
Phone: (416) 921-2329

Chapters are also located in Vancouver, British Columbia, and Ottawa, Ontario. Several others will be forming in the near future.

National Alliance for the Mentally Ill
(Check local telephone book.)

Overeaters Anonymous
Central Ontario Intergroup
175 St. Clair Avenue, West, Suite 25
Toronto, Ontario M4V 1P7
Phone: (416) 929-5361

The Parkinson Foundation of Canada
55 Bloor Street, West, Suite 232
Toronto, Ontario M4W 1A6
Phone: (416) 964-1155

Patients' Rights Association
40 Homewood Avenue, Suite 315
Toronto, Ontario M4Y 2K2
Phone: (416) 923-9629

Hot Lines

AIDS Hot Line
Phone: (800) 342-AIDS [342-2437] [8:30 AM to 5:30 PM EST]

Sponsored by the US Public Health Service and operated by the American Social Health Association. Gives a recorded informational message on AIDS. If the caller stays on the line, someone will be available to answer questions or respond to concerns.

Alcohol Hotline
Phone: (800) ALCOHOL [252-6465]

Operated by the Ad Care Hospital in Worcester, Massachusetts. Provides information on alcohol- and drug-related problems.

Alcoholics Anonymous
Local phone books in the United States and Canada list the number of the closest 24-hour answering service.

Alzheimer's Disease and Related Disorders Association
Phone: (800) 621-0379; in Illinois (800) 572-6037

Counseling for families and friends of those with Alzheimer's disease and related disorders.

National Cocaine Helpline
Phone: (800) COCAINE [262-2463]

A 24-hour nationwide referral and information service for cocaine users, nonuser victims, and health care professionals. Based at Fair Oaks Hospital in Summit, New Jersey.

National Gay Task Force Crisis Line
Phone: (800) 221-7044; in New York (212) 807-6016 [5–10 PM EST]; in San Francisco (800-FOR-AIDS); in Los Angeles (800-922-AIDS)

Provides up-to-date information on AIDS.

National Institute on Drug Abuse—Cocaine Hotline
Phone: (800) 662-HELP [662-4357]

National Runaway Switchboard—Adolescent Suicide Hotline
Phone: (800) 621-4000

New York City Gay and Lesbian Antiviolence Project
Phone: (212) 807-0197

Parents Anonymous
Phone: (800) 421-0353; in California (800) 352-0386 [24 hours]

Provides confidential assistance with possible child abuse cases. Offers referrals to local chapters for help or information.

PRIDE Drug Information System
Phone: (800) 241-7946 [8:30 AM to 5 PM EST]

Sponsored by Parents' Resource Institute for Drug Education. Taped message after 5 PM.

Sleep Helpline
Sleep Disorder Center
Thomas Jefferson University Hospital
Philadelphia, PA
Phone: (215) 928-8019

Glossary

Abreaction A process in which repressed material, particularly a painful experience or conflict, is brought back to a person's awareness. The person then not only recalls but also relives the repressed material, which is accompanied by affective response.

Accommodation Adjustment of the organism to an object in the environment; incorporation of an experience as it is.

Acquaintance (or date) rape Rape by an acquaintance, friend, lover, boyfriend, or husband.

Acquired immune deficiency syndrome (AIDS) A contagious and fatal condition of immune system depression for which there is no known cure.

Acting out Term used to describe a recreation of the client's life experiences, relationships with significant others, and resultant unresolved conflicts. Acting out may include, but is not limited to, destructive actions.

Adaptation The result of interchange between the organism and environment involving modification of the organism that enhances its ability for further interchange; involves assimilation and accommodation.

Addiction A cluster of cognitive behavioral and physiologic symptoms that indicate that a person has impaired control of psychoactive substance use. Called psychoactive substance dependence in DSM-IIIR.

Adrenocorticotropic hormone (ACTH) Brain hormone that is not suppressed in depressed clients, reflecting a limbic system dysfunction associated with disturbances in mood, affect, appetite, sleep, and autonomic nervous system activity.

Adult ego state In transactional analysis theory, the ego state responsible for the objective appraisal of reality and the capacity to process data.

Affect Emotion or feeling; the tone of one's reaction to persons and events.

Affection need The interpersonal need to establish and maintain a satisfactory relation between self and other people with regard to intimacy and liking.

Affective disorders A specific group of psychiatric diagnoses that are predominantly characterized by disturbances in mood accompanied by a full or partial manic or depressive syndrome. Called mood disorders in DSM-IIIR.

Agism Negative, hostile attitudes toward the elderly.

Agnosia Difficulty recognizing everyday objects.

Agoraphobia The fear of being in places or situations from which escape might be difficult or embarrassing or in which help might not be available in the event of a panic attack.

AIDS-related complex (ARC) The condition of having some clinical symptoms diagnosed as AIDS-related, but without the formal indicators of AIDS as defined by the Centers for Disease Control.

Akathisia One of the classes of side-effects caused by neuroleptic drugs. Signs of this condition include motor restlessness and a subjective sense of anxiety.

Alcoholic In popular usage, one whose continued or excessive drinking results in impairment of personal health, disruption of family and social relationships, and loss of economic security. Alcoholism is believed by many to be a disease with strong genetic links.

Alcoholics Anonymous (AA) A self-help organization that uses a twelve-step program to assist alcoholics in achieving and maintaining sobriety; Al-Anon is concerned with spouses of alcoholics; Alateen is concerned with teenage children of alcoholics.

Algorithms Behavioral steps, or step-by-step procedures, for the management of common problems to provide structured, standardized guidelines for decision making.

Alternate nostril breathing A general relaxation exercise that helps a person reduce tension and sinus headaches by inhaling and exhaling through alternate nostrils one at a time.

Alzheimer's disease A progressive brain atrophy, usually fatal within a few years; may be known as "senile" and "presenile dementia." With the progression of the condition there is often memory and judgment loss, loss of interest, and carelessness. Symptoms worsen until disorientation, epileptiform attacks, and contractures are evident. The cause of this disease is unknown, and there is no known treatment. Diagnosis is based ultimately on histopathologic changes in the brain, including plaques and neurofibrillary tangles. Is recorded as a physical disease on Axis III of DSM-IIIR.

Ambivalence Simultaneous conflicting feelings or attitudes toward a person or object.

American Law Institute's Model Penal Code (ALI) States that a person is not held responsible for his or her behavior if he or she lacks the capacity to appreciate the wrongfulness of the act or to conform his or her behavior to the requirements of the law. Used in more than half the states and all federal circuits.

American Nurses' Association (ANA) Classification of the Phenomena of Concern for Psychiatric/Mental Health Nursing A refinement of psychiatric nursing diagnoses developed by an ANA appointed panel of specialists and termed "PND-I" by the authors of this text.

Amnestic syndrome A category of OMS in which relatively selective areas of cognition (short and long-term memory) are impaired.

Anger rape Rape distinguished by physical violence and cruelty to the victim. The ability to injure, traumatize, and shame the victim provides the rapist with an outlet for his rage and temporary relief from his turmoil.

Anhedonia The inability to experience pleasure.

Animism In a child's cognition, attributing human attributes to objects.

Anorexia nervosa Refusal to maintain body weight over a minimal normal for age and height accompanied by disturbance in body image.

Antabuse (disulfiram) A drug given to alcoholics that produces nausea, vomiting, dizziness, flushing, and tachycardia if alcohol is consumed.

Anterograde amnesia Amnesia for short-term memories; remote memories remain intact. Present in blackouts, a symptom of alcoholism.

Anticholinergic side-effects Side-effects caused by the use of neuroleptic medications, including symptoms such as dry mouth, constipation, urinary retention, blurred vision, and dry mucous membranes.

Anticipatory guidance A process that aims to help persons cope with a crisis by discussing the details of the impending difficulty and problem solving before the event occurs.

Antidepressant medications Psychopharmacologic preparations used to treat symptoms of depression and depressive equivalents. Most common antidepressants come from the tricyclic or monoamine oxidase inhibitor classes.

Antipsychotic medications Psychopharmacologic preparations used to treat symptoms of disintegrated thought, perception, and affect; also called neuroleptics, they include the following classes: phenothiazine, thioxanthene, butyrophenone, dihydroindolone, dibenzoxazepine.

Antisocial Behavior that is counterproductive or hostile to the well-being of society in general.

Antisocial personality disorder A personality disorder with the essential feature of a pattern of irresponsible and antisocial behavior.

Anxiety Nonspecific, unpleasant feeling of apprehension and discomfort that can be communicated interpersonally and that prompts the person to take some action to seek relief.

Anxiety disorders Patterns in which anxiety is either the predominant disturbance or a secondary disturbance that is confronted if the primary symptom is taken away.

Anxiolytic medications Psychopharmacologic preparations used in the abatement of anxiety-related symptoms. Drug classes in this group include benzodiazepines, beta-blockers, antihistamine sedatives, sedatives with hypnotic effects, and propanedides.

Apathy Lack of feeling, concern, interest, or emotion.

Aphasia Difficulty searching for words.

Appropriate death A way of living to the end of life, maintaining function at as high a level as possible, being as pain free as possible, and being able to make choices, resolve conflicts, and fulfill wishes.

Apraxia Inability to perform previously known, purposeful, and skilled activities.

Assault A physical attack that results in physical injury.

Assertiveness Asking for what one wants or acting to get what one wants in a way that respects the other person.

Assertiveness training An approach to therapy that is usually accomplished in groups to help people who tend either to be passive and discount themselves or to be too aggressive. Assertiveness techniques and exercises are designed to teach individuals to ask for what they want and to refuse requests from others without feeling guilty.

Assimilation Adjustment of an object in the environment to the organism; taking in experience to the extent that one can integrate it.

Attention-deficit hyperactivity disorder Developmentally inappropriate inattention, impulsiveness, and hyperactivity.

Autistic Relating to private, individual affects and ideas that are derived from internal drives, hopes, and wishes. Most commonly refers to the private reality of persons labeled schizophrenic as opposed to the shared reality of the external world.

Autistic disorder A severe pervasive developmental disorder with onset in infancy or childhood characterized by impaired social interaction, impaired communication, and a markedly restricted repertoire of activities and interests.

Autogenic training A systematic training program of structured exercises to reduce stress-related conditions, modify the reaction to pain, and reduce or eliminate stress disorders.

Avoidant personality disorder A personality disorder with the essential feature of a pervasive pattern of social discomfort, fear of negative evaluation, and timidity.

Axon The part of the neuron that conducts impulses away from the cell body.

Barrio Hispanic neighborhood.

Beck's Depression Inventory A twenty-one item multiple choice questionnaire on which clients rate themselves on variables related to depression, such as sadness, weight loss, fatigue, guilt, suicidal ideas, social withdrawal, insomnia, etc.

Behavior modification A method of reeducation or treatment mode based on the principles of Pavlovian conditioning and further developed by B. F. Skinner; an effort to change behavior patterns through techniques that manipulate stimuli.

Behavioral contract An agreement between client and staff that clearly identifies expected client behaviors and expected staff behaviors.

Behaviorist model of psychiatry A model, based on the research of Ivan Pavlov and J. B. Watson, that is sometimes called "stimulus-response learning" or "behavioral conditioning." It assumes that psychiatric symptoms are clusters of learned behaviors that persist because they are rewarding to the individual.

Bestiality See zoophilia.

Bioenergetics Techniques for reducing muscular tension by releasing feelings, consisting of physical exercises and verbal techniques.

Bioethics A philosophic field that applies ethical reasoning to issues and dilemmas in the area of health care.

Biofeedback   A technique for gaining conscious control over unconscious body functions such as blood pressure and heartbeat to achieve relaxation or the relief of stress-related physical symptoms; involves the use of self-monitoring equipment.

Bioperiodicities   Biologic rhythms ranging from microseconds of biochemical reactions for nerve activity to the menstrual cycle or the entire life span.

Bipolar disorders   One or more manic episodes accompanied by one or more depressive episodes.

Bisexuality   Sexual preference for same or opposite sex interactions; has sexual activity with either.

Bizarre delusion   Belief involving a phenomenon that a person's culture would regard as totally implausible, e.g., thought broadcasting or being controlled by a dead person.

Blackouts   A term for anterograde amnesia experienced by alcoholics; some believe blackouts are an acute brain syndrome due to dehydration of brain tissue.

Blended family   A family in which one or both marital partners have previously been divorced or widowed and bring with them their children from the former relationship.

Blind spot (psychologic)   An area of a person's personality of which the person is totally unaware. Unperceived areas are often hidden by repression so that one can avoid painful emotions.

Blunted affect (emotions)   An extreme restriction in emotional expression; only minor degrees of emotional intensity are evident.

Body dimorphic disorder   Preoccupation with an imagined defect in appearance, or grossly excessive concern over a slight physical anomaly.

Body image   An individual's concept of the shape, size, and mass of his or her body and its parts; the internalized picture that a person has of the physical appearance of his or her body.

Body scanning   Focusing separately on all parts of the body to note the location of any tension or tightness.

Borderline personality disorder   A personality disorder with the essential feature of a pervasive pattern of unstable self-image, interpersonal relationships, and mood.

Bulimia nervosa   Recurrent episodes of binge eating accompanied by purging and persistent overconcern with body shape and weight.

Burnout   A condition in which health professionals lose their concern and feeling for the clients they work with and begin to treat them in detached or dehumanizing ways. It is an attempt to cope with the intense stress of interpersonal work by distancing.

Cao gio   Also called "coining," this folk practice is used by people from the Far East for treatment of fever or headache. The caregiver rubs a coin up and down the person's body with great pressure until red marks appear.

Cardiac neurosis   A combination of anxiety, tension, and the signs and symptoms of cardiac disease in the absence of underlying cardiovascular pathology; a type of hypochondriasis.

Care-partners   A term coined by gay persons to describe those persons to whom they are emotionally committed in a long-term relationship.

Catalysts   Unconflicted members of a group who are able to move the group on to the next phase of group work.

Catatonia   A disturbance in psychomotor behavior that can either take the form of stupor, in which the client appears unaware of the environment, or rigidity, in which the client may maintain a rigid posture and resist efforts to be moved.

Catatonic   A term used to describe an unusual behavioral state where the disordered person assumes a fixed position and may remain in that state for hours; most commonly related to specific forms of schizophrenia.

Catchment area   A geographically circumscribed area identified as the service area for a community mental health center.

Catharsis   A basic process in psychotherapy, in which the client freely puts personal feelings, thoughts, daydreams, and interpersonal problems into words. The process usually produces a feeling of relief.

Cathexis   In psychoanalysis, the attachment of emotion to an object, person, or idea. It may be positive or negative emotion (love or hate).

Cephalocaudal principle   Physical development begins with the head and progresses to lower body parts.

Cerebellum   The second largest portion of the human brain, which is divided into two sections and is located posterior to the cerebrum.

Cerebrum   The most superiorly located, largest section of the brain; divided into two connected hemispheres.

Certification   A method of attesting to competence, usually by a professional organization.

Checking perceptions   A communication skill in which the therapist shares how he or she perceives and hears the client and asks the client to verify these perceptions. Perception checks are used to make sure that one person understands the other.

Child ego state   In transactional analysis theory, the ego state that represents the archaic relics of early childhood.

Chronic disorders   Diagnostic categories that carry a high potential for persistent and severe impairment; clients often called "the chronically mentally ill" (CMI).

Chronically mentally ill   The population whose continuing or episodic functional impairment may be attributed to serious psychiatric disorder, regardless of specific diagnosis or living situation.

Chronobiology   The study of biorhythms or periodic processes. Disturbances in biorhythms are thought to influence some mental disorders.

Circadian rhythms   Cycles of approximately twenty-four-hour duration in humans that control diurnal fluctuations in sleep, body temperature, plasma concentration of cortisol and other hormones.

Circularity   A characteristic of family system behavior in which each person's behavior is viewed as cause and effect at the same time.

Circumstantial communication   See circumstantiality.

Circumstantiality   A disturbance in associative thought processes in which a person digresses into unnecessary details and inappropriate thoughts before communicating a central idea.

Clarifying   Asking the client to give an example to clarify a meaning in order to understand the basic nature of the client's statement.

Client government   Strategy of milieu therapy in which hospitalized clients use the democratic process to govern themselves.

Clinical ecology   An alternative to traditional environmental medicine; entails assessment/treatment of physical/psychologic disorders that have been triggered secondary to exposure to certain foods, chemicals, and inhalants in the environment.

Clinical specialist in psychiatric nursing   A graduate of a master's program providing specialization in the clinical area of psychiatric/mental health nursing.

Cohesion   A sense of belonging, the result of all the forces acting on members to remain in a group.

Commitment The legal process by which a person is confined to a mental hospital, usually associated with involuntary hospitalization. Also a sense of dedication and responsibility.

Communal family A family in which many people band together in a living arrangement. Members may or may not be married and typically negotiate rights and responsibilities in regard to their roles, material possessions, economic concerns, sexual expression, and parenting activities.

Community mental health center The executive locus for applying community mental health concepts. Centers include in-patient facilities, partial hospital facilities (day, night, or weekend), out-patient department, emergency services, consultation, and education programs.

Community Mental Health Systems Act 1963 legislation authorizing 150 million dollars in federal funds over three years to construct comprehensive community mental health centers.

Competitive frame of reference A system in which no two people can be thinking, feeling, or doing the same thing at the same time.

Complementary relationships Relationships based on the enjoyment of differences and interdependence. They may deteriorate when one partner controls what the complementarity is and how it is maintained.

Complementary transactions Transactions in which the transactional stimulus and the transactional response occur on identical ego levels.

Complex partial seizure A seizure that usually originates in the temporal lobe and involves limbic system structures; these seizures consist mainly of automatisms that last up to five minutes.

Compulsion An uncontrollable, persistent urge to perform an act repetitively in an attempt to relieve anxiety; performed in response to an obsession, according to certain rules, or in a stereotyped fashion.

Concepts Abstractions that categorize observations based on commonalities and differences.

Conceptual framework (conceptual model) A preliminary stage of a theory in which interrelated concepts offer a framework for conducting research. Sometimes called a theoretical framework.

Concrete communication Overly symbolic communication or inability to think and communicate abstractly; thought to be a sign of preoccupation with unreal or delusional material.

Conditioned response Behavior that occurs as a consequence of rewarding conditions that act as a stimulus.

Conduct disorder A persistent pattern of conduct in which the basic rights of others and major age-appropriate societal norms or rules are violated.

Confidentiality Treating as private the information clients provide about themselves so that no harm will befall the client for having disclosed the information; includes releasing information about clients only with their permission.

Conflict A clash between opposing forces. It may be conscious or unconscious, intrapersonal or interpersonal.

Conflicted member A member of a group whose posture toward authority or intimacy is inflexible, rigid, or compulsive.

Confounding variable Other variables in addition to the independent variable that might affect the dependent variable. Can confuse the interpretation of a study's results if not controlled for in the study's design or procedures. Also called extraneous variable.

Confrontation A communication that deliberately invites another to self-examine some aspect of behavior in which there is a discrepancy between what the person says and does.

Conjugal family A family with marriage ties.

Consultation-liaison The provision of psychiatric and mental health expertise regarding a client or problem area at the request of another health professional.

Contract A set of expectations agreed on by two or more people about what each will contribute to the relationship.

Control need The interpersonal need to establish and maintain a satisfactory relation between self and others with regard to power and influence.

Conversion disorder Alteration or loss of physical functioning that cannot be explained by any known pathophysiologic mechanism; apparently an expression of a psychologic conflict or need.

Coping behavior The behaviors persons under stress use in struggling to improve their situations.

Coprolalia Repeating socially unacceptable, usually obscene, words or phrases; a complex phonic tic.

Cotherapy The sharing of responsibility for therapeutic work, usually in groups or with families.

Counterdependency Behavior that stems from a need to deny dependence longings. May be displayed as aggressiveness, extreme independence, or other maneuvers that distance others.

Countertransference Sigmund Freud's term for irrational attitudes taken by an analyst toward a patient. It may create problems in psychotherapeutic work. The therapist needs to become aware of countertransference and seek consistent supervision to intervene when it occurs.

Couples therapy A contemporary term for what used to be known as marital therapy. Acknowledges the existence of interactional dyads not necessarily based on marriage.

Creutzfeldt-Jakob's disease Presenile dementia affecting the cerebral cortex through cell destruction and overgrowth; shortens life expectancy; documented as a slow-acting viral agent.

Crisis A situation in which customary problem-solving or decision-making methods are no longer adequate; a state of psychologic disequilibrium. A crisis may be a turning point in a person's life.

Crisis counseling A counseling strategy designed to be brief (five to six sessions) and issue oriented. It may be individual, group, or family therapy.

Crossed transaction A transaction in which a change in ego state occurs terminating a complementary relationship.

Cultural relativism The belief that all cultures are equally valued and that they can be evaluated based only on their own values.

Cultural stereotyping Assuming that all members of one ethnic group are alike.

Culture Abstract values, beliefs, and perceptions of the world that lie behind behavior and are reflected by behavior. Culture is *learned* behavior.

Culture-bound syndromes Concepts of mental disorders that exist only within a given culture, such as windigo psychosis.

Culture broker A person who functions as a mediator between two people or groups from different cultures.

Culture shock The feelings of depression and frustration that are the result of being immersed in a totally different environment.

Curanderismo A folk healing system in Hispanic cultures derived from Aztec Indian and Spanish cultures.

Curandero(a) A folk healer in Hispanic cultures who is able to treat susto (fright) and other folk illnesses.

Custodial care   The process of maintaining people in an institution though not for treatment purposes.

Cyclothymia   Chronic mood disturbance of at least two years' duration involving numerous hypomanic episodes and numerous periods of depressed mood or loss of interest and pleasure that is not sufficient to meet the criteria of major depression or a manic episode.

Death anxiety   A paralyzing fear of death that deprives one of the desire to live.

Decanoate   A form of injectable neuroleptic that is released into the body over a period of approximately two weeks.

Decline/deterioration   The third phase of dying, according to Weisman, when the symptoms and progression of the disease are increasingly obvious.

Deep breathing   Moving the diaphragm downward in order to fill the lungs completely with air.

Defense mechanisms   Operations outside of a person's awareness that the ego calls into play to protect against anxiety; the psychoanalytic term for coping mechanisms; also called mental mechanism. A glossary of terms containing defense mechanisms and their definitions is included in DSM-IIIR (1987).

Dehumanize   To detract from or interfere with unique human qualities to think, plan, create, relate to others, and experience a sense of autonomy and separateness from others.

Deinstitutionalization   A humanitarian philosophy committed to community-based care for the mentally ill, which has resulted in decreased census of the state mental hospitals and emergence of community-based treatment facilities.

Delirium   A reversible, acute confusional state that usually appears within hours or days.

Delirium tremens (DTs)   An acute psychotic state usually occurring after a prolonged and copious intake of alcohol.

Delusional disorder   Termed paranoid disorder in DSM-III; mental disorder with essential feature of persistent, nonbizarre delusion that is not due to any other mental disorder; hallucinations are not prominent; delusions may be erotomanic, grandiose, jealous, persecutory, and somatic.

Delusions   An important personal belief that is almost certainly not true and resists modification.

Dementia   An organic mental syndrome that is often chronic. Onset is usually acute although it may be gradual. Recent memory becomes impaired first; personality change is apparent and brain damage is evident.

Dementia praecox   Kraepelin's term for schizophrenia, meaning "early senility."

Dendrite   The part of the neuron that conducts impulses toward the cell body.

Denial   A defense mechanism, or coping mechanism, by which the mind refuses to acknowledge a thought, feeling, wish, need, or reality factor.

Dependent personality disorder   A personality disorder with the essential feature of a pervasive pattern of dependent and submissive behavior.

Depersonalization   An alteration in the perception or experience of the self in which the usual sense of one's reality is temporarily lost or changed; feeling as if one is in a dream, detached, or an outside observer of one's body or mental processes.

Depersonalization disorder   The occurrence of persistent or recurrent episodes of depersonalization severe enough to cause marked distress.

Depressive disorder   One or more major depressive episodes without the history of a manic or hypomanic episode.

Derealization   A feeling of being disconnected from the environment; sometimes manifested by a feeling that the environment has changed.

Desensitization   A counterconditioning technique used by behaviorists to overcome fears by gradually increasing exposure to the fearful stimuli.

Devaluation   Sustained criticism used to defend against feelings of inadequacy.

Developmental/maturational crisis   A turning point during which usual coping patterns are inadequate; a crisis that occurs in response to stress common to a particular period in human life cycle.

Developmental phases/stages   Universally experienced series of biologic, social, and psychologic events that occur on a timetable and include specific tasks or challenges to be met.

Developmental task   A challenge that arises during predictable life periods calling for the person to use skills, resources, and supports to achieve the goal inherent in the task.

Dexamethasone suppression test (DST)   Test used in diagnoses of endogenous depression (chronic depression not caused by external factors like grief or loss). Involves administering a single dose of dexamethasone followed by blood and/or urine monitoring of cortisol levels. In depressed people the dexamethasone does not suppress adrenocortical functioning.

Diencephalon   Consists of the portions of the brain located between the cerebral hemisphere and the midbrain, its main structures include the thalamus and hypothalamus.

Disengagement   A family pattern characterized by unresponsive and unconnected interactions between members. Structure, order, and authority may be absent or weak.

Disinhibition   A condition seen in conjunction with benzodiazepine administration in which a person demonstrates irritability, often verbal hostility, and possibly violent outbursts.

Displacement   A defense or coping mechanism in which a person discharges pent-up feelings on persons less threatening than those who initially aroused the emotion.

Disruptive behavior disorders   Behavior disturbances that are distressing to others and interfere with the child's social functioning.

Dissociation   A defense or coping mechanism that protects the self from a threatening awareness of uncomfortable feelings by denying their existence in awareness.

Dissociative disorders   Characterized by a disturbance or alteration in the normally integrative functions of identity, memory, or consciousness.

Dopamine hypothesis (DA)   The biochemical hypothesis that schizophrenia may be related to overactive neuronal activity that is dependent on dopamine; increased dopamine activity is associated with increased schizophrenic symptoms.

Double bind   A complex series of paradoxical interactions in which one person demands a response to a message containing mutually contradictory signals while the other person is not able to comment on the incongruity or to escape from the situation.

DRGs (diagnostically related groups)   The list of conditions on which prospective hospital cost payment is calculated; intended to predict resource use.

Drug holidays   Planned and carefully executed withdrawals from psychotropic medications; especially common in cases where neuroleptic medications are used.

DSM-IIIR   Abbreviation for the revised third edition of the *Diagnostic and Statistical Manual of Mental Disorders* published by the American Psychiatric Association in 1987.

Dual diagnosis   The simultaneous existence of a major psychiatric condition and a medical condition.

Dualism   A philosophic perspective that views an individual as two irreducible elements: mind and body.

Dumping   Moving the chronically mentally disordered from an institution into the community without providing for continuity of care.

Dyspareunia   Pain with sexual activity, commonly associated with sexual intercourse.

Dysphoria   A sense of disquiet or restlessness.

Dysthymia   Chronic disturbance of mood involving depressed mood for at least two years.

Ego   A concept of the organized part of personality that screens stimuli from the outside world and controls internal demands. As intermediary between the unconscious and the world, it includes defensive, cognitive, and executive functions. Consciousness resides in the ego, but some of its operations are out of the person's awareness.

Egocentric thought   In a child's cognition, everything is considered from child's point of view.

Ego-dystonic homosexuality   Homosexual arousal that is distressing to the individual who explicitly states a desire for heterosexual arousal patterns.

Elder abuse   Maltreatment of an older individual ranging from passive neglect of physical and emotional needs to overt physical, mental, or sexual assault.

Electra complex   In psychoanalytic theory, incestuous attachment of girls to their fathers during the phallic stage (from 3 to 6 years of age). Parallels the Oedipus complex for boys.

Elimination disorders   Disorders that involve a child or adolescent's inability to achieve bowel or bladder training at the appropriate age level.

Elopement   The departure or flight of a client from a psychiatric hospital.

Empathy   The ability to feel the feelings of other people so that one can respond to and understand their experiences on their terms. It is distinguished from sympathy by lack of condolence, agreement, or pity.

Enabler   Family member in an alcoholic's or addict's life whose behavior contributes to the continuation of chemical use.

Enmeshment   A family pattern characterized by a fast tempo of interpersonal exchange, overcontrol, and intrusiveness, usually from parent to child.

Epigenetic principle   The concept, adapted from embryology by Erikson, that physical and psychosocial growth are regulated by innate capacities of the person and arise in response to relations with others.

Espiritismo   A religious cult of European origin that can counteract or prevent mal de ojo and is concerned with moral behavior.

Espiritista   A spiritualist in Hispanic cultures who is able to put people in touch with the dead.

Ethnocentrism   The belief that one's own culture is more important than, and preferable to, any other culture.

Euthanasia   The intentional termination of a life of such poor quality that it is considered not worth living; can be active or passive.

Evocative memory   The ability to understand that an unseen object or person still exists when out of sight.

Excess disability   The increased cognitive impairment seen when depression and/or delirium occurs in a demented individual.

Excitement phase   Phase of sexual response marked by vaginal lubrication and penile erection.

Exhibitionism   Intentional exposure of one's genitals to a stranger or unsuspecting person accompanied by sexual arousal and masturbation either during or after the experience.

Existential plight   The first phase of dying identified by Weisman, encompassing the numbness and shock experienced at the realization that one's life is coming to a foreseeable end.

Extended family   All persons related by birth, marriage, or adoption to the nuclear family.

Extraneous variable   See confounding variable.

Extrapyramidal side-effects (EPS)   Side-effects caused by the use of neuroleptic medications, including three separate classes: parkinsonism, dystonias, and akathisia.

Extrapyramidal system   A system of descending motor tracts that originate from various regions of the cerebral cortex and subcortical areas. Because these tracts do not travel through the pyramids of the medulla, they are called extrapyramidal.

Factitious disorders   Physical or psychologic symptoms that are consciously and voluntarily produced by the client.

Faith healers   Religious people who deal with illness ascribed to spiritual or supernatural causes.

Family burden   The stress created in a family caring for a demented individual.

Family life-style   A family's biased perception of the outside world and its automatic means of coping with this world. It is the front or facade the family presents to others.

Family myths   Well-integrated unchallenged beliefs, shared by all family members, about each other and their positions in family life.

Family of origin   The family in which an individual grew up.

Family theme   A family's perception of its development and history.

Fantasized nurturing parent   An internal construct of a loving and benevolent person developed by the child as a means of dealing with the experience of inconsistent or abusive parenting.

Fantasy   A defense mechanism that is a sequence of mental images, like a daydream. It may be conscious or unconscious. It is considered by some to be an individual's attempt to resolve an emotional conflict.

Feedback   The process by which performance is checked and malfunctions corrected; a regulatory function in the communication process, requiring two persons—one to give and one to receive it.

Female sexual arousal disorder   Failure to attain or maintain adequate lubrication during sexual activity and/or lack of a subjective sense of sexual excitement during sexual activity.

Fetal alcohol syndrome (FAS)   Physical and mental defects found in babies of alcoholic women.

Fetishism   Requiring the presence of a nonliving object such as shoes, hair, or panties for sexual arousal.

Fight-flight   Aggression (fight)–withdrawal (flight) response to stress.

Fisting   The insertion of finger(s), hand, or fist into the rectum.

Flat affect (emotions)   A lack of emotional expression.

Folk domain of health care   Nonprofessional healers such as root doctors, faith healers.

Frail elder   Dependent, chronically ill older person.

Frotteurism   Intense sexual arousal associated with acts or fantasies of rubbing against a nonconsenting partner.

Functional encopresis   Repeated involuntary or intentional passage of feces into places not appropriate for that purpose.

Functional enuresis   Repeated involuntary or intentional voiding of urine into bed or clothes after an age at which continence is expected.

Gender identity   The sex role assignment as masculine, feminine, or ambivalent; generally based on external genital identification at birth.

Gender role   The socialization and demonstration of the sexual behaviors expected of a given sex.

General adaptation syndrome (GAS)   The objectively measurable structural and chemical changes produced in the body when stress affects the whole body. The GAS occurs in three stages: (1) alarm, (2) resistance, and (3) exhaustion.

General systems theory   A conceptual framework that can be applied to living systems or people and that integrates the biologic and social sciences logically with the physical sciences.

Generalized anxiety disorder   A disorder characterized by "free-floating" unrealistic or excessive anxiety about two or more life circumstances; manifested by autonomic hyperactivity (sweating, dizziness), irritability, and musculoskeletal tension.

Gerontophobia   Fear of contact and dealing with the elderly.

Ghettoization   Movement of the mentally ill to restricted areas such as central business areas offering single room rentals.

Global assessment of function (GAF)   A ninety-point scale used as Axis V of DSM-IIIR to assess a client's psychologic social and occupational function. Ratings are made for the current level at the time of evaluation and for the highest level in the past year.

Group dynamics   The interactions among members of a group; the forces that underlie group interaction.

Group therapy   Psychotherapy of several clients at the same time in the same session. It may emphasize examination of the interpersonal relationships of members of the group to see how they usually interact with others.

Groupthink   The mode of thinking engaged in by people who are members of a highly cohesive in-group in which uniformity and agreement are given such priority that critical thinking is impossible or unacceptable; term coined by Irving Janis.

Guerrilla AIDS clinics   Informal clinics that provide alternative drugs, chemicals, or nutritional additives for the treatment of AIDS.

Hallucination   A false perception, the most common of which are auditory and involve hearing voices; other types of hallucinations are tactile, somatic, visual, gustatory, and olfactory. A sensory impression in the absence of external stimuli that occurs during the waking state.

Here-and-now   Interpersonal and intrapersonal responses and reactions as they occur on the spot.

Heterosexuality   Preference for sexual activity with a partner of the opposite sex.

Hidden agenda   A personal goal that is unknown to others and is at cross-purposes with dominant group goals.

Histrionic personality disorder   A personality disorder with the essential feature of a pervasive pattern of excessive emotionality and attention seeking.

HIV-seropositive   Having blood serum that tests positive for the HIV antibody, but not necessarily having a diagnosis of AIDS or ARC.

Holism   A philosophic perspective that views the person as an integrated whole whose parts share an organic and functional relationship.

Homelessness   Absence of housing. In an extreme form, homelessness refers to street dwellers. A more moderate type of homelessness involves movement between temporary forms of housing such as emergency shelters.

Homeostasis   The principle that all organisms react to changing conditions in an effort to maintain a relatively constant internal environment; in general systems theory, the characteristic of systems to strive to maintain a dynamic equilibrium, or balance, among various forces that operate within and on it.

Homophobia   The unrealistic fear of homosexuality and homosexuals that stems from myths and stereotypes associated with homosexuality.

Homosexuality   Preference for sexual activity with a partner of the same sex.

Hoodoo men/women   See root doctors.

Hot line   A telephone crisis counseling service often used in crisis intervention centers to provide immediate contact between a person in crisis and a counselor.

Human immunodeficiency virus (HIV)   The extremely tiny but virulent retrovirus that causes AIDS. It consists basically of a double-layered shell or envelope full of proteins, surrounding a bit of ribonucleic acid (RNA).

Humanism   A view of human beings that values the individual's freedom of choice. In psychiatric nursing practice, a philosophy of devotion to the interests of human beings wherever they live and whatever their status. It reaffirms the spirit of compassion and caring for others and constructively and wholeheartedly affirms the joys, beauties, and values of human living.

Huntington's disease   A genetically transmitted disease involving both motor and cognitive changes; an example of a condition with subcortical dementia.

Hypertensive crisis   Dangerously high blood pressure, precipitated by the combination of monoamine oxidase inhibitor antidepressants and foods rich in tyramine.

Hypoactive sexual desire disorder   Persistent or recurrent lack of interest or drive in sexual expression or sexual fantasies

Hypervigilance   Increased state of guardedness or watchfulness.

Hypochondriasis   Preoccupation with the fear of having or the belief that one has a serious disease despite medical reassurance.

Hypomanic episode   A distinct period in which the predominant mood is elevated, expansive, or irritable but less severe than manic episode and without delusions.

Hypothesis   Statement of relationship between two or more study concepts or variables.

Id   In psychoanalytic theory, all inherited psychic properties of the person, most notably the instincts and drives.

Identification   A defense mechanism; the wish to be like another person and to assume the characteristics of that person's personality.

Identity diffusion   The failure to integrate various childhood identifications into a harmonious, adult, psychosocial identity; the "as if" personality.

Illusions   Misperceptions and misinterpretations of externally real stimuli. Visual and auditory illusions are much more common than tactile, olfactory, and gustatory illusions.

Imparting information   A communication skill in which the nurse makes statements that give needed data to the client and therefore encourages further clarification based on additional input.

Inappropriate affect   Affect that is discordant with the content of a client's speech or ideas.

Incest   Sexual relations between blood relatives or members of the same socialization unit other than husband and wife.

Inclusion need   The interpersonal need to establish and maintain relationships with others.

Induced psychotic disorder   A mental disorder with the essential feature of a delusional system that develops in a second person as a result of association with a first person who already has a psychotic disorder (historically known as *folie à deux*).

Informational confrontation   Describing the visible behavior of another person.

Infradian   Biorhythms longer than twenty-four hours.

Inhibited female orgasm   Persistent or recurrent failure to attain orgasm during sexual activity.

Inhibited male orgasm   Delay or lack of ejaculation even with intense sexual stimulation over a lengthy period of time.

Insanity   An obsolete medical term for psychosis or mental illness. Continues to be used in legal terminology.

Institutionalization   The process of decline in functioning characterized by dependency, apathy, resignation, and inability to manage daily living outside an institution and created by an environment that controls all individual decision making, negates independence and autonomy, and segregates inmates from the mainstream community.

Intellectualization   A defense mechanism in which intellectual processes are overused to avoid closeness or affective experience and expression. It is closely related to rationalization.

Interpersonal communication   Communication that takes place between two persons and in small groups; person-to-person communication.

Interpretive confrontation   Expressing thoughts and feelings about another's behavior and drawing inferences about the meaning of the behavior.

Intoxication   Maladaptive behavior and substance-specific syndrome due to ingestion of a psychoactive substance.

Intrafamily physical abuse   Violence within the family.

Intrafamily sexual abuse   Inappropriate sexual behavior, instigated by an adult family member or surrogate family member, whose purpose is to arouse the adult or a child sexually. Behaviors can range from exhibitionism, peeping, and explicit sexual talk to touching, caressing, masturbation, and intercourse.

Involuntary commitment   The legal process by which a person is confined without consent to a mental hospital. There are three categories: (1) emergency, (2) temporary, and (3) extended. Criteria vary from state to state.

Irrational self-talk   In rational-emotive therapy, the untrue thoughts with which one describes and interprets the world to oneself; usually catastrophic interpretations of an event or the need to live up to an absolute standard.

Irresistible impulse   The inability of a person to control his or her behavior as a result of a mental disorder even though he or she may know it is wrong. Supplements M'Naghten rule in an insanity plea in a few states.

Kaposi's sarcoma   An opportunistic malignancy that is the second most common opportunistic condition among persons with AIDS. May affect the skin and several internal organs including the brain.

Kinesics   The study of body movement (for example, facial expressions, gestures, and eye movements) as a form of nonverbal communication.

Kluver-Bucy-like syndrome   A syndrome occurring in the ter-

minal phase of Alzheimer's disease including hyperorality, blunting of emotions, bulimia, and attempts to touch objects in sight.

La belle indifférence   An inappropriate lack of concern about a disability. Seen in certain clients with conversion disorder. Literally means "beautiful indifference."

Labile affect   A pattern of observable behaviors that express emotion characterized by repeated, rapid, abrupt shifts.

Learned helplessness (excessive dependence)   A condition in which a person attempts to establish and maintain contact with another by adopting a helpless, powerless stance.

Least restrictive alternative   Imposition of the least amount of limitation or interference on an individual's thought and decision-making, physical activity, and sense of self as necessary to provide both maintenance care and active treatment.

Lesbianism   A form of sexual behavior between females.

Lethality assessment   A systematic method of assessing a client's suicide potential.

Lethality index   The ratio of suicide attempts to successful suicides.

Libido   In psychoanalytic theory, the sexual drive; see sexual desire.

Life script   Expectations for the client's life that have evolved over time due to the client's life experiences and relationships with significant others. The life script can affect numerous areas of living, e.g., the client's choices for career, life mate (to have or not to have), and patterns of behavior.

Life space interview   Assessment of the child during normal daily activities and routines over a period of time.

Limbic system   Is considered to be the "emotional brain." The parts of the limbic system include the hippocampus, lingulate gyrus, isthmus, hippocampal gyrus, and uncus.

Limit-setting   The reasonable and rational setting of parameters for client behavior that provide control and safety.

Linking   A communication skill in which the nurse responds to the client in a way that ties together two events, experiences, feelings, or people. It may be useful in connecting the past with current behaviors.

Loose associations   Thinking characterized by speech in which ideas shift from one subject to another that is unrelated.

Looseness of associations   A phenomenon commonly observed in schizophrenia where an apparently unrelated idea or experience reminds a person of some other experience or idea.

Magical thinking   The belief that one's thoughts, words, or actions will produce an outcome that defies normal laws of cause and effect.

Maintenance roles   Group roles oriented toward building group-centered attitudes among the members and maintaining and perpetuating group-centered behavior.

Major depressive episode   Depressed mood or loss of interest or pleasure in all or almost all activities for a period of at least two weeks.

Mal de ojo   "The evil eye" thought to be the result of a witch purposefully casting a spell or a person involuntarily injuring a child by looking admiringly at it.

Male erectile disorder   Persistent or recurrent difficulty attaining or maintaining an erection during sexual activity and/or a lack of a subjective sense of sexual excitement during sexual activity.

Malleus Maleficarum (The Witches' Hammer)   A 1487 textbook of both pornography and psychopathology that labeled dissenters and the mentally ill as witches and recommended burning at the stake to destroy the devil's host or witch.

Malpractice   Negligent act of professionals when they fail to act in a responsible and prudent manner in carrying out their professional duties.

Manic episode   A distinct period during which the predominant mood is elevated, expansive, or irritable.

Mantra   A syllable, word, or name that is chanted over and over during meditation.

Masochism   See sexual masochism.

Masturbation   Manual stimulation of genital organs or other body parts. The act may be for the purpose of erotic stimulation commonly resulting in orgasm but is not limited to that (e.g., may be a conscious expression of hostility toward the nurse or may be an unconscious expression of the client's anxiety).

Mediators   Cognitive cues to enhance memory and learning.

Medical-biologic model of psychiatry   A model based on classification that emphasizes systematic observation, naming, and classification of symptoms, and views emotional-behavioral disturbances as diseases like any other disease. Abnormal behavior is assumed to be directly attributable to a disease introduced from outside the body or an internally developed biochemical change.

Meditation   A method of achieving a state of deep rest and increasing alpha wave brain activity enabling one to focus on one thing at a time in order to achieve inner peace and harmony.

Medulla oblongata   The specialized segment of neurologic tissue that attaches the brain to the spinal cord.

Mental disorder   A clinically significant behavioral or psychologic syndrome or pattern that occurs in a person and is associated with distress or disability or with an increased risk of suffering death, pain, disability, or an important loss of freedom; is not an expectable response to a particular event or experience.

Mental hygiene movement   The development of preventive psychiatry and the formation of child guidance clinics based on the social consciousness of the early 20th century.

Mental status examination   Usually a standardized procedure with the primary purpose of gathering data to determine etiology, diagnosis, prognosis, and treatment.

Midbrain   Lies between the cerebral hemispheres and the pons. Within the midbrain are specialized centers for vision, hearing, and the modulation of wakeful/sleepful periods.

Midlife crisis   Period of disequilibrium between 35 and 45 years of age during which people discover visible signs of aging and experience feelings of boredom, dissatisfaction with the way life has developed, and uncertainty about the future.

Milieu therapy   The purposeful use of people, resources, and events in the patient's immediate environment to promote optimal functioning in activities of daily living, development/improvement of interpersonal skills, and capacity to manage outside the institutional setting.

Minnesota Multiphasic Personality Inventory (MMPI)   Complex, lengthy psychologic test consisting of 550 questions and yielding a clinical profile of the client's personality structure.

Mirroring   Imitating the client's behavior.

Mitigation/accommodation   The second phase of dying according to Weisman, representing the attempt to maintain function, balance, and control in the face of the reality of foreshortened life expectancy.

Mixed message   Communication in which the verbal and the nonverbal aspects contradict one another.

M'Naghten rule   Legal rule to determine whether a psychiatrically ill person is responsible for a criminal act he or she committed. Based mainly on whether the person knew the "nature and quality" of the act and that doing it was "wrong." Used in about one-third of the states.

Mnemonic disturbances   Inability to remember recent events; may extend to profound memory loss for both recent and past events.

Monistic view   A philosophy that asserts that the mind and body are one.

Mood   A prolonged emotion that colors the whole psychic life.

Mood disorders   A group of disorders with the essential feature of disturbance of mood accompanied by a full or partial manic or depressive syndrome. Previously called affective disorders in DSM-III.

Moral treatment   A movement for psychiatric reform that considered mental illness a disease and proposed its "moral management" in therapeutic surroundings; humane treatment rather than punishment for the mentally ill.

Multiaxial system   The five axes of DSM-III and DSM-IIIR.

Multi-infarct dementia   Dementia due to significant cerebrovascular disease; patchy deterioration.

Multiple personality disorder   The existence of two or more distinct personalities or personality states within a person that recurrently take control of the person's behavior.

Multiplex relationships   Relationships that have two or more functions or activities, in contrast to uniplex relationships.

Mutual self-help groups   A type of social support provided through group interaction by persons currently undergoing the same type of event or situation.

Narcissistic personality disorder   A personality disorder, the essential feature of which is a pervasive pattern of grandiosity, hypersensitivity to the evaluation of others, and lack of empathy.

Narcoanalysis   Psychotherapeutic treatment to uncover repressed memories and affects under partial anesthesia induced by intravenous barbiturates, for example.

Negative reinforcement   In behaviorist/learning theory, alteration of an adversive stimuli to increase the probability that a behaviorial response will occur.

Negative transference   Client reactions in therapeutic work based on negative feelings (hate, bitterness, contempt, annoyance, etc.) left over from unsatisfying past relationships.

Negotiated reality   The creation of a mutually understood, common ground.

Neologism   A private, unshared meaning of a word or term. Neologisms are frequently characteristic of the language of schizophrenic individuals.

Network density   The extent to which other members in the focus person's network know one another. *Interconnectedness* is a parallel term.

Neuroleptic   Medications also known as "antipsychotics."

Neuroleptic malignant syndrome (NMS)   An infrequent yet extreme condition that occurs in clients who are severely ill and is believed to be the result of dopamine blockade in the hypothalamus. Symptoms of this syndrome include: diaphoresis, muscle rigidity, and hyperpyrexia.

Neurolinguistic programming (NLP)   A communication model derived from theory in linguistics, neurophysiology, psychology, cybernetics, and psychiatry.

Neuron   The cell that transmits electrical impulses throughout the body, but specifically characteristic of the nervous system.

Neurosis   A pre–DSM-IIIR category of mental disorders characterized by anxiety and avoidance behavior.

Neurosyphilis   Dementia that is the direct result of primary syphilis that has gone untreated; usually fatal in three years.

Neurotic conflict   In psychoanalytic theory, the consequence of a traumatic experience in which client experiences ideas or feelings that are incompatible with his or her ego; believed to generate anxiety and use of defense mechanisms.

Neurotransmitter   A highly specialized neurochemical that allows transmission of an electrical impulse from one neuron to the next across the synapse.

New chronic patient   Term applied to younger, community-based clients who appear difficult to treat in conventional services.

Nonoxynol-9   A spermicidal agent believed to inactivate the AIDS virus.

Nonverbal communication   Communication between two or more people without the use of words. Facial expressions, gestures, and body postures are examples.

Normal pressure hydrocephalus   A presenile dementia affecting 5 percent of those diagnosed as demented; may be incorrectly diagnosed as Parkinson's disease.

Norms   The set of unwritten rules of conduct or prescriptions of behavior established by members of a group.

North American Nursing Diagnosis Association (NANDA)   Nursing organization responsible for reviewing, studying, and accepting specific nursing diagnoses that cover all clinical practice areas.

NSGAE (Nursing Adaptation Evaluation)   A proposed alternative to Axis V or additional Axis VI for DSM-IIIR or DSM-III.

Nuclear family   The "traditional" family consisting of two parents in a time-limited, two-generational relationship consisting of a married couple and their children by birth or adoption. A relatively recent development in human history.

Nursing   "The diagnosis and treatment of human responses to actual or potential health problems" (ANA 1980).

Nursing diagnosis   The conceptualization of a client's need, problem, or situation from the unique perspective of the theoretical constructs in the discipline of nursing.

Nursing process   The conscious, systematic set of cognitive behavioral steps that comprise the clinical act in nursing practice.

Objective data   Verifiable information collected from other sources than client and significant family, including psychologic test results and laboratory test findings.

Object permanence   The capacity to understand that an absent person or object will return.

Object relation   The emotional attachment one person has for another as opposed to feelings for oneself.

Obsession   A persistent idea, thought, or impulse that cannot be eliminated from consciousness by logical effort even though the person recognizes it as the product of his or her own mind.

Obsessive compulsive personality disorder   A personality disorder with the essential feature of a pervasive pattern of perfectionism and inflexibility.

Occulogyric crisis   One of the manifestations of an acute dystonic reaction in which the affected person demonstrates a fixed gaze, often upward.

Oedipal conflict/Oedipus complex   In psychoanalytic theory, the major process of the phallic stage from 3 to 6 years of age in which incestuous feelings are attached to the opposite sex parent and aggressive feelings are directed to the same sex parent.

Omnipotence   Fantasies of greatness or power.

One-to-one relationship   A mutually defined, collaborative, goal-directed client-therapist relationship for the purpose of crisis intervention, counseling, or individual psychotherapy.

Opisthotonos   A manifestation of an acute dystonic reaction in which the affected person demonstrates spasms of the neck and back, forcing the back to arch and the neck to bend backward.

Opportunistic infection   Infection caused by an organism that may be common in the environment but causes disease only in a person with a poorly functioning immune system.

Oppositional defiant disorder   A pattern of negative, hostile, and defiant behavior (without violation of the rights of others) to an extent more common than in others of the same mental age.

Oral character   The individual with unresolved conflicts of the earliest life stage of development (a sense of trust as theoretically defined by Erik Erikson). These insatiable needs may be displayed through overeating, verbal pessimism, sarcasm, and mistrust of others.

Organic anxiety syndrome   Prominent, recurrent panic attacks or generalized anxiety caused by a specific organic factor.

Organic delusional syndrome   Presence of delusions due to a specific organic factor.

Organic hallucinosis   Presence of prominent persistent or recurrent hallucinations due to a specific organic factor.

Organic mental disorders   Designate particular organic mental syndromes in which the etiology is known or presumed.

Organic mental syndromes (OMS)   Refers to a constellation of psychologic or behavioral signs and symptoms without reference to etiology.

Organic mood syndrome   Prominent and persistent depressed, elevated, or expansive mood due to a specific organic factor.

Organic personality syndrome   Persistent personality disturbance due to a specific organic factor.

Orgasm phase   Extremely pleasurable phase of sexual response marked by contractions of the sexual organs and pelvic muscles.

Orientation phase   The beginning phase of a one-to-one relationship characterized by the establishment of contact with the client.

Overload   In communication theory, sensory input that exceeds a person's tolerance level or capacity.

Pace   To go with or match the patient at whatever rate he or she is moving, talking, or feeling.

Panic   An acute attack of anxiety associated with personality disorganization.

Panic disorder with agoraphobia   Recurrent panic attacks accompanied by the fear of being in a situation from which escape might be difficult or embarrassing or help might not be available.

Panic disorder without agoraphobia   Recurrent panic attacks without the avoidance behavior that results from agoraphobia.

Paradox   A self-contradictory communication; for example, the demand "Stand up for yourself!"

Paranoid personality disorder   A personality disorder with the essential feature of a pervasive and unwarranted tendency to interpret the actions of people as deliberately demeaning or threatening.

Paraphilia   Persistent or necessary association of a specific non-human object activity that involves giving or receiving pain, or activity with a nonconsenting partner, to experience full sexual arousal and satisfaction.

Paraphrasing   An activity or communication skill in which the nurse restates what she or he has heard the client communicating. It offers an opportunity to test the nurse's understanding of what the client is attempting to communicate.

Parataxic mode   Earliest experiences of the infant in which all the baby knows consists of momentary experiences, undifferentiated feeling states without connections, or sense of self as a separate being.

Parens patriae   Enables the state to take the role of protector and involuntarily hospitalize individuals "for their own good."

Parent ego state   In transactional analysis theory, the ego state that incorporates the feelings and behaviors learned from parents or authority figures.

Parkinson's disease   A condition involving tremors and rigidity without cognitive involvement, recently associated with ultimate dementia for one in three clients over time.

Passive-aggressive personality disorder   A personality disorder with the essential feature of a pervasive pattern of resistance to demands for adequate social-occupational performance.

Pedophilia   The sex object is a child. Manipulation or fondling of the child's genitals is usually involved.

Perception   The experience of sensing, interpreting, and comprehending the world; a highly personal and internal act.

Perseveration   Persistent repetition of words, ideas, or subjects.

Personal space   The "invisible bubble" of territory around a person's body into which intruders may not come.

Personality   Deeply ingrained patterns of behavior that include the way one relates to, perceives, and thinks about the environment and self.

Personality disorders   Enduring patterns of perceiving, relating to, and thinking about the environment and oneself that become inflexible and maladaptive and cause either significant functional impairment or subjective distress; coded on Axis II of DSM-IIIR.

Pervasive developmental disorders   See autistic disorder.

Phantom experience   The sensation of feeling a part of the body that is no longer there.

Phantom pain   Perception of pain in a body part that has been surgically or accidentally separated.

Phenothiazines   One of the classes of neuroleptic or antipsychotic medications.

Phobia   An excessive, persistent, irrational fear of an object or situation that causes the person to avoid the object or situation.

Pick's disease   Presenile dementia with age onset in the mid fifties; possibly a genetic predisposition.

Pinpointing   Calling attention to statements, inconsistencies among statements, or similarities or differences in points of view, feelings, or actions.

Plateau phase   Phase of sexual response after excitement; marked by increased levels of muscle tension and vasocongestion; precedes orgasm.

Play therapy   Therapy used with children, usually of preschool and early latency ages. The child reveals problems on a fantasy level with dolls, toys, and clay. The therapist may intervene with explanations about the child's responses and behavior in language geared to the child's comprehension.

Pleasure principle   In psychoanalytic theory, the tendency for the id to seek pleasure and avoid pain. The demands of the plea-

sure principle become modified by the reality principle, and the individual thereby develops the capacity to delay immediate release of tension or achievement of pleasure.

Pneumocystis carinii pneumonia   A common opportunistic infection in persons with AIDS and the most frequent cause of death.

Polypharmacy   The mixing and matching of medication seen in elderly persons who often have a variety of chronic medical problems.

Pons   The neurologic structure that is located above the medulla; contains the centers for cranial nerves 5, 6, 7, and 8 and aids in the regulation of respirations.

Poppers   Volatile amyl and butyl nitrates in breakable glass capsules inhaled to enhance sexual pleasure.

Popular domain of health care   Family and friends who function in the role of healer by offering health information, emotional support, prayers, and advice.

Positive reinforcement   In behaviorist theory and operant conditioning, an environmental event that rewards and thus increases the probability of a behavioral response.

Positive transference   Client reactions in therapeutic work based on positive feelings (love, affection, respect, trust) from satisfying past relationships.

Post-traumatic stress disorder   Reexperiencing with intense terror, fear, and helplessness a psychologically distressing event that is outside the range of usual human experience.

Postural hypotension   A clinical phenomenon in which, after receiving certain psychotropic medications, the affected person's blood pressure decreases, especially when standing up from a lying or sitting position. Hypotension is most common with aliphatic and piperidine antipsychotic preparations.

Poverty of content of speech   Speech that is adequate in amount but conveys little information because of vagueness, empty repetitions, or use of stereotyped or obscure phrases.

Power rape   Rape distinguished by the rapist's intent to command and master another person sexually, not to injure the victim.

Premature ejaculation   Ejaculation occurring in sexual activity with minimal stimulation and before the individual wishes it to occur.

Preterminality/terminality   According to Weisman, the fourth and final phase of dying, when the imminence of death is apparent.

Primary data source   The client himself or herself as the provider of assessment information.

Primary degenerative dementia, Alzheimer's type   See Alzheimer's disease.

Primary prevention   Elimination of factors that cause or contribute to development of disease or disorder.

Primitive idealization   Assigning unrealistic powers to an individual on whom one is dependent.

Privileged communication   Legal term, established by state statute to protect possibly incriminating disclosures made by the client. The privilege is the client's, the professional can reveal the information at the client's request.

Problem solving   A specific form of intellectual activity used when an individual faces a situation he or she is unable to handle in terms of past learning. Problem-solving strategies are considered crucial in any psychotherapeutic endeavor. They consist of the following sequential steps: observation, definition, preparation, analysis, ideation, incubation, synthesis, evaluation, and development.

Processing   A complex and sophisticated communication skill in which direct attention is given to the interpersonal dynamics of the nurse-client experience. Process comments focus on the content, feelings, and behavior experienced within the nurse-client relationship.

Professional domain of health care Traditional Western institutionally sanctioned health care workers such as a psychiatrist, nurse, and social worker.

Professional Service (Standards) Review Organization (PSRO) Required by Congress to implement quality control methods in health care delivery systems; a mode of evaluation.

Progressive relaxation A method of deep muscle relaxation based on the premise that muscle tension is the body's physiologic response to anxiety-provoking thoughts and muscle relaxation blocks anxiety.

Progressive supranuclear palsy (PSP) A presenile subcortical dementia resulting from cell atrophy in the midbrain portions of the brain; no known cause or treatment.

Projection An unconscious defense mechanism in which what is emotionally unacceptable to the individual is rejected and attributed to others.

Projective identification The placement of one's aggressive feelings onto another, thereby justifying expressions of anger and self-protection.

Prospective payment A shift in American health care policy initiated by Medicare in 1983 away from cost-based retrospective reimbursement for hospital costs toward fixed payment based on diagnostically related groups (DRGs).

Prototaxic mode Process of perceiving experience that appears as the infant matures so that parts are recognized; however, there is still no ability to see logical connections (follows parataxic mode).

Proxemics The study of the space relationships maintained by people in social interaction, including the dimensions of territoriality and personal space.

Proximal-distal principle Governs infant's physical progress; mastery proceeds in an inward to outward direction.

Pseudodementia A syndrome in which dementia is mimicked by a functional illness; a more current concept is that of a depression-induced organic mental disorder.

Pseudohostility Chronic conflict, alienation, tension, and inappropriate remoteness among members of a family. The problems of family life are denied in an attempt to negate the hostility among the members.

Pseudomutuality A method of family functioning in which the members act "as if" it is a close, happy family when in fact it is not.

Psychiatric audit A means of evaluation in which criteria for quality care are compared with actual practice as recorded on the client's chart.

Psychiatric history A set of interview questions oriented to the medical model, designed to elicit information about an individual's present and previous psychiatric experiences. Information may be provided by family, friends, and others about the client, resulting in a variety of perceptions.

Psychiatric nurse According to the American Nurses' Association, a registered nurse in a psychiatric setting who possesses a minimum of a bachelor's degree.

Psychiatric nursing A specialty within the nursing profession in which the nurse directs efforts toward the promotion of mental health, the prevention of mental disturbance, early identification of and intervention in emotional problems, and follow-up care to minimize long-term effects of mental disturbance.

Psychiatric Nursing Diagnoses, ed 1 (PND-I) Used in this text to refer to The American Nurses' Association classification system

of specific nursing diagnoses that comprise the phenomena of concern for generalist and specialist psychiatric-mental health nursing (1987).

Psychic determinism In psychoanalytic theory, the tenet that none of human behavior is accidental, that emotional and behavioral events do not happen randomly or by chance. Each psychic event is believed to be determined by the ones that preceded it.

Psychoanalysis A theory of human development and behavior and a form of psychotherapy developed by Sigmund Freud and his followers. It is a form of insight therapy that relies on the technique of free association to explore the dynamic, psychogenic, and transference aspects of a client's personality.

Psychoanalytic model of psychiatry An approach founded by Sigmund Freud, holding that all psychologic and emotional events are understandable. The meanings behind behavior are sought from childhood experiences that are believed to cause adult neurosis. Therapy in this model consists of clarifying the psychologic meanings of events, feelings, and behavior and thereby gaining insight.

Psychobiology The study of the biochemical foundations of thought, mood, emotion, affect, and behavior.

Psychodrama A form of group psychotherapy, developed by Jacob Moreno, that uses dramatic techniques and the language and setting of theatrical productions to achieve psychotherapeutic goals.

Psychoeducation An approach used with family caregivers that emphasizes goals of (1) decreasing client vulnerability to environmental stimulation through educated maintenance chemotherapy; (2) increasing family stability by increasing both knowledge and coping strategies.

Psychoendocrinology The study of the relationships between behavior, endocrine function, and human biology.

Psychogenic amnesia A sudden inability to recall important personal information that is too extensive to be explained by ordinary forgetfulness.

Psychogenic fugue Sudden, unexpected travel away from home or customary work locale with assumption of a new identity and inability to recall one's previous identity.

Psychogerontology Study of mental health and illness in later life.

Psychoimmunology An exploration of relationships between the central nervous system, the immune system, behavior, and human biology.

Psychophysiologic disorders Disorders having both physiologic and psychologic components.

Psychosis A state in which a person's mental capacity to recognize reality, communicate, and relate to others is impaired, thus interfering with the person's capacity to deal with life demands.

Psychotic transference A situation in which the relationship with the therapeutic person supersedes all other relationships.

Questioning A very direct communication activity that may be useful when the nurse needs specific information from the client. There are two types: (1) Open-ended questioning focuses on the topic but allows freedom of response; and (2) closed-ended questioning limits the client's responses to yes or no. When used to excess, questioning acts to control the nature and extent of the client's responses.

Rape   Any forced sex act with the key factor being lack of adult consent.

Rape trauma syndrome   A syndrome of specific responses to the experience of being raped; also a nursing diagnosis.

Rationalization   A defense or coping mechanism in which a person falsifies experience by constructing logical or socially approved explanations of behavior.

Reaction formation   A defense or coping mechanism in which unacceptable feelings are disguised by repression of the real feeling and reinforcement of the opposite feeling.

Reactive drinking   Late-onset alcohol abuse associated with developmental transitions and life losses in the elderly.

Reality principle   In psychoanalytic theory, largely a learned ego function whereby people develop the capacity to delay immediate release of tension or achievement of pleasure. This is Sigmund Freud's term for the practical demands of society, which are often in conflict with the individual's own wishes.

Recidivism   A tendency to relapse into a previous mode of behavior. For psychiatric clients, recidivistic concerns focus on relapse of psychiatric illness with a reemergence of symptoms.

Reciprocity   In social support, the extent to which each person gives and receives in the exchanges that occur between the two people.

Reflected appraisals   In Harry Stack Sullivan's interpersonal theory of psychiatry, the means by which one's self-view is learned through interaction with significant others.

Reflecting   A communication skill in which the nurse reiterates either the content or the feeling message of the client. In "content" reflection, the nurse repeats basically the same statement as the client. In "feeling" reflection, the nurse verbalizes what seems to be implied about feelings in the client's comment.

Reinforcement   Term from behaviorist or learning theory that refers to altering environmental stimuli to increase the probability that a behavioral response will occur; can be positive as a reward or negative as a removal of adversive stimuli.

Reliability   A quality of a research instrument important in evaluating its worth. It means that the instrument produces consistent results or data on repeated use, usually because the investigator has standardized the process for using it. Also used to describe data or study design.

Repression   A coping mechanism in which unacceptable feelings were kept out of awareness.

Residual deviance   Term from sociologist Thomas Schiff's theory of mental disorder referring to diverse forms of deviance that do not fit under any other explicit label.

Resistance   All the phenomena that interfere with and disrupt the smooth flow of feelings, memories, and thoughts. In the traditional psychoanalytic sense, anything that inhibits the client from producing material from the unconscious. Resistance is often cited by psychotherapists to "explain" unsuccessful treatment of a client.

Resolution phase   Phase of sexual response where body organs return to their prearoused state.

Reticular activating system   Located within the reticular formation; receives information from the cord and relays it via the thalamus to all parts of the cerebral cortex. It plays a major role in states of consciousness.

Revolving door syndrome   Short hospital stays with rapid turnover and a pattern of readmission.

Rigidity   Lacking in flexibility; unyielding; a need to be precise and accurate.

Rimming   Oral-anal contact

Role taking   A process through which people are able to sense the feelings of another because they have aroused in themselves the attitude of the person to whom they are relating.

Rolfing   Structural realignment of the body in proper relationship to the field of gravity; a body-mind therapy.

Root doctors (hoodoo men/women)   Folk health practitioners who use plants, ground fibers, and various herbs to put an evil spell on another or to neutralize an evil spell.

Rorschach test (inkblot test)   A personality test in which a person says whatever comes to mind as he or she looks at a series of ten standardized cards with inkblots on them. It is believed to reveal many aspects of the individual's personality structure and emotional functioning.

Sadism   See sexual sadism.

Sadistic rape   Rape distinguished by brutality as a necessary ingredient for the rapist to become sexually excited.

Santeria   In Hispanic cultures, a religion comprised of a unique blend of Catholicism and mysticism. A Santero(a) is a practitioner/priest of Santeria.

Scapegoating   A process by which an individual or group of individuals are identified as different from others and become the object of the group's fears, frustrations, or anger.

Schema (_plural, schemata_**)**   Internal representation of some specific action, according to Piaget's cognitive theory. Beginning in infancy, they evolve to operational schemata of higher order in adolescence when abstract thinking occurs.

Schismatic family   A family in which the children are forced to join one or the other camp of two warring spouses.

Schizoaffective disorder   A mental disorder that appears to be both schizophrenia and a mood disturbance but does not meet DSM-IIIR criteria for either.

Schizoid personality disorder   A personality disorder with the essential feature a pattern of indifference to social relationships and a restricted range of emotional experience and expression.

Schizophrenia   A mental disorder with essential features of characteristic psychotic symptoms during the active phase of the illness, functioning below highest level previously achieved, failure in social development, and a duration of at least six months.

Schizophreniform disorder   A mental disorder that shares all essential features with schizophrenia except that the duration, including all phases, is less than six months.

Schizotypal personality disorder   A personality disorder with the essential feature of a pervasive pattern of peculiarities of ideas, appearance, and behavior and deficits in interpersonal relatedness.

Seasonal affective disorder (SAD)   A major depressive episode with seasonal pattern.

Secondary data source   Charts, test results, and family members who provide assessment information about a client.

Secondary prevention   The early detection and treatment of disease and disorder.

Seduction of the nurse   An attempt by the client to manipulate the nurse to relate in a nontherapeutic way. This manipulation and the end result may be of a sexual nature, but it usually takes the form of nonsexual behaviors. For example, it may involve flattery to get the nurse to do special favors for the client or to ignore maladaptive behavior usually warranting limit setting.

Selective inattention   A filtering out of stimuli under conditions of moderate and severe anxiety.

Self-actualizing people   According to Maslow, people who make full use of their talents and potentialities; those doing the best they can understand themselves better than other people, and do not allow their own desires to distort their judgment.

Self-awareness A sense of knowing what one is experiencing. It is a major goal of all therapy.

Self-disclosure Being open to personal feelings and experiences; sharing information and feelings with others.

Self-fulfilling prophecy An idea or expectation that is acted out, largely unconsciously, thus "proving" itself.

Self-hypnosis Putting oneself into a hypnotic state, often used to achieve significant relaxation, to make positive suggestions for changes in one's life, or to uncover forgotten events that continue to influence the person.

Self-system (self-dynamism) One of Harry Stack Sullivan's central concepts—that the self is a construct built out of the child's experience. It is made up of "reflected appraisals" learned in contacts with other significant people.

Separation-individuation The process of identifying oneself as different from the primary caretaker while maintaining an emotional attachment to that person.

Sexual aversion disorder Persistent or recurrent extreme aversion to and avoidance of all or almost all genital sexual contact with a sexual partner.

Sexual desire (libido) The motivation to seek out or be receptive to sexual activity or interaction.

Sexual masochism The need to experience emotional or physical pain in reality or fantasy to have sexual arousal.

Sexual sadism The need to inflict emotional or physical pain or humiliation in activity or fantasy to have sexual arousal.

Shaman Medicine man.

Shaping An intervention procedure in behaviorist/learning theory in which reinforcement is manipulated to bring the client closer and closer to a desired behavior.

Ships of fools Boatloads of mad people set out to sea during the early Renaissance period.

Simple phobia Persistent fear of a specific stimulus object or situation accompanied by an immediate anxiety response.

Skewed family A family in which one spouse is severely dysfunctional and the other spouse, usually aware of the dysfunction of the partner, assumes a passive, peacemaking stance to preserve the marriage.

Social-interpersonal model of psychiatry A model of psychiatry whose advocates believe that crucial social processes are involved in the development and resolution of disturbed behavior. It focuses on the larger and more general context of deviant behavior and on the processes by which an individual comes to be labeled or identified as deviant.

Social network A social network of an individual refers to all those persons known personally by the focus person.

Social phobia Persistent fear of one or more social situations in which the person is exposed to scrutiny by others and fears acting in a way that will be humiliating or embarrassing.

Social support Emotional and tangible support given and received through interpersonal interactions among people who know one another.

Somatization Excessive preoccupation with physical symptoms often associated with depression in the elderly.

Somatization disorder Recurrent and multiple somatic complaints for which medical attention has been sought; apparently not due to physical disorders.

Somatoform disorder A disorder in which physical symptoms suggest the presence of a physical disorder in the absence of organic findings; there may be positive evidence or a strong presumption of associated psychologic factors.

Splitting A defense mechanism that prevents one from uniting

the good (love) and bad (hate) aspects of oneself or of one's image of another person. The person views himself or herself as all good or all bad, failing to integrate the positive and negative qualities of the self and others into a cohesive image.

Stanford-Binet Scale A commonly used intelligence test for children, consisting of a series of tasks of increasing difficulty.

Stimulus Term from behaviorist or learning theory that refers to an event, condition, or situation that precedes a response or behavior.

Stress A broad class of experiences in which a demanding situation taxes a person's resources or capabilities causing a negative effect.

Stressor The source of stress, the demanding situation.

Stress-vulnerability models Models that look at relapses among the chronically mentally ill in terms of an interaction between individual vulnerability and environmental stressors.

Structuring An attempt to create order or evolve guidelines.

Subjective data Information reported by the client and significant others in their own words.

Subsystem In family systems theory, a triad, dyad, or other group of members who are linked together in some special association in the family.

Suicidal attempt A serious suicide try involving definite risk. The outcome frequently depends on the circumstances and is not under the person's control.

Suicidal cluster A contagion of suicides in which one suicide appears to set off another.

Suicidal gesture A more serious warning than a suicidal threat. May be followed by a carefully planned suicidal act that attracts attention without seriously injuring the subject.

Suicidal threat A statement of suicidal intent accompanied by behavior changes indicative of suicidal ideation.

Suicide The taking of one's own life. It is considered destructive aggression turned inward.

Summarizing A communication skill in which main ideas are highlighted. Summarizing reviews for client and nurse what the main themes of the conversation were. It is useful in helping the client to focus thinking.

Superego In psychoanalytic theory, a special agency of the ego that embodies rules (conscience) and values (ego ideal) resulting from influences of parental figures.

Suppression A defense or coping mechanism in which unacceptable feelings and thoughts are consciously kept out of awareness.

Suspiciousness An attitude of doubt about the trustworthiness of objects or people.

Susto Fright sickness present in some Hispanic groups, believed to be from a natural cause such as viewing something very unpleasant.

Symbiosis From about 4 to 5 months of age, the infant's psychologic fusion with the mothering person; a reciprocal process.

Symbolic interactionism A distinctive approach to the study of human conduct based on the premises that (1) human beings act toward things on the basis of the meaning that the things have for them, (2) the meaning of things in life is derived from the social interactions a person has with others, and (3) people handle and modify the meanings of the things they encounter through an interpretive process.

Symmetrical relationships   Relationships based on maintaining equality between members. They allow for respect and trust but may deteriorate into competition.

Synapse   The microscopic gap between neurons.

Synaptic vesicles   Small liquid filled sacs located on the membranes of neurons at the synapse. The synpatic vesicles contain neurotransmitter substances.

Synergy   The characteristic of a system such as a family that the whole is greater than the sum of its parts.

Syntaxic mode   A process of perceiving experience in which a child learns to use language in a consensually validated way, i.e., with reference to meaning accepted by the listener (follows parataxic mode).

Systematic desensitization   A process in which a person is exposed serially to a predetermined list of anxiety-provoking situations, graded in a hierarchy from the least to the most frightening, with the goal of reducing the anxiety these situations cause.

Tangential communication   Expressions or responses that are irrelevant to the content of the topic at hand.

Tangential response   An inappropriate response to a statement in which the content of the statement is disregarded. The reply is directed toward either an incidental aspect of the initial statement, the type of language used, the emotions of the sender, or another facet of the same topic.

Tardive dyskinesia   Usually a nonreversible and late-onset complication of antipsychotic medications. Characteristically, this condition is evidenced by the presence of abnormal, involuntary movements.

Task roles   Group roles that facilitate group efforts in the selection, definition, and solution of a group problem.

Termination phase (of one-to-one)   The end phase of the one-to-one relationship characterized by the termination of contact with the client.

Territoriality   The assumption of a proprietary attitude toward a geographic area by a person or a group.

Tertiary prevention   Reducing impairment and disability associated with disease and disorder

Tetrahydroaminoacridine (THA)   A potent anticholinesterase drug undergoing trials for restoration of some cognitive function in early Alzheimer's disease.

Thematic Apperception Test (TAT)   A projective psychologic test using a series of ambiguous pictures that are shown to the client so they can be described.

Theory   A set of interrelated constructs or propositions that present a systematic explanation of phenomena.

Therapeutic alliance   A conscious relationship between a helping person and a client in which each implicitly agrees that they need to work together to help the client with personal problems and concerns.

Therapeutic community   Creation of an environmental milieu in which the hospitalized client can have a corrective interpersonal experience by recreating and resolving obstacles to constructive social relationships; traditional hierarchical roles and authority structures are minimized; originally attributed to Maxwell Jones.

Therapeutic contract   The client's definition of personal goals for treatment, plus the nurse's professional responsibilities.

Therapeutic touch   The specific transfer of energy in a therapeutic manner in which some of the excess energies of the healer are directed to the client, or energy is transferred from one place to another in the client's body.

Therapeutic use of self   The ability of the psychiatric nurse to use theory and experiential knowledge along with self-awareness and the ability to explore one's personal impact on others.

Thought blocking   Stopping the expression of a thought midway.

Thought broadcasting   Belief that thoughts, as they occur, are broadcast from one's head to the external world.

Thought insertion   The belief that thoughts that are not one's own are being inserted into one's mind.

Thought stopping   A method of overcoming obsessive and phobic thoughts by first concentrating on the unwanted thoughts and, after a short time, stopping or interrupting the unwanted thoughts.

Thought withdrawal   The belief that thoughts have been removed from one's head.

Tic disorders   Disorders characterized by involuntary, sudden, rapid, recurrent, nonrhythmic, stereotyped, motor movement or vocalization.

Tort   A wrongful act resulting in injury for which the injured party is requesting compensation through a civil suit.

Torticollis   One of the manifestations of an acute dystonic reaction characterized by an uncontrollable twisted neck.

Tourette's disorder   Multiple motor and one or more vocal tics; may involve touching, squatting, twirling, grunts, barks, sniffs, and coprolalia.

Traits (personality traits)   Enduring patterns of perceiving, relating to, and thinking about the environment and oneself.

Transactional analysis (TA)   A system introduced by Eric Berne that has four components: (1) structural analysis of intrapsychic phenomena, (2) transactional analysis proper, (3) game analysis, and (4) script analysis—used in both individual and group psychotherapy.

Transference   In psychoanalytic theory, an unconscious phenomenon in which feelings, attitudes, and wishes originally linked with significant figures in one's early life are projected onto others who have come to represent these figures in one's current life.

Transinstitutionalization   Movement from one custodial setting to another.

Transsexualism   Persistent discomfort and sense of inconsistency between psychologic gender identity and anatomic gender.

Transvestic fetishism   Cross dressing required for sexual arousal prior to masturbation or coitus.

Triangulation   In family systems theory, the process of forming a triad. Dysfunctional triangulation is a major concept in the Bowen approach to family therapy.

Trust   Feeling confident that another person will behave in ways that will bring beneficial consequences.

Type A personality   A highly competitive, driving personality often associated with coronary disease, angina pectoris, and myocardial infarction.

Type I schizophrenia   A type of schizophrenia characterized by "positive symptoms" of schizophrenia, including hallucinations, delusions, and thought disorder; thought to be associated with biologic abnormality of dopamine receptors; responds well to psychotropic medications.

Type II schizophrenia   A type of schizophrenia characterized by "negative symptoms" of flattening of affect, loss of motivation, and poverty of speech; shows little response to neuroleptic treatment.

Ulterior transaction   A transaction that occurs on both overt (social) and covert (psychologic) levels.

Ultradian   Biorhythms shorter than 24 hours.

Unconflicted member (independent member)   A group member who is able to assess situations and alter roles or behavior appropriately.

Unconscious   In psychoanalytic theory, the part of the mind that is out of awareness and helps to determine personality.

Underload   A situation that occurs when delay or lack of information interferes with one person's ability to comprehend the message of another.

Uniplex relationship   Relationships that have only one function or activity, in contrast to multiplex relationships.

Vaginismus   Sexual disorder marked by involuntary spasm of the vaginal muscles making sexual intercourse difficult or impossible.

Validity   A quality of an instrument important to evaluating its worth. It means that the instrument measures what it is supposed to measure.

Values clarification   A systematic, widely applicable method of helping learners become aware of their beliefs and values, choose among alternatives, and match stated beliefs with actions.

Victimatology   The study of victims of violent assault.

Violence   Behavior by an individual that threatens or actually does harm or injury to people or property.

Visualization   Using a person's own imagination and positive thinking to reduce stress or promote healing.

Voluntary commitment   A legal process by which a person chooses to be admitted to a mental hospital; requires written application by the person or someone acting in his or her behalf, such as a parent or guardian.

Volunteer linking   A social support intervention that involves using a person who has experienced a similar event or situation to provide temporary support and assistance to someone currently undergoing the same type of event or situation.

Voyeurism   Watching an unsuspecting person while that person is undressing, grooming, or having sexual activity; associated with masturbation during or after the activity.

Wernicke-Korsakoff syndrome   A syndrome usually associated with alcoholism and characterized by confusion, disorientation, and amnesia with confabulation.

Working phase   The middle phase of the one-to-one relationship characterized by the maintenance and analysis of contact.

Works   The intravenous drug user's needle and syringe.

World view   Refers to how a group of people (culture or subculture) see their social world, symbolic system, and physical environment and their own place in each of them.

Writ of habeas corpus   A means by which a person can challenge the legality of his or her detention.

Yin and yang   In Oriental philosophy, two opposing forces that must be in perfect balance for physical and mental health and social harmony to be maintained.

Zoophilia (bestiality)   Selection of animals as actual or fantasized sexual partners.

Index

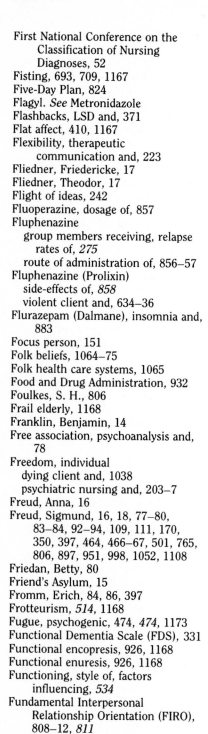

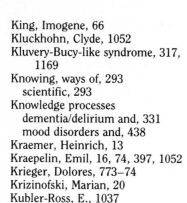